HANKEY'S CLINICAL NEUROLOGY

SECOND EDITION

Editors

Philip B. Gorelick
MD, MPH, FACP, FAHA, FAAN, FANA
Medical Director, Mercy Health Hauenstein Neuroscience Center at Saint Mary's
Professor, Translational Science & Molecular Medicine
Michigan State University College of Human Medicine
Grand Rapids, Michigan, USA

Fernando D. Testai
MD, PhD, FAHA
Assistant Professor in Neurology
University of Illinois College of Medicine at Chicago
Chicago, Illinois, USA

Graeme J. Hankey
MBBS, MD, FRACP, FRCP, FRCPE
Winthrop Professor of Neurology, School of Medicine and Pharmacology
The University of Western Australia
Consultant Neurologist, Department of Neurology
Sir Charles Gairdner Hospital
Perth, Australia

Joanna M. Wardlaw
MBChB, MRCP, DMRD, FRCR, MD, FRCP, FMedSc
Professor of Applied Neuroimaging
Division of Clinical Neurosciences, University of Edinburgh,
Western General Hospital,
Edinburgh, UK

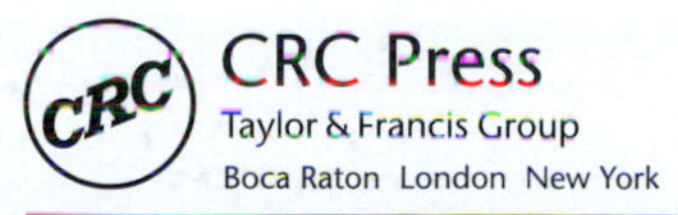

CRC Press
Taylor & Francis Group
Boca Raton London New York

CRC Press is an imprint of the
Taylor & Francis Group, an **informa** business

Book design by Ayala Kingsley; illustration by Cactus Design and Ayala Kingsley.

CRC Press
Taylor & Francis Group
6000 Broken Sound Parkway NW, Suite 300
Boca Raton, FL 33487-2742

Printed and bound in India by Replika Press Pvt. Ltd.

Printed on acid-free paper
Version Date: 20131119

International Standard Book Number-13: 978-1-84076-193-1 (Hardback)

Visit the Taylor & Francis Web site at
http://www.taylorandfrancis.com

and the CRC Press Web site at
http://www.crcpress.com

CONTENTS

CONTRIBUTORS

Annu Aggarwal
Centre for Brain and Nervous System,
Kokilaben Dhirubhai Ambani Hospital and Medical Research Institute,
Mumbai, India

Venkatesh Aiyagari
Professor,
Departments of Neurosurgery and Neurology and Neurotherapeutics;
Director, Neurocritical Care Division,
University of Texas Southwestern Medical Center,
Dallas, TX, USA

Vibhav Bansal
Diplomate of the American Board of Psychiatry and Neurology,
Vascular/Interventional Neurology Stroke Fellow,
Sparrow Health Systems/Michigan State University,
Department of Neurology,
East Lansing, MI, USA

Brandon R. Barton
Assistant Professor,
Department of Neurological Sciences,
Movement Disorders Section,
Rush University Medical Center,
Jesse Brown VA Medical Center,
Chicago, IL, USA

Alma R. Bicknese
Department of Pediatrics,
Division of Pediatric Neurology,
University of Illinois at Chicago College of Medicine,
Chicago, IL, USA

James L. Cook
Director, Division of Infectious Diseases,
Loyola University Medical Center;
Professor of Medicine and Co-Director,
Infectious Disease and Immunology Institute,
Loyola University Chicago, Stritch School of Medicine;
Chief, Infectious Diseases, Edward Hines, Jr. Veterans Administration Hospital,
Chicago, IL, USA

Wilson Cueva
Clinical Associate,
Department of Neurology,
University of Chicago,
Chicago, IL, USA

Robert P. Dinapoli
Department of Neurology,
Mayo Clinic,
Rochester, MN, USA

John Dunne
Department of Neurology,
Royal Perth Hospital,
Perth, WA, Australia

Robert Edis
Department of Neurology,
Royal Perth Hospital,
Perth, WA, Australia

Victor Fung
Department of Neurology,
Westmead Hospital,
Sydney, NSW, Australia

Molly E. Gilbert
Department of Ophthalmology and Visual Science,
University of Illinois at Chicago College of Medicine,
Chicago, IL, USA;
Captain James A. Lovell Federal Health Care Center,
North Chicago, IL, USA

Sid Gilman
Professor (retired),
Department of Neurology,
University of Michigan Health System,
Ann Arbor, MI, USA

Peter J. Goadsby
Professor, Headache Group,
Department of Neurology,
University of California,
San Francisco, CA, USA

Julie E. Hammack
Department of Neurology,
Mayo Clinic,
Rochester, MN, USA

Graeme J. Hankey
Winthrop Professor of Neurology,
School of Medicine and Pharmacology,
The University of Western Australia;
Consultant Neurologist,
Department of Neurology,
Sir Charles Gairdner Hospital,
Perth, WA, Australia

Robert Henderson
Department of Neurology,
Royal Brisbane and Women's Hospital,
Brisbane, QLD, Australia

Daniel B. Hier
Professor of Neurology and Rehabilitation,
Department of Neurology and Rehabilitation Medicine,
University of Illinois at Chicago College of Medicine,
Chicago, IL, USA

John H. Jacobsen
Department of Neurology,
University of Chicago Medical Center,
Chicago, IL, USA

Qin Li Jiang
Clinical Assistant Professor,
Department of Neurology and Rehabilitation Medicine,
University of Illinois at Chicago College of Medicine,
Chicago, IL, USA

Andres M. Kanner
Director, International Comprehensive Epilepsy Center;
Head, Epilepsy Section;
Professor of Clinical Neurology and Psychiatry,
University of Miami, Miller School of Medicine,
Miami, FL, USA

Jorge Kattah
Professor and Head of Neurology,
Department of Neurology,
University of Illinois College of Medicine at Peoria,
Peoria, IL, USA

Octavia Kincaid
Assistant Professor,
Department of Neurology and Rehabilitation Medicine,
University of Illinois at Chicago College of Medicine,
Chicago, IL, USA

Michael Kohrman
University of Chicago Medicine, Comer Children's Hospital,
Chicago, IL, USA

James A. Mastrianni
Associate Professor of Neurology,
Director, Center for Comprehensive Care and Research on Memory Disorders,
University of Chicago,
Chicago, IL, USA

William McAuliffe
Clinical Associate Professor (Medicine), University of Western Australia;
Interventional Neuroradiologist,
Neurointervention and Imaging Service of WA,
Sir Charles Gairdner Hospital,
Royal Perth Hospital,
Perth, WA, Australia

Edward A. Michals
Assistant Professor of Radiology and Director of Radiology,
Residency Program,
Department of Radiology,
University of Illinois at Chicago College of Medicine,
Chicago, IL, USA

Paul V. Motika
Assistant Professor,
Department of Neurology,
Comprehensive Epilepsy Center,
Oregon Health and Science University,
Portland, OR, USA

Peter Pytel
Assistant Professor of Pathology,
Department of Pathology,
University of Chicago,
Chicago, IL, USA

Kourosh Rezania
Department of Neurology,
University of Chicago,
Chicago, IL, USA

Julie Rowin
Department of Neurology and Rehabilitation Medicine,
University of Illinois at Chicago College of Medicine,
Chicago, IL, USA

Helene Rubeiz
Department of Neurology,
University of Chicago,
Chicago, IL, USA

Sean Ruland
Associate Professor,
Department of Neurology,
Loyola University Medical Center,
Stritch School of Medicine,
Maywood, IL, USA

Neil Scolding
Burden Professor and Director of the Bristol Institute of Clinical Neurosciences,
Department of Neurology,
Frenchay Hospital,
Bristol, UK

Vikram Shakkottai
Assistant Professor,
Department of Neurology,
University of Michigan Health System,
Ann Arbor, MI, USA

Kathleen M. Shannon
Professor,
Department of Neurological Sciences,
Movement Disorders Section,
Rush University Medical Center,
Chicago, IL, USA

Betty Soliven
Department of Neurology,
University of Chicago,
Chicago, IL, USA

Judy Spies
Department of Neurology,
Royal Prince Alfred Hospital,
Camperdown, NSW, Australia

James L. Stone
Departments of Neurosurgery and Neurology,
University of Illinois at Chicago College of Medicine,
Chicago, IL, USA

Andrea Swenson
Department of Neurology,
University of Iowa Hospitals and Clinics,
Iowa City, IA, USA

Fernando D. Testai
Assistant Professor in Neurology,
University of Illinois College of Medicine at Chicago,
Chicago, IL, USA

Philip Thompson
Professor of Neurology, The University of Adelaide;
Head, Department of Neurology, Royal Adelaide Hospital,
Adelaide, SA, Australia

Peter Todd
Assistant Professor,
Department of Neurology,
University of Michigan Health System,
Ann Arbor, MI, USA

James H. Tonsgard
Associate Professor,
Pediatric Neurology,
University of Chicago Medicine,
Chicago, IL, USA

Prasad S.S.V. Vannemreddy
Department of Neurosurgery,
University of Illinois at Chicago College of Medicine,
Chicago, IL, USA

Jeremy D. Young
Assistant Professor of Clinical Medicine
Section of Infectious Diseases, Immunology, and International Medicine,
Department of Medicine,
University of Illinois at Chicago College of Medicine,
Chicago, IL, USA

PREFACE

A DECADE HAS PASSED since the first edition of *Clinical Neurology*. Those who have embraced it have encouraged us to update it. The explosion of rigorous scientific evidence for interventions in clinical neurology, coupled with astonishing advances in the clinical neurosciences, have further inspired us to undertake a second edition. As the initial authors (GJH and JMW) are now a decade older and have gravitated toward greater subspecialization, another couple of fellow enthusiasts (PBG and FT) from Grand Rapids and Chicago, USA have joined to facilitate a re-energized, comprehensive, and more global, rather than Anglo–Australian, effort. Together we have enlisted the generosity and specialist expertise of our friends and colleagues throughout the world who are recognized leaders in their field and who have kindly agreed to enlighten us with a chapter on the subject to which they are dedicated.

The subjects and format of the first edition have been maintained and are complemented by the addition of a new chapter on sleep disorders. The chapter covering degenerative diseases of the nervous system has now been subdivided into three main sections, dementias, Parkinson's disease and parkinsonian syndromes, and hereditary ataxias. The cranial neuropathies chapter now includes an entirely new section on neuro-ophthalmology. In addition there are over 440 new illustrations.

The perspective for each chapter is also fresh, as each chapter (with the exception of the chapter on stroke) has been written by one or more of our new contributors, in contrast to the first edition which represented the perspective of GJH and JMW. The purpose of the book, nevertheless, continues to focus on the essentials for students of clinical neurology, particularly neurologists-in-training and practicing neurologists, who wish to have ready access to a comprehensive, up-to-date, and evidence-based guide to the understanding, diagnosis, and management of common and important neurologic disorders.

Many of the illustrations are images taken from our own patients, whom we would like to thank for allowing us to photograph them or the outcome of their investigations. Furthermore, we would also like to thank all the current and past contributors of figures (too many to list individually here) for providing illustrations, as indicated throughout the book. Finally, we would like to thank our families and colleagues for supporting us in this endeavor. We hope you enjoy it and we welcome any comments and criticisms.

Graeme J. Hankey
Joanna M. Wardlaw
Philip B. Gorelick
Fernando D. Testai

DEDICATIONS

I dedicate this book in honor of Mr. Ralph Hauenstein for service to his country and his many generous commitments to the neuroscience programs at Saint Mary's Health Care and the Western Michigan area, and to Sister Myra Bergman for her dedication, devotion and spirited work as a missionary and religious leader in our region and beyond.

Philip B. Gorelick

To my wife, Flavia, for her love, patience, and endless support; to our beautiful children, Sofia and Martin, for being continuous examples of enthusiasm and dedication; to my parents, Ruben and Stella, and sisters, Alejandra and Naiara, for their motivation and support throughout the years; to our neurology residents for having chosen one of the most amazing paths in the medical sciences; and foremost, to our most brilliant mentors – our patients.

Fernando D. Testai

To the memory of my father, the late Dr. John Hankey

Graeme J. Hankey

I am grateful to my family for ongoing support and so dedicate this work to them.

Joanna M. Wardlaw

ABBREVIATIONS

5HT 5-hydroxytryptamine
AA anaplastic astrocytoma
AAD atlantoaxial dislocation
AASM American Association of Sleep Medicine
Aβ amyloid-β
Aca aceruloplasminemia
ACE angiotensin-converting enzyme
ACE-R Addenbrooke's Cognitive Examination Revised
AChR acetylcholine receptors
ACTH adrenocorticotropic hormone
AD Alzheimer's disease
ADAMTS a disintegrin and metalloprotease with thrombospondin motif
ADC apparent diffusion coefficient
ADCA autosomal dominant cerebellar ataxia
ADEM acute disseminated encephalomyelitis
ADHD attention deficit hyperactivity disorder
ADL activities of daily living/adrenoleukodystrophy
ADLP adrenoleukodystrophy protein
ADP adenosine diphosphate
AED antiepileptic drug
AF atrial fibrillation
AFB acid-fast bacilli
AFP alpha-fetoprotein
AHI apnea/hypopnea index
AICA anterior inferior cerebellar artery
AIDP acute inflammatory demyelinating polyradiculoneuropathy
AIDS aquired immunodeficiency syndrome
AION anterior ischemic optic neuropathy
AIP acute intermittent porphyria
ALD adrenoleukodystrophy
ALDP adrenoleukodystrophy protein
ALS amyotrophic lateral sclerosis
ALT alanine aminotransferase
AMAN acute motor axonal neuropathy
AML angiomyolipoma
AMN adrenomyeloneuropathy
(c)AMP (cyclic) adenosine monophosphate
AMSAN acute motor and sensory axonal neuropathy
ANCL adult neuronal ceroid lipofuscinoses
AO anaplastic oligodendroglioma
AOA oligoastrocytoma
ApoE apolipoprotein E
APP amyloid precursor protein
APS antiphospholipid syndrome
aPTT activated partial thromboplastin time
ARAS ascending reticular activating system
ARDS adult respiratory distress syndrome
ARI absolute risk increase
ARR absolute risk reduction
ARSA arylsulfatase A
ARSACS autosomal recessive spastic ataxia of Charlevoix–Saguenay
ARX Aristaless-related homeobox
ASA atrial septal aneurysm
ASD atrial septal defect
AST aspartate aminotransferase
AT ataxia telangiectasia
ATM acute transverse myelitis
AVM arteriovenous malformation
AVS acute vestibular syndrome
AZA azathioprine
BAEP brainstem auditory evoked potential
BAL British anti-Lewisite
BBS Bardet–Biedl syndrome
BDNGF brain-derived nerve growth factor
BF blood flow
bFGF basic fibroblast growth factor
BHC benign hereditary chorea
BMD Becker's muscular dystrophy
BMI body mass index
BNCT boron neutron capture therapy
BP blood pressure
BPAP bilevel positive airways pressure
BPPV benign paroxysmal positional vertigo
BSE bovine spongiform encephalopathy
BSK Barbour–Stoenner–Kelly
BWSTT body weight supported treadmill training
CADASIL cerebral autosomal dominant arteriopathy with subcortical infarcts and leukoencephalopthy
CAM computer assisted myelography
CAS carotid artery stenting
CBD corticobasal degeneration
CBF cerebral blood flow
CBS corticobasal syndrome/cystathionine β-synthase deficiency
CBT cognitive behavioral therapy
CDC Centers for Disease Control and Prevention
CEA carotid endarterectomy/carcinoembryonic antigen
cEEG continuous electroencephalography
CE-MRA contrast-enhanced magnetic resonance angiography
CGRP calcitonin gene-related peptide
CI confidence interval/cholinesterase inhibitor
CIDP chronic inflammatory demyelinating polyneuropathy
CIM critical illness myopathy
CIMT constraint-induced movement therapy
CIP critical illness polyneuropathy
CIS clinically isolated syndrome
CISC clean intermittent self-catheterization

(f/i/s/v)CJD	(familial/iatrogenic/sporadic/variant) Creutzfeldt–Jakob disease
CK	creatine kinase
CLAM	cholesterol-lowering agent
CM	congenital myopathy
CMAP	compound muscle action potential
CMD	congenital muscular dystrophy
CMT	Charcot–Marie–Tooth disease
CMV	cytomegalovirus
CNS	central nervous system
COACH	cerebellar vermis hypo/aplasia, oligophrenia, ataxia congenital, coloboma, and hepatic fibrosis
COMT	catechol-O-methyltransferase
CORS	cerebello-oculo-renal syndrome
COX	cyclo-oxygenase
CPA	cerebello-pontine angle
CPAP	continuous positive airway pressure
CPK	creatine phosphokinase
CPM	central pontine myelinolysis
CPP	cerebral perfusion pressure
Cr	creatinine
CRAO	central retinal artery occlusion
CRP	C-reactive protein
CRVO	central retinal vein occlusion
CS	Cowden's syndrome
CSA	central sleep apnea
CSF	cerebrospinal fluid
CT	computed tomography
CTA	computed tomography angiography
CTV	computed tomography venography
CV	color vision
CVA	cerebrovascular accident
CVT	cerebral venous thrombosis
DAI	diffuse axonal injury
DALY	disability-adjusted life year
DBS	deep-brain stimulation
DFA	direct immunofluorescent antibody
DGC	dystrophin glycoprotein complex
DIC	disseminated intravascular coagulation
DLB	dementia with Lewy bodies
DMD	Duchenne's muscular dystrophy
DNA	deoxyribonucleic acid
DNET	dysembryoplastic neuroepithelial tumor
DRPLA	dentato-rubro-pallido-luysian atrophy
DSA	digital subtraction cerebral angiography
DSPN	distal symmetric polyneuropathy
DUB	deubiquitinating enzyme
DVT	deep vein thrombosis
DWI	diffusion-weighted imaging
EACA	epsilon-aminocaproic acid
EBRT	external beam radiation therapy
EBV	Epstein–Barr virus
ECG	electrocardiogram/electrocardiography
ECT	electroconvulsive therapy
EDH	extradural hematoma
EEG	electroencephalography
EGF(R)	epidermal growth factor (receptor)
EIAC	enzyme-inducing anticonvulsant
EITB	enzyme-linked immunoelectrotransfer blot assay
ELISA	enzyme-linked immunosorbent assay
EM	erythema migrans
EMD	Emery–Dreifuss muscular dystrophy
EMG	electromyography
EOG	electro-oculogram
EPP	endplate potential
EPT	enhanced physiologic tremor
ER	extended-release
ERG	electroretinography
ESR	erythrocyte sedimentation rate
ESRD	end-stage renal disease
ET	essential tremor
EV	Eustachian valve
EVD	extraventricular drain
FA	Friedreich's ataxia
FAST	Functional Assessment Staging Test
FDA	Food and Drug Administration
FES	functional electrical stimulation
FFI	fatal familial insomnia
FHM	familial hemiplegic migraine
FIESTA	fast imaging employing steady state acquisition sequence
FLAIR	fluid attenuated inversion recovery
FMD	fibromuscular dysplasia
FSHD	facioscapulohumeral muscular dystrophy
FTA	fluorescent treponemal antibody
FTD	frontotemporal dementia
FTLD	frontotemporal lobar degeneration
FVC	forced vital capacity
FXTAS	fragile X-associated tremor/ataxia syndrome
GABA	gamma-aminobutyric acid
GAD	glutamic acid decarboxylase
GALC	galactocerebrosidase
GBM	glioblastoma multiforme
GBS	group B streptococci/Guillain–Barré syndrome
GCI	glial cytoplasmic inclusion
GCS	Glasgow Coma Scale
GCSE	generalized convulsive status epilepticus
GCT	undifferentiated germinoma
GFR	glomeruler filtration rate
Glut 1	glucose transporter type 1 (deficiency)
GMP	guanosine monophosphate
GPi	globus pallidus internus
GSS	Gerstmann–Straüssler–Scheinker syndrome
GTN	glyceryl trinitrate
GTP	guanosine triphosphate
H&E	hematoxylin and eosin
HAART	highly-active antiretroviral therapy
HAM/TSP	HTLV-associated myelopathy/tropical spastic paraparesis
HANAC	hereditary angiopathy, nephropathy, aneurysm, and muscle cramps
HARP	hypoprebetalipoproteinemia, acanthocytes, retinitis pigmentosa, pallidal degeneration
HCD	hepatocerebral degeneration
HCG	human chorionic gonadotropin
HCP	hereditary coproporphyria

HD Huntington's disease
HDL Huntington disease-like
HE hepatic encephalopathy
HELLP hemolysis, elevated liver enzymes, low-platelet count syndrome
HHT hereditary hemorrhagic telangiectasia (Osler–Rendu–Weber syndrome)
HHV human herpesvirus
hIBM hereditary inclusion body myopathy
HIF hypoxia-inducible factor
HIS head impulse sign
HIT horizontal head impulse test
HIV human immunodeficiency virus
HLA human leukocyte antigen
HNPP hereditary neuropathy with liability to pressure palsies
HPE holoprosencephaly
HR hazard ratio/heart rate
HRIG human rabies immune globulin
HSP hereditary spastic paraparesis
HSV herpes simplex virus
HTIG human tetanus immune globulin
HTLV human T-lymphotropic virus
hyperPP hyperkalemic periodic paralysis
hypoPP hypokalemic periodic paralysis
HZV herpes zoster virus
IBM inclusion body myositis
IBPN immune-mediated brachial plexus neuropathy
ICA internal carotid artery
ICCA infantile convulsions and choreoathetosis
ICH intracerebral hemorrhage
ICP intracranial pressure
ICU Intensive Care Unit
ICVT intracranial cerebral venous thrombosis
IF intrinsic factor
Ig immunoglobulin
IGF insulin-like growth factor
IGRA interferon-γ release assay
IIH idiopathic intracranial hypertension
IL interleukin
ILAE International League against Epilepsy
ILOCA idiopathic late onset cerebellar ataxia
INO internuclear ophthalmoplegia
INR international normalized ratio
ION ischemic optic neuropathy
IOP intraocular pressure
IPC intermittent pneumatic compression
IPV inactivated poliovirus vaccine
IRIS immune reconstitution inflammatory syndrome
IVIG intravenous immune globulin
JCV John Cunningham virus
JME juvenile myoclonic epilepsy
KBS Klüver–Bucy syndrome
KD Krabbe disease
KSS Kearns–Sayre syndrome
LAA left atrial appendage
LCMV lymphocytic choriomeningitis virus
LD Lhermitte–Duclos disease
LDL low-density lipoprotein
LEMS Lambert–Eaton myasthenic syndrome
LFT liver function testing
LGG low-grade glioma
LGMD limb-girdle muscular dystrophy
LGV lymphogranuloma venereum
LHON Leber's hereditary optic neuropathy
LITAF lipopolysaccharide-induced tumor necrosis factor-alpha factor
LLN lower limit of normal
LMN lower motor neuron
LNS Lesch Nyhan syndrome
LNSS linear nevus sebaceous syndrome
LMWH low-molecular weight heparin
LOC loss of consciousness
LP lumbar puncture
LS Leigh syndrome
LTBI latent tuberculous infection
MAO monoamine oxidase
MAP mean arterial pressure
MAPT microtubule-associated tau gene
MBP myelin basic protein
MCA middle cerebral artery
MCI mild cognitive impairment
MCP middle cerebellar peduncle
MCPH microcephaly
MCTD mixed connective tissue disease
MEG magnetoencephalography
MELAS mitochondrial encephalomyopathy, lactic acidosis, and stroke-like episodes
MEP motor evoked potential
MERRF myoclonic epilepsy with ragged red fibers
MFAP muscle fiber action potential
MFS Miller–Fisher syndrome
MHA-TP microhemagglutination for antibodies to *Treponema pallidum*
MG myasthenia gravis
MGMT methylguanine-DNA methyltransferase
MIP maximum intensity projection/maximal inspiratory pressure
MJD Machado–Joseph disease
MLD metachromatic leukodystrophy
MLF medial longitudinal fasciculus
MMF mycophenolate mofetil
MMR mumps, measles, rubella
MMSE Mini Mental State Examination
MND motor neuron disease
MoCA Montreal Cognitive Assessment
MOTSA multiple overlapping thin-slab acquisition
MPR multi-planar reformat
MRA magnetic resonance angiography
MRI magnetic resonance imaging
mRS Modified Rankin Score
MRSA methicillin-resistant *Staphylococcus aureus*
MRV magnetic resonance venography
MS multiple sclerosis
MSA multiple system atrophy
MSLT Multiple Sleep Latency Test

MSM men who have sex with men
MSPNST malignant peripheral nerve sheath tumor
MTHFR methylenetetrahydrofolate reductase
MTR methionine synthase
MUP motor unit action potential
MuSK muscle-specific receptor tyrosine kinase
MUT methylmalonyl-CoA mutase
MWT Maintenance of Wakefulness Test
MZ monozygotic/marginal zone
NAAT nucleic acid amplication testing
NAc neuroacanthocytosis
NAD nicotinamide adenine dinucleotide
NADP nicotinamide adenine dinucleotide phosphate
NAION nonarteritic anterior ischemic optic neuropathy
NARP neurogenic weakness with ataxia and retinitis pigmentosa
NBIA neurodegeneration with brain iron accumulation
NCL neuronal ceroid lipofuscinosis
NCS nerve conduction studies
NCSE nonconvulsive status epilepticus
NDT neurodevelopmental therapy
NF neuroferritinopathy
NF-1 neurofibromatosis 1
NFT neurofibrillary tangle
NFG nerve growth factor
NFLE nocturnal frontal lobe epilepsy
NGGCT nongerminoma
NHL non-Hodgkin's lymphoma
NIF negative inspiratory pressure
NIH-SS National Institutes of Health Stroke Scale
NIID neuronal intranuclear inclusion disease
NMDA *N*-methyl-D-aspartate
NMJ neuromuscular junction
NMO neuromyelitis optica
NMS neuroleptic malignant syndrome
NO nitrous oxide
NPC Niemann–Pick type C
NPH normal pressure hydrocephalus
NPHP nephronophthisis
NSE neuron-specific enolase
NTD neural tube defect
O-AA organic amino aciduria
OAA oculomotor apraxia
OCD obsessive compulsive disorder
ONH optic nerve head
OP opening pressure
OPCA olivopontocerebellar atrophy
OPV oral poliovirus vaccine
OR odds ratio
OSA obstructive sleep apnea
OTR ocular tilt reaction
PA pernicious anemia
PACI partial anterior circulation infarct
PACS partial anterior circulation syndrome
PAF pure autonomic failure
PAM potassium aggravated myotonia
PAS para-aminosalicylic acid/periodic acid–Schiff
PC phase contrast
PCD paraneoplastic cerebellar degeneration
PCNSL primary CNS lymphoma
PCom posterior communicating artery
PCR polymerase chain reaction
PCV vincristine
PD Parkinson's disease
PDD Parkinson's disease dementia
PDGF platelet-derived growth factor
PDW proton density-weighted
PE plasma exchange
PEG percutaneous endoscopic gastrostomy
PEM paraneoplastic encephalomyelitis
PEO progressive external ophthalmoplegia
PET positron emission tomography
PFK phosphofructokinase
PFO patent foramen ovale
PION posterior ischemic optic neuropathy
Pi-TON posterior indirect traumatic optic neuropathy
PKAN pantothenate kinase-associated neurodegeneration
PLED periodic lateralized epileptiform discharge
PLEX plasmapheresis
PLM periodic leg movement
PLMD periodic leg movement disorder
PMA progressive myoclonic ataxia
PME progressive myoclonic epilepsy
PML progressive multi-focal leukoencephalopathy
PMN polymorphonuclear
PMzD Pelizeaus–Merzbacher disease
PNET primitive neuroectodermal tumor
PNFA progressive nonfluent aphasia
POCI posterior circulation infarct
POCS posterior circulation syndrome
POEMS polyneuropathy, organomegaly, endocrinopathies, M-protein, skin changes including thickening and hyperpigmentation, clubbing of the fingers
POST positive occipital sharp transients of sleep
POVL postoperative visual loss
PP preplate zone/perfusion pressure
PPA primary progressive aphasia
PPRF paremedian pontine reticular formation
PRES posterior reversible encephalopathy syndrome
PRG pontine respiratory group
PrP prion protein
PSN paraneoplastic sensory neuropathy
PSP progressive supranuclear palsy
PSV peak systolic velocity
PSWC periodic sharp wave complex
PTH parathyroid hormone
PTSD post-traumatic stress disorder
PWI perfusion-weighted imaging
PXA pleomorphic xanthoastrocytoma
PXE pseudoxanthoma elasticum
RBC red blood cell
RCT randomized controlled trial
RCVS reversible cerebral vasoconstriction syndrome
RDI respiratory disturbance index
REM rapid eye movement
RERA respiratory event-related arousal

RF resistance to flow
rFVIIa recombinant activated factor VII
RLS right-to-left shunt/restless legs syndrome
RMSF Rocky Mountain spotted fever
RNA ribonucleic acid
RNS repetitive nerve stimulation
ROM range-of-motion
RPR rapid plasma reagin
RR risk ratio/relative risk
RRR relative risk reduction
(r)-tPA (recombinant) tissue plasminogen activator
SAM S-adenosyl-methionine
SC Sydenham's chorea
SCA spinocerebellar ataxia
SCC semicircular canal
SCD subacute combined degeneration
SCI spinal cord injury
SCLC small-cell lung carcinoma
SCN suprachiasmatic nucleus
$ScvO_2$ central venous oxygen saturation
SD semantic dementia
SDB sleep-related breathing disorder
SDS Shy–Drager syndrome
SE status epilepticus
SEGA subependymal giant cell astrocytoma
SFEMG single fiber electromyography
SGCT subependymal giant cell tumor
SIADH syndrome of inappropriate antidiuretic hormone
SIBM sporadic inclusion body myositis
SIS second impact syndrome
SISCOM subtraction ictal SPECT coregistered to MRI
SLE systemic lupus erythematosus
SMA spinal muscular atrophy
SMN survival of motor neuron
SNAP sensory nerve action potential
SND striatonigral degeneration
SOD septo-optic dysplasia
SOREMP sleep onset REM period
SPECT single photon emission tomography
SSCP single-stranded conformational polymorphism
SSEP somatosensory evoked potential
SSPE subacute sclerosing panencephalitis
SSRI selective serotonin-reuptake inhibitor
SSS superior sagittal sinus/Scandinavian Stroke Scale
SUDEP sudden unexplained death in epilepsy
SVV subjective visual vertical
SVZ subventricular zone
SW Sturge–Weber syndrome
SWI susceptibility-weighted imaging
TA temporal arteritis
TAB temporal artery biopsy
TACI total anterior circulation infarct
TACS total anterior circulation syndrome
TAO thyroid-associated ophthalmopathy
TB tuberculosis
TBI traumatic brain injury
TCD transcranial Doppler ultrasonography
TCS tuberous sclerosis complex
TGF transforming growth factor
THB tetrahydrobiopterin
TIA transient ischemic attack
TMJ temporomandibular joint
TMP–SMX trimethoprim–sulfamethoxazole
TN trigeminal neuralgia
TNF tumor necrosis factor
TOAST Trial of Org 10172 in Acute Stroke Treatment
TOE trans-esophageal echocardiography
TOF time-of-flight
TPHA *Treponema pallidum* particle agglutination assay
TS Tourette's syndrome
TSE turbo spin echo/transmissible spongiform encephalopathy
TSH thyroid stimulating hormone
TST thermoregulatory sweat test
TTE transthoracic echocardiography
TTR time in therapeutic range/transthyretin
UBO unidentified bright object
UFH unfractionated heparin
ULN upper limit of normal
UMN upper motor neuron
VA visual acuity
VaD vascular dementia
VAPP vaccine-associated paralytic poliomyelitis
VLDL very low-density lipoprotein
VDRL Venereal Disease Research Laboratory
V-EEG video electroencephalography
VEGF vascular endothelial growth factor
VEMP vestibular evoked potential
VEP visual evoked potential
VF visual field
VGCC voltage-gated calcium channel
VHL von Hippel–Lindau disease
VKA vitamin K antagonist
VLCFA very long-chain fatty acid
VLM ventrolateral medulla
VNG video-nystagmography
VNS vagal nerve stimulation
VOR vestibulo-ocular reflex
VP vascular parkinsonism/variegate porphyria
VPM ventral posteromedial
VR volume rendered
VSGP vertical supranuclear gaze palsy
VSR vestibulospinal reflex
VTE venous thromboembolism
vWF von Willebrand factor
VWFCP von Willebrand factor-cleaving protease
VZ ventricular zone
VZV varicella-zoster virus
WBC white blood cell
WBRT whole brain radiation therapy
WD Wilson's disease
WHO World Health Organization
WNV West Nile virus
XP xeroderma pigmentosum

NEUROLOGIC DIAGNOSIS

John Dunne, Robert Edis, William McAuliffe

INTRODUCTION

Neurologic diagnosis is now often made with greater certainty, facilitated by the advent of sophisticated neurodiagnostic tests. Combined with the constant growth in neurologic knowledge and portable access to it via the internet, there has been a debate about the relevance of teaching traditional neurologic assessment. It is evident to neurologist educators, however, that 'the clinical neurologic assessment is not obsolete', but that it must be informed by new technologies and be enhanced by teaching better internal medicine, psychiatry, and communication skills in a societal context[1,2].

Internet teaching sites can demonstrate examination techniques, and show examples of neurologic conditions when 'once seen, are easier to recognise a second time around' (for example, unusual eye movement disorders)[3,4]. The role of Google as a diagnostic tool is increasingly being utilized. It can be both educational and helpful in formulating a differential diagnosis in neurology[5]. Using online medical literature search engines such as Cochrane Library and Pubmed is now the key to rapidly accessing relevant knowledge and evidence-based guidelines and protocols.

A mobile phone video can play a vital diagnostic role, when taken by an observer documenting an episode of altered behavior or loss of consciousness[6]. A small digital camera (or mobile phone) in the neurologist's examination bag is helpful in capturing images for teaching and documentation.

Tele-neurology, where the neurologist takes a history and may be able to watch an examination by video-link, is now being incorporated into outpatient clinics because of increasing demands on resources, and this requires a modified approach to the neurologic consultation[7].

Tip

► *Despite these technological advances the clinical history remains the most important and productive part of the neurologic assessment as it generates the diagnostic possibilities and directs the examination, investigations, and information search.*

Precise clinical findings are often needed to guide investigations and their interpretation, for example when directing the radiologist where to look for the magnetic resonance imaging (MRI) signs of a brainstem stroke or a possible vertebral artery dissection. In addition, the neurologist is now often asked to interpret the clinical significance of surprise MRI imaging findings such as a Chiari I malformation, multiple white matter lesions (possible multiple sclerosis [MS]), or an enlarged cerebrospinal fluid (CSF) space (possible stroke).

The acquisition of superior clinical neurologic skills through sufficient experience requires several years of apprenticeship, and a demonstration that certain key competencies have been achieved. This needs practice, with the regular commitment of the history, the physical examination findings, and diagnostic formulation to paper, for presentation and review to diverse mentors, who in turn can teach unique skills and insights. A flexible neurology curriculum which includes inpatient care, sufficient ambulatory outpatient exposure (as well as some formal terms in internal medicine and psychiatry if possible) as an initial general training is ideal. Learning from, and communicating with colleagues, including allied health practitioners and nurses, is integral to a neurologic education, particularly as neurologists are now often members of multidisciplinary teams.

THE DIAGNOSTIC PROCESS IN NEUROLOGY

Depending on the presentation, the process is based on two different pathways:

- Pattern recognition: this refers to recognizing something that one has seen before, relying on past experience or a pattern of symptoms and signs which have meaning (such as trigeminal neuralgia, carpal tunnel syndrome, Parkinson's disease). It is intuitively used by experts who have a wide experience and knowledge but is more difficult for the inexperienced trainee.
- Hypothetico-deductive system: clinical reasoning in unfamiliar conditions depends on early hypothesis formation from clues in the history, which may then be modified by further deductive reasoning as new data are collected from the history and examination.

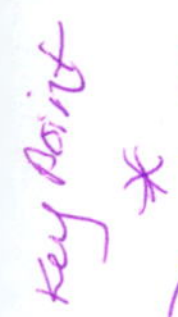

In the situation of an evolving organic neurologic dis order, the history and signs lead to an anatomical localization and a differential diagnosis of pathologies and causes which may need targeted investigation to clarify (for example, a spinal MRI with gadolinium in an ascending myelopathy with pain).

Diagnostic questions

There are six basic diagnostic questions to be answered:

1. *Is there a neurologic problem present?* This requires good internal medicine, psychiatric, and neurologic knowledge.
2. *Where is the problem?* This requires knowledge of anatomy and physiology.
   - Localization: focal, multifocal, diffuse.
   - Cortical (supratentorial).
   - Brainstem (infratentorial).
   - Spinal cord (extrinsic or intrinsic).
   - Peripheral (nerve, neuromuscular junction, muscle).
   - More than one level.
3. *What has caused the problem?*
   - Factors: hereditary, congenital, infective, inflammatory, traumatic, degenerative, neoplastic, vascular, metabolic, toxic, social/psychiatric.
4. *How bad is the problem?* This needs an appreciation of how the patient is functioning at home and at work.
5. *What is the likely outcome?* The prognosis will influence investigation and treatment.
6. *What can be done about it?* Treatment and management options.

Tip

▶ *Answers to the six basic diagnostic questions must be actively sought throughout the history and examination, with early, broad hypothesis generation tested and refined by goal-directed questioning, while simultaneously considering the consequences for the patient.*

Important elements of the consultation process

- Be friendly throughout, and after introducing yourself by name and making sure that the patient knows your role, spend some minutes in general conversation to begin to establish rapport. Use humour when possible and appropriate throughout.
- Clarify with the patient what they expect from the consultation, and that this is in accord with what you can deliver, as sometimes inappropriate referral or expectations need to be addressed early.
- Ask whether the symptoms are better, worse, or unchanged since the referral, to bring yourself up to date.
- A contribution from family members or friends is essential if a presentation suggests dementia, altered behavior, or loss of consciousness.
- If necessary, at the time of the interview, telephone to clarify information or to get a witness description.
- Write down brief notes (especially verbatim statements), particularly timelines, as well as diagnostic, investigation, and treatment thoughts as they come to mind.

How to improve communication

Patients are now more informed and demanding, armed with ideas from family, friends, alternative health practitioners, and the internet. To use the consultation as a positive intervention in its own right requires honest open dialogue with the patient and family. This patient-centered approach means that rather than 'taking the history' we want to 'build a history' and a joint understanding with the patient through an interactive conversation. Communication skills need to be learnt and practiced and they include core skills of a) appropriate questioning, b) active listening, c) facilitating, d) keeping the patient relevant, and e) summarizing[8].

Questioning

- Use open questions as often as possible, particularly at the beginning of an interview.
- For example, '*Begin from when you were last perfectly well*'.
- '*Tell me what is worrying you the most*'.
- '*Tell me about your headaches*'.
- Then when necessary, obtain specific information by using focused and goal-directed questions as you formulate hypotheses.
- Use probing questions to clarify, for example, '*What do you mean by dizziness?*', and accuracy of information, for example, '*What were you doing exactly at the time your symptoms came on?*', '*What was the very first thing you noticed?*', '*Then what happened next?*'.
- Avoid asking several questions at once or giving multiple options.

Active listening

- Allow the patient to talk about the presenting problem(s) without interruptions (usually takes less than 2 minutes!).
- Make empathic statements and show sympathy when appropriate, for example, '*That must have been difficult for you*'.
- Permit pauses and silences to encourage the patient to reveal more.

Facilitating

Encourage more information with verbal ('*Tell me more*'; '*Go on*'; '*Hmm*'), and physical (head nodding) cues.

Relevance

It is important to use time effectively and this may involve redirecting the interview at certain times in the history.

Summarizing

Paraphrasing the story back to the patient is helpful at times during and at the end of the consultation. This confirms that you have been listening and allows the patient to agree, clarify, or add further information.

The structure of a neurologic history

Practicing a systematic approach to the interview makes sure that all relevant information has been gathered. Flexibility in how this information is gathered, and the importance of some aspects over others in any one patient, comes with experience. Often some elements of the history cannot be raised during the consultation because of time constraints, new diagnostic thoughts, or because it may be best to seek sensitive information away from an accompanying person.

Presenting problem/complaint

The chief problem(s) should be clear from the referral but must be confirmed with the patient by asking, depending on the context: '*What is it that you have come to see me about?*'; or '*Tell me the story of your problem*'; or '*What is it you hope I will be able to do for you today?*'. It is often helpful early in the consultation to get a sense of the patient and their world, by enquiring about their work, where they live, daily activities, and family responsibilities, to provide a context for the symptoms.

There may be one or a number of symptoms ('problem list') which need to be analyzed. For each relevant symptom find out the circumstances, timing, content, and its relationship to other symptoms.

- Onset ('*When exactly did it begin?*'; '*What were you doing at the time?*'; '*Did it begin suddenly/gradually and over what time period?*'. If long-standing, '*Why are you presenting now?*').
- Constant or intermittent ('*How long does it last for?*'; '*Any particular time of day?*'; '*Is it the same each time or does it vary in content or intensity?*').
- Triggering factors (such as cough or sneeze-induced arm pain, and paresthesia with radiculopathy; exercise or overheating causing visual blurring in optic neuropathy; situational syncope due to prolonged standing, pain, defecation, micturition, coughing, or swallowing).
- Relieving/exacerbating factors (such as shaking the hand/driving the car in carpal tunnel syndrome; hand on the head relieving nerve root compression pain).
- Any associated symptoms (pallor, sweating, nausea, postictal confusion, tongue biting when evaluating syncope *vs.* seizure, one of the most common presentations to neurologists where a detailed history in evaluating convulsive syncope is pivotal in making the diagnosis)[9].
- Timing of the onset and evolution of the problem is often a clue to a cause:
  - Intermittent or episodic symptoms with full recovery can suggest migraine, syncope, epilepsy, transient ischemic attacks (TIA), myasthenia gravis, periodic paralysis.

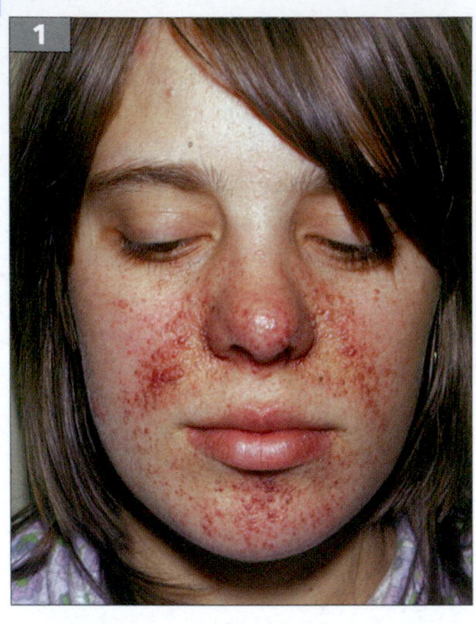

1 Typical facial adenoma sebaceum rash in a patient with tuberous sclerosis.

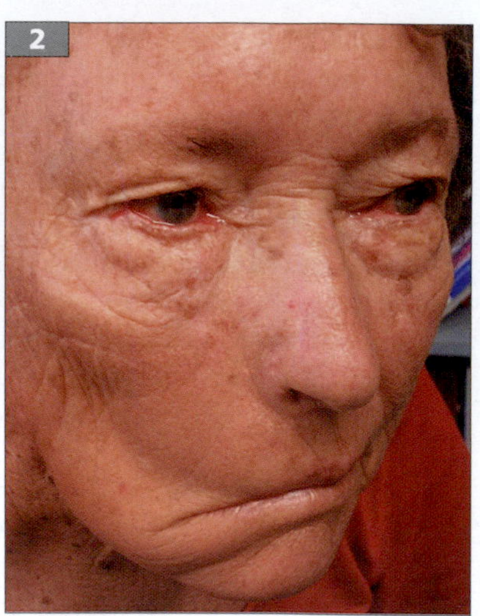

2 VII nerve palsy due to local spread of a basal cell carcinoma.

- A fluctuating and chronic course over years may point to MS, autoimmune, or functional symptoms.
- A chronic progressive history points to an inflammatory or neurodegenerative disorder.
- Acute or subacute progressive course may indicate a neoplastic, inflammatory, paraneoplastic, or infective problem.
- Acute onset single event with recovery may suggest an epileptic, inflammatory, or vascular cause.

Remember that 10–30% of patients seen by neurologists have symptoms which are thought to have a psychologic basis. Psychiatric causes are important in some cases (conversion, panic disorder, depression). However, many patients do not have a psychiatric disorder, but psychologic factors such as past life experiences, erroneous beliefs and anxiety, amplify their minor physical sensations. These symptoms have attracted many different labels (medically unexplained, psychogenic), but the most accepted and useful term is 'functional symptoms'. They are within the domain of neurology rather than psychiatry[10].

Tip

► *In diagnostic hypothesis formation, mentally refer to useful criteria sets in your own mind which characterize different conditions (e.g. carpal tunnel syndrome* vs. *cervical radiculopathy; seizure* vs. *syncope; trigeminal neuralgia* vs. *atypical facial pain; functional* vs. *organic symptoms; different headache/epilepsy syndromes).*

Review of body systems

The purpose of this review is to look for further evidence to test a hypothesis already generated or to elicit information that may be overlooked by the patient. Questions briefly probe particularly appetite; weight change; sleep; chest tightness, palpitations, shortness of breath if suspecting chronic hyperventilation or amplification of normal bodily sensations; sphincter function; skin lesions (**1**); the musculoskeletal system; exercise patterns; and mood.

Smoking and alcohol intake

Record the patient's smoking, alcohol, and other drug habits, and any attempt to modify these habits.

Medications

Record current and recent past medication intake. This is particularly important in patients with epilepsy and headache, and should include dose and length of use, side-effects, and the patient's attitude to medication. Patients should be specifically asked about the use of the oral contraceptive, complementary and alternative medicines, nutritional supplements, and over-the-counter drugs. These are commonly taken in conjunction with conventional medication and may be relevant to the patient's symptoms or to a proposed treatment (for example, direct toxicity from high-dose pyridoxal; or toxicity from interaction with conventional mediation).

Past medical history

Enquiry into previous illness, operations, accidents, and admissions to hospital may give information relevant to the current illness (multiple admissions with unexplained illnesses suggesting somatization; previous skin cancer surgery with query incomplete skin cancer removal [**2**]).

Family history

The current family members' ages and health; age of death and cause in first degree relatives should be documented. Patients may be suffering from an unsuspected genetic disorder (for example, hereditary spastic paraplegia or late-onset familial peripheral neuropathy) or the patients' concerns may relate to the experience of others in the family (dementia or brain tumor). An ever increasing number of neurologic disorders are being recognized of genetic origin.

Social history

Details of the domestic, social, and business background (e.g. the patient's relationship with family, friends, employer, and workmates, attitude to work, when they last took holidays, hobbies, living arrangements, financial state, and sexual preference) may be keys to understanding the patient's presentation. It is often helpful to run through the course of a typical day with the patient. This may also give an insight into unrecognized or denied stress factors which can relate in particular to functional disorders, chronic tension-type headache, 'dizziness', and relapse of seizures. Mononeuropathies could be due to hobbies or daily activities that put nerves at risk of pressure or stretch, such as repeated leaning on an elbow while at the computer, causing a compressive ulnar neuropathy. It is important to know of the impact of the illness on other family members.

Concluding the history

By the end of the history make sure you have the answers to the questions: '*What do you think is causing your problem*?' and '*Is there anything else you would like to discuss*?'.

You should have a working diagnosis with perhaps several alternatives, and these are usually correct in well over two-thirds of cases. It is often appropriate briefly (and broadly, without committing yourself, if uncertain) to discuss initial diagnostic thoughts with the patient and what you would now like to examine.

Tip

▶ *Not obtaining a sufficient and detailed history is the most common cause of failure to make the correct diagnosis. If time is short, skimp on the examination rather than the history.*

NEUROLOGIC EXAMINATION

The bedside neurologic examination is a powerful portable low-cost diagnostic tool. A 'focused neurologic examination' is designed to look for abnormal signs relevant to a diagnostic hypothesis generated from the history. For example, in a case of an acute ascending paralysis with reduced limb reflexes, attention will be given to the plantar responses, the pattern of any sensory loss in the limbs and trunk, and of weakness including whether there is mild facial weakness, in considering a differential diagnosis of the Guillain–Barré syndrome or a myelopathy.

A 'screening neurologic examination' is designed to detect abnormalities that may not be apparent to the patient, such as mild pyramidal/extrapyramidal motor signs, gait abnormality, visual field loss, pupillary change, papilledema, cortical sensory loss, and reflex changes (e.g. fundoscopy in all headache patients to detect papilledema in the rare case of idiopathic intracranial hypertension).

Incorporate a relevant general examination into the sequence of the neurologic examination by initially taking and examining the patient's hand, looking for general health clues (**3**), taking the pulse and blood pressure (BP) in the sitting position (rechecking at the end of the examination if it is high; lying and standing BP if looking for postural hypotension in syncope, and in parkinsonian syndromes on treatment and as a clue to a multisystem atrophy where postural hypotension may be asymptomatic).

Tip

▶ *Perform an examination focused on functions relevant to the presenting problem, both for diagnosis and because a careful examination helps the therapeutic relationship. It also continually reinforces an appreciation of the range of normal responses. If you do not perform an examination, explain why you do not think it is necessary.*

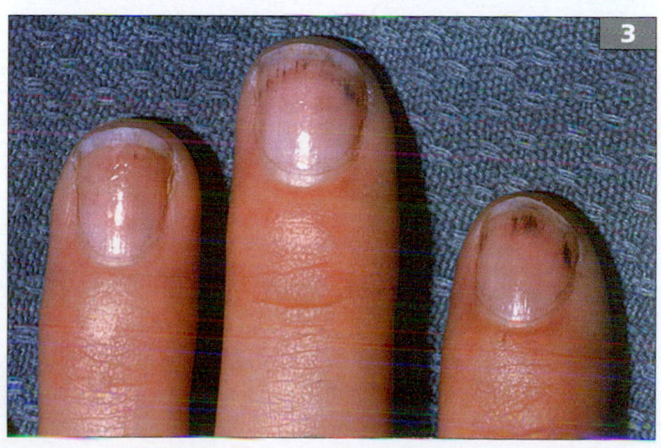

3 Splinter hemorrhages in a patient with infective carditis and an embolic stroke.

Look at the skin for a rash (4), or markers of associated neurologic disease (e.g. tuberous sclerosis [1], Fabry's disease) and in headache patients, the range of joint and neck movement, tenderness over the greater occipital nerves at the base of the skull, and temporal artery pulsation. Auscultate the heart, neck, and orbits for bruits if there is pulsatile tinnitus, a TIA, or stroke. Record the patient's weight at the end of the examination when possible.

Although there are traditional clinical methods for examining the nervous system, every neurologist develops their own style influenced by mentors, clinical experience, and from texts[1–4].

First impressions

Some diagnoses are apparent immediately by pattern recognition (e.g. parkinsonism, hypothyroidism, hemifacial spasm, essential head or voice tremor, chorea, a patient sitting crossed-leg presenting with a foot drop). Behavioral hyperventilation may be evident with the patient sighing frequently during the history and is often a clue to the cause of their symptom. Looking frequently to their spouse to answer questions points to a cognitive problem.

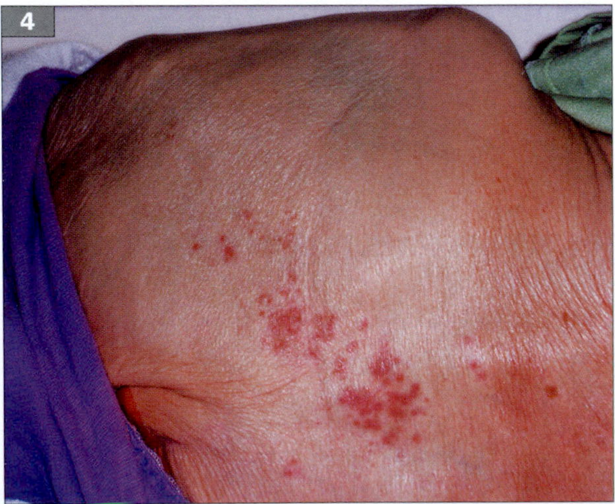

4 A left lumbar nerve root (motor and sensory) herpes zoster, presenting with a painful quadriceps weakness and a subtle paraspinal rash.

MENTAL STATE (HIGHER MENTAL FUNCTION)

Screening tests

History taking is part of mental status testing. Observations can be made about the patient's:

- Attention and cooperation.
- Language and memory functions reflected by responses to questions.
- Behaviour and awareness of the consultation purpose and context.

The Mini-Mental State Examination (MMSE) (*Table 1*) is the most widely used screening test but it is not sensitive in detecting mild cognitive impairment, focal deficits, and frontal lobe disorders, where patients may score almost perfectly.

Formal tests

- If suspicions are aroused during the history or the presenting complaint is of loss of memory, language errors, behavioral change, or hallucinations, then do more detailed higher function testing.
- Correlations can be made between failure on certain tests and brain localization of function.
- When testing for a possible dementia, mental test batteries can be useful particularly if following a patient over time. The purpose of the testing must be explained to the patient to get them to participate; administer in an encouraging nonjudgmental manner. The MMSE can be used but supplement with bedside tests looking for focal cognitive impairments.
- A more useful comprehensive sensitive cognitive battery is the Addenbrooke's Cognitive Examination Revised (ACE-R), which takes 20 minutes to administer. There are good normative data. It can help detect mild cognitive impairment, early Alzheimer's disease, and frontotemporal dementia; a MMSE score is recorded as a subset score. The ACE-R with a scoring guide and accompanying-person interview proforma is available free from the authors and from the internet[5,6].
- In a pseudo-dementia of depression, the patient usually gives up on test items, and if suspected, it is worth applying a depression screening test (e.g. Geriatric Depression Scale; Patient Health Questionnaire PHq-9).

Supplementary or alternative mental function tests

- Orientation:
  - Establish the patient's orientation to time (year, month, day, date, time of day, season); place (city, building, floor, ward); person (name, date of birth, age, marital status); reason for consultation.
- Attention:
  - Repeat an irregular series of numbers between 1 and 9 of increasing length (abnormal is <5 forward; <3 backwards).
  - Serial recitation of months of the year backwards; days of the week; serial subtraction of 7 from 100.
- Memory:
  - Anterograde: recall of recent events (hours, days); recall of three items after 3 minutes; learning of a word list (e.g. *tulip, seventeen, belt, Toyota, cabbage, camel, goose, river*) read to the patient for the list to be recalled immediately; this is repeated five times and scored. After 20 minutes a delayed free recall is tested (normal is at least six items) and then recalled with cues.
  - Retrograde: names of family members; politicians; sports events; precise chronologic details about personal events in the patient's life; '*What has been in the news lately*?'.
  - Semantic: naming pictures; pointing at named pictures; defining words or pictures; semantic fluency in naming from categories in 1 minute (e.g. animals or fruits; normal is >15); draw objects (e.g. a pyramid).

TABLE 1 **MINI-MENTAL STATE EXAMINATION**

	Maximum score
ORIENTATION	
What is the time / day / month / year / season?	5 points
What is the name of this ward / hospital / town / state / country?	5 points
REGISTRATION	
Name three objects (e.g. *car, dog, book*) and then ask patient to repeat these.	3 points
The number of objects repeated correctly is the score. Endeavor, by further attempts and prompting, to have all three repeated, so as to test recall later.	
ATTENTION AND CALCULATION	
Subtract 7 from 100, and then 7 from the result.	5 points
Repeat this five times, scoring 1 point for each correct subtraction. If the patient cannot/will not do this: spell '*world*' backwards.	
RECALL	
Name the three objects repeated in the registration test.	3 points
Score 1 point for each correct answer.	
LANGUAGE	
Name two objects (e.g. a pencil and a watch).	2 points
Repeat a short phrase (e.g.'*No ifs, ands or buts*').	1 point
Execute a three-stage command, scoring 1 point for each stage (e.g.'*With the index finger of your left hand touch the tip of your nose and then your left ear.*').	3 points
Read and obey the following '*Close your eyes*'.	1 point
Write a sentence of your own choice (the sentence must make sense and contain a subject and verb).	1 point
Copy a diagram showing two intersecting pentagons.	1 point
Total score	30 points

Scoring 23 or less denotes cognitive impairment (76% detection rate, 4% false positive).
(Adapted from Dick *et al.*, *J. Neurol. Neurosurg. Psychiatry*, 1984; **47**:496)

Frontal lobe functions

The clinical evaluation of frontal lobe functions depends at least as much on the history and behavioral observation as on the results of bedside tests. Evaluate in suspected dementia or behavioral change.

Attention and behavior abnormality

Patient is easily distracted and shows facetiousness and punning (witzelsucht); or apathy and poor initiation and social interaction (abulia).

Verbal fluency

This may be impaired in dysphasia or frontal dysfunction; ask the patient to say as many words as possible excluding names of people and places in 1 minute each with the letters F, A, and S; perseveration of names is abnormal (most people get 15 words at least per letter; <30 for FAS is usually abnormal); '*Tell me the names of as many animals as you can in 1 minute*' (around 20 is normal; 15 is low average; 10 is impaired).

Abstraction

Concrete interpretation is seen in frontal lobe damage. Proverbs, e.g. '*too many cooks spoil the broth*', '*make hay while the sun shines*'; similarities, e.g. apple and banana; table and chair; praise and punishment.

Response inhibition and set shifting

The ability to shift from one cognitive task to another and to inhibit inappropriate responses can be tested by:

- Motor sequencing – Luria three-step test. Demonstrate the series of three hand movements 'fist–edge–palm' three times without verbal cues and ask the patient to repeat the sequence three times with you, and then alone (5). Patients with frontal deficits often fail even a two-step sequence of fist–palm without prompts.
- The alternating hand movements test. The examiner demonstrates the test by having one hand with fingers extended and the other with clenched fist; then the hand positions are reversed by alternately opening and closing each hand in a rhythmical sequence. Ask the patient to perform this sequence.

Frontal release signs

These reflexes are released from normal inhibition in frontal lobe disease. The grasp reflex is the most specific while the glabella tap and palmomental responses may occur in the normal elderly.

- Grasp reflex: To elicit lightly stroke your hand across the patient's palm while distracting the patient with casual conversation. A positive response is an involuntary grasping, which can be forceful or subtle (do not instruct the patient 'not to grasp'). Usually a contralateral finding to the abnormal frontal lobe in the alert patient, and bilateral in dementias with frontal involvement and in metabolic/infective encephalopathies.
- Utilization behavior is when the patient reaches out to pick up and uses objects around them inappropriate to the social setting, with a limited capacity to over-ride such actions. It may occur spontaneously (e.g. fiddling with your stethoscope or a sheet) or if on handing the patient an item without instruction, they unusually toy with it. This is seen in frontal lobe disorders but not in Alzheimer's disease.

Paratonia (gagenhalten)

This is an abnormal variable resistance in limb muscles found contralateral to a mesial frontal lobe lesion, where there seems to be an inability to relax with an inclination to resist, increasing with more rapid movement; it affects the whole limb.

Tip

▶ *The FAB, a frontal assessment battery at the bedside, is a series of standardized frontal lobe tests (as above) with a scoring system, taking 10 minutes to administer*[7].

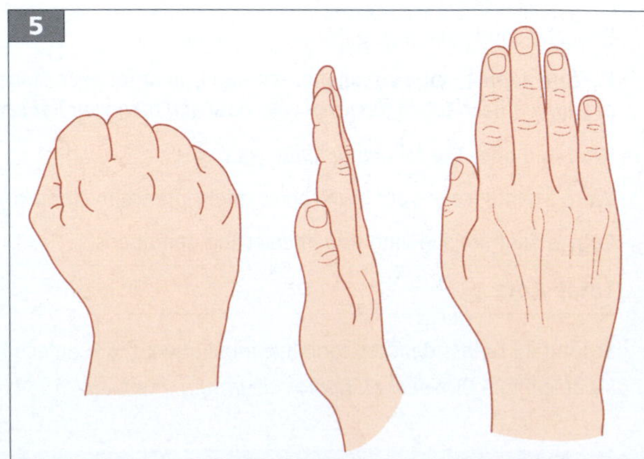

5 Luria three-step test sequence of hand positions (fist–edge–palm).

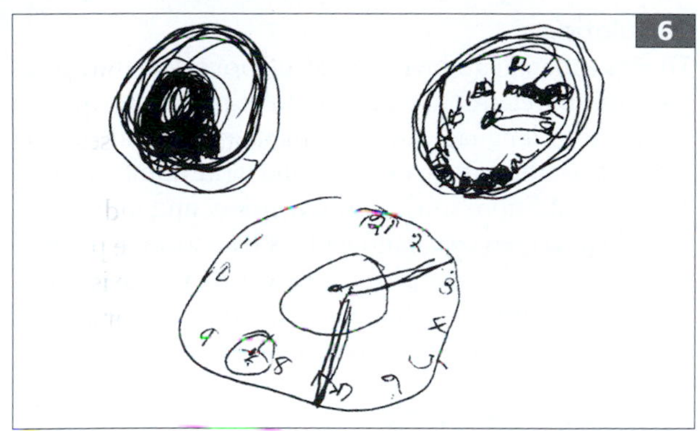

6 A patient with a right temporal–parietal stroke with left spatial neglect showing clock drawing improving over a number of weeks. *Courtesy of the late Dr. M. Sadka, Consultant Neurologist, Royal Perth Hospital, Western Australia.*

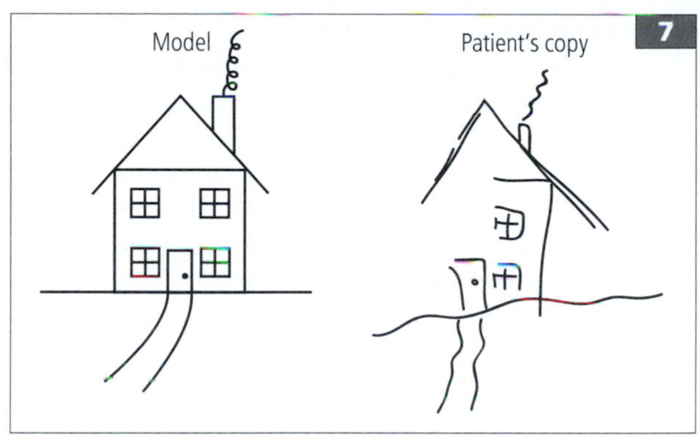

7 A similar patient's response when asked to copy a drawing of a house.

Right hemisphere function

Functions associated with the nondominant right hemisphere (in the right handed) should be tested in a patient with a left hemiparesis or sudden change in behavior.

Sensory visual and tactile neglect

This is tested by:

- Questions such as '*Describe what you see in this picture*', showing, for example, a picture in a magazine.
- Sensory extinction to simultaneous bilateral stimulation, when the patient consistently ignores the touch stimulus to the affected side but which is felt on unilateral touch.

Hemispatial neglect

This is tested by:

- Instructions such as '*Draw a clock face and put the numbers in at ten past five*'; '*Copy this house*'; '*Draw a stick man*' (**6**, **7**).
- Line bisection, when the examiner draws a series of overlapping horizontal lines down a piece of paper and asks the patient to bisect each of the lines, whereupon an obvious bias to one side may be evident.

Dressing dyspraxia

This is best detected by questioning the family or nursing staff and by observing the patient putting on a shirt/blouse which has been turned inside out.

Object and facial recognition (prosopagnosia)

- Prosopagnosia can be tested by showing objects to be named and face recognition of politicians and celebrities from a magazine.

Dominant left hemisphere function (in right-handed patients)

Dysphasia is impairment of language function caused by brain damage and may be obvious or subtle in spontaneous speech. Testing at the bedside requires a simple sequence of observations.

Language

- Spontaneous speech during conversation and picture description (e.g. from a magazine); note if it is nonfluent and agrammatical or fluent but full of syllable substitutions (phonemic paraphasias) or word confusions (semantic paraphasias), and if there are nonsense words (neologisms).
- Naming: show a mixture of common and uncommon items (e.g. a watch face, coin, paperclip, key).
- Comprehension is tested in conversation but formally by:
  - Pointing to command: '*Point to the window, watch, key, coin*'; '*Close your eyes*'; '*Stick out your tongue*'.
  - Then more complex instructions: '*Touch your left ear with your right hand*'; '*Point to the ceiling, the door, and the window*'. It is normal to be able to do four -step commands.
- Repetition is tested with a series of words and sentences of increasing complexity (e.g. red, caterpillar, hippopotamus; the dog chased the cat; who did what to whom).

- Reading aloud and comprehension:
  - Write a command for the patient to follow, e.g. '*Close your eyes*'; '*Place your hands on your head*'.
  - Get the patient to read a passage from a test-type book or magazine and ask about the content.
- Writing: ask the patient to write several sentences or a paragraph about their job or home and look for errors in spelling and grammatical composition.

Document the above responses as a description of their dysphasia; the results may fit a profile that can be specified (e.g. Broca's, Wernicke's, conduction, nominal, transcortical dysphasia).

Praxis

Dyspraxia is an inability to carry out complex motor acts despite intact motor and sensory systems, coordination, and comprehension of the task. Praxis is tested in left hemisphere parietal lesions (mainly stroke patients), suspected early dementia, or other neurodegenerative syndromes.

Test first to command and if not able to do, by asking the patient to imitate your actions:

- '*Show me how you would*' (symbolic gestures) – blow out a match; lick your lips; wave goodbye; salute; brush your teeth; hammer a nail. A common error is the use of 'body-part as object' e.g. forefinger used as a toothbrush.
- '*Copy these hand gestures*' (meaningless nonsymbolic gestures) as demonstrated by the examiner. The interlocking finger test is a recent validated bedside praxis screen for parietal lobe dysfunction[8]. Ask the patient to imitate each of the four interlocking finger figures, one at a time, as you demonstrate them. Failure on any one is significant (8).

Calculation

To make mental and written calculations demands comprehension, retention, and manipulation of information and involves language, working memory, and calculation skills (check the patient can read and write numbers first). Test oral addition, subtraction, division, and multiplication; then written calculations. This is abnormal in dominant parietal lobe pathology, where it may be associated with an inability to distinguish left from right, to write, and to name fingers, i.e. Gerstmann's syndrome.

CRANIAL NERVES

Screening tests

- Ask about vision and visual acuity.
- Observe eyelid position for each eye.
- Test the visual fields of each eye and for visual inattention.
- Observe visual fixation in the primary position.
- Range of horizontal and vertical eye movement.
- Pupil size and reaction to direct light.
- Fundoscopy each eye.
- Facial power by the patient closing their eyes tightly and then showing their teeth.
- Hearing by finger rubbing outside each ear.
- Protrude tongue; voice quality.

Formal tests

Nerve I (olfactory nerve)

- This is only tested if there is a complaint of a disturbed taste or smell or a closed head injury or fracture. The examiner can use coffee grounds; a cut orange; peppermint; vanilla to each nostril with the patient's eyes closed.

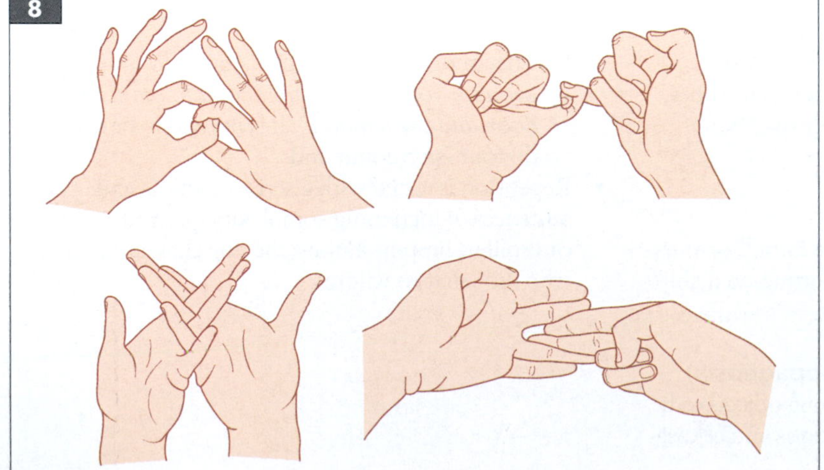

8 Examiner's hands demonstrating the four interlocking finger positions.

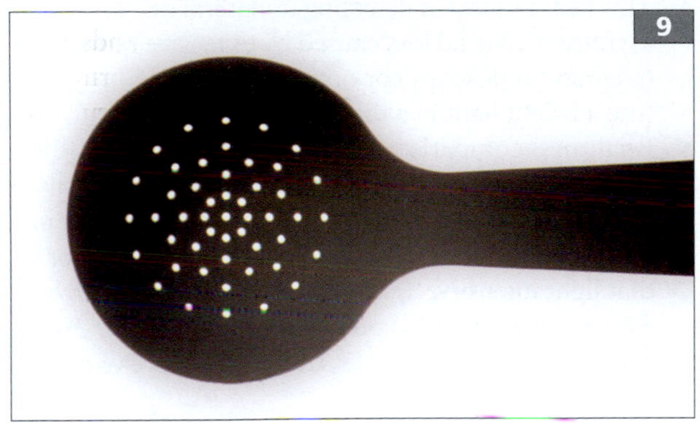

9 Multi-pinhole tester for visual acuity testing.

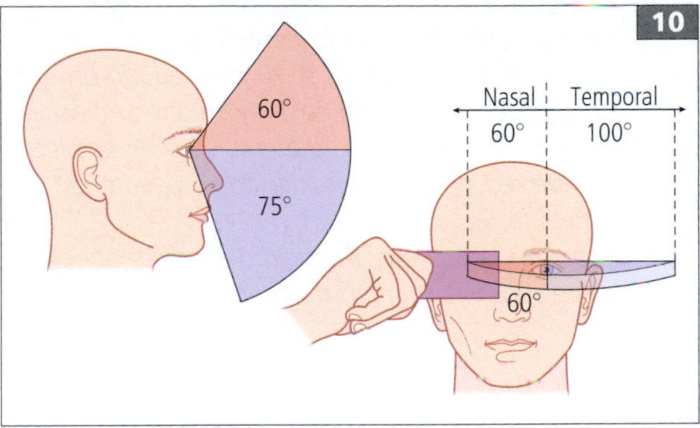

10 Extent of the normal visual field.

Nerve II (optic nerve)

Visual acuity

Record the best visual acuity (VA) with glasses, if necessary, at least for near vision, such as reading type book/hand-held card. Also test distance vision if a Snellen Chart is available.

Tip

▶ *Testing with a 1–2 mm pinhole to reduce the blur circle on the retina is essential if vision is impaired (distance or near) because if VA is significantly improved with the pinhole then there is an uncorrected refractive error or early cataract, and not an optic neuropathy (9).*

Colour vision

Testing of colour vision (CV) is most useful in assessing optic nerve function. CV errors with only a minimal reduction in VA support an optic nerve basis for visual loss. CV is most easily tested by Ishihara colour plates (a 14 plate set), by recording how many are correctly read by each eye. However, about 10% of males and 1% of females have some colour blindness. A subjective comparison of brightness of a red target (red pin or, for example, a Mydriacyl [tropicamide] bottle top) viewed alternately with each eye may show a desaturation in an eye with a optic nerve lesion.

Confrontation testing of visual fields

It is necessary to know the VA to select the size of the test object. For example, if vision is poor then it may be a hand movement only. The examination performed is related to the particular clinical problem:

- If testing for a monocular visual loss with pain on eye movement, then test for a central or paracentral, absolute or relative scotoma with a 5 mm and 10 mm pin head.
- If testing for a retrochiasmal lesion, look for a homonymous quadrantic, hemianopic defect, or visual inattention (**10**).
- If there is a complaint of a visual field (VF) loss, then it is helpful to get the patient to look at a picture, at your face, and to try to read, and to describe any bits 'blurred or missing'.
- Test each eye's VF individually at 0.5 m while the patient holds one hand over the other eye and fixes gaze on your eye; use finger counting by flicking up one, two, or three fingers in the four quadrants 10–20° from fixation, testing your VF against theirs.
- Visual inattention is tested for with both eyes open, by holding both hands up in the bilateral peripheral upper and lower quadrants, moving one or both simultaneously, and asking '*Tell me if you see one or both hands move*?' or testing monocularly by finger counting simultaneously across each upper and lower hemifield.
- When a patient is lying in bed and cannot sit up a 'facial-outline perimery' technique can be used, where the VF of each eye is tested (the other eye covered); while fixing on the examiner's eye or nose, the patient is asked to notify the examiner of the first appearance of a small (5–10 mm) pin or other small target moved from behind the patient forward in each quadrant (8–12 meridians), a few inches (2–3 cm) from their face. This is testing the patient's VF against the facial outline and VF defects can be easily recognized.
- Central VF testing. Place a red pin head in each of the four quadrants of the VF, close to its center. If it disappears into a scotoma or is gray or pink (i.e. desaturated) then this can help detect an optic nerve or chiasmal lesion.
- Record VF findings and label left and right as conventions differ.

Tips

▶ *The most sensitive method of detecting VF defects by confrontation is to use a small 5–10 mm red pin brought in from the periphery, testing each eye alone and asking when the pin is first seen as red (it will be seen as black initially as the red VF is smaller than the movement/ white VF)*[9].

▶ *Do automated perimetry if a field defect is suspected as it is more sensitive than confrontation tests.*

Pupillary responses

- Note the size and shape of each pupil, while the patient fixes on a distant target.
- Shine a bright light into one eye from below in a dimly lit room and note the pupil reaction in the eye (direct response) and in the other eye (consensual response) while the patient looks into the distance. Repeat for the other eye.
- Accommodation (near response) is tested only if there is no light reaction, by asking the patient to look into the distance and then to a near target 20 cm from the patient's nose and observe pupil constriction. A better near response than to direct light (light–near dissociation) is seen in small syphilitic Argyll Robertson pupils, some diabetics, and as a tonic response in the Adie's pupil.
- The swinging flashlight test is used to test for a relative afferent pupillary defect (**11**).

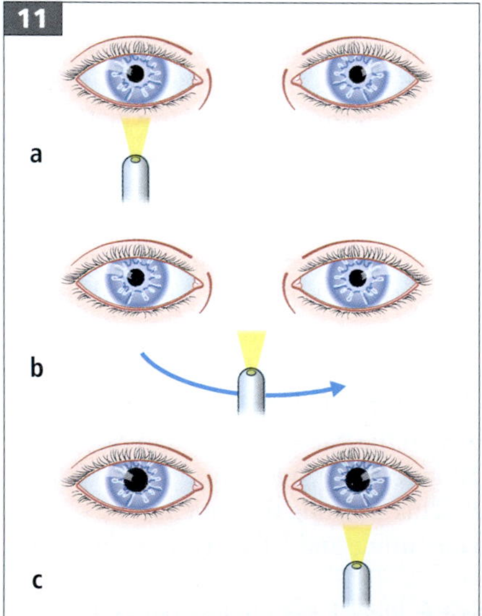

11 Pupil testing in a left optic neuropathy by a swinging flashlight test. (a) Both pupils constricted as a result of direct and consensual light reflex. (b) Pen moved toward affected left eye. (c) Both pupils dilate as less light is interpreted by the affected eye.

- This test is useful in detecting unilateral or asymmetric visual loss caused by extensive retinal (seen on fundoscopy) or optic nerve disease (use a bright light in a dimly lit room).
- Brightness comparison test. If the above test is equivocal, then shine the light alternately into each eye and ask if it is the same in each eye or brighter in one eye, and ask a 'price' the patient would pay for that light intensity, '*If this amount of light is worth $1 how much would you pay for it in the other eye?*'. The light is significantly less bright in an eye with an optic neuropathy.

Tips

▶ *Up to 20% of the normal population will have a pupil size difference of up to 1 mm (simple anisocoria) and no investigation is necessary if light reactions are normal and there is no ptosis on the smaller pupil side.*

▶ *These tests help detect optic neuropathy with visual loss, especially in acute retrobulbar optic neuritis, where the optic disc appears normal on fundoscopy.*

Fundoscopy

Perform fundoscopy in all patients with the direct ophthalmoscope (patient sitting or lying down). The ability to see the fundus (or at least the optic disc) through an undilated pupil is a necessary skill. Dim the light and ask the patient to fix on a distant target and to continue to keep their head still even as your head gets in the way. Adjust the ophthalmoscope focus for your refraction if necessary. Use the narrow light beam and a less intense light setting to access small pupils, and if it is difficult to see the fundus in patients with a high refractive error, then view while the patient is wearing their glasses. The red-free light highlights hemorrhages, drusen, cotton wool spots, and the retinal fiber layer. Use mydriatic drops (e.g. tropicamide 1% 30 mins to act fully, lasts 3 hours) to get a good view of the fundus if required[10].

- The red reflex: approach from about 50 cm (20 inches) away at a 15° angle from the side with the focus set on '0', shining the light through the pupil to see the 'red reflex' reflection from the retina (**12**). This is diminished or absent if there is a opacity between the cornea and retina (**13**). For example, a cataract may appear as a dark web. Then move forward, changing the lens focus close to the eye and locate the blood vessels of the retina to lead you to the optic disc.

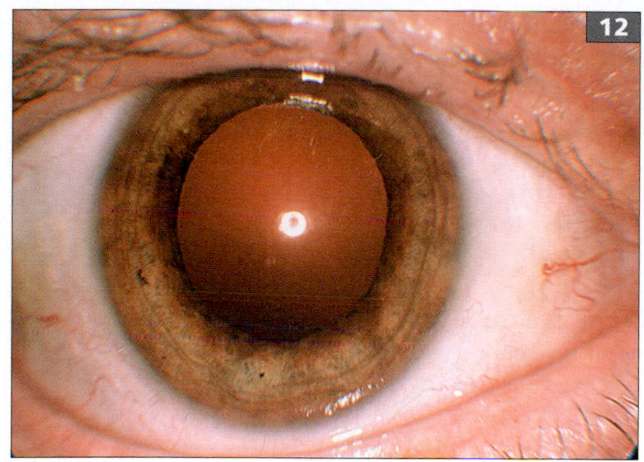

12 Normal red reflex.

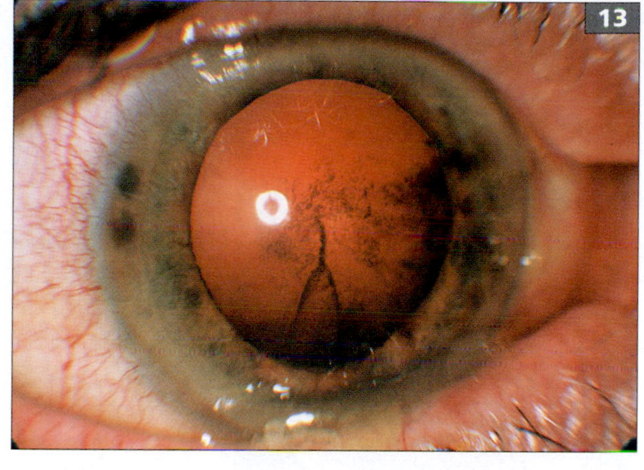

13 A red reflex with a lens opacity.

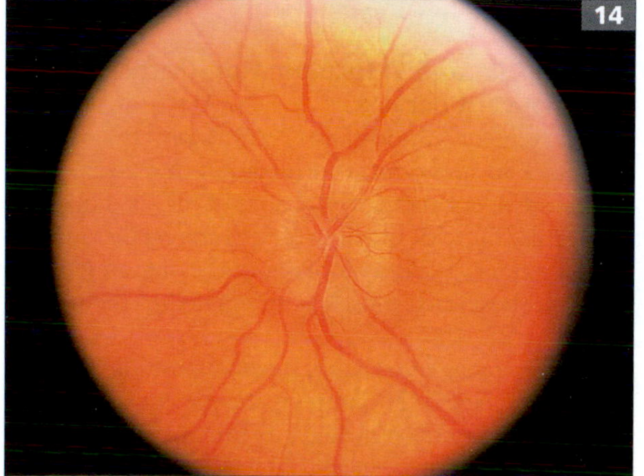

14 Ocular fundus showing papilledema in a patient with headache due to idiopathic intracranial hypertension. Note the congested swollen optic disc, loss of the physiological cup, blurred disc margins, and engorged retinal veins. *Courtesy of the late Mr M Wade, Department of Medical Illustrations, Royal Perth Hospital, Western Australia.*

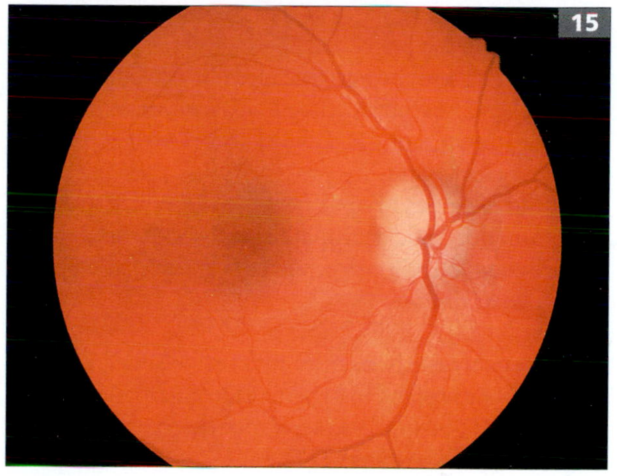

15 A 16-year-old male with vague intermittent blurring of right vision, visual acuity 20/20 (6/6), normal color vision, no relative afferent pupillary reflex defect, disc has a swollen appearance due to buried optic nerve head drusen.

- Optic disc: note its colour: pale in optic atrophy, pink and congested in papilledema where dilated veins and adjacent retinal hemorrhages are often present due to raised intracranial pressure (ICP) (**14**):
  - Optic cup: cup/disc ratio size 0.1–0.3 is diminished in papilledema and enlarged in glaucoma.
  - Spontaneous venous pulsation as the vein enters the disc or disc margin. Identifying venous pulsations is worthwhile, as if they are present, raised ICP is unlikely. However, pulsation is absent in 20% of the normal population.
- Disc margins: blurred in papilledema or by 'bubbles' of optic nerve head drusen (benign). Drusen buried in the optic nerve head may be a cause of anxiety as 'pseudo-papilledema' (**14, 15**).

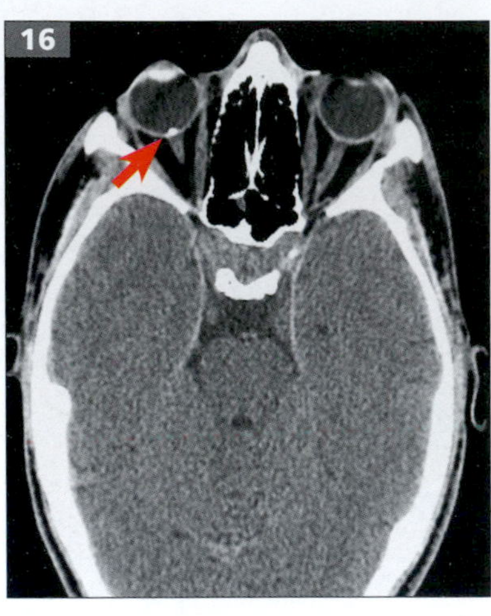

16 CT scan showing optic nerve head calcification due to buried drusen (arrow).

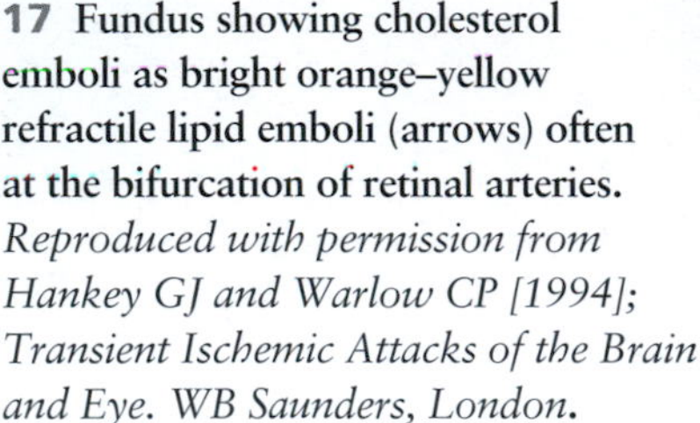

17 Fundus showing cholesterol emboli as bright orange–yellow refractile lipid emboli (arrows) often at the bifurcation of retinal arteries. *Reproduced with permission from Hankey GJ and Warlow CP [1994]; Transient Ischemic Attacks of the Brain and Eye. WB Saunders, London.*

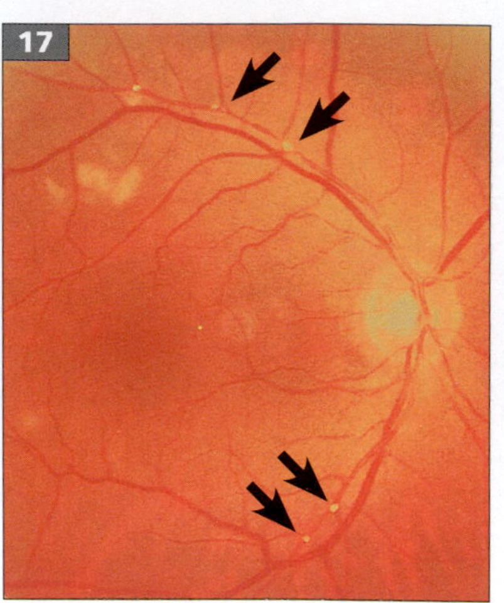

    - As the optic nerve head is often calcified, this can be confirmed on thin-slice computed tomography (CT) head scan (**16**) or orbital ultrasound.
  - Other causes of optic nerve head swelling include anterior optic neuropathies (inflammatory, ischemic, infiltrative, and compressive) as well as ocular disease.
- Retina:
  - Retinal vessels: narrow and tortuous with arterio-venous nipping in hypertension; microaneurysms with diabetes; cholesterol, platelet, or calcific emboli in arterioles (**17**).
  - Venous sheathing away from the disc can be seen in MS or inflammatory disorders.
  - Retinal pigmentation may be present in retinitis pigmentosa, mitochondrial cytopathy, and spino-cerebellar ataxias.
- Macula: is two disc diameters away lateral in the temporal retina or ask the patient to look directly at the light if the pupil has been dilated.

PanOptic ophthalmoscope (Welch Allyn)

This novel hand-held direct ophthalmoscope (**18**) gives a larger view of the fundus (25° *vs.* 5°] and more magnification. Because of the patient eyecup it is easier to see through small pupils. It is more expensive than the conventional ophthalmoscope but some neurologists now use it exclusively.

Nerves III, IV, and VI (oculomotor, trochlear, and abducens nerves)

Eye movement abnormalities are important as they give clues to anatomical localization and to possible causes[11]. Understanding the actions of the six individual extraocular muscles and how they work together in yoke muscle pairs is aided by looking at the anatomy of the orbit and how each muscle is orientated in the muscle cone (**19**).

When moving into the six cardinal positions of gaze, tested by tracing a 'H' figure as the patient follows the target, one muscle of each eye is primarily responsible (yoke muscles), e.g. the right (R) superior rectus and left (L) inferior oblique in gaze up to the right. Knowing the yoke muscles in each of the six cardinal directions of gaze is essential in diplopia analysis (**20**). Adding the primary position, straight full up and down positions (multiple muscles responsible) makes the nine diagnostic positions of gaze.

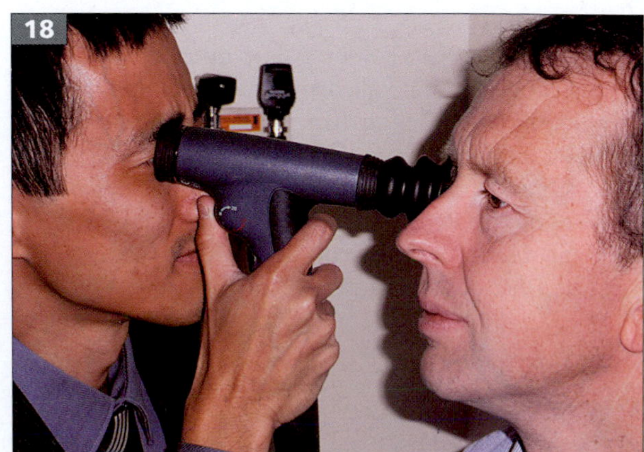

18 PanOptic ophthalmoscope. *Reproduced with permission.*

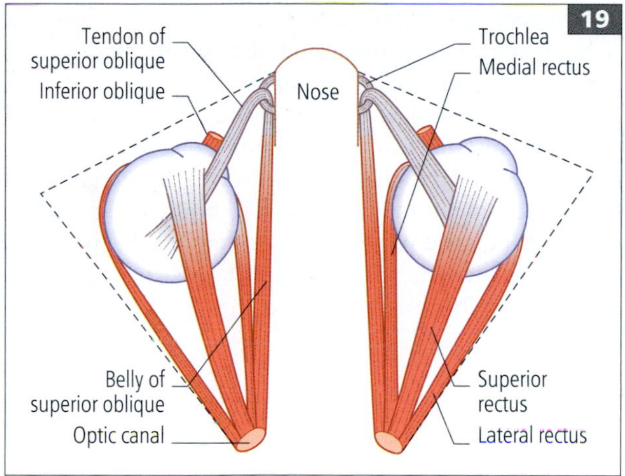

19 Schematic representation of extraocular muscles.

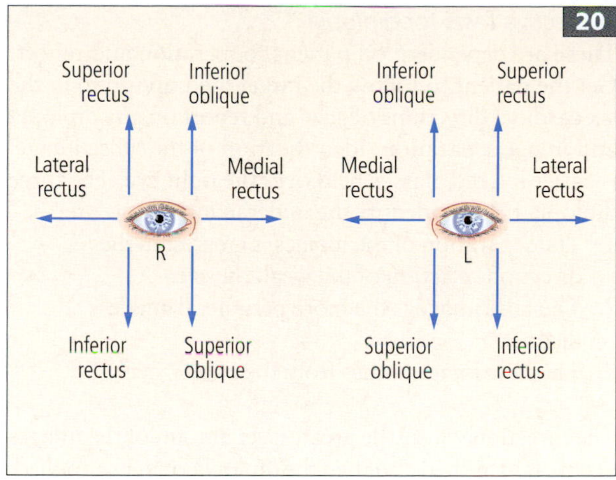

20 The six cardinal positions of gaze.

Test procedure

- Ask the patient to look at a target for near (e.g. a pen tip) and distance, and examine the eyes in the primary position of gaze looking straight ahead, noting the position of each eye (whether the eyes are conjugate), whether there are any involuntary movements of the eyes (e.g. nystagmus, fixational instability), pigmented corneal rings (Kayser–Fleischer ring), ptosis, or lid retraction on one or both sides.
- Ask if the patient sees one or two targets and then check with monocular occlusion that the double vision is binocular. If monocular diplopia, then usually there is an ocular cause which can disappear using a pinhole, if due to an early cataract; or functional; if monocular diplopia is in each eye, then it is likely due to an occipital cortex lesion accompanied by VF defects (cerebral polyopia).
- If the eyes are clearly misaligned, the degree of misalignment varies with gaze position in noncomitant strabismus (due to recent paretic or restrictive cause), but not in comitant strabismus (childhood strabismus or a decompensation of a long-standing phoria). The term 'phoria' refers to a deviation normally kept in check by binocular fusion mechanisms (a latent deviation); a 'tropia' is a deviation not kept in check by fusion and is present at all times (a manifest deviation).

The cover–uncover test

This is the basic test for a manifest eye deviation (tropia).

- The patient wears glasses appropriate for the distance being tested (near or far) and looks straight ahead at a target.
- Briefly cover and uncover the right eye several times while watching the left eye (an occluder can be used or thumb with fingers resting on the forehead). If the left eye moves out to fixate, it was turned in (esotropia); if it moves in: exotropia; if it moves downward: hypertropia; if upward: hypotropia.
- If no movement of the left eye occurs, then briefly cover and uncover the left eye while watching the right eye to see if it moves.

The alternate cover test

This is done if the cover test is normal and you are looking for a latent deviation (phoria) as a cause of an intermittent diplopia when fusion breaks down. The test is as above: briefly swinging the occluder or thumb alternately between the two eyes to break fusion and observe any movement of the uncovered eye as it tries to fixate, to reveal a horizontal phoria (common in normals) or vertical phoria (uncommon in normals).

Testing individual eye movements (ductions)

Test the range of movement for each eye individually to observe any reduction in movement. Normal is about 10 mm for adduction, abduction, and elevation, and about 7 mm for depression. Note any limitation by mm or % of normal on the H diagram. Limitation of movement rarely can be restrictive due to a muscle infiltration or entrapment and if suspected, the patient should be referred to an ophthalmologist to do forced ductions to detect this.

Subjective tests for diplopia

These are dependent on patient cooperation and report. Get the patient to follow the target (pen tip/torch) in the six cardinal directions of gaze and report on any diplopia and image separation. Identification of the 'false image' is easier if a red glass is held over the right eye. The three diplopia rules to identify the underacting muscle are:

1. The separation of the images is greatest in the direction of action of the weak muscle.
2. The false image is the more peripheral and less distinct.
3. The false image comes from the paretic eye.

The direction where the greatest separation of the images occurs is identified and then the diplopia rules are applied, occluding each eye alone to identify the false image. If more than one extraocular muscle is weak then direct observation or range of movement (ROM) is required to identify them.

Abducens (VI) nerve palsy

- Double vision with images side by side, worse towards the abduction defect and in the distance than near, due to weakness of the lateral rectus.
- Usually an esotropia (convergent squint).
- Will be other brainstem signs if nuclear; may be nerve or neuromuscular junction.

Trochlear (IV) nerve palsy

- Double vision on looking down, vertically separated due to weakness of the superior oblique muscle.
- If one horizontal image is tilted in one eye on monocular viewing, then the palsy is in this eye.

Oculomotor (III) nerve palsy

- A complete palsy causes a severe ptosis, and absent adduction with impaired elevation and depression, the eye being down and out in position with a dilated pupil unreactive to light.
- A partial palsy will have less weakness of the involved muscles (medial rectus, superior rectus, inferior rectus, inferior oblique) and there may be sparing of the pupil with an incomplete ptosis. It is typically a complication of diabetes mellitus.
- Beware myasthenia gravis mimicking the pupil-sparing IIIrd nerve palsy.

Internuclear ophthalmoplegia

A brainstem medial longitudinal fasciculus lesion will impair adduction of the ipsilateral eye associated with abducting nystagmus of the opposite eye on horizontal gaze. The internuclear ophthalmoplegia (INO) may be unilateral or bilateral, subtle or obvious. Rapid horizontal eye movements may be needed to bring out an adduction slowing. The patient may or may not be aware of diplopia to one side. The INO may be an isolated sign or accompany other brainstem signs.

Skew deviation

This is a small vertical deviation of the eyes that results from a prenuclear lesion in the brainstem or cerebellum associated with a vestibular pathway lesion. It is usually comitant, and often associated with an INO or other brainstem signs and causes vertical diplopia.

Testing movements of both eyes

The observation of slow eye movements (pursuit), rapid eye movements (saccades), convergence, and the vestibulo-ocular reflex gives insights into widely distributed central oculomotor pathways and vestibular functions.

Smooth pursuit

This is tested when the patient follows the target slowly moved (5°/sec) horizontally and vertically. If 'cogwheel or catch-up saccades' occur in both directions, this is a nonspecific sign; it may indicate a cerebellar problem but can be seen in diffuse cerebral problems, medication, or just aging. If only found in one direction, it indicates an ipsilateral parietal cortical or subcortical problem.

Saccades

Saccades are rapid eye movements to an eccentric target tested by getting the patient to look rapidly from side to side and up and down. Look at initiation, velocity, and accuracy of the eye movement. In some diseases saccades may be abnormal early while pursuit is normal (e.g. in progressive supranuclear palsy). Saccades can be used to accentuate a mild limitation of eye movement to make it easier to see (e.g. an abduction defect).

Test convergence

Convergence should be tested if there is a complaint of diplopia for near. Wearing glasses if necessary, the patient looks at a target 30 cm away and the target is brought in slowly to the 'near point of convergence' where the patient sees double (normally around 10 cm).

Vestibulo-ocular reflex (VOR)

If the vestibulo-ocular system is functioning normally, passive rotation of the patient's head when the patient looks straight ahead results in a slow eye movement so that the eyes move in the opposite direction to that of the head movement. The test for this is known as the oculocephalic maneuver and is done both in the horizontal and vertical directions. This test can help distinguish nuclear gaze palsies, where it is lost, from supranuclear, where it is retained. When tested rapidly with a sudden brief head impulse to right and left, while holding the patient's head on both sides and the patient fixing on your nose, a lag in the eye movement and a refixation saccade to the nose indicates a peripheral vestibular deficit to that side. It can be unilateral or bilateral. (See Chapter 5, Vertigo.)

The ability of the visual system to suppress the VOR during head movement while visually fixing can be tested by sitting the patient in a swivel chair, getting them to fix on their outstretched thumb, while the chair is oscillated. Normally the eyes will stay fixed on the thumb; if there is nystagmus to one or both sides then there is a breakdown in the central vestibulo-ocular pathway (ipsilateral cerebellar or parietal lobe if only in one direction; bilateral if in both directions).

Nystagmus and other ocular oscillations

Nystagmus can be defined as repetitive to-and-fro eye movements which may be asymptomatic (sometimes only seen on fundoscopy) or large enough in amplitude for the patient to be aware of 'jumping vision' (oscillopsia).

- Examine initially in the primary position, then on following a target to extreme left and right (always maintaining binocular vision to avoid end-point physiologic nystagmoid jerks), and then full up and down gaze.
- Describe whether the movement in each direction is the same amplitude and speed (pendular), or if there is a fast phase in one direction and a slow phase in another (jerk). The direction of the nystagmus is described by the fast phase (e.g. right-beating jerk nystagmus).

Tip

▶ *Nystagmus is an important clinical sign helpful in localization. It is a complex topic with physiologic, voluntary, congenital, and pathologic causes, including drug effects, peripheral and central vestibular disorders, cerebellar, and brainstem disease*[12].

Other ocular oscillations

Become familiar with other uncommon movements intruding on steady fixation, including square wave jerks, macrosaccadic oscillations, ocular flutter, and superior oblique myokymia.

Eyelids

Observe if there is a ptosis or lid retraction on one or both sides, assessing the lid position with respect to the cornea (normally covering the upper 1 mm). Distinguishing levator palpebrae superioris dehiscence (aponeurotic ptosis) from other causes of ptosis is important, as this can be confused with myasthenic ptosis as it may be in one or both eyes. Levator palpebrae superioris dehiscence is characterized by:

- A high upper lid skin crease (normally 6–7 mm above the lid margin).
- Good levator function (over 10 mm).
- Increased excursion of the lid on downgaze (lower than the other eye).
- Ptosis worsens only a little at the end of the day.

If myasthenia gravis is suspected, there is almost always weakness of the orbicularis oculi in forced eye closure, shown by a careful examination.

Ptosis fatiguablity should be sought by asking the patient to maintain upgaze for up to 2 minutes at a target, trying as hard as possible not to blink. If the ptosis increases then ask the patient to rest their eyes by gently closing them for 30 seconds, and then reopen. If the ptosis at least partially recovers there is no need for a Tensilon/neostigmine test.

Lid retraction can occur in progressive supranuclear palsy (Collier's sign), and hyperthyroidism. Lid-lag on looking up and down can occur with eyelid myotonia in the hypo/hyperkalemic periodic paralyses.

Nerve V (trigeminal nerve)

Corneal reflex (V_1 reflex)

- Not tested routinely.
- Performed only if there are facial sensory symptoms, or a suspected acoustic neuroma.
- After warning the patient, use a cotton wool 'whisp'; ask the patient to look up and away, gently touching each cornea in turn to observe the blink; ask if it felt the same each side.

Facial sensation

Light touch and pinprick (or use the cold of a tuning fork blade) is tested on the forehead, cheek, and chin on each side and ask '*Did that feel the same each side*?'.

Masticatory muscles

These are only tested when there is trigeminal sensory impairment, dysarthria, or dysphagia. Pterygoid power is tested by asking the patient to open the mouth fully. A unilateral trigeminal motor neuropathy will manifest with deviation of the lower jaw (chin) to the weak side.

Tips

▶ *Functional complaints of facial sensory symptoms are common; true sensory impairment is usually persistent 'like a dental anesthetic', requires consistent findings on repeated testing conforming to trigeminal sensory anatomical boundaries, and/or a reduced corneal reflex.*

▶ *With facial weakness there may appear to be also a deviation of the jaw and tongue because of the facial asymmetry; holding up the weak side will clarify a pseudo-deviation or not.*

Jaw jerk

Tested in the context of a suspected pseudobulbar dysarthria, and in distinguishing limb hyper-reflexia due to a cervical lesion from a higher level, i.e. above mid pons. Ask the patient to let their mouth hang open while you place your index finger over the middle of their chin and tap it with a reflex hammer. A brisk upward jerk of the mandible is a positive response.

Nerve VII (facial nerve)

Muscle power

To test facial muscle power the examiner generally needs to demonstrate these tests to the patient and request the patient to mimic.

- Ask the patient to '*Look up to the ceiling*'; the frontalis muscle is spared in contralateral upper motor neuron (supranuclear) lesions due to bilateral hemispheric representation.
- Test the power of the orbicularis oculi by urging the patient '*Close your eyes as tightly as possible and don't let me open them*'. Failure to bury the eyelashes as well on one or both sides can indicate weakness. Try to pry the eyes open using the fingers of both hands. This is normally difficult and finding weakness can be a very important sign when suspecting myasthenia gravis with associated ptosis or diplopia or other cause of a lower motor neuron facial weakness.
- Ask the patient to '*Show me your teeth*'. When there is a weak lower face there is often a relative preservation of facial symmetry in upper motor neuron weakness when smiling, compared to a voluntary movement.
- Ask the patient to whistle and then to blow their cheeks out holding the air in.
- To test the platysma, ask the patient to clench their teeth while stretching their mouth sideways; this response is weak in both upper and lower motor neuron lesions.

Tips

▶ *Beware bifacial weakness, as it is easy to miss on casual observation as the facial features are symmetric; it should be suspected if the patient is expressionless, unblinking, or has a 'transverse smile' (e.g. in some patients with myopathies, myasthenia gravis, Guillain–Barré syndrome). Facial muscle strength needs to be tested formally.*

▶ *Mild facial asymmetry without weakness is common; check with the patient, or a companion, as to whether it is new or not. They may need to look in a mirror.*

Examination of taste

Altered taste may be a symptom of a lower motor neuron facial palsy or, rarely, an isolated chorda tympani lesion (e.g. with a carotid artery dissection). Testing taste is rarely required; however, in a peripheral facial palsy if taste is impaired, the lesion is proximal to the junction with the chorda tympani; if preserved, then distal to the stylomastoid foramen. Testing can be done with a swab stick dipped in sugar placed on to the side of the protruded tongue while it is held with gauze; the mouth is then rinsed, and salt next applied.

Nerve VIII (auditory and vestibular nerve)

Bedside hearing tests

- Rub your thumb and middle finger together repetitively, about 2–3 cm (0.8–1.2 in) away from the ear. Ask the patient if they hear the sound; check both ears. Alternatively, rub your thumb and middle finger together next to one ear (to produce a masking sound) and quietly whisper numbers (ninety-nine, fifty-three) at varying distances.
- Screening for a high frequency loss with a pocket watch (tick) held outside the ear can also be useful.
- Deafness can be further tested by:
  - The Rinne test: involves striking the 256 or 512 Hz tuning fork and holding the vibrating tuning fork about 2–3 cm (0.8–1.2 in) from the ear. Ask the patient if they can hear it. Then place the base of the vibrating tuning fork behind the ear, on the mastoid process and ask whether the sound is louder 'in the front' (outside the ear) or 'at the back' (on the mastoid process). It is normally louder in the front, as air conduction is better than bone conduction; if not, then this suggests conductive hearing loss, due to blocked ears or a middle ear defect. Auroscopy is required.
  - The Weber test: involves placing the vibrating tuning fork over the vertex of the head in the midline and asking the patient where they hear the sound loudest. Normally, it is heard in the middle of the head. If it lateralizes to one side, this suggests a conductive hearing loss on that side (more masking of external sounds); in a sensorineural hearing loss it is heard best in the normal ear. The Rinne and Weber tests are not always reliable.

Nerves IX and X (glossopharyngeal and vagus nerves)

- Ask the patient to open their mouth and to say '*Ah*'. Inspect the palate and uvula, using a tongue depressor if necessary, and if the palate moves to one side this indicates a lesion of the vagus nerve (motor to the soft palate) on the contralateral side. If the palate does not move well this may be due to a bilateral supranuclear, nuclear, or infranuclear vagus nerve lesion, a disturbance of the neuromuscular junction, or muscle function. The gag reflex occurs with touching the back of the throat each side with a tongue depressor.

Tip

▸ *Only test the gag reflex if it is relevant to the presenting complaint.*

Nerve XI (accessory nerve)

The sternocleidomastoid muscle both flexes the head and rotates it to the opposite side. Note that the cerebral hemisphere innervates the contralateral trapezius and the ipsilateral sternocleidomastoid.

Muscle power

- Place the palm of your right hand over the patient's left mandible and ask the patient to turn their head to the left against your resistance to test the power of the right sternocleidomastoid. Observe the muscle for atrophy or hypertrophy. Repeat on the other side with your left hand.
- Place your hand on the patient's forehead to test head flexion, asking them to push forward. This can be performed with the patient supine or in a sitting position.

Tip

▸ *When the arm is actively held in abduction, winging of the scapula occurs in trapezius weakness more than when pushed forward against resistance (i.e. opposite to the winging of the scapula from serratus anterior weakness due to a long thoracic nerve palsy).*

Nerve XII (hypoglossal nerve)

- Unilateral weakness of the tongue may cause few symptoms as speech and swallowing are little affected.
- Nuclear or infranuclear lesions cause wasting and fasciculation and deviation to the side of the lesion when protruded, because of the action of the genioglossis muscle.
- Ask the patient to:
  - Open their mouth. Inspect the tongue while it is at rest in the floor of the mouth, noting any wasting or fasciculation.
  - Poke out their tongue, observe any deviation.
  - Wiggle their tongue from side to side and then in and out as fast as possible; this is slowed with a bilateral pyramidal tract lesion without wasting; also in severe lower motor neuron weakness.

Tip

▸ *Don't overcall possible isolated fasciculation of the tongue; if it is really present, there should be other signs or symptoms of tongue weakness.*

MOTOR SYSTEM

Assessing limb function for a motor abnormality is pivotal, as complaints of weakness, 'dropping things', clumsiness, and imbalance are common. Request the patient disrobe sufficiently for your test requirements (e.g. to look widely for fasciculation and wasting in suspected motor neuron disease).

Screening tests

Posture of outstretched hands

Ask the patient to extend their arms forward with palms uppermost, and then close their eyes. Postural tremor can appear, or rest tremor cease; a downward pronator drift of the forearm after 30 seconds is a early sign of a pyramidal tract lesion; a progressive downward fall of the arm may indicate proximal weakness. Chorea or asterixis may become apparent.

Rapid finger and foot tapping

Doing rapid repetitive skilled finger and foot movement is an important test for disturbed motor function and this may be present even if there is minimal or no weakness. Alternating two finger (index and middle) tapping as quickly as possible on the back of the other hand or a desk top, and sustaining this for 15–20 seconds, is a sensitive test for a pyramidal tract lesion affecting the hand when slowing is evident. Slowing with a diminishing amplitude tap is also seen in extrapyramidal disease (e.g. Parkinson's disease) but not in cerebellar disorders when it is irregular with retained amplitude, or lower motor neuron weakness as long as strength remains to do the test[13].

Slowed foot tapping also occurs in pyramidal and extrapyramidal disorders and is helpful to correlate with results of reflex, tone, power, and plantar responses.

The forearm and finger-rolling tests

These tests can be sensitive in detecting a subtle upper motor neuron lesion, sometimes even when tone, power, and reflexes are normal. In each test the forearms or index fingers are first rapidly rotated around each other separated by 5 cm for about 5 seconds in one direction and then reversed. The affected limb will remain relatively stationary while the normal forearm rotates around it. It is also affected with a decreased excursion in extrapyramidal disorders. The sensitivity and specificity of these tests has been reviewed[14].

Power

Arm muscle-power screening is shoulder abduction, elbow flexion and extension, finger extension and flexion. Leg proximal and distal muscle power can be screened by getting the patient to get up from a squat and to walk on toes and heels.

Tone

Muscle tone is the resistance to passive stretch and it is assessed by the resistance encountered on stretching the muscles at increasing velocities through a range of movement by the examiner. This resistance can only be gauged when the patient is fully relaxed. They may need to be distracted by conversation while doing the testing.

Arms

Passively pronate and supinate the patient's forearms, and flex and extend the fingers, wrists, and elbows, noting a steady resistance that is insensitive to the velocity of stretch ('lead pipe' rigidity) and may be interrupted by tremor ('cog-wheel' rigidity) found in extrapyramidal disorders (the hallmark of Parkinson's disease); or an increased resistance in proportion to the velocity with which the muscle is stretched (spasticity), often towards the end of the range in the forearm (pronator catch) or across the wrist or finger flexors.

Tip

▶ *In Parkinson's disease, rigidity in one arm may only be detectable or accentuated on passive movement when the other arm is moved at the same time voluntarily (activation) such as when drawing a circle in the air or moving it up and down.*

Legs

With the patient lying down, and the legs relaxed, grasp the knee with one hand and roll the leg briskly to-and-fro about the hip. Normally, the foot flops in and out passively. If tone is decreased, as in lower motor neuron disorders, the passive movement is increased. If tone is increased (as in spasticity and extrapyramidal rigidity), the foot excursions are decreased.

- A brisk flick at the knee with the legs resting in extension can reveal a spastic catch in the quadriceps, lifting the foot off the bed. Normally the foot will remain on the bed.
- Clonus is a rhythmic series of muscle contractions in response to maintained stretch that may be elicited at the ankle by supporting the patient's knee, flexed about 15°, and then suddenly and forcefully dorsiflexing the patient's foot with the palm of the examiner's right hand. Clonus is a sign of a pyramidal tract lesion to the calf muscles. However, up to three beats can be normal.

- Myotonia is a disorder of the muscle membrane where the tone is normal at rest but where contraction produces a temporary persistence of muscle contraction with slow relaxation, best seen after getting the patient to 'make a fist, then open fast' with then a slow opening of the fingers; also 'percussion myotonia' may be detected by tapping with a reflex hammer the thenar eminence or the extensor digitorum communis in the dorsal forearm, resulting in a brief abnormal sustained muscle contraction.

Formal tests

Power

Testing power and being confident of detecting a true mild weakness is the most difficult skill to achieve in the neurologic examination. It requires the routine application of a standardized method of testing muscles[15], done in an orderly sequence usually from proximal to distal muscles. The test techniques are designed in such a way, that in most cases the muscle will only be overcome if it is weak. Comparing muscle strength with the same muscle in the opposite limb can help confirm mild weakness.

Factors that need to be considered include whether the patient understands the instructions (you may need to demonstrate the postures you require and encourage maximal effort), pain limiting the response, or brief contractions with then 'give-way' weakness of poor effort or functional weakness. Always using the same power-testing techniques will lead to consistency and will give confidence in detecting minimal weakness (*Table 2*).

Some neurologists prefer just the descriptive terms of 'normal, mild, moderate, or severe weakness' (more helpful in describing pyramidal tract weakness after a stroke).

Tip

▶ *Grade power to the maximum response, even if it was for a second or two before the muscle 'giving way'.*

Which muscles are examined depends on whether you are doing a screening examination for weakness or examining to test various diagnostic possibilities. Learning the patterns of weakness in pyramidal lesions of motor pathways, peripheral neuropathies, mononeuropathies, radiculopathies, myopathies, and functional weakness takes study and exposure to patients with these conditions.

TABLE 2 **MUSCLE POWER GRADES ACCORDING TO THE MEDICAL RESEARCH COUNCIL (MRC) SCALE**

Grade	Description
0	No contraction
1	A flicker or trace of contraction
2	The muscle can move the limb with gravity eliminated (e.g. support the limb if necessary)
3	The muscle can maintain the limb against gravity
4−	The muscle can move the limb against gravity and slight resistance by the examiner
4	Active movement against gravity and moderate resistance
4+	Active movement against gravity and strong resistance
5	Normal power

The calf muscles are usually too strong to be tested lying down and are tested by getting the patient to walk on their toes; then take all the body weight on one forefoot; and finally if necessary, by jumping on one leg alone and not allowing the heel to hit the floor (the patient will require a supporting hand).

Beevor's sign of a lesion around T10 spinal level is sought if there is proximal leg weakness or difficulty in getting up from the couch. Ask the patient to try to sit up from the lying position without using their arms. If this is not possible, the abdominal muscles are weak. The upper 'motor level' can sometimes be ascertained by noting the position of the umbilicus with the patient supine and then asking the patient to lift their head off the bed against your hand, to contract the rectus abdominis. If the umbilicus deviates upwards, this indicates that the lower abdominal muscles are weaker than the upper muscles.

Coordination

These tests are usually equated with testing for cerebellar function but must be interpreted in light of any coincidental weakness or sensory ataxia in the limbs which can affect their performance.

Screening tests

- Rebound in arms.
- Finger–nose test.
- Rapid alternating movements of the hands and feet.
- Heel–knee–shin test.
- Tandem walking.

Formal tests

Arms

- Finger–nose test: ask the patient to touch the tip of their nose, then your finger which is held at arm's length in front of the patient making the patient stretch, then their nose again. You may have to demonstrate how to do this. Look for an intention tremor increasing in amplitude as the target is approached, or dysmetria where the finger falls short of the target or exceeds it ('past-pointing').
- Rapid alternating movements: test by asking the patient to alternately slap their palm and back of the hand on the dorsum of the other hand or on the thigh. A slow and clumsy response is called 'dysdiadochokinesis'.
- Rebound phenomenon: gentle downward pressure on the wrists, followed by a release, can reveal an asymmetric excessive rebound upwards in a cerebellar lesion affecting that arm.

Legs

- Heel–knee–shin test: the patient lifts one leg, places the heel of the foot on the opposite knee, and runs it up and down the front of the shin several times. Abnormality is a side-to-side jerkiness.
- Rapid tapping movement of the foot against the examiner's hand, which may be slow and irregular.

Deep tendon reflexes

Screening tests

Biceps, triceps, brachioradialis, knee, ankle reflexes; plantar response.

Formal tests

It is important to use a relatively heavy hammer (e.g. Tromner, Queen Square) and to deliver a brief sharp blow to the tendon (finger only over the biceps tendon), with a flexible wrist movement. The patient can be sitting or lying; ankle reflexes are best tested supine with the hips slightly externally rotated, knee slightly flexed, and the Achilles tendon under a little stretch. If elicited in kneeling, the test is even more sensitive. If a reflex is absent or depressed then a 'reinforcement maneuver' (other hand squeeze or 'grit your teeth' for arm reflexes; a Jendrassik 'monkey grip' of the hands for leg reflexes) should be tried to see if it enhances the reflex (*Table 3*).

Absent and asymmetric reflexes are usually pathologic; depressed or only on reinforcement may not be abnormal; brisk reflexes are sometimes difficult to interpret since they may be normal, but pathologic if also sustained clonus is present.

- An absent or depressed reflex can be very helpful in the diagnosis of a nerve root lesion.
- An absent reflex may be accompanied by hyperactive reflexes below the spinal level if there is spinal cord involvement (e.g. an 'inverted brachioradialis reflex' with reflex loss but with brisk finger jerks instead.
- Superficial abdominal reflexes: these are contractions of the abdominal muscles pulling towards the stimulus, elicited by a light stroke directed towards the umbilicus in the upper and lower quadrants bilaterally. They are unreliable, and rarely useful.

The plantar response (Babinski sign or extensor plantar response)

The value and the reliability of eliciting the plantar response has been questioned but when done properly and interpreted in light of other signs, it is a valuable sign of pyramidal tract involvement.

The outer border of the sole of the foot (S1 dermatome) is stimulated from the heel, up to and across the metatarsal heads, by a light stroke with a blunt-point stimulus such as a key or a wooden stick, after warning the patient of the impending test (**21**). The great toe normally plantar-flexes, but after damage to the pyramidal pathways that inhibit flexor reflexes, the great toe extends (dorsiflexes) with or without abduction of the toes. Universally there will also be a flexion synergy contraction of the tensor fascia lata and the hamstrings (seen or palpated). If there is a withdrawal response then adapt the

TABLE 3 **REFLEX TESTING**

Symbol	Description	Interpretation
0	Absent despite reinforcement	Usually abnormal
1+/−	Present with reinforcement	May or may not be abnormal
1+	Present	
2+	Brisk	
3+	Very brisk	Usually abnormal (UMN lesion)
Clonus	Clonus	Sustained clonus for more than 3 beats
Deep tendon reflexes	**Main spinal segment**	
Biceps	C5, 6	
Brachioradialis/supinator	C5, 6	
Triceps	C6, 7, 8	
Finger flexion	C8	'Finger jerks' increased in C8/T1 UMN spasticity
Hip adductors	L2, 3	Increased and 'crossed adductor' in a pyramidal UMN lesion above this level
Knee	L3, 4	
Internal hamstrings	L5*	
External hamstrings	S1*	*Unilateral depression may be useful in diagnosis of an L5 or S1 radiculopathy
Ankle	S1, 2	Absent or reduced in an S1 root lesion or a peripheral neuropathy
Superficial abdominal relexes		May help in UMN/LMN lesion localization
Upper	T7, 8, 9	
Lower	T10, 11, 12	

LMN: lower motor neuron; UMN: upper motor neuron.

stimulus to what the patient can tolerate: a short scratch may only be required to elicit the response; or as an alternative, scratching the lateral side of the foot may be better tolerated. A true upgoing toe is reproducible, unlike voluntary withdrawal.

Tips

- *It should be noted that sometimes a pyramidal lesion will affect the leg without an extensor plantar response being present; and that an extensor plantar response may be present as a transient sign in metabolic coma, such as hypoglycemia, or in a postictal state.*
- *The initial upward movement of the big toe is the most important movement to observe.*
- *There is often a correlation of an extensor plantar response with a slowed foot tap rate as a sign of a pyramidal lesion*[16]*.*

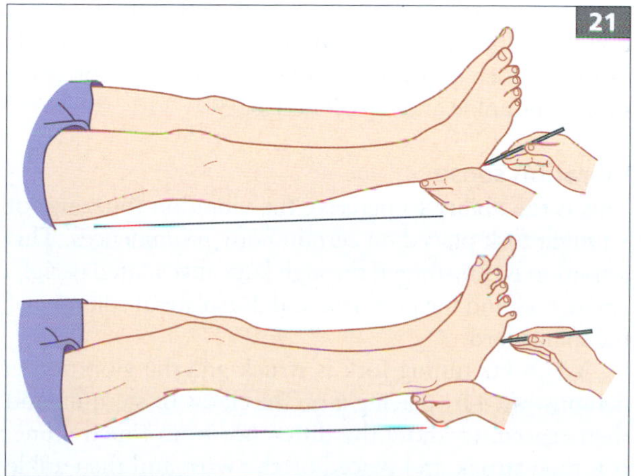

21 Babinski sign.

SENSATION

Screening tests

Ask about any sensory symptoms or area of persistent altered or loss of sensation. Check for sensory inattention in every case of a hemiparesis.

Formal tests

The focus of the examination is guided by whether the sensory symptoms suggest a peripheral mononeuropathy, peripheral neuropathy, nerve root, spinal cord, a brainstem, or cortical lesion.

The patient may be able to map out accurately the distribution of sensory loss (e.g. lateral cutaneous nerve of thigh). The area in question can be examined with a piece of cotton wool for light touch; a disposable pin or a cold metal tuning fork blade as a pin substitute for pain and temperature appreciation. Test from the area of sensory impairment toward the normal area until a line of demarcation is reached where sensation becomes normal. More weight is given to sensory loss than just altered sensation (i.e. interpret apparent subtle sensory change with caution).

Proprioception

Arm

Proprioception in the arm is tested by taking the sides of one of the patient's distal interphalangeal joints and passively moving the distal phalanx up or down, requesting 'up, down, or don't know' responses with eyes open initially to show the test; then with eyes closed. Only small movements (1 mm) are required to be detected. If not, try larger movements and, failing that, proceed proximally to the interphalangeal joints, wrist, and elbow if necessary.

Leg

Proprioception in the leg is tested in the great toe metatarsophalangeal joint by holding the toe on the sides and first demonstrating to the patient with eyes open, making minimal movements (usually 1 mm) and requesting 'up, down, or don't know' responses with the eyes closed. If incorrect, then larger movements are made with progression to the ankle and knee if necessary.

Vibration sense

This is the ability to perceive the vibration (buzzing) of a tuning fork placed on certain bony prominences. This sensation is transmitted through large myelinated peripheral nerves and the posterior and dorsolateral columns of the spinal cord.

A 128 Hz tuning fork is struck and the vibration is demonstrated by placing it on the elbow or sternum and then ceased, to show the difference from touch alone. It is then struck and placed on the wrist and then ankle medially, and held until the patient (with eyes closed) no longer feels the vibration. A few trials of prematurely stopping the vibration are worthwhile to confirm the reliability of the patient's reports. If impaired, the stimulus point is moved proximally (elbow, shoulder, knee, hip) to see when it can be felt, and for how long. Judgment about abnormality can be difficult and depends on a regular technique and experience, and should account for the normal decline with age (compare with your own ability to feel the stimulus in the same area if necessary).

Cortical-based discriminative sensation

This is tested with the eyes closed after demonstrating the first two tests to the patient. The opposite hand can be compared as a 'control'.

- Two-point discrimination (normally >3 mm [>0.1 in] on the pulps of the fingers) using a two-point discriminator is helpful when asymmetric but difficult to interpret and is not often done now.
- Graphesthesia: recognition of number writing 1–9 on the palm or finger pulps.
- Stereognosis: ability to distinguish the nature, size, and texture of small objects such as coins, paper clips, keys, dice placed sequentially in the hand.
- Sensory attention: ability to detect simultaneous stimuli at similar sites on two sides of the body. Tell the patient you will touch one or both arms or legs and to report 'one or both sides touched'; sensation is ignored contralateral to a usually parietal lobe lesion.

If there has been a slowly developing mononeuropathy, palpation along individual peripheral nerves may reveal focal thickening of a neuroma or a hypertrophic mononeuropathy (perineuroma).

STANCE AND GAIT

Screening tests

Observe walking slow and fast; walking on toes and heels; tandem walk; standing on each leg alone; Romberg test.

Formal tests

- Either at the beginning (particularly if there is a gait or balance complaint) or at the end of the examination, ask the patient to walk up and down slowly, then faster over at least six paces.
- Note the initiation of gait, the trunk posture (erect or flexed), stride length, heel strike, and extent and symmetry of arm swing. As the patient turns, pay attention to any overbalancing or extra little steps that may occur with hydrocephalus, extrapyramidal, or cerebellar conditions.

- Dystonic movements, chorea, and parkinsonian tremor are enhanced by walking. Pyramidal tract lesions cause the foot to drag and the toes to scuff, and a spastic leg may be made more obvious by rapid walking or an attempted run; a 'scissoring gait' if both legs are spastic.
- Flaccid foot drop is usually obvious.
- An ataxic broad-based unsteady gait is likely to be cerebellar ataxia.
- An apraxic gait with ignition failure shows 'feet stuck to the floor' with small steps, improved when you walk beside the patient getting them to match your stride.
- Ask the patient to (you may need to demonstrate the test):
  - Walk 'heel-to-toe' to test tandem gait. Patients with a lesion of the midline cerebellar vermis may only manifest truncal ataxia and have no evidence of limb ataxia on coordination testing.
  - Stand on one leg alone and keep their balance.
  - Stand still with feet together, first with eyes open, and then shut (Romberg test), and notice any significant change in stability where the patient shows a tendency to actually fall (needs your support) that reflects impaired joint position sense from a spinal dorsal column deficit or severe sensory polyneuropathy. Some normal subjects and those with other balance problems will show a nonsignificant small–moderate body sway; functional patients may show an exaggerated response.
- Postural (righting) reflexes are examined in parkinsonian syndromes or if there have been unexplained falls. Explain that this test has both diagnostic and falls-risk assessment value. Start with gentle pushes forwards, sideways, and backwards while supporting the patient. Once they have accepted the idea, repeat while standing behind the patient so they can't anticipate the timing or direction of the push or pull (the Pull test) to the shoulders, but reassure them that you will protect them from a fall (it is best to have a wall behind you!). A normal response is a body sway or a step to control balance; abnormality is a distinct tendency to fall.

INTERPRETATION OF CLINICAL SIGNS

- The examination techniques should be performed in a consistent manner to gain an appreciation of the range of normal and abnormal responses; a lack of consistency can produce uncertainty and error in interpretation of the signs.
- Distinguish between hard and soft signs: 'hard signs' are objective and do not depend on the patient's cooperation (e.g. pupillary changes, eye movement disorders [apart from voluntary nystagmus and convergence spasm], muscle wasting, reflex changes, fasciculation); 'soft signs' include sensory signs, variable or 'give-way' weakness, endpoint nystagmus, mild facial asymmetry, tongue fasciculation. More weight must be given to hard than soft signs.
- Uncertainty whether findings are normal or abnormal can be a problem for inexperienced examiners (e.g. a questionable reflex asymmetry or mild weakness). Both errors of commission and omission can occur. Recheck the examination or ask for help to elicit or interpret a sign from a mentor or colleague.
- Functional signs include: give-way weakness; weakness with normal tone and reflexes; whole limb anesthesia; hemisensory loss for all modalities to the midline; dragging a foot slowly; a dramatically positive Romberg test with position sense testing normal at the toes; a variety of nonepileptic seizure manifestations.
- False localizing signs are where the signs reflect dysfunction distant or remote from the expected anatomical locus of pathology, which can confuse a traditional clinicoanatomical correlation unless taken into consideration. This can occur as a consequence of raised ICP, and with spinal cord lesions[17].

CONCLUDING THE EXAMINATION

By the end of the consultation, a definite diagnosis or a working diagnosis with a limited differential will usually be possible. Be honest about uncertainty and, if needed, offer a further review consultation to help clarify the diagnosis. Discuss with the patient how conclusions were reached, avoiding medical jargon, and explain the rationale of any investigations.

Draw diagrams, and use models or illustrations (e.g. of peripheral nerves or of the brain) as part of your explanation and give patients key phrases to 'Google' their diagnosis. Give educational material from self-help organizations if appropriate, such as the Parkinson's Disease Society or the Multiple Sclerosis Society. If the diagnosis is serious, make sure a support person for the patient will be present before any definitive discussion. When giving such news it is important first to find out what the patient was thinking, and then to follow the 'giving of bad news' protocol.

When the diagnosis is of a functional problem explain how the symptoms may have arisen from a disturbance of brain function and offer a helpful patient website such as 'www.neurosymptoms.org'. Emphasize the capacity for the patient to get better and how this can be achieved; if severe or persistent symptoms are present, a referral to a clinical psychologist or consultation liaison psychiatrist may be recommended (but not always accepted!).

If the patient seems uncertain at the end of the consultation ask them to repeat back what has been discussed to confirm that there is a mutual understanding. Finally, you may send the patient a copy of the consultation letter with an explicit 'Conclusions and Recommendations' paragraph in simple language, so that they have a record of the consultation outcome.

LUMBAR PUNCTURE AND CSF EXAMINATION

With the advent of modern imaging, lumbar puncture (LP) is less needed, and is done only for specific diagnostic and therapeutic indications. It is recognized that risks of the procedure can be substantial and even life threatening.

Performing a successful LP requires a knowledge of relevant anatomy and correct technique and should not be undertaken casually or by inexperienced operators without proper supervision[1]. The procedure should be explained to the patient and the reason why it is being done; written consent should be sought where possible.

Indications

- Diagnosis of suspected meningitis and encephalitis.
- Studies for blood products to diagnose a subarachnoid hemorrhage when a CT head scan is normal (3–5% of proven cases). Delay LP 12 hours to allow bilirubin to form from red blood cell lysis[2].
- To measure CSF pressure in the diagnosis of idiopathic intracranial hypertension.
- As an aid to diagnose various conditions, e.g. MS, neurosyphilis, sarcoidosis, meningeal neoplastic involvement, demyelinating peripheral neuropathies, CSF vasculitis, various dementias, and immune antibody-mediated encephalopathies.
- Removal of CSF therapeutically (e.g. idiopathic intracranial hypertension; normal pressure hydrocephalus testing).
- Intrathecal injection of drugs or contrast media.

Contraindications

- Intracranial space-occupying lesion (e.g. abscess, hematoma, tumor).
- Obstructive hydrocephalus.
- Generalized brain edema with obliteration of the cisterns around the upper brainstem.

Do a CT head scan if the above conditions are suspected before doing a LP; if a CT scan is unavailable, an LP is contraindicated in patients with clinical features of the above three conditions (e.g. papilledema and/or of focal neurologic signs and/or coma). If bacterial meningitis is suspected, and if no CT scan can be done urgently, it is essential to treat the patient immediately and empirically with broad spectrum antibiotics (after collecting blood cultures), rather than risking brain herniation in order to isolate an organism in the CSF.

- Infection of the skin in the lumbar region.
- Bleeding diathesis (e.g. platelets below 40×10^9/l; anticoagulant drugs).

Technique

For diagnostic LP, the left lateral recumbent position (for right handed doctors) is preferred.

- Ask the patient to try and touch the flexed knees with his/her chin. Place a pillow between the knees and ensure the shoulders and pelvis are perpendicular to the floor. For patient comfort, maximally flex the patient to widen the gap between the spinous processes only when you're ready to insert the needle.
- Identify and mark the L4 and L5 vertebral spinous processes, the former of which lies between the anterior superior iliac spines; the caudal part of the spinal cord ends about the level of the interspace between the first and second lumbar vertebrae.
- Wash your hands and put on a sterile gown and gloves.
- Sterilize a large area of skin over the lumbosacral spine and drape the area.
- Draw up 5 ml of 1–2% lignocaine and inject the skin and subcutaneous tissue down to the supraspinous ligament between the L4 and L5, or L3 and L4, vertebral bodies.
- Wait a few minutes for the local anesthetic to work; during this time assemble the three-way tap to the manometer. Alternatively, the manometer can be directly connected to the LP needle.
- Insert the LP needle (22 gauge standard needle with stylet) at the superior aspect of the spinous process that lies inferior to the space entered. When the L3/4 or L4/5 interspace is used the needle should be directed towards the umbilicus (15° cephalad) (**22**). Advance the needle (and bevel) in the sagittal plane, parallel to the floor, steadying the needle shaft with

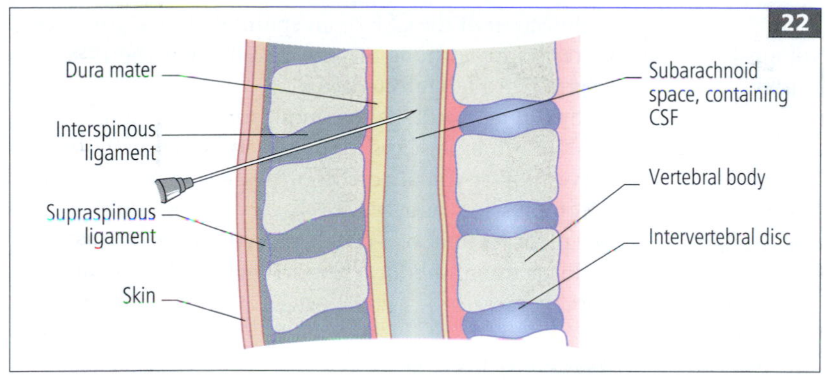

22 Midline sagittal section through the mid-lumbar spine to show the course of a lumbar puncture needle.

your other hand. Resistance may be felt as the needle penetrates the ligamentum flavum, that in young people has the consistency of soft toffee, and again at the dura, where you may feel a popping sensation. At this point, remove the stylet and if the needle is in the subarachnoid space, CSF will flow out of the needle.

- Attach the three-way tap and manometer and wait a minute or so for the CSF to rise up and stabilize before recording the CSF pressure (normal less than about 200 mm of CSF). Check that the CSF moves up and down with respiration or with relaxing the legs a little (i.e. extending the hips a little).
- Empty the CSF from the manometer into one sterile bottle for biochemical examination (protein, glucose, oligoclonal bands) and then allow another 3–5 ml to run into a sterile bottle for microbiological examination (cells, Gram stain, culture) and another bottle for DNA analysis (e.g. polymerase chain reaction [PCR]), antigen testing, spectrophotometry, or cytology. Label the bottles first, second, and third (*Table 4*).
- Replace the stylet and remove the needle, then place a band-aid/plaster over the skin puncture.
- It is traditional to advise the patient to lie down for 1 hour before getting up, but there is no evidence that this decreases the incidence of post-LP headache and early ambulation is acceptable.
- Take a simultaneous blood glucose test.
- Send the CSF and blood specimens to the appropriate laboratories immediately. Otherwise refrigerate them at 4°C (39.2°F).
- If a LP needs to be repeated within 1 or 2 weeks, do not use the same interspace as it may be into an epidural CSF collection.

TABLE 4 **MINIMUM VOLUMES OF CSF REQUIRED FOR COMMON DIAGNOSTIC TESTS**[3]

Test	Volume required	Comments
Cell count and differential	0.5–1 ml	
Glucose and protein	0.5 ml	+ Simultaneous serum sample
Gram stain and bacterial culture	2–5 ml	Larger volumes → ↑ yield
Viral PCR ± culture	1–2 ml	
Cytospin or flow cytometry	2–5 ml	
Mycobacterial and/or fungal culture	~20 ml	Low yield for smaller volumes
PCR for mycobacteria	1–2 ml	
Cryptococcal antigen	0.5 ml	+ Simultaneous serum sample
VDRL or Wasserman	0.5 ml	+ Simultaneous serum sample
Oligoclonal bands and/or serology	>2 ml	+ Simultaneous serum sample

PCR: polymerase chain reaction; VDRL: Venereal Disease Research Laboratory.

Problems

- If the needle hits bone or nerve root, evoking pain down the leg, withdraw the needle to the subcutaneous tissue, check the alignment of the needle in the sagittal, coronal, and axial planes, and reinsert it.
- If CSF does not flow, despite the needle seeming to be in the subarachnoid space, try rotating the open needle slightly as it may be abutting a nerve root. Never attempt to aspirate CSF. A 'dry tap' is usually due to incorrect positioning of the patient and needle placement.
- If fresh blood emerges from the needle, it may be in the epidural venous plexus, the needle being too far lateral or advanced too far anteriorly (or it may be a subarachnoid hemorrhage). The presence of a clot strongly favors a 'traumatic tap'. Try again through another disc space (e.g. L3/4 or L4/5 but never L2/3).
- If the LP fails, try again through another interspace (L3/4 or L4/5). If a pencil-point atraumatic needle was tried first, then use a standard needle.
- In difficult patients (e.g. obese patient with poor landmarks) seek a radiologist to carry out the LP under fluoroscopic screening either initially or after one failed attempt.

Complications

Herniation of the medial temporal lobe through the tentorial opening (transtentorial herniation) or of the medulla through the foramen magnum (coning) leads to medullary compression and death. This rare tragic complication can be avoided by never doing a LP if there is evidence for raised ICP with focal signs, or obstructed CSF flow or brain shift laterally on CT scan. The decrease in pressure in the spinal canal by removal of CSF in these situations will cause downward brain movement with herniation. On the other hand, if there is diffusely raised ICP with free flow of CSF through all parts of the intracranial and spinal CSF compartments, which can be discerned with CT or MRI scan, then LP should be safe (e.g. idiopathic intracranial hypertension).

Spinal nerve root damage can be caused, usually by inserting the needle lateral to the midline.

Low-pressure headache occurs in up to 40% of LPs and is thought to be due to low CSF pressure consequent on leakage from the dura. The headache is characteristically postural (relieved by lying flat), usually occurs within 48 hours of LP (although onset in some is 72 hours later), and rarely lasts more than a week. The incidence decreases with the use of a smaller gauge or atraumatic LP needle (but there is a lower successful LP rate if used). If headache persists then an autologous epidural blood patch can be used to block the CSF leak; or as a last resort, by open surgery to seal the dural leak.

Infection of the CSF or an epidural abscess can occur, if sterile precautions are not taken, or if the needle is inserted through infected skin.

Spinal hemorrhage (epidural, subdural, or subarachnoid) may manifest as severe back and/or nerve root pain, nerve root or spinal cord compression requiring urgent decompression surgery. This is very rare unless there is a low platelet count or a coagulation defect.

Intracranial subdural hemorrhage or VIth nerve palsy are very rare.

Assessing the CSF

Decisions on what tests should be done, and with what priority, depend on the clinical situation; discussion with a pathologist and/or infectious disease specialist may be appropriate prior to doing the LP[3]. The following parameters are measured:

- Pressure. Less than 250 mm of CSF/water, and usually less than 200 mm if the patient is relaxed (must be measured vertically from the needle hub in the lateral decubitis position).
- Red blood cells. Normally the CSF is clear with no red blood cells. If the CSF is bloody it should be centrifuged immediately and the supernatant examined by eye and spectrophotometry if a subarachnoid hemorrhage is suspected. Yellow (xanthochromic) pigmentation is due to breakdown of products of hemoglobin (e.g. oxyhemoglobin and bilirubin), and is seen in subarachnoid hemorrhage at least 12 hours before, jaundice, and very high CSF protein (>1.5 g/l [150 mg/dl]).
- White blood cells. CSF cell count ideally should be done within 30 minutes of sampling, since cell counts diminish after this time due to settling and lysis. Normally CSF contains <5 lymphocytes/ml and usually no neutrophils (although one or two may be found in otherwise normal CSF). In the event of a traumatic tap, a correction of 1 white blood cell per 700 red blood cells/ml allows some estimation of CSF pleocytosis, but cannot be relied upon in the presence of anemia or leukocytosis.
- Glucose. Normally 50–65% of a simultaneous serum glucose (CSF:blood glucose ratio ≥0.6). It is depressed (usually ≤0.4) in ~50% of patients with bacterial meningitis; most patients with tuberculosis and fungal meningitis; ~25% with mumps and herpetic meningitis.
- Protein. 0.15–45 g/l (15–45 mg/dl), depending on the laboratory. Increased protein is the most common and least specific of CSF alterations in disease. Levels above 2 g/l (200 mg/dl) suggest bacterial infections; above 5 g/l (500 mg/dl) in tuberculous meningitis, arachnoiditis, and spinal block. Red blood cells in the CSF may raise protein by roughly 10 mg/l (1 mg/dl) per 1000 red blood cells.

- Oligoclonal IgG bands. Present in the CSF but not in the serum, suggests an immune response within the CNS, and may be seen in a variety of acute and chronic CNS conditions including MS.
- PCR testing. Requires a specialized and experienced molecular laboratory, giving results in hours to days. PCR is widely available for viruses (enteroviruses, herpes simplex 1 and 2, varicella zoster, cytomegalovirus, Epstein–Barr, JC virus, human immunodeficiency virus [HIV], Japanese encephalitis, Murray Valley encephalitis, West Nile virus). Also for *Neisseria meningitidis*, *Streptococcus pneumoniae*, *Haemophilus influenzae*, *Mycobacterium tuberculosis*, *Tropheryma whippelii* (Whipple's disease) with variable availability and sensitivity according to the local laboratory.
- Antigen testing. Mainly of use in cryptococcal CNS infection, with a sensitivity of 80–90% and good specificity. Specific bacterial antigen testing may be of use in partially treated meningitis in which initial Gram stain and culture are negative.
- Antibody testing. May be useful in cases of possible subacute sclerosing panencephalitis (SSPE; measles antibody), neurosyphilis, and in anti-*N*-methyl-D-aspartate receptor antibody autoimmune limbic encephalitis, where the antibody may be present in the CSF but not detected in the serum.
- Detection of 14-3-3 protein in CSF. This is a marker for Creutzfeldt–Jakob disease (CJD) in an appropriate clinical setting but may also be present in other neurologic conditions.

NEUROPHYSIOLOGIC EXAMINATION

Electroencephalography (EEG)

The EEG is a recording of the electrical activity of the cerebral cortex. It reflects the summated excitatory and inhibitory post-synaptic potentials of the upper layers of cerebral cortex, especially the pyramidal cells because of their vertical orientation and large apical dendritic trees. This activity is influenced by subcortical structures, especially the thalamus and rostral brainstem reticular formation.

Technique

Surface electrodes (usually 21), metal or silver–silver chloride discs, are placed equidistantly over the scalp according to an international convention (10–20 System) (23). They are attached to the scalp with an adhesive material such as collodion, using conductive paste under the electrodes to ensure good electrical contact with the scalp. As with electrocardiogram (ECG), electromyogram (EMG), nerve conduction, and other biologic recordings, pairs of electrodes are then connected to differential amplifiers that reject in-phase activity common to both input electrodes. The output of a differential amplifier reflects the difference between the two input electrodes. This approach is required because each electrode records not only physiologically relevant activity but also large amounts of environmental electrical noise. By combining pairs of electrodes, hopefully the environmental noise common to both electrodes will cancel out. Filtering highlights activity that is biologically relevant, for EEG a bandpass of 0.5–70 Hz, but filtering distorts raw data to a degree and is no substitute for good technique.

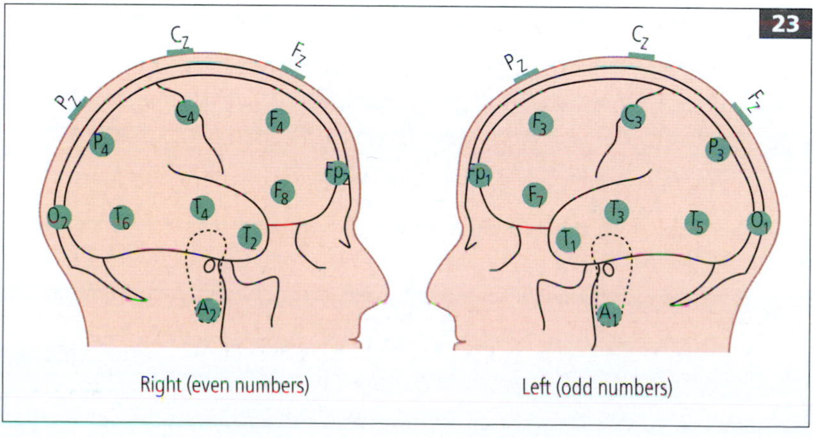

23 The international 10–20 electrode system of electrode placement. Each electrode site is identified by a letter indicating the lobe and a number indicating the hemispheric location. F: frontal lobe; T: temporal lobe; C: central lobe; P: parietal lobe; O: occipital lobe; z: midline. Note: F_7 and F_8 mainly record anterior temporal lobe activity.

Each differential amplifier output forms one derivation or 'channel', with EEG displays showing multiple channels called montages, either chains of adjacent electrode pairs (bipolar montages) or sometimes choosing a single reference electrode for all other electrodes (referential montage). The channels forming a montage are displayed in a vertical array on a digital screen or a paper trace moving at a standard speed of 3 cm/s, with voltage change on the vertical axis *vs*. time on the horizontal axis. By convention, if the active electrode of a channel is relatively negative to the reference electrode (or the reference electrode is relatively positive to the active electrode), then the trace deflection will be up.

Patients are usually in the awake state, lying or sitting down in a quiet room with their eyes closed. The resting EEG is recorded for about 30 minutes. Careful clinical observation, video recording, or both are required throughout the recording. A number of 'activating' procedures are usually carried out:

- Sleep: the patient is allowed to fall asleep, because sleep may enhance epileptiform abnormalities.
- Hyperventilation: the patient is asked to breathe deeply 20 times a minute for at least 3 minutes, evoking hypocapnia, alkalosis, and cerebral vasoconstriction. The EEG normally increases in amplitude and rhythm slows (**24**), and epileptiform and other abnormality may be induced.
- Photic stimulation: a powerful flashing light (stroboscope) is placed about 40 cm (16 in) from the patient's eyes using varying frequencies of 1–50 per second (Hz) with the patient's eyes open and closed. The normal EEG may show occipital waves evoked by each flash of light (visual evoked response or 'photic driving'), and patients with a predisposition to seizures may show epileptiform abnormalities (a photoparoxysmal response), and sometimes a subtle myoclonic or absence seizure. The most potent stimulus is usually between 10 Hz and 30 Hz and during eye closure or shortly after eye closure (**25**). Photic stimulation may also evoke forehead and eyelid muscle artifact (a photomyogenic response) that may be misinterpreted as being of significance.

Other techniques that can be used to identify epileptic foci include:

- Sleep recordings, which may reveal abnormalities not evident when the subject is awake or in light sleep. A single routine EEG recording will show definite epileptiform abnormalities in only 20–40% of adults who have epilepsy[1,2]. Sleep deprivation is the most effective way of obtaining a sleep recording, which doubles the sensitivity of EEG.
- Prolonged (6–8 hours) telemetric recordings.
- Video EEG monitoring in order capture and analyze the patient's symptoms, if sufficiently frequent.

Tips

▶ *Adequate EEG recordings require well-trained and skilled neurophysiology technicians. Excessive filtering and gain reduction make the EEG look nice, but distort and reduce data. Filter EEG with your brain instead. Don't forget the accompanying ECG recording, important in exploration of episodes of unconsciousness.*

▶ *EEG reading Zen: prepare yourself (EEG reading requires careful training), clear your mind and focus on the waves (not on your watch or the request form), go with the flow (not too fast), know and change montages.*

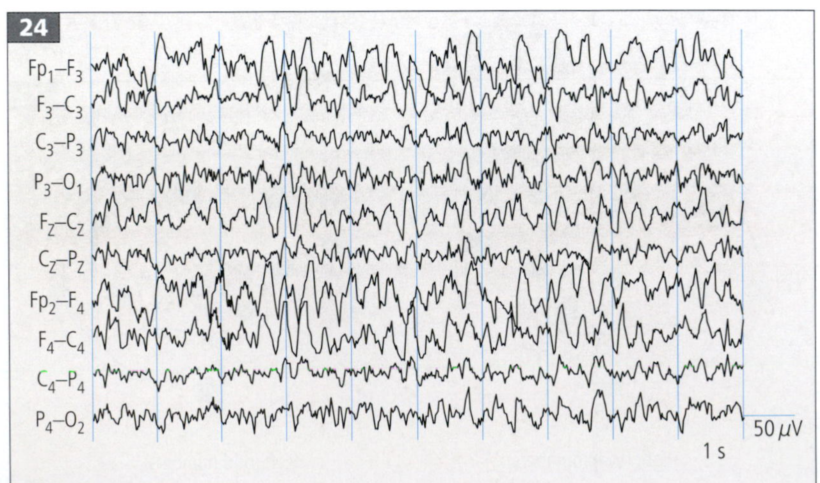

24 **Normal EEG during hyperventilation. The EEG is of high amplitude, with prominent anterior delta slowing and a jagged admixture of other faster frequencies. The subject is a normal 19-year-old male.**

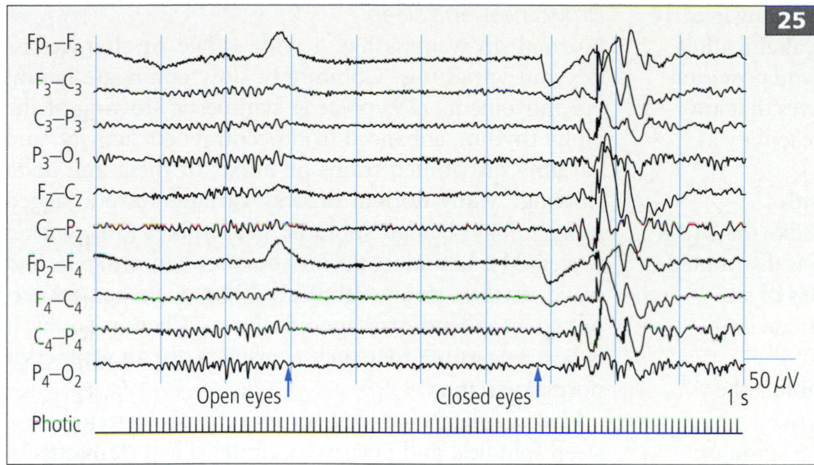

25 10 Hz photic stimulation. The normal alpha rhythm attenuates upon eye opening. With eyes open normal low amplitude 10 Hz bilateral photic driving responses are seen. After eye closure a brief and self-limited photoparoxysmal response occurs, with a burst of generalized spikes and delta slowing. The subject is a 17-year-old male.

26 EEG wave frequencies.

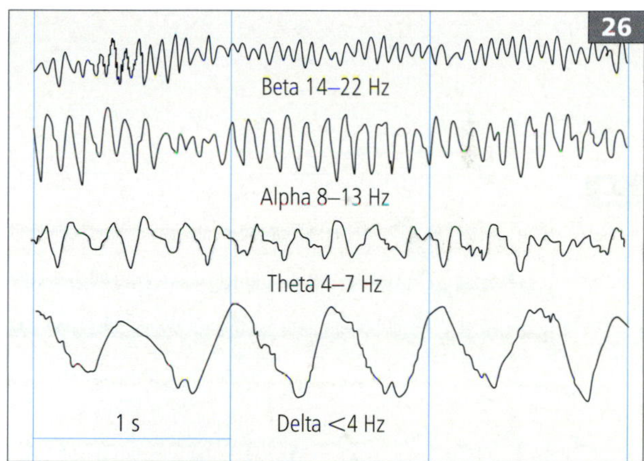

Normal EEG recordings

Age and state dependency dramatically influence the normal EEG, and there are many variations of normal.

Awake

- Amplitude: 10–200 µV.
- Wave forms/rhythms (**26**):
  - Alpha waves: 8–13 per second (Hz). 'Alpha rhythm' is sinusoidal alpha activity recorded over the occipital regions, present when the eyes are closed and attenuated by eye opening or mental activity (**25, 27**). A small proportion of adults have little or no alpha rhythm, and both slow (4–5 Hz) and fast (14–16 Hz) normal variants of alpha rhythm may be seen. Temporal and frontal alpha activity also forms part of the background.
  - Beta waves: 14–22 Hz, low amplitude (10–20 µV) are recorded diffusely, maximal over the frontal and midline regions.
  - Theta waves: 4–7 Hz, are prominent diffusely in children, gradually diminishing during adolescence and adulthood. Theta activity also emerges with drowsiness in adults, especially over the temporal or frontotemporal regions.

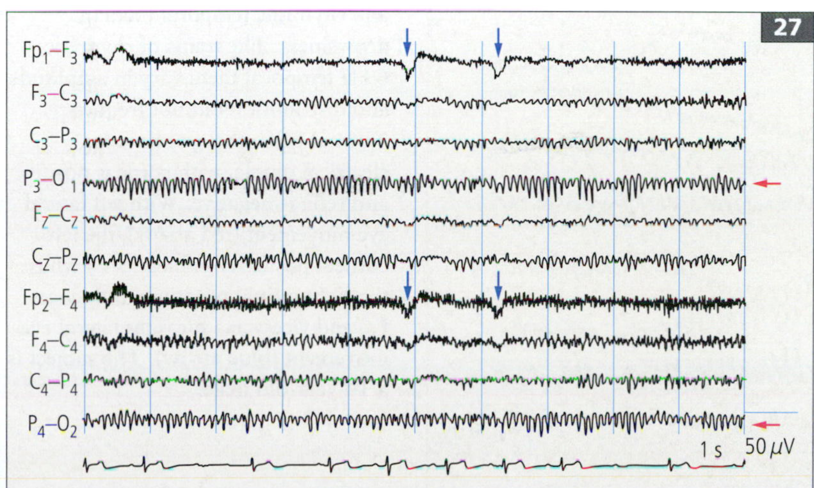

27 Normal awake EEG, but not ECG, shows atrioventricular dissociation. Patient has cardiogenic syncope rather than epileptic seizure. The EEG shows symmetrical 10–11 Hz alpha rhythm (red arrows). The frontopolar delta waves are eye-blink artifacts (blue arrows). The frontal beta activity, best seen in the Fp_2–F_4 channel, is a scalp muscle artifact. The subject is a 25-year-old female.

- Delta waves: <4 Hz, are a normal finding in early childhood, but not in the normal wakeful adult save for hyperventilation-induced and posterior slowing of youth, 2–4 Hz delta waves that are admixed with and have the same reactivity as alpha rhythm.
- Mu rhythm: alpha activity often with characteristic arciform appearance like the Greek letter μ or the top of a picket fence, is distributed asymmetrically in the central regions of the head, and attenuates with contralateral limb movement.
- Lambda waves: a waveform resembling the Greek letter lambda λ, that is an evoked response to actively viewing a visual stimulus, generated in the occipital region by saccadic eye movements (28).

Drowsiness and sleep

Normal drowsiness has a wide range of characteristics and variations. Commonly slow conjugate lateral eye movements (29) precede symmetric slowing of the alpha rhythm, enhanced frontocentral beta activity, and variably distributed trains or bursts of theta and delta slowing. Many normal drowsy variants have a jagged morphology: benign sporadic sleep spikes (30), wicket waves (31), 14 and six positive bursts, phantom spike and wave, rhythmic temporal theta (29) that can be misinterpreted as epileptiform abnormalities. When in doubt, it is best to assume that such transients are an artifact or normal variant.

During sleep characteristic waveforms (vertex waves, sleep spindles, and positive occipital sharp transients of sleep) appear (32). They may have a striking a jagged contour, and may be misinterpreted as epileptiform abnormalities. Benzodiazepine or barbiturates may induce prominent beta during both sleep and wakefulness.

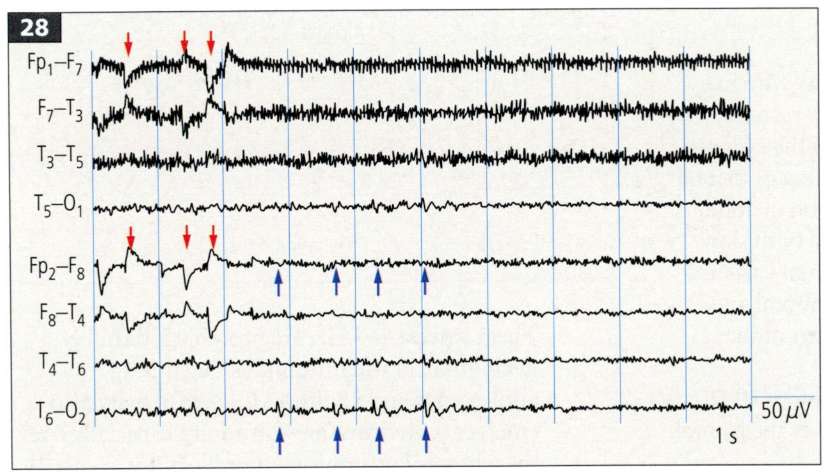

28 Normal EEG. Saccadic lateral eye movements (red arrows); lambda waves (blue arrows).The prominent beta activity in multiple channels on the left is muscle artifact. The subject is a 41-year-old female.

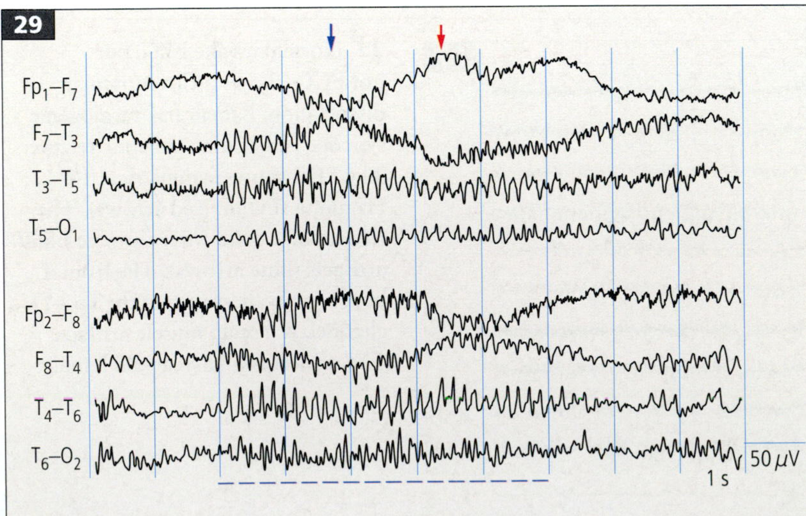

29 Slow bilateral eye movements and rhythmic temporal theta of drowsiness. The trains of rhythmic 6 Hz temporal theta vary in amplitude and distribution but not frequency. Normal EEG: the eyes have an electrical dipole, with corneas positive and retinas negative. With left lateral eye movement (red arrow), the left corneal positivity influences F_7 whilst the right retinal negativity influences F_8, and vice-versa for right lateral eye movement (blue arrow). The subject is a 14-year-old male.

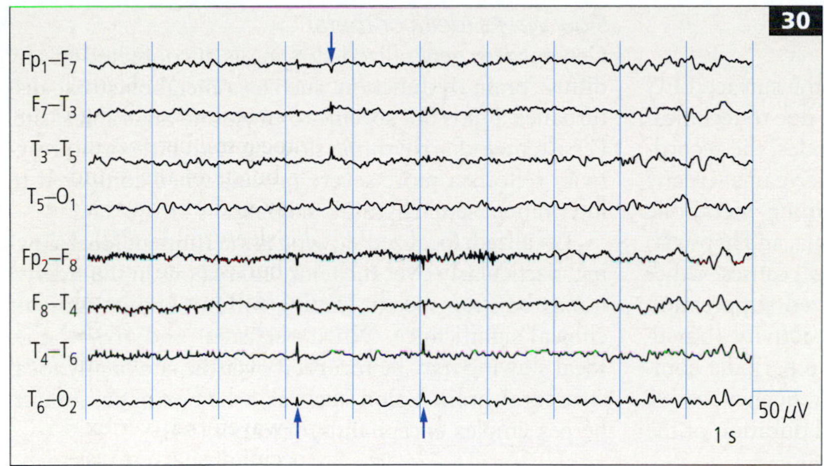

30 Normal EEG. Benign sporadic sleep spikes (arrows) are brief, diphasic, have no or little aftercoming slow wave and do not disrupt the background.

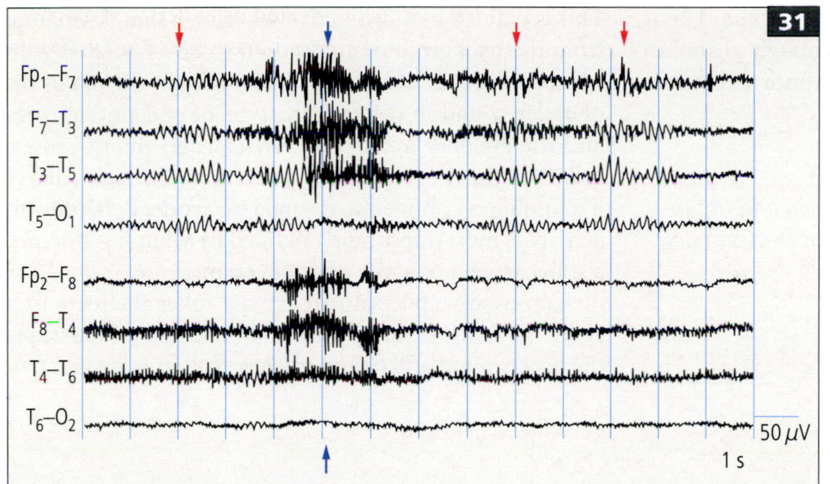

31 Left temporal wicket waves (red arrows). Normal EEG.Wicket waves comprise unilateral or bilateral and shifting trains of sometimes notched 6–11 Hz temporal waves, without aftercoming slowing or background disturbance.During a swallow (blue arrows), enhanced bilateral scalp muscle and underlying tongue movement (the glossokinetic potential) artifacts may be seen.

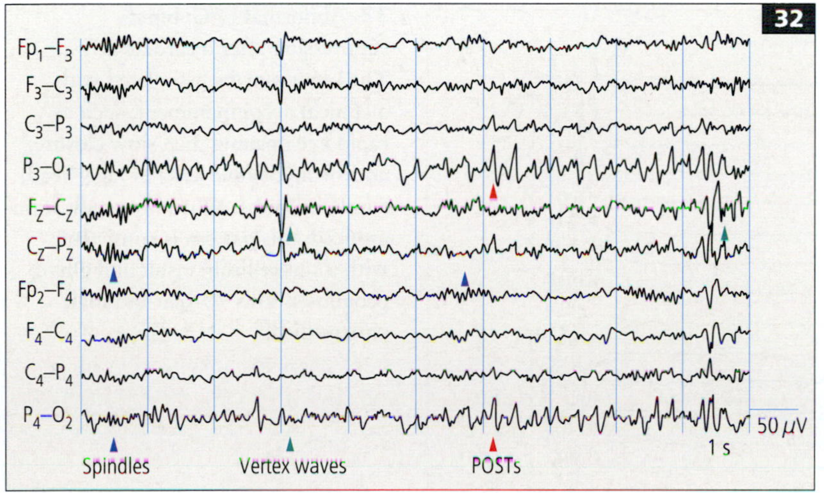

32 Normal sleep with vertex waves (green arrowheads), sleep spindles (blue arrowheads), and positive occipital sharp transients of sleep (POSTs; red arrrowheads).

Tip

▶ *Background slowing is normal in drowsiness/sleep, and every sharply contoured wave is an artifact or normal variant until proven otherwise.*

Abnormal EEG recordings

Absent brain waves

In generalized 'electrocerebral silence', the surface EEG is absent or less than 2 μV. This may be due to technical problems (identified by checking electrodes, the recording system, and then increasing amplifier gains) or any cause of severe encephalopathy including metabolic (e.g. hypothermia, diffuse cerebral ischemia, and hypoxia) and toxic (anesthetic levels of many drugs) causes. Other severe coma patterns include generalized suppression admixed with brief bursts of cortical activity (burst–suppression; **33**), generalized unreactive periodic complexes, and unreactive single or mixed frequency waves. Prognosis is determined by etiology and duration of the coma rather than by the EEG pattern itself.

Localized absent waves indicate a large area of brain softening, tumor, or extra- or subdural hematoma. This is rare because most lesions are not large enough to abolish brain waves or prevent recording of abnormal waves arising from the borders of the lesion.

Tip

▶ *Brain death is first and foremost a clinical and not an EEG diagnosis. Clinical neurophysiology at best can only be an adjunct to the clinical assessment.*

Slow waves (delta or theta)

Generalized: generalized slowing is encountered in any diffuse brain dysfunction, such as a metabolic/toxic disturbance, but is not specific to cause and anatomical site. Persistent and arrhythmic slowing with little or no reactivity reflects a more severe process when compared to intermittent semi-rhythmic slowing.

Localized: localized slowing is intermittent focal slowing, particularly over the temporal regions in the elderly; it may be a nonspecific finding without known cause or clinical significance. When persistent and arrhythmic, focal slowing may be recorded over the site of any focal structural brain lesion such as a hemorrhage, infarct, herpes simplex encephalitis, or tumor (**34**).

Epileptiform activity

This is defined as a distinctive waveform that is separate from the background and known to be associated with epilepsy. EEG is of critical importance in the diagnosis of epilepsy and in defining the type of epileptic seizures and the epilepsy syndrome. Artifact has many causes, may mimic almost any EEG pattern, and is highly likely if a finding is confined to a single electrode. Epileptiform activity is most importantly defined by what it is not; not a spiky artifact or spiky normal variant.

Commonly epileptiform activity takes the form of a spike (≤70 ms) or sharp wave (70–200 ms) that disrupts the background and has an aftercoming slow wave.

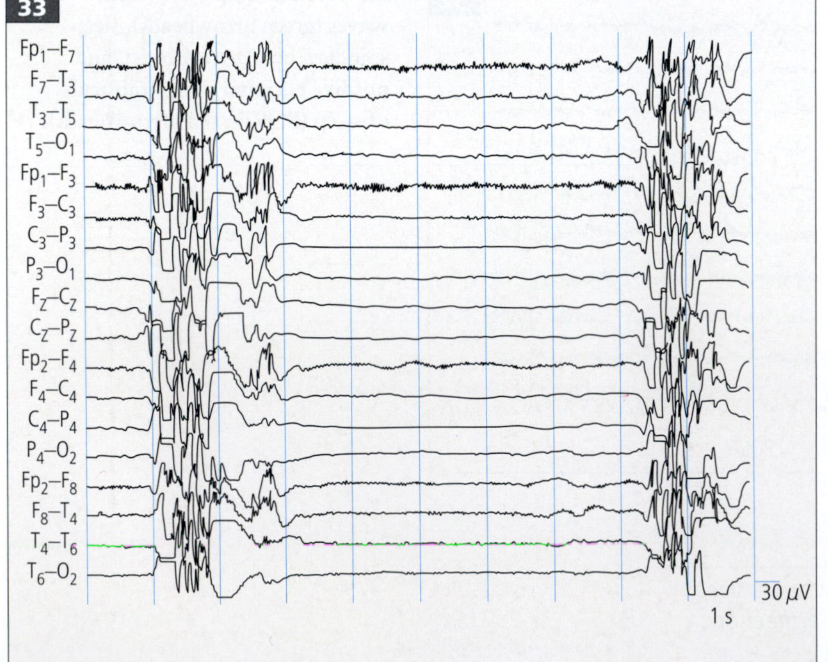

33 Abnormal EEG: burst–suppression after a cardiac arrest. The burst may be associated with a clinical accompaniment, such as rapid eye opening then slow closure, and/or myoclonic jerks of face, head, trunk, or limbs. When not medication-induced, this pattern is consistent with a severe brain insult and grave prognosis. This 70-year-old male patient died.

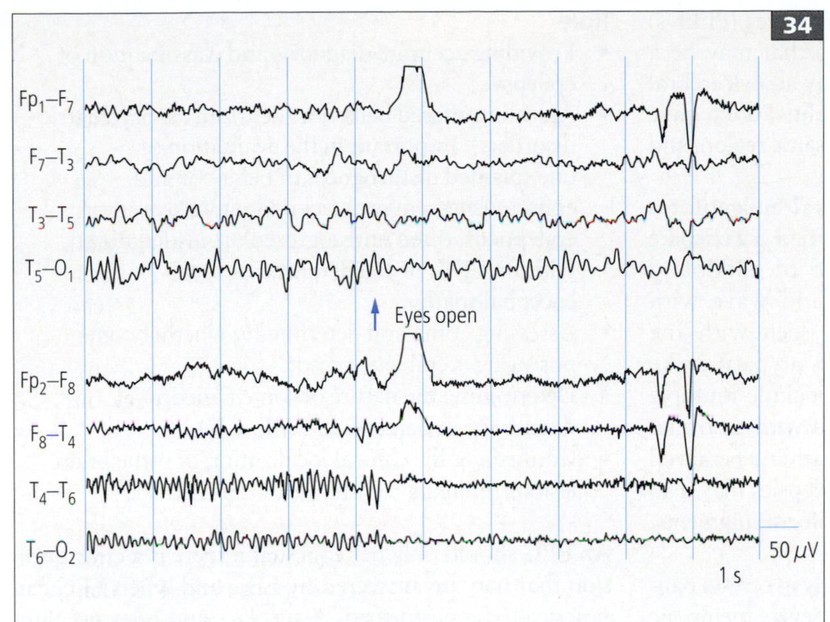

34 **Persistent left-sided slowing and reduced reactivity after stroke. The subject is a 38-year-old female with dysphasia and a right hemiparesis after a left middle cerebral artery territory stroke 2 years previously. The EEG findings reflect this, with persistent focal delta slowing seen in structural lesions with subcortical white matter involvement.**

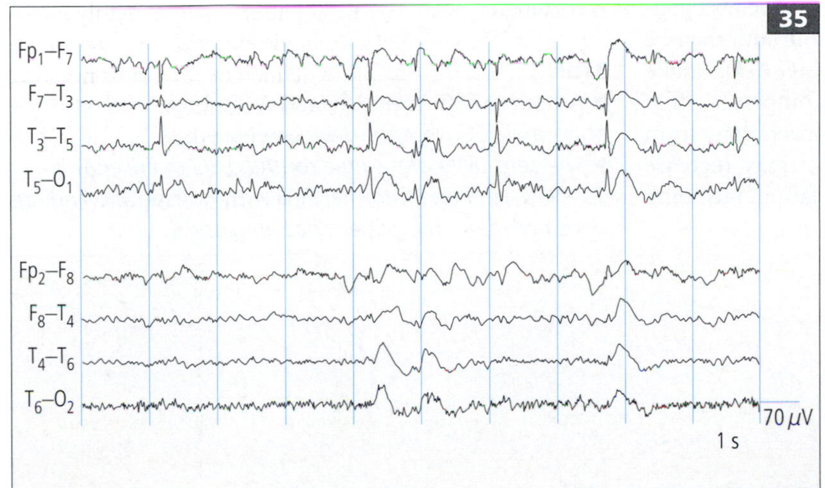

35 **Frequent predominately left temporal spike and wave complexes. The spikes are maximal in the anterior (F_7) and mid-temporal (T_3) electrodes, and the configuration of the bipolar montage displays this as a 'phase-reversal' around these electrodes. The spikes have a negative polarity and consistently have an aftercoming slow wave. The subject is a 23-year-old female with left temporal lobe epilepsy.**

Tip

▶ *Artifact can mimic almost any EEG pattern of cerebral origin. Watch accompanying video (routine if possible) as needed to assess possible artifact.*

Spike and wave or sharp waves

Localized: localized epileptiform abnormalities indicate a potentially epileptogenic focus (35). However, focal epilepsy (particularly extratemporal) may manifest as widespread or generalized spikes.

Periodic lateralized epileptiform discharges (PLEDs) are ongoing semiperiodic sharp waves that may be a postictal finding or can be seen after any acute cerebral insult such as stroke or herpes encephalitis, often have associated attenuation or slowing in the same region, and indicate a predisposition to seizures (**36**).

Generalized: Several types of general epileptiform abnormalities are recognized. Well-formed 3 Hz spike and wave ('typical') is characteristic of childhood absence epilepsy; slow 2 Hz sharp and wave with an abnormally slow background is seen with the symptomatic generalized epilepsies; and 'atypical' spike and wave, other than 3 Hz and may include multiple spikes (polyspike wave complexes), and with a normal background (**37**) is seen with other idiopathic generalized epilepsies. However, the generalized epilepsies may also show asymmetric and even focal epileptiform fragments, particularly during drowsiness.

Periodic discharges may occur regularly in certain pancortical diseases such as CJD, SSPE, and severe metabolic encephalopathies. Generalized triphasic complexes (**38**) are commonly seen with metabolic and toxic encephalopathies; they may have a jagged contour and then be misinterpreted as generalized spike and wave (**39**). Unlike spike and wave complexes, triphasic complexes often have a lag in phase and/or changes in morphology from front to back and are state-dependent (may increase with arousal [**39**], and decrease with sedation, including medications) rather than state-dictating.

Role

- Providing accurate diagnosis and classification of epilepsy.
- Assessing altered behavior (delirium *vs*. psychiatric disorders). Important in the evaluation of unexplained disturbances of behavior and consciousness; may detect nonconvulsive status epilepticus, often unrecognized or misdiagnosed without EEG, or a generalized or focal encephalopathy.
- Assessing coma and determining whether coma posturing is epileptic or not.
- Determining the nature of some pancortical disturbances: dementias, SSPE, CJD.
- Confirming the clinical localization of some brain lesions (imaging techniques do this better).

An EEG should only be requested if there is a clear question that may be answered by EEG and when EEG can practically be performed. A succinct and relevant clinical history is crucial to accurate interpretation of the recording.

Tips

▶ *A normal EEG does not exclude epilepsy, and an abnormal EEG may not diagnose epilepsy.*

▶ *The sensitivity of a single routine EEG in epilepsy is 25–56%, and an abnormal EEG with nonspecific findings does not mean the patient has epilepsy*[1,2].

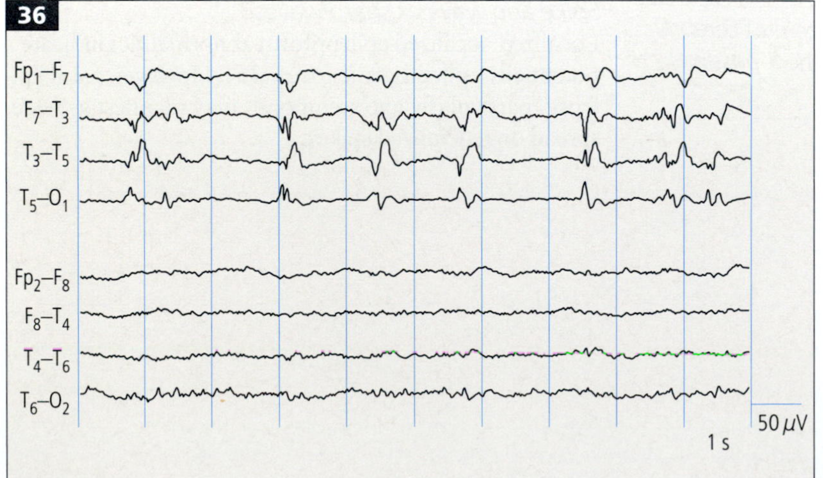

36 Left temporal periodic lateralized epileptiform discharges in a patient with herpes encephalitis. Semiperiodic sharp and slow waves are present over the left temporal region. The subject is a 79-year-old female who presented with a fever and dysphasia, related to encephalitis involving the left temporal lobe.

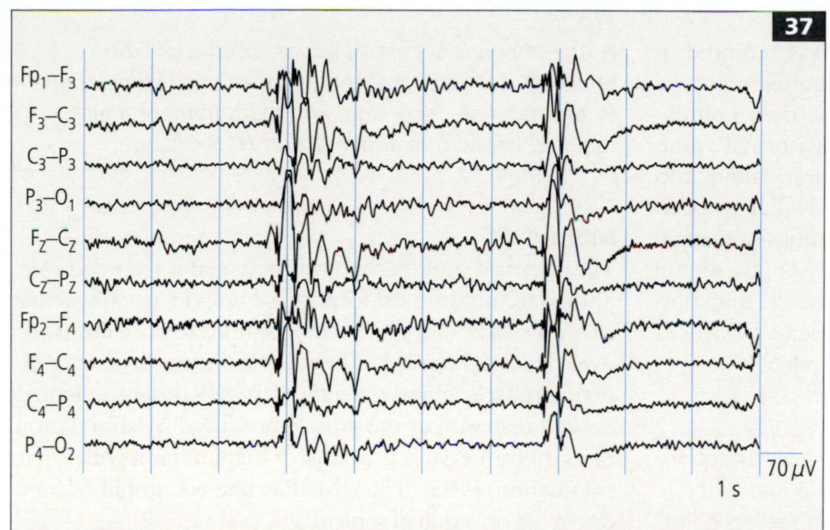

37 Patient with idiopathic generalized epilepsy. Bursts of generalized spike and wave on a normal background. The subject is a 17-year-old female.

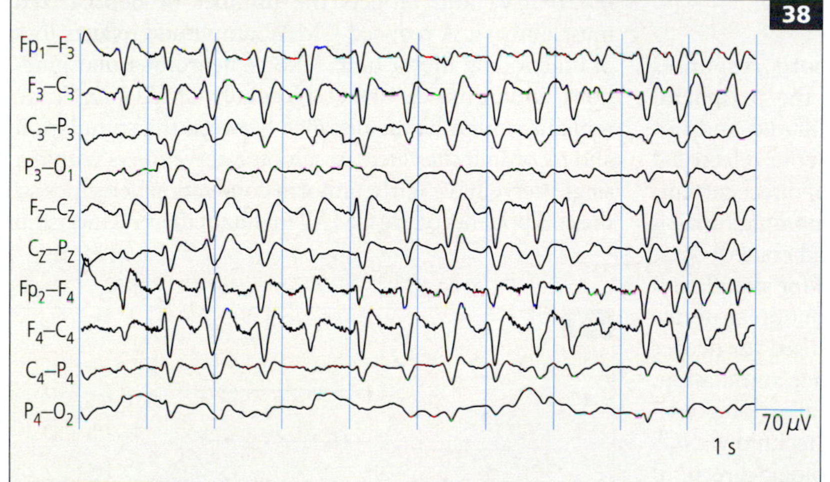

38 Patient with hepatic encephalopathy. The EEG shows generalized and anteriorly dominant triphasic waves (small negative first phase, a prominent second positive phase and then a broader negative third phase) with a 1–2 Hz periodicity and anteroposterior phase lag. No normal background frequencies are present. The subject is a 61-year-old female.

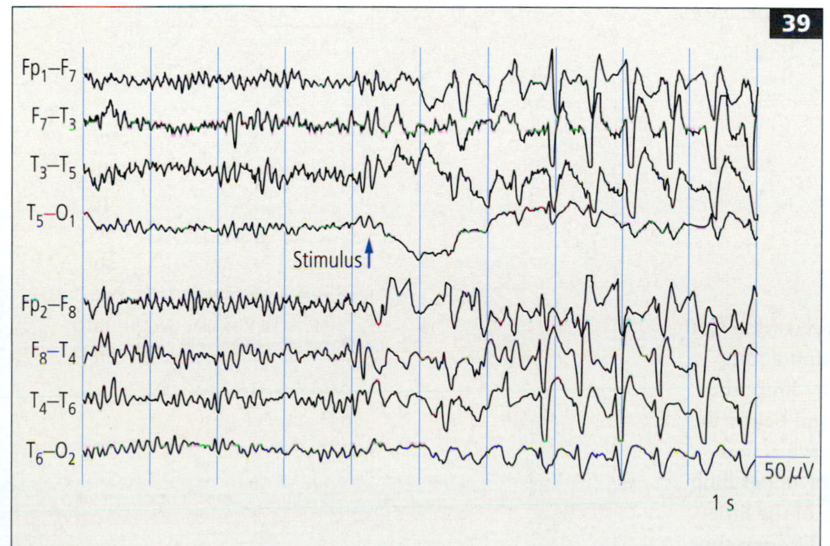

39 Triphasic waves showing state-dependent reactivity. The subject is a 69-year-old female with a metabolic encephalopathy due to renal failure. Arousal (blue arrow) evokes generalized triphasic complexes, with the jagged first phase resembling sharp waves. Triphasic waves are suppressed by benzodiazepines, and so is consciousness and respiration. Such suppression does not help the patient, and triphasic waves may be misinterpreted as epileptiform abnormality responding to treatment.

Interpretation

Considerable training, skill and caution is required to interpret EEG accurately. The EEG requires objective analysis independent of clinical biases, then contextual interpretation. There is considerable normal variation dependent on age and state of alertness, and all too often normal variations can be erroneously diagnosed as abnormal or, even worse, nonspecific findings or normal variants diagnosed as indicative of epilepsy or other brain disorders. Epileptiform activity is better missed than misdiagnosed. Furthermore, a normal interictal EEG does not have sufficient sensitivity to exclude epilepsy.

Tip

▶ *Be an advocate for the recording, with a presumption of innocence until proven otherwise. When in doubt, give the benefit of the doubt – you will do far less harm.*

Nerve conduction studies

Nerve conduction studies (NCS) record responses of nerve or muscle to stimulation of the peripheral nerve. Routine NCS assess large, myelinated and not small, unmyelinated axons. Percutaneous electrical stimuli stimulation (a square wave pulse of direct current) is usually used, ensuring the stimulus is supramaximal in order to allow comparison of patient and control data. Surface bipolar prong electrodes are used for stimulation of accessible nerves, but a near-nerve monopolar needle referenced to a surface electrode can be used for deeper structures or when edema impairs surface stimulation. Nerve stimulation produces a bidirectional action potential, and so depending on the recording technique NCS may be described as orthodromic (physiologic direction) or antidromic (opposite direction). Recording employs surface electrode pairs (small metal discs or adhesive electrodes) applied to the skin where possible.

Tip

▶ *Age-dependent control values, control of limb temperature, and consistent techniques of stimulation (supramaximal), recording, and measurement are required to perform and interpret NCS reliably.*

Motor NCS

The electrical (not mechanical) potential is recorded over a standard anatomical location of muscle, usually active electrode over end-plate region, and reference electrode over the distal tendon. The recorded orthodromic compound muscle action potential (CMAP) is the summated evoked response of the muscle produced by stimulation of its motor nerve (e.g. abductor digiti minimi with ulnar stimulation) (**40a**). The CMAP is filtered, amplified, and displayed on a digital screen.

The amplitude of the CMAP is measured in millivolts (2–20 mV) and reflects the number of depolarized muscle fibers. A reduced CMAP amplitude reflects loss of functioning motor units (axons, neuromuscular junctions, and/or muscle fibers). Normally CMAP amplitude remains similar as the distance between the stimulation and recording sites increases; motor nerve fibers within a single nerve have fairly uniform conduction velocities so the components of the CMAP maintain their relationship

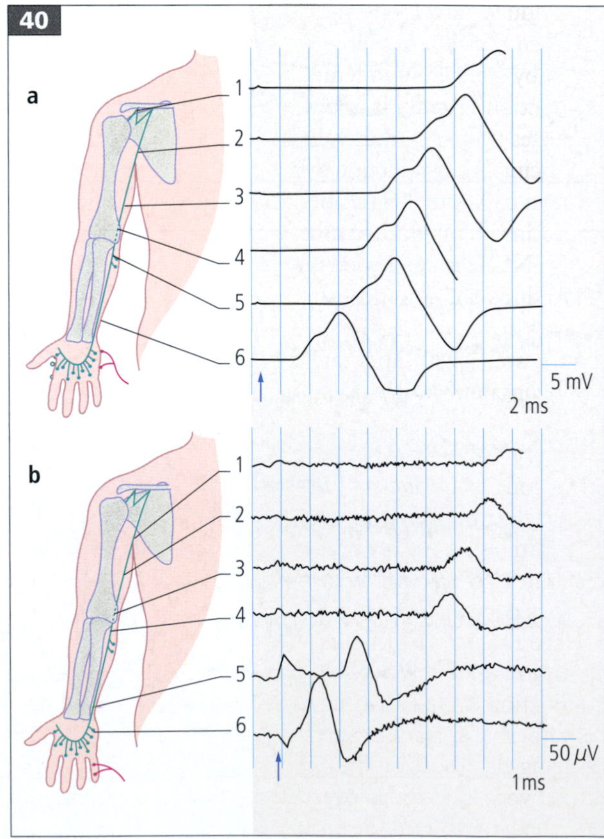

40 (a) Compound muscle action potential recorded from the hypothenar eminence after electrically stimulating the ulnar nerve at various points in the upper limb: the supraclavicular fossa (1), axilla (2), above and below the elbow (3, 4, 5) and wrist (6). (b) Sensory nerve action potential recorded from various points in the upper limb after electrically stimulating the ulnar nerve in the little finger (orthodromic conduction). Note the different time and voltage scale compared with motor nerve conduction studies in (a).

(**40**). When CMAP amplitude significantly decreases (usually by more than 50% in area and amplitude) along the nerve (e.g. ulnar CMAP amplitude reduced after stimulation above the elbow when compared to stimulation at the wrist) then 'conduction block' may be present. This may reflect slowing or block of conduction of some nerve fibers between the two stimulus sites. However, caution is required since physiologic anomalies of innervation can mimic conduction block.

Tip

▶ *Physiologic anomalies of innervation and inadequate proximal stimulation can mimic conduction block.*

The delay (latency) between stimulus delivery and onset of the CMAP is measured in milliseconds (e.g. the distal motor latency for median nerve stimulation at the wrist may be 3.6 ms, and the latency for more proximal stimulation at the cubital fossa may be 7.6 ms) (*Table 5*). The measured distance between the two stimulus sites (e.g. 200 mm) can be divided by the differences in latency (7.6 ms – 3.6 ms = 4 ms) to produce a conduction velocity in meters/second (e.g. 50 m/s). For reliable conduction velocity estimation, the two stimulus locations should be at least 10 cm apart.

Normal limb nerve conduction velocities are of the order of 40–70 m/sec (*Table 5*). Onset latencies are used, so conduction velocity measures the fastest conducting fibers in the nerve. Nerve conduction velocity is influenced by age and limb temperature. In infants the motor conduction velocity is about one-half that of adults and increases to reach adult values at about 3–5 years. With advancing age conduction then slows. Cooling slows conduction by about 1.9 m/s per °C below normal temperature. Limb temperature must be known and controlled before NCS can be carried out and interpreted reliably.

Reduction of conduction velocity, when mild, reflects loss or narrowing of large, fast conducting axons, and when moderate to severe reflects segmental demyelination.

Sensory NCS

Antidromic conduction can be assessed in accessible sensory or mixed sensorimotor nerves by electrically stimulating the sensory nerve proximally (e.g. the median or ulnar nerve at the wrist) and recording the resulting sensory nerve action potential (SNAP) distally (e.g. from surface ring electrodes placed around the index or little fingers respectively) (**40b**). Alternatively, orthodromic conduction can be assessed by stimulating the distal sensory fibers (e.g. median nerve with electrodes on the palm and ring electrodes on the index finger) and recording the SNAP with electrodes over the nerve more proximally (e.g. median nerve at the wrist; **41**).

TABLE 5 **NORMAL PARAMETERS IN NERVE CONDUCTION STUDIES**

Distal motor latency to onset of compound muscle action potential (CMAP) (ms)	
Median nerve (wrist to abductor pollicis brevis)	<4.2
Ulnar nerve (wrist to abductor digiti minimi)	<3.5
Peroneal nerve (ankle to extensor digitorum brevis)	<6.5
Tibial nerve (ankle to abductor hallucis)	<5.8
Normal motor conduction velocities (m/s)	
Median nerve in forearm	>49
Ulnar nerve in forearm	>51
Common peroneal nerve	>41
Tibial nerve	>40

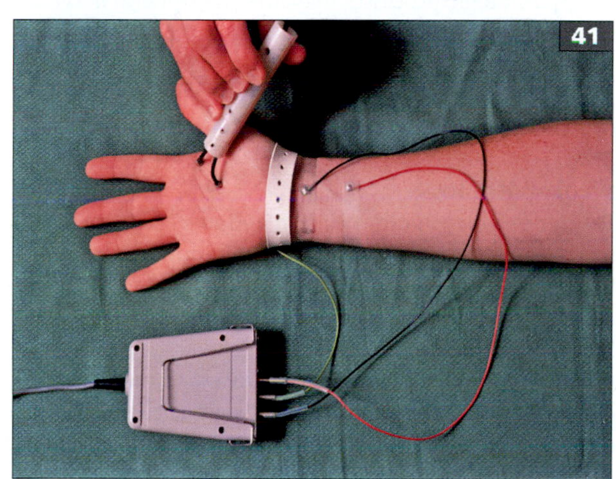

41 Orthodromic median sensory conduction: stimulation of the palm, recording over the median nerve at the wrist.

The amplitudes of SNAPs are much smaller than CMAPS, are measured in microvolts (5–150 μV), and reflect the number of nerve fibers that have responded to the stimulus. A reduced SNAP amplitude reflects loss of functioning axons due to lesions of the sensory nerves distal to the dorsal root ganglia. Unlike motor fibers, the sensory fibers within a single nerve have variable conduction velocities; so increasing temporal dispersion of the sensory fibers causes the SNAP amplitude to decrease as the distance between the stimulation and recording sites increases (**40**) (*Table 6*). Sensory nerve conduction velocities are therefore more technically demanding and less reliable, but can be calculated by recording the SNAP onset latencies at two separate points over a nerve.

Sensory distal latencies are recorded as peak negative rather than onset latencies, because they are more reliably measured. Control values are age dependent, require control of limb temperature, and consistent techniques of supramaximal stimulation, recording, and measurement.

TABLE 6 **NORMAL SENSORY ACTION POTENTIALS**

	Latency to peak (ms)	**Amplitude** (μV)
Median nerve (wrist to index finger)	<3.5	>15
Ulnar nerve (wrist to little finger)	<3.1	>10
Sural nerve (calf to ankle, 14 cm)	<4.0	>6

Pathologies

Four pathologic processes may affect peripheral nerves.

Wallerian degeneration

This follows mechanical injury (e.g. transection or crush) or ischemia (e.g. vasculitis) of nerve fibers (**42**).

Neuropathology

Within 4–5 days, both the axon and myelin distal to the site of injury degenerate. The degenerating myelin forms linear arrays of ovoids and globules along the degenerating axon. The axon of the proximal segment regenerates forming sprouts that grow distally, and some reinnervate the surviving distal neurilemmal tubes of the Schwann cell basement membrane, inside which the Schwann cells have divided and arranged themselves in line. The regenerating axons are then myelinated by the Schwann cells but the nerve fibers are smaller in diameter and have shorter internodal lengths than originally.

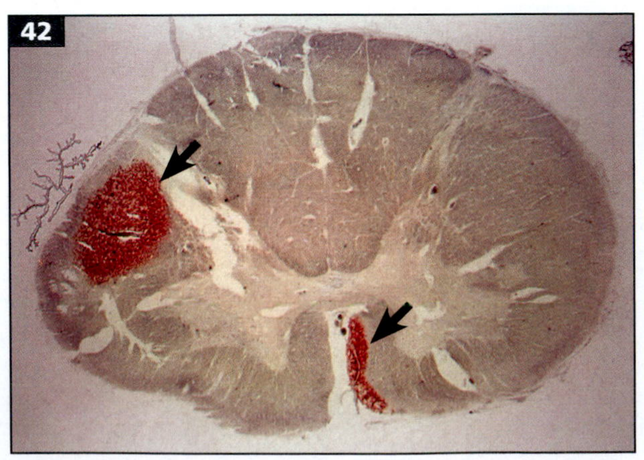

42 Autopsy specimen of the thoracic spinal cord in cross-section showing evidence of Wallerian degeneration of the contralateral and ipsilateral corticospinal tracts (arrows), secondary to a more proximal corticospinal tract lesion (i.e. internal capsule lacunar infarct).

Neurophysiology

Following nerve transection, the fibers continue to conduct impulses at normal or near normal conduction velocities until about 1–4 days later, when the fibers become totally unexcitable and conduction ceases. Nerve function may slowly be restored over many months following nerve fiber regeneration, but CMAP and SNAP amplitudes and conduction velocities are rarely restored completely.

Axonal degeneration

This follows most metabolic, toxi, and nutritional diseases of peripheral nerves, a disturbance of the metabolism of the cell body or perikaryon. It impedes fast axonal transport and other functions so that the most distal parts of the axon (which may be up to 1 m [3.3 ft] from the cell body) are affected first and die back from the periphery ('dying-back neuropathy').

Neuropathology

Axonal degeneration of the distal portion of the nerve fiber, similar to the Wallerian degeneration.

Neurophysiology

The intact proximal segments function normally but CMAP and SNAP amplitudes decrease and conduction slows and may fail over the distal degenerating part of the axon similar to Wallerian degeneration. Conduction slowing tends to be mild since the remaining intact axons maintain myelination and saltatory conduction.

Segmental demyelination

This follows primary damage of the myelin sheath by a disturbance of Schwann cell metabolism (e.g. some hereditary neuropathies), a direct immune-mediated attack on the myelin or the Schwann cell (e.g. Guillain–Barré syndrome), or toxic damage to the myelin sheath (e.g. diphtheria toxin).

Neuropathology

Demyelination usually begins paranodally and tends to affect peripheral nerves proximally (e.g. the roots) and very distally at the nerve terminal more than (or, as much as) intervening regions. The axon remains intact unless demyelination is severe, causing secondary axonal degeneration. Remyelination occurs when Schwann cells divide and form new internodes of irregular length with thin myelin sheaths. Repeated episodes of demyelination and remyelination result in the formation of concentric layers of Schwann cell cytoplasm around the axon ('onion-bulb' formations).

Neurophysiology

Demyelination may result in marked slowing of conduction, conduction block, and increased susceptibility to changes in temperature. In normal myelinated fibers, impulses conduct rapidly from one node of Ranvier to the next by saltatory conduction. In demyelinated nerve fibers conduction between nodes is delayed or, as with unmyelinated nerve fibers, conduction becomes nonsaltatory and continuous, therefore much slower across the demyelinated segments. The delay in conduction may result in markedly prolonged distal latencies, marked slowing of segmental conduction velocity, and temporal dispersion and a lower amplitude of the action potential across the involved segment.

Conduction block is present when a proportion of nerve fibers fails to transmit any electric impulses, and CMAP amplitude drops across a demyelinated segment. Segmental conduction slowing and conduction block may be caused by focal demyelination caused by nerve compression and inflammatory neuropathies.

Neuronopathy or primary nerve cell degeneration

Primary destruction of nerve cell bodies occurs in the anterior horn cells (e.g. spinal muscular atrophy, poliomyelitis, amyotrophic lateral sclerosis) or dorsal root ganglia (e.g. Friedreich's ataxia, paraneoplastic).

Neuropathology

The peripheral sensory axons degenerate distally and the ascending sensory tracts in the posterior columns and other spinal tracts degenerate proximally. As the cell bodies are destroyed, there is no recovery.

Neurophysiology

With anterior horn cell loss the CMAP amplitude decreases or is lost. Intact motor units continue to conduct normally, and SNAP amplitudes remain normal unless superimposed peripheral compression neuropathies are present. With dorsal root ganglion loss the SNAP amplitude decreases or is lost.

Late responses

F-wave

The F-wave is a late motor response evoked by a supramaximal stimulus of a motor nerve (e.g. the median nerve at the wrist). Nerve stimulation produces a bidirectional action potential in the motor axons, traveling orthodromically to produce the initial direct CMAP (the M-wave) but also traveling antidromically to activate some anterior horn cells that then produce a later CMAP (the F-wave). The F-wave is much smaller (1–5% of the M-wave) and more variable than the M-wave. The name derives from its first recordings from foot muscles by Magladery and McDougal in 1950. The F-wave latency is a measure of the motor conduction time from stimulation site to the anterior horn cell and then back again to the recording site, so can test conduction in the proximal segments of nerves and spinal roots. F-waves may be delayed or lost with proximal disturbances of conduction, but are rarely a diagnostic finding in isolation.

H-reflex

The H-reflex is a late motor response evoked by a low intensity, submaximal stimulus to the motor nerve. It is regularly present in the calf muscles after stimulation of the posterior tibial nerve, but not other nerves. It is named in honour of Hoffman's description in 1918. When present, the response is of smaller amplitude than the supramaximal M-wave, but, unlike the F-wave, is of consistent latency, configuration, and occurrence. It is thought to be due to a monosynaptic spinal reflex, with selective activation of the Ia sensory fibers from the muscle spindles ascending to the spinal cord, then synapsing with and activating the anterior horn cells.

The H-reflex is decreased or absent in most peripheral neuropathies, and increased in upper motor neuron disorders. It directly correlates with the presence of a deep tendon reflex, so is rarely of additional usefulness to clinical examination.

The long loop reflex

Stimulation of a nerve during a muscle contraction causes a brief pause in muscle activity (the silent period) within which a long loop reflex response, or 'C' response, lies. It is not normally present at rest, and is thought to have a circuit that extends above the spinal cord and may involve the cerebral cortex, hence the choice of the terms. Hyperactivity of this long loop reflex may be involved in the production of certain abnormal movements; a 'C' response at rest may be seen in disorders with cortical myoclonus.

Repetitive stimulation studies

Repetitive stimulation of motor nerves is helpful for testing for disorders of neuromuscular transmission. Normally, with repeated supramaximal electric stimuli to a nerve (e.g. the ulnar nerve at the wrist) at rates of up to 25 Hz (which most patients would not be able to tolerate), each CMAP will have the same form and amplitude. Fatigue occurs only after sustaining rapid rates of stimulation for over 60 seconds. The distribution and severity of symptoms and accessibility determine which nerve–muscle groups are tested. More proximal groups (e.g. accessory–trapezius, axillary–deltoid) are usually more sensitive.

A 2–3 Hz repetitive supramaximal stimulation for four or more responses is usually used, and in normals produces no decrement in the CMAP amplitude. A consistent (usually >10%) decrement in CMAP amplitude, when performed without technical problems such as movement of the stimulating or recording electrodes, is a marker of a disturbance of neuromuscular transmission (myasthenia gravis, myasthenic syndrome, and early reinnervation with immature neuromuscular junctions) (**43**).

Post-activation facilitation (transient resolution of the decremental response after 10 seconds of exercise) or post-activation exhaustion (a decremental response revealed or enhanced after prolonged exercise for 60 seconds, with the decremental response emerging after the exercise over several minutes) may also be present.

Tip

▶ *A meaningful decrement in CMAP amplitude to repetitive stimulation requires exclusion of technical problems such as movement of the stimulating or recording electrodes.*

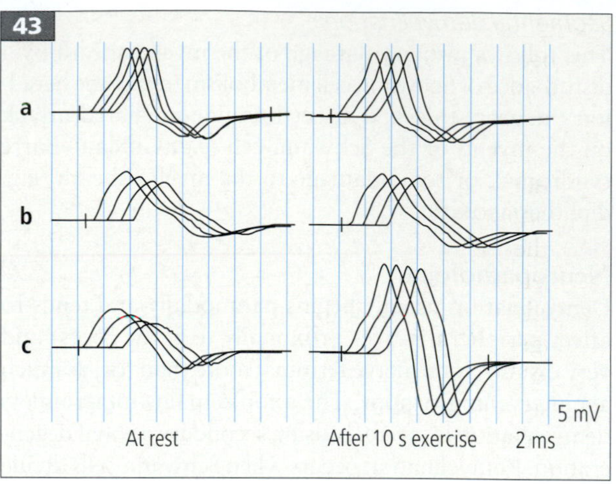

43 Motor responses to 2 Hz repetitive stimulation, with no decrement in a normal subject (a), with decremental responses in myasthenia gravis (b) and Lambert–Eaton myasthenic syndrome (c), then with post-activation facilitation (especially prominent with Lambert–Eaton myasthenic syndrome).

In the Lambert–Eaton myasthenic syndrome and botulism, acetylcholine release from the nerve terminal is disturbed. The initial resting CMAP is usually of reduced amplitude, 2-Hz repetitive stimulation reveals a decremental response, and brief exercise for 10 seconds evokes striking post-activation facilitation with a two or more times increase in CMAP amplitude. The rapid stimulation of the nerve terminal caused by brief exercise temporarily facilitates acetylcholine release from the nerve terminal.

Electromyography

Electromyography (EMG) is the recording through a needle, or surface electrodes, of electric activity from muscles. Bipolar concentric needle electrodes have an inner active wire core separated from the outer shaft reference by insulation material. Monopolar needle electrodes are Teflon-coated with an active bare tip referenced to an adjacent surface electrode. Standard bipolar needle electrodes have an effective recording range of about 2 mm. The signals are amplified, filtered, and displayed visually on an oscilloscopic screen and more importantly are broadcast audibly through a loudspeaker. The audio output by far delivers the most useful information. Qualitative and, less commonly, quantitative needle EMG techniques can be used.

Tip

▶ *For needle EMG, listening to the audio output is far more important than looking at the oscilloscope screen.*

Normal muscle activity

Insertional activity

When the needle is moved gently within the muscle, there is a brief irregular burst of electric activity lasting a few hundred milliseconds (**44**). Insertional activity may be prolonged in denervated muscle, myotonic disorders, and as a normal variant, and may be reduced in periodic paralysis and if muscle is replaced by connective tissue or fat (e.g. chronic, end-stage myopathy).

At rest with no needle movement (spontaneous)

No electric activity arises from muscle fibers at rest, save for mechanical activation of motor end-plates and small intramuscular nerves (end-plate noise from miniature end-plate potentials and end-plate spikes from muscle fiber activation), and occasional fasciculation potentials (**45**).

Muscle activation

Much of what can be learnt depends on understanding the motor unit: the anatomical unit of an anterior horn cell, its axon, the neuromuscular junctions, and all of the muscle fibers innervated by the axon. With slight voluntary muscle activation the smallest motor unit in the pool will begin to fire slowly, producing a stereotyped recurrent individual motor unit action potential (MUP) on the screen and over the loudspeaker. A MUP is the summated electrical activity of that part of a single motor unit that is within the recording range of the electrode.

The configuration, amplitude, duration, number of phases (number of baseline crossings + 1), and variability can be assessed. Normal findings vary with muscle, age, and temperature.

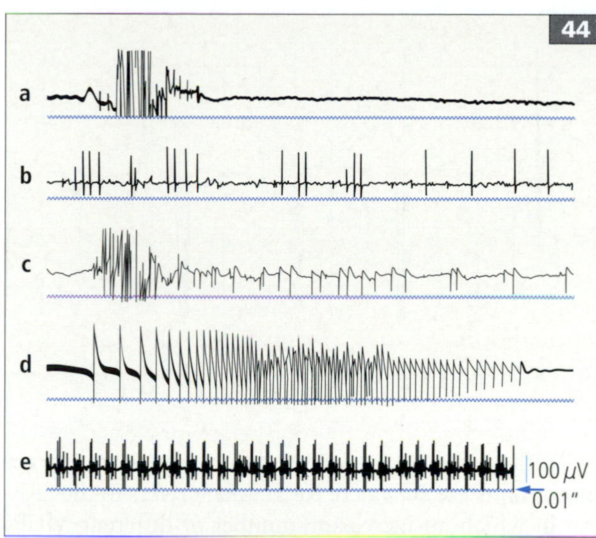

44 Insertional activity; the electric activity that may be evoked by insertion of a needle electrode into muscle. (a) Normal brief discharge of electric activity (insertion potentials that last little longer than the movement of the needle); (b) 'end-plate noise' and associated muscle fiber action potentials are electric activity evoked when the needle is in contact with motor end-plates and irritates small intramuscular nerves; (c) 'positive waves' are a form of fibrillation potential evoked in denervated muscle; (d) 'myotonic discharges' are the action potentials of muscle fibers firing in a prolonged fashion after external excitation. They take two forms (positive waves and brief spikes) depending on the relationship of the recording electrode to the muscle fiber, and wax and wane in amplitude and frequency (20–100 Hz); (e) 'complex repetitive discharges' (bizarre repetitive potentials), are action potentials of groups of muscle fibers discharging regularly in near synchrony at high rates (5–100 Hz). They typically begin and end abruptly.

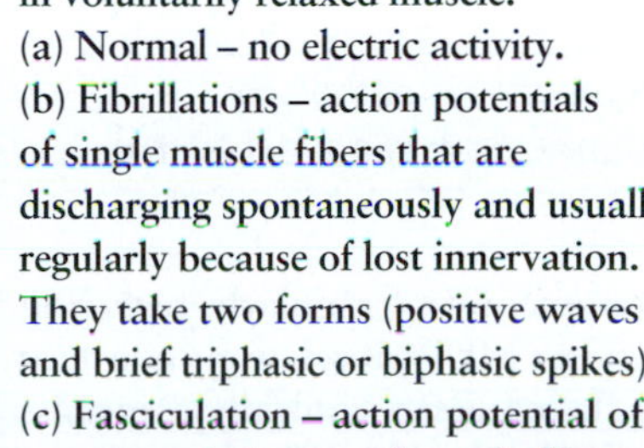

45 Spontaneous electric activity in voluntarily relaxed muscle. (a) Normal – no electric activity. (b) Fibrillations – action potentials of single muscle fibers that are discharging spontaneously and usually regularly because of lost innervation. They take two forms (positive waves and brief triphasic or biphasic spikes). (c) Fasciculation – action potential of a motor unit (group of muscle fibers innervated by an anterior horn cell) that discharges in a random, irregular fashion.

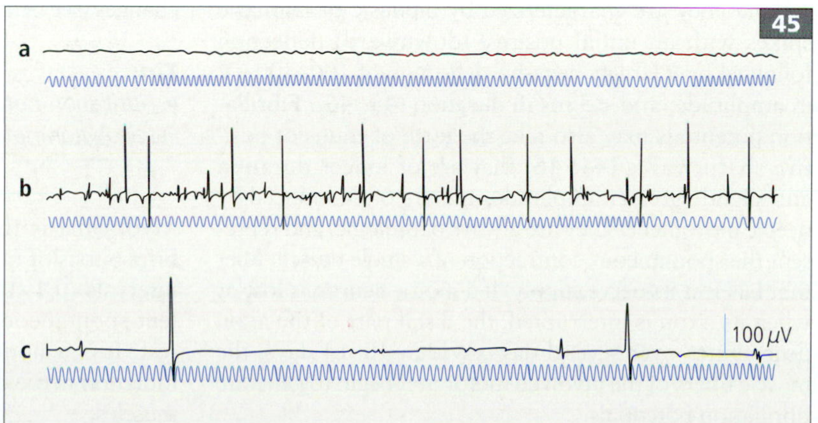

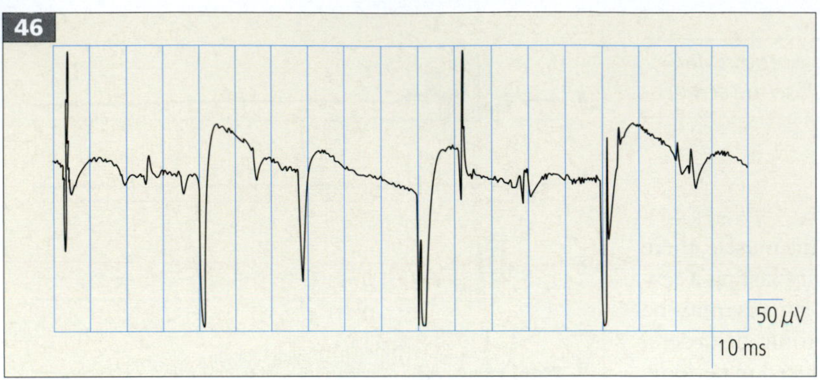

46 Needle EMG recording of a resting muscle, showing spontaneous fibrillation potentials (upward spikes) and positive sharp waves (downward spikes), always a pathologic finding.

With increasing voluntary effort, more and larger motor units are activated. Recruitment refers to the fashion in which an increasing number of different MUPs (each representing a different motor unit) are brought into the firing pattern with increased voluntary muscle activation. Normal recruitment varies with the muscle.

Maximum voluntary effort produces an 'interference pattern' in which no individual MUPs can be identified. The interference pattern can be used to assess recruitment indirectly, but this inferior approach can be painful and confounded by incomplete voluntary activation.

Abnormal muscle activity

Insertional activity

Activity is increased when muscle fibers are irritable, seen in denervation and many forms of muscle disease, including muscle inflammation and muscle membrane instability. Activity is decreased in advanced denervation or myopathy where muscle fibers have been largely replaced by fat and connective tissue, and when muscle fibers are inactive (e.g. periodic paralysis during an episode of paralysis).

At rest (spontaneous)

Fibrillation potentials are the spontaneous discharges of single muscle fibers, are usually repetitive and regular, sometimes decelerating or even accelerating before cessation. They are characterized by biphasic or triphasic spikes with an initial positive (downward) deflection followed by a largely negative deflection of 100–300 μV in amplitude, and <5 ms in duration (**45, 46**). Fibrillation potentials may also take the form of trains of positive sharp waves (**44, 46**) that are of longer duration and slightly greater amplitude, and are often induced by needle movement. They are always pathologic, and represent the spontaneous contraction of a single muscle fiber that has lost its nerve supply. If a motor neuron is lost or when its axon is interrupted, the distal part of the axon degenerates over several days. Within 10–14 days, the muscle fibers of the involved motor unit begin to generate fibrillation potentials.

These denervation potentials may also be recorded in some primary necrotizing muscle diseases with muscle fiber splitting, inflammation, or vacuolation (e.g. Duchenne muscular dystrophy, polymyositis, inclusion-body myositis, muscle trauma including surgery), because the terminal innervation of some muscle fibers is damaged by the disease process. Fibrillation potentials continue until the muscle fiber is reinnervated by regeneration of the interrupted motor axon if the motor neuron remains intact, by the outgrowth of new axons from remaining healthy nerve fibers (collateral sprouting), or until the atrophied muscle fibers degenerate and are replaced over years by connective tissue.

Fasciculation potentials are the spontaneous discharges of single motor units. They are usually random and nonrhythmic, and since all muscle fibers of the involved motor unit depolarize, they are several millivolts in amplitude and 5–>15 ms in duration (**45**). Such contractions of a motor unit may be large enough to cause a brief visible twitching or dimpling under the skin. They are evidence of motor nerve fiber irritability and not necessarily denervation. They may occur in normal people in the calves and hands, and may be induced by exercise, low temperature, and low serum calcium levels. However, they also occur in denervation, especially anterior horn cell loss, and this can be confirmed by the presence of associated fibrillation potentials and certain MUP changes (see below).

Tip

▶ *Fibrillation potentials are always pathologic. Fasciculation potentials may occur in normal people.*

Myokymia is the phenomenon of regularly recurring brief bursts of rapidly firing MUPs at relatively constant intervals (0.1–10 Hz). It manifests clinically as persistent spontaneous rippling and quivering of muscles at rest. It is a nonspecific finding, often associated with radiation nerve damage, and commonly benign in eyelid muscles.

Myotonia: prolonged discharge of single muscle fibers firing spontaneously and at high frequency. They generally have a positive sharp waveform and regular firing pattern that waxes and wanes in frequency (20–100 Hz) and amplitude, producing a 'dive-bomber' sound over the audio (**44**). Myotonia is elicited by voluntary muscle contraction and mechanically by movement of the needle electrode. After muscle contraction, myotonia may occur for up to several minutes, corresponding clinically to failure of voluntary muscle relaxation after forceful contraction. Myotonia occurs due to an abnormality in the muscle fiber membrane, and causes include myotonic dystrophy, myotonia congenita, paramyotonia, cholesterol-lowering agents (CLAM), hyperkalemic periodic paralysis, and acid maltase deficiency.

Complex repetitive discharges are action potentials of groups of adjacent muscle fibers discharging regularly in near synchrony at high rates (5–100 Hz). They typically start and stop abruptly. A nonspecific sign of chronicity (>6 months) in a wide range of neurogenic (e.g. poliomyelitis, motor neuron disease, spinal muscular atrophy, radiculoneuropathies) and myopathic processes (e.g. chronic polymyositis, Duchenne dystrophy, limb-girdle dystrophy), they are thought to be due to ephaptic and cyclical excitation of adjacent muscle fibers.

Continuous muscle fiber activity (neuromyotonia) is high frequency (150–300 Hz) repetitive MUP discharges of varying morphology and complexity, often starting or stopping abruptly. They may occur spontaneously, with needle movement, or voluntary effort. Successive discharges show decrements in amplitude. These discharges probably originate in the distal peripheral nerve, where activity of afferent nerve fibers excites distal motor terminals. They may be seen in Isaac's syndrome, anticholinesterase poisoning, tetany, and during intraoperative EMG monitoring when a nerve is irritated.

Voluntary muscle activation

Upper motor neuron lesion

Poor drive from the upper motor neuron results in poor voluntary activation of a few motor units. If voluntary activation is sufficient to assess recruitment of MUPs, this remains normal. This pattern of poor voluntary activation may also be seen in patients who do not (e.g. hysteria), or cannot (e.g. due to joint pain), make an adequate voluntary effort.

Lower motor neuron lesion

After recent denervation of muscle fibers and motor units within a muscle, reduced recruitment is seen (**47**). The loss of motor units imposes on the remaining motor units a need to fire more rapidly unaided to generate the required force, i.e. the recruitment of additional MUPs is reduced. Initially these remaining MUPs are of normal morphology. From day 10 associated fibrillation potentials emerge.

Over the following weeks and months undamaged axons from surviving motor units within the muscle begin to sprout new nerve twigs from nodal points and terminals, and reinnervate some or all of the adjacent denervated fibers. Thus more muscle fibers are added to the surviving motor units, creating a higher density of muscle fibers innervated by a single motor unit within recording range.

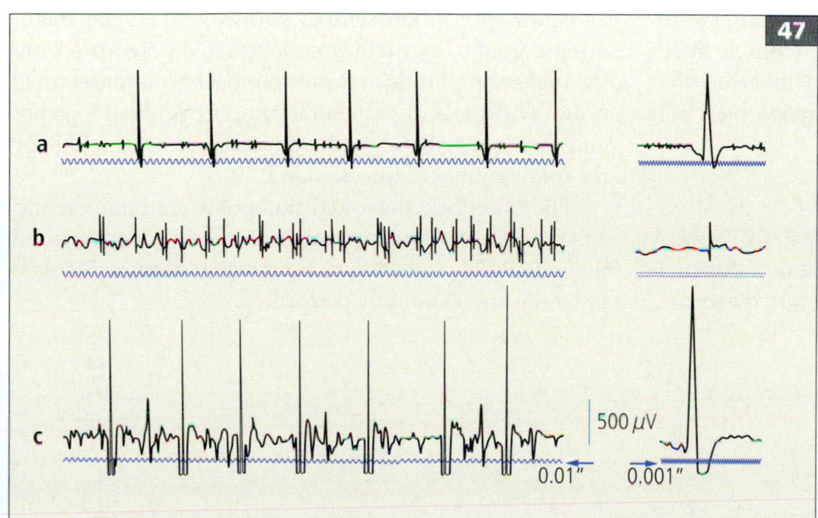

47 Motor unit action potentials during weak voluntary contraction of the biceps brachii in (a) a normal person; (b) a patient with muscular dystrophy showing increased recruitment of low amplitude, short-duration motor unit potentials; (c) a patient with motor neuron disease with high amplitude, long-duration motor unit potentials. The time base for the action potentials recorded on the left is slower (7.7 s sweep) than those on the right (0.2 s sweep).

These expanding MUPs initially appear on the EMG as of normal amplitude but long duration and complex (polyphasic) potentials, since the newly reinnervated muscle fibers are 'stragglers' because of immature connections with variable and slower conduction. Then the MUP gradually remodels to become of higher amplitude, with lesser duration and lesser polyphasia, as reinnervation matures and the muscle fibers of the motor unit activate more synchronously. If reinnervation is complete, fibrillation potentials disappear, but the reduced recruitment and large MUPs remain. This evolution in acute neurogenic insult provides a means of determining the chronology of some processes.

Neuromuscular junction disease

During sustained weak voluntary contraction, a single MUP may vary in amplitude and duration as neuromuscular transmission to individual muscle fibers within the motor unit either fails or is delayed. Specialized EMG recording of repetitive activation of pairs of single muscle fibers belonging to the same motor unit may show excessive variation of their firing interval ('jitter'), due to variability in synaptic delay at the disordered neuromuscular junction. This may increase to the point of actual block in conduction, and one or other fiber fails to fire. If severe, a functional denervation may occur, and associated fibrillation potentials can emerge.

Muscle disease (myopathy)

Muscle fibers are destroyed resulting in fewer functional muscle fibers in each motor unit. Affected MUPs are therefore of reduced amplitude and of short duration, and are commonly polyphasic because the MUP is fragmented because of missing muscle fibers and slower activation of affected muscle fibers (**47**). With voluntary muscle activation, recruitment is increased and is more rapid. More of these small motor units need to be recruited to generate the force required. Necrotizing myopathies have associated fibrillation potentials. Needle EMG mainly assesses low-threshold type I muscle fibers, so myopathies with mainly type II muscle fiber involvement (e.g. steroid and other endocrine myopathies) may show little change.

Movement disorders

Multichannel muscle recordings using pairs of surface electrodes can be valuable in the assessment of disorders of movement such as tremor, myoclonus, and dystonia.

Role

EMG is an extension of the neurologic examination. There is no completely 'routine' procedure, since what is performed relies heavily on the clinical findings, the specific question being asked, and the ongoing interpretation of results.

- To characterize disease type: neuropathy (axonal *vs*. demyelinative), myopathy, disorder of neuromuscular junction.
- To localize the pattern or level of abnormality(diffuse *vs*. focal, root *vs*. plexus *vs*. peripheral nerve).
- To define severity and duration/course of disease.
- To assess a patient sometimes who cannot be tested clinically.

Like EEG, an EMG should only be requested if there is a clear question to be answered, the question is answerable by means of EMG, and the EMG can practically be performed, with the patient informed about what to expect. A succinct and relevant clinical history is crucial to accurate planning and interpretation of the recording.

Tip

▶ *Always start with a brief history and examination. This will optimize the study and ultimately save time.*

Interpretation

Like EEG, considerable training, technical skill, and caution are required to interpret EMG accurately.

Evoked potentials

Evoked potentials are the recorded electrical responses of the nervous system to stimulation. A single sensory or motor pathway is usually tested, and the modality tested defines the study. For sensory evoked potentials, stimulation of sensory organs or peripheral nerves produces small time-locked, event-related responses (or potentials) along the appropriate sensory pathway. Averaging methods are used to extract the small evoked potentials from the higher amplitude and random background electrical noise. The traces of sequential stimuli are added together and then normalized by dividing the summed traces by the total number of traces added.

The time-locked evoked potentials are retained and enhanced by averaging while the random background noise hopefully cancels out. Four types of sensory evoked potential are commonly performed.

Visual evoked potentials

Visual evoked potentials (VEPs) assess primarily activity originating in the central 3–6° of the visual field. The patient fixes with one eye (other eye covered) on the center of a screen displaying a black and white checkerboard of high contrast and luminance with pattern reversal at 2 Hz. The size of the checkerboard is increased if visual acuity is poor. Retinal stimulation evokes a response that travels through the optic nerve, optic chiasm, and optic radiations to the occipital cortices. Surface EEG recording electrodes are placed over the occipital region, usually O_Z is referenced to the ear or vertex. Normalized averaging of ≥100 stimuli reveals a characteristic potential (~1–10 μV) over the occipital region with a major positive peak at about 100 ms (P1 or P100), often preceded by a negative peak (N1) and followed by another negative peak (N2): the pattern-reversal VEP (**48**). VEP amplitudes vary far more than latencies in normal subjects. Impaired visual acuity has little effect on the latency, but reduces the amplitude of the VEP. Other important influences include age, sex, and poor visual fixation.

Demyelinating lesions of the optic nerve in particular delay conduction and lead to an increase in the P100 latency. Neurophysiologic evidence of delayed conduction in the visual pathways is found in about 90% of patients with clinically definite MS, including about one-third of patients with MS who have no history or clinical evidence of optic nerve involvement.

An abnormal VEP is not specific for MS, and may be produced by many other diseases of the anterior visual pathway affecting the optic nerve (compressive and intrinsic) and optic chiasm, and occasionally retinal disease and glaucoma.

Refractive errors, ocular opacities, and visual inattention, and lesions posterior to the optic chiasm do not usually prolong the latency of the VEP but tend to affect the amplitude of the VEP. Some laboratories use hemifield rather than full-field stimulation and other specialized techniques to localize retrochiasmal lesions.

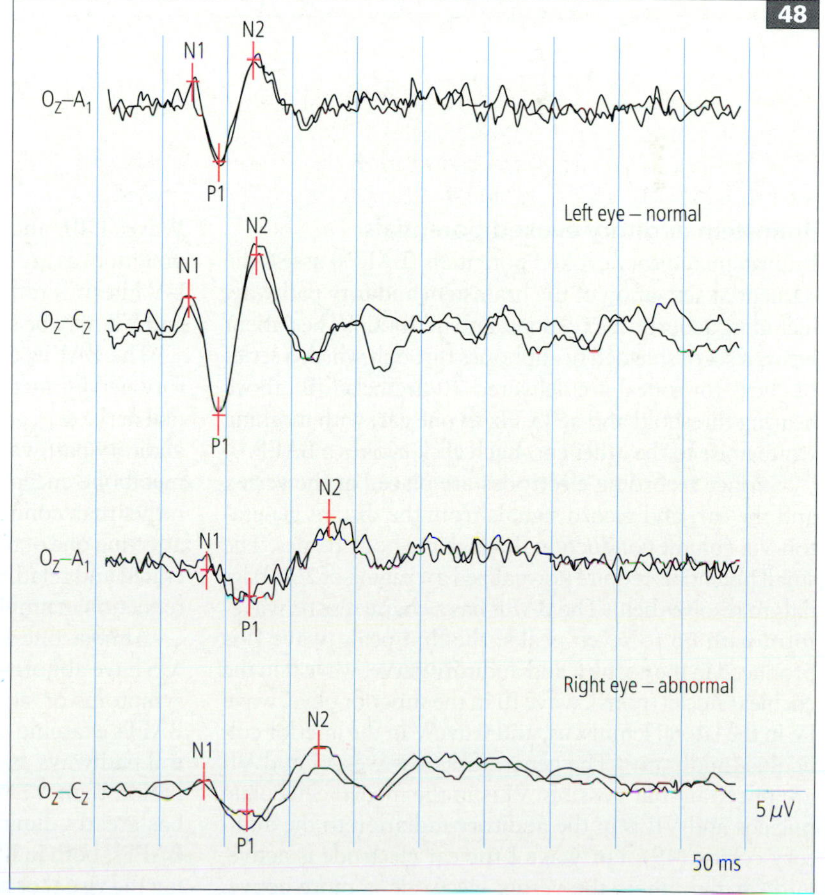

48 Visual evoked potentials from a 36-year-old female with multiple sclerosis and right optic neuropathy. The left eye (top two traces) shows normal, well-formed responses with a P1 latency <115 msec. The right eye (bottom two traces) shows attenuated responses (<50% amplitude compared to the left) with a prolonged P1 latency.

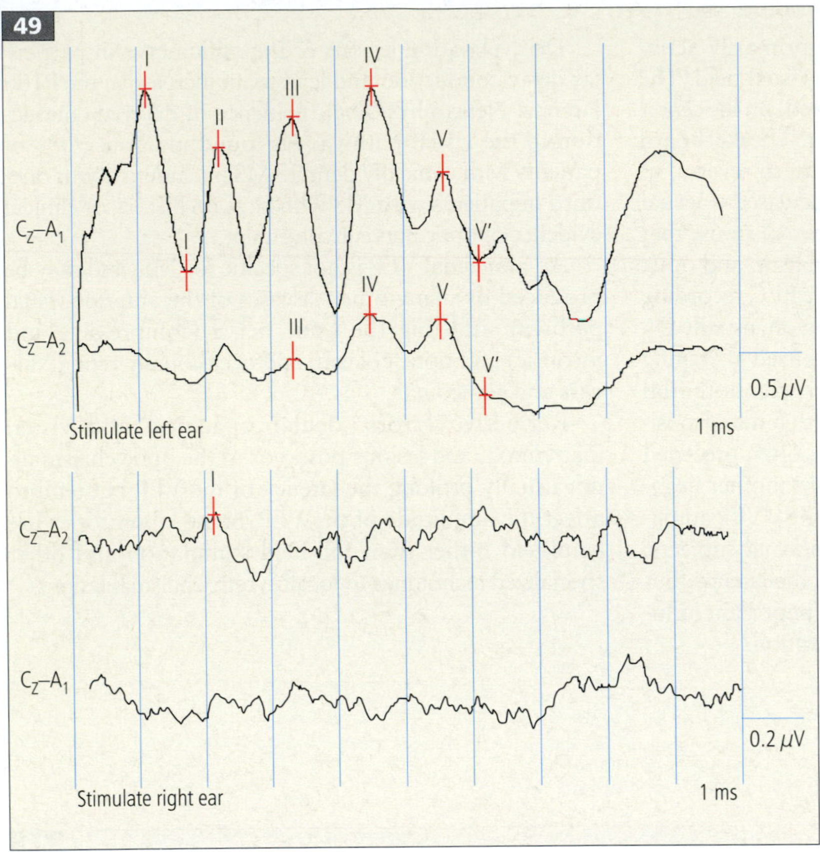

49 **Brainstem auditory evoked potentials in a patient with acoustic neuroma. Recording electrodes at the vertex (C_Z) and the ear (left: A_1, right: A_2), showing up to seven waves within 10 ms of the click stimuli. Wave I is recorded by the ear electrode, and the others by the vertex. By convention, vertex positivity is displayed as an upward deflection and the individual waves are labeled by their positive peaks. The normal left ear stimulation shows trials recording from C_Z–A_1 (the ipsilateral ear), upper trace showing waves I–VII, and from C_Z–A_2 (the contralateral ear), lower trace showing the later waves recorded from C_Z. The abnormal right ear shows an attenuated or absent Wave I, but no subsequent waves.**

Brainstem auditory evoked potentials

Brainstem auditory evoked potentials (BAEPs) assess the sequential activation of the brainstem auditory pathway, including acoustic nerve, pons, and midbrain. The patient wears a set of shielded headphones through which a series of clicks (or tones) are delivered 70 decibels (dB) above hearing threshold and at 11 Hz to one ear, with masking white noise to the other ear. Each click evokes a BAEP.

Surface recording electrodes are placed at the vertex and the ear, and record signals from the distant generators via volume conduction through the body tissues. The small potentials require normalized averaging of 2000 signals to resolve them. The BAEP has a characteristic waveform with up to seven peaks: the first peak (wave I) is produced in the cochlea and auditory nerve, wave II in the cochlear nuclei (pons), wave III in the superior olive, wave IV in the lateral lemniscus, and wave V in the inferior colliculus (midbrain). The generators of waves VI and VII are uncertain but possibly VI is in the medial geniculate nucleus and VII is in the auditory radiation to the auditory cortex (**49**). For wave I the ear electrode is active, and for the others the vertex electrode is more active. Waves I, III, and V are the most reliable for BAEP interpretation, as are interpeak intervals (most importantly the I–V interval) rather than absolute latencies. Waves II, VI, and VII may be absent in normal subjects.

The BAEPs can be used to assess cochlea and auditory nerve function and detect lesions of the VIIIth cranial nerve (e.g. acoustic neuromas, **49**) and the brainstem auditory pathways. BAEPs are also resistant to toxic and metabolic encephalopathies, and may be used to refute rather than confirm the diagnosis of brain death. A lesion affecting one of the relay stations attenuates the wave generated and relatively delays its latency, with an absence or reduction in amplitude of subsequent waves.

Almost one-half of patients with clinically definite MS have abnormal BAEPs, even in the absence of clinical symptoms or signs of brainstem dysfunction. However, BAEPs examine only a relatively short segment of the central pathways and are less sensitive in detecting demyelination than VEPs and MRI imaging of the brain. MRI has greatly diminished the diagnostic role of VEPs and BAEPs, both in MS and in the detection of lesions involving the visual or auditory pathways.

Somatosensory evoked potentials

Somatosensory evoked potentials (SSEPs) assess large diameter, fast-conducting sensory fibers (group Ia muscle and group II cutaneous afferents) which ascend mainly in the dorsal columns, medial lemniscus, and thalamus to the parietal cortex.

Consecutive electric stimuli are applied, at frequencies of 1–3 Hz (offset slightly from a whole number to avoid 60 Hz harmonics) to sensory or mixed peripheral nerves (e.g. the posterior tibial, median, and ulnar nerves) while tracking the ascending evoked potentials from multiple electrode pairs: for the upper limb over the cubital fossa, Erb's point above the clavicle, the cervical spine, and the scalp overlying the contralateral parietal cortex; and for the lower limb over the popliteal fossa, the lumbar and cervical spines, and the contralateral sensory cortex.

Characteristic waveforms, designated by the symbol P (positive) or N (negative) and a number indicating the expected interval of time from stimulus to recording (e.g. N20), are recorded, and averaged by computer (**50, 51**). Amplitudes, absolute latencies, and interpeak intervals can be assessed, if the potentials are of sufficient amplitude and are not obscured by muscle and other artifacts. Delay between the stimulus site and Erb's point or lumbar spine indicates peripheral nerve disease, and relative delay from Erb's point (or lumbar spine) to the cortex implies an abnormality in the appropriate nerve roots or in the posterior columns.

Performing median, ulnar, or tibial SSEPS with side-to-side comparisons can assist in detecting and sometimes localizing disturbances of central somatosensory conduction. SSEPs are used in suspected MS and cervical spondylitic myelopathy, in the evaluation of suspected psychogenic sensory loss, and in surgical monitoring of spinal cord function during operations such as scoliosis surgery. They are abnormal in up to 70% of patients with clinically definite MS, but are not as sensitive as VEPs and MRI in detecting central demyelination.

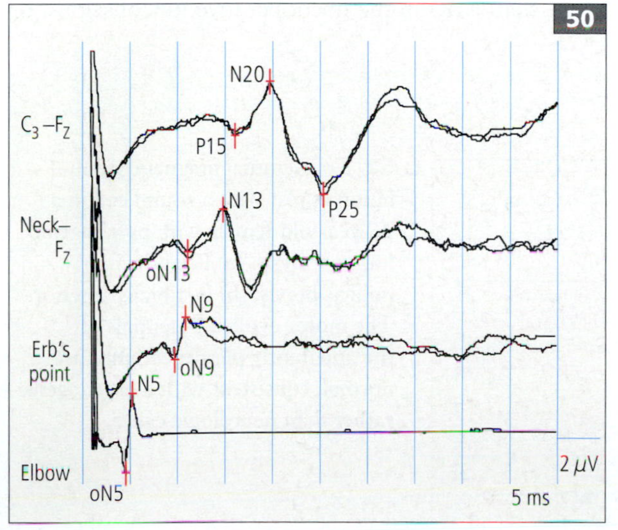

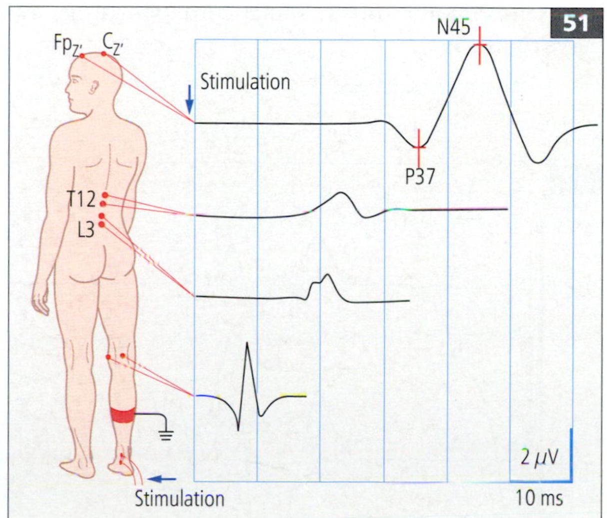

50, 51 Normal somatosensory evoked potentials (SSEPs). (50) Stimulation of the median nerve at the wrist evokes prominent peripheral potentials over the elbow and Erb's point. The neck trace shows a surface negative peak (N13) over the fifth cervical vertebra (C5). Finally, a polyphasic potential is recorded over the contralateral parietal somatosensory cortex (C_3–F_Z), with a negative peak at about 20 ms (N20) and a positive wave at about 25 ms (P25); (51) stimulation of the posterior tibial nerve at the ankle and SSEPs recorded at the popliteal fossa, spine, and scalp.

Motor evoked potentials (MEPs)

Central motor conduction down the corticospinal tract can be measured by transcranial surface electrical or magnetic stimulation of the motor cortex, then recording CMAP amplitudes and latencies in limb muscles (usually thenar eminence and tibialis anterior; 52). Magnetic stimulation uses a coil producing a time-varying magnetic field, inducing current flow in deeper tissues. It is preferred in awake subjects, because it easily activates the motor cortex without the pain electrical stimulation causes. When possible, slight voluntary activation of the muscle to be tested markedly enhances the MEP. MEPs are used for similar purposes to SSEPs, particularly the evaluation of suspected psychogenic paralysis, and for intraoperative spinal cord and brain monitoring. During surgical monitoring, transcranial electrical rather than magnetic stimulation is used because it produces far more reliable MEPS.

Role

Evoked potentials retain a diagnostic role, but this has been greatly diminished since the advent of MRI, which has a higher sensitivity in lesion detection. Evoked potentials remain important in assessing patients who cannot be tested clinically, such as those suspected of having psychogenic loss of function and most particularly in intraoperative monitoring.

Evoked potentials can make surgery safer by monitoring the functional integrity of structures at risk (e.g. spinal cord, facial and acoustic nerves), and by identifying important structures that need to be preserved (e.g. sensorimotor cortex, spinal cord, cranial nerves, nerve roots).

IMAGING THE BRAIN AND SPINE

Computerized tomography (CT) and magnetic resonance imaging (MRI) are the two major modalities for imaging of the brain. Their utility, strengths, and weaknesses will vary between patients and pathologies. Before requesting an image investigation on a specific patient it is important to ask the following questions:

1. Which test will give me the most accurate information?
2. Which will be able to be tolerated by this particular patient and can be performed in a timely fashion?
3. Which investigation minimizes irradiation to the patient?

Sometimes the resultant request will be formed and modified because of the above thought processes. It is important to remember that the gold standard image investigation which takes 1 week to get is not necessarily the best investigation for the patient, depending on the acuity of the illness.

CT imaging of the brain

The most important advance in CT imaging in the last decade has been the advent of multi-slice CT technology. This has transformed the investigation from a series of 16–22 axial, 7–10 mm thick slices to a volume dataset (240–300 images). It is a tremendous diagnostic tool, rapidly acquired in an environment that is well tolerated by the patient. It is widely available in major hospitals, often at all hours. The result is often obtained more quickly than most blood test results. It is a safer technique than MRI in the uncooperative, unconscious, or

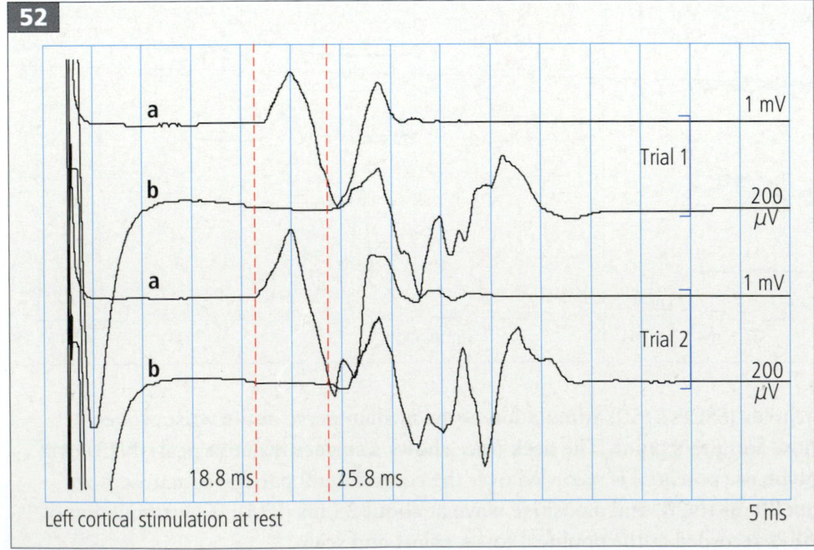

52 Transcranial magnetic stimulation at rest with a round coil in a 26-year-old female with psychogenic limb paralysis. (a) R. abductor pollicis brevis; (b) R. tibialis anterior. The motor evoked potentials of the apparently paralyzed limbs are normal, consistent with a psychogenic rather than neurologic cause.

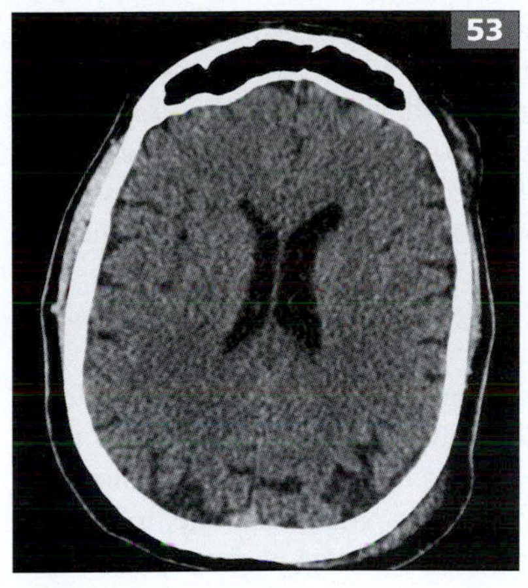

53 Axial thin section (0.625 mm) CT from a helical acquisition at the level of the lateral ventricles. Note the grainy appearance with relatively poor gray/white differentiation due to a low signal-to-noise ratio. The patient was not scanned straight in the scanner because of her poor conscious state.

54–56 5-mm reconstructions of the thin-volume dataset from the patient in 53: (54) axial, (55) coronal, (56) sagittal. Note the improved gray/white differentiation and the visualization of small structures such as the optic chiasm (arrow). The images can be manipulated so that the original dataset, acquired obliquely, is now reconstructed straight (54).

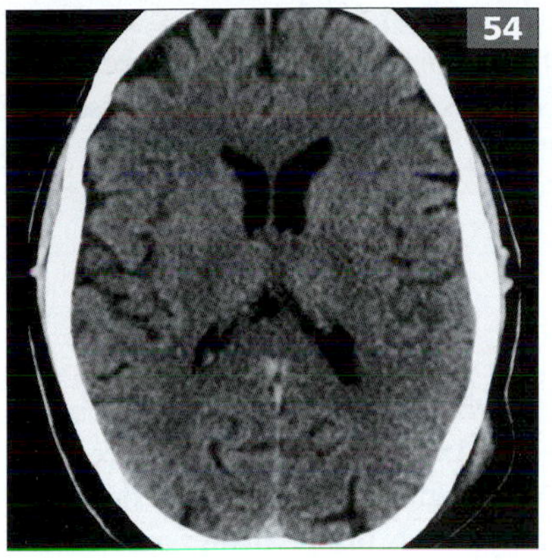

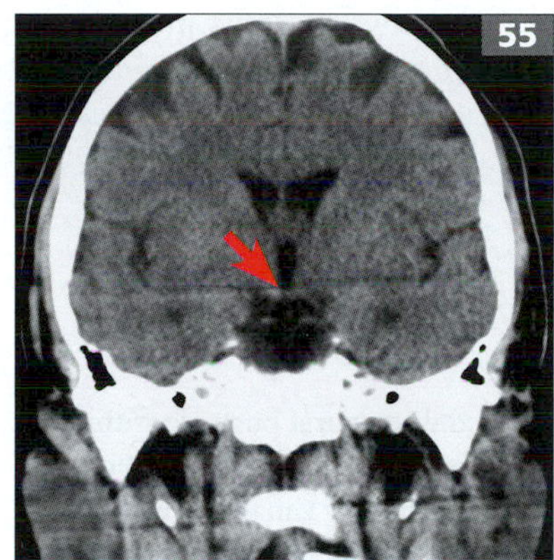

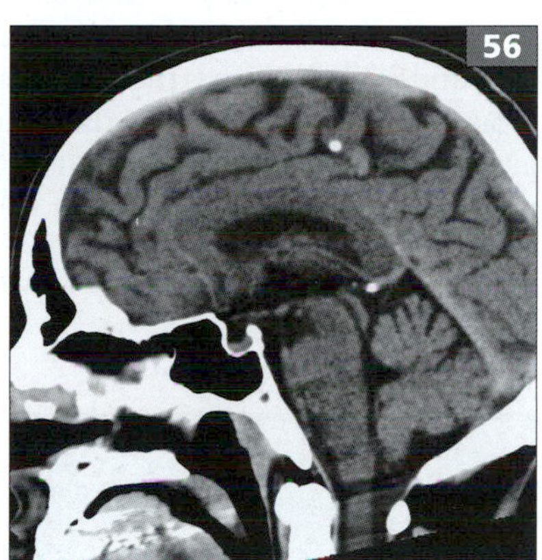

intubated patient. It remains the investigation of choice in patients with trauma, suspected subarachnoid hemorrhage (SAH) and prior to lumbar puncture. CT is still the major tool of triage for patients with suspected stroke for thrombolysis. The quality of images continues to improve with new advances.

Technique

Orthodox nonhelical CT scanners perform axial slices (5–7 mm thick) acquiring 16–24 slices per brain study. Multi-slice (helical) CT scanners commonly still are asked to perform axial nonhelical CT slice technique because of radiation considerations, particularly in routine follow-up scans. Multi-slice volume techniques are used for multi-planar reformations or in a restless patient. Rapid, thin, (0.5–0.625 mm) overlapping axial slices provides 200–300 images of the brain which have a grainy appearance (53). This volume dataset however, can be post-processed into slices of any orientation (sagittal, axial, coronal, or oblique) of any thickness, resulting in multi-planar reformats (MPR). These thicker slices give increased signal to noise and the multi-planar nature of the images give valuable information (**54–56**).

A helical brain scan takes 8–10 seconds to perform, although time must be taken to prepare the patients and move them in and out of the scanner. The radiation source and the radiation detectors are arrayed in a 'donut' configuration around the patient. Both the radiation detectors and the radiation source spin around as the patient moves on a sliding table through the scanner during the acquisition. Each tiny piece of tissue (voxel) in the patient is represented by a pixel which is assigned a number. This number is on the Hounsfield (HU) gray scale with –1000 assigned black and +3000 assigned white. This gives contrast separation of various tissues depending on how much irradiation a specific tissue absorbs. Tissues such as bone which block radiation will be assigned a high HU (1000–3000) while tissue which radiation passes through without impediment (air) will be assigned a negative HU (–1000) and appear very black. Water (CSF) is zero. Differentiation between gray matter (HU 45) and white matter (HU 30) shows a small amount of contrast separation between these differing structures. CT is very good at detecting large contrast ranges, for example delineating air within a frontal sinus (HU –1000) and the thin ethmoidal septi (HU +1000).

When a scan is processed, the information is passed through an algorithm to highlight preferred structures. For example, a bone algorithm is used to look at the cervical spine whereas temporal bone algorithm (high spatial resolution) will be used specifically to look at the petrous temporal bone (57). A soft algorithm will be used to assess brain parenchyma (53). In addition, individual settings of a brain scan can be altered at a PACS console or on the computer scanner by adjusting the center and the window width. By changing the window one can highlight bone structures or use this to examine closely the brain parenchyma (58–60).

Disadvantages of CT

A major disadvantage is irradiation of the patient. Axial slice nonhelical brain CT has an effective dose of between 1.65 and 2 mSv, which is the equivalent to 1 year of background radiation. This has a risk of inducing one cancer in every 10,000 patients studied. Helical (volume acquisition) has a higher effective dose of 1.9 mSv.

A second disadvantage is that low contrast tissue resolution, for example the difference between gray and white matter, is not nearly as good as seen in MRI. Assessment of white matter diseases, such as MS, is therefore much less accurate with CT compared with MRI. Posterior fossa assessment continues to be suboptimal when compared to MRI.

Precautions

Patients who are pregnant or potentially pregnant should not undergo CT unless absolutely essential. Elective CT in a female should be delayed until either a negative pregnancy test is confirmed or the patient is in the first half of the menstrual cycle. If contemplating performing a CT on any patient it is important to assess whether MRI would give more accurate information. If this results in a delay in the imaging test being performed, this may well be in the patient's best interest unless a rapid diagnosis is essential for the patient's safety.

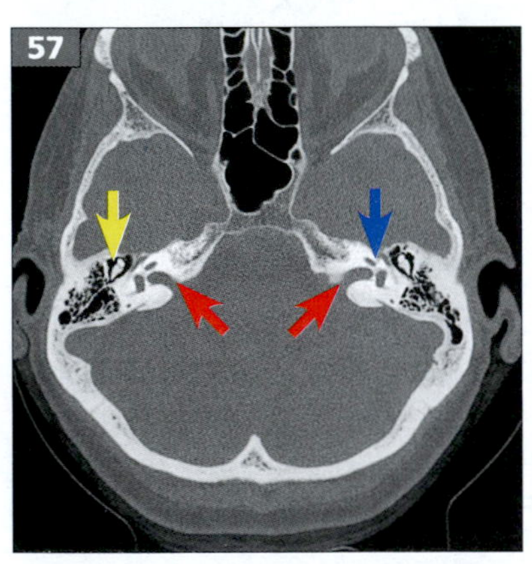

57 Axial temporal bone algorithm with bone windows at the level of the internal auditory canal (red arrows) gives exquisite detail of the ossicles in the middle ear (yellow arrow) and the geniculate fossa (blue arrow). Note the lack of visualization of the brainstem and temporal lobes.

58–60 CT soft tissue windows. (58) Axial soft tissue window (center 40, width 80) of the brain at the level of the body of the lateral ventricle. Subtle signs of acute infarction and loss of gray/white differentiation (arrow) are present; (59) same image with narrowed windows (center 45, width 55) demonstrates this more clearly. This replicates the findings on a delayed CT scan (60) (center 40, width 80) performed at 24 hours.

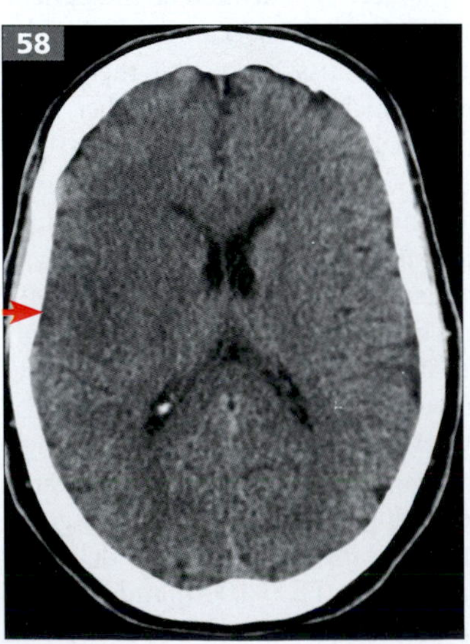

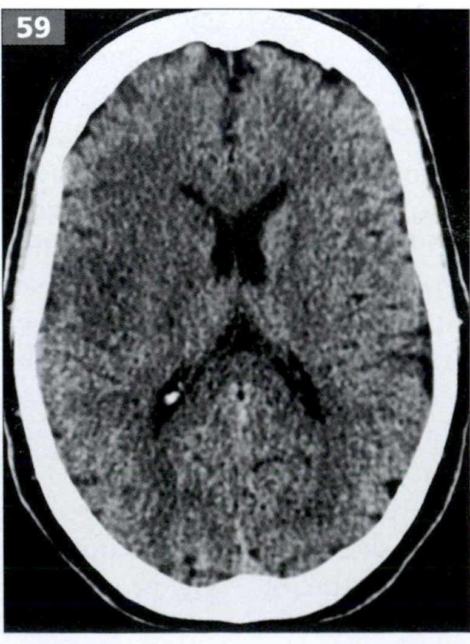

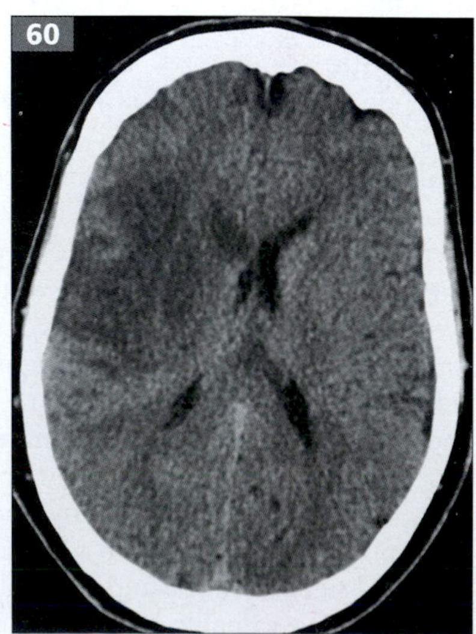

Modern non-ionic contrast has a very low risk of significant reaction (1:40,000) but it is important to ask if the patient has any atopy, asthma, or previous contrast reaction. It is important to define what the reaction to the previous contrast was and whether the patient required steroids, adrenaline, or admission to hospital. Renal impairment is a relative contraindication. Patients should be well hydrated and consider test replacement if creatinine (Cr) >150 μmol/l (1.7 mg/dl) or glomerular filtration rate (GFR) <40 ml/min/1.73 m^2.

Contrast-induced nephropathy can result in metformin accumulation and, rarely, precipitate metformin-related lactic acidosis. Therefore metformin should be ceased for 48 hours after intravenous (IV) contrast. It is wise to discuss this with a radiologist prior to the request being allocated a time. Finally, when filling in a request form, it is vital that all relevant clinical information, including the time of illness onset, is given to the neuroradiologist so that they can potentially refine the protocol and look for specific pathology. It is in the patient's interest for the neuroradiologist to have all the information and it can be important to limit the number of request forms that say 'stroke for investigation'. Finally, if uncertain which is the best test, discuss this with your neuroradiologist.

How to review a brain imaging scan

There is increasing flexibility in viewing images, with films being progressively replaced by electronic media such as a PACS unit or CD on a personal computer. Classically, the images are projected from the base of the skull to the top of the head, from the frontal sinus to the occiput in the coronal plane, and from left to right in the sagittal plane. If you are uncertain, look at the scanogram which will label the images in numerical order. Check the date and the name of the patient to ensure that you are looking at the right study. The key to looking at an imaging study is to compare left with right and look for asymmetry.

Electronic media allow the viewer to alter the windows to maximize the opportunity to see CT signs of early stroke (**58–60**) or subtle subdural hematomas. Widening the windows to look at bony structures, such as the sinuses and for skull fractures, may be important. Reviewing the scans with the neuroradiologist as often as possible can be the best way of increasing your knowledge base and diminishing the number of lesions that you miss. It is a great teaching opportunity which you should use as often as possible. Finally, if you can't see anything abnormal in the brain parenchyma, remember to review the skull, orbits, nasopharynx, and pituitary fossa.

Tip

▶ *Remember to use the flexibility of a PACS station to rewindow scans to look for subtle signs of early stroke or skull fracture on CT.*

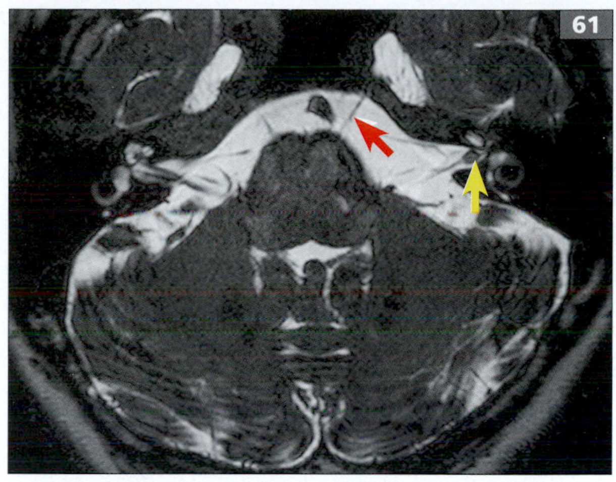

61 Axial heavily T2-weighted image at the level of the internal auditory canal demonstrates the VII and VIII nerve complexes in the internal auditory canal on the left, with a tiny vestibular neuroma (yellow arrow). Note the VI nerve (red arrow).

MRI

Advantages

The three major advantages of magnetic resonance imaging compared with CT are:

- Lack of radiation.
- Increased low tissue contrast resolution.
- Ability to define recent stroke.

The ability to see large differences in contrast between gray and white matter and to be able to assess the posterior fossa and pituitary fossa without streak artifact has been a tremendous boon in neuroimaging. Initially, when MRI was introduced, its multi-planar attributes were also a unique major advantage over CT, although this has been largely negated by multi-slice CT. The ability to define very small structures such as the VI and VIII nerves (**61**), and to assess the substance of the spinal cord are also major advances. MRI machines have different magnetic strength, with most machines being at 1.5 or 3 tesla (T). 3-T machines may have advantages in increased spatial and contrast resolution in some neuroimaging applications such as temporal lobe imaging and assessment of subtle gray matter abnormalities.

Contraindications

Cardiac pacemaker, intraocular metallic foreign body, cochlear implant, some types of heart valve and incompatible aneurysm clips are absolute contraindications. All devices compatible with 1.5 T need re-evaluation prior to subjecting the patient to a higher field-strength 3-T machine. Some patients are claustrophobic and others are too obese to fit in the unit. MRI-compatible general anesthetic equipment is available, but is more costly than a normal general anesthetic set-up. The physical isolation and removal of the patient from ready visual and physical access to the anesthetist does cause concern on occasion. MRI is a very safe tool, but is usually not available to pregnant women in the first two trimesters unless there is specific life-threatening indication. Patients with GFR <40 ml/min/1.73 m^2 are at risk of nephrogenic systemic sclerosis and gadolinium contrast is contraindicated, unless contrast is absolutely indicated. If GFR is <50 ml/min/1.73 m^2 consider macrocyclic gadolinium agents instead.

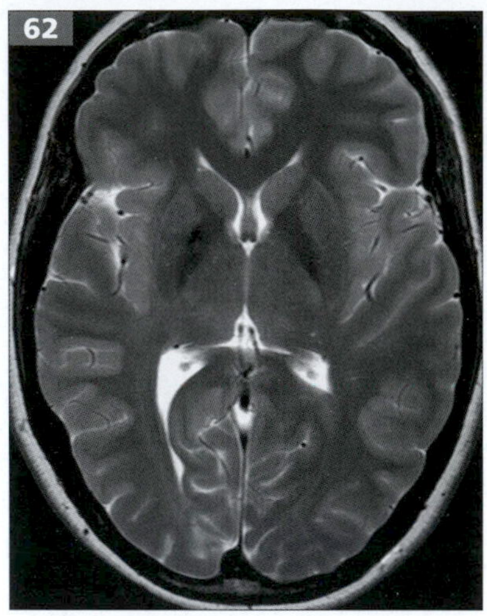

62 Axial fast spin echo T2-weighted image at the level of the third ventricle. Note the white CSF, black white matter, gray cortex, and fat is still white.

The appearances of various tissues using MRI

Broadly speaking there are a wide number of variations on two types of basic sequences. T2-rated sequences have white CSF, cortex appears pale gray, and white matter appears dark gray (**62**). Fat can appear white or black depending upon the sequence and whether it is fat suppressed. T1-weighted sequences result in the CSF looking black, cortex appears gray, and white matter appears pale gray. Fat and subacute blood are white. These scans look more anatomical in nature (**63**).

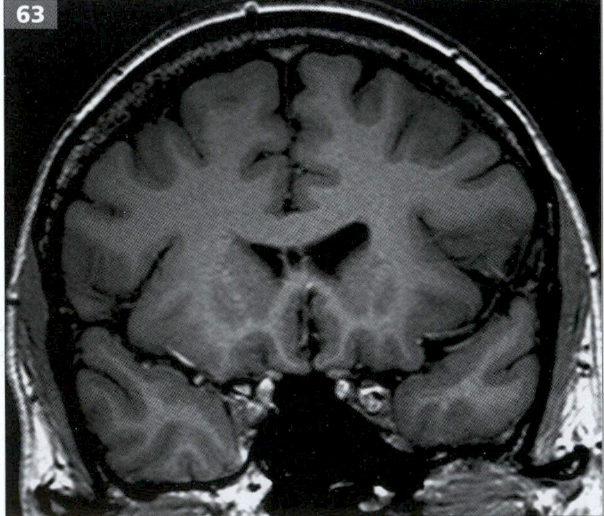

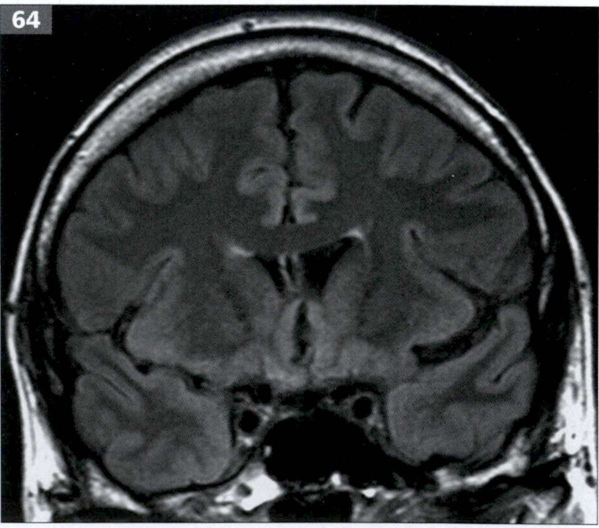

63, 64 MRI at the level of the anterior horns of the of the lateral ventricles. (63) Coronal T1 image. CSF is black, the white matter is white, the cortex is gray, and fat is white. In the coronal FLAIR image at the same level (64), the CSF is nulled (black) and fat remains white. As this is a T2-weighted signal sequence, note the contrast differentiation between gray and white matter.

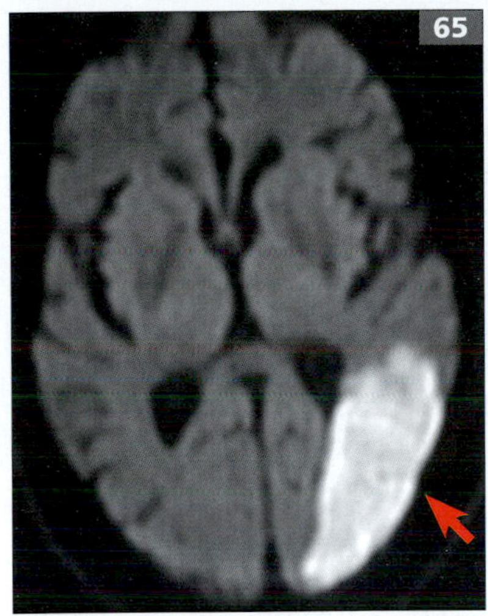
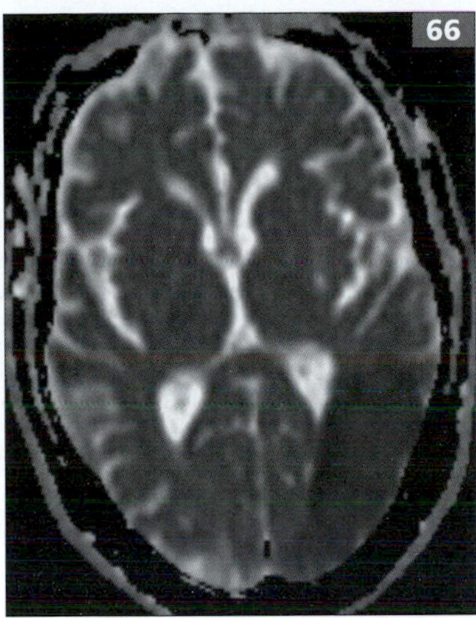
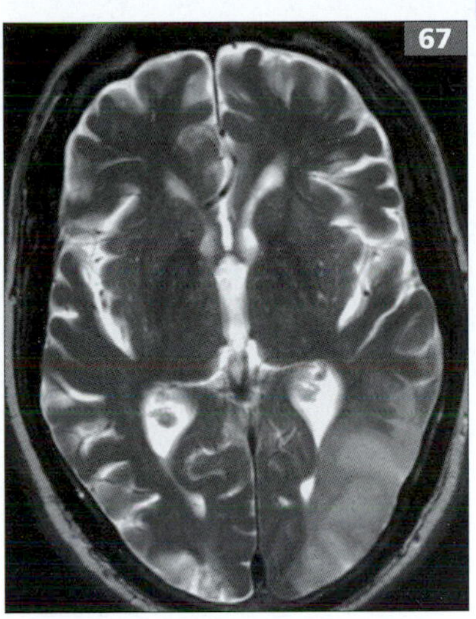

65–67 MRI of infarct. (65) Diffusion image (B1000) demonstrates restricted diffusion in the left parieto-occipital region (arrow). This indicates cytotoxic edema and is matched by a loss of signal intensity on the apparent diffusion coefficent (ADC) map (66). This is a reliable sign of an acute infarction and can be recognized at 2 hours and, in this case, the infarct is demonstrable on the axial T2-weighted image (67).

An important sequence is the fluid-attenuated inversion recovery sequence (FLAIR), where CSF is black. It is otherwise T2-weighted and excellent in detecting white matter lesions in MS, as well as assessing the cortex (**64**).

The number and types of MR sequences are complex and used in different situations. For instance, T2-weighted sequences, looked at initially for areas of abnormality (which are usually white), can then be correlated with T1-weighted sequences. Intravenous contrast is given largely with T1-weighted sequences, which may be fat suppressed.

Gradient images are useful for looking for blood products. Diffusion image maps measure restriction of movement of water in tissue and B1000 images will show very bright signal in areas of recent infarction with cytotoxic edema. These B1000 images are compared with apparent diffusion coefficient (ADC) maps, which will show areas of corresponding blackness, confirming an acute infarct (**65–67**). These changes are positive within 2–4 hours and fade over 5–14 days and can accurately date infarcts, a major advantage over CT.

Tip

► *CT is still the investigation of choice in acute brain injury and cases of suspected subarachnoid hemorrhage.*

Other miscellaneous MR techniques

Functional MRI

Functional MRI is an advanced high-end tool, used for the assessment of speech, vision, motor function, and sensory function in patients as a noninvasive localization of cerebral function. There are a variety of techniques used, but most employ a paradigm that the patient will follow with the MR sequence, picking up very subtle changes in the level of blood deoxygenation, which is portrayed as a colour map overlaid by an anatomical MRI image. MR perfusion is similar to CT perfusion, but more difficult to access in the acute stroke patient where test immediacy is paramount.

MRI spectroscopy

MRI spectroscopy (MRS) is used in the assessment of tumor, radiation necrosis, and hepatic encephalopathy.

Miscellaneous imaging techniques

Both positron emission tomography (PET) and single photon emission tomography (SPECT) are nuclear medicine isotope techniques used in the evaluation of dementia, post-radiation necrosis, cerebral vascular disease, neurologic paraneoplastic syndromes, and investigation of temporal lobe epilepsy. They are very useful, but have boutique roles in neurologic imaging.

Imaging the cerebral circulation

There has been a major shift in imaging of the cerebral vascular circulation in the last 10 years with the advent of noninvasive techniques, including contrast-enhanced CT angiography (CTA), noncontrast and contrast MR angiography (MRA), duplex carotid angiography, and transcranial Doppler. The application of high-end post-processing techniques, using work stations to manipulate and present angiographic image sets mimicking intra-arterial angiography, is a big advance.

Doppler ultrasound

Colour Doppler ultrasound is the method of choice for screening patients for significant carotid artery disease in stroke, but reliable consistent results are only obtained in laboratories with a large volume of work and experienced operators. Ultrasound displays exquisite detail of the wall of the cervical carotid artery from just above the angle of the mandible to the sternal inlet, which is the major site of atheromatous formation and stenosis in western society. It is an innocuous examination without radiation and takes between 15 and 25 minutes to perform. A combination of B mode (anatomical), colour, and Doppler traces is used to assess the presence of atheroma and the degree of stenosis (**68, 69**). The mainstay of stenosis assessment is peak systolic velocity, with peak diastolic velocity and peak systolic ratios and colour imaging playing secondary roles.

CT angiography (CTA)

High-end volume data acquisition scanners can acquire images of the aortic arch, neck, and intracranial vessels with approximately 20 seconds scanning time; 75 ml of contrast is injected via the arm and scanning is triggered by the detection of contrast in the aortic arch. The rapidity of the volume acquisition results in minimal enhancement of the veins. Various post-processing techniques are applied, which takes time. MPR (**70, 71**) and volume rendered (VR) reformats (**72–74**) are processed in a workstation which produces reconstructions of arteries with exquisite detail. Radiation for a neck carotid CTA is in the order of 6.5 mSv whereas a circle of Willis has a radiation dose of 1.2 mSv. Remember to assess GFR and renal function prior to asking for this study.

CT venography

CT venography (CTV) is acquired using the same technique as CTA with a further delay prior to acquiring the information so that the contrast has reached the venous phase. It is a great technique for problem solving equivocal MR venography or in patients who are unsuitable for a MR examination.

68, 69 Ultrasound imaging of blood vessels. (68) B-mode imaging gives a grayscale appearance with black blood and intermediate echogenicity of the wall of the vessel (yellow arrows). Increased echogenicity can be seen in the wall of the vessel indicating an area of calcific or fibrotic atheroma at the carotid bifurcation (red arrow). (69) A combination of B-mode, colour, and Doppler imaging is represented to further evaluate this area for stenosis. Note the peak systolic velocity (red arrows) is within normal limits.

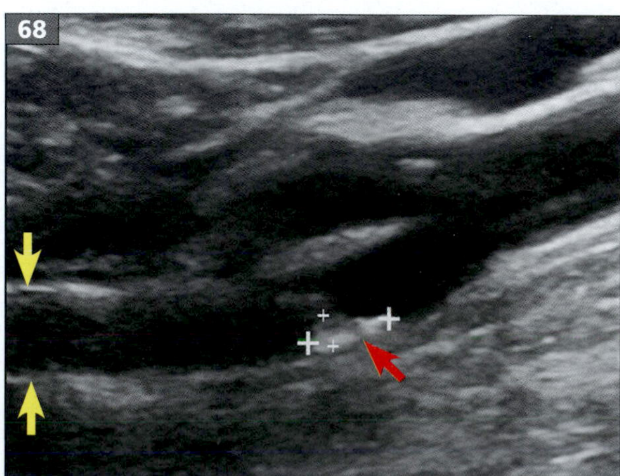

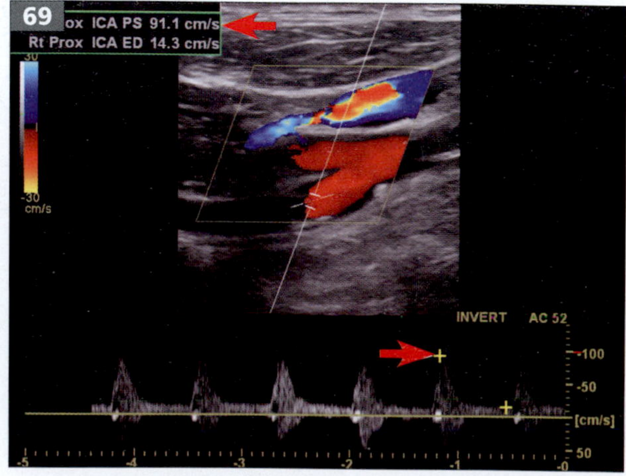

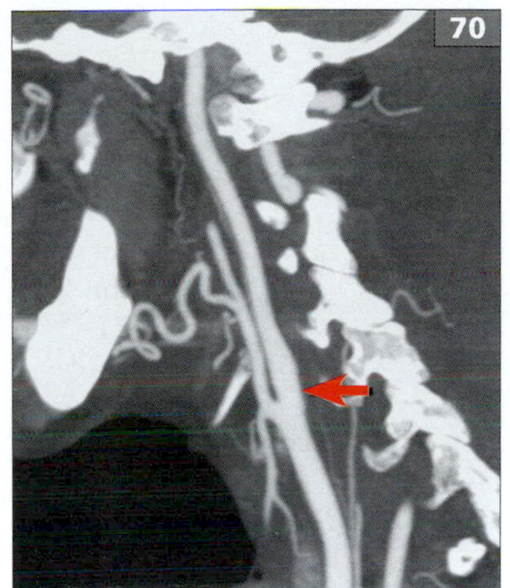

70, 71 CT angiography.
(70) Multi-planar reformat (MPR) CTA image of the carotid bifurcation in the sagittal plane (arrow).
(71) Axial MPR CTA reconstruction of a previously clipped anterior communicating artery aneurysm (red arrow) and coiled middle cerebral artery bifurcation aneurysm (yellow arrow). Note the lack of streak artifact, due to the metal reduction algorithm being used.

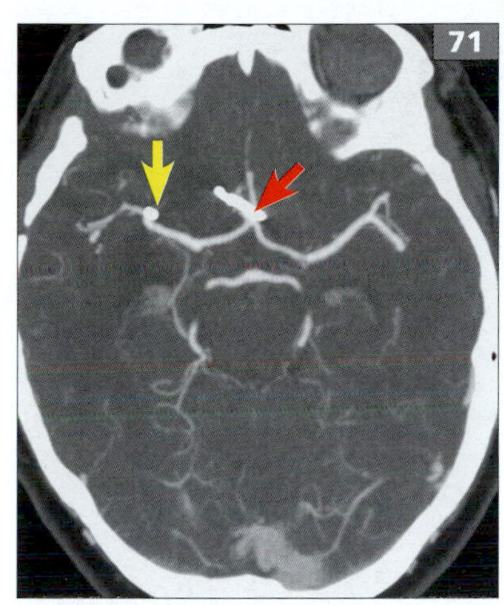

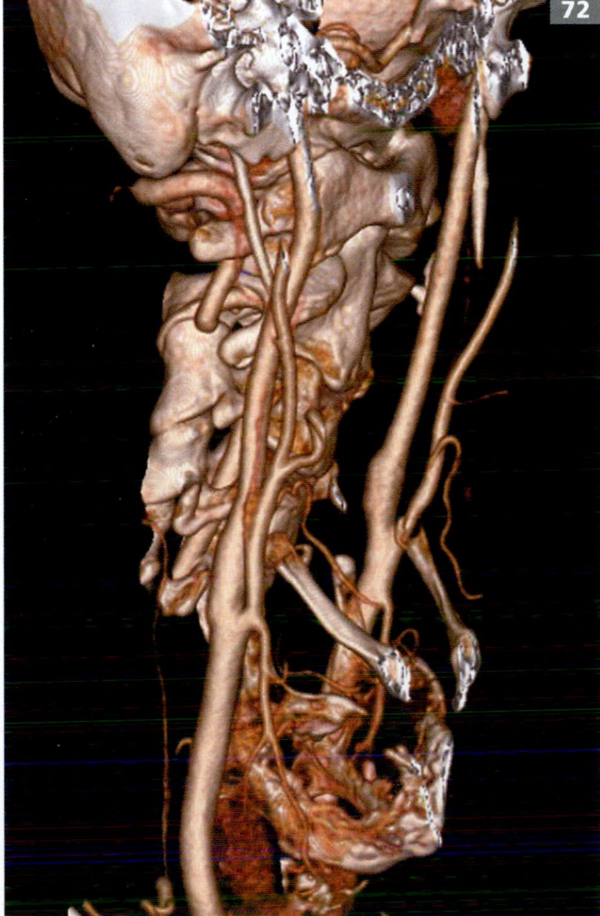

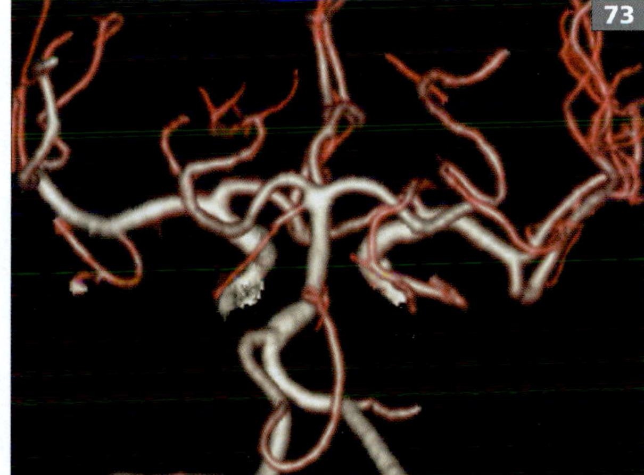

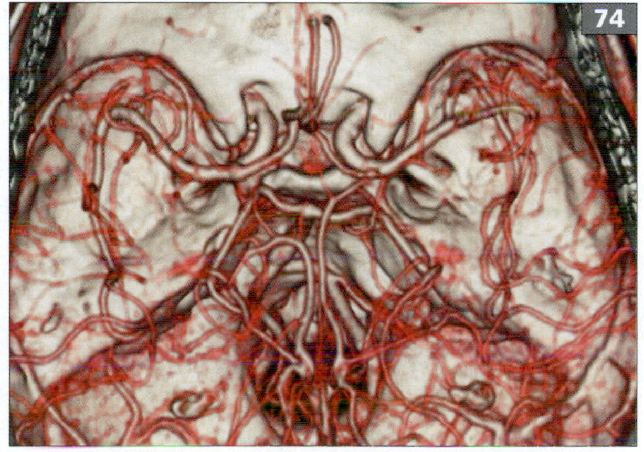

72–74 An alternative algorithm for reconstructing a CTA is colour volume-rendered (VR) imaging, in which a similar dataset to (70) is manipulated and represented in a different manner. This can be rotated on a work station to maximize information (72). Similar techniques can be used intracranially to look at the circle of Willis (73). An overview image of the same dataset can also be displayed with the skull base intact for further neurosurgical planning (74).

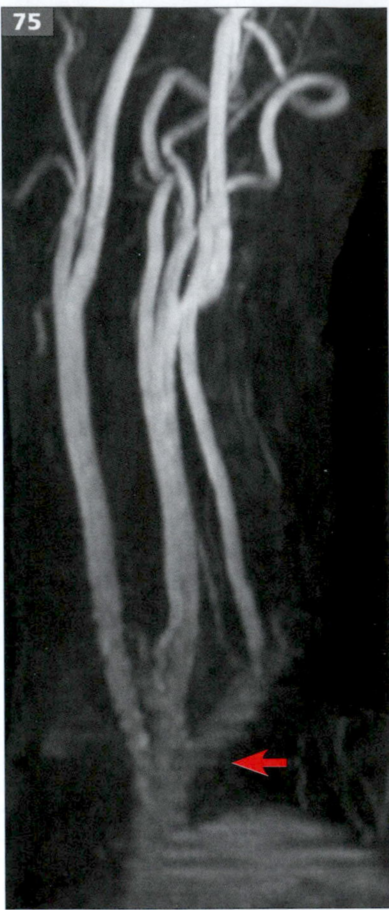

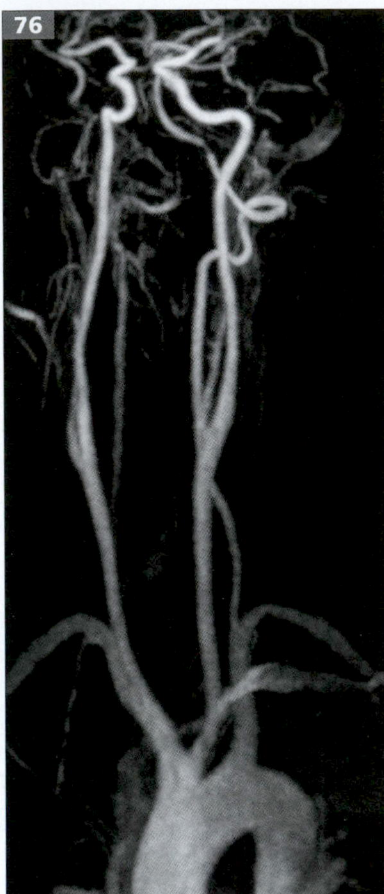

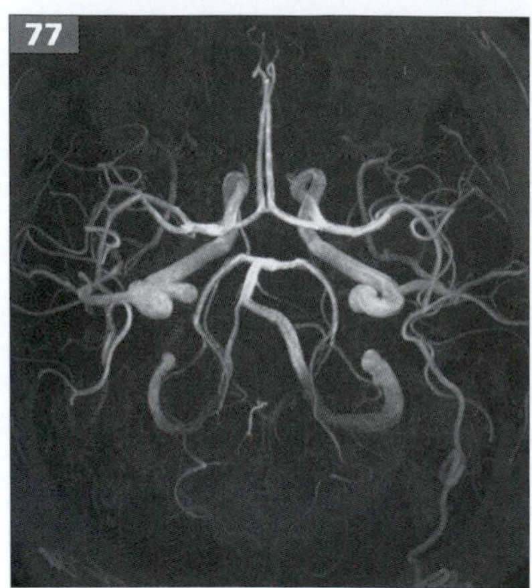

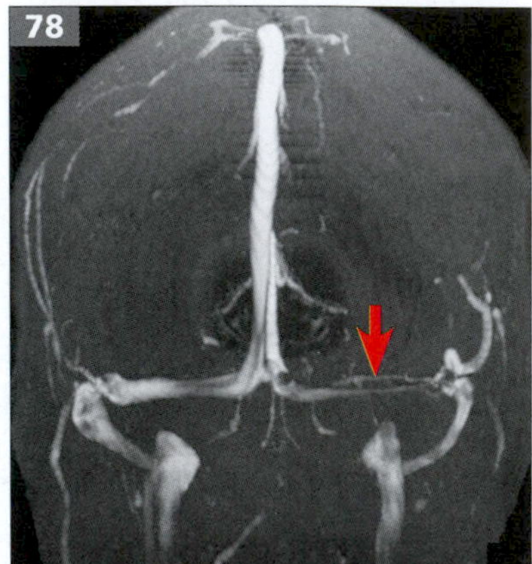

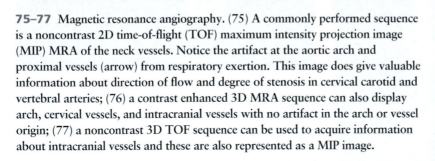

75–77 Magnetic resonance angiography. (75) A commonly performed sequence is a noncontrast 2D time-of-flight (TOF) maximum intensity projection image (MIP) MRA of the neck vessels. Notice the artifact at the aortic arch and proximal vessels (arrow) from respiratory exertion. This image does give valuable information about direction of flow and degree of stenosis in cervical carotid and vertebral arteries; (76) a contrast enhanced 3D MRA sequence can also display arch, cervical vessels, and intracranial vessels with no artifact in the arch or vessel origin; (77) a noncontrast 3D TOF sequence can be used to acquire information about intracranial vessels and these are also represented as a MIP image.

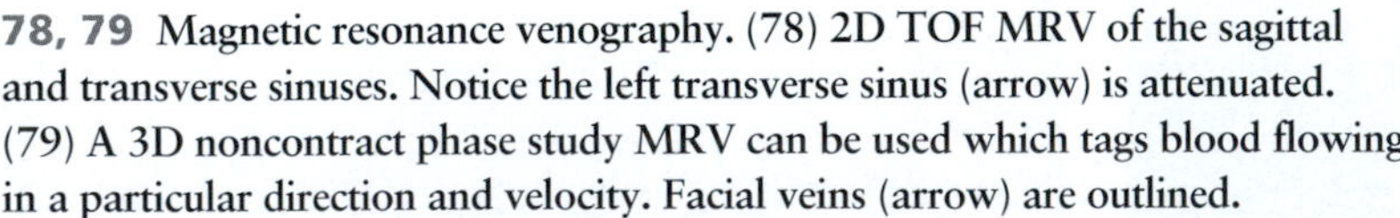

78, 79 Magnetic resonance venography. (78) 2D TOF MRV of the sagittal and transverse sinuses. Notice the left transverse sinus (arrow) is attenuated. (79) A 3D noncontract phase study MRV can be used which tags blood flowing in a particular direction and velocity. Facial veins (arrow) are outlined.

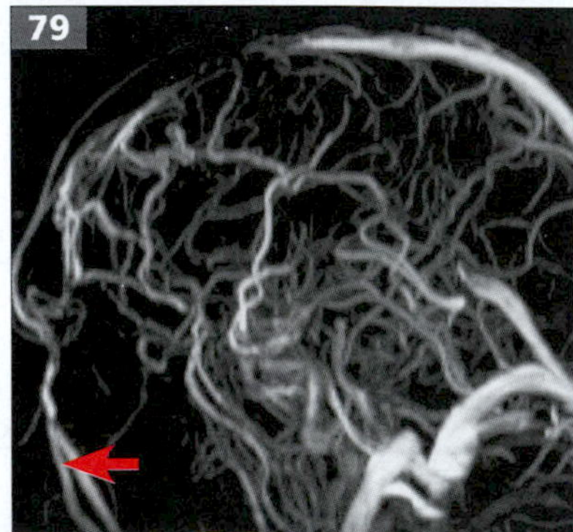

Magnetic resonance angiography

A variety of techniques are used to assess the carotid artery, intracranial circulation, and aortic arch (75–77). Noncontrast images provide very valuable information, without the risks of contrast or radiation from CTA. As a consequence, magnetic resonance angiography (MRA) is the investigation of choice in all patients, if it is freely available. CTA is probably slightly more sensitive for detection of aneurysms of <3 mm intracranially. Contrast-enhanced MRA of the arch and great vessels can be used, but is contraindicated with a GFR of <40 ml/min/1.73 m^2 .

Magnetic resonance venography

Magnetic resonance venography (MRV) is a noninvasive way of assessing flow in the dural sinuses and deep veins. It is acquired using a variety of noncontrast techniques. A similar noncontrast technique to the 2D TOF MRA used to depict images of the carotid artery can be employed to look at venous structures in the brain. TOF and phase contrast (PC) techniques relate to blood flow-related enhancement (78, 79). Gadolinium contrast-enhanced MRV can be used for problem-solving cases.

Digital subtraction cerebral angiography

Contrast digital subtraction angiography (DSA) is a minimally invasive technique which is used to obtain exquisite images of the cerebral vessels. It is still the gold standard in assessment of carotid and intracranial disease and requires admission to hospital as a day case, insertion of a catheter into the femoral artery, an injection of intra-arterial contrast, and radiation as contrast passes through the blood vessels (80–82). It gives a dynamic assessment of intracranial circulation, with the trade-off being that there is a very small risk (1%) of damaging a vessel, which could result in a stroke. In addition, there is the cost of admission, radiation, and contrast burden to be considered.

Noninvasive imaging has largely replaced the need for DSA in the study of cervical carotid artery stenosis, unless the patient is undergoing carotid stenting. It is still the gold standard in assessment of intracranial vasculitis. DSA is widely used in the assessment and endovascular treatment of intracranial aneurysms, which is now the treatment of choice. It is also used extensively in the treatment of dural fistulas, cerebral arteriovenous malformation, epistaxis, tumor embolization, and carotid test occlusion. DSA is also used in WADA testing in the preoperative assessment of patients with epilepsy.

Tip

▶ *Doppler gives a very accurate display of the carotid bifurcation wall, for detection of very early atheroma, whereas standard MRA, DSA and, to a certain extent, CTA, study the patent lumen. This additional information may potentially be used to decide how aggressive to be when considering antilipid medication in a younger patient.*

80–82 Angiographic imaging. (80) Digital angiogram in a frontal projection of the right internal carotid artery (ICA). Note the coil mass in the region of the anterior communicating artery aneurysm (arrow) that has been treated, and the presence of the skull; (81) identical image using digital subtraction (DSA). The bone and the coils are removed but the underlying angiographic detail remains. The middle cerebral artery (blue arrow) and the position of the subtracted coils (red arrow) are demonstrated; (82) lateral view of a left vertebral artery (red arrow) angiogram, depicting basilar artery (blue arrow).

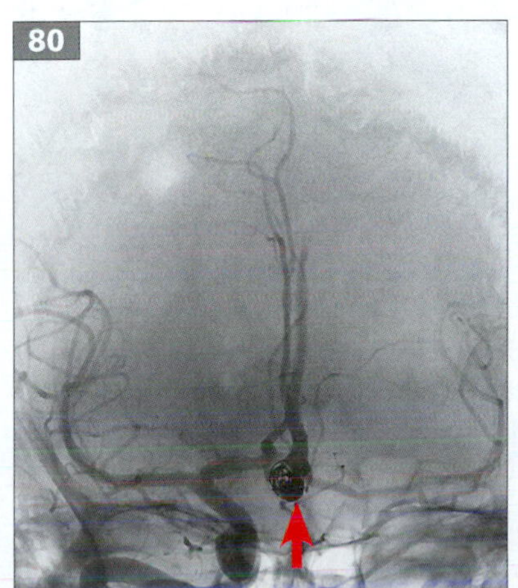

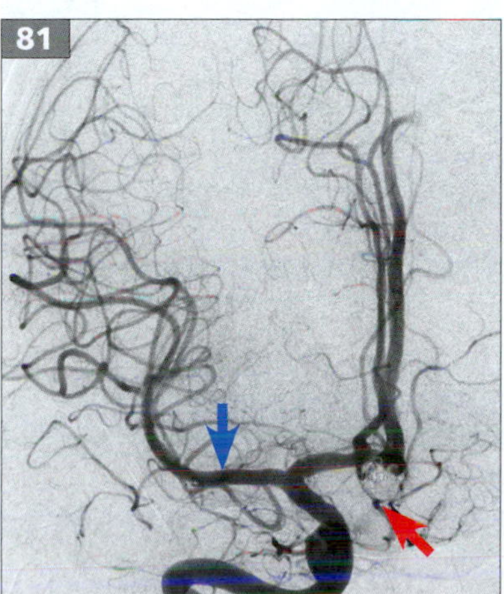

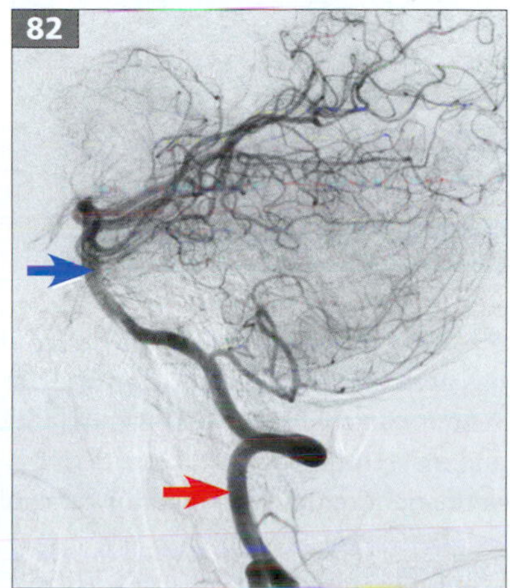

CT perfusion

CT perfusion is a technique that looks at cerebral blood flow to the brain, by assessing contrast uptake in the feeding artery and draining vein (**83**). From this information, calculations can be made and flow maps produced of cerebral blood volume, cerebral blood flow, and mean transit time (**84, 85**). This is very useful in the assessment of patients with acute stroke, vasospasm, or hypoperfusion. It has not been subjected to rigorous assessment with respect to large volume trials in the care of patients with stroke and thrombolysis.

CT cisternography

Contrast is instilled via LP as for a myelogram. Contrast is run up through the spinal canal looking for foci of CSF leak. The contrast is then run into the brain cisterns. The patient is quickly transferred to CT for high resolution images of the skull base to assess for leak through the cribriform plate or other site. This is also used in patients with recurrent meningitis, spontaneous cerebral hypotension, or in post-traumatic CSF leak.

Imaging the spine

Plain films and CT are still essential in the assessment of patients with trauma (**86, 87**) supplemented by MRI where indicated. For elective patients with radiculopathy or spinal stenosis, MRI is the investigation of choice. CT or CT myelography is reserved for patients who have contraindications to MRI, previous surgery making MRI impracticable, or claustrophobic patients who are considered high risk for general anesthetic.

MRI of the spine

Multiplanar T1- and T2-weighted images are used to assess the disc, vertebral bodies, spinal canal, cord, foramina, facet joints, and supporting structures (**88–91**). Look logically at all these structures for each spinal level so you don't miss anything. Intravenous gadolinium contrast is used in post-operative cases (scar *vs.* recurrent disc) or where a tumor is suspected. Exquisite detail about the state of hydration of the disc, the presence of spinal stenosis, disc protrusion, spinal cord anatomy, and pathology are well demonstrated.

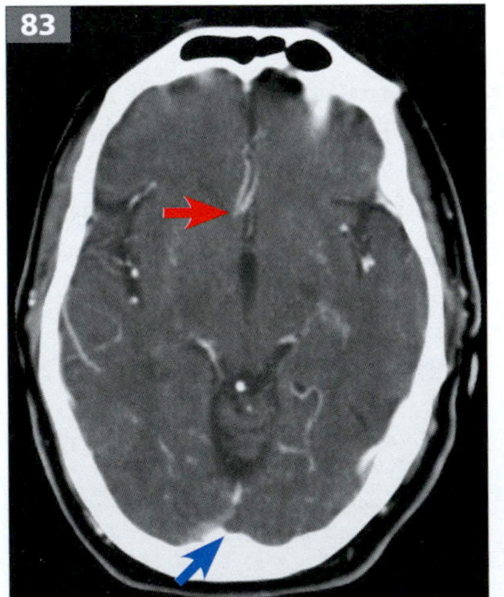

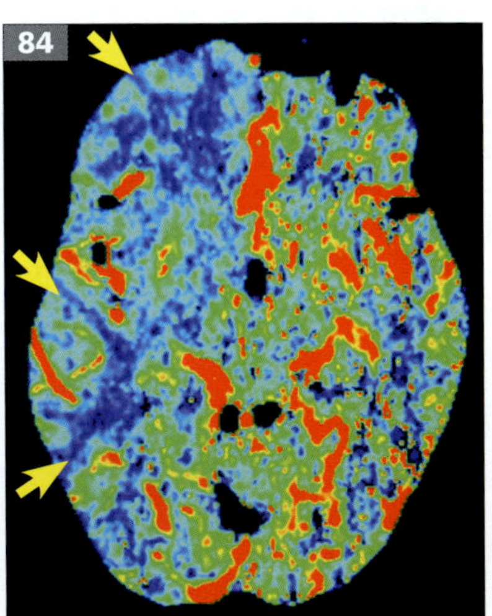

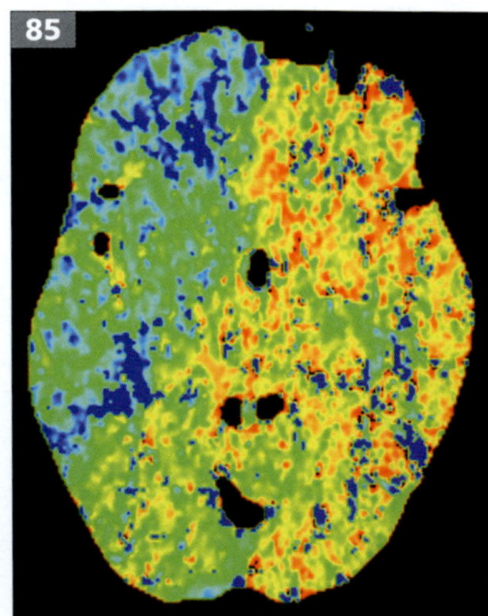

83–85 CT perfusion data are derived from repeatedly imaging at a defined level in the cerebral hemisphere where contrast has been injected. The anterior cerebral artery marks the arterial input function (red arrow) and the torcula marks the venous control factor (blue arrow). Calculations are made from which cerebral blood volume, cerebral blood flow (84) and mean transit time (85) are derived. A qualitative assessment is made and the findings in this instance represent ischemia in the right middle and anterior cerebral artery distribution (yellow arrows).

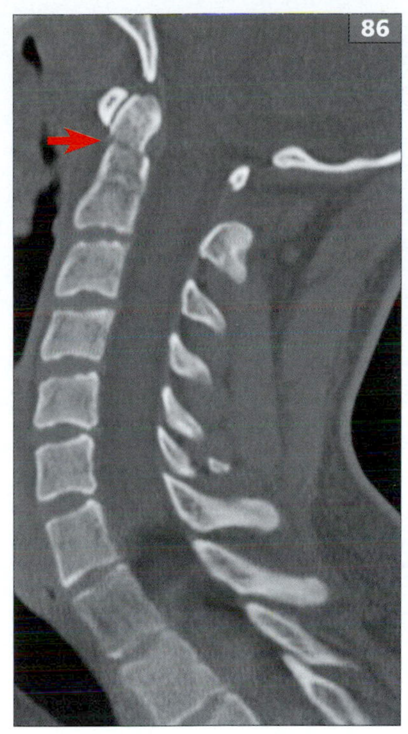

86 A sagittal CT reconstruction of the cervical spine in a bone algorithm. A C2 fracture is demonstrated (arrow).

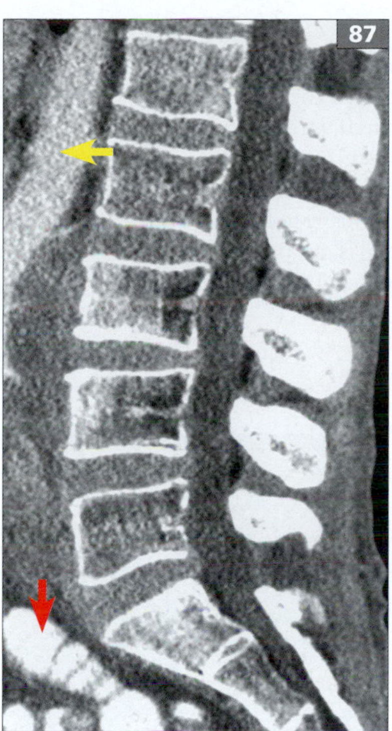

87 A sagittal CT lumbar spine image with a soft tissue algorithm and soft tissue windows in a multitrauma patient. Note the oral contrast in the gut (red arrow) and in the aorta (yellow arrow).

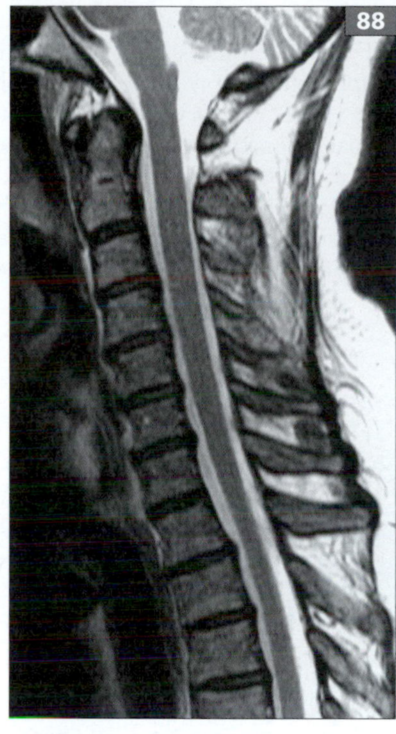

88 A sagittal fast spin echo T2-weighted sequence of the cervical and upper thoracic spine. Note the detail of the cord, which is not visible on a usual CT scan. CSF is white.

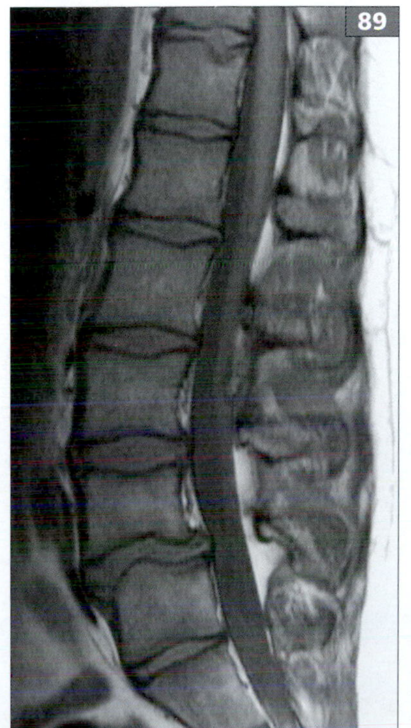

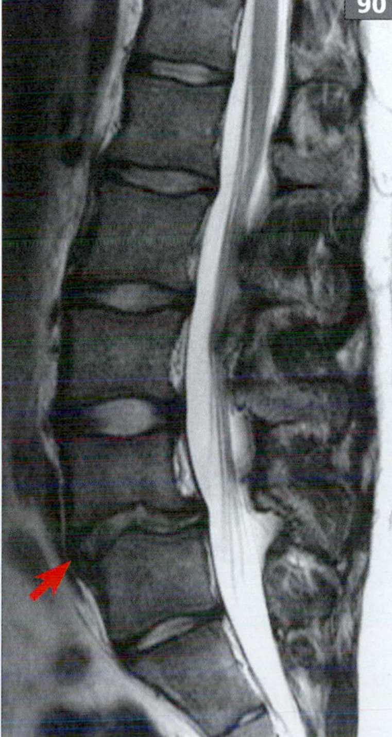

89, 90 Sagittal T1-weighted image of the lumbar spine (89) with black CSF, gray cord, and gray discs. The corresponding T2-weighted image (90) demonstrates white CSF. The degenerate discs become dark (arrow).

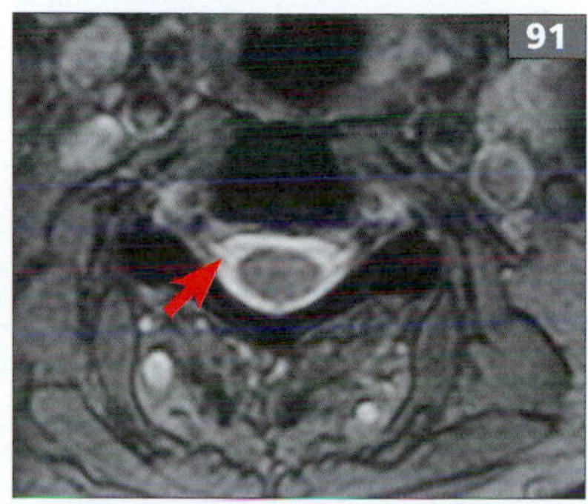

91 An axial gradient T2-weighted image where bone is black, CSF is white, and the nerve roots are discernible (arrow).

CT myelography

CT myelography is used in conjunction with myelography after X-ray contrast is instilled into the spinal CSF via LP. Helical CT datasets are acquired with multiplanar reconstructions. Excellent detail is given in relation to the intrathecal nerve roots and the bony anatomy (92–95). The outline of the cord is demonstrated, but intrinsic signal abnormality within the cord is not perceptible and is much more easily defined with MRI.

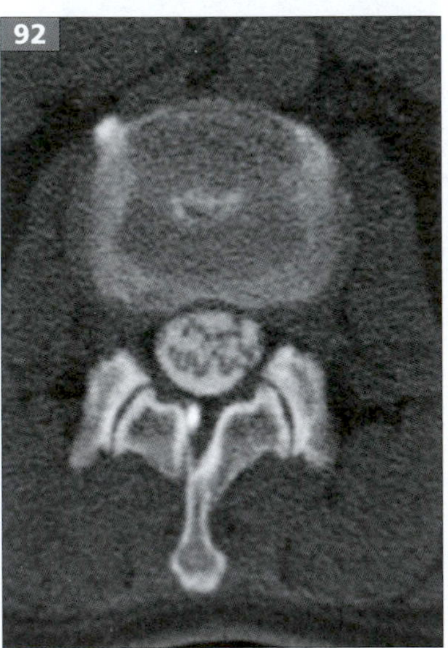

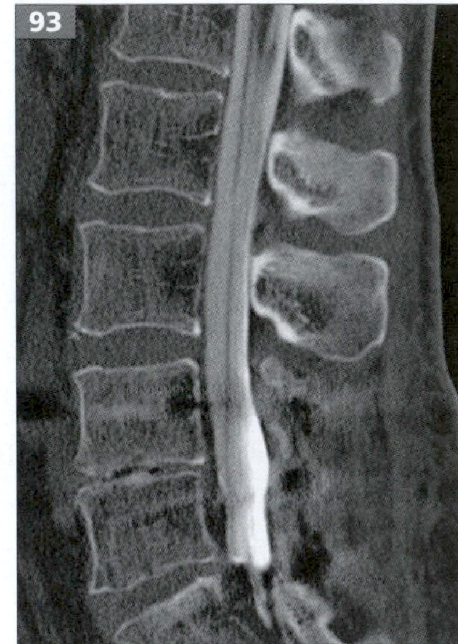

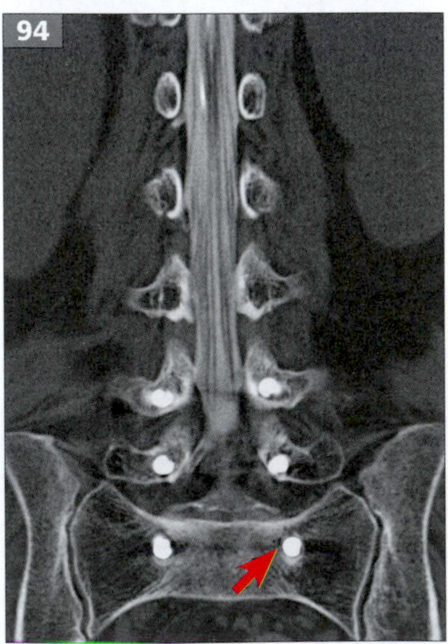

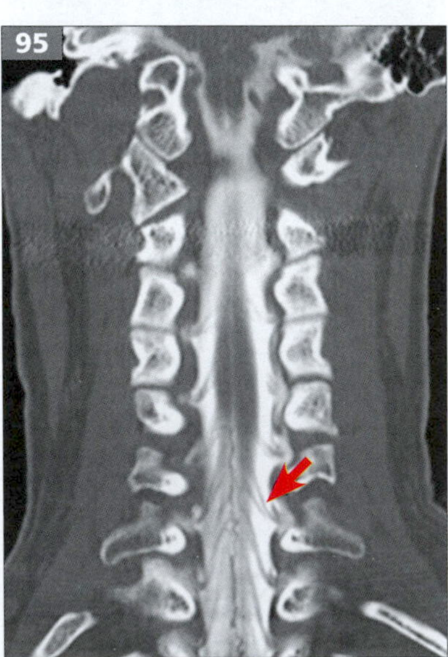

92–95 Axial bone algorithm image (92) of the cauda equina at the level of L2 can be reconstructed in the sagittal (93) or coronal plane (94). The cauda equina and cord are perfectly demonstrated. Notice the lack of artifact from the pedicular screws (arrow). Post-myelogram cervical CT (95) demonstrates a coronal reconstructed image of a cervical myelogram with excellent demonstration of the intradural rootlets (arrow).

REFERENCES

Introduction

1 Aminoff MJ (2008). Training in neurology. *Neurology* 70:1912–1915.
2 Elkind MSV (2009). Teaching the next generation of neurologists. *Neurology* 72:657–663.
3 www.richmondeye.com/eyemotil.asp.
4 www.neuroexam.com.
5 Tang H, Ng JHK (2006). Googling for a diagnosis – use of Google as a diagnostic aid: internet based study. *BMJ* 333:1143–1145.
6 Zeiler SR, Kaplan PW (2009). Our digital world: camera phones and the diagnosis of a seizure. *Lancet* 373:2136.
7 Patterson V, Wooton R (2006). How can teleneurology improve patient care? *Nature Clin Pract Neurol* 2(7):346–347.
8 Lloyd M, Bor R (2004). *Communication Skills for Medicine*, 2nd edn. Churchill Livingstone, Edinburgh.
9 Lempert T (1996). Recognizing syncope: pitfalls and surprises. *J R Soc Med* 89:372–375.
10 Stone J (2009). Functional symptoms in neurology. *Pract Neurol* 9(3):179–189.

Neurologic examination

1 Fuller G (2008). *Neurological Examination Made Easy*, 4th edn. Churchill Livingstone, Edinburgh.
2 Campbell WW (2005). *De Jong's The Neurologic Examination*, 6th edn. Lippincott Williams & Wilkins, Phildelphia.
3 Mayo Clinic and Mayo Foundation (1997). *Clinical Examinations in Neurology*, 7th edn. WB Saunders, Philadelphia.
4 Gates P (2010). *Clinical Neurology: a Primer*. Churchill Livingstone, Elsevier.
5 Mioshi E, Arnold R, Dawson K, Hodges J R, Mitchell J (2006). The Addenbrooke's Cognitive Examination Revised (ACE-R) : a brief cognitive test battery for dementia screening. *Int J Geriatr Psychiatry* 21:1078–1085.
6 Hodges JR (2007). *Cognitive Assessment for Clinicians*, 2nd edn. Oxford University Press, Oxford.
7 Dubois B, Litvan I, Pillon B, Slachevsky A (2000). The FAB: A frontal assessment battery at the bedside. *Neurology* 55:1621–1626.
8 Moo LR, Hart J, Slotnick SD, Tesoro MA, Zee DS (2003). Interlocking finger test: a bedside screen for parietal lobe dysfunction. *J Neurol Neurosurg Psychiatry* 74:530–532.
9 Cooper SA, Metcalfe RA (2009). How to do it: assess and interpret the visual fields at the bedside. *Pract Neurol* 9(6):324–334.
10 Acierno MD (2001). Ophthalmoscopy for the neurologist. *Neurologist* 7(4):234–251.
11 Rucker JC, Tomsak RL (2005). Binocular diplopia: a practical approach. *Neurologist* 11(2):98–110.
12 Serra A, Leigh R J (2002). Diagnostic value of nystagmus: spontaneous and induced ocular oscillations. *J Neurol Neurosurg Psychiatry* 73:615–618.
13 Blessing WW (2000). Alternating two finger tapping as part of the neurological motor examination. *Aust NZ J Med* 30:506–507.
14 Anderson NE (2010). The forearm and finger rolling tests. *Pract Neurol* 10(1):39–42.
15 O'Brien M (2010). *Aids to the Examination of the Peripheral Nervous System*, 5th edn. Elsevier Saunders, Edinburgh.
16 Miller TM, Johnston C (2005). Should the Babinski sign be part of the routine neurologic examination? *Neurology* 65:1165–1168.
17 Larner AJ (2003). False localising signs. *J Neurol Neurosurg Psychiatry* 74:415–418.

Lumbar puncture and CSF examination

1 Boon JM, Abrahams PH, Meiring JH, Welch T (2004) Lumbar puncture: anatomical review of a clinical skill. *Clin Anat* 17:544–553.
2 Beetham R (2004). Recommendations for CSF analysis in subarachnoid haemorrhage. *J Neurol Neurosurg Psychiatry* 75:528.
3 Lawrence RH (2005). The role of lumbar puncture as a diagnostic tool in 2005. *Crit Care Resusc* 7:213–220.

Neurophysiologic examination

1 Salinsky M, Kanter R, Dasheiff RM (1987). Effectiveness of multiple EEGs in supporting the diagnosis of epilepsy: an operational curve. *Epilepsia* 28:331–334.
2 Sundaram M, Hogan T, Hiscock M, *et al.* (1990). Factors affecting interictal spike discharges in adults with epilepsy. *Electroencephalogr Clin Neurophysiol Suppl* 75:358–360.

Neurophysiologic examination

Further reading

Binnie CD, Prior PF (1994). Electroencephalography. *J Neurol Neurosurg Psychiatry* 57:1308–1319.

Blume WT, Holloway GM, Kaibara M, Young GB (2010). *Blume's Atlas of Pediatric and Adult Electroencephalography*, 1st edn. Lippincott Williams & Wilkins, Philadelphia.

Ebersole JS, Pedley TA (eds) (2003). *Current Practice of Clinical Electroencephalography*, 3rd edn. Lippincott Williams & Wilkins, Philadelphia.

Kimura J (2001). *Electrodiagnosis in Diseases of Nerve and Muscle: Principles and Practice*, 3rd edn. Oxford University Press, USA.

Neal PJ, Katirji B (2011). *Nerve Conduction Studies: Practical Guide and Diagnostic Protocols*. American Association of Neuromuscular & Electrodiagnostic Medicine, Rochester, USA.

Perotto A (2005). *Anatomical Guide for the Electromyographer: the Limbs and Trunk*, 4th edn. Charles C Thomas, Springfield, Illinois.

Preston DC, Shapiro BE (2005). *Electromyography and Neuromuscular Disorders*, 2nd edn. Butterworth-Heinemann, Boston.

Santamaria J, Chiappa KH (1987). The EEG of drowsiness in normal adults. *J Clin Neurophysiol* 4:327–382.

Imaging the brain and spine

Further reading

Atlas SW (2009). *Magnetic Imaging of the Brain and Spine*, 4th edn. Lippincott, Williams & Wilkins, Philadelphia.

Grossman RI (2003). *Neuroradiology: The Requisites*, 2nd edn. Mosby, St Louis.

Osborn AG (2007). *Diagnostic Imaging of Brain*. Amirsys Inc, Salt Lake City.

DISORDERS OF CONSCIOUSNESS

Vibhav Bansal, Sean Ruland, Venkatesh Aiyagari

IMPAIRED CONSCIOUSNESS

Definition

Consciousness is a state in which a person is awake, alert, and aware of his/her surroundings.

Classification

Consciousness exists on a continuum ranging from an alert cognitively intact state, to one in which there is complete unresponsiveness to any environmental stimuli (i.e. coma). Many terms have been used to describe impaired consciousness which may lead to confusion when applied inconsistently between observers. A detailed description of the patient's clinical state including motor postures and responses to various applied stimuli (e.g. verbal, tactile, noxious, etc.) is preferred. Detailed descriptions may not only prevent misinterpretation errors but may also have localizing value.

Impaired level of arousal and attention defines disorders of consciousness. As the level of consciousness declines, increasing levels of stimulation are required to elicit and maintain attention until coma is encountered. Various terms have been utilized to describe these stages and are described as follows:

- Normal consciousness/alert and awake: refer to a state where consciousness is intact.
- Obtundation/drowsiness/lethargy/confusion/clouded consciousness/delirium: refer to decreased responsiveness whereby patients are arousable to minor applied stimuli such as verbal or light tactile. Although arousal may be maintained for varying lengths of time following cessation of the stimulus, difficulty is encountered in maintaining a consistent state of attention.
- Stupor/profound somnolence: refer to a severely depressed level of consciousness such that vigorous and noxious stimulation is required to achieve arousal. Upon cessation of stimulation, these patients immediately lapse back into a more deeply impaired state.
- Coma: refers to a state of unresponsiveness whereby a patient is incapable of purposefully responding to the most vigorous and noxious stimuli. However, occasional eye opening, flexion or extension of the limbs, grimacing, grunting, or groaning in response to pain, and primitive reflexes may be present.

TABLE 7 **GLASGOW COMA SCALE**

	Score
EYES OPEN	
Nil	1
To pain	2
To verbal stimuli	3
Spontaneously	4
BEST VERBAL RESPONSE	
No response	1
Incomprehensible sounds	2
Inappropriate words	3
Disorientated and converses	4
Orientated and converses	5
BEST MOTOR RESPONSE	
No response	1
Extension (decerebrate rigidity)	2
Abnormal flexion of upper limbs (decorticate rigidity)	3
Flexion – withdrawal to pain	4
Localizes pain	5
Obeys commands	6
Total	**15**

Standardized scoring systems such as the Glasgow Coma Scale (see *Table 7*), originally developed and validated for trauma patients, may have clinical and prognostic value in patients with selected etiologies of impaired consciousness. However, the Glasgow Coma Scale has several limitations and a newly devised coma score called FOUR (Full Outline of UnResponsiveness) Score has been developed, that incorporates respiratory patterns and brainstem reflexes but does not incorporate verbal responses[1].

Pathophysiology

Consciousness depends on an intact and interacting brainstem reticular formation and cerebral hemispheres. The reticular formation (from the Latin word 'reticulum', meaning 'a net') consists of a network of small and large cells and their connections throughout the brainstem from the medulla to the thalamus. All major sensory pathways project to the reticular formation where they interact before proceeding to the sensory cortex. The ascending reticular activating system (ARAS) originates in the midbrain and projects through the intralaminar nuclei of the thalamus bilaterally and diffusely to the cerebral cortex. It influences arousal and maintains wakefulness. When the ARAS pathways in the brainstem and/or the bilateral cerebral hemispheres are disrupted, impaired consciousness occurs.

While diffuse brain injuries and dysfunction affect the ARAS in an intuitively obvious manner, focal injuries and dysfunction leading to impaired consciousness are more complex:

- A focal injury to the upper brainstem will adversely affect ARAS function at its origin.
- Cerebellar mass lesions may cause obstructive hydrocephalus leading to transtentorial herniation and upper brainstem compression or ischemia from vascular torsion. Direct brainstem compression, upward herniation through the tentorial notch, and downward herniation through the foramen magnum from cerebellar mass lesions may also occur.
- Hemispheric lesions must be multiple and bilateral to cause ARAS dysfunction in both hemispheres, or have substantial mass effect to cause remote injury to the ARAS within the contralateral hemisphere or brainstem. In the case of space-occupying supratentorial lesions, the exact mechanism of remote dysfunction is uncertain and several possibilities alone or in combination may occur:
  - Direct compression of the contralateral hemisphere or upper brainstem (96–98).
  - Contralateral ischemia due to vascular impingement against the tentorium as the vessels emerge through the tentorial notch.
  - Brainstem ischemia or hemorrhage due to brainstem displacement and vascular torsion (99).
  - Large and small isolated hemisphere lesions may impair consciousness due to contralateral spread of convulsive and nonconvulsive seizure activity adversely affecting the ARAS.

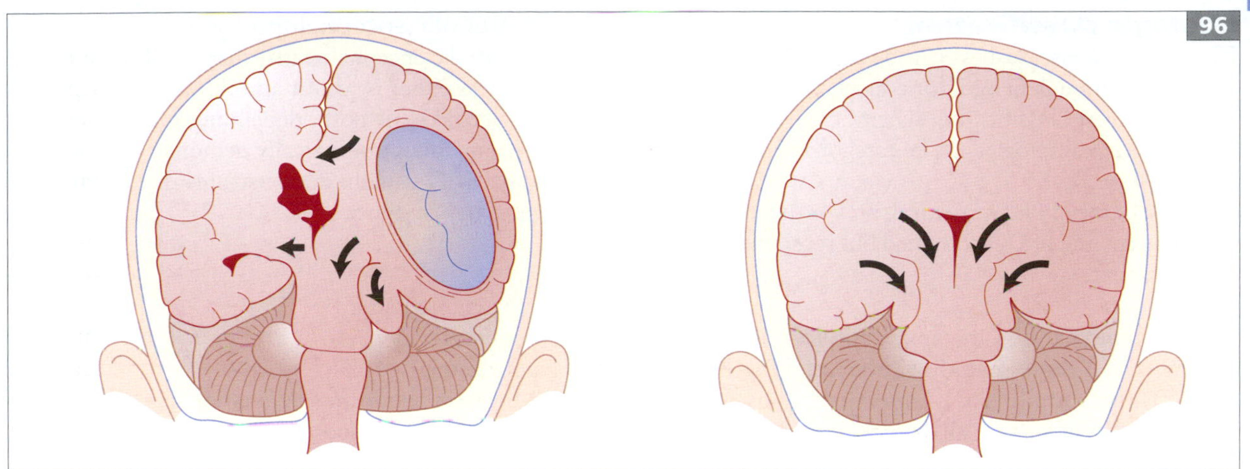

96 Herniation of the brain. *Left:* Uncal and transtentorial herniation. A mass such as a cerebral hemorrhage, cerebral infarct or hemorrhagic infarct in one cerebral hemisphere displaces the diencephalon and mesencephalon horizontally and caudally. The cingulate gyrus on the side of the lesion herniates under the falx cerebri (top arrow). The uncus of the ipsilateral temporal lobe herniates under the tentorium cerebelli (lower arrows) and becomes grooved and swollen and may compress the ipsilateral oculomotor (IIIrd cranial) nerve causing pupillary dilatation (Hutchinson's sign). The cerebral peduncle opposite the supratentorial mass becomes compressed against the edge of the tentorium, leading to grooving (Kernohan's notch) and a paresis homolateral to the cerebral mass lesion. Central downward displacement also occurs but is less marked than in the adjacent figure on the right. *Right:* Central transtentorial herniation. Diffuse or multifocal swelling of the cerebral hemispheres (or bilateral subdural or epidural hematomas) compress and elongate the diencephalon from above. The mamillary bodies are displaced caudally. The cingulate gyrus is not herniated. *Adapted from Plum F, Posner JB (1985). The Diagnosis of Stupor and Coma, 3rd edn. FA Davis, Philadelphia.*

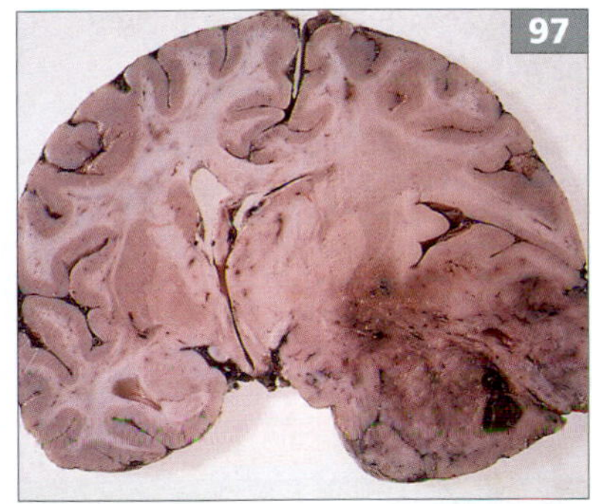

97 Herniation of the brain. Coronal section of the brain of a patient with a massive right temporal lobe glioblastoma multiforme who died after developing the syndrome of uncal herniation.

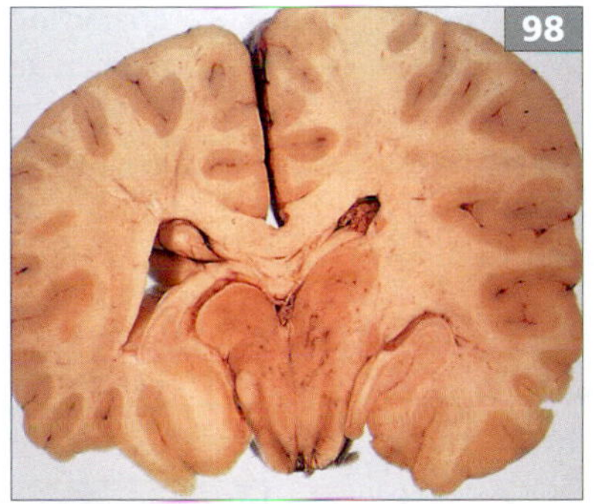

98 Coronal section of the brain of a patient with multiple cerebral metastases causing brain swelling, raised intracranial pressure, and compression, elongation, and caudal displacement of the diencephalon and medial temporal lobes.

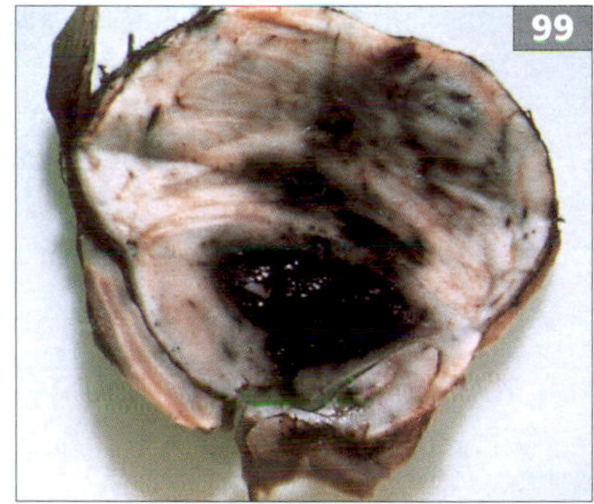

99 Axial section through the mid pons showing Duret hemorrhages in the central core of the brainstem of a patient who died after rapid expansion of an acute lobar intracerebral hemorrhage causing transtentorial herniation, downward displacement of the midbrain and pons, and stretching of the medial perforating arteries of the basilar artery (which is tethered to the circle of Willis and cannot shift downward).

Etiologic classification

Disorders of consciousness can be categorized in different ways. Although helpful for considering a differential diagnosis, these classification schemes may have considerable overlap. Etiologies can be categorized as:

- Diffuse or focal.
- Toxic or metabolic, structural, and/or functional.
- Transient and brief, protracted but reversible, or permanent.

Clinical examination, imaging, and electroencephalography (EEG) are essential in differentiating between these. Diffuse etiologies of impaired consciousness account for up to 70% of all disorders of consciousness.

Hypoxic–ischemic encephalopathy

The mechanism is diffuse cerebral hypoxia resulting from:

- Global ischemia due to cardiopulmonary arrest or severe hypotension.
- Hypoxemic respiratory failure.
- Carbon monoxide exposure.

The pathology is characterized by diffuse neuronal necrosis:

- Cortex often shows laminar necrosis which may be more severe in depths of sulci than on gyral crests (**100**).
- Severity increases from anterior to posterior – the occipital lobe is most sensitive.
- Hippocampus and amygdala also tend to be affected.
- Thalamic structures are often involved; however, changes are usually appreciated after 3 months.
- Deep subcortical white matter tracts are often affected as well, especially those leading to and away from the thalamus.

Less commonly there may be focal injury:

- When present it is typically seen after hypotension.
- Necrosis may involve watershed areas or borderzones between large vessel distributions.
- Patients with pre-existing cerebral arterial stenosis tend to have greater neuronal loss in flow-dependent regions.

Toxic metabolic encephalopathy[2]

Toxic metabolic encephalopathy may result in impaired consciousness either by direct and diffuse neuronal suppression, seizures, or both, depending on the etiology. Neuroimaging does not typically demonstrate any acute pathology. EEG usually demonstrates diffuse theta or delta frequency rhythms.

Electrolyte disturbances

- Severe hyponatremia.
- Hypernatremia.
- Hypocalcemia:
  - May have tetany on examination (e.g. Chvostek's sign, carpopedal spasm, etc.).
  - Seizures may occur.
- Hypercalcemia.
- Seizures may occur in disorders of sodium, calcium, severe hypomagnesemia, and severe hypophosphatemia.

Endocrine dysfunction

- Hypoglycemia: seizures and focal deficits may occur.
- Hyperosmolar hyperglycemia with or without acidosis: breath odor of ketones suggests ketoacidosis.
- Hypopituitarism.
- Hypothyroidism/myxedema coma:
  - It may be precipitated by cold, infection, or abrupt discontinuation of thyroid replacement hormone.
  - Clinical signs may include low body temperature, coarse facies, obesity, bradycardia, nonpitting edema, and delayed relaxation of tendon reflexes.
- Hypoadrenalism.

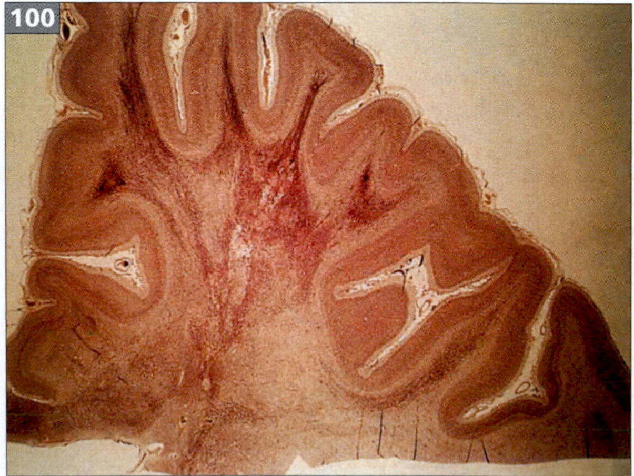

100 Microscopic section of a cerebral hemisphere showing laminar necrosis and demyelination in the white matter due to carbon monoxide poisoning. *Courtesy of Professor BA Kakulas, Royal Perth Hospital, Western Australia.*

Renal failure[3]

- Hypotension may occur during dialysis.
- Severe electrolyte disturbances.
- Uremia:
  - May have asterixis (i.e. flapping tremor) and fetid breath odor on examination.
  - EEG may reveal prominent frontal triphasic waves.
- Metabolic acidosis.
- Impaired excretion of drugs and other toxins.

Hepatic failure[4]

- Decreases endogenous toxin clearance.
- Associated with elevated serum ammonia levels.
- Impairs drug metabolism.
- May have asterixis (i.e. flapping tremor) and fetid breath odour on examination.
- EEG may reveal prominent frontal triphasic waves.

Sepsis

Cytokine-mediated[5].

Acute thiamine depletion (i.e. Wernicke's encephalopathy)

- Impaired consciousness or confusion, opthalmoplegia (including nystagmus), and ataxia.
- Chronic thiamine deficiency due to alcoholism and malnutrition predisposes to an acute encephalopathy.
- Encephalopathy may become manifest after intravenous (IV) dextrose-containing solutions.
- Parenteral thiamine 100 mg should be administered prior to IV dextrose.

Intoxication and pharmacologic causes

- Alcohol ingestion:
  - Patient odor may suggest alcohol intoxication.
  - Alcohol intoxication does not preclude concomitant drug abuse, seizures/postictal state, and/or intracranial hemorrhage.
- Sedative/hypnotic drug use/abuse (e.g. benzodiazepines, barbiturates, opiates, phenothiazines, and tricyclic antidepressants alone or in combination):
  - Naloxone may be given diagnostically and therapeutically in suspected opiate toxicity. However, its half-life is comparatively shorter than most opioids and prolonged monitoring is required.
  - Flumazenil may acutely reverse suspected benzodiazepine toxicity although it carries a risk of provoking seizures and should be avoided in most circumstances.
- Prescription drugs in usual dosages may result in an encephalopathy in those with impaired metabolism or clearance such as in the elderly and those with renal or hepatic dysfunction, or when a new agent is introduced with a drug–drug interaction.
- Neuroleptic malignant syndrome[6]:
  - Assess for history of neuroleptic use.
  - Clinical signs may include fever, tachycardia, rigidity, bradykinesia, elevated creatine kinase, and leukocytosis.
  - Treatment includes discontinuing the offending agent and fever control. Benzodiazepines and dopamine agonist therapy (e.g. bromocriptine) may be useful.
- Serotonin syndrome[6]:
  - Can be seen in patients who were on serotonergic agents in the past 5 weeks. Implicated agents include selective serotonin reuptake inhibitors, monoamine oxidase inhibitors, tricyclic antidepressants, opiate analgesics, over-the-counter cough medications, antibiotics, weight-reduction agents, herbal products, antiemetics, antimigraine agents, and drugs of abuse.
  - Clinical triad of mental status changes, autonomic hyperactivity, and neuromuscular abnormalities.
  - The rapid onset of symptoms and hyperkinesia (in contrast to bradykinesia) can help distinguish this from neuroleptic malignant syndrome.
  - Management includes removal of the offending agents, supportive measures including management of hyperthermia, agitation, and autonomic instability, and the use of 5-hydroxytryptamine (5-HT) 2A antagonists such as cyproheptadine.

Meningoencephalitis (101)[7]

- Assess history of sick contacts, insect bites, and recent travel.
- Fever may be absent.
- Nuchal rigidity may be absent with deep coma.
- Meningoencephalitis may also present with focal signs due to focal predilection (e.g. herpes simplex virus [HSV]) or secondary cerebral infarction.
- Secondary obstructive hydrocephalus may also be present and must be excluded prior to performing a lumbar puncture (LP).

Seizures

- Assess for history of epilepsy, evidence of tongue-biting, and incontinence.
- Primary or secondary generalized status epilepticus.
- Post-ictal state: transient and resolves over minutes to several days proportionate to seizure duration.
- Nonconvulsive status epilepticus due to a primary seizure disorder or from other diffuse and focal etiologies of impaired consciousness has been reported in up to 30% of those monitored with continuous EEG.

101 **Ventral surface of the brain of a patient who died from acute meningoencephalitis.**

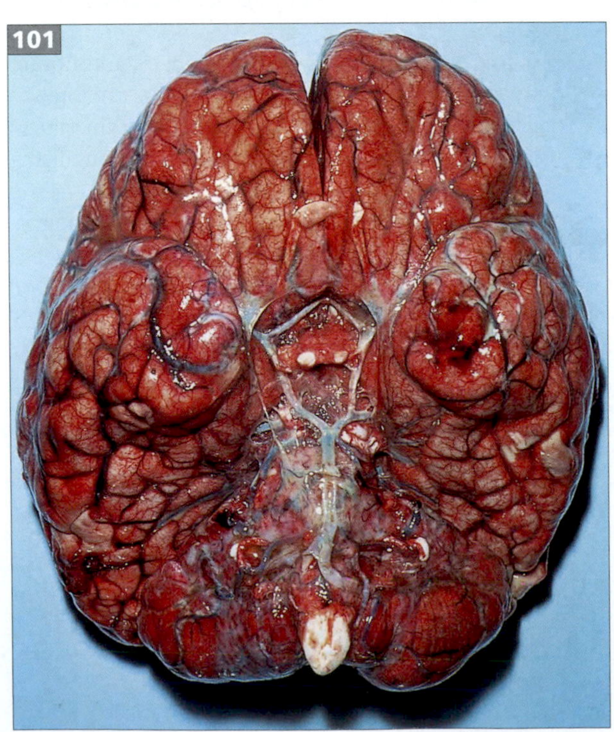

Vascular causes

Subarachnoid hemorrhage (SAH)

Increase in intracranial pressure (ICP) from an acute increase in intracranial blood volume or obstructive hydrocephalus may decrease cerebral perfusion.

Cerebral vein thrombosis

- Superior sagittal sinus (SSS) occlusion may cause bilateral cortical injury (i.e. infarction or hemorrhage) and/or increase ICP.
- Occlusion of the vein of Galen or straight sinus may cause bilateral thalamic infarction.
- Cerebral venous thrombosis (including SSS) may be associated with seizures.

Reversible cerebral vasoconstriction syndrome (RCVS)[8]

- Associated with serotonergic medication, cannabinoids.
- Post-partum vasculopathy.
- Posterior reversible encephalopathy syndrome (PRES):
  - Hypertensive encephalopathy.
  - Eclampsia.
  - Chemotherapy (e.g. cyclosporine A, FK506, etc.).

Non-neurologic etiologies

Clinical assessment includes:

- Normal rate and depth of respiration, pupillary reactions, muscle tone, deep tendon and abdominal reflexes, and downgoing plantar responses.
- Forced resistance of eye opening.
- Slow, roving eye movements and oculocephalic reflex are not present due to suppression from an intact cortex.
- Optokinetic nystagmus may be present.
- Irrigation of the ears with ice-cold water is noxious and evokes nystagmus with the fast component beating away from the side of the irrigated ear. Associated nausea with vomiting may occur.

Psychogenic causes

Assess for a history of psychiatric disorder:

- Conversion disorder.
- Catatonia.
- Malingering.

Structural lesions resulting in impaired consciousness

These account for up to 30% (15% supratentorial and 15% infratentorial) of all disorders of consciousness.

Patterns of supratentorial brain shift (96–99, 102)

Cingulate hernation (97)

- Occurs when the expanding hemisphere forces the cingulate gyrus under the falx cerebri.
- Compression and displacement of the anterior cerebral arteries leading to infarction in the territory of the anterior cerebral artery may occur.

Uncal hernation (98)

- Occurs when expanding lesions in the temporal fossa cause the basal edge of the uncus and hippocampal gyrus to bulge over the incisural edge and displace the adjacent midbrain contralaterally.
- The posterior cerebral artery may be caught between the overhanging uncus and the incisural edge causing ipsilateral medial temporal and occipital lobe infarction.
- In addition to impaired consciousness, initial signs include contralateral motor deficits and ipsilateral IIIrd nerve dysfunction (e.g. fixed and dilated pupil), either from direct compression or ischemia due to vascular torsion.
- Ipsilateral motor signs may develop if the contralateral cerebral peduncle is compressed against the contralateral incisura (i.e. Kernohan's notch) (**102**).

*Central or transtentorial herniation (**102**)*

- Occurs when the hemispheres, basal nuclei, and diencephalon are displaced through the tentorial notch into the adjoining midbrain.
- The vein of Galen is compressed causing venous congestion, edema, and even infarction which lead to more mass effect and further herniation.
- The cerebral aqueduct may be compressed compromising cerebrospinal fluid (CSF) circulation.
- Obstructive hydrocephalus may also contribute to further herniation.
- Stretch of the brainstem vascular supply may cause vascular torsion and avulsion leading to brainstem ischemia and hemorrhage.

Tips

► *While traditional teaching emphasized downward displacement of the brain as being responsible for worsening level of sensorium, more recent evidence suggests that horizontal displacement of brainstem correlates better with the level of the sensorium than vertical displacement[9,10].*

► *Pupillary changes from supratentorial expanding mass lesions may also be due to distortion of the midbrain rather than compression of the IIIrd nerve by the uncus of the temporal lobe.*

102 The under-surface of the forebrain at autopsy in a patient who died after transtentorial herniation, showing swelling and grooving of the uncus of the left medial temporal lobe (arrows), which has herniated through the tentorium cerebelli and compressed the midbrain. *Courtesy of Professor BA Kakulas, Royal Perth Hospital, Australia.*

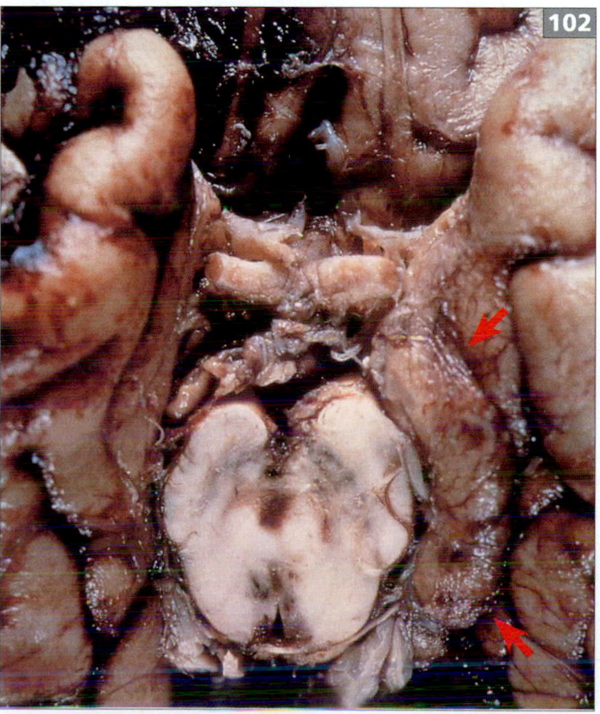

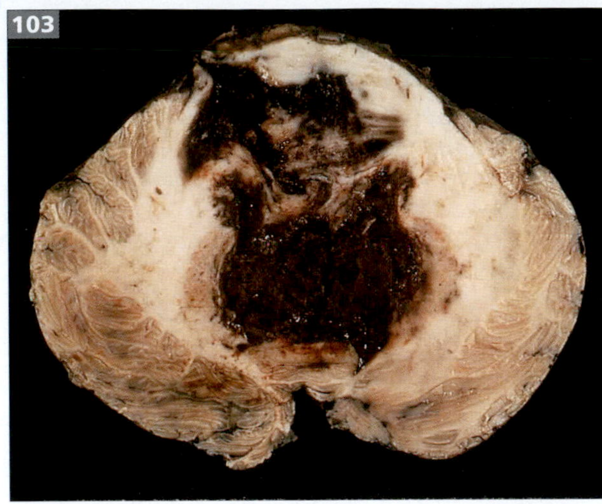

103 Section through the pons and cerebellar hemispheres, axial plane, showing massive fatal pontine hemorrhage extending into the fourth ventricle. *Courtesy of Professor BA Kakulas, Royal Perth Hospital, Australia.*

Intracranial hemorrhage
- Intracerebral (supratentorial, brainstem, or cerebellar) hemorrhage, subdural and epidural hemorrhage, and SAH with associated intracerebral hemorrhage and/or obstructive hydrocephalus (**99, 103**).
- Surgical evacuation and/or ventriculostomy may be life-saving early in the course.

Cerebral infarction
- Malignant middle cerebral artery infarction: decompressive hemicraniectomy may improve outcome in selected patients.
- Brainstem infarction: occlusion of the basilar artery can lead to coma or a 'locked-in syndrome' (see below).
- Cerebellar infarction:
  - Typically occurs with posterior inferior cerebellar artery infarction.
  - Early ventriculostomy and suboccipital decompressive craniotomy should be considered.

Cerebral vein thrombosis
- May be unilateral or bilateral.
- Impaired consciousness may be due to mass effect from congestion, infarction, or hemorrhage leading to herniation.
- Seizures may also occur.

Cerebral infections
- Brain abscess:
  - A solitary supratentorial abscess may cause mass effect.
  - Multiple cerebral abscesses are common and may affect both cerebral hemispheres.
  - Cerebellar abscesses may efface the fourth ventricle and cause obstructive hydrocephalus.
- Encephalitis:
  - Herpetic encephalitis has a predilection for the frontal and temporal lobes.
  - Impaired consciousness may result from mass effect or seizures.

Intracranial neoplasm
- Brain tumors may be primary or metastatic and affect the hemispheres, cerebellum, and brainstem.
- Posterior fossa tumors may obstruct the fourth ventricle leading to obstructive hydrocephalus.
- Metastastic tumors may be multiple and affect both hemispheres.
- Seizures may occur.

Head trauma
- Head trauma may cause intracranial hemorrhage in the intracerebral, subarachnoid, subdural, and epidural compartments (see above).
- Clinical signs may be focal or diffuse.
- Acute bilateral cerebral cortical, subcortical, and thalamic structural injury may result from shear stress (i.e. diffuse axonal injury [DAI]):
  - DAI Grade 1: nonfocal involvement of white matter structures.
  - DAI Grade 2: focal lesion in the corpus callosum in addition to widespread white matter damage.
  - DAI Grade 3: focal lesions in the dorsolateral rostral brainstem, focal corpus callosum injury, and widespread white matter damage.
- A secondary process of axotomy taking up to 6 hours to occur involving axonal and mitochondrial swelling, the appearance of nodal blebs, loss of microtubule structure and neuronal architecture, retraction bulb formation, and subsequent axonal rupture has been proposed.
- Secondary damage from ischemia has been consistently found in patients who die from high-force blunt trauma (rather than angulated traumatic injury). Hypoxemia due to ventilatory failure and decreased cerebral perfusion due to increased ICP may be contributory.

Clinical assessment

While assessing a comatose patient, the diagnostic evaluation and management should occur simultaneously.

Tips

▶ *Subjects with a Glasgow Coma Scale score of 9 are probably unable to protect their airway and should be intubated.*

▶ *Before lowering an elevated blood pressure with pharmaceutical agents, the effect on cerebral perfusion in case of raised intracranial pressure should be considered.*

Physical examination

The history and physical examination may often yield important clues to the underlying etiology of impaired consciousness. Obtain the history from as many collateral sources as possible (e.g. family, friends, Emergency Medical Services personnel, bystanders, etc.). In addition to a detailed general examination looking for evidence of acute and chronic systemic diseases which may cause or contribute to impaired consciousness, pay particular attention to the following:

Respiratory

- Assess adequacy of airway and respiratory effort. Intubate if necessary.
- Breathing rate and pattern may suggest the level of brain injury:
  - Post-hyperventilation apnea: bilateral hemisphere dysfunction.
  - Long-cycle crescendo–decrescendo (i.e. Cheyne Stokes): diencephalic injury.
  - Central hyperventilation: midbrain or upper pons injury.
  - Periodic breathing: pontine injury.
  - Ataxic or short-cycle Cheyne Stokes breathing: medullary injury.
  - Slow and shallow breathing: drug intoxication.
  - Deep and rapid breathing: metabolic acidosis (i.e. Kussmaul breathing with diabetic ketoacidosis).
  - Periodic breathing, yawning, or hiccoughs: brainstem injury.

Vital signs

- Temperature:
  - Fever: meningitis, encephalitis, brain abscess, septic encephalopathy due to systemic infection, anticholinergic and neuroleptic medications, and seizures.
  - Hypothermia: exposure to low environmental temperature, alcohol or sedative intoxication, or hypothyroidism.
- Heart rate:
  - Sinus tachycardia: sepsis, alcohol withdrawal, seizures, neuroleptic malignant syndrome.
  - Atrial fibrillation: cerebral infarction.
  - Bradyarrhythmia: global hypoperfusion – intravenous atropine 0.5–1 mg or pacing may be required.
- Blood pressure:
  - Hypotension: sepsis, hypoxic ischemic encephalopathy, Addison's disease, sedative/hypnotic intoxication. Resuscitate with volume expansion and vasopressors as needed. Intravenous hydrocortisone 100 mg q8 hours or 50 mg q6 hours may be required in patients with adrenal insufficiency.
  - Hypertension may be secondary such as due to seizures or alcohol withdrawal, or it may be primary such as with hypertensive encephalopathy. In patients with hypertensive encephalopathy, judiciously lower mean arterial pressure by no more than 10% in the first hour and 25% in the first 2–3 hours.

General appearance

- Cyanosis: hypoxemia or shock.
- Cherry red mucous membranes: carbon monoxide poisoning.
- Jaundice: hepatic failure.
- Petechiae and purpura: bleeding diathesis, intracranial hemorrhage.
- Hyperpigmentation: Addison's disease.
- Needle punctures: diabetes or illicit drug abuse.

Neurologic function

- Position, posture, and spontaneous movements.
- Level of consciousness:
  - Glasgow Coma Scale (*Table 7*).
  - Noxious stimuli above (e.g. supraorbital and temporomandibular joint pressure) and below (e.g. sternal rub and nail-bed pressure) the neck: observe for facial grimacing and the amplitude, quality, and symmetry of extremity movement (e.g. localization, flexion, extension, or withdrawal).
- Brainstem function:
  - Pupillary size and reactivity:
    - A unilateral dilated and nonreactive pupil is a sign of uncal herniation until proven otherwise.
    - Nonreactive (fixed) pupils: midbrain dysfunction, anesthesia, anticholinergic (e.g. atropine) medication effect.
    - Small (pin-point) pupils: opiate intoxication, pontine injury, pilocarpine ophthalmic drops.
    - Horner's syndrome: brainstem infarct with or without cerebellar infarction, hypothalamic injury, and carotid dissection.
  - Fundoscopy:
    - Papilledema: increased ICP.
    - Subhyaloid hemorrhages: SAH.
    - Retinal emboli, diabetic or hypertensive retinopathy.

The absence of papilledema does not exclude raised intracranial pressure particularly early after onset, as papilledema may not become manifest for several hours.

- Eye position and movement:
  - A minor degree of ocular divergence is normal in unconscious patients.
  - Roving eye movements indicate cortical dysfunction with intact brainstem function.
  - Conjugate horizontal gaze deviation: ipsilateral frontal lobe dysfunction or contralateral low pontine injury or status epilepticus.
  - Conjugate downgaze: midbrain tectal lesion or compression (e.g. pineal mass and/or hydrocephalus).
  - Skew deviation: brainstem injury.
  - Dysconjugate eyes: nuclear or infranuclear oculomotor or abducens nerve injury, or internuclear ophthalmoplegia (i.e. medial longitudinal fasciculus). Bilateral abducens nerve injury may be falsely localizing and due to hydrocephalus or a supratentorial mass lesion causing downward brainstem shift and stretch of the bilateral abducens nerve fibers as they enter the cavernous sinuses.
  - Ocular bobbing: low pontine injury.
  - Saccadic eye movements suggest functioning frontal cortical gaze centers, vestibular pathways, and oculomotor system. Therefore, spontaneous nystagmus is unlikely in comatose patients.
  - Oculocephalic reflex (i.e. 'doll's eye' maneuver): rotating an unconscious patient's head from side to side elicits conjugate eye movement in the opposite direction when the vestibular pathways and oculomotor system are intact. Absence of eye movement(s) suggests brainstem injury. Do not perform this maneuver when cervical spine injury is suspected.
  - Oculovestibular reflex (i.e. cold caloric testing): instillation of 50 ml of ice-cold water into a patent external acoustic meatus of an unconscious patient with intact vestibular pathways and oculomotor system elicits tonic conjugate gaze deviation toward the irrigated ear. Conscious patients or those with psychogenic unresponsiveness with intact corticopontine fibers will have a saccadic component that attempts to drive the eyes back to mid-position, thus generating the fast phase of nystagmus away from the irrigated side. A dysconjugate or absent response is likely due to brainstem injury. Test both ears independently; testing both ears simultaneously may evoke conjugate downward movement (with upward saccades in a conscious patient).
  - Corneal responses: may be suppressed in drug intoxication or deep toxic metabolic coma.
- Cough and gag reflexes:
  - Presence indicates intact function of the medulla.
  - Asymmetric palatal rise indicates ipsilateral medulla injury.
  - Absence of adequate cough and gag reflexes suggests poor airway protection and intubation should be considered.
- Motor function:
  - Spontaneous movement:
    - Purposeful
    - Focal or generalized tonic, clonic, or tonic–clonic movements suggesting seizures.
    - Multifocal myoclonus: diffuse cortical irritation due to anoxia or metabolic disturbances; may be induced by tactile stimulation; when not inducible, it may be difficult to distinguish clinically from generalized seizure activity and EEG may be helpful.
  - Muscle tone: can be increased in neuroleptic malignant syndrome.

- Provoked movements:
  - Localizing noxious stimulation.
  - Unilateral or bilateral upper extremity flexion (i.e. decorticate posturing) or extension (i.e. decerebrate posturing).
  - Withdrawal.
  - Absent.
- Deep tendon reflexes: amplitude, quality, and symmetry.
- Plantar responses.

Investigations

Brain imaging (computed tomography [CT] or magnetic resonance imaging [MRI]) should be performed in patients with focal neurologic signs or evidence of head injury. Brain imaging may also be useful when lateralizing signs are absent and the etiology is uncertain, as some structural etiologies may present without lateralizing signs (e.g. acute obstructive hydrocephalus, SAH, bilateral subdural hematomas, multiple abscesses, and metastases).

Laboratory assessment

- Serum glucose: hypoglycemia may produce profound lateralizing signs.
- Electrolytes including sodium, magnesium, phosphorus, and calcium.
- Serum urea nitrogen and creatinine: uremia.
- Complete blood count: infection and thrombocytopenia.
- Prothrombin time and partial thromboplastin time (aPTT): bleeding diathesis.
- Blood or urine toxicology screening.
- Arterial blood gas: acidosis, hypoxemia.
- Carboxyhemoglobin level; carbon monoxide exposure.
- Serum ammonia and hepatic transaminases: hepatic encephalopathy.
- Red blood cell transketolase: Wernicke's encephalopathy.
- Thyroid function tests: myxedema coma.
- Plasma and urine osmolality.
- Random serum cortisol and cosyntropin stimulation test: adrenal insufficiency.

LP and CSF analysis

CSF analysis (cell count, protein, glucose, Gram stain, cultures, and cytology in selected patients) should be performed to assess for infection, inflammation, or neoplasm (i.e. carcinomatous meningitis or intracerebral neoplasm with possible shedding of tumor cells into CSF). Impaired consciousness is not likely to be due to SAH that is beyond the resolution of contemporary brain imaging.

LP is contraindicated in the presence of space-occupying lesions that may increase the pressure gradient between intracranial compartments or across the foramen magnum, as it may exacerbate this pressure gradient and precipitate a herniation syndrome, particularly brainstem 'coning'.

EEG

- Diffuse or focal slow waves are common.
- Frontal triphasic slow waves suggest hepatic or uremic encephalopathy.
- Continuous EEG monitoring may reveal nonconvulsive status epilepticus in up to 30% of patients with impaired consciousness.

Prognosis

The prognosis for patients with impaired consciousness ranges from full recovery to death, and depends on the etiology, duration, and treatment of impaired consciousness and the presence of comorbid disease states. In general, patients with toxic metabolic disorders typically show improvement within a few days of correction of the underlying abnormality. However, irreversible brain injury can occur when the metabolic disturbance is severe and/or prolonged. Hypoxic–ischemic and other structural etiologies are more likely to cause permanent brain injury. A detailed discussion of prognosis for each cause of impaired consciousness is beyond the scope of this chapter. However, prognostic indicators for selected disorders will be described in the forthcoming sections.

BRAIN DEATH

Definition

The absence of clinically detectable brain functions when the proximate cause is known and demonstrably irreversible. Neuroimaging may be necessary in most circumstances to exclude potentially reversible causes. The clinical diagnosis of brain death requires the absence of potentially confounding factors such as neuromuscular blocking agents, deep sedation, severe metabolic disturbances, and hypothermia.

Etiology and pathophysiology

Severe injury to the entire brain, including the brainstem and both cerebral hemispheres, leads to irreversible whole brain destruction. Etiology includes:

- Traumatic brain injury.
- Hypoxic–ischemic injury.
- Stroke: hemorrhagic, malignant hemisphere infarction.
- Intracranial infection: encephalitis, meningitis.

Clinical features

- Coma without cerebral motor response to pain below and above the neck (i.e. sternal rub, nail-bed pressure, pressure over the supraorbital notch or temporomandibular joint).
- Absent pupillary response to bright light.
- No oculocephalic and oculovestibular reflexes. Oculocephalic maneuvers should not be performed in patients with suspected cervical spine injury.
- Absent corneal reflexes.
- Absent jaw jerk reflex.
- Absent grimace to noxious stimuli.
- Absent pharyngeal reflexes (i.e. gag or cough to deep tracheal suctioning).
- Apnea. Apnea must be confirmed by formal testing:
  - Prerequisites:
    - Core temperature ≥36°C (≥97°F).
    - Systolic blood pressure ≥100 mmHg.
    - Normal PO_2 (may be in the presence of supplemental oxygen).
    - PCO_2 >35 mmHg.
  - Connect a pulse oximeter.
  - Pre-oxygenate with 100% O_2 for at least 10 minutes and discontinue ventilator support.
  - Supplemental oxygen may be administered through a cannula inserted through the endotracheal tube and placed at the level of the carina.
  - Visually monitor for chest wall movement.
  - Draw arterial blood gas approximately 8–15 minutes and reconnect the ventilator.
  - If respiratory movements are absent and arterial PCO_2 is >60 mmHg, the apnea test supports the diagnosis of neurologic death. If the patient's baseline PCO_2 is ≥40 mmHg, then the PCO_2 must increase by 20 mmHg before the test is deemed positive.
  - If respiratory movements are observed, the apnea test is inconsistent with the clinical diagnosis of brain death.
  - If the PCO_2 is <60 mmHg or the PCO_2 is <20 mmHg over baseline PCO_2, the result is indeterminate and the test should be repeated or an ancillary test should be considered if the patient is not able to tolerate a longer period of apnea.
  - Terminate the test and reconnect the ventilator immediately if spontaneous respiratory movements or signs of hemodynamic instability (e.g. hypotension, hypoxemia, arrhythmia) are observed.
- Clinical observations compatible with the diagnosis of neurologic death. These manifestations are occasionally seen and should not be misinterpreted as evidence for brainstem function:
  - Spontaneous extremity movements (i.e. spinal reflexes and not to be confused with decorticate or decerebrate posturing).
  - Shoulder elevation and adduction, back arching, intercostal expansion without significant tidal volumes.
  - Autonomic responses such as sweating, blushing, and tachycardia.
  - Hemodynamic stability without pharmacologic support.
  - Absence of diabetes insipidus.
  - Preserved deep tendon reflexes or triple flexion response.
  - Up-going plantar responses.

Diagnosis

The protocol for determining brain death may vary by country and by institution. In some institutions, the diagnosis of death by neurologic criteria may be made on the basis of repeated assessments as described above after an interval of no less than 6 hours for adults. More prolonged periods of interval observation may be required for children and neonates. Inability to exclude reliably potentially confounding conditions or complete the full clinical assessment including the apnea test requires confirmation by an ancillary test.

Established ancillary tests for brain death confirmation

- Conventional catheter-based cerebral angiography, showing absent intracranial flow above the skull base.
- Radionuclide brain imaging, showing absent brain blood flow.
- Transcranial Doppler ultrasound, showing oscillating flow or short systolic spikes in both hemispheres and across the foramen magnum.
- EEG, showing electrocerebral silence (no cerebral activity over 2 μV from symmetrically placed electrode pairs at least 10 cm apart). However, deep pharmacologic sedation may also produce electrocerebral silence, and EEG is susceptible to artifacts in the intensive care setting that may be confused with brain activity.
- Maintain open and ongoing communication with the family or family spokesperson. Remain compassionate but precise when describing the underlying condition, brain death determination process, and final diagnosis, and provide emotional and practical support.
- Notify organ procurement organization as per any applicable legal requirement. Maintain advocacy for the patient at all times. The decision to donate organs is a personal one. Refrain from imposing any preconceived bias into the organ procurement process so as to avoid perception of conflict of interest.

PERSISTENT/PERMANENT VEGETATIVE STATE

Definition and clinical features

A condition of unawareness of self and the environment in which there may be periods of eye opening simulating a sleep/wake cycle. External stimuli fail to consistently elicit any behavioral responses beyond reflex reactions. Reflex reactions include reflex limb withdrawal, facial grimacing and smiling, laughing and weeping, blink to threat, and transient changes in autonomic tone in response to noxious stimuli or spontaneously. Nonsustained visual pursuit may be seen after tactile stimulation, although reproducible optokinetic response or tracking are absent. Other spontaneous movements, including roving eye movements, chewing, teeth grinding, groaning, grunting, and swallowing, may occur.

Diagnostic criteria[11]

- Absent awareness of self or environment and an inability to interact with others.
- No evidence of sustained, reproducible, purposeful, or voluntary behavioral responses to visual, auditory, tactile, or noxious stimuli.
- Lack of language compression and expression.
- Intermittent wakefulness.
- Sufficiently preserved hypothalamic and brainstem autonomic functions to permit survival with medical and nursing care.
- Bowel and bladder incontinence.
- Variably preserved brainstem and spinal reflexes.

Other features include the following:

- Spontaneous or provoked decorticate or decerebrate posturing may be present.
- Brainstem reflex function is usually preserved.
- Primitive reflexes such as pouting, sucking, grasp, and withdrawal may be present.
- Plantar reflexes are commonly extensor.
- Absence of cortical integrity indicating awareness: clinical or electrophysiologic seizures are compatible with a vegetative state.
- The vegetative state may be transient in the early recovery from coma or it may persist until death[11]:
  - The persistent vegetative state: a vegetative state for a minimum of 1 month duration.
  - The permanent vegetative state: defined as permanent 3 months after nontraumatic brain injury and 1 year after traumatic brain injury.
    - Likelihood of meaningful recovery is very low beyond these time periods.
    - Important for prognostication and informed decision-making by the patient's legally authorized representative.

Any unambiguous sign of clinical perception or deliberate action is incompatible with the vegetative state and prolonged observation is required before concluding that apparent wakefulness is unaccompanied by awareness. The diagnosis of vegetative state should only be rendered by medical practitioners with appropriate training and experience in assessing the nervous system.

Etiology and pathophysiology

- Traumatic brain injury.
- Hypoxic–ischemic injury (usually post-cardiac arrest).
- Stroke: hemorrhagic, malignant hemispheric infarction.
- Hypoglycemia.
- Intracranial infection: encephalitis, meningitis.
- Brain tumor.
- End stage of neurodegenerative disorder: Alzheimer's disease.

TABLE 8 **DIFFERENTIAL DIAGNOSIS OF VEGETATIVE STATES**

	Locked-in syndrome	Minimally conscious state	Vegetative state	Coma	Brain death
Awareness	Intact but difficult to confirm	Intact but impaired	Absent	Absent	Absent
Wakefulness	Intact	Intact	Intact	Absent	Absent
Motor function	Quadriplegic	Variable with purposeful movements	Reflexive, nonpurposeful	Absent or reflex posturing	Absent or spinal reflexes only
Brainstem and respiratory function	Intact breathing, preserved vertical eye movement and eyelid movement	Intact	Intact	Variably impaired	Absent
EEG activity	Usually normal	Nonspecific slowing	Delta, theta, or slow alpha	Polymorphic delta or theta, burst suppression	Electrocerebral silence
Evoked potentials	Brainstem evoked responses variable, cortical evoked responses usually normal	Brainstem evoked responses and cortical evoked responses usually normal	Brainstem evoked responses normal, cortical evoked responses variable	Brainstem evoked responses variable, cortical evoked responses often absent	Absent
Brain metabolism	Normal or nearly normal	Reduced, secondary areas can be stimulated	≥50% reduction	≥50% reduction	Absent cortical metabolism
Prognosis	Depends on cause	Variable	Variable	Depends on cause	No recovery

The pathophysiology involves:

- Severe diffuse injury of cortical neurons, thalami or white matter tracts connecting the thalami and cortex, sparing the brainstem and hypothalamus.
- Traumatic injuries in general affect the white matter more than the gray matter, nontraumatic injuries generally have the opposite trend.

Differential diagnosis *(Table 8)*

- Locked-in syndrome (see below): usually a brainstem lesion disrupting voluntary control of extremity, facial, and horizontal ocular movement but awareness is preserved.
- Coma: usually evolves into the vegetative state when prolonged.
- Brain death: irreversible loss of all brain functions including the brainstem.
- Akinetic mutism: a state of profound apathy with evidence of awareness and attentive visual pursuit that is usually due to lesions involving the medial frontal lobes.
- Minimally conscious state (see below).

Prognosis

Prognosis for regaining awareness is worse if the vegetative state is due to a nontraumatic injury as compared to traumatic brain injury. The longer the vegetative state persists, the lesser the chance of recovery. The probability of recovery of awareness is <1% after 3 months in nontraumatic vegetative states and after 12 months in post-traumatic vegetative states.

MINIMALLY CONSCIOUS STATE[12]

Definition

A state of impaired consciousness where patients are in a chronic state of impaired responsiveness but retain some demonstrable awareness.

Clinical criteria

- Global impaired responsiveness.
- Limited but unequivocal evidence of awareness of self and environment as indicated by the presence of one or more of the following behaviors:
  - Following simple commands.
  - Gestural or verbal responses to yes/no questions.
  - Intelligible verbalization.
  - Purposeful behavior: movements or behaviors that occur in response to environmental stimuli that are not reflexive, e.g. reaching for objects, touching and holding objects in a way that accommodates the size and shape of the object, sustained visual tracking of moving objects, smiling or crying appropriately to linguistic or visual content.

Etiology and pathophysiology

Similar to persistent vegetative state but less extensive.

Prognosis

There are few reliable indicators of prognosis in the minimally conscious state. Among patients who are initially in a minimally conscious state after traumatic brain injury, up to 50% will regain independent function at 1 year.

LOCKED-IN SYNDROME

Definition

A de-efferented state in which patients are aware of themselves and their environment but are unable to respond due to loss of motor and speech function.

Etiology and pathophysiology

Ventral brainstem lesion

- Infarction or hemorrhage (commonly hypertensive patients) (**104, 105**).
- Tumor.
- Demyelination (multiple sclerosis).
- Central pontine myelinolysis, following profound hyponatremia.
- Head injury.

Polyneuropathy

- Critical illness polyneuropathy.
- Acute onset post-infectious polyradiculoneuropathy (Guillain–Barré syndrome).

Pathophysiology involves:

- A supranuclear (upper motor neuron) lesion of the descending corticospinal tracts, usually in the ventral portion of the brainstem (commonly the pons), below the level of the IIIrd cranial nerve nuclei, causes paralysis of the muscles innervated by the lower cranial nerves and peripheral nerves.
- A widespread nuclear or infranuclear (lower motor neuron) disease of motor nerves.

104 Plain (non-contrast) cranial CT scan showing high density in the basilar artery (due to thrombus, red arrow) and an area of low density in the ventral pons and due to ventral pontine infarction (yellow arrow) in a patient who presented 'locked-in'.

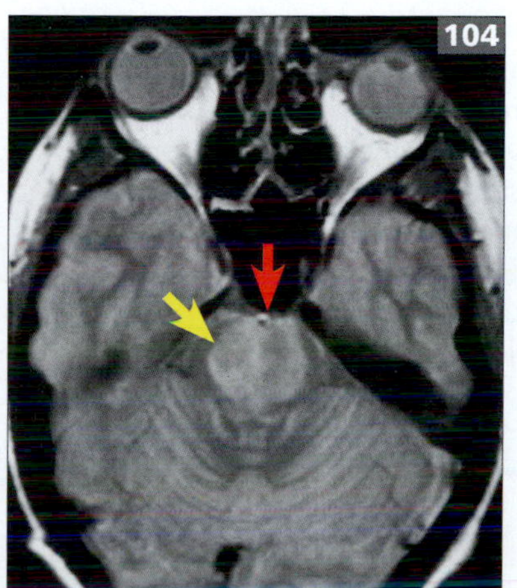

105 Autopsy specimen of a cross-section of the midpons and cerebellum in the axial plane of a patient who was 'locked-in' showing hemorrhagic infarction in the ventral pons bilaterally.

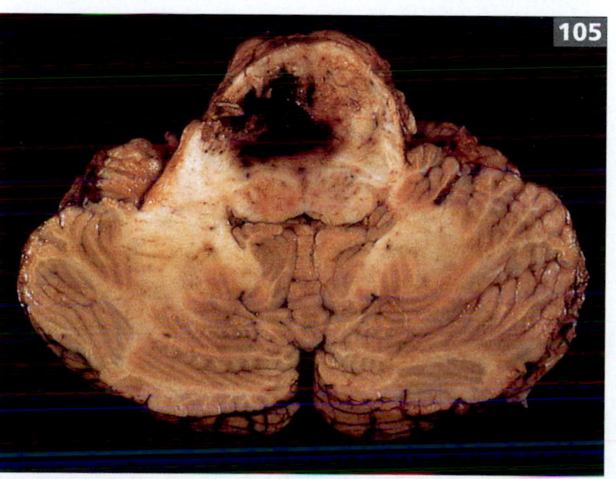

Clinical features

- Unable to speak.
- Unable to move the limbs.
- Awareness and consciousness are preserved because the brainstem tegmentum, including the reticular formation, and oculomotor nerves and pathways are spared.
- Able to open the eyes and move them (particularly in the vertical plane) and blink, in order to try to communicate.

Investigations

- CT or MRI brain scan: ventral pontine or midbrain lesion.
- Other investigations, as appropriate, to ascertain the cause (e.g. serum sodium, EEG, electromyography [EMG]).

Diagnosis

Diagnosis is clinical, based on the presence of total paralysis of the limbs and muscles innervated by the lower cranial nerves, but with the ability of the patient to open and close the eyes voluntarily and in response to commands, and to respond to verbal and sensory stimuli by blinking or by vertical eye movements.

Treatment

Caregivers should be aware that patients can see, hear, and feel and are sensitive to what staff are saying. They are also very frustrated that they cannot move. Prevention of complications of immobility is important, such as pneumonia, deep vein thrombosis, contractures, and urinary tract infection. Rehabilitation includes physiotherapy, swallowing and speech therapy, occupational therapy, and psychologic support and therapy. Computerized devices can be used to facilitate communication. Specific treatment involves treating the underlying cause.

Prognosis

Prognosis is poor. Some patients recover, usually with residual limb spasticity.

SYNCOPE

Definition and epidemiology

A transient loss of postural tone and consciousness resulting from an acute reduction in blood flow to the brain.

- Incidence: 6.2/1000 person-years in the Framingham study.
- Prevalence: 19% among adults. The most common nonepileptic cause of loss of consciousness.
- Age and gender: any age and either sex.

Pathophysiology

Basic neurophysiology

The conscious state depends on the integrity of the brainstem reticular activating system interacting (through its ascending pathways) with both cerebral hemispheres. Therefore, to disturb consciousness, the function of the brainstem or both cerebral hemispheres needs to be disturbed (see 'Approach to impaired consciousness').

Basic vascular physiology

Blood flow to the brain depends on the mean arterial blood pressure and the ICP. Blood pressure (BP) is the product of the cardiac output (heart rate × stroke volume) and total peripheral resistance. Blood flow in the brain is maintained by autoregulation in response to minor changes in systemic BP. However, sudden, dramatic reductions in BP below a mean arterial BP of about 6.5 kPa (50 mmHg) result in a parallel fall in brain perfusion, resulting in a loss of consciousness.

Etiology

In descending order of frequency:

- Neurally mediated reflex syncope:
  - Vasovagal syncope.
  - Carotid sinus syndrome.
  - Situational faints (e.g. pain, coughing, micturition, post-prandial, brass instrument playing).
  - Post-exercise.
  - Glossopharyngeal and trigeminal neuralgia.
- Orthostatic syncope:
  - Secondary autonomic failure (e.g. diabetic or amyloid neuropathy, drugs, alcohol).
  - Hypovolemia (e.g. dehydration, hemorrhage, Addison's disease).
  - Primary autonomic failure (e.g. autoimmune dysautonomia, Shy–Drager syndrome, or multisystem atrophy).
  - Postural intolerance syndrome.

- Cardiac arrhythmias:
  - Sinus node dysfunction
  - Atrioventricular conduction defects.
  - Paroxysmal supraventricular or ventricular arrhythmias (including long QT syndrome, Brugada syndrome, short QT, arrhythmogenic right ventricular dysplasia).
  - Device (pacemaker or implanted cardioverter-defibrillator) dysfunction or proarrhythmogenic drugs.
- Structural cardiopulmonary disease:
  - Acute myocardial infarction or ischemia.
  - Valvular heart disease.
  - Obstructive cardiomyopathy.
  - Acute aortic dissection.
  - Pumonary embolism/pulmonary hypertension.
  - Atrial myxoma.
  - Pericardial tamponade/ constrictive pericarditis.
- Cerebrovascular:
  - Basilar migraine.
  - Vascular steal syndromes.

Clinical assessment

History

The history should be directed firstly toward confirming that the patient has syncope, and secondly towards finding the cause. Interview the patient and a witness if available.

Precipitating/contributory factors

- Venesection, acute pain or emotional shock, prolonged standing, overcrowding, heat (vasovagal syncope).
- Valsalva maneuver: deliberate or during weight lifting, playing a wind or brass musical instrument, or straining at stool.
- Coughing.
- Micturition.
- Changes in posture (e.g. standing after sitting or lying in bed for a prolonged period) and head position.
- Drugs (nitrates, α-adrenoreceptor blockers [venodilators]; diuretics [low blood volume]).
- Hot environment (vasodilatation of cutaneous vessels).
- Large meal (vasodilatation of splanchnic vessels).

Pre-syncopal symptoms

- Lightheadedness.
- Faintness.
- 'Dizziness' (not vertigo).
- Dimming or loss of vision in both eyes (not to be confused with lone bilateral blindness), sounds seem to be distant/muffled.
- Generalized weakness.
- Symptoms of adrenergic activity such as nausea, hot and cold feelings, and sweating.
- Palpitations and chest pain may indicate a cardiac cause, but palpitations are also common in panic attacks and overbreathing.
- Absence of prodromal symptoms and sudden onset may be suggestive of a cardiac conduction defect rather than vasovagal syncope.

Associated features during the attack

- Pale (rather than cyanosed).
- Sweaty/clammy.
- Floppy (rather than rigid).
- Pulse: absent or difficult to feel (but this cannot be relied upon).
- Incontinence of urine may occur.
- Motor symptoms, such as a brief tonic contraction of the trunk, tonic–clonic movements, and multifocal, arrhythmic, myoclonic jerks may occur, particularly if an upright or semi-upright posture is maintained.

Duration

Syncope lasts seconds to 1 or 2 minutes, provided the patient assumes the recumbent position, and isn't held upright (by someone or an obstacle).

Sequelae

As consciousness is regained quickly there is very little mental confusion or difficulty recalling the warning symptoms (unless there has been head trauma), in contrast to the prolonged confusion, drowsiness, and myalgia that may be seen after a generalized seizure. Convulsive syncope may occur following prolonged vagal stimulation (causing pronounced bradycardia or asystole) with or without a prolonged upright posture. The patient becomes pale and falls limply, followed by a stiffening of the body or opisthotonous, clonic movements, upward deviation of the eyes, and urinary incontinence. It is common, particularly in children and young adults, and affects girls more commonly than boys.

Systemic enquiry

- Autonomic symptoms: bladder, bowel, sexual, and thermoregulatory dysfunction.
- Extrapyramidal symptoms: slowness, stiffness, tremor.
- Polyneuropathy: altered sensation, weakness.
- Medications/drugs: hypotensive agents.

Physical examination

The physical examination is commonly normal. Skin and mucous membranes are dry with reduced tissue turgor if dehydrated, pigmented buccal mucosa if Addison's disease.

Cardiovascular

- Pulse: rate, rhythm, character.
- BP: supine and standing. A fall in diastolic BP of 1.3 kPa (10 mmHg) and systolic BP of 2.7 kPa (20 mmHg) or more in the standing position is defined as postural hypotension.
- Jugular venous pressure: low if hypovolemic, raised if pulmonary embolism or cardiac failure.
- Heart: auscultation for features of aortic stenosis and other causes of outflow obstruction (e.g. hypertrophic obstructive cardiomyopathy).
- Serial pulse and standing BP over 30 minutes. Normally, the pulse increases to a maximum at the 15th beat after standing but with autonomic failure, loss of consciousness may occur without a recordable increase in the peripheral pulse rate or the presence of skin vasoconstriction.

Neurologic

- Extrapyramidal dysfunction: rigidity, bradykinesia, tremor.
- Brainstem dysfunction.
- Peripheral neuropathy: muscle wasting, weakness, areflexia, sensory loss.

TABLE 9 **DIFFERENTIAL DIAGNOSIS SYNCOPE vs. EPILEPTIC SEIZURE**

	Syncope (faints)	Seizures (fits)
Onset	Often gradual	Sudden
Circumstances	Special	Nonspecific
Relation to upright posture	Common	No
Symptoms	Lightheaded/ faint	Amnesic
	Blurred/dimmed vision	
	Sounds seem distant	
	Tinnitus	
	Weakness	
	Nausea	
	Hot and cold	
	Sweating	
Skin colour	Pale	Blue or normal
Respiration	Shallow	Stertorous
Aura or premonitory symptoms	Usually	Sometimes
Tone	Floppy*	Rigid
Convulsion	Rare	Common
Urinary incontinence	Rare**	Common
Tongue biting	Rare	Common
Post-ictal confusion	Minimal	Common and prominent
Focal neurologic symptoms	No	Occasional
Clues to underlying cause	Cardiac arrhythmia	
	Aortic stenosis	
	Cardiomyopathy	
	Postural hypotension	

* A tonic phase is common in convulsive syncope.

** Traditionally not a feature, but actually not uncommon.

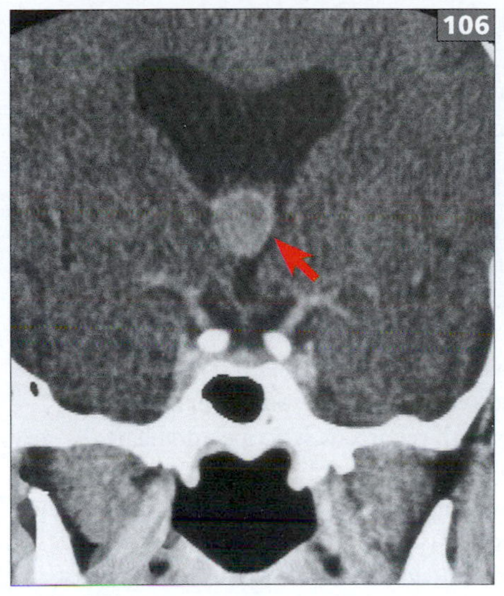

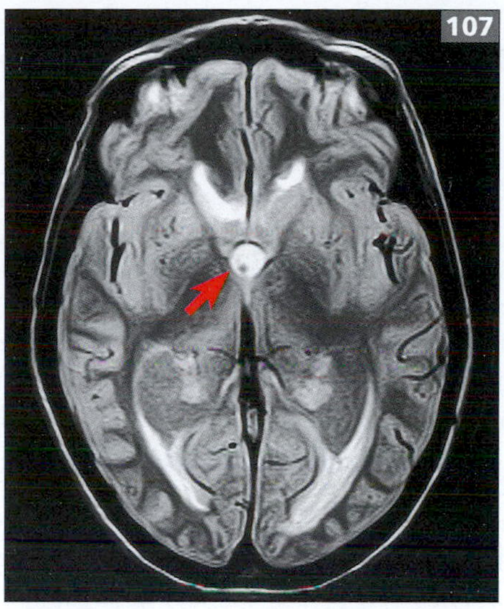

106 Contrast-enhanced CT brain scan, coronal plane, showing a colloid cyst of the third ventricle as a round hyperintense mass lesion (arrow), causing obstructive hydrocephalus.

107 MRI brain scan, coronal plane, showing a colloid cyst of the third ventricle (arrow).

Differential diagnosis

- Epilepsy (see *Table 9*).
- Vertebrobasilar artery territory ischemia: seldom causes isolated loss of consciousness; other symptoms of focal brainstem ischemia coexist: vertigo, diplopia, ataxia. Carotid territory ischemia does not cause loss of consciousness unless bilateral and severe.
- Drop attacks:
  - Spontaneous episodic raised ICP may impair brain perfusion (e.g. colloid cyst of the third ventricle [106, 107], posterior fossa tumor). Usually associated headache and visual obscurations.
  - Cryptogenic drop attacks: abrupt episodes of falling to the ground without any warning, precipitating factor, or loss of awareness. Usually in middle-aged women and benign.
- Metabolic disorders:
  - Hypoglycemia: usually in diabetics but may be caused by insulinoma, Addison's disease, and post-gastrectomy. Tends to occur after fasting. Associated symptoms may include sweating and a sensation of hunger.
  - Pheochromocytoma: episodic release of catecholamine may lead to transient palpitations, headache, sweating, and hypotension. Many patients have postural hypotension due to chronic excess secretion of catecholamines, but rarely causes syncope.
  - Hyperventilation-induced alkalosis.
- Sleep disorders:
  - Narcolepsy: excessive daytime sleepiness.
  - Cataplexy: sudden onset of focal or generalized loss of muscle tone, often precipitated by emotion such as laughter, and resulting in either episodic limb weakness or sudden collapse from an upright position.
  - Obstructive sleep apnea.
- Psychiatric: pseudoseizures.

Investigations

The history, physical examination, and electrocardiogram (ECG) are the core of the diagnostic work-up. In most patients, there is an obvious precipitant and no investigations are required, or at most an ECG and hemoglobin. For example, syncope in the elderly often results from polypharmacy and abnormal physiologic responses to daily events. The need for further investigations is determined by the certainty of the clinical diagnosis and nature of the clinical findings.

Cardiologic

These are indicated in patients with known or suspected heart disease (e.g. history of congestive heart failure or ventricular arrhythmia), exertional syncope, and recurrent syncope.

Noninvasive

- ECG: to exclude complete heart block, an aberrant conduction pathway, and an acute cardiac event (**108, 109**).
- 24-hour ambulatory or patient-activated ECG recording (Holter monitoring) can be useful if the attacks are frequent enough to be captured and the patient is known to have, or is suspected of having, heart disease. However, it may fail to detect arrhythmias if they do not occur during the monitoring period, and increasing the period of monitoring only slightly improves sensitivity. If an arrhythmia is detected (e.g. frequent ventricular ectopic beats) but it is associated with no symptoms, it does not prove that the arrhythmia is the cause of the syncope. Nevertheless, the arrhythmia may point to an underlying structural heart disease.
- Implantable loop recorder: is extremely valuable when events are infrequent.
- Echocardiography: if valvular heart disease, outflow obstruction, or cardiomyopathy is suspected.
- Carotid sinus stimulation under ECG control: aims to detect carotid sinus hypersensitivity but is of limited use. It should be performed with the patient lying supine. A period of more than 3 seconds of asystole on ECG monitoring is positive, although this response is nonspecific, being present in up to 20% of the asymptomatic population.
- Upright tilt table testing: a method of diagnosing vasovagal syncope in patients with frequent recurrent undiagnosed syncopal events but no heart disease, and patients with recurrent syncope and heart disease but no evidence of arrhythmias. The technique involves constant ECG recording and BP monitoring while the patient is brought from a supine to an upright position(e.g. 70° head-up tilt) in a series of stages, and maintained in that position, in the absence of drugs, for up to 40 minutes.

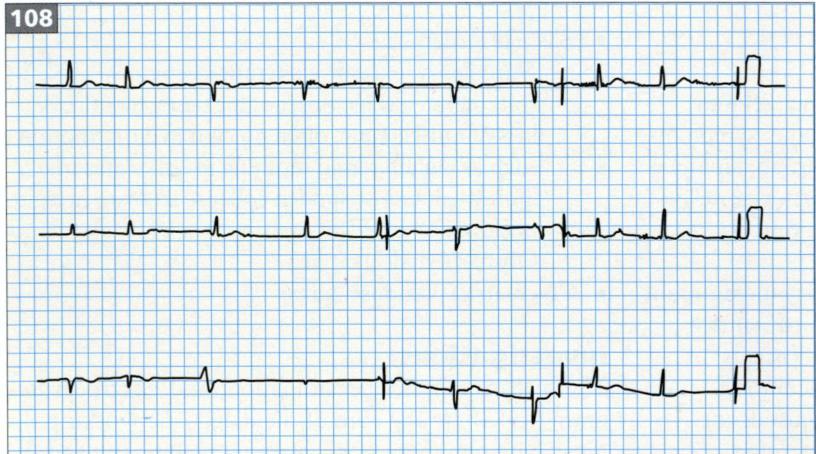

108 Electrocardiograph (ECG) showing slow atrial fibrillation with a ventricular rate of about 45 per minute.

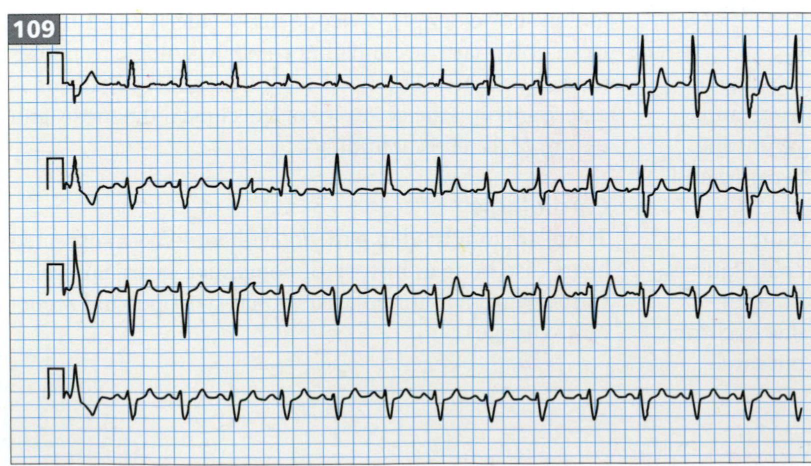

109 Electrocardiograph (ECG) showing bifascicular block (a combination of right bundle branch block and left anterior hemiblock) due to coronary artery disease in a 70-year-old man who presented with three episodes of collapse due to cardiac syncope related to paroxysmal bradycardia. Electrophysiologic studies failed to induce clinically significant tachycardia and the patient responded well to permanent pacemaker insertion. Bifascicular block can develop into complete conduction block due to trifascicular block or complete AV block.

- The test is positive if there is syncope or presyncope in association with hypotension and/or bradycardia.
- The sensitivity of this test is up to 70%, but the specificity is uncertain. If there is no abnormal response, an isoprenaline (isoproterenol) infusion can be given to improve sensitivity further (at the expense of specificity). It is begun at 1 µg per minute and the rate progressively increased every 5 minutes by a further microgram per minute at successive tilts. The isoprenaline (isoproterenol) infusion initially increases the heart rate and then the rhythm may change from sinus to another rhythm (e.g. junctional rhythm), resulting in a fall in BP and symptoms of syncope. The symptoms resolve with resumption of the supine posture.
- The test is again positive if there is syncope or presyncope in association with hypotension and/or bradycardia.

Invasive

- Electrophysiologic studies directly assess intracardiac conduction and the presence of inducible supraventricular and ventricular arrhythmias by intracardiac stimulation. Although invasive, the morbidity is low (1–2%) and mortality very low. It may be indicated if recurrent and disabling syncopal episodes, clinical suspicion of an arrhythmia, abnormal resting ECG, arrhythmias on Holter monitoring, and structural heart disease are identified.
- Blood: basic laboratory tests are not usually helpful and should be minimized:
  - Hemoglobin level may reveal anemia.
  - Serum urea and electrolytes and glucose may reveal the most common metabolic causes.
  - Prolonged fast to exclude hypoglycemia.
  - Short tetracosactrin (cosyntropin) test to exclude Addison's disease.
- Urine: 24-hour urine collection for vanillylmandelic acid to exclude pheochromocytoma.
- Neurologic: this is rarely helpful unless additional neurologic symptoms or signs are present:
  - CT or MRI brain scan: if there are drop attacks or a suspected Arnold–Chiari malformation, hydrocephalus, colloid cyst of the third ventricle, or subdural hematoma.
  - EEG (combined with simultaneous ECG monitoring) if there is a suspected seizure disorder. A positive EEG may support the diagnosis of epilepsy but a negative study does not exclude it.
  - Nerve conduction studies and EMG if neuropathy is suspected.
  - Autonomic function tests.
- Biopsy: rectal, if amyloidosis is suspected (rare).
- Psychiatric: occasionally a psychiatric assessment may be useful in patients with otherwise unexplained frequent syncopal events and no injury, as patients with anxiety disorders, panic reaction, and somatization disorders may report syncope as a symptom.

TABLE 10 **FINDINGS RAISING A SUSPICION OF CARDIAC SYNCOPE**

HISTORY
Acute or prior myocardial infarction
Heart failure
Syncope on exertion or in supine position
Palpitations
PHYSICAL EXAMINATION
Irregular heart beat
Evidence of structural heart disease or heart failure
ELECTROCARDIOGRAM
Second or third-degree atrioventricular block
Severe bradycardia
Pre-excitation syndrome (e.g. Wolff–Parkinson–White syndrome)
Prolonged or short QT interval
Brugada pattern
Findings suggestive of a myocardial infarction, Brugada syndrome, or arrhythmogenic right ventricular dysplasia.

Diagnosis

The key to the diagnosis of syncope is a sound clinical history from the patient and an eyewitness. Findings raising a suspicion of cardiac causes of syncope are listed in *Table 10.*

Treatment

Treatment aims to identify and correct the specific underlying cause. In most patients with infrequent episodes, whose syncope was due to the simultaneous occurrence of several predisposing factors (e.g. dehydrated, tired, hot and stuffy room), an explanation and reassurance is all that is required. Any metabolic and hormonal deficiencies should be corrected.

Neurally mediated reflex syncope

Patients should be educated about recognizing and responding to prodromal symptoms to avoid injury. Patients with recurrent syncope who are aware of prodromal symptoms may benefit from physical counter measures such as squatting, arm-tensing, leg-crossing, and leg-crossing with lower-body tensing. Strategies to reduce long-term recurrence of syncope include:

- Physical techniques to improve orthostatic tolerance, such as home 'tilt-training' techniques, where patients are instructed to stand and place only the upper back against the wall, starting with 3–5 minutes daily and progressively increasing the duration over the next 10–12 weeks.
- Pharmacologic interventions, including volume expanders such as fludrocortisone and vasoconstrictors such as midodrine.
- Cardiac pacing is indicated in carotid sinus syndrome and older patients with documented asystole during the episode.

Orthostatic hypotension

- Any drugs that may cause postural hypotension should be stopped (if possible), particularly in the elderly. These include diuretics (particularly in hot weather), α-adrenoreceptor blockers (e.g. prazosin), psychotropic drugs with α-adrenoreceptor blocking activity (tricyclic antidepressants, antipsychotics, including prochlorperazine), α-methyldopa, nitrovasodilators (e.g. glyceryl trinitrate, including long-acting formulations), and antiparkinsonian drugs (L-dopa, bromocriptine).
- Avoid large meals, especially when accompanied by alcohol.
- Change posture, from supine to standing, slowly (avoid sudden changes).
- Waist-high supportive garments (e.g. elasticated stockings) or antigravity suits may be helpful for venous pooling, but can be uncomfortable.
- Elevate the head of the bed at night.
- High-salt diet.
- Prophylactic medication such as the mineralocorticoid fludrocortisone in low dose; sympathomimetics such as ephedrine and midodrine; caffeine; nonsteroidal anti-inflammatory drugs such as indomethacin, if there is no contraindication; ergot alkaloids, theophylline, β-adrenoreceptor antagonists with intrinsic sympathomimetic activity; disopyramide and octreotide (somatostatin analogue).

Cardiac arrhythmias

Treatment is based on the underlying abnormality. Pacemakers are effective for bradyarrhythmias, while for tachyarrhythmias, invasive electrophysiologic mapping studies followed by ablation can be effective. If not possible, a combination of antiarrhythmic drugs and implanted pacemakers or cardiovertor-defibrillator must be considered.

Structural cardiopulmonary disease

Severe valvulopathies, such as critical aortic stenosis or mitral stenosis, can be treated with surgery. Medical management and possibly cardiac pacing may be indicated for patients with hypertrophic obstructive cardiomyopathy.

Cerebrovascular syncope

Cerebrovascular steal syndromes can be treated with surgical or endovascular techniques.

Prognosis

Prognosis depends upon the underlying cause; it is benign in many cases, a warning sign of sudden death in a minority of others. Sudden death occurs within the next year in about 20% of patients with syncope, due to ischemic or structural heart disease. The spontaneous remission rate is high and the rate of sudden death is low in patients with unexplained syncope after intensive investigation.

HYPOXIC–ISCHEMIC ENCEPHALOPATHY

Definition and epidemiology

Brain dysfunction caused by a global lack of oxygen and blood flow to the brain as a result of failure of the circulation or respiration.

- Incidence: uncommon.
- Age: middle-aged and elderly.
- Gender: either sex.

Pathophysiology

Acute, global brain hypoxia (110–112)

- Laminar cortical necrosis (**110**): extensive, multifocal or diffuse, and almost invariably involving the hippocampus.
- Scattered small areas of infarction or neuronal loss may be present in the deep forebrain nuclei, hypothalamus, or brainstem. Sometimes, relatively selective thalamic necrosis occurs.
- Most, if not all, of the gray matter of the cerebral, cerebellar, and brainstem structures, and even the spinal cord, is severely damaged if the hypoxia is severe enough and prolonged.

Delayed post-anoxic encephalopathy

- Demyelination throughout the subcortical white matter of the cerebral hemispheres.
- Necrosis of the globus pallidus.

Tip

► *The above features can occur in any patient with hypoxia and are not predictors of delayed anoxic encephalopathy.*

Etiology

- Reduced oxygen saturation of hemoglobin.
- Suffocation:
  - Aspiration of blood or vomitus.
  - Compression of the trachea by hemorrhage or a surgical pack.
  - Obstruction of the trachea by a foreign body.
  - Drowning.
  - Status asthmaticus.
  - Strangulation.
  - Altitude sickness.

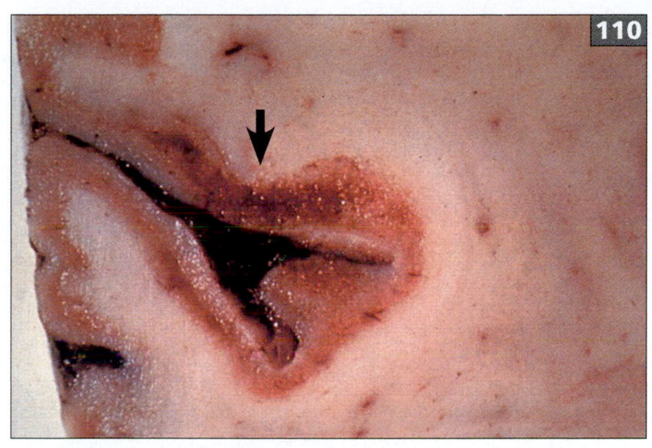

110 Section of the cerebral cortex showing laminar necrosis due to cerebral hypoxia (arrow). *Courtesy of Professor BA Kakulas, Royal Perth Hospital, Western Australia.*

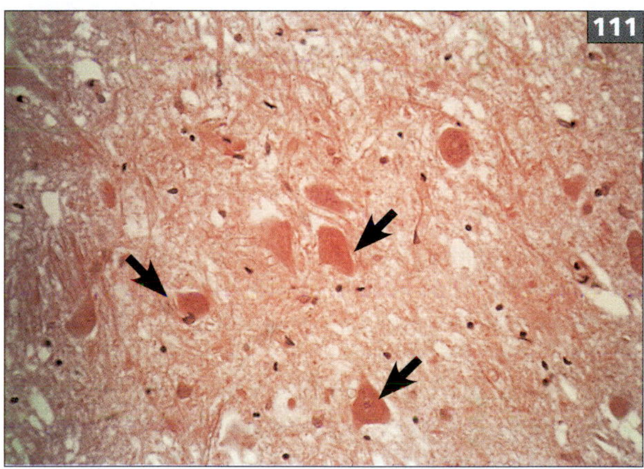

111 Hypoxic neurons in the brain (arrows): swollen, more eosinophilic, indistinct outline, faint-staining nuclei, and loss of Nissl substance.

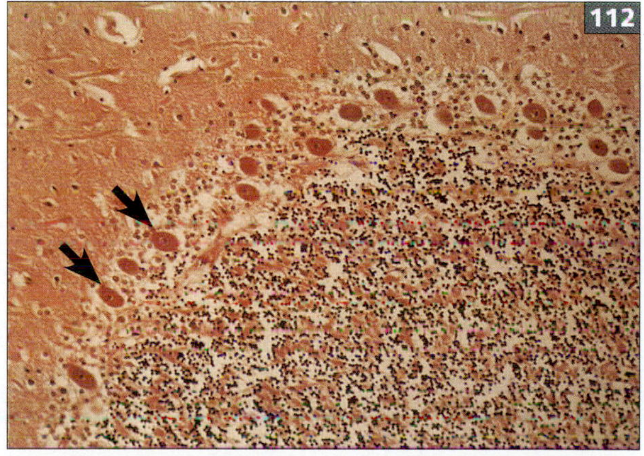

112 Hypoxic, eosinophilic Purkinje cells in the cerebellum (arrows).

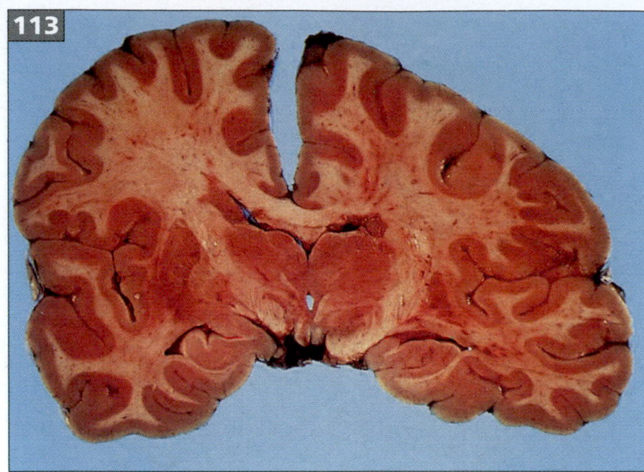

113 **Cross-section of the brain in the coronal plane at post mortem, showing a diffuse pink coloration due to vasodilatation induced by cerebral anoxia in a patient who died from carbon monoxide poisoning.** *Courtesy of Professor BA Kakulas, Royal Perth Hospital, Western Australia.*

- Carbon monoxide poisoning (**113**): carbon monoxide binds to hemoglobin 200 times more avidly than oxygen. It is obtained from:
  - Car exhaust fumes.
  - Fumes from incomplete combustion of fossil fuels, particularly in poorly ventilated heating systems.
  - Household gas where natural gas is not used.
  - Metabolic conversion of methylene chloride that is found in paint strippers.
- Respiratory paralysis:
  - Guillain–Barré syndrome.
  - Poliomyelitis.
- Diffuse central nervous system (CNS) disease (trauma, vascular disease, metabolic/toxic encephalopathy, including drug overdose).
- Reduced cerebral perfusion.
- Shock:
  - Cardiac arrest during inhalation or spinal anesthesia.
  - Myocardial infarction.
  - Massive systemic hemorrhage.
  - Septicemia.
- Delayed post-anoxic demyelination.
- Partial arylsulphatase A deficiency predisposes susceptible individuals to delayed post-hypoxic leukoencephalopathy and implicates lactic acidosis in its pathogenesis.

Pathophysiology

Although the brain only weighs 1300–1400 g (46–49 oz) (2% of total adult body weight), it consumes about 20% of the total oxygen consumption of the body at rest. If the brain is deprived of any oxygen for longer than about 5 minutes, some brain cells become permanently damaged. The persistence and severity of the neurologic damage reflect the site of ischemia, the duration and severity of the anoxic insult, and the metabolic demands of the cells (e.g. hypothermia lowers metabolism and prolongs the tolerable period of hypoxia).

The brain cells which are most vulnerable to hypoxia are neurons, followed in order of decreasing sensitivity by oligodendroglia, astrocytes, and endothelial cells. The most vulnerable neurons to mild hypoxia are the pyramidal neurons in the CA1 and CA4 zones of the hippocampus, followed by neurons in the cerebellum, striatum, and neocortex. Consequently, cerebral anoxia manifests itself as clinical features of dysfunction of these neurons (i.e. amnesia, bradykinesia, rigidity, dystonia, choreoathetosis, and bilateral corticospinal tract involvement).

Clinical features

Mild hypoxia

Mild hypoxia can occur from insults such as mountaineering or chronic low level carbon monoxide poisoning. Symptoms and signs include:

- Inattentiveness, irritability, fatigue, headache, nausea, and mild confusion.
- Poor judgment.
- Motor incoordination.

There are no lasting clinical effects other than a slight decline in visual and verbal long-term memory and mild aphasic errors in some people. Degrees of hypoxia that at no time abolish consciousness rarely, if ever, cause permanent damage to the nervous system.

Moderate hypoxia

After a short period of coma, consciousness is regained and some patients pass quickly through an acute post-hypoxic phase, characterized by variable degrees of confusion, visual agnosia, or any one of several types of movement disorder (e.g. action or intention myoclonus, extrapyramidal rigidity, choreoathetosis) and proceed to make a complete recovery. Others, however, are left with permanent neurologic sequelae of various combinations of one of the post-hypoxic syndromes:

- Persistent coma or stupor (see below).
- Visual agnosia.
- Dementia with or without extrapyramidal signs.
- Extrapyramidal (parkinsonian) syndrome with or without cognitive impairment.

- Choreoathetosis.
- Cerebellar ataxia.
- Action or intention myoclonus.
- Korsakoff amnesic state.
- Seizures may or may not persist.

Severe but not sustained hypoxia

Initially patients are comatose with eyes slightly divergent and motionless, pupils reactive, limbs inert and flaccid or rigid, and tendon reflexes that are diminished. Within a few minutes of restoring cardiac action and breathing, generalized convulsions and muscle twitches (myoclonus) may occur. Coma and decerebrate postures persist, or the latter occur in response to painful stimuli, and bilateral extensor plantar responses can be elicited.

After about 1 week or more, the eyes open, initially in response to pain and later spontaneously, the eyelids blink in response to any threat to the eye, and the eyes rove around inattentively. The patient is unaware of the surroundings and may manifest chewing movements and grinding of teeth, and groan and grunt. Swallowing is possible. Body posture may be decorticate or decerebrate. Primitive reflexes such as pouting and sucking reflexes, grasp reflex, and withdrawal reflexes to pain are present. Plantar responses are extensor. The individual may survive in this vegetative state (mute, unresponsive, and unaware of the environment) for weeks, months or years (see p. 93).

Severe and sustained hypoxia

This occurs after insults such as cardiac arrest. It may result in brain death.

Special forms

Delayed post-anoxic encephalopathy[13]

Encephalopathy usually manifests 1–4 weeks after acute anoxic exposure, though the interval may be as short as 1 day and as late as 7 weeks.

- Epidemiology: rare; middle-aged and elderly are usually affected.
- Etiology: most commonly reported with carbon monoxide exposure.
- Pathophysiology: uncertain. There is pseudodeficiency of arylsulphatase A, and reversible alteration of CSF γ-aminobutyric acid (GABA) and dopamine concentrations following recovery, which may have pathogenic implications.
- Clinical features: most patients have severe anoxia with deep coma when found, but regain consciousness within 24 hours and resume full activity in 4–5 days. One to 4 weeks later, the clinical triad develops of mental deterioration (apathy, confusion, irritability, and occasionally agitation or mania), sphincteric incontinence, and gait disturbances consequent to frontal lobe and basal ganglia dysfunction. Examination reveals dementia, pseudobulbar palsy, and parkinsonism, and other frontal lobe signs of grasp reflex, glabella tap, and retropulsion, and extrapyramidal signs of short steppage gait, masked face, and rigidity.
- Differential diagnosis: many cases are mistakenly diagnosed as suffering from psychiatric disturbances.
- Investigations. Imaging: CT and MRI show bilaterally symmetric extensive hemispheric subcortical demyelination. Symmetric lesions in the region of the globus pallidus suggest a poor outcome.
- Pathology: there is characteristic subcortical white matter demyelination with necrosis of globus pallidus.
- Treatment and prognosis: no specific therapy is known, but the majority (50–75%) recover spontaneously. Some patients experience persisting late sequelae including memory disturbances and parkinsonism; in others the neurologic syndrome progresses with weakness, shuffling gait, diffuse rigidity and spasticity, incontinence, coma, and death after 1–2 weeks; rarely, the hypoxic episode is followed by a slow deterioration over weeks to months until the patient is mute, rigid, and helpless.

Differential diagnosis

- Anesthesia.
- Drug intoxication.
- Hypothermia.
- Psychiatric disturbance.

Investigations

- Blood: carboxyhemoglobin level (<10% is not symptomatic).
- EEG: may be normal or show a spectrum of diffuse generalized polymorphic theta or delta activity which may be of very low voltage and not attenuated by sensory stimulation. The EEG may become isoelectric. Epileptiform activity is unusual.

Imaging

CT may show diffuse white matter low density, low density in the globus pallidus, and parenchymal atrophy. Carbon monoxide poisoning produces a similar picture but with more basal ganglia involvement, seen as symmetric low density.

MRI brain shows increased signal throughout the white matter on T2-weighted imaging and proton density-weighted (PDW) imaging. Carbon monoxide poisoning produces a similar picture but with more basal ganglia involvement, seen as symmetric increased signal in the globus pallidus (**114**).

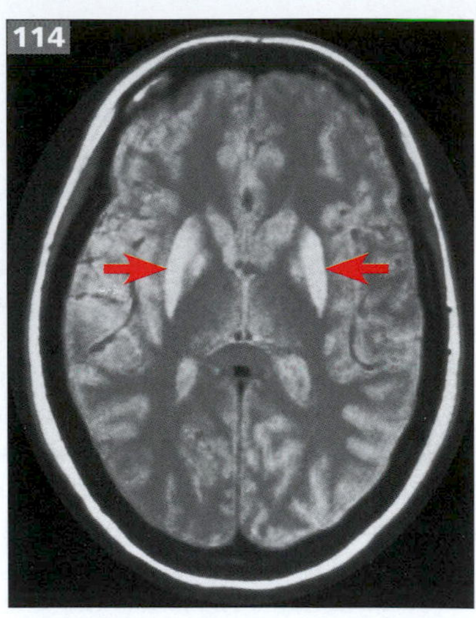

114 PDW axial MRI through the basal ganglia showing increased signal (arrows) typical of carbon monoxide poisoning. *Courtesy of Dr R Sellar, Department of Neuroradiology, Western General Hospital, Edinburgh, UK.*

Diagnosis

Hypoxic encephalopathy

A history of a hypoxic episode with evidence of a cardiac arrest, sustained BP below 9.3 kPa (70 mmHg) systolic, reduced oxygenation of arterial blood, or carbon monoxide poisoning (cherry red colour of skin) and the typical clinical sequence of events as outlined above aids the diagnosis.

Carbon monoxide poisoning

The diagnosis is made by measuring the blood carboxyhemoglobin level (<10% is not symptomatic) in patients with any of the above symptoms from chronic headache to coma, if unexplained.

Treatment

Post-cardiac arrest

- General measures include standard intensive care treatment.
- Monitoring includes:
  - General intensive care monitoring, e.g. BP, O_2 saturation, continuous ECG, urine output, temperature, and so on.
  - Advanced hemodynamic monitoring, e.g. echocardiography and cardiac output monitoring.
  - Cerebral monitoring, e.g. EEG, CT/MRI.
- Hemodynamic optimization: the aim is to achieve a mean arterial BP of 65–100 mmHg, central venous pressure of 8–12 mmHg, central venous oxygenation saturation ($S_{cv}O_2$) >70%, urine output >1 ml/kg/hr, and normal or decreasing serum lactate. O_2 saturation is ideally maintained at 94–96% and normocarbia achieved.
- Treat dysrhythmias, hypotension, and low cardiac index.
- Consider coronary angiography and percutaneous coronary intervention if indicated.

Two randomized clinical trials and a meta-analysis showed improved outcome in comatose survivors of out-of-hospital ventricular fibrillation cardiac arrest who underwent therapeutic hypothermia[14,15]. Patients were cooled to a range of 32–34°C (89.6–93.2°F) for 12–24 hours. Induction of hypothermia can be instituted with IV ice-cold fluids or ice packs on the groin, armpits, neck, and head. Surface or intravenous cooling devices can also be used. Maintenance of hypothermia is best achieved with external or internal cooling devices with continuous temperature feedback to achieve the desired target temperature. Slow rewarming at 0.25–0.5°C per hour is recommended. Shivering can be treated with sedation and neuromuscular blockade.

Complications, including electrolyte abnormalities, arrhythmias, hyperglycemia, coagulopathy, and immune suppression, should be anticipated and managed appropriately. Seizures should be treated as appropriate, if they occur.

Carbon monoxide poisoning

Hyperbaric oxygen may restore consciousness more rapidly and completely than normobaric oxygen.

Prognosis

Degrees of hypoxia that at no time abolish consciousness rarely, if ever, cause permanent damage to the nervous system. Prognostication has been best studied in coma after cardiac arrest.

Clinical factors

The bedside neurologic examination is one of the most reliable and widely validated predictors of functional outcome. Previous studies have concluded that absent pupillary or corneal reflexes at 72 hours have a 0% false-positive rate (95% CI: 0–9%), and absent motor response at 72 hours has a 5% false-positive rate (95% CI: 2–9%) for poor outcome[16]. However, these estimates may not be applicable to post-cardiac arrest patients treated with hypothermia[17].

Status myoclonus is associated with poor outcome.

Neurophysiologic tests

Bilaterally absent N20 component of the median nerve somatosensory evoked potentials (SSEP) from 24 hours to 1 week after cardiac arrest is a predictor of poor outcome. EEG patterns associated with poor outcome include generalized voltage suppression to <20 μV, burst suppression pattern with generalized epileptiform activity, and generalized periodic complexes on a flat background.

Neuroimaging

Diffuse cortical abnormalities on diffusion-weighted imaging or fluid attenuated inversion recovery (FLAIR) sequences are associated with poor outcome when considered in the context of clinical factors.

Biochemical markers

Elevated levels of biochemical markers, such as neuro-specific enolase and S100β at days 1–3, have also been used as predictors of outcome. However, the exact cut-off values for accurate prognosis have not yet been fully validated.

The prognostic indicators discussed above have not been validated in patients treated with therapeutic hypothermia.

CENTRAL PONTINE MYELINOLYSIS

Definition and epidemiology

Central pontine myelinolysis (CPM) is a disorder characterized by rapidly developing quadriparesis and a large, symmetric, demyelinating lesion of the greater part of the basis pontis. It may also affect extrapontine brain areas.

- Prevalence: up to 0.25% of autopsies.
- Age: any age; reported in children (particularly those with severe burns) as well as adults.
- Gender: either sex.

Etiology and pathophysiology

CPM is sporadic. Specific regions of the brain, such as the centers of the basis pontis, have a special susceptibility to acute osmotic shifts (possibly to rapid correction or to overcorrection of hyponatremia, and possibly hyperosmolality), analogous perhaps to the selective vulnerability of the corpus callosum and anterior commissure in Marchiafava–Bignami disease.

Myelinolysis is more likely to occur after the treatment of chronic rather than acute hyponatremia, and is more likely to occur with a rapid rate of correction. The exact pathogenesis has not been determined but rapid osmotic shifts are thought to be responsible.

Risk factors

- Hyponatremia: with rapid correction of severe hyponatremia (<130 mEq/l [<130 mmol/l]) to normal or higher than normal levels of serum sodium.
- Extreme serum hyperosmolality.
- Nutritional deficiency.
- Serious, often life-threatening, medical illness including sepsis, renal failure, and organ transplantation.

Clinical features

Patients are usually already very ill.

Predisposing illness

- Vomiting.
- Cachectic patients from a variety of causes.
- Chronic alcoholics.
- Chronic renal failure treated by dialysis.
- Hepatic failure.
- Advanced malignancy.
- Severe bacterial infection.
- Dehydration and electrolyte disturbances, particularly hyponatremia.
- Acute hemorrhagic pancreatitis.
- Pellagra.

Variable clinical illness

CPM has a subacute onset with a biphasic course over several days, usually after correction of hyponatremia, of:

- Mental changes ranging from mild confusion to coma, followed by a second phase occurring 2–7 days later, comprising of:
  - Pseudobulbar palsy.
  - Flaccid or spastic quadriparesis.
  - Extensor plantar responses bilaterally.
  - Conjugate eye movements may be limited and nystagmus may be present.
  - Pupillary reflexes, eye movements, corneal reflexes, and facial sensation are spared.
- Locked-in syndrome:
  - Absent or transient mild neurologic symptoms and signs may be all that are seen if the pontine lesion is small, extending only 2–3 mm on either side of the median raphe nucleus and involving only a small portion of the corticopontine or pontocerebellar fibers.
  - Coma may be present due to underlying metabolic or other associated disease which obscures the presence of central pontine myelinolysis.

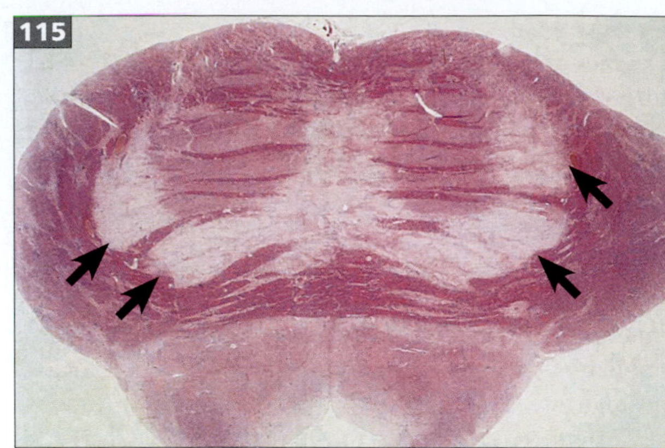

115 Transverse section of the pons showing demyelination of corticospinal tract fibers in the center of the basis pontis (arrows) with preserved neurons on the pontine nuclei and no evidence of inflammation.

Differential diagnosis

- Stroke due to brainstem infarction:
  - Sudden onset or step-like progression.
  - History of vascular risk factors (atheroma) or neck trauma (dissection).
  - Asymmetry of long tract signs.
  - Caused by basilar artery occlusion.
  - More extensive involvement of tegmental structures of pons as well as midbrain and thalamus.
- Multiple sclerosis (MS): massive pontine demyelination in acute or chronic relapsing MS may rarely produce a pure basis pontis syndrome, but other features of this disease provide the clue to the correct diagnosis (see Ch. 14).
- Post-infectious encephalomyelitis.
- Hyponatremic encephalopathy: a generalized encephalopathy without localizing motor signs. Usually there is a distinct interval between the occurrence of a generalized hyponatremic encephalopathy initially which improves with elevation of the sodium level and then, about 2–3 days after hyponatremia is corrected, the neurologic syndrome of myelinolysis evolves. However, sometimes the hyponatremic encephalopathy does not improve before focal myelinolytic symptoms emerge and it can be difficult to recognize that two separate disease processes are occurring sequentially.
- Psychiatric illness: the common initial symptoms of myelinolysis (mutism, dysarthria, lethargy, and affective changes) may be mistaken for psychiatric/psychologic illness.

Investigations

- Full blood count: for infection.
- Urea and electrolytes: for hyponatremia, renal failure.
- Liver function tests: for chronic alcoholism, liver failure.
- Amylase: for pancreatitis.
- CT brain scan: there may be low density throughout the pons, basal ganglia, hemispheric white matter, without mass effect or enhancement.
- MRI brain scan is more sensitive than CT. Increased signal is visible in the pons, with a thin rim of normal signal around the margins of the pons and possible sparing of the corticospinal tracts, which leaves two rounded normal signal areas within the high signal of the pons. There may also be increased signal in the thalami, putamen, caudate nuclei, amygdala, and hemispheric white matter. Diffusion-weighted imaging can demonstrate abnormalities as early as 24 hours after symptom onset.
- Brainstem auditory evoked potentials.

Diagnosis

- Clinical: a gravely ill patient with a general medical disease who develops a quadriplegia, pseudobulbar palsy, and locked-in syndrome over a few days.
- Radiologic: a lesion in the center of the basis pontis consistent with demyelination.

Pathology

Demyelination occurs in the center of the pons (**115**) and occasionally other parts of the brainstem.

Macroscopic

Grayish discoloration and fine granularity are seen in the center of the basis pontis. The lesion may be only a few millimeters in diameter or it may occupy almost the entire basis pontis. The lesion may extend posteriorly to involve the medial lemnisci and, in most advanced cases, other tegmental structures as well: superiorly to encroach on the midbrain, inferiorly to the pontomedullary junction; and anteriorly, but there is always a rim of intact myelin between the lesion and the surface of the pons.

Particularly extensive pontine lesions may be associated with identical myelinolytic foci symmetrically distributed in the thalamus, subthalamic nucleus, striatum, internal capsule, amygdaloid nuclei, lateral geniculate body, white matter of the cerebellar foliae, and deep layers of the cerebral cortex and subjacent white matter ('extrapontine myelinolysis').

Microscopic

Destruction of myelin is seen throughout the lesion, with relative sparing of the axis cylinders and neuronal cell bodies. These changes always begin and are most severe in the geometric center of the lesion, where they may proceed to frank necrosis of tissue. Macrophages containing cytoplasm laden with myelin debris are present throughout the demyelinative focus, with loss of oligodendroglia and no significant inflammatory response.

Treatment

Treatment is mainly supportive (be aware that 'locked-in' patients can see, hear, and feel everything [including pain and itch] but are incredibly frustrated that they cannot move). There should be active treatment of the underlying medical illness, and prevention of complications of immobility, including pneumonia, deep vein thrombosis, contractures, and urinary tract infection.

Rehabilitation includes physiotherapy, swallowing and speech therapy, occupational therapy, and psychologic support and therapy.

Prevention

Optimal management of hyponatremia patients involves weighing the risk for illness and death from untreated hyponatremia against the risk for myelinolysis due to correction of hyponatremia. Chronic hyponatremia should be corrected by no more than 10 mEq/l (10 mmol/l) in any 24-hour period.

Prognosis

The outcome of CPM varies. Some patients die, many make a gradual but partial recovery with residual sequelae that include bulbar dysfunction, spastic quadriparesis, movement disorders, behavioral changes, and alterations in cognition, while others recover completely. Some patients remain in a state of mutism and paralysis with relatively intact sensation and comprehension, i.e. the 'locked-in' syndrome.

REFERENCES

1 Wijdicks EFM, Bamlet WR, Maramattom BV, *et al.* (2005). Validation of a new coma scale: The FOUR score. *Ann Neurol* **58**:585–593.
2 Frontera JA (2012). Metabolic encephalopathies in the critical care unit. *Continuum* (Minneap Minn) **18**:611–639.
3 Brouns R, De Deyn PP (2004). Neurological complications in renal failure: A review. *Clin Neurol Neurosurg* **107**:1–6.
4 Munoz SJ (2008). Hepatic encephalopathy. *Med Clin North Am* **92**:795–812.
5 Young GB (1995). Neurological complications of systemic critical illness. *Neurol Clin* **13**:645–658.
6 Perry PJ, Wilborn CA (2012). Serotonin syndrome vs. neuroleptic malignant syndrome: a contrast of causes, diagnoses, and management. *Ann Clin Psychiatry* **24**:155–162.
7 Davies NW, Sharief MK, Howard RS (2006). Infection-associated encephalopathies: their investigation, diagnosis, and treatment. *J Neurol* **253**:833–845.
8 Ducros A (2012). Reversible cerebral vasoconstriction syndrome. *Lancet Neurol* **11**:906–917.
9 Ropper AH (1986). Lateral displacement of the brain and level of consciousness in patients with an acute hemispheral mass. *N Engl J Med* **314**:953–958.
10 Fisher CM (1995). Brain herniation: a revision of classical concepts. *Can J Neurol Sci* **22**:83–91.
11 Quality Standards Subcommittee of the American Academy of Neurology (1995). Practice Parameters: assessment and management of patients in the persistent vegetative state. *Neurology* **45**:1015–1018.
12 Giacino JT, Ashwal S, Childs N, *et al.* (2002). The minimally conscious state: definition and diagnostic criteria. *Neurology* **12**:349–353.
13 Custodio CM, Basford JR (2004). Delayed post-anoxic encephalopathy: a case report and literature review. *Arch Phys Med Rehabil* **85**:502–505.
14 Bernard SA, Gray TW, Buist MD, *et al.* (2002). Treatment of comatose survivors of out-of-hospital cardiac arrest with induced hypothermia. *N Engl J Med* **346**:557–563.
15 The Hypothermia After Cardiac Arrest (HACA) study group (2002). Mild therapeutic hypothermia to improve the neurologic outcome after cardiac arrest. *N Engl J Med* **346**:549–556.
16 Levy DE, Caronna JJ, Singer BH, *et al.* (1985). Predicting outcome from hypoxic-ischemic coma. *JAMA* **253**(10):1420–1426.
17 De Georgia M, Raad B (2012). Prognosis of coma after cardiac arrest in the era of hypothermia. *Continuum* (Minneap Minn) **18**:515–531.

Further reading

Coma

Bateman DE (2001). Neurological assessment of coma. *J Neurol Neurosurg Psychiatry* **71**(Suppl 1):il3–il7.

Bates D (1993). The management of medical coma. *J Neurol Neurosurg Psychiatry* **56**:589–598.

Stevens RD, Bhardwaj A (2006). Approach to the comatose patient. *Crit Care Med* **34**:31–41.

Zeman A (2001). Consciousness. *Brain* **124**:1263–1289.

Brain death

Heran MKS, Heran NS, Shemie SD (2008). A review of ancillary tests in evaluating brain death. *Can J Neurol Sci* **35**:409–419.

Wijdicks EFM, Varelas PN, Gronseth GS, *et al.* (2010). Evidence-based guideline update: Determining brain death in adults: Report of the Quality Standards Subcommittee of the American Academy of Neurology. *Neurology* **74**:1911–1918.

Persistent vegetative state and minimally conscious state

Bernat JL (2010). Current controversies in states of chronic unconsciousness. *Neurology* **75**(S1):S33–S38.

Bernat JL (2006). Chronic disorders of consciousness. *Lancet* **367**:1181–1192.

Syncope

Benditt DG, Nguyen JT (2009). Syncope: therapeutic approaches. *J Am Coll Cardiol* **53**:1741–1751.

Wieling W, Thijs RD, van Dijk N, Wilde AAM, Benditt DG, van Dijk JG (2009). Symptoms and signs of syncope: a review of the link between physiology and clinical cues. *Brain* **132**:2630–2642.

Hypoxic encephalopathy

Holzer M, Bernard SA, Hachimi-Idrissi S, *et al.* (2005). Hypothermia for neuroprotection after cardiac arrest: Systemic review and individual patient data meta-analysis. *Crit Care Med* **33**:414–418.

Neumar RW, Nolan JP, Adrie C, *et al.* (2008). Post-cardiac arrest syndrome: epidemiology, pathophysiology, treatment, and prognostication. A Consensus Statement from the International Liaison Committee on Resuscitation (American Heart Association, Australian and New Zealand Council on Resuscitation, European Resuscitation Council, Heart and Stroke Foundation of Canada, InterAmerican Heart Foundation, Resuscitation Council of Asia, and the Resuscitation Council of Southern Africa); the American Heart Association Emergency Cardiovascular Care Committee; the Council on Cardiovascular Surgery and Anesthesia; the Council on Cardiopulmonary, Perioperative, and Critical Care; the Council on Clinical Cardiology; and the Stroke Council. *Circulation* **118**:2452–2483.

Central pontine myelinosis

Kleinschmidt-DeMasters BK, Rojiani AM, Filley CM (2009). Central and extrapontine myelinolysis: Then ... and now. *J Neuropathol Exp Neurol* **65**:1–11.

Kumar S, Fowler M, Gonzalez-Toledo ED, Jaffe SL (2006). Central pontine myelinolysis, an update. *Neurol Res* **28**:360–366.

EPILEPSY

Paul V. Motika
Andres M. Kanner

DEFINITION

Epilepsy is a disease that has been recognized in all cultures for millennia as evidenced by the multiple references to epileptic patients and seizures throughout written history. The word epilepsy itself is derived from the Greek *epilambanein* or *epilamvanein*, meaning to 'seize' or 'be seized,' or to be 'attacked'. In *The Sacred Disease*, Hippocrates and his contemporaries describe epilepsy in detail, including the cardinal clinical features of epileptic seizures that are recognized in modern medicine. Accurate descriptions of epilepsy and ictal psychoses have been identified in ancient Babylonian texts, and descriptions of epilepsy are also found in ancient Byzantium, ancient China, ancient India, and the Bible, amongst others.

Epilepsy is a heterogeneous disorder of the central nervous system (CNS) characterized by recurrent seizures (at least two seizures, or one seizure in the presence of electrographic evidence of epileptiform activity). Seizure is the term used to describe a paroxysmal event characterized by stereotypic signs and symptoms resulting from abnormal electrical brain activity. The clinical manifestations can vary widely, depending on the source and propagation pattern of the epileptic activity and engagement of eloquent cortex, resulting in motor, sensory, psychic, emotional, autonomic, and cognitive signs and symptoms. Epilepsy must be distinguished from acute symptomatic seizures which result from a provoking factor, in the absence of which seizures will cease to occur.

The lifetime risk of individuals (expected to live up to the age of 80) to develop epilepsy is approximately 3.4%[1]. While the occurrence of seizures is the primordial clinical manifestation of epilepsy, comorbid psychiatric and cognitive disturbances are frequent clinical expressions of this disease, and their treatment is as important as that of the actual seizures.

EPIDEMIOLOGY

A number of studies have been published world-wide estimating epilepsy prevalence and incidence in various populations. There are inherent difficulties in performing these studies including variations in terminology and classification, reporting biases, access to health-care, and social stigma. Additionally, the methodology for such studies ranges from examination of records to self-reporting or interviews.

In the USA, a population-based study of epilepsy in Rochester, Minnesota, from 1940–1980 estimated a prevalence from 2.7/1000 in 1940 to 6.8/1000 in 1980, adjusted to 1980 population numbers[2]. In Mississippi in 1978, Haerer *et al.* estimated active prevalence by door-to-door survey at about 6.8/1000[3], and in a multi-racial and multi-ethnic community in New York City in 2007, Kelvin *et al.* reported prevalence of self-reported active epilepsy at 5.2/1000[4]. In South America, Lavados *et al.* estimated the overall prevalence of epilepsy in Chile in 1988 at 17.7/1000[5]. Other prevalence studies in Europe and Asia have found comparable figures using a variety of methodologies.

Incidence studies are similarly variable in methodology and classification. The incidence in some of the North American studies discussed above range from approximately 16 to 61 per 100,000. Higher values are seen (112 per 100,000) if the incidence of all afebrile seizures is measured. Incidence also varies widely in studies performed outside the USA, though are generally comparable. In both incidence and prevalence, differences are often seen in subcategories such as gender (males being typically more affected) and age, though the differences are not always statistically significant.

PATHOPHYSIOLOGY

Epilepsy can be divided into lesional and nonlesional forms, with the former representing those epilepsy syndromes that occur as a result of pathologic mechanisms identifiable with either structural or functional neuroimaging studies (e.g. magnetic resonance imaging [MRI] and positron emission tomography [PET]), while the latter consists of the (many) forms of epilepsy with no obvious identifiable underlying lesion. Many of these are thought to have underlying genetic pathogenic mechanisms.

Epileptic activity is thought to result from an imbalance of synaptic excitation (mediated by neurotransmitters such as glutamate) and inhibition (modulated by neurotransmitters such as gamma aminobutyric acid [GABA]), though the pathogenic role played by other neurotransmitters such as serotonin, norepinephrine, and dopamine has been recently recognized.

Ion channel disturbances (sodium, potassium, chloride, calcium) have been identified as important pathogenic mechanisms in the epilepsies, which may act in parallel with the neurotransmitter disturbances cited above and which have become the target of pharmacologic therapy. For example, rapid sodium channel blockade constitutes one of the most frequent mechanism of action of a large number of antiepileptic drugs (AEDs) (e.g. phenytoin, carbamazepine, lamotrigine). Any insult to the brain and/or genetic disturbance that disrupts the normal flow of electrochemical signals is a potential generator of seizure activity.

Genetic disturbances may be associated with generalized epilepsies (e.g. idiopathic generalized epilepsies) or epilepsies of focal origin (e.g. adult nocturnal frontal lobe epilepsy or familial temporal lobe epilepsy). Genetic disturbances associated with a progressive encephalopathic process may lead to treatment-resistant epilepsies (e.g. progressive myoclonic epilepsies), while those that occur in the absence of an encephalopathic process are often identified in epilepsies of benign prognosis (e.g. idiopathic generalized epilepsy presenting as childhood absence epilepsy or juvenile myoclonic epilepsy [JME]).

Some common acquired lesions which may lead to seizures include: 1) ischemia/stroke (particularly when hemorrhagic); 2) neoplasms (both benign and malignant); 3) arteriovenous malformations (including cavernous angiomas); 4) infection; 5) malformations of cortical development; 6) CNS trauma (**116–118**).

The severity of the seizure disorder is a function of age, location and extent of insult or epileptogenic lesion, and course of the etiologic process. Pathologies vary between developed and developing countries, as well as between geographic regions. For instance, in India and central and south American countries, neurocystercircosis is the most frequent cause of seizures. Epileptic disorders presenting as generalized epilepsies are more common in children while those resulting from a focal insult to the CNS are more frequent in adults.

Seizures can occur in the context of systemic processes such as drug and alcohol intoxication or withdrawal, metabolic derangements, and eclampsia of pregnancy. In these cases, seizures may be considered provoked, and may not necessarily indicate future risk of developing epilepsy.

Epilepsy in special age groups

Children

Among pediatric populations, a wide range of epilepsy syndromes is seen which is not present in other age groups. Pediatric epilepsy syndromes vary from the benign and often self-limited epilepsies (e.g. Rolandic epilepsy of childhood, benign neonatal familial convulsions) to the extremely severe and devastating syndromes and epileptic encephalopathies (e.g. West syndrome, Ohtahara syndrome [early infantile epileptic encephalopathy with suppression burst], Landau–Kleffner syndrome [acquired epileptic aphasia]).

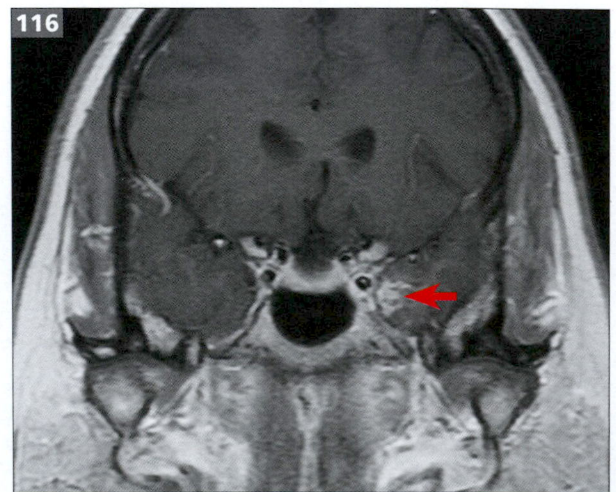

116 Coronal MRI showing left temporal cavernous hemangioma (arrow).

Several of the idiopathic generalized epilepsy syndromes (e.g. childhood absence epilepsy, juvenile absence epilepsy, JME) are age-related (and differentiated by age of onset), and most commonly diagnosed in childhood, adolescence, or early adult years. These syndromes are typically characterized by the absence of focal neurologic symptoms and signs, and a normal interictal electrographic background. Prognosis and treatment is generally favorable. Genetic factors are thought to play a large role in these syndromes.

Localization-related epilepsy syndromes in pediatric populations, unlike in adults, often tend to be extratemporal in nature.

The elderly

The incidence of epilepsy in the elderly is higher than in any other age group, and continues to increase. It is estimated that 1–2% of the aging population has epilepsy, and this may be under-recognized[6].

Diagnosis may be more difficult as seizures may present atypically in this population; symptoms may be vague, and include memory problems, confusion (episodic or prolonged), syncope, sleep disturbances, mood disorders (such as anxiety and panic), and so on. These symptoms are often misdiagnosed as other neurologic and medical conditions (such as transient ischemic attack [TIA] or cardiovascular disease) that are more common in this population. Accordingly, it is important for the treating neurologist to recognize the possibility of unusual presentations of seizures.

Often the first seizure may occur in the setting of cognitive and psychiatric changes. In addition to treatment of the seizure, a neuropsychologic and neuropsychiatric evaluation should also be undertaken, due to the increased risk of this type of morbidity. Up to 70% of seizures in this population are partial (simple or complex), with or without secondary generalization. New-onset epilepsy tends to be more commonly frontal, whereas in younger adults it is often temporal. In some cases, status epilepticus may be the initial presenting event.

The most common cause of newly diagnosed epilepsy in the elderly is stroke. Other common causes include infection, metabolic etiologies, neoplasm (primary or metastatic), and medication side-effect. Other risk factors include dementia (particularly Alzheimer's disease), head injury, hypertension, and cerebrovascular disease in general. Epilepsy in the elderly typically has a more benign course than in younger adults (depending on the etiology), but is associated with relatively higher mortality.

Special consideration should be given to changes in the pharmacokinetics of AEDs in the elderly. This necessitates alteration of treatment dosing and regimen. In general, treatment should be started at lower doses and titrated more slowly. Care should be given to the selection of AEDs, as side-effects and the risks of drug–drug interactions are higher in this population.

Tip

▶ *Seizures may present with atypical symptoms in elderly patients.*

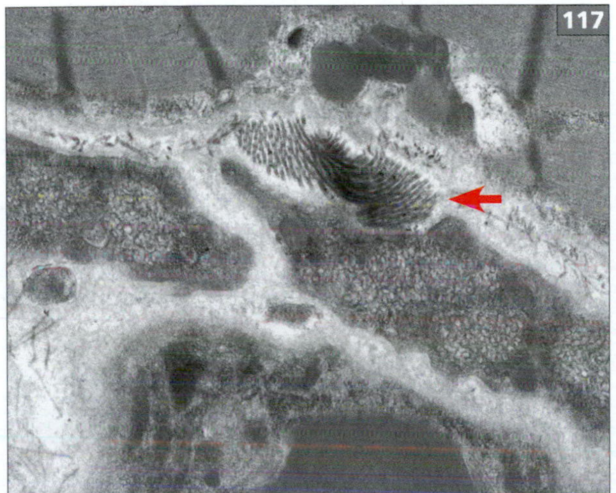

117 Electron microscopy showing curvilinear bodies (arrow) as seen in neuronal ceroid lipofuscinoses.

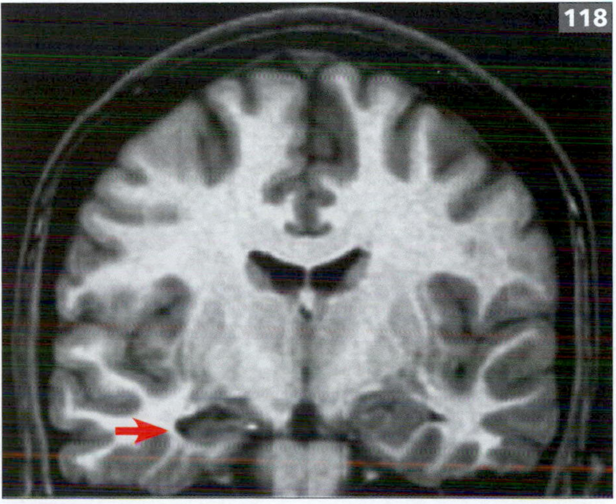

118 Coronal MRI showing right hippocampal atrophy (arrow).

CLASSIFICATION

A clinically useful and accepted classification system for epilepsy is that of the International League Against Epilepsy (ILAE)[7]. This system divides epilepsy into two major divisions: 1) epilepsies of generalized; and 2) of focal onset (localization-related, also known as partial). These divisions are then further divided and separate epilepsies of known etiologies, referred to as symptomatic or 'secondary' epilepsies from those that are idiopathic or 'primary'; a third subdivision refers to 'cryptogenic' epilepsies, where the cause has not been identified. Four classes of syndromes are then derived, which include: 1) localization-related (focal, partial, local) epilepsies and syndromes; 2) generalized epilepsies and syndromes; 3) undetermined epilepsies and syndromes; and 4) special syndromes (**119**).

- Epilepsies of known or suspected etiology are termed 'symptomatic,' and are thought to be the result of (or 'secondary to') another CNS condition, such as a structural lesion or trauma.
- 'Idiopathic' epilepsies have no identifiable underlying cause other than a familial or hereditary etiology (e.g. juvenile absence epilepsy).
- 'Cryptogenic' epilepsies refer to seizure disorders which are presumed to be symptomatic but in which no etiology has been identified (Lennox–Gastaut syndrome is thought to often fit into this category).
- Within this system also exist categories of special syndromes and syndromes whose classification is not yet determined (e.g. Landau–Kleffner syndrome and neonatal seizures).

It is becoming more apparent that these terms ('focal', 'generalized') may be less accurate as we learn more about the genetic, pathophysiologic, anatomic, and neurobiologic factors underlying seizures. For example, high resolution MRI studies in the brain of patients with 'idiopathic' generalized epilepsies have revealed subtle cortical abnormalities in the frontal lobes.

119 Classification of epilepsies[7].

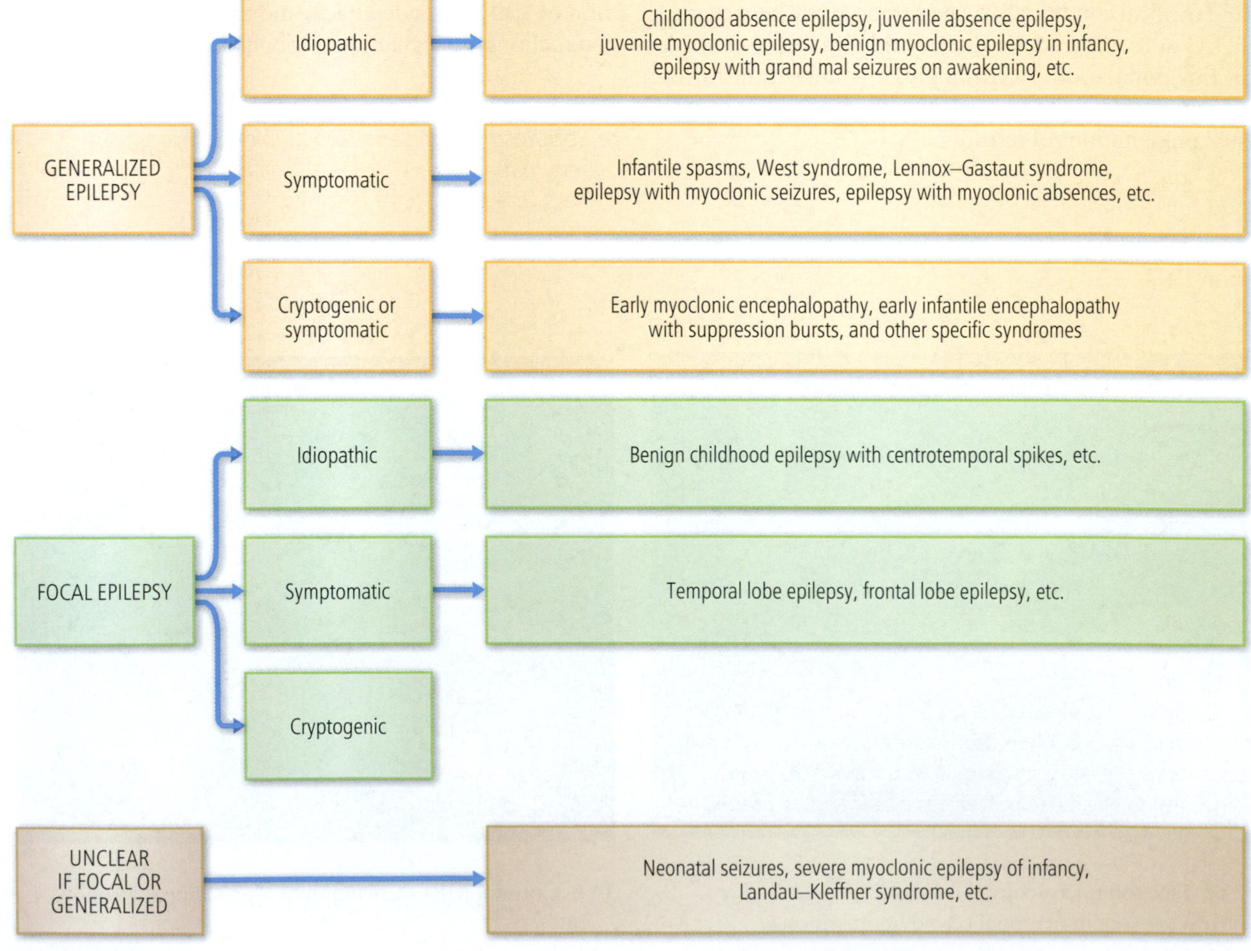

Recent updated guidelines propose the revision of the 1989 classification to be replaced with an approach that emphasizes organization of syndromes and epilepsies in a 'flexible, multi-dimensional manner as appropriate for the specific purpose'. A more fluid approach of classification emphasizing specific features (genetic, molecular, structural, electrographic) of the epilepsy can then be constructed[8]. An excellent review of the precise terminology for describing different types of seizures and clinical manifestations thereof was recently published by Blume and the ILAE[9].

CLINICAL FEATURES

The anatomic and pathophysiologic variation that accounts for the different underlying seizure etiologies also helps to explain their varied clinical presentations and semiologies. Much of our understanding of human neuroanatomy and function is derived from observations made of the anatomic localization of the epileptogenic and symptomatogenic zones. If one uses the basic classification system described, it is apparent that in many cases, the clinical features of seizures can be explained readily based on the location of onset and subsequent propagation of the epileptic activity into adjacent and distant eloquent cortices (**120**). Having said that, this may be an oversimplification, as many seizures are the result of, or contribute to, complex interactions among various neural networks, often making localization based on semiology alone difficult.

Seizures are transient events (excluding recurrent seizures or status epilepticus) which have paroxysmal features. Seizures are extremely variable, and may exist in more than one form even in an individual patient, but should have a somewhat stereotypic presentation. Focal (partial) seizures arise from a distinct area of the brain. They may remain localized, spread to adjacent cortical regions or subcortical structures in the ipsilateral hemisphere, spread to homologous structures in the contralateral hemisphere, or to the entire brain.

Depending on the eloquent cortex (or cortices and subcortical structures engaged by the epileptic activity), focal or partial seizures may have various clinical manifestations including motor, sensory, psychic, and autonomic signs and symptoms. While signs and symptoms are primarily positive, negative signs and symptoms have also been described.

'Simple' partial seizures do not involve any alteration of consciousness. They are often referred to as 'auras'. Auras can be sensory (e.g. a sensation of tingling or numbness), psychic (e.g. feelings of *déjà vu* or *jamais vu*), motor, autonomic (e.g. palpitations or flushing), cognitive, or combinations of all.

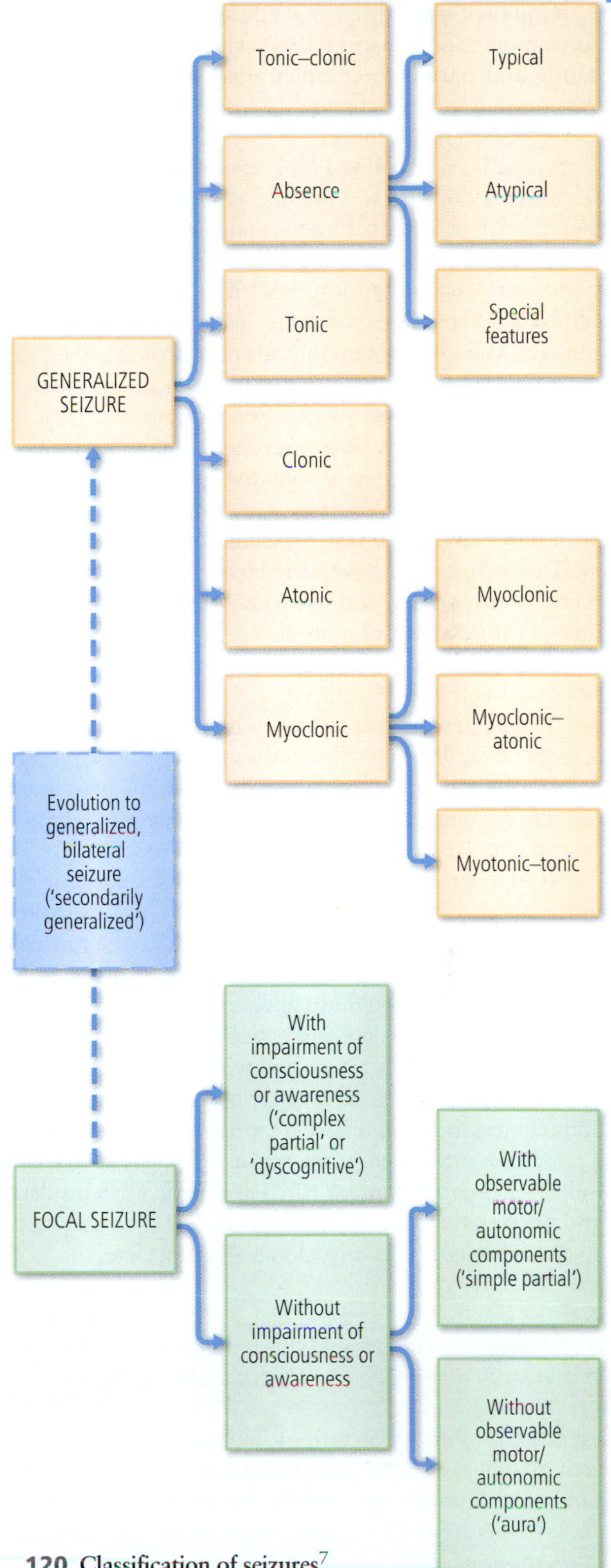

120 Classification of seizures[7].

'Complex' partial seizures affect awareness of one's surroundings or 'consciousness', which may range from subtle and partial to complete loss of consciousness. Patients may fail to recognize the loss of awareness when it is very short in duration.

Secondarily generalized tonic–clonic seizures are focal seizures that may present initially as simple partial, complex partial, or both, before the epileptic activity spreads to the entire brain. Often, however, secondary generalization is very fast and a focal onset may not be identified clinically. Idiopathic or secondary generalized seizures are thought to begin throughout the entirety of the brain at once and can present with motor phenomena (e.g. tonic, clonic, myoclonic, tonic–clonic) or without (e.g. typical and atypical absence). Generalized seizure activity always involve loss or alteration of cognitive function.

Status epilepticus (SE), which will be discussed further, is an important and severe presentation of seizure activity. Definitions of SE have varied over the years, but current consensus is that approximately 5 minutes of continuous seizure activity, or multiple seizures (two) without a return to baseline, constitutes SE. SE may be convulsive or nonconvulsive. Generalized convulsive status epilepticus (GCSE) may present initially with tonic and/or clonic activity, as well as loss of consciousness, but these motor features may become less clinically apparent over time (despite ongoing electrographic seizure activity). Convulsive SE may evolve into nonconvulsive SE (NCSE).

NCSE refers to ongoing electrographic seizure activity in the absence of obvious clinical signs. This can make the diagnosis extremely difficult. NCSE may be further divided into absence, complex partial, and myoclonic SE. Absence SE is thought to have a more benign course, and may respond to less aggressive treatment, whereas complex partial SE is associated with higher morbidity and mortality, as well as underlying neuronal damage, and requires more aggressive treatment. Myoclonic SE is a condition often seen in the setting of severe global or multifocal neuronal injury (such as anoxic CNS insult), and often portends a very poor prognosis. The utility of aggressive treatment of myoclonic SE is not clear.

Tip

▶ *The underlying etiology of status epilepticus is often important in determining treatment and prognosis.*

Pseudo-SE refers to a state of continuous seizure-like activity that is nonepileptic (e.g. psychogenic) in origin. This may be recognized clinically, but continuous electroencephalography (EEG) is often necessary for proper evaluation, as there may be a comorbid occurrence of psychogenic nonepileptic events in patients with actual epilepsy.

It is important from a treatment standpoint to distinguish between the above forms of SE. Continuous EEG (c-EEG) monitoring is virtually always necessary for appropriate diagnosis and treatment, though acquisition of c-EEG should not delay treatment. c-EEG should be continued until there is complete remission of electrographic activity.

DIFFERENTIAL DIAGNOSIS

- Seizures are discrete, paroxysmal events that can result in a variety of clinical symptoms and signs.
- Other neurologic and psychiatric disorders may also present with recurrent episodic events that mimic epileptic seizures, and must be included in the differential diagnosis of any patient being evaluated for a 'presumed' epileptic seizure disorder (*Table 11*).
- One of every four to five patients referred to epilepsy centers around the world with a diagnosis of treatment-resistant epilepsy does not suffer from epilepsy!

Tip

▶ *Nonepileptic events, including psychogenic nonepileptic events, are commonly misdiagnosed as epileptic seizures.*

INVESTIGATION AND DIAGNOSIS

The diagnosis of seizures should be based first and foremost on clinical data. Auxiliary tests should be used as diagnostic tools to confirm or rule out a diagnosis. A complete history of 'presumed' seizures and/or other paroxysmal episodes requires detailed descriptions from the patient whenever possible, and just as importantly from family members or friends that may have witnessed the seizure. Practitioners can often utilize technology to their advantage, asking family members to record the events with video cameras. Family members can also be educated about the typical clinical symptoms associated with seizures and can test the patient during a typical event. A clear description of the events in question, including such elements as positive and negative phenomena ('*Was the patient subsequently able to recall a phrase given during the event?*' '*Was ictal or post-ictal speech present or absent?*') and the reproducible or variable nature of the events is often the most helpful investigational tool.

TABLE 11 COMMON ENTITIES TO BE CONSIDERED IN THE DIAGNOSIS OF SEIZURE

PSYCHOGENIC AND/OR PSYCHIATRIC DISORDERS

Nonepileptic psychogenic spells
- Conversive disorders
- Dissociative disorders
- Factitious disorders
- Panic attacks

ORGANIC NONEPILEPTIC EVENTS

Transient CNS ischemic events
Migraine headaches
Movement disorders:
- Nonepileptic myoclonic syndromes
- Paroxysmal dystonias

Sleep disorders:
- Cataleptic events
- Sleep paralysis
- Obstructive sleep apnea
- Parasomnias
- REM behavior disorder

Syncopal events (vasovagal, cardiogenic)
Cardiac abnormalities (for example, long QT syndrome)
Breath holding spells in children
Laryngospasm secondary to gastroesophageal reflux
Cyclical vomiting
Transient global amnesia
Delirium/encephalopathy
Iatrogenic (tardive dyskinesia)

The first and often most difficult step in the investigation is to establish whether or not the episodes of concern are epileptic or nonepileptic. The clinical history and examination can often sort this out, but other forms of testing can help to support a diagnosis. The second step is to determine what type of epileptic syndrome the patient has. This information is pivotal to plan a rational pharmacologic treatment.

It is important to determine whether the seizure that brings the patient to medical attention is the first epileptic seizure ever experienced by the patient. It is not unusual for patients with a first generalized tonic–clonic seizure to have had unrecognized seizures of a different type for some time (e.g. myoclonic seizures in patients with JME or simple partial seizures in patients with temporal lobe epilepsy). Misdiagnosis of epilepsy as other diseases is not uncommon. One example is the patient presenting with symptoms of recurrent anxiety and 'panic attacks' which are, in fact, the expression of simple partial seizures arising from the mesial temporal structures. If the early signs of seizures are not recognized, then treatment may be delayed.

Auxiliary tests used in the diagnosis of epilepsy include neurophysiologic studies such as EEGs and video-EEG monitoring studies, structural (brain MRI) and functional studies (PET, ictal single photon emission tomography with or without interictal imaging [SPECT], proton magnetic resonance [H1 MRS]). In addition, one should consider evaluating for the presence of comorbid cognitive deficits with a neuropsychologic evaluation, and psychiatric comorbidities with a neuropsychiatric evaluation. These tests should be tailored to the individual clinical situation, and further testing may be required to identify more clearly and treat the epileptic (or nonepileptic) syndrome.

Electroencephalography

EEG is a test that helps to confirm the diagnostic impression made by clinical data. It should never be used as the sole diagnostic tool in the diagnosis of epilepsy (**121–124**, next page). The recordings of interictal epileptiform discharges and of ictal activity are the two electrographic representations of epileptiform activity. Of note, scalp EEG recordings will only detect epileptiform activity that activates (in a synchronous manner) an area equivalent to 6–10 cm^2 of cortex.

A routine EEG is the initial auxiliary test in patients suspected of having epileptic seizures. Any routine EEG ordered for this purpose must include awake and sleep recordings, as epileptiform activity may be activated by sleep. Any EEG study carried out in patients with suspected seizures without sleep recordings is an incomplete study and must be repeated. EEG can be easily obtained in most situations and can quickly confirm the presence or absence of focal abnormalities, including epileptogenic discharges.

The absence of epileptic activity on routine EEG does not preclude the presence of seizures. In fact, EEG recordings of 50% of patients with known epilepsy may not have epileptiform activity in the first EEG study. Epileptiform activity can be identified in 70% of people with epilepsy with a second study, done under sleep-deprived conditions with 2-hour recordings. Between 5 and 10% of EEG recordings of patients with known epilepsy will not reveal epileptiform activity.

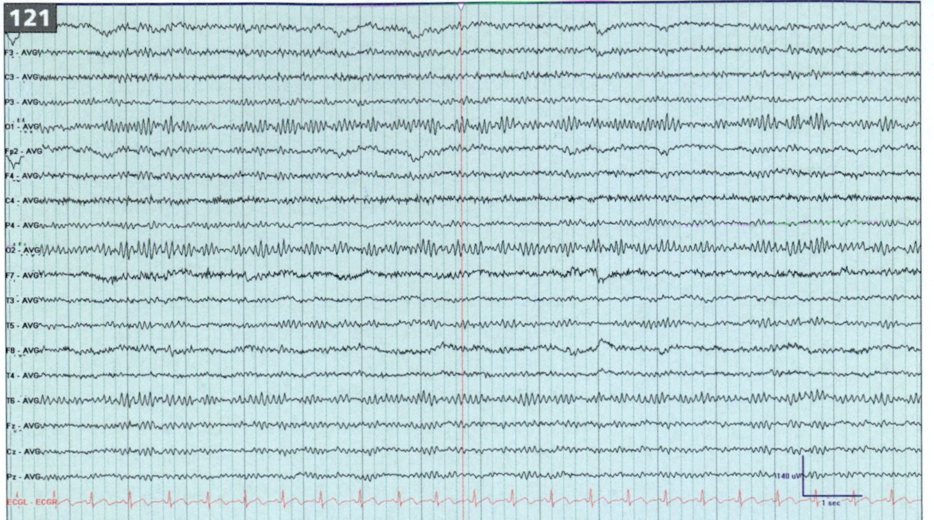

121 Adult EEG (normal) during wakefulness. This recording demonstrates a normal posterior background activity, no slowing, and low voltage, fast (beta) activity in bifrontal regions

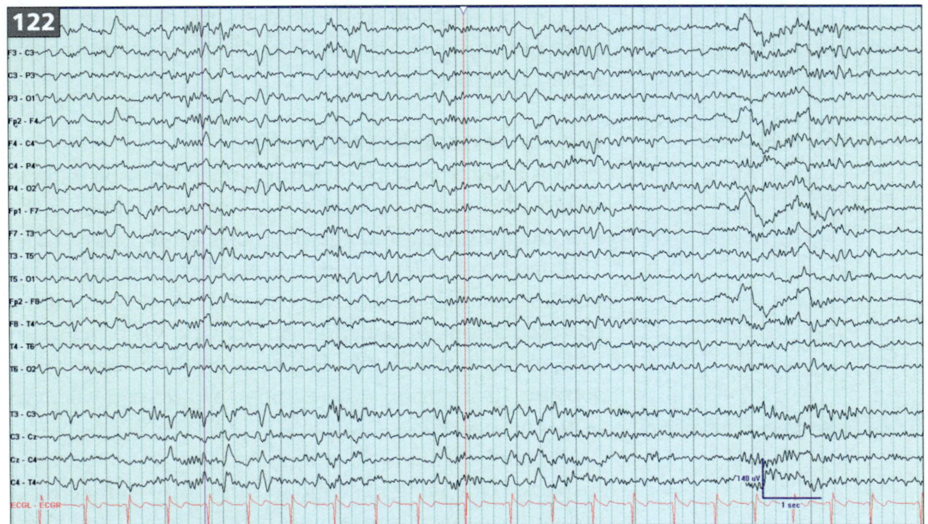

122 Adult EEG (normal) during stage II of sleep, which demonstrates K-complexes and sleep spindles.

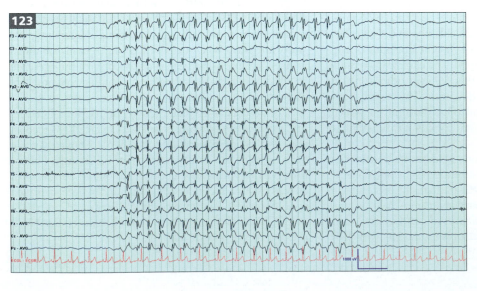

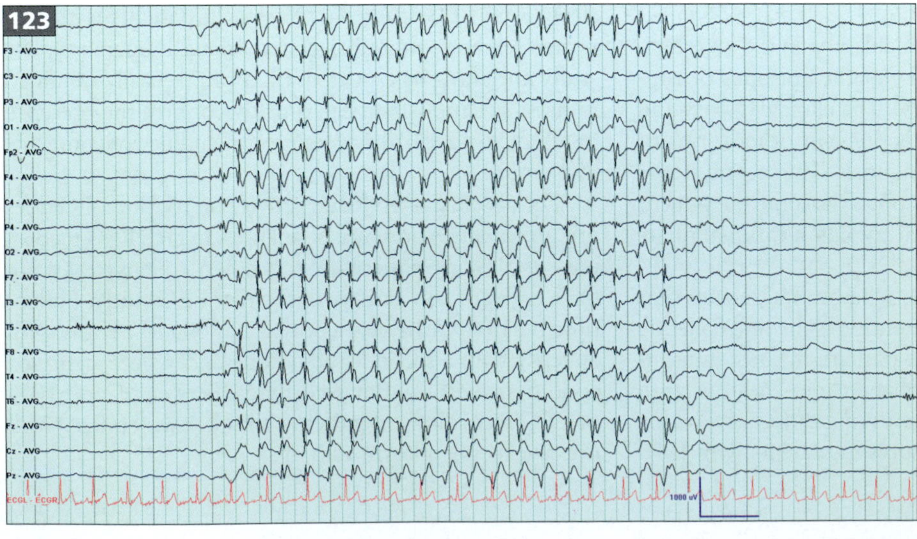

123 EEG demonstrating generalized 3 Hz spike and wave discharges consistent with primary generalized epilepsy and suggestive of absence seizures.

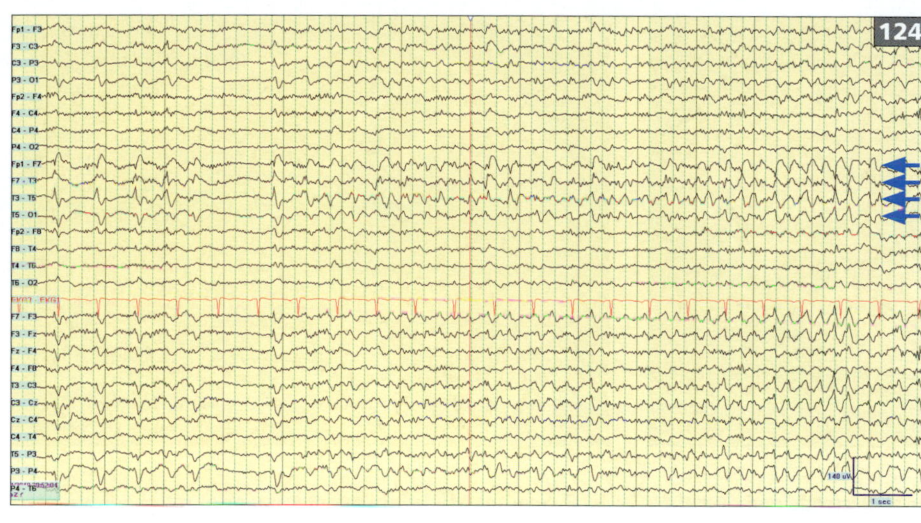

124 EEG demonstrating left temporal seizure activity (arrows).

The presence of epileptiform discharges on EEG does not necessarily confirm a diagnosis of epilepsy, as false positives do occur. It has been estimated that epileptiform activity can be identified in up to 2% of people in the general population who have never had any epileptic seizure. This may include people with migraines, first relatives of people with certain types of idiopathic generalized epilepsy, children with benign focal epileptiform discharges of childhood, and patients with autistic spectrum disorders. Furthermore, epileptiform discharges can be identified in elderly people who suffered from a stroke, but never had an epileptic seizure. Thus, clinical correlation is of the essence and AED therapy should not be started solely on the basis of EEG data.

The detection of epileptiform activity on scalp recordings is a function of the following variables: 1) extent of cortical area synchronously activated (see above); and 2) the angle subtended by scalp electrodes to the source of the epileptic activity and its propagation. Epileptiform activity originating in mesial frontal, mesial temporal, mesial parietal, and mesial occipital regions may often go undetected, unless it propagates to distant structures. In such cases, the addition of more electrodes (i.e. antero-temporal or supra-orbital electrodes) or closely spaced electrodes (also known as 10–10 system electrodes) can significantly improve the yield.

When routine EEG studies with awake and sleep recordings done under sleep deprivation and for at least 2 hours of recording with the use of special electrodes (antero-temporal electrodes when epilepsy of mesial temporal origin is suspected or supra-orbital electrodes in case of frontal lobe epilepsy) do not provide adequate information to confirm a diagnosis, continuous EEG monitoring (cEEG) may be considered. A 24-hour cEEG recording has a 90–95% probability of recording interictal epileptiform activity in people with epilepsy.

cEEG monitoring can be done as an ambulatory or in-hospital study. The former may or may not have concurrent video recordings and may be performed for 24 to up to 72 hours. The latter is typically a video-EEG (V-EEG) monitoring study which may be obtained over several hours to an entire day in an outpatient EEG laboratory. It may also involve inpatient admission of several days' duration.

The advantages of doing an outpatient cEEG include lower cost and the ability to record from the patients' homes, where they are exposed to their usual stressors and triggers of events. The disadvantages include the frequent muscle and motion artifact that make EEG recordings unreadable and, if no video is available, the inability to distinguish epileptic seizures that mimic psychogenic nonepileptic events (e.g., seizures of mesial frontal origin) from nonepileptic events proper. This has led to frequent false-negative misdiagnoses.

The use of inpatient V-EEG is an important ancillary tool as it allows the addition of extra electrodes that lead to higher localization yield of ictal and interictal epileptiform activity and the ability to correlate clinical events with electrographic activity. V-EEG allows for the recording of the typical paroxysmal events in question and establishing with high certainty a diagnosis of epileptic *vs.* nonepileptic seizures. The recording of paroxysmal events with V-EEG is still the gold standard to reach a diagnosis. cEEG is also standard in the localization of epileptogenic zone as part of pre-surgical evaluations in patients with treatment-resistant epilepsy.

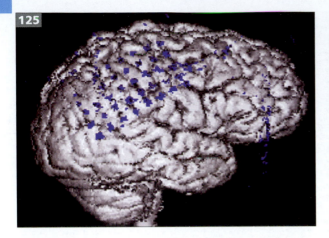

125 CT reconstruction of subdural electrode pad over the right hemisphere.

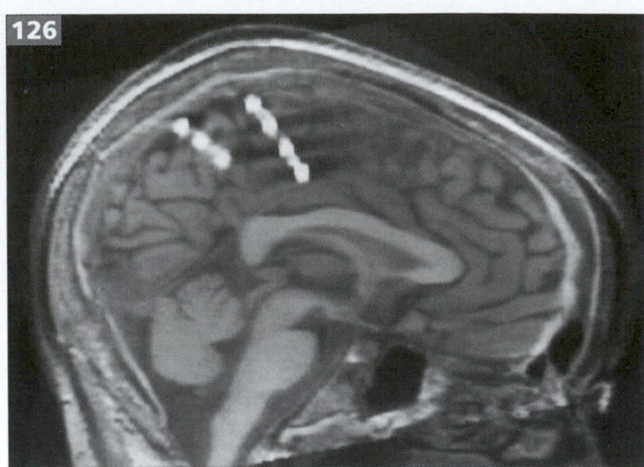

126 Sagittal MRI showing placement of interhemispheric electrodes.

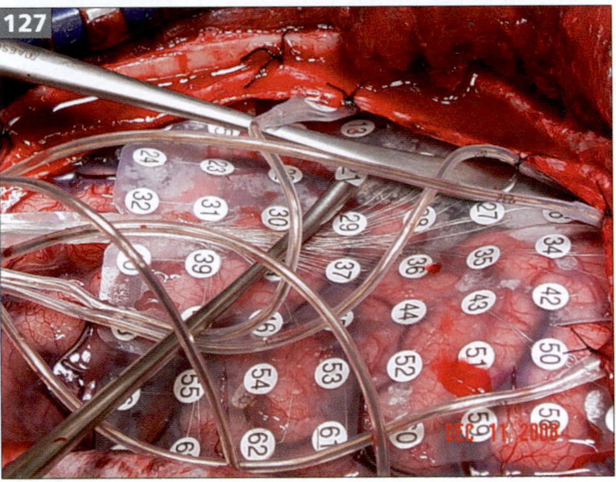

127 Operating room photo showing placement of electrodes for electrocorticography.

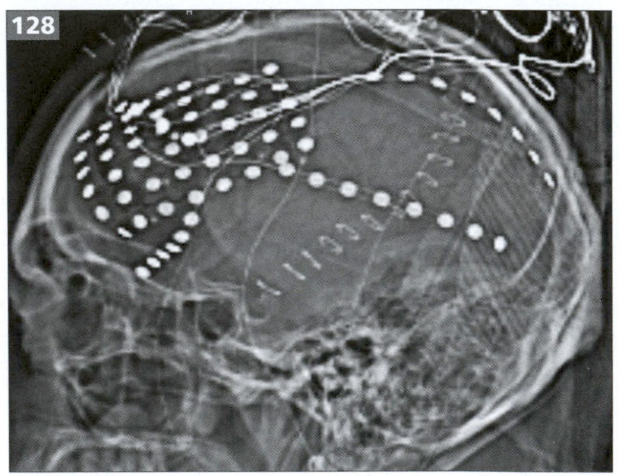

128 Post-operative X-ray of implanted electrodes.

In pre-surgical evaluations, V-EEG studies are the initial diagnostic studies, coupled with high resolution brain MRI, functional neuroimaging studies (PET, ictal SPECT), neuropsychological studies, and neuropsychiatric evaluations. When data from all of these studies yields nonconcordant information or EEG recordings fail to identify the epileptogenic zone, V-EEG with a variety of intracranial electrodes (subdural grids, strips, intraparenchimal depth electrodes) is carried out (**125–128**).

Other neurophysiologic studies include magnetoencephalography (MEG), which is used to demonstrate magnetic dipoles of individual epileptic discharges, and can help to identify the source of the epileptic activity, particularly when originating in deep structures.

Imaging

With most cases of new-onset seizure activity, some form of imaging of the CNS is recommended, despite the fact that in a large proportion of patients with epilepsy, imaging is normal. To rule out acute etiologies or large structural abnormalities, computed tomography (CT) with or without contrast may be useful. CT is less useful at providing detailed anatomic information, and in up to 30% of cases, CT can miss a variety of neoplasms such as low-grade gliomas, hamartomas, and focal dysplasias. For further evaluation MRI is recommended.

Epilepsy protocol MRI (for example with higher strength magnet or thin continuous slices through the regions of interest) should be considered. In patients suspected to have temporal lobe epilepsy, a high resolution brain MRI with coronal cuts done perpendicular to the long axis of the hippocampal formations is of the essence to identify the presence of mesial temporal sclerosis, the most frequent cause of treatment-resistant epilepsy in adults. The exact recommendations for imaging in various presentations of seizures may vary. For example, new-onset childhood absence epilepsy may not necessarily require imaging of the CNS.

As stated above, other forms of specialized functional imaging techniques have been developed and employed particularly in pre-surgical evaluations of treatment-resistant epilepsy. In fact, the diagnostic value of these techniques is paramount in nonlesional epilepsies. Ictal and interictal SPECT, and subtraction ictal SPECT coregistered to MRI (SISCOM) can show regions of significant blood flow change at the onset of seizure activity (**129–131**). PET may show asymmetries of metabolic activity, which may be particularly helpful in localization of seizures to the temporal lobes.

Other diagnostic considerations

Depending on the suspected etiology of the seizures, other diagnostic testing should be entertained. This may include analysis of cerebrospinal fluid (CSF) for infection, hemorrrhage, or other abnormalities; genetic or metabolic analysis; vascular imaging; brain biopsy, and so on.

Common comorbid disorders in epilepsy

Epilepsy involves not just seizures but a host of comorbid medical, cognitive, psychiatric, and psychosocial conditions. These often vary by gender and age.

Psychiatric and psychosocial comorbidities

Among the psychiatric comorbidities, mood and anxiety disorders are the most common in patients with epilepsy, identified in approximately 25–40% of patients. In children, attention deficit hyperactivity disorder (ADHD) is the most frequently recognized psychiatric comorbidity, although mood and anxiety disorders are being identified with increasing frequency.

Psychiatric comorbidites have a significant impact on quality of life. In fact, in patients with treatment-resistant epilepsy, the presence of comorbid mood and anxiety disorders has a worse impact on measures of quality of life than the actual seizure frequency and severity. Patients with chronic epilepsy are also at higher risk of suicide. In population-based studies, patients with epilepsy and without psychosocial problems have a two- to threefold higher risk of committing suicide compared to the general population. In the presence of a mood disorder, the risk increases by 32-fold, and by 12-fold in the presence of anxiety disorders[10,11]. Accordingly, it is important to screen for these conditions and to treat them appropriately, or refer the patient to a mood disorders specialist.

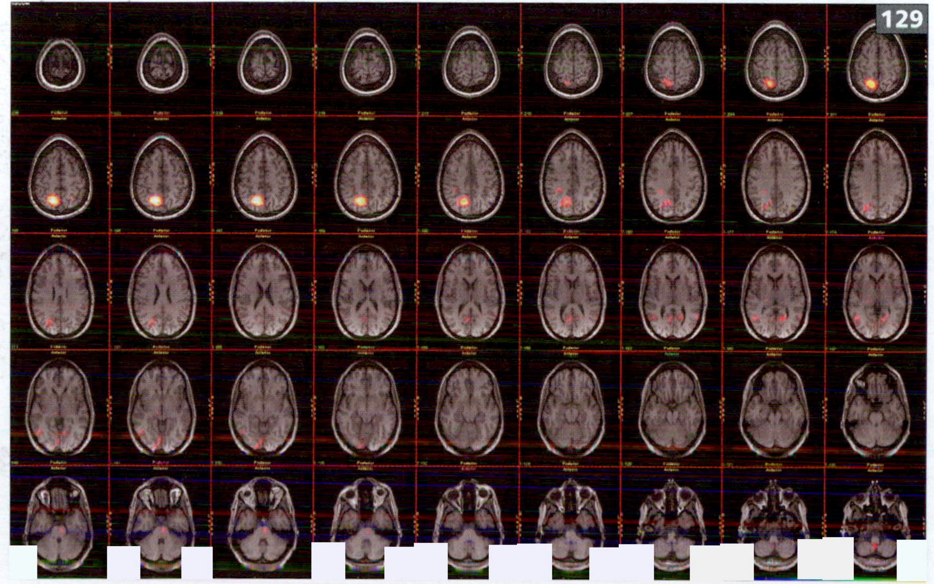

129 Axial SISCOM showing area of increased activity in the right parietal region.

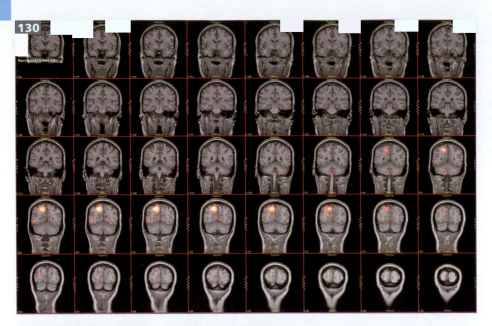

130 Coronal SISCOM of the patient in 129. This study reveals an area of hyperperfusion in the right mesial parietal region, representing a possible epileptogenic area that needs to be confirmed with intracranial ictal recordings.

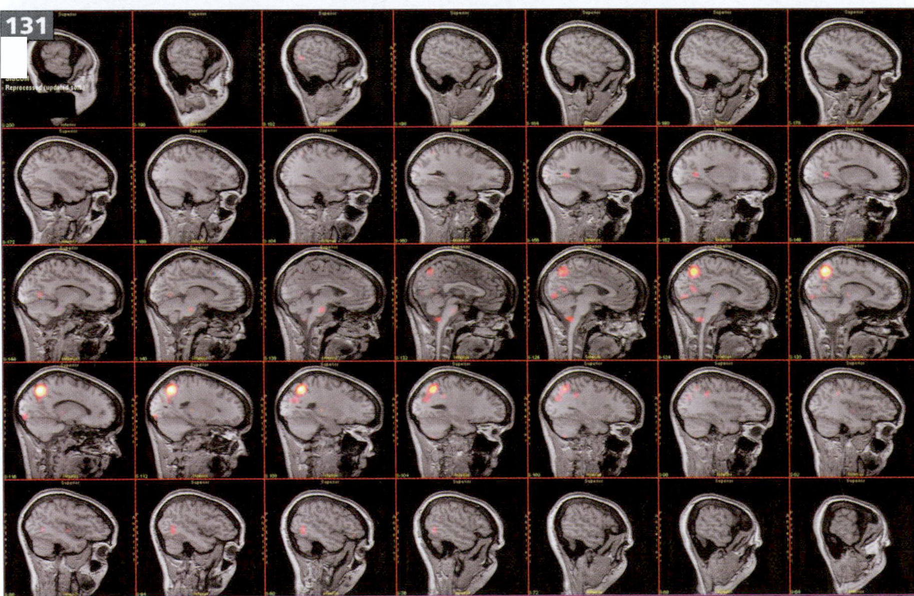

131 Sagittal SISCOM of the patient in 129.

Some psychiatric disorders, such as mood ADHDs have been found to have a bidirectional relationship. In other words, not only are patients with epilepsy at higher risk of experiencing these disorders, but patients with depressive disorders have a 3–7-fold higher risk of developing epilepsy[12,13].

The presence of psychiatric disorders and in particular epilepsy has been associated with a higher risk of developing treatment-resistant epilepsy and in patients undergoing epilepsy surgery, a lifetime history of depression is predictive of a lower probability of achieving complete seizure freedom after temporal lobectomy.

Commonly encountered psychosocial issues when treating patients with epilepsy relate to loss of employment and income, loss of driving privileges (which vary by country and state), emotional and social stigmata, and injuries related to seizures.

Tip

▶ *Psychiatric comorbidities in patients with epilepsy are commonly under-recognized and undertreated by physicians, including neurologists.*

Gender and sexual comorbidities

Sexual disturbances have been identified in up to 30% of men and women with epilepsy and include decreased sexual drive and anorgasmia in both genders, penile erectile and ejaculatory disturbances in men, and vaginismus and dyspareunia and lack of vaginal lubrication in the face of normal desire and experience in women. These problems have been associated with lower pregnancy rates in women with epilepsy compared to the general population.

The causes of sexual disturbances are multifactorial and include endocrine disturbances, the type of epilepsy (temporal lobe epilepsy being the most frequent type of epilepsy associated with these disturbances), as well as the presence of comorbid depressive and anxiety disorders.

Menstrual disturbances

Up to 30% of women with epilepsy suffer from a variety of menstrual disturbances, including dysmenorrhea and amenorrhea, anovulatory cycles, polycystic ovaries, and polycystic ovarian syndrome. These disturbances have been associated with abnormal secretion patterns of follicular stimulating and luteinizing hormones that yield abnormal estrogen and testosterone serum concentrations. Furthermore, AEDs with enzyme-inducing properties (e.g. phenytoin, carbamazepine, phenobarbital, primidone, topiramate, and oxcarbazepine) can lower the free fraction of testosterone and estrogen by inducing the synthesis of sex hormone-binding globulin.

Seizures may occur around the menstrual cycle and/ or ovulation in about 20–30% of women with epilepsy. This is known as catamenial epilepsy and is defined by the occurrence of >70% of seizures during these two periods. In such cases, treatment with natural progesterone (e.g. prometrium) has yielded significant improvement in seizure frequency.

Sudden unexplained death in epilepsy

Sudden unexplained death in epilepsy (SUDEP) is the most frequent cause of death in people with epilepsy. The rate has been estimated to be 1/1500 patient years in patients with rare seizures and 1/200 patient years in patients with treatment-resistant epilepsy. The causes of SUDEP remain unknown but cardiac arrhythmia occurring during seizures and sudden pulmonary edema have been postulated as potential mechanisms. Generalized tonic–clonic seizures during sleep and poor compliance with AEDs have been also associated with the occurrence of SUDEP.

Comorbidities in elderly patients

In the elderly, thought should be given to the comorbid conditions that often accompany or contribute to seizures, including cardiovascular disease (stroke in particular), and hypertension. Seizures have also been identified as a risk factor for stroke in the elderly, and may be the presenting symptom. The dosage of AEDs in the elderly also requires careful consideration due to decreased metabolism and excretion of these medications.

TREATMENT

There are a variety of treatments available for epilepsy. While the majority of these are pharmacologic in nature, surgical treatments are becoming increasingly common and in some cases the standard of care for refractory seizures. New technologies, genetic analysis, and targeted pharmacogenomics hold great promise for the future.

To plan a meaningful treatment, it is imperative to establish an accurate diagnosis of the seizure type and epileptic syndrome in question. Clinicians must always answer the following questions before starting any AED:

- What type of epileptic seizure does the patient present?
- What is the epileptic syndrome in this patient?
- Am I sure that these events are epileptic?

Characterization of the type of seizure, syndrome, and cause of epilepsy is of the essence to establish the therapeutic expectations of pharmacologic treatments. For example, seizure-freedom can be expected in 80–90% of patients with idiopathic generalized epilepsy, 50% of focal epilepsy, but only 30% of mesial temporal sclerosis.

The goal of therapy is to reach complete seizure-freedom, as even one seizure per year is associated with increased morbidity and mortality, and precludes patients from driving and engaging in other activities that significantly affect their quality of life.

Pharmacologic treatment

The vast majority of epilepsy patients will receive treatment with AEDs. Population-based studies done in patients who never received treatment for their seizure disorder have estimated a spontaneous seizure remission of approximately 50%. A number of population-based studies have been performed to date which indicate that the majority of patients (60–70%) will achieve complete seizure remission with therapy.

However, in 30–40% of patients, seizures will remain refractory to pharmacologic treatment. The exact numbers have been difficult to interpret as these patients have tended to be identified at tertiary facilities where there may be some element of referral bias. Additionally, medical intractability (or remission) has been defined differently in various studies, sometimes without specific parameters.

Studies by Kwan and Brodie[14] confirmed findings in prior large studies and indicated that while almost 50% of patients with newly diagnosed epilepsy will respond to treatment with the first AED, only about 11% of those patients who fail initial treatment with an appropriate AED will become seizure-free with additional monotherapy trials.

A report from the ILAE proposed a definition of treatment-resistant epilepsy as the persistence of seizures after two trials with the appropriate AEDs at optimal doses[15]. The importance of this proposal is that it will allow for the early identification of patients who are unlikely to respond to AED therapy and hence should be referred to epilepsy centers to determine if they can be candidates for surgical or other therapies.

The decision to start pharmacologic therapy is one that should be made jointly with the patient. This decision may be influenced by a variety of factors, such as the risk of recurrent seizures, the side-effect profile of the medication in question, and other medical and social issues (such as the restrictions on driving for patients with epilepsy in most areas). It is important to consider other factors such as the side-effect profile of the AED (e.g. teratogenicity in women), pharmacokinetic and pharmacodynamic interactions with concomitant medications, and potential for poor compliance.

In recent years, the increasing use of generic substitutions has become a source of concern among clinicians and patients. These stem from variations in bioavailability resulting in worse efficacy and potential toxicity when switched from brand to generic formulations and among different generic formulations. The professional societies in the USA and Europe have recommended that seizure-free patients be maintained on brand formulations. Prospective trials are underway at this time to evaluate these concerns. In addition, the American Epilepsy Society has issued a statement supporting strong guidelines concerning medication substitutions, and has recommended that generic substitution not take place without physician and patient approval[16]. For patients who cannot stay on brand formulations due to cost implications, dispensation of the generic formulations should be limited to the same manufacturer.

Risk/benefit decisions

The clinician should have some idea of the risk of recurrent seizure activity, as this can influence the risk/benefit decision when considering medical treatment. One factor to consider is whether the seizure is 'provoked'. A provoked seizure, or acute symptomatic seizure, is that occurring 'in close temporal association with an acute systemic, metabolic, or toxic insult or in association with an acute CNS insult (infection, stroke, cranial trauma, intracerebral hemorrhage, or acute alcohol intoxication or withdrawal)'. Other common causes include fever, medication exposure, recreational drugs, neoplasm, post-cranial surgery, acute withdrawal from seizure medications, and numerous other medical conditions. Provoked seizures typically only occur in the presence of the acute etiology and thus may not be characterized as epilepsy. This differs from other forms of symptomatic seizures which may have different prognoses. Acute symptomatic seizures may be repeated.

One estimate of the risk of experiencing an acute symptomatic seizure over an 80-year life span is approximately 3.6%, which varies by sex and etiology. The risk of recurrence with acute symptomatic seizures is relatively low, and may not require prolonged treatment. A recent study on acute symptomatic seizures and unprovoked seizures due to CNS infection, stroke, and traumatic brain injury found that individuals with a first acute symptomatic seizure were about 80% less likely to experience a subsequent unprovoked seizure compared with individuals with a first unprovoked seizure[17].

Over the years a number of studies have looked at the risk of recurrent seizures after a first unprovoked seizure, though relatively few prospective randomized trials (without treatment after the first seizure) have been published. A meta-analysis by Berg and Shinnar of numerous different trials estimated the 2-year risk of seizure recurrence after a single unprovoked seizure at 36–47%[18].

Two large prospective European trials were recently completed. Overall, the estimated 2-year risk of recurrence after nontreatment of a first unprovoked seizure was approximately 40–50%. The risk of recurrent seizure appears to be greatest immediately following the first seizure, with a drop-off over time. Factors which increase the risk of recurrence include abnormal EEG (particularly focal or epileptiform abnormalities), an abnormal neurologic examination, or a symptomatic cause for the seizure. Interestingly, in one study, initial presentation with multiple seizures did not necessarily increase risk of recurrence, suggesting that these should be considered as a single event, though those patients were treated more frequently in part due to other variables such as perceived etiology. An excellent review of the risk of seizure recurrence and mitigating factors was recently published by Berg[19].

Relative efficacy of AEDs

The AEDs are commonly grouped into two categories: the 'first' generation of AEDs (carbamazepine, valproate, phenobarbital, phenytoin, ethosuximide, primidone, benzodiazepines) and the relatively newer 'second' generation AEDs (felbamate, gabapentin, tiagabine, lamotrigine, oxcarbazepine, topiramate, zonisamide, rufinamide, levetiracetam, pregabalin, lacosamide). There was an approximately 15-year gap between the release of valproate and the approval of the first newer generation AED in 1993. While there is substantial research demonstrating efficacy in these medications, there have been relatively few head-to-head randomized trials conducted that demonstrate superiority of one AED over another. While the USA Food and Drugs Administration (FDA) indications for the older medications are vaguely worded, those for the newer generation AEDs specify use for seizure type as well as indication for use as monotherapy, conversion to monotherapy, or adjunctive therapy. *Table 12* presents a summary of commonly used AEDs.

A number of studies have examined the relative efficacy of AEDs for treatment of different forms of epilepsy. A practice parameter published in 2004 by the American Academy of Neurology examined the available evidence published in peer-reviewed scientific literature on the efficacy and tolerability of the newer AEDs for treatment of children and adults with newly diagnosed partial and generalized epilepsies, including gabapentin, lamotrigine, topiramate, tiagabine, oxcarbazepine, levetiracetam, and zonisamide (*Table 13*)[20]. Of note, the demonstration of equivalence between two drugs in these studies was accepted as effectiveness by the authors, though the USA FDA requires a demonstration of superiority against placebo.

In newly diagnosed epilepsy:

- Lamotrigine, topiramate, and oxcarbazepine were found to be effective in a mixed population of newly diagnosed partial and generalized tonic–clonic seizures.
- There was insufficient evidence to evaluate tiagabine, zonisamide, or levetiracetam. The tolerability may be superior in the newer medications in many cases.
- It was recommended that patients with newly diagnosed epilepsy may be started on any of the standard AEDs (carbamazepine, valproic acid, phenytoin, phenobarbital) or on lamotrigine, oxcarbazepine, gabapentin, or topiramate.
- With respect to idiopathic generalized epilepsies, lamotrigine was found to be effective in the treatment of children with newly diagnosed absence seizures, though insufficent information was available to evaluate effectiveness in newly diagnosed primary or secondarily generalized epilepsy for topiramate, oxcarbazepine, tiagabine, zonisamide, or levetiracetam.
- Similar guidelines developed for the treatment of refractory epilepsy have found that gabapentin, lamotrigine, oxcarbazepine, tiagabine, levetiracetam, topiramate, and zonisamide are effective as add-on therapy in treatment-resistant partial epilepsy and topiramate, lamotrigine, and oxcarbazepine are effective as monotherapy in this form of epilepsy[21].

In the more recent SANAD (Standard and New Antiepileptic Drugs) trial in the UK, the efficacy and safety of carbamazepine was compared with that of lamotrigine, gabapentin, and oxcarbazepine in the treatment of newly diagnosed partial seizure disorders, while valproic acid was compared with topiramate and lamotrigine in the treatment of newly diagnosed idiopathic generalized epilepsy[22]. The data suggested that lamotrigine may be a clinical and cost-effective alternative to carbamazepine in the treatment of partial seizures. In patients with idiopathic generalized epilepsy or epilepsy that was difficult to classify, valproate was considered to be the most cost-effective medication, though topiramate could be considered as an alternative in some cases.

An excellent review of many of the randomized trials to date comparing efficacy in monotherapy was recently completed by Stephen and Brodie[23]. A multicenter randomized controlled trial has demonstrated efficacy and safety of levetiracetam monotherapy in new-onset focal and idiopathic generalized epilepsy. In addition, add-on levetiracetam and lamotrigine have been shown to be efficacious in refractory JME and idiopathic generalized tonic–clonic seizures, respectively.

TABLE 12 **CHARACTERISTICS OF COMMONLY USED ANTIEPILEPTIC DRUGS (AEDS)**

AED	**Seizure type** (FDA indications may vary)	**Additional notes**	**Major mechanism of action**	**Primary metabolism**	**Protein binding** (%)	V_d (l/kg)
Phenytoin	Partial, tonic–clonic	Zero-order kinetics	Sodium channel blockade	Hepatic	85–95	0.6–0.8
Valproate	Partial, tonic–clonic, absence, myoclonic, LGS, IS	Free fraction increases above concentrations of 70 µg/ml	Increases GABA activity	Hepatic (glucoronidation and beta-oxidation	85–95	0.14–0.23
Carbamazepine	Partial, tonic–clonic, mixed	Auto-induction, may worsen certain types of generalized seizures	Sodium channel blockade	Hepatic	76	0.8–2
Phenobarbital	Partial, tonic–clonic, absence, perhaps LGS		Increases GABA activity	Hepatic	20–45	0.5–0.75
Ethosuximide	Absence, perhaps myoclonic/atonic		Decreased (T type) calcium channel activity	Hepatic	<10	0.6–0.7
Primidone	Partial, tonic–clonic		Similar to phenobarbital	Hepatic	20–30	0.64–0.86
Felbamate	Partial, tonic–clonic, LGS	Associated with severe bone marrow suppression	NMDA receptor antagonist; sodium channel blockade	Hepatic	20–25	0.73–0.85
Topiramate	Partial, tonic–clonic, myoclonic, LGS		Sodium channel blockade, increased GABA activity, AMPA/glutamate antagonism, carbonic anhydrase inhibitor	Hepatic	9–41	0.6–0.8
Zonisamide	Partial, tonic–clonic, perhaps absence/myoclonic/LGS/IS		Sodium channel blockade, carbonic anhydrase inhibitor	Hepatic (acetylation)	40–60	1.45
Lamotrigine	Partial, tonic–clonic, absence, myoclonic, LGS, IS	May exacerbate myoclonic seizures; increased risk of Stevens–Johnson syndrome	Sodium channel blockade	Hepatic	55	0.9–1.3
Levetiracetam	Partial, tonic–clonic, myoclonic, absence, perhaps LGS/IS	Relatively few medication interactions	Unclear	Enzymatic hydrolysis; hepatic (minimal)	<10	0.7
Ezogabine	Partial, tonic–clonic	May be associated with urine retention, skin discoloration, retinal pigment changes, QT prolongation	Potassium channel (KCNQ family) potentiation	Hepatic (glucoronidation and acetylation)	Ezogabine: 80%; NAMR (major active metabolite): 45%	2–3

TABLE 12 continued

AED	**Seizure type** (FDA indications may vary)	**Additional notes**	**Major mechanism of action**	**Primary metabolism**	**Protein binding** (%)	V_d (l/kg)
Pregabalin	Partial, tonic–clonic, perhaps absence/IS/LGS/myoclonic		GABA analog; binds to $\alpha 2\delta$ site of Ca^{2+} channel	Minimal	0	0.5
Gabapentin	Partial, tonic–clonic	60% maximum bioavailability; nonlinear absorption	Unknown; likely similar to pregabalin and increases GABA transmission	None	<3	N/A
Tiagabine	Partial, tonic–clonic, perhaps myoclonic/LGS		Blocks GABA uptake to presynaptic neurons	Hepatic; glucoronidation	96	
Oxcarbazepine	Partial, tonic–clonic		Unknown; presumed blockade of voltage-sensitive sodium channels	Hepatic	40–60	
Lacosamide	Partial		Sodium channel slow inactivation and binds to CRMP-2	Biotrans-formation; demethylation	<15	0.6
Rufinamide	Partial, tonic–clonic, LGS, perhaps absence/myoclonic		Unknown; may pro-long inactive state of sodium channel	Hepatic, primar-ily hydrolysis	34%	Varies
Clonazepam	Partial, tonic–clonic, myoclonic, perhaps LGS/IS		Enhanced GABA activity	Hepatic	85	
Clobazam	Partial, tonic–clonic, myoclonic, LGS, perhaps IS	May have fewer psychomotor side-effects than other benzodiazepines	Enhanced GABA activity	Hepatic	Extensive	0.87–1.37
Vigabatrin	IS, partial, per-haps tonic–clonic	May worsen absence, myoclonic seizures; may cause irreversible visual field deficits	Unknown; thought to be irreversible inhibition of GABA transaminase	Minimal	0	0.8–1.1

AMPA: alpha-amino-3-hydroxy-5-methyl-4-isoxazole propionic acid; CRMP-2: collapsing response mediator protein-2; GABA: gamma-aminobutyric acid; FDA: (US) Food and Drug Administration; IS: infantile spasms; LGS: Lennox–Gastaut syndrome; NMDA: *N*-methyl-D-aspartate; Vd: volume of distribution.

Sources: Micromedex, (Stein and Kanner 2009, Stephen and Brodie 2009[23], Azar and Abou-Khalil 2008).

NB: FDA indications may vary depending on formulation and individual drug and seizure type.

Combinations of different AEDs (e.g. valproate + lamotrigine) may display synergistic efficacy.

AEDs may have multiple mechanisms of action.

Values are for adults unless otherwise specified.

TABLE 13 **AMERICAN ACADEMY OF NEUROLOGY GUIDELINES[20,21] FOR THE EFFICACY AND TOLERABILITY OF THE NEW ANTIEPILEPTIC DRUGS IN TREATMENT OF NEW-ONSET AND REFRACTORY EPILEPSY, USING *LEVEL A OR B RECOMMENDATIONS**

New-onset epilepsy		**Refractory epilepsy**				
Monotherapy for partial or mixed seizure types	*Absence seizures*	*Adult partial adjunct*	*Partial monotherapy*	*Primary generalized*	*Symptomatic generalized*	*Pediatric partial adjunct*
Gabapentin	Lamotrigine	Gabapentin	Lamotrigine		Lamotrigine	Gabapentin
Lamotrigine		Lamotrigine	Topiramate	Topiramate†	Topiramate	Lamotrigine
Topiramate		Topiramate	Oxacarbazepine			Topiramate
Oxacarbazepine		Tiagabine				Oxacarbazepine
		Oxacarbazepine				
		Levetiracetam				
		Zonisamide				

*Level A: established as useful/predictive or not useful/predictive for the given condition in the specified population; level B: probably useful/predictive or not useful/predictive for the given condition in the specified population.

This summary is independent of the FDA-approved indications for each medication.

†Generalized tonic–clonic seizures only

As stated above, when choosing an antiepileptic medication, accurate classification of the epilepsy or epileptic syndrome is crucial. While there is often little objective difference in efficacy amongst AEDs for similar seizure types, there are some exceptions.

For example, in some cases the use of carbamazepine can exacerbate primary generalized seizure activity such as JME. If the seizure type or syndrome cannot be accurately identified, a rule of thumb is to use an AED with broad mechanisms of action. While there are no specific guidelines, it is generally recommended that monotherapy be a goal if possible.

Other factors to consider include pharmacokinetic and pharmacodynamic properties and interactions with other medications (including other AEDs), side-effect profile, allergic reactions and cross-reactivity, metabolism (especially in patients with abnormal renal or hepatic function), teratogenicity, age and weight, ease of titration, ease of formulation, and possibility of treatment of comorbid conditions with the same medication (e.g. depression or mood disorders).

Status epilepticus

SE is a neurologic emergency which carries a risk of significant mortality and morbidity. The proposed definition of SE has varied over time, from 30 minutes to 10 minutes, and recently to 5 minutes of continuous seizure duration. In practice, 5 minutes of seizure duration or recurrent seizures without a return to baseline mental status generally constitutes SE.

The distinction between convulsive and nonconvulsive SE (SE in the absence of clinically obvious seizure activity) is an important one, as it affects management and prognosis. NCSE should be suspected in patients with recent cessation of clinically obvious seizure activity but without a return to baseline mental status (including after treatment). It should also be suspected in patients with altered mental status with no other obvious etiology for the symptoms. Several studies have shown that nonconvulsive or subclinical SE is more prevalent in medical intensive care unit settings than previously thought.

An EEG (preferably continuous monitoring) should be ordered immediately in these patients, and in general in all patients being treated for SE. The distinction between simple and complex partial status *vs.* generalized SE is also an important one, as the benefit of very aggressive treatment in the former conditions is not as clear as for generalized SE, and in some studies has been shown to be associated with increased morbidity.

Treatment protocols vary between institutions, but some generally agreed upon guidelines exist. First, treatment should be instituted rapidly (within minutes). There is some evidence that delay in treatment can result in worsened outcomes and decreased likelihood of seizure control. Proper emergency stabilization of the patient, including airway management, breathing evaluation, and circulatory evaluation is key. Oxygen should be administered. Intravenous access should be established. If the latter is not possible, treatment should proceed by using medications that can be administered via other modes (i.e. intramuscular, rectal, nasal).

Basic laboratory values should be obtained, including arterial blood gases in many cases, and any metabolic or medical derangements should be corrected. Blood glucose should be obtained and intravenous glucose given if the level is not available or if hypoglycemia is suspected. Intravenous thiamine should be administered. Any obvious precipitating factors should be eliminated.

Anticonvulsant therapy should be initiated as soon as possible and with stabilization of the airway. First-line treatment consists of benzodiazepines, such as lorazepam in increasing doses up to 0.1 mg/kg given at 2 mg/minute. In most cases, the patient is concurrently started on a second-line therapy for prevention of withdrawal. Most algorithms suggest phenytoin (usually administered as fosphenytoin due to the lower risk of cardiovascular side-effects) at 20 mg/kg loading dose. If seizures continue, an additional 10 mg/kg may be given. Should seizures continue, most practitioners will next load phenobarbital 20 mg/kg IV, or proceed directly to anesthesia with propofol or midazolam depending on the clinical scenario.

Sedation with pentobarbital (to burst suppression on EEG or seizure cessation) may be necessary if seizures continue despite aggressive management. Intravenous valproate has been suggested as an alternative and has shown some promising results. Other antiepileptic medications (levetiracetam, topiramate) have been used depending on the clinical scenario.

Virtually all patients at this stage should be admitted to an intensive care unit for close clinical monitoring and ideally continuous V-EEG monitoring. It is important to ensure that maintenance dosing is initiated right away and is adequate and that levels are followed when possible to ensure therapeutic dosing. Other clinical symptoms such as hyperthermia, metabolic derangements, and infections, need to be managed. Refractory SE may require more aggressive treatment and required an intensive care unit setting and EEG monitoring.

Iatrogenic considerations of pharmacotherapy

The side-effects of AEDs are a significant concern. Patients who are prescribed these medications should be aware of the potential side-effects, and should have routine screening as indicated. The effects of enzyme-inducing AEDs in particular should be noted, particularly with respect to their effects on the efficacy of other medications and on accelerated bone density loss. Calcium and vitamin D_3 supplementation is now being recommended for patients on long-term use of enzyme-inducing AEDs.

Of particular importance is the discussion of teratogenicity in women who are on AEDs, and the need for appropriate choice of AED, institution of contraceptive techniques, and folate supplementation in women with child-bearing potential. Practice guidelines recently published through the American Academy of Neurology are available for issues related to women with epilepsy[24–26].

Nonpharmacologic therapy

Epilepsy surgery is increasingly considered the standard of care for treatment-resistant, localization-related epilepsy in those patients who meet appropriate criteria. Not all patients meet these criteria, thus evaluation at an epilepsy surgery center is mandatory. In general, it is felt that patients who fail trials of two to three appropriate AEDs be evaluated for surgical therapy.

The goals of surgery are generally to stop seizures entirely, though in some patients this is not possible and palliative surgery can be offered. The most common type of epilepsy surgery is temporal (anterior) lobectomy, usually for cases involving mesial temporal sclerosis, though extratemporal resection, corpus callosotomy, hemispherectomy, topectomy, and multiple subpial transection are also performed.

The success rate of epilepsy surgery varies based on several factors, including the presence or absence of an identifiable structural lesion that correlates with the epileptogenic region, the complete resection of the epileptogenic area (not only the most interictally active tissue), temporal *vs.* extratemporal resection, and ictal/interictal data that are (preferably) unifocal and concordant to the region in question.

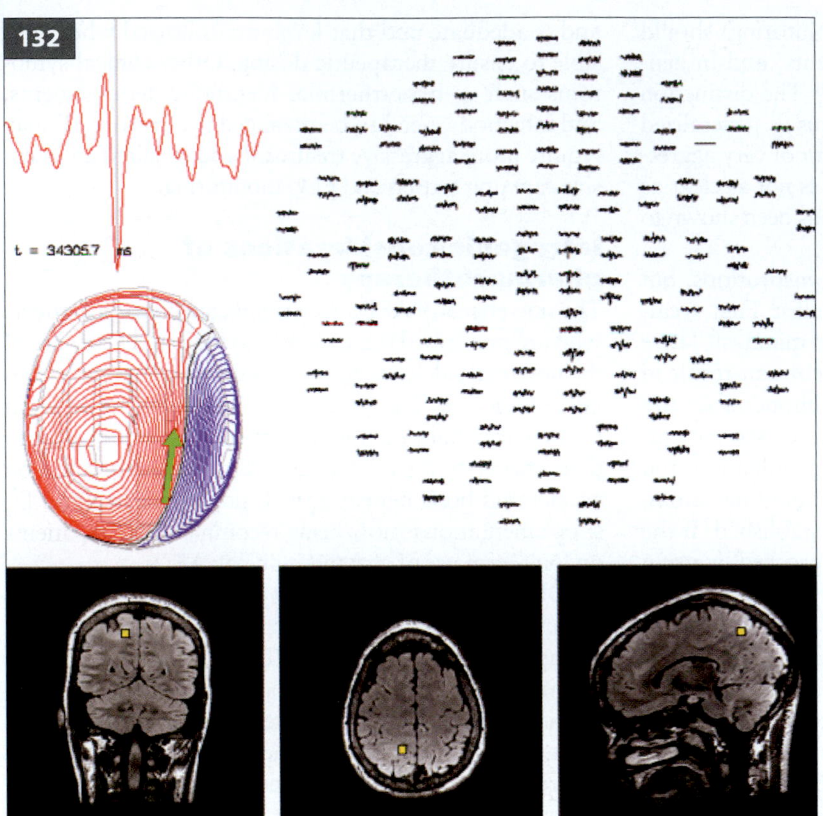

132 MEG studies showing abnormal activity in the right parietal region.

Functional neuroimaging studies such as ictal SPECT, SISCOM, PET, and MEG (**132, 133**) are used to help confirm the region that is hypothesized to be epileptogenic.

In terms of outcome, a number of studies have been published, primarily looking at the efficacy of temporal lobe surgery. One randomized controlled study by Wiebe and colleagues[27] demonstrated superiority of surgery for temporal lobe epilepsy over prolonged medical therapy, with 58% compared to 8% of medically-treated patients (cumulative) being free of seizures impairing awareness at 1 year. The proportion of actual surgery patients (36) who were free of disabling seizures at 1 year was close to 64%. A review paper by Spencer *et al.*[28] looked at reported seizure-freedom for at least 1 year across several studies and found seizure-freedom rates for temporal lobe surgeries of 48–84%. Other studies (with differing criteria and organization) have found similar results with seizure freedom from disabling seizures in temporal lobe surgery in approximately two-thirds of patients.

Anterior temporal lobectomy in appropriate patients is recommended by the American Academy of Neurology. Results are typically better in those patients with identifiable structural lesions. Other forms of epilepsy surgery have slightly less favorable outcomes; however, this should not prevent evaluation and treatment as even a modest improvement in seizures may dramatically affect quality of life.

There is increasing evidence that successful surgery can have a beneficial impact on other factors related to quality of life, including mood and numerous other psychosocial and cognitive concerns. There is also some evidence that overall health-care costs decline following successful temporal lobe epilepsy surgeries.

The risks of epilepsy surgery can be significant, and include focal neurologic deficits (such as motor, sensory, language function) depending on the region of resection, complications related to surgery, and longer-term concerns such as declines in cognitive function (in particular memory). It is increasingly possible with the aid of such tools as improved EEG and imaging protocols, cortical mapping, neuropsychological testing, functional MRI, and WADA testing, to evaluate and predict these risks beforehand to ensure proper informed consent. Additionally, consensus is growing that in patients with temporal lobe epilepsy and already impaired memory function, surgery may offer very little further risk. In those patients at higher risk for memory decline following surgery, some evidence suggests that avoiding surgery may not prevent memory loss over time, thus surgery should still be considered, and may be appropriately planned to minimize risk.

Corpus callosotomy remains a surgical option in certain patient populations. This procedure has been used for many seizure syndromes over the years though there are significant variations in outcome for different seizure types. The theory is that this procedure interrupts propagation of seizure activity between the hemispheres, thus preventing bilateral electrical synchrony and stopping unilateral seizures from generalizing. Corpus callosotomy has been shown to be most effective in patients (often children) with intractable atonic or tonic seizures which have resulted in falls ('drop attacks') and injuries, and do not respond to treatment with medication or vagal nerve stimulation. Corpus callosotomy is recognized as a palliative (not curative) procedure, though may have a significant positive impact on quality of life.

Other alternatives

New options for seizure treatment are becoming increasingly available. Apart from medications and surgery, several viable and approved treatment options may be considered, depending on the patient and type of epilepsy.

- The ketogenic diet and similar modified, high fat and high protein diets have been demonstrated to be successful in several kinds of epilepsy, particularly in children.
- Vagal nerve stimulation (VNS) is also approved as a recommended adjunct therapy for pharmacoresistant partial onset seizures in adults and adolescent children. VNS is the only currently approved device for epilepsy treatment, however other forms of neurostimulation are being investigated, some of which are static and some responsive, and may hold promise for patients with refractory seizures in the near future (Medtronic, NeuroPACE, SANTE).

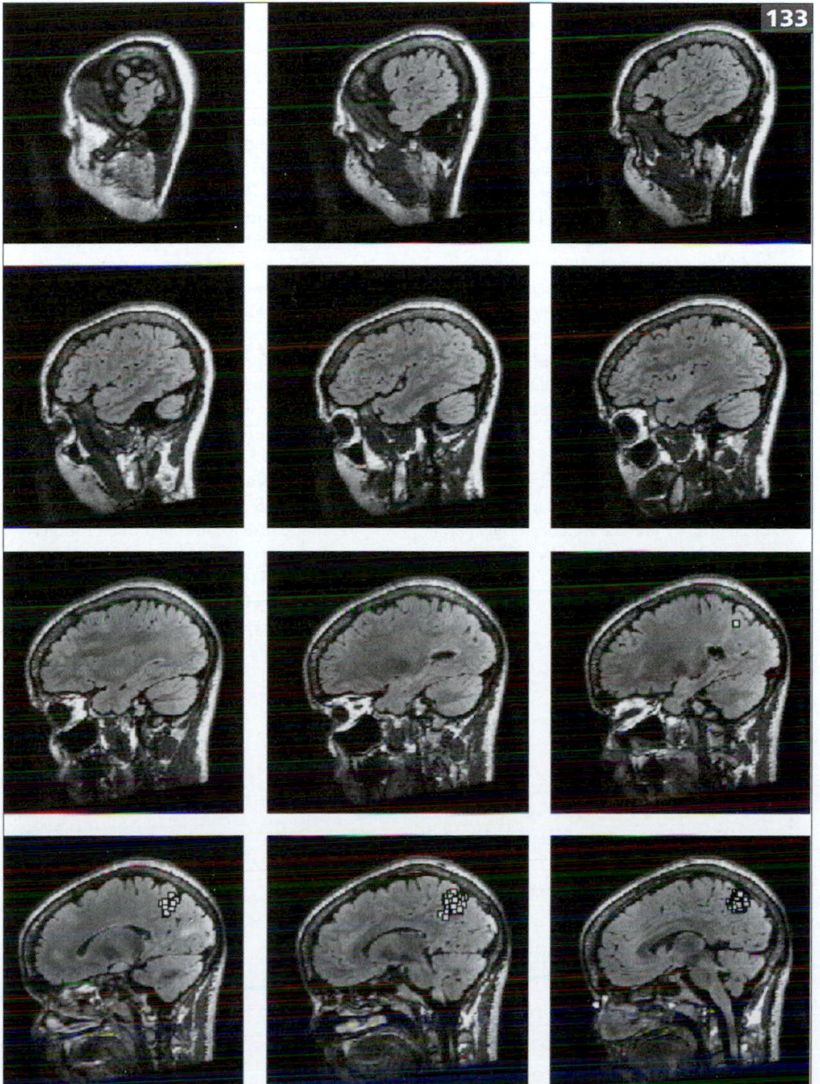

133 MEG studies showing abnormal activity in the right parietal region.

REFERENCES

1 Hesdorffer D, Logroscino G, Benn E, Katri N, Cascino G, Hauser W (2011). Estimating risk for developing epilepsy: a population-based study in Rochester, Minnesota. *Neurology* 76(1):23–27.

2 Hauser W, Annegers J, Kurland L (1991). Prevalence of epilepsy in Rochester, Minnesota: 1940–1980. *Epilepsia* 32:429–445.

3

4 Kelvin E, Hesdorffer D, Bagiella E, *et al.* (2007). Prevalence of self-reported epilepsy in a multiracial and multiethnic community in New York City. *Epilepsy Res* 77:141–150.

5 Lavados J, Germain L, Morales A, Campero M, Lavados P (1992). A descriptive study of epilepsy in the district of El Salvador, Chile, 1984–1988. *Acta Neurol Scand* 85:249–256.

6 Hauser WA, Annegers JF, Kurland LT (1993). Incidence of epilepsy and unprovoked seizures in Rochester, Minnesota 1935–1984. *Epilepsia* 34:453–458.

7 ILAE (1989). Proposal for revised classification of epilepsies and epileptic syndromes. Commission on Classification and Terminology of the International League Against Epilepsy. *Epilepsia* 30:389–399.

8 Berg A, Berkovic S, Brodie M, *et al.* (2010). Revised terminology and concepts for organization of seizures and epilepsies: report of the ILAE Commission on Classification and Terminology, 2005–2009. *Epilepsia* 51:676–685.

9 Blume W, Lüders H, Mizrahi E, Tassinari C, van Emde Boas W, Engel JJ (2001). Glossary of descriptive terminology for ictal semiology: report of the ILAE task force on classification and terminology. *Epilepsia* 42:1212–1218.

10 Christensen J, Vestergaard M, Mortensen P, *et al.* (2007). Epilepsy and risk of suicide: a population-based case–control study. *Lancet Neurol* 6:693–698.

11 Tellez-Zenteno JF, Patten SB, Jette N, *et al.* (2007) Psychiatric comorbidity in epilepsy: a population-based analysis. *Epilepsia* 48:2336–2344.

12 Forsgren L, Nystrom L (1999). An incident case referent study of epileptic seizures in adults. *Epilepsy Res* 6:66–81.

13 Hesdorffer DC, Hauser WA, Annegers JF, *et al.* (2000). Major depression is a risk factor for seizures in older adults. *Ann Neurol* 47:246–249.

14 Kwan P, Brodie M (2001). Effectiveness of first antiepileptic drug. *Epilepsia* 42:1255–1260.

15 Berg A (2009). Identification of pharmacoresistant epilepsy. *Neurol Clin* 27:1003–1013.

16 Position statement on the substitution of different formulations of antiepileptic drugs for the treatment of epilepsy. Available at: www.aesnet.org.

17 Hesdorffer D, Benn E, Cascino G, Hauser W (2009). Is a first acute symptomatic seizure epilepsy? Mortality and risk for recurrent seizure. *Epilepsia* 50:1102–1108.

18 Berg A, Shinnar S (1991). The risk of seizure recurrence following a first unprovoked seizure: a quantitative review. *Neurology* 41:965–972.

19 Berg A (2008). Risk of recurrence after a first unprovoked seizure. *Epilepsia* 49(Suppl 1):13–18.

20 French J, Kanner A, Bautista J, *et al.* (2004). Efficacy and tolerability of the new antiepileptic drugs I: treatment of new onset epilepsy: report of the Therapeutics and Technology Assessment Subcommittee and Quality Standards Subcommittee of the American Academy of Neurology and the American Epilepsy Society. *Neurology* 62:1252–1260.

21 French J, Kanner A, Bautista J, *et al.* (2004). Efficacy and tolerability of the new antiepileptic drugs II: treatment of refractory epilepsy: report of the Therapeutics and Technology Assessment Subcommittee and Quality Standards Subcommittee of the American Academy of Neurology and the American Epilepsy Society. *Neurology* 62:1261–1273.

22 Marson A, Jacoby A, Johnson A, Kim L, Gamble C, Chadwick D; M. R. C. M. S. Group (2005). Immediate versus deferred antiepileptic drug treatment for early epilepsy and single seizures: a randomised controlled trial. *Lancet* 365:2007–2013.

23 Stephen L, Brodie M (2009). Selection of antiepileptic drugs in adults. *Neurol Clin* 27:967–992.

24 Harden C, Hopp J, Ting T, *et al.* (2009). Practice parameter update: management issues for women with epilepsy; focus on pregnancy (an evidence-based review): obstetrical complications and change in seizure frequency: report of the Quality Standards Subcommittee and Therapeutics and Technology Assessment Subcommittee of the American Academy of Neurology and American Epilepsy Society. *Neurology* 73:126–132.

25 Harden C, Meado K, Pennell P, *et al.* (2009). Practice parameter update: management issues for women with epilepsy; focus on pregnancy (an evidence-based review): teratogenesis and perinatal outcomes: report of the Quality Standards Subcommittee and Therapeutics and Technology Assessment Subcommittee of the American Academy of Neurology and American Epilepsy Society. *Neurology* 73:133–141.

26 Harden C, Pennell P, Koppel B, *et al.* (2009). Practice parameter update: management issues for women with epilepsy; focus on pregnancy (an evidence-based review): vitamin K, folic acid, blood levels, and breastfeeding: report of the Quality Standards Subcommittee and Therapeutics and Technology Assessment Subcommittee of the American Academy of Neurology and American Epilepsy Society. *Neurology* 73:142–149.

27 Wiebe S, Blume W, Girvin J, Eliasziw M, E. a. E. o. S. f. T. L. E. S. Group (2001). A randomized, controlled trial of surgery for temporal-lobe epilepsy. *N Engl J Med* 345:311–318.

28 Spencer S, Huh L (2008). Outcomes of epilepsy surgery in adults and children. *Lancet Neurol* 7:525–537.

Further reading

ILAE (1993). Guidelines for epidemiologic studies on epilepsy. Commission on Epidemiology and Prognosis, International League Against Epilepsy. *Epilepsia* **34**:592–596.

First Seizure Trial Group (1993). Randomized clinical trial on the efficacy of antiepileptic drugs in reducing the risk of relapse after a first unprovoked tonic-clonic seizure. *Neurology* **43**:478–483.

Annegers J, Hauser W, Elveback L (1979). Remission of seizures and relapse in patients with epilepsy. *Epilepsia* **20**:729–737.

Annegers J, Hauser W, Lee J, Rocca W (1995). Incidence of acute symptomatic seizures in Rochester, Minnesota, 1935–1984. *Epilepsia* **36**:327–333.

Arif H, Hirsch L (2008). Treatment of status epilepticus. *Semin Neurol* **28**:342–354.

Azar N, Abou-Khalil B (2008). Considerations in the choice of an antiepileptic drug in the treatment of epilepsy. *Semin Neurol* **28**:305–316.

Banerjee P, Filippi D, Allen Hauser W (2009). The descriptive epidemiology of epilepsy – a review. *Epilepsy Res* **85**:31–45.

Beghi E, Tognoni G (1988). Prognosis of epilepsy in newly referred patients: a multicenter prospective study. Collaborative Group for the Study of Epilepsy. *Epilepsia* **29**:236–243.

Boylan L, Flint L, Labovitz D, Jackson S, Starner K, Devinsky O (2004). Depression but not seizure frequency predicts quality of life in treatment-resistant epilepsy. *Neurology* **62**:258–261.

Budrys V (2007). Neurology in holy Scripture. *Eur J Neurol* **14**:e1–6.

Claassen J, Lokin J, Fitzsimmons B, Mendelsohn F, Mayer S (2002). Predictors of functional disability and mortality after status epilepticus. *Neurology* **58**:139–142.

Claassen J, Mayer S, Kowalski R, Emerson R, Hirsch L (2004). Detection of electrographic seizures with continuous EEG monitoring in critically ill patients. *Neurology* **62**:1743–1748.

Cockerell O, Johnson A, Sander J, Shorvon S (1997). Prognosis of epilepsy: a review and further analysis of the first nine years of the British National General Practice Study of Epilepsy, a prospective population-based study. *Epilepsia* **38**:31–46.

DeLorenzo R, Hauser W, Towne A, *et al.* (1996). A prospective, population-based epidemiologic study of status epilepticus in Richmond, Virginia. *Neurology* **46**:1029–1035.

Devinsky O (1999). Patients with refractory seizures. *N Engl J Med* **340**:1565–1570.

Devinsky O, Barr W, Vickrey B, *et al.* (2005). Changes in depression and anxiety after resective surgery for epilepsy. *Neurology* **65**:1744–1749.

Economou N, Lascaratos J (2005). The Byzantine physicians on epilepsy. *J Hist Neurosci* **14**:346–352.

Engel J, Pedley TA (2008). *Epilepsy: A Comprehensive Textbook*. Wolters Kluwer Health/Lippincott Williams & Wilkins, Philadelphia.

Engel JJ, Wiebe S, French J, *et al.* (2003). Practice parameter: temporal lobe and localized neocortical resections for epilepsy: report of the Quality Standards Subcommittee of the American Academy of Neurology, in association with the American Epilepsy Society and the American Association of Neurological Surgeons. *Neurology* **60**:538–547.

Gilliam F, Kuzniecky R, Faught E, Black L, Carpenter G, Schrodt R (1997). Patient-validated content of epilepsy-specific quality-of-life measurement. *Epilepsia* **38**:233–236.

Glauser T, Ben-Menachem E, Bourgeois B, *et al.* (2006). ILAE treatment guidelines: evidence-based analysis of antiepileptic drug efficacy and effectiveness as initial monotherapy for epileptic seizures and syndromes. *Epilepsia* **47**:1094–1120.

Jones J, Hermann B, Barry J, Gilliam F, Kanner A, Meador K (2003). Rates and risk factors for suicide, suicidal ideation, and suicide attempts in chronic epilepsy. *Epilepsy Behav* **4**(Suppl 3):S31–S38.

Jordan K (1999). Continuous EEG monitoring in the neuroscience intensive care unit and emergency department. *J Clin Neurophysiol* **16**:14–39.

Kho L, Lawn N, Dunne J, Linto J (2006). First seizure presentation: do multiple seizures within 24 hours predict recurrence? *Neurology* **67**:1047–1049.

Kwan P, Brodie M (2000). Early identification of refractory epilepsy. *N Engl J Med* **342**:314–319.

Lai C, Lai Y (1991). History of epilepsy in Chinese traditional medicine. *Epilepsia* **32**:299–302.

Langfitt J, Holloway R, McDermott M, *et al.* (2007). Health care costs decline after successful epilepsy surgery. *Neurology* **68**:1290–1298.

Logroscino G, Hesdorffer D, Cascino G, Annegers J, Hauser W (2001). Time trends in incidence, mortality, and case-fatality after first episode of status epilepticus. *Epilepsia* **42**:1031–1035.

Lowenstein D, Alldredge B (1993). Status epilepticus at an urban public hospital in the 1980s. *Neurology* **43**:483–488.

Lowenstein D, Alldredge B (1998). Status epilepticus. *N Engl J Med* **338**:970–976.

Manyam B (1992). Epilepsy in ancient India. *Epilepsia* **33**:473–475.

Mazarati A, Baldwin R, Sankar R, Wasterlain C (1998). Time-dependent decrease in the effectiveness of antiepileptic drugs during the course of self-sustaining status epilepticus. *Brain Res* **814**:179–185.

Ramos Lizana J, Cassinello Garciá E, Carrasco Marina L, Vázquez López M, Martín González M, Muñoz Hoyos A (2000). Seizure recurrence after a first unprovoked seizure in childhood: a prospective study. *Epilepsia* **41**:1005–1013.

Ramsay RE, Rowan AJ, Pryor FM (2004). Special considerations in treating the elderly patient with epilepsy. *Neurology* **62**:S24–S29.

Reynolds E, Kinnier Wilson J (2008). Psychoses of epilepsy in Babylon: the oldest account of the disorder. *Epilepsia* **49**:1488–1490.

Sperling M, O'Connor M, Saykin A, Plummer C (1996). Temporal lobectomy for refractory epilepsy. *JAMA* **276**:470–475.

Stein MA, Kanner AM (2009). Management of newly diagnosed epilepsy: a practical guide to monotherapy. *Drugs* **69**:199–222.

Todman D (2008). Epilepsy in the Graeco-Roman world: Hippocratic medicine and Asklepian temple medicine compared. *J Hist Neurosci* **17**:435–441.

Towne A, Waterhouse E, Boggs J, *et al.* (2000). Prevalence of nonconvulsive status epilepticus in comatose patients. *Neurology* **54**:340–345.

Téllez-Zenteno J, Dhar R, Hernandez-Ronquillo L, Wiebe S (2007). Long-term outcomes in epilepsy surgery: antiepileptic drugs, mortality, cognitive and psychosocial aspects. *Brain* **130**:334–345.

HEADACHE

Peter J. Goadsby

HEADACHE

Definition and etiology

Table 14 presents the clinical classification and prevalence of different types of headache in the general population. The etiologies of headache are presented in *Table 15*.

Clinical history

- Length of history of headache: is this a new headache or not; has it changed in character, severity or frequency? Why seek care now?
- Assess frequency: how many headache days a month or per week? Check by asking how many completely headache-free days per week. It is often easier in frequent headache to say how often it is not there.

TABLE 14 **CLINICAL CLASSIFICATION AND PREVALENCE OF HEADACHE IN THE GENERAL POPULATION (%)**

Primary	%
Tension-type headache	69
Primary stabbing headache (ice-pick headache)	33
Migraine	16
Exertional headache	1
Cluster headache	0.1
Secondary	%
Systemic infection	63
Head injury	4
Drug-induced headache	3
Vascular disorders	1
Subarachnoid hemorrhage	<1
Brain tumour	0.1

TABLE 15 **ETIOLOGY OF HEADACHE**

	Children/ adolescents (3–17 years)	**Adults** (18–65 years)	**Adults** (65+ years)
Tension-type headache	++	+++	+
Migraine	++	+++	+
Idiopathic stabbing headache	+	+	+
Exertional headache	+	++	–
Cluster headache	+	++	+
Post-traumatic	++	+++	+
Medication overuse headache	–	++	++
Cervicogenic (referred from neck)	–	+	+++
Cranial arteritis	–	+	+++
Subarachnoid hemorrhage	+	++	+
Subdural hematoma	+/–	++	++
Brain abscess	+	+	+
Brain tumor	+	++	++
Idiopathic intracranial hypertension	+/–	++	–
Glaucoma	–	+	++
Paget's disease of the skull	–	+	++
Cerebral venous sinus thrombosis	+/–	+	+
Arnold–Chiari malformation	+/–	+	+/–

- Features of the headache itself:
  - Location/site of headache.
  - Onset.
  - Type/quality of headache (throbbing, steady).
  - Timing including duration.
  - Severity.
  - Radiation.
  - Associated features:
    - Nausea, photophobia, phonophobia.
    - Aura: neurologic symptoms such as visual disturbance, weakness, diplopia, clumsiness, disturbance of balance.
    - Fever, altered consciousness.
    - Cranial autonomic features: lacrimation, conjunctival injection, periorbital swelling, nasal symptoms, ptosis.
  - Exacerbating factors (e.g. physical activity, bright light, noise).
  - Relieving factors.
  - Triggers: changes in sleep pattern, eating, exertion, stress (especially relaxation after stress), menses, alcohol.
  - Premonitory features: neck discomfort, tiredness, yawning, cognitive impairment, mood change, polyuria, food cravings.
- Family history.
- Medications/drugs.

Physical examination

- Fever or other signs of systemic illness (e.g. temporal artery tenderness [**134**, **135**]).
- Conscious state.
- Neck stiffness.
- Upper cervical spine facet joints.
- Papilledema (**136**).
- Subhyaloid hemorrhage (**137**).
- Eye movements.
- Facial weakness.
- Limb weakness or incoordination.
- Gait disturbance.

Differential diagnosis

Primary headaches

See *Table 16*.

Secondary headaches

- Meningitis: fever, meningismus (stiff neck).
- Temporal arteritis (**135**): elderly, scalp tenderness, jaw claudication, high erythrocyte sedimentation rate (ESR).
- Idiopathic (benign) intracranial hypertension (**136**): young, obese women, papilledema.
- Subarachnoid hemorrhage (SAH) (**137**): sudden onset, severe headache, stiff neck, subhyaloid hemorrhage).

TABLE 16 **DIFFERENTIAL DIAGNOSIS OF PRIMARY HEADACHES**

	Tension-type headache	**Migraine**	**Cluster headache**
Gender	Male = female	Female predominance (3:1)	Male predominance (3:1)
PAIN			
Location	Bilateral	2/3 hemicranial orbit or frontal	Unilateral orbit or temple
Type	Steady tightness	Throbbing	Boring
Severity	Moderate	Severe	Very severe
Duration	Chronic, usually daily	Hours to days	15–180 minutes, often nocturnal
Aura	None	One-third	Rare
Nausea/vomiting	None	Often	Uncommon
Photophobia, phonophobia	None	Often	Less common
Ipsilateral autonomic features	None	One-third	Typical
Periodicity	Episodic or chronic, usually daily	Episodic, may be chronic	Clusters (weeks to months) 1–8 attacks/day

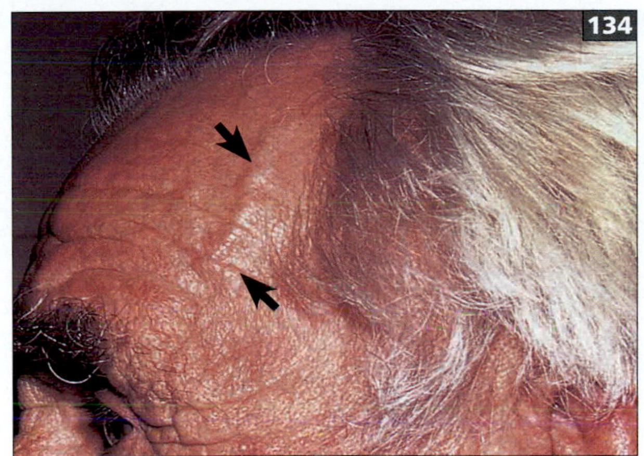

134 Lateral photograph of the forehead of a patient with giant cell arteritis showing a visibly enlarged, tender, temporal artery (arrows).

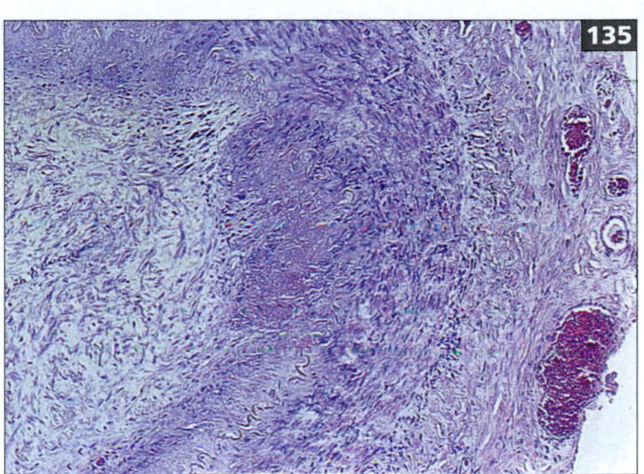

135 Temporal artery in cross-section showing features of active giant cell arteritis with fibroblastic proliferation in the intima (on the left of the photograph), fibrinoid necrosis in the subintima, disruption of the internal elastic lamina, histiocytic proliferation, multinucleated giant cells, and infiltration of adventitia by lymphocytes and plasma cells.

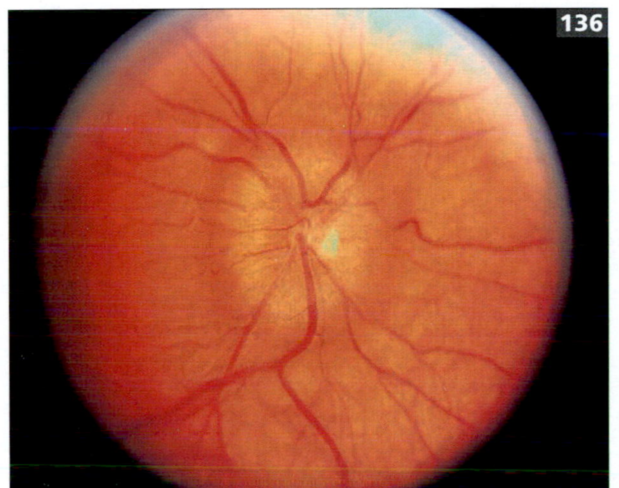

136 Ocular fundus showing papilledema in a patient with idiopathic intracranial hypertension. *Courtesy of Mr M. Wade, Department of Medical Illustrations, Royal Perth Hospital, Australia.*

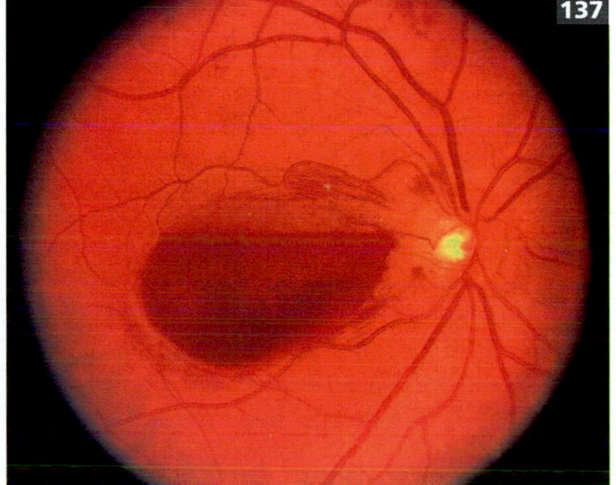

137 Ocular fundus showing subhyaloid hemorrhage in a patient with subarachnoid hemorrhage. *Courtesy of Mr M. Wade, Department of Medical Illustrations, Royal Perth Hospital, Australia.*

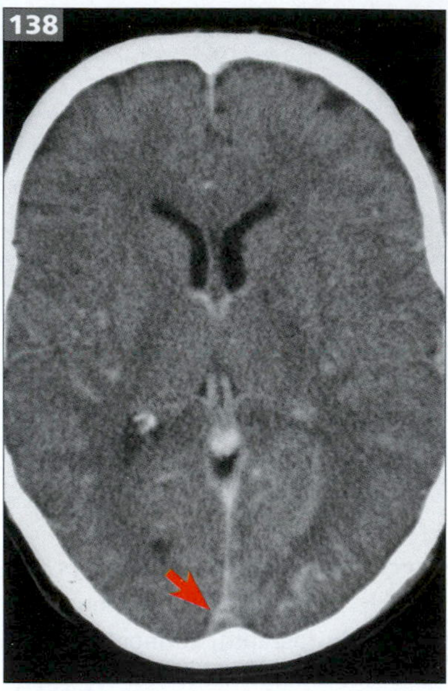

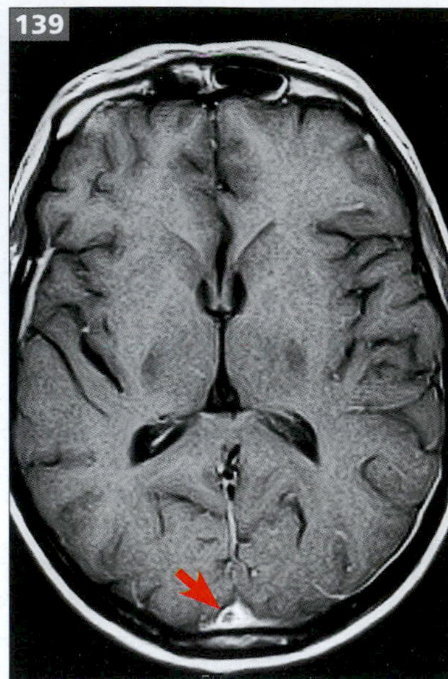

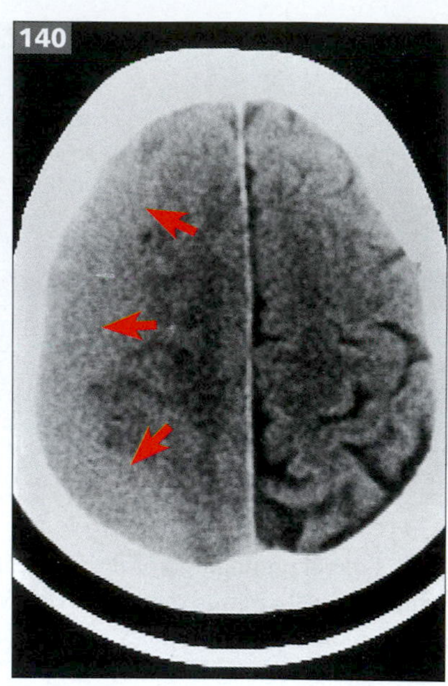

138, 139 CT brain scan with contrast (138) and MRI brain scan (139), T1W post contrast axial images showing a filling defect at the torcula due to venous sinus thrombosis (the empty delta sign, arrows).

140 CT brain scan, axial image, showing a right subdural haematoma as slight hyperdensity over the convexity of the right cerebral hemisphere (arrows).

- Cerebral venous sinus thrombosis (**138, 139**).
- Subdural hemorrhage (**140**).
- Cerebral tumor: headache in early morning, neurologic signs often present, personality change, seizures.
- Arnold–Chiari malformation (**141**): orthostatic – low cerebrospinal fluid (CSF) pressure/volume headache, better when recumbent, worse when upright and at the end of the day. Magnetic resonance imaging (MRI) with gadolinium demonstrates diffuse meningeal enhancement (**142**).

Restrict to patients presenting with:
- Atypical symptoms or signs indicative of organic pathology.
- Certain physical signs, such as papilledema or a red tender scalp vessel.

Diagnosis and investigations

Before a primary type of headache such as tension-type headache or migraine is diagnosed, secondary headaches should be considered and eliminated on clinical grounds or by appropriate investigations (see *Table 17*). If there is suspicion of secondary headache consider:
- Full blood count.
- ESR in patients over 50 years old.
- Blood biochemistry.

Computed tomography (CT) or MRI brain scan

Use of CT and MRI (**138–141**) depends on the type of headache and any associated features. For example, sudden onset headache associated with loss of consciousness suggests probable SAH or pituitary apoplexy, in which case CT brain scanning is the initial investigation of choice. Headache coming on over several weeks which is worse in the morning and on coughing suggests raised intracranial pressure, in which case a contrast enhanced CT scan (?brain tumor) or MRI scan (?venous sinus thrombosis), perhaps followed by angiography would be appropriate. If an Arnold–Chiari malformation is suspected, then the craniocervical junction and brain needs to be imaged by high resolution CT or MRI scan. Arnold–Chiari can be seen in low CSF pressure headache. The imaging requirements of headache with localizing features require a little more thought; for example, pituitary disease (MRI), ear disease (MRI for internal auditory meatus, CT for middle and external ear problems), or sinus disease (CT to diagnose plus look at the ostia), but in any case it is essential to state all the relevant history on the request card or the investigation may not answer the problem.

Treatment

- Explain the problem to the patient.
- Identify and avoid any precipitating factors.
- Institute appropriate specific treatment.

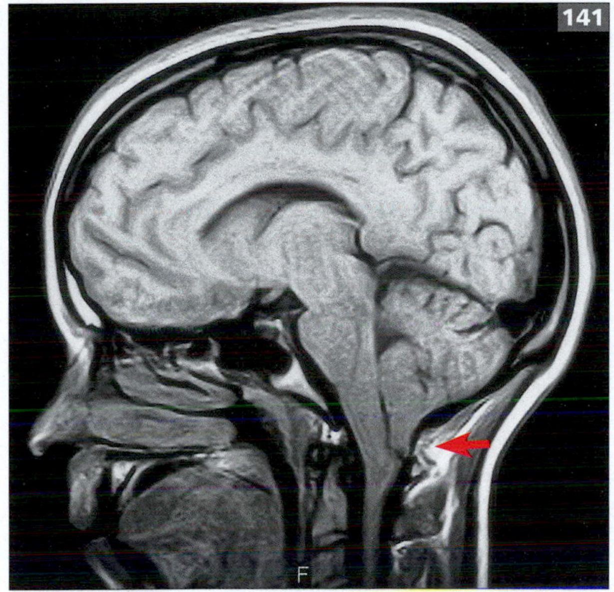

141 MRI brain scan, sagittal image, showing an Arnold–Chiari malformation (arrow).

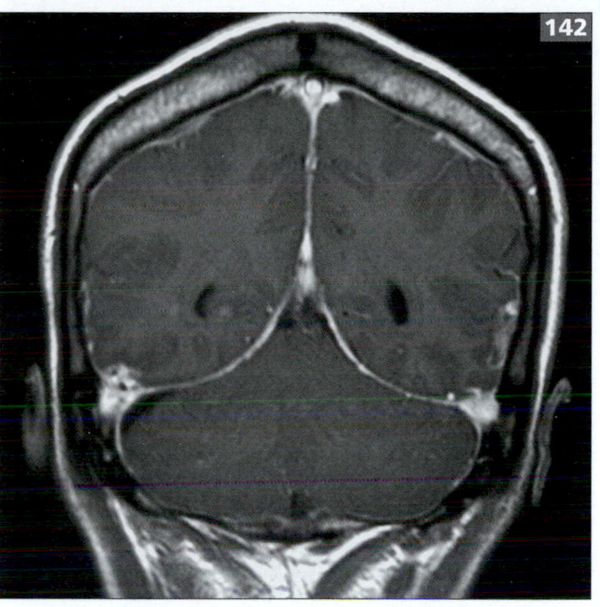

142 MRI brain scan, coronal plane, showing diffuse enhancement (whiteness) of the meninges in a patient with headache due to low cerebrospinal fluid pressure.

MIGRAINE

Definition, epidemiology, and etiology

A neurologic disorder that manifests as discrete episodes of headache associated with other features of sensory sensitivity.

Tip

▶ *Migraine is the most common form of primary headache that comes to physicians, accounting for 90% of presentations, as it is much more disabling than tension-type headache.*

- Prevalence[1]:
  - Lifetime:
    - Women: 33% (95% CI: 31–37%).
    - Men: 13% (95% CI: 12–16%).
  - 1 year:
    - Women: 25% (95% CI: 23–29%).
    - Men: 7.5% (CI: 7–9%).
    - Higher in Caucasians than African-Americans, than Asians.
- Age:
  - Onset is nearly always (90%) before age 50 years; 25% begin in childhood/adolescence.
  - Peak incidence at age 10–12 for males and 14–16 years for females.
  - Peak prevalence at age 50 years for men and 35 years for females.
  - Attacks commonly increase in frequency at the menopause for some years and then settle. Aura without headache may begin at that time (sometimes called acephalgic migraine).
- Gender:
  - Children: M = F.
  - Adolescents and adults: F>M = 2–3:1.

Etiology is unknown.

TABLE 17 **INVESTIGATION OF THE PATIENT PRESENTING WITH HEADACHE**

Headache onset	**Abrupt**	**Subacute** (hours)	**Subacute** (hours to days)	**Progressive** (days to weeks)	**Intermittent** (may be abrupt)
ASSOCIATED FEATURES*					
Unilateral headache	o	o	o	+	+
Bilateral headache	+	+	+	+	+
Visual symptoms	o	o	o	+	+
Photophobia	+	o	o	o	+
Family history	o	o	o	o	+
Personality change	⩽	o	o	+	o
Seizures	o	o	+	+	o
Focal neurologic symptoms and signs	o	o	+	+	+
Fever	o	+	+	o	o
Neck stiffness	+	+	o	o	o
Papilledema	o	o	o	+	o
Subhyaloid blood	+	o	o	o	o
Coma	+	+	+	+	o
Rash	o	+	o	o	o
Recurrent		o	o	o	+
SUSPECT**	Subarachnoid hemorrhage	Meningitis	Viral encephalitis	Structural intra-cranial lesion	Migraine

Think: *Is there a high index of suspicion for bacterial meningitis? Are immediate blood cultures and empirical antibiotics required?*

Imaging (CT or MRI)	Subarachnoid blood or normal	Normal (meninges may enhance)	May be normal	Lesion: subdural haematoma tumour, abscess	Normal; not indicated except to exclude other causes

Lumbar puncture: *May be unsafe if there is evidence of raised intracranial pressure, a mass, lesion, a swollen brain, a bleeding diathesis or sepsis at the site of the lumbar puncture. Needs to be delayed at least 12 hours after onset of suspected subarachnoid hemorrhage, and if CT brain scan is negative. If done, always record the opening pressure.*

* Not all need to be present.

** Tension-type headache is the most common cause of headache, though as it is rarely disabling it only infrequently presents to doctors, and even less so in emergent situations.

\+ Present

o Absent

TABLE 17 continued

CEREBROSPINAL FLUID	**Subarachnoid hemorrhage**	**Meningitis**	**Viral encephalitis**	**Structural intra-cranial lesion**	**Migraine**
Appearance	Xanthochromia	Turbid	Clear or turbid	Contraindicated	Not indicated
RBC	+	o	o		o
WBC	<3 (normal)	Polymorphs	Lymphocytes		<3 (normal)
Gram stain	Negative	Organisms	Negative		Negative
Protein	Normal or raised	Raised	Raised		Normal
Glucose	Normal	Low	Normal or low		Normal
Management	Consult Neurosurgery and Neuroradiology (Surgery? GDC coil?) Cerebral angiography	Antibiotics	Acyclovir, EEG, HSV, PCR	Consult Neurosurgery	Consider fluids Antiemetics Treat headache: non-specific-NSAIDS, prochlorperazine; specific: triptans, dihydroergotamine **Note:** *opioid analgesics are generally a poor choice.*

Migraine without aura

A combination of genetic factors (possibly involving ion channel function) and environmental factors (e.g. stress); first-degree relatives of probands with migraine without aura have a twofold increased risk of migraine without aura compared with the general population; the proband-wise concordance rate is higher in monozygotic (MZ) than dizygotic twins (0.43 [95% CI: 0.36–0.49] *vs.* 0.31 [95% CI: 0.26–0.36])[2].

Migraine with aura

Largely genetic; first-degree relatives of probands with migraine with aura have a fourfold increased risk of migraine with aura compared with the general population; the proband-wise concordance rate is higher in MZ than dizygotic twins (0.50 [95% CI: 0.38–0.62] *vs.* 0.21 [95% CI: 0.12–0.30]). However, environmental factors are also important as the pairwise concordance rate is less than 100% in MZ twin pairs (i.e. it is about 34% [95% CI: 23–45%])[2].

Familial hemiplegic migraine

Familial hemiplegic migraine (FHM) is a rare autosomal dominant subtype of migraine with aura. Genes for FHM include *CACNA1A*, *ATP1A2*, and *SCN1A*. The *CACNA1A* gene at 19p13 encodes the alpha1A subunit (the ion conducting part) of a brain specific P/Q type voltage-dependent calcium channel, suggesting that migraine aura may be a 'cerebral calcium channelopathy'.

Pathophysiology

Migraine is triggered by the effect of a range of putative environmental and biochemical factors on the brain or hypothalamus (the latter of which, in turn, is modulated by seasonal patterns, diurnal and biological clocks, and hormonal factors and coitus); the premonitory symptoms of elation, yawning, or a craving for sweet foods, experienced by about three-quarters of patients, suggest hypothalamic involvement.

Triggers

- Emotional stress and tension.
- Relaxation after stress.
- Altered sleep patterns.
- Hormonal changes: fall in estradiol levels at menstruation and midcycle.
- High dose estrogen-containing contraceptives.
- Strong sensory stimulation: bright or flickering light; loud noise; strong smells; nerve compression (e.g. 'swim-goggle migraine').
- Head trauma, such as heading the ball in soccer ('footballer's migraine').
- Food idiosyncrasies/allergies: alcohol, perhaps specific dietary amines (cheese).
- Missing meals.
- Meteorologic changes.
- Nitrates.
- Medication overuse.

Tip

▶ *Regularity of habit is the key advice to patients with migraine.*

Migraine and the brain[3]

Subcortical structures, such as hypothalamus and brainstem nuclei, dorsal raphe nuclei (which contain serotonin), and locus ceruleus (containing noradrenaline) are initially dysfunctional leading to increased afferent input through the trigeminovascular system and cortical over-activity due to dyshabituation (**143**).

Axons of the first division of the trigeminal nerve, which innervate the pain-producing intracranial structures, depolarize as a result of direct neuronal activation or vasodilatation of dural and cerebral arteries, or both, leading to central transmission of nociceptive pain signals to bipolar neurons in the trigeminal ganglion and on to the trigeminal nucleus in its most caudal extent in the caudal medulla and the dorsal horn of the spinal cord at C1 and C2: the trigeminocervical complex, which accounts for the commonly reported neck pain with migraine. Impulses are then transmitted to the ventroposteriomedial nucleus of the thalamus via the quintothalamic tract, from where they are relayed to the cortex.

Stimulation of the trigeminal ganglion leads to the release of powerful vasodilator neuropeptides such as calcitonin gene-related peptide (CGRP) from trigeminal neurons that innervate the cranial circulation. This peptide is not only a vasodilator but is a crucial transmitter in the trigeminovascular system in the trigeminocervical complex and the thalamus[4].

Tip

▶ *Migraine is a disorder of the brain's perception of the environment: light, sound, movement, and so clinicians need a broad view when unusual symptoms are encountered.*

Migraine aura and headache

At the onset of aura, regional cerebral blood flow to the clinically involved part of the brain is reduced by about 20%, and reduced neuronal activity spreads in a wave across the cerebral cortex, usually beginning in the occipital region and slowly moving forward (spreading depression of Leao). Migraine headache begins while regional cerebral blood flow is reduced. During the headache, the level of a vasodilator peptide, CGRP, increases in the external jugular venous blood.

Migraine attacks can be ameliorated by activating serotonin (5-hydroxytryptamine) 5-HT 1B/1D receptors that are found on cranial vessels, pre-junctional nerves, in the trigeminocervical complex, and in other brain areas such as trigeminothalamic neurons and in the ventrolateral periaqueductal gray matter.

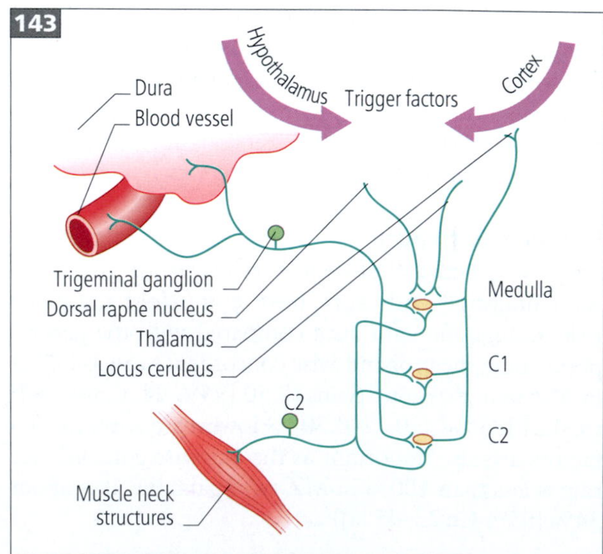

143 **Diagram showing how the trigeminovascular pathway may be activated to produce migraine headache.**

Clinical features

For precipitating factors, see Triggers, above.

Pattern

Phase one: premonitory:

- Occurs in 75% of migraineurs.
- Gradual onset and evolution over up to 72 hours.
- Tiredness, neck discomfort, yawning, lightheadedness, dulled perception, irritability, withdrawal, cravings for particular foods (particularly sweet foods), polyuria, elation and speech difficulties.

Phase two: aura

- Present in only 25% of patients: aura.
- Visual symptoms most commonly: blurred vision, flashing lights (photopsia) or shimmering zigzag lines of light (fortification spectra), sometimes around an area of impaired vision or blindness (scintillating scotoma) in a part of the visual field of one or both eyes (**144**).
- Somatosensory: tingling or pins and needles, or less commonly numbness, in the face, arm, hand, or leg.
- Dysphasia: difficulty understanding and expressing speech.
- Gradual onset, symptoms 'build up' or progress over 5–10 minutes, then subside within 5–60 minutes.
- Followed within 60 minutes by headache; the aura may continue into the headache phase.

Phase three: headache

Present in most, but not all migraine attacks (cf. migraine aura without headache, previously known as acephalgic migraine).

Site

- Unilateral in two-thirds of patients, and bilateral in one-third.
- Frontotemporal region commonly, spreading to occipital region.

Quality

- Throbbing/pulsatile.
- Moderate to severe.

Tip

▶ *Migraine presents as a syndrome; not all manifestations are present in all patients.*

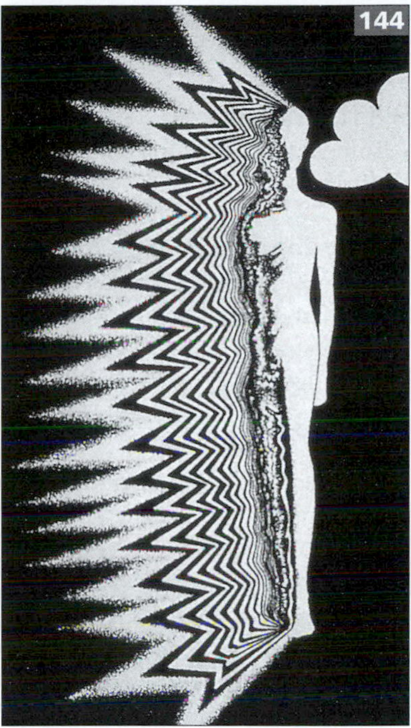

144 Illustration of the type of visual aura a migraineur may describe; in this case shimmering zigzag lines of light (fortification spectra).

Attack features include

- Scalp tenderness on the affected side (about two-thirds of cases): allodynia.
- Nausea (90% of patients).
- Vomiting (10%).
- Physical activity/movement.
- Light (photophobia, 80%).
- Sound (phonophobia, 75%).
- Diarrhea (10%).
- Duration is 4–72 hours; commonly 2–6 hours in children, and 6–24 hours in adults.

Phase four: post-drome

For up to 24 hours after the headache has subsided, most migraineurs feel tired and 'drained' or 'washed-out', with aching muscles. Others however, become euphoric for a period of time.

Periodicity with recurrence: migraine is paroxysmal; clearly defined episodes may recur many times each month. Family history of migraine is present in more than one-half of patients.

Special forms

Migraine variants occur in less than 1% of migraineurs.

Retinal migraine

Monocular, rather than binocular hemianopic visual disturbance.

Ophthalmoplegic migraine

This is not currently considered a form of migraine, rather an ophthalmic cranial neuropathy[5]:

- Paralysis of one of the ocular cranial nerves, usually the IIIrd nerve, at the height of a migraine headache.
- The paralysis usually resolves but may persist after recurrent episodes.
- This entity does not embrace a transient dilatation or constriction (Horner's syndrome) of one pupil as this is quite commonly seen during severe migraine attacks.
- The cause of the cranial neuropathy in ophthalmoplegic migraine is probably transient ischemia of the cranial nerve.

Vertebrobasilar or basilar-type migraine

Now called migraine with brainstem aura. Gradual onset and evolution over several minutes of brainstem, cerebellar, and visual disturbances, often accompanied or followed by headache and syncope.

Hemiplegic migraine[6,7]

Hemiparesis preceding or occurring with a migraine headache. A family history of hemiplegic migraine is often present and the gene is located on chromosome 19 or 1.

Migrainous infarction

Permanent focal neurologic symptoms persisting beyond 24 hours after the cessation of migraine headache. Cranial CT or MRI scan shows features consistent with cerebral infarction. The cause is probably arterial thrombosis, provoked by arterial spasm and a procoagulant state (e.g. cigarette smoking and the oral contraceptive pill).

Menstrual migraine

Just before menstruation, plasma estradiol (rather than progesterone) levels fall rapidly below about 20 ng/ml which sets in motion a series of changes (perhaps through prostaglandins) that culminate in the onset of migraine in about 60% of women migraineurs and exclusively at that time in about 14%. Migraine is relieved by pregnancy in about 60% of women, many, but not all, of whom have a history of menstrual migraine.

Migraine in childhood

- Headache and vomiting are common but the child may be unable to describe the symptoms and may simply appear pale, ill, limp, and inert, complaining of poorly localized abdominal pain.
- Fever up to 38.5°C (101.3°F) may be present so that the suspicion of appendicitis or mesenteric adenitis often arises.
- Rather than accept a label of 'bilious attacks' or 'periodic syndrome', recurrent headaches or vomiting attacks in children which may develop at times of excitement or stress should be considered as possibly migrainous and not psychosomatic.

Differential diagnosis

Abrupt onset of headache ('thunderclap headache')

Tip

▶ *Thunderclap headache should be treated as secondary until investigated.*

Primary

- Cluster headache.
- Primary exertional headache.
- Primary sex headache.
- Idiopathic stabbing headache.

Secondary

- SAH.
- 'Sentinel headache' (enlargement of a cerebral aneurysm without rupture).
- Intracerebral hemorrhage (ICH).
- A precipitous rise in blood pressure: drug-induced headache.
- Head injury.
- Acute obstruction of the CSF pathways.

Unilateral headache

- Cluster headache.
- Temporal arteritis.
- Glaucoma.
- Temperomandibular joint disease.
- Internal carotid or vertebral artery dissection.
- Structural intracranial lesion.

Continuous or daily headache

(Headache on 15 days or more per month for more than 3 months.)

Tip

▶ *The presence of features, such as lateralization, light, sound, or movement sensitivity, differentiates migraine from tension-type headache.*

Primary

- Tension-type headache: just headache with no other features of sensory sensitivity.
- Chronic migraine: migrainous biology manifest on 15 days or more per month.

Secondary

- Rebound headache: a periodic daily bilateral headache that has gradually increased in frequency, and changed in character from the typical migraine headaches, in concurrence with increasing consumption and overuse of analgesic drugs, particularly those which also contain caffeine.
- Systemic infection.
- Giant cell arteritis.
- Raised intracranial pressure: idiopathic intracranial hypertension, brain tumor.

Migraine aura without headache

(acephalgic migraine)

- Transient ischemic attack (TIA).
- Epileptic seizure.
- Arteriovenous malformation.
- Mitochondrial deoxyribonucleic acid (DNA) disorders (e.g. mitochondrial encephalomyopathy, lactic acidosis, and stroke -like episodes [MELAS]).
- Cerebral autosomal dominant arteriopathy with subcortical infarction and leukoencephalopathy (CADASIL).

Investigations

Investigation should only be necessary if headache is suspected to be secondary to another disorder. 'Alarm symptoms' include:

- Onset above age 50 years.
- Aura without headache.
- Aura symptoms of acute onset without spread.
- Aura symptoms that are very brief (<5 min) or unusually long (>60 min – prolonged aura).
- Aura symptoms that are stereotyped (i.e. always at the same body site).
- Sudden increase in migraine frequency or change in migraine characteristics.
- High fever.
- Abnormal neurologic examination.

The role of imaging in patients with suspected migraine is to exclude structural causes for the headache such as arteriovenous malformations (AVMs) or tumors. A contrast-enhanced CT scan is satisfactory for this, and is usually normal (unless there is an AVM or tumor). If MRI is performed, the T2-weighted image occasionally shows areas of altered signal in the white matter which have recently been shown to have no long-term consequences[8], or may rarely be due to CADASIL. The appearance is nonspecific, however.

Diagnosis

Diagnosis is clinical, and includes the following:

- At least five attacks.
- Attacks last 4–72 hours if untreated or unsuccessfully treated.
- At least two of:
    - Unilateral headache.
    - Pulsating headache.
    - Moderate or severe headache.
    - Headache aggravated by routine physical activity.
- At least one of:
    - Nausea, with or without vomiting.
    - Photophobia.
    - Phonophobia.

Tip

▶ *Migraine presents as a syndrome; not all features are necessary for the diagnosis.*

Treatment[1,9]

The patient should avoid precipitating/triggering factors, and identify these by keeping a diary, if necessary.

Treatment of the acute migraine attack

Ancillary measures:

- Rest in a quiet dark room.
- Intravenous fluids if severely dehydrated.

Nonspecific analgesics and antiemetic/prokinetic compounds

- Aspirin 2 or 3 × 300 mg chewable tablets (600–900 mg) orally.
- Paracetamol (acetaminophen) 2 × 500 mg tablets (1 g) orally.
- Compound codeine-containing analgesic (e.g. codeine 15–30 mg) may cause or exacerbate nausea and tend to make other medicines such as triptans not as effective, thus opioids should be avoided.
- Nonsteroidal anti-inflammatory drugs:
  - Ibuprofen.
  - Naproxen: oral, rectal.
  - Diclofenac: oral (potassium salt-rapid absorption), intramuscular.
  - Ketorolac: intramuscular.
- Other nonspecific drugs:
  - Chlorpromazine: intramuscular, but long term considerations (e.g. tardive dyskinesia).
  - Opioid/narcotic analgesic use is highly controversial, not evidence-based, and is associated with prominent adverse effects, a high risk of dependency, and the tendency to make future attacks harder to treat.

Treat as early as possible (e.g. aspirin 600–900 mg or ibuprofen 400–800 mg, together with domperidone 10 mg, ondansetron 4 mg, or metoclopramide 10 mg), and wait 40 minutes. If headache persists, try a specific treatment such as sumatriptan 50 mg tablet, and wait >1 hour. If headache persists, repeat. Antiemetic and prokinetic compounds (e.g. metoclopramide 10 mg, domperidone 10–20 mg, or ondansetron 4 mg) can be used if nausea and vomiting are a problem. If vomiting is severe, suppositories of domperidone, prochlorperazine, or chlorpromazine may be helpful.

Specific antimigraine agents

Ergot alkaloids are no longer considered first-line agents[10]. However, some patients with frequent and highly disabling migraine may require inpatient management, and IV dihydroergotamine can be extremely useful in this context.

Triptans

Triptans are selective and potent agonists of 5-HT 1B/1D receptors; some are active at the 5-HT 1F receptor, which probably contributes to the neural components of their action. Antimigraine effects are mediated by some part of combination of:

- Inhibition of firing of cells in trigeminal nuclei (5-HT 1B/1D receptors in the brainstem: second generation triptans).
- Inhibition of dural presynaptic 5-HT 1D receptors.
- Vasoconstriction of meningeal, dural, cerebral, or pial vessels (stimulation of presynaptic vascular 5-HT 1B receptors).
- Inhibition of trigeminothalamic neurons (5-HT 1B/1D).
- Modulation of ventrolateral periaqueductal gray modulatory neurons (5-HT 1B/1D).

Tip

▶ *One approach is to start oral sumatriptan and if a patient has an issue use the comparative data to work out where to go next.*

First-generation triptans[11]

Sumatriptan is a specific and selective 5-HT 1B/1D/1F receptor agonist. It is available as subcutaneous injection (4 and 6 mg), oral tablets (25, 50, and 100 mg), nasal spray (20 mg), and rectal preparations (25 mg).

Subcutaneous sumatriptan injection (4 and 6 mg):

- Bioavailability: 96%.
- Therapeutic plasma levels: within 10 minutes.
- For 6 mg, 79% of patients improved at 2 hours after injection ('therapeutic gain' [TG]: active minus placebo = 52%); 71% (TG: 51%) improved within 1 hour.
- 60% of patients pain-free at 2 hours after injection (TG: 42%); 43% (TG: 35%) pain-free after 1 hour.

Oral sumatriptan tablets (2, 50, and 100 mg):

- Bioavailability: 14%.
- Therapeutic plasma levels: within 30–90 minutes.
- For 100 mg, 59% (95% CI: 57–60%) of patients improved at 2 hours after tablets (TG: 33%); 29% (27–30%) of patients pain-free at 2 hours (TG: 26%).

Oral sumatriptan is more effective than conventional treatment with aspirin and metoclopramide or oral ergotamine plus caffeine, particularly in the second and third attacks, suggesting greater consistency for sumatriptan. Recurrence of headache occurs within 24–48 hours in about one-third of responders to sumatriptan (and any other acute antimigraine drug).

Repeated drug administration is usually effective, but the headache may recur again. Recurrence can be reduced by about one-third by the coadministration of naproxen 500 mg[12].

Adverse effects of sumatriptan are common but are usually mild and short-lived. The most frequent are tingling, paresthesias, and warm sensations in the head, neck, chest, and limbs; less frequent are dizziness, flushing, and neck pain or stiffness. The risk and intensity is greater with the fixed subcutaneous formulation. 'Chest-related symptoms' include short-lived heaviness or pressure in the arms and chest, shortness of breath, chest discomfort, anxiety, palpitations, and, very rarely, chest pain. The mechanism is unknown. The risk of sumatriptan-induced myocardial ischemia in the absence of coronary artery disease appears to be acceptable (e.g. no greater than the risk of exercise-induced myocardial ischemia in sportsmen)[13].

Second-generation triptans

- Zolmitriptan 2.5 mg, 5 mg: similar to oral sumatriptan.
- Naratriptan 2.5 mg: slower action and perhaps fewer and less severe adverse effects, but lower efficacy.
- Rizatriptan 10 mg, 40 mg: better efficacy and consistency, and similar tolerability.
- Almotriptan 12.5 mg: similar efficacy, better consistency and tolerability.
- Eletriptan 20 mg, 40 mg, and 80 mg; 80 mg orally is more effective than sumatriptan 100 mg orally with similar consistency but lower tolerability.
- Frovatriptan: lower initial efficacy rates than oral sumatriptan.

None of these agents is consistently effective in all patients and all attacks, and some cause disturbing adverse effects. Moreover, given individual variation each triptan has a role in particular patients, and this can only be determined by use. In general terms, rizatriptan 10 mg and eletriptan 80 mg provide the highest likelihood of success. Ergotamine and sumatriptan should not be prescribed for patients with suspected coronary artery disease, Prinzmetal variant angina, or uncontrolled hypertension.

Prevention

Nonpharmacologic

The patient should avoid precipitating factors: these must be individually determined although in general alcohol and nitrates are reliable triggers. Stress reduction through relaxation exercises and CDs, meditation, yoga, swimming, and similar strategies will reduce migraine frequency in many patients. Regular exercise such as swimming is helpful. Acupuncture in short courses by an experienced therapist can be a useful adjunct to other strategies in some patients.

Pharmacologic

The indication for prophylactic therapy is when the patient needs it. This is usually when the migraine attacks are frequently interfering with their life and recurring every 2 weeks or so, and not responding quickly and adequately to acute treatment. Efficacy is limited: at most about one-half of patients will have a reduction in attack frequency of 50% or more.

The choice of prophylactic agent is primarily determined by the patient and which potential adverse effects are most acceptable (*Table 18*, next page). Adverse effects occur commonly. Discuss the adverse effect profile of each drug with the patient and determine their preference. Asthma (beta blockers), weight gain (pizotifen [pizotyline] and valproate) and cognitive dysfunction (topiramate) are major and common concerns. Botulinum toxin type A has been licensed in many countries specifically to treat chronic (frequent) migraine (*Table 18*)[14].

Establish realistic expectations with the patient before starting: the medication may reduce the frequency of attacks but uncommonly abolishes attacks, and so occasional breakthrough attacks requiring acute treatment will occur. Start slowly, with dosage increments every 7–10 days to minimize adverse effects. Encourage patients to persist for at least 3 months to trial the drug adequately and because most adverse effects become less prominent with time. Follow on with a drug-free interval to reassess the frequency and severity of migraine attacks.

Some patients with frequent and highly disabling migraine may require inpatient management. Intravenous dihydroergotamine can be extremely useful in this context[15].

Tip

► *Start low, go slow with preventives to allow patients to tolerate them better.*

Menstrual migraine

Standard prophylactic (interval) therapy, as above, should be used before hormone manipulation.

Nonsteroidal anti-inflammatory drugs, such as naproxen 500 mg twice daily for 1–2 days prior to menses, may be helpful, as can application of a gel containing 1.5 mg estradiol to the skin 48 hours before the expected onset of menstruation.

Subcutaneous implantation of estradiol pellets, starting with 100 mg, inhibits ovulation and maintains estradiol levels, while regular monthly periods can by induced by cyclical oral progestogens. IM progesterone or 3 monthly cycles of the oral contraceptive pill are alternative strategies.

TABLE 18 ADVERSE EFFECTS OF PREVENTIVE AGENTS IN MIGRAINE

Agent	Dose	Adverse effects
β-ADRENORECEPTOR BLOCKERS		
Propranolol	40–240 mg/day	Tiredness, exercise intolerance, postural hypotension, vivid dreams, probably contraindicated in asthmatic patients
Metoprolol	100–200 mg/day	
ANTI-EPILEPTIC DRUGS		
Sodium valproate	400–800 mg/day	Drowsiness, tremor, weight gain, abnormal liver enzymes, risk of teratogenicity in pregnant women
Topiramate	50–200 mg/day	Paresthesias, cognitive dysfunction, weight loss
5-HT RECEPTOR ANTAGONISTS		
Pizotifen	0.5–3 mg nocte	Drowsiness, sedation, weight gain
Methysergide	1–4 mg/day	Drowsiness, leg cramps, small (0.5%) risk of retroperitoneal or pleural fibrosis if treatment is not stopped for 1 month every 4–6 months and screened with physical examination, CXR, and renal function
NON-SELECTIVE CALCIUM CHANNEL BLOCKERS		
Flunarizine	5–15 mg daily	Constipation; rare extrapyramidal adverse effects with flunarizine Effective in preventing cluster headache
Verapamil	40–120 mg tds	
VITAMINS		
Riboflavin (vitamin B2)	400 mg/day	Diarrhea, polyuria
HERBAL MEDICINES		
Feverfew	–	–
NON-STEROIDAL ANTI-INFLAMMATORY DRUGS		
Naproxen	–	Small risk of peptic ulceration
ANTIDEPRESSANTS		
Amitriptyline	50–150 mg/day	Useful for concurrent tension-type headaches
Dothiepin		Drowsiness, dry mouth, blurred vision
NEUROTOXINS		
Botulinum toxin type A	155U bu PREEMPT protocol	Ptosis, swallowing problems

Prognosis

Migraine is generally paroxysmal, and even in patients with daily headache, worsenings on top are the rule. Clearly defined episodes of migraine recur as often as three or six times each month but sufferers remain symptom-free between attacks. Migraine symptoms frequently change over time.

The frequency of migraine attacks may increase until it develops into chronic migraine, in many patients as a result of acute attack medicine overuse (probably at 10 days or more per month). The severity of the attacks often diminishes with time and in some patients the attacks cease in later years, particularly after the menopause in women. In some women however, attacks increase in frequency at the menopause.

Remission occurs in 70% of pregnancies. For young women, below the age of 45 years, the relative risk of ischemic stroke among migraineurs is increased (compared with age-matched controls), particularly among those taking the oral contraceptive pill, but the absolute risk is extremely small (17–50 per 100,000 per year).

TENSION-TYPE HEADACHE

Definition and epidemiology

An episodic or chronic headache of unclear etiology. While common in the community, careful diary-supported studies show that <10% of patients coming to see a primary care physician/general practitioner have tension-type headache, while 92% have migraine.

- Prevalence:
  - Episodic tension-type headache: 38% 1 year period prevalence.
  - Chronic tension-type headache: 2.2% 1 year period prevalence.
- Age:
  - Any age.
  - Onset before 10 years of age in 15%.
  - Peak prevalence 30–39 years of age.
- Gender: F>M: 1.2:1.

Tip

► *Less than 10% of patients presenting to general practitioners with disabling headache have tension-type headache.*

Etiology and pathophysiology

Unknown. Perhaps, at least in part, a disorder of the central nervous system (CNS) with probable trigeminal activation and sensitization of second-order trigeminal neurons and some peripheral component. Generation of nitric oxide may have a role in central sensitization. Of headache disorders, tension-type headache is the least well understood[16].

Predisposing factors

Genetic factors

First-degree relatives of probands with chronic tension-type headache have about three times the risk of chronic tension-type headache than the general population, suggesting the importance of genetic factors in chronic tension headache[17,18].

Physical abnormalities

- Cervical spondylosis: degenerative changes in the cervical spine are said to be related to this form of headache; however, the evidence is poor.
- Eye strain: refractive errors or ocular imbalance may be a source of tension and should be corrected. At school or at work, the patient should sit in a comfortable chair which is adjusted to the height appropriate for the desk (to ensure good posture) with light adjusted to the correct angle for comfort.

Psychologic factors

- Stress may be clearly associated with exacerbations of headache in some patients and may be helped by readjustment of stresses, alteration of life-style, or psychologic counseling.
- Sleep disturbance is a major perpetuating factor in patients with intermittent muscle contraction headache, which contributes to it becoming chronic.
- Chronic tension-type headache is usually, but not always, related to or exacerbated by anxiety or depression (as well as sleep disturbance).

Psychogenic mechanisms are said to be relevant in some patients, but the evidence is poor. Some form of sensitization with second-order trigeminal neurons is likely to be involved.

Clinical features

- Site: usually bilateral and diffuse or at the vertex of the head, around the head, or in the neck or occiput.
- Nature: nonpulsatile, tight, pressing, heavy or band-like sensation.
- Onset: may occur during times of fatigue, stress, or anxiety.
- Timing: episodic, but may become constant, occurring all day, every day, for months and even years.
- Exacerbating and relieving factors: episodic headache may be relieved by relaxation or analgesics.
- Associated symptoms: for a clear diagnosis of tension-type headache features such as nausea, light or sound sensitivity, or sensitivity to movement should not be present at all.

Differential diagnosis

- Migraine headache is feature-full, i.e. attacks have some combination of nausea, light or sound sensitivity, or sensitivity to movement, with typical change physiology triggers: sleep, eating, exertion. None of these are features of tension-type headache.
- Tension-type headache does not stop normal daily activities but is an irritation.
- Cervicogenic pain: pain referred from the neck.
- Medication overuse headache.
- Raised intracranial pressure.

Investigations and diagnosis

Investigations are not necessary unless a secondary headache is suspected. Diagnosis is based on the history: episodic tension-type headache is featureless headache on <15 days a month; chronic tension-type headache is featureless headache on 15 days a month for ≥3 months.

Treatment

Nonpharmacologic

Reassurance must be prompt and convincing! A course in relaxation training may be highly beneficial in a well-motivated patient. They are now conducted by psychologists, physiotherapists, and many hospitals and community health centers. Various forms of biofeedback may assist relaxation but do not make a substantial impact.

Consider discontinuing or minimizing heavy analgesic intake. For patients in whom episodic tension-type headache or, less frequently, migraine becomes transformed into chronic tension-type headache, overuse of analgesic drugs frequently plays a role in aggravating the disorder, and discontinuation of daily drug intake often results in improvement.

Pharmacologic[19]

Tricyclic antidepressants: amitriptyline, in particular, may be very helpful, commencing with one-half of a 25 mg tablet at night and gradually increasing to three tablets (75 mg) as a single nocturnal dose, provided there are no adverse effects such as drowsiness and confusion. If effective, an improvement will usually be noticed within 2 weeks. Treatment should be continued for about 6 months and then gradually phased out to see whether it is still necessary or whether improvement can be maintained with relaxation alone.

Anxiolytics, such as the benzodiazepines, have a limited role. They should be used for short periods only, and under supervision, because of the risk of habituation, dependency, and drug-induced headache.

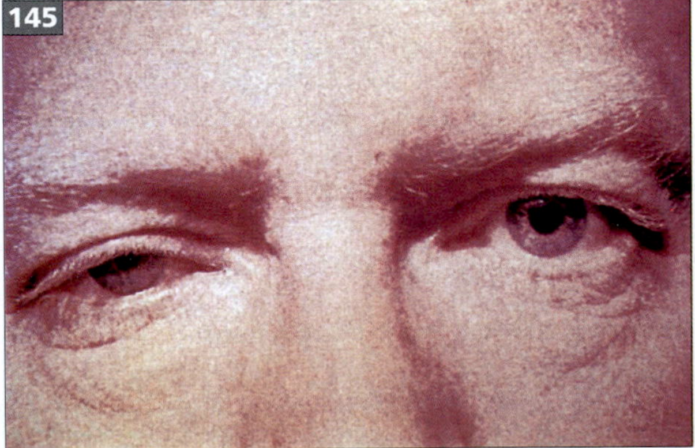

145 Facial photograph during an attack of cluster headache showing unilateral eyelid edema, ptosis, miosis, and conjunctival injection.

CLUSTER HEADACHE

Definition and epidemiology

A relatively rare form of primary headache marked by recurrent episodes, lasting 15–180 minutes, of excruciating unilateral periorbital pain and associated autonomic features, that tend to occur once or twice a day in bouts or clusters, lasting from weeks to months at a time, separated by remission periods of months or 1–2 years.

- Incidence: 6 (3–10)/100,000/year.
- Lifetime prevalence: 0.3 (95% CI: 0.2–0.6)/1000.
- Age: any age, but unusual in children and most common at 20–50 years of age.
- Gender: mainly men (ratio 3:1).

Etiology and pathophysiology[20]

Cluster headache is a neurovascular disorder, which is hypothesized to be generated in the CNS in pacemaker or circadian regions of the hypothalamic gray matter. The trigeminal autonomic reflex is central to the pathogenesis (see Migraine, p. 139). Activation of the trigeminovascular system (i.e. release of CGRP from peripheral terminals of trigeminal nociceptive neurons, which supply cephalic blood vessels) underlies symptoms of cluster headache. Increases in neuropeptide markers of this system rapidly return to normal after treatment with sumatriptan.

The mechanism by which nitroglycerine can induce an attack of cluster headache is at least partly due to activation of the trigeminovascular system.

Clinical features

- Severe, boring, unilateral periorbital pain that may radiate upwards over the frontotemporal region and downwards to the face, jaw, neck, and shoulder.
- Edema of the ipsilateral eyelid.
- Redness of the ipsilateral eye (conjunctival injection).
- Watering of the ipsilateral eye (lacrimation).
- Miosis with or without ptosis ipsilaterally in about 20% of cases (**145**); permanent partial Horner's syndrome (ptosis and miosis) ipsilaterally in about 5% of patients.
- Swelling, dilatation, and tenderness of the superficial temporal vessels occasionally.
- Rhinorrhea and a blocked nostril ipsilaterally.
- Temporal spacing of attacks: the pain usually lasts 30 minutes to 2 hours and recurs once or twice a day, often at night at the same time, for several weeks (active periods), followed by an attack-free period (remission period).
- Alcohol and nitrates may precipitate attacks during the active period, but not in remission periods.

Tip

▶ *Most (90%) of patients with acute cluster headache are agitated and move about while less than 10% of migraineurs behave that way.*

Differential diagnosis

- Other trigeminal autonomic cephalalgias (TACs)[21].
- Pituitary tumors.

Primary short-lasting headaches with prominent cranial autonomic features

Paroxysmal hemicrania (PH)[22]

- Frequent brief attacks of excruciating unilateral orbital, supraorbital, or temporal pain (distribution of ophthalmic division of trigeminal nerve) that last 2–45 minutes and recur five or more times daily (periods with lower daily frequency may occur). The pain is usually stabbing or boring, but may be throbbing as it builds up.
- At least one associated autonomic symptom, such as conjunctival injection, lacrimation, nasal congestion, rhinorrhea, ptosis, or eyelid edema.
- Attacks always resolve rapidly within days of initiating treatment with indomethacin in an adequate dose of up to 225 mg/day orally.
- Age of onset: usually in the twenties, but may occur in children.
- Gender distribution: F = M.
- Pathophysiology: activation of structures in the hypothalamic region and ventral midbrain shown on functional imaging.
- May have chronic or episodic (remitting) course.
- Secondary causes include cavernous sinus meningioma, gangliocytoma of the sella turcica, frontal lobe tumor, AVM, intracranial hypertension, connective tissue disease, and pancoast tumor.
- Distinguished from cluster headache by the shorter duration and higher frequency of attacks, the female preponderance, and the selective response to indomethacin.

Short-lasting unilateral neuralgiform headache attacks with conjunctival injection and tearing (SUNCT) syndrome[23]

- Rare.
- Males predominate: M>F (1.5:1).
- Paroxysms of unilateral moderate or severe orbital or temporal stabbing or throbbing pain lasting between 5 and 250 seconds (i.e. <5 minutes).
- Average about 28 attacks a day (range 3–100).
- Conjunctival injection and lacrimation are present and prominent; other cranial autonomic features may occur such as periorbital swelling, nasal symptoms, or sweating of the forehead and rhinorrhea.
- Pathogenesis: functional imaging demonstrate posterior hypothalamic region involvement.
- SUNCT syndrome may be secondary to posterior fossa lesions such as homolateral cerebellopontine angle AVMs.
- Lamotrigine, topiramate, and gabapentin are useful treatments in many patients.
- Primary short-lasting headaches without prominent cranial autonomic features.

Primary stabbing headache

- Gender: F>M.
- Pain: any part of the head, stabbing, and severe.
- Attack duration: less than 1 second.
- Attack frequency: few to many/day.
- Responds to indomethacin.

Hypnic headache[24]

- Rare.
- Age: elderly (67–84 years).
- Gender: M>F (5:3).
- Pain: generalized, throbbing, and moderately severe.
- Attack duration: 15–30 minutes.
- Attack frequency: 1–3 per night, often awakening patient from sleep.
- Responds to lithium carbonate 600 mg at bedtime, or paradoxically to caffeine taken before bed.

Primary cough headache[25]

A bilateral headache of sudden onset, lasting less than 1 minute, and precipitated by coughing, in the absence of any intracranial disorder, such as a Chiari type I malformation.

Primary exertional headache

A bilateral throbbing headache, lasting from 5 minutes to 24 hours, specifically provoked by physical exercise and unassociated with any systemic or intracranial disorder, such as SAH, sinusitis, and brain metastases.

Headache associated with sexual activity

- Bilateral headaches precipitated by masturbation or coitus, in the absence of any systemic or intracranial disorder, such as SAH.
- Two primary types are recognized:
  - A dull ache in the head and neck that intensifies as sexual excitement increases.
  - A sudden, severe, explosive headache occurring at orgasm.
- A postural headache, resembling that of low CSF pressure, developing after coitus is likely to be due to a CSF leak.

Other secondary or longer-lasting unilateral headaches[26]

Migraine

- Women are affected more commonly than men.
- Headache often lasts a lot longer, up to 72 hours.
- Migraine causes people to want to remain still in a quiet dark room, whereas cluster headache is so severe that patients often pace the floor restlessly or wander outdoors to seek relief in the cold night air.

Giant cell (cranial) arteritis

- Age >50 years at onset.
- New onset of localized headache, which may be unilateral, bilateral, or occipital.
- Claudication of the jaw or tongue during eating.
- Symptoms of systemic upset (fever, sweats, malaise, weight loss, polymyalgia).
- Scalp and temporal artery tenderness or decreased temporal artery pulse.
- Elevated ESR >50 mm/hour.
- Biopsy showing necrotizing arteritis.
- Responds within 24 hours of commencing prednisolone 60 mg/day.

Glaucoma

- Recurrent attacks of pain in the eye and forehead, that may be precipitated by sitting in the dark, mydriatics, or emotional upset.
- Accompanying features include vomiting, visual impairment, cloudiness of the cornea, discoloration of the iris, a dilated pupil, and circumcorneal injection.
- An arcuate scotoma and pallid cupped disc are characteristic of narrow-angle glaucoma, which is often familial.
- Tonometry is necessary to confirm elevated intraocular pressure.

Acute sinusitis (frontal, ethmoidal, maxillary)

- A dull, aching, throbbing pain over the affected sinus, worse on bending or with the head in a certain position in bed.
- The pain is temporarily eased by decongestant nasal drops and antibiotics and seldom lasts more than 1–2 weeks.
- Usually associated with coryza and purulent nasal discharge.

Other conditions

- Cervicogenic headache.
- Facial trauma with soft tissue injury.
- Pituitary adenoma[27,28].
- Pseudoaneurysm within the cavernous sinus.
- Ipsilateral vertebral artery aneurysm.
- Occipital lobe arteriovenous malformation.
- Upper cervical meningioma.

Investigations

Nil usually, unless secondary causes of headache need to be excluded: blood count (thrombocythemia), ESR (cranial arteritis), chest X-ray (pancoast tumor), vasculitic investigations, and CT or MRI brain scan. Should the pain become bilateral, a lumbar puncture may be indicated to exclude intracranial hypertension.

Diagnosis

Episodic

1. At least five attacks fulfilling criteria 2–5.
2. Severe, unilateral orbital, supraorbital and/or temporal pain lasting 15–180 minutes if untreated.
3. Headache associated with at least one of the following signs which have to be present on the painful side: conjunctival injection, lacrimation, nasal congestion, rhinorrhea, forehead and facial sweating, miosis, ptosis, eyelid edema.
4. Incidence of attacks ranging from one attack on alternate days to eight attacks/day.
5. History and/or physical and neurologic examinations do not suggest other disorders associated with head trauma.

Chronic

Attacks occur for more than 1 year without remission, or with remission lasting less than 14 days. The attacks are clinically indistinguishable from episodic cluster headache.

Treatment

Acute attack

- Oxygen 100% at 12–15 l/min often affords relief within 15 minutes[29].
- Sumatriptan, 6 mg subcutaneous injection, or 20 mg nasal spray, or zolmitriptan, 5 mg nasal spray; each has randomized placebo-controlled evidence for an effect in acute cluster headache[30–32].

Prophylactic

During the susceptible period, regular medication can be taken in anticipation of attacks:

- Verapamil in doses up to 960 mg daily with careful monitoring of the electrocardiogram is very effective in cluster headache[33].
- Prednisone 50 mg daily, for 3 days and then reduced rapidly to a dose (usually about 25 mg a day) that is just sufficient to prevent the attacks. This is effective in about 80% of cases in whom it should be maintained for the duration of the bout before weaning off slowly. It should be used no more than once a year to avoid aseptic necrosis.

Chronic cluster headache

- Verapamil as above.
- Lithium carbonate, 250 mg two or three times daily, the dose being adjusted to maintain a blood level of 0.5–1.2 mmol/l. Adverse effects include confusion and tremor.
- Methysergide 1–2 mg three times daily with treatment limited to 6 months and then a 1 month break to avoid fibrotic complications.

Paroxysmal hemicrania

- Indomethacin, 25 mg three times daily, increasing to 75 mg three times daily for 2 weeks to ensure there is an effect.
- Topiramate is a reasonable second-line choice.

Prognosis

The headaches usually recur once or twice a day, often at night, for a period of 4 weeks to 4 months. Remission is then usual, until the next cluster ensues, months or 1–2 years later.

REFERENCES

1 Goadsby PJ, Lipton RB, Ferrari MD (2002). Migraine- current understanding and treatment. *N Engl J Med* **346**:257–270.

2 Gervil M, Ulrich V, Kaprio J, Olesen J, Russell MB (1999). The relative role of genetic and environmental factors in migraine without aura. *Neurology* **53**:995–999.

3 Akerman S, Holland P, Goadsby PJ (2011). Diencephalic and brainstem mechanisms in migraine. *Nature Rev Neurosci* **12**: 570–584.

4 Ho TW, Edvinsson L, Goadsby PJ (2010). CGRP and its receptors provide new insights into migraine pathophysiology. *Nature Rev Neurol* **6**:761–766.

5 Gelfand AA, Gelfand JM, Prabhakar P, Goadsby PJ (2012). Ophthalmoplegic 'migraine' or ophthalmoplegic cranial neuropathy: new cases and a systematic review. *J Child Neurol* **27**:759–766.

6 Haan J, Kors EE, van den Maagdenberg AM, *et al.* (2004). Toward a molecular genetic classification of familial hemiplegic migraine. *Curr Pain Headache Rep* **8**:238–243.

7 Ducros A, Denier C, Joutel A, *et al.* (2001). The clinical spectrum of familial hemiplegic migraine associated with mutations in a neuronal calcium channel. *N Engl J Med* **345**:17–24.

8 Palm-Meinders IH, Koppen H, Terwindt GM, *et al.* (2012). Structural brain changes in migraine. *JAMA* **308**:1889–1897.

9 Goadsby PJ, Sprenger T (2010). Current practice and future directions in the management of migraine: acute and preventive. *Lancet Neurol* **9**:285–298.

10 Tfelt-Hansen P, Saxena PR, Dahlof C, *et al.* (2000). Ergotamine in the acute treatment of migraine – a review and European consensus. *Brain* **123**:9–18.

11 Ferrari MD, Roon KI, Lipton RB, Goadsby PJ (2001). Oral triptans (serotonin, 5-HT1B/1D agonists) in acute migraine treatment: a meta-analysis of 53 trials. *Lancet* **358**:1668–1675.

12 Brandes JL, Kudrow D, Stark SR, *et al.* (2007). Sumatriptan-naproxen for acute treatment of migraine: a randomized trial. *JAMA* **297**:1443–1454.

13 Dodick D, Lipton RB, Martin V, *et al.* (2004). Consensus Statement: Cardiovascular safety profile of triptans (5-HT1B/1D agonists) in the acute treatment of migraine. *Headache* **44**:414–425.

14 Dodick DW, Turkel CC, DeGryse RE, *et al.* (2010) Onabotulinumtoxin A for treatment of chronic migraine: pooled results from the double-blind, randomized, placebo-controlled phases of the PREEMPT clinical program. *Headache* **50**:921–936.

15 Nagy AJ, Gandhi S, Bhola R, Goadsby PJ (2011). Intravenous dihydroergotamine (DHE) for inpatient management of refractory primary headaches. *Neurology* **77**:1827–1832.

16 Goadsby PJ (1999). Chronic tension-type headache: where are we? *Brain* **122**: 1611–1612.

17 Ostergaard S, Russell MB, Bendtsen L, Olesen J (1997). Comparison of first degree relatives and spouses of people with chronic tension-type headache. *BMJ* **314**: 1092–1093.

18 Russell MB, Ostergaard S, Bendsten L, Olesen J (1999). Familial occurrence of chronic tension-type headache. *Cephalalgia* **19**:207–210.

19 Holroyd KA, O'Donnell FJ, Stensland M, Lipchik GL, Cordingley GE, Carlson BW (2001). Management of chronic tension-type headache with (tricylic) antidepressant medication, stress-management therapy and their combination: a randomized controlled trial. *JAMA* **285**:2208–2215.

20 May A (2005). Cluster headache: pathogenesis, diagnosis, and management. *Lancet* **366**:843–855.

21 Goadsby PJ, Lipton RB (1997). A review of paroxysmal hemicranias, SUNCT syndrome and other short-lasting headaches with autonomic features, including new cases. *Brain* **120**:193–209.

22 Cittadini E, Matharu MS, Goadsby PJ (2008). Paroxysmal hemicrania: a prospective clinical study of thirty-one cases. *Brain* **131**:1142–1155.

23 Goadsby PJ, Cittadini E, Cohen AS (2010). Trigeminal autonomic cephalalgias: paroxysmal hemicrania, SUNCT/SUNA and hemicrania continua. *Sem Neurol* **30**:186–191.

24 Evers S, Goadsby PJ (2003). Hypnic headache – a literature review on clinical features, pathophysiology, treatment. *Neurology* **60**:905–909.

25 Pascual P, Iglesias F, Oterino A, Vazquez-Barquero A, Berciano J (1996). Cough, exertional, and sexual headache. *Neurology* **46**:1520–1524.

26 Headache Classification Committee of the International Headache Society (2013). The International Classification of Headache Disorders, 3rd edition (beta version). *Cephalalgia* **33**:629–808.

27 Levy M, Jager HR, Powell MP, Matharu MS, Meeran K, Goadsby PJ (2004). Pituitary volume and headache: size is not everything. *Arch Neurol* **61**:721–725.

28 Levy M, Matharu MS, Meeran K, Powell M, Goadsby PJ (2005). The clinical characteristics of headache in patients with pituitary tumours. *Brain* **128**:1921–1930.

29 Cohen AS, Burns B, Goadsby PJ (2009). High flow oxygen for treatment of cluster headache. A randomized trial. *JAMA* **302**:2451–2457.

30 van Vliet JA, Bahra A, Martin V, *et al.* (2003). Intranasal sumatriptan in cluster headache – randomized placebo-controlled double-blind study. *Neurology* **60**:630–633.

31 Cittadini E, May A, Straube A, Evers S, Bussone G, Goadsby PJ (2006). Effectiveness of intranasal zolmitriptan in acute cluster headache. A randomized, placebo-controlled, double-blind crossover study. *Arch Neurol* **63**:1537–1542.

32 Rapoport AM, Mathew NT, Silberstein SD, *et al.* (2007). Zolmitriptan nasal spray in the acute treatment of cluster headache: a double-blind study. *Neurology* **69**:821–826.

33 Cohen AS, Matharu MS, Goadsby PJ (2007). Electrocardiographic abnormalities in patients with cluster headache on verapamil therapy. *Neurology* **69**:668–675.

Further reading

General

Goadsby PJ (2003). Headache (chronic tension-type). *Clin Evid* Dec:1538–1546.

Lance JW, Goadsby PJ (2005). *Mechanism and Management of Headache*, 7th edn. Elsevier, New York.

Lipton RB, Bigal M (2006). *Migraine and Other Headache Disorders*, 1st edn. Marcel Dekker, Taylor & Francis Books, New York.

Olesen J, Tfelt-Hansen P, Ramadan N, Goadsby PJ, Welch KMA (2005). *The Headaches*. Lippincott, Williams & Wilkins, Philadelphia.

Silberstein SD, Lipton RB, Goadsby PJ (2002). *Headache in Clinical Practice*, 2nd edn. Martin Dunitz, London.

Silberstein SD, Lipton RB, Solomon S (2001). *Wolff's Headache and Other Head Pain*, 7th edn. Oxford University Press, Oxford.

Migraine

Bahra A, Matharu MS, Buchel C, Frackowiak RSJ, Goadsby PJ (2001). Brainstem activation specific to migraine headache. *Lancet* **357**:1016–1017.

Goadsby PJ (2007). Emerging therapies for migraine. *Nature Clin Pract Neurol* **3**:610–619.

Hand PJ, Stark RJ (2000). Intravenous lignocaine infusions for severe chronic daily headache. *Med J Aus* **172**:157–159.

Lipton RB, SIlberstein SD, Saper J, Bigal ME, Goadsby PJ (2003). Why headache treatment fails. *Neurology* **60**:1064–1070.

Silberstein SD (2000). The US Headache Consortium Report of the Quality Standards Subcommittee of the American Academy of Neurology Practice parameter: evidence-based guidelines for migraine headache (an evidence-based review). *Neurology* **55**:754–763.

Sprenger T, Goadsby PJ (2010). What has functional neuroimaging done for primary headache…and for the clinical neurologist? *J Clin Neurosci* **17**:547–553.

Trigeminal autonomic cephalalgias

Bussone G, Leone M, Peccarisi C, *et al.* (1990). Double blind comparison of lithium and verapamil in cluster headache prophylaxis. *Headache* **30**:411–417.

Cohen AS, Matharu MS, Goadsby PJ (2006). Short-lasting unilateral neuralgiform headache attacks with conjunctival injection and tearing (SUNCT) or cranial autonomic features (SUNA). A prospective clinical study of SUNCT and SUNA. *Brain* **129**:2746–2760.

Ekbom K, The Sumatriptan Cluster Headache Study Group (1991). Treatment of acute cluster headache with sumatriptan. *N Engl J Med* **325**:322–326.

Goadsby PJ, Edvinsson L (1994). Human *in vivo* evidence for trigeminovascular activation in cluster headache. *Brain* **117**:427–434.

Leone M, D'Amico D, Attanasio A (1999). Verapamil is an effective prophylactic for cluster headache: results of a double-blind multicentre study versus placebo. In: Olesen J, Goadsby PJ (eds). *Cluster Headache and Related Conditions*. Oxford University Press, Oxford, pp. 296–299.

Leone M, D'Amico D, Frediani F, *et al.* (2000). Verapamil in the prophylaxis of episodic cluster headache: a double-blind study versus placebo. *Neurology* **54**:1382–1385.

May A, Bahra A, Buchel C, Frackowiak RS, Goadsby PJ (1998). Hypothalamic activation in cluster headache attacks. *Lancet* **352**:275–278.

May A, Goadsby PJ (1999). The trigeminovascular system in humans: pathophysiological implications for primary headache syndromes of the neural influences on the cerebral circulation. *J Cereb Blood Flow Metab* **19**:115–127.

Nesbitt AD, Goadsby PJ (2012). Cluster Headache. *British Medical Journal* **344**:e2407

Other primary headache disorders

Cittadini E, Goadsby PJ (2010). Hemicrania continua: a clinical study of 39 patients with diagnostic implications. *Brain* **133**:1973–1986.

Dodick DW, Brown RD, Britton JW, Huston J (1999). Nonaneurysmal thunderclap headache with diffuse, multifocal, segmental, and reversible vasospasm. *Cephalalgia* **19**:118–123.

Pareja JA, Ruiz J, Deisla C, Alsabbah H, Espejo J (1996). Idiopathic stabbing headache (jabs and jolts syndrome). *Cephalalgia* **16**:93–96.

Schwartz BS, Stewart WF, Simon D, Lipton RB (1998). Epidemiology of tension-type headache. *JAMA* **279**:381–383.

Secondary headaches

van Gijn J (1997). Slip-ups in diagnosis of subarachnoid hemorrhage. *Lancet* **63**:1492.

Wijdicks EFM, Kerkhoff H, van Gijn J (1988). Long-term follow up of 71 patients with thunderclap headache mimicking subarachnoid hemorrhage. *Lancet* **2**:68–70.

VERTIGO

Jorge Kattah

INTRODUCTION

The purpose of this chapter is to provide clinicians with a diagnostic and management algorithm for the evaluation of patients with vertigo, to classify the type of vertigo according to the timing (duration of the event) and possible triggers, to localize the lesion responsible within the peripheral or central vestibular system, and to treat the specific cause of vertigo in relation to the underlying pathophysiology. Vertigo represents a frequent complaint in general neurologic practice and emergency medicine. In this text a new approach to the evaluation of vertiginous patients is presented. In addition, significant advances in clinical, epidemiologic, and imaging in the field have increased our understanding of the pathogenesis of vertigo and its management. A secondary goal is to discuss vestibular abnormalities such as the superior canal dehiscence, vestibular paroxysmia, and the simultaneous acute and chronic bilateral vestibular loss syndromes that have become better understood in the last decade. By virtue of their symptoms these patients frequently visit the neurologist as the initial specialist or in expert consultation.

Definition

- *Vertigo*: a spontaneous pathologic perception of spinning or tilting that builds up over a time period ranging from seconds to minutes, and is the result of an acute peripheral or central vestibulopathy, typically occurring spontaneously and potentially exacerbated by motion. Nausea and vomiting and motion intolerance are commonly associated with vertigo.
- *Motion sickness*: an intense vasovagal reaction in response to linear or angular movement associated with land, air, or sea transport and not necessarily the result of a vestibulopathy.
- *Lightheadness or presyncope*: impending faint often related to arterial hypotension or cardiac arrhythmia.
- *Imbalance*: unsteadiness, disequilibrium.
- *Dizziness*: it may be characterized by any of the above definitions or a nonspecific complaint. Recent clinical epidemiologic data support the concept that the type of sensation described by the patient may be potentially misleading, when it is intermittent, timing (duration) of the episode, and triggers are more relevant for proper syndrome classification.
- *Oscillopsia*: a 'to and fro' movement of the visual environment which is either due to failure of the vestibulo-ocular reflex (VOR) or to fixation nystagmus causing unsteady visual fixation.

Tip

▶ *The subjective description of the terms listed above may be quite variable; therefore, an emphasis on the triggers for a specific complaint and duration of symptoms may prove more efficient.*

TABLE 19 **CLASSIFICATION OF VERTIGO ACCORDING TO TIMING (DURATION)**

Syndrome	Duration	Clinical findings	Pathophysiology
Paroxysmal positional vertigo Posterior SCC	Seconds	Positional nystagmus duiring Dix–Hallpike manuever	Canalolithiasis of the posterior SCC
Tullio's phenomenon	Seconds	Noise-induced vertigo	Perilymphatic fistula; superior canal dehiscence
Vestibular paroxysmia	Seconds to minutes	Nsytagmus prompted by positional changes	Compression of the vestibular nerve by an arterial loop
Horizontal paroxysmal positional vertigo	Seconds but present with any lateral head turn	Paroxysmal horizontal nystagmus with lateral head turn	Canalolithiasis or cupulolithiasis
Transient ischemic attack	Minutes	Pattern of nystagmus may be peripheral or central	Ischemia of labyrinth, vestibular nerve, brainstem, or cerebellum
Migraine	Minutes	Nystagmus may be present; headache usually present	Unknown mechanism
Ménière's Syndrome	Hours	Nystagmus present, direction depends on the stage of the attack; usually tinnnitus, ear fullness, and hearing fluctuations	Endolymphatic hydrops
Labyrinthitis	Days	Horizontal nystagmus with contralesional fast phase; severe acute hearing loss; abnormal HIT	Inflammation presumably viral, ischemia, or autoimmune process
Vestibular neuritis	Days	Horizontal nystagmus contralesional; hearing not affected; abnormal HIT	Presumably viral or ischemia
Vestibular root entry stroke/ lateral pontine stroke	Days	As above; skew and direction-changing nystagmus may be present; abnormal HIT; facial weaknesss may be present	Ischemia; less likely multiple sclerosis plaque or tumor
Lateral medullary stroke	Days	Horizontal, rotary, or vertical nystagmus; may be direction-changing; normal HIT	Ischemia lateral medulla; less frequently multiple sclerosis plaque or tumor
Medial medullary stroke	Days	Horizontal or vertical nystagmus; hemiparesis; pyramidal tract signs	Ischemia medial medulla
Cerebellar stroke	Days	Direction-changing nystagmus; normal HIT and skew	Ischemia in several locations in the cerebellum, mostly ventral vermis

HIT: horizontal head impulse test; SCC: semicircular canal.

Classification according to timing

Table 19 presents the classification of vertigo on the basis of timing (duration). Duration of the attack of vertigo is a key question if the episode has subsided at the time of initial examination:

- Episodic, brief, lasting seconds: typically, very brief episodes of vertigo (seconds) may occur in benign paroxysmal positional vertigo (BPPV) and noise-induced vertigo, and a few minutes duration is frequently found in transient ischemic attacks (TIA) and vestibular paroxysmia. Episodic disequilibrium and presyncope with or without a sensation of rotation may occur with nonvestibular pathology, in particular orthostatic hypotension and other cardiovascular disorders and endocrine disorders.
- Episodic of intermediate duration lasting minutes to hours: Ménière's syndrome, vestibular migraine, and TIAs will be the main considerations.
- Acute prolonged, nonremitting vertigo: this is known as the acute vestibular syndrome (AVS), which is continuous and unremitting, lasts typically from several days to an average of 1–2 weeks, and may be caused by a labyrinthitis (if associated with hearing loss) or vestibular neuritis. Stroke, affecting the labyrinth, vestibular nerve, brainstem vestibular pathways, and cerebellum, can cause either pseudolabyrinthitis or pseudoneuritis, depending on whether hearing is affected or spared. Although cerebrovascular disease is the most common cause of pseudoneuritis, this clinical picture may also be reported by patients with multiple sclerosis (MS), vasculitis, and inflammatory/infectious diseases affecting either the base of the skull or the brainstem[1]. In individual patients, a history of an initial AVS followed months later by brief BPPV may be found. Generally speaking, complete unilateral vestibular periphery or central lesions compensate in a matter of a few weeks; typically, the acute symptoms subside and are generally superseded by a sensation of unsteadiness and visual blurring with rapid gaze shifts or head movement.

Tips

► *The duration of the attack is typically very brief in BPPPV, lasts hours in Ménière's syndrome and migraine, and days in vestibular neuritis and stroke.*

► *In BPPV patients there is an associated feeling of unsteadiness when upright which may be incorporated in the patient's description as an attack of prolonged duration.*

Epidemiology

Dizziness is a frequent complaint in both acute emergency and neurologic practice. In emergency medicine, the most common cause of dizziness relates to a cardiovascular etiology; 30% of patients with dizziness who seek medical attention have vestibular vertigo with an otoneurologic cause, most commonly paroxysmal positional vertigo (33%), Ménière's syndrome (1%), or vestibular migraine (14%)[2,3]. Approximately 3.3% of emergency department visits in the US are related to dizziness/vertigo and 5 % of them probably represent acute vestibular neuritis or labyrinthitis[2,4].

Annual incidence: among 2.6 million emergency department annual visits in the US for dizziness, 150,000 cases are due to vestibular neuritis[4,5]. Vertigo is frequently caused by cerebrovascular disease, primarily cerebellar and brainstem disorders. Stroke involving basilar artery circulation accounts for a total of 20% of all annual cerebrovascular events and may be associated with vertigo[4].

A prospective study of life-threatening disorders manifested initially with an AVS is not currently available. A pseudoneuritis presentation with either fatal outcome or severe morbidity was reported in 15 young patients (less than age 40) with an acute stroke manifested by an AVS[6].

A psychosomatic etiology and side-effects of medications are also frequent causes of dizziness.

Given this epidemiologic picture, clinicians evaluating patients with dizziness confront a spectrum of disorders that vary in prognosis from benign to potentially life-threatening. A thorough history and examination are the only options for providers to triage these patients properly. A practical algorithm for the diagnosis and management of vertiginous patients is suggested (**146**, next page).

Tip

► *The AVS patient evaluation by frontline providers is particularly challenging. Recommendations for effective triaging of AVS patients with stroke who may be at risk of additional brainstem and cerebellar embolism and post-ischemic malignant cerebellar edema is provided.*

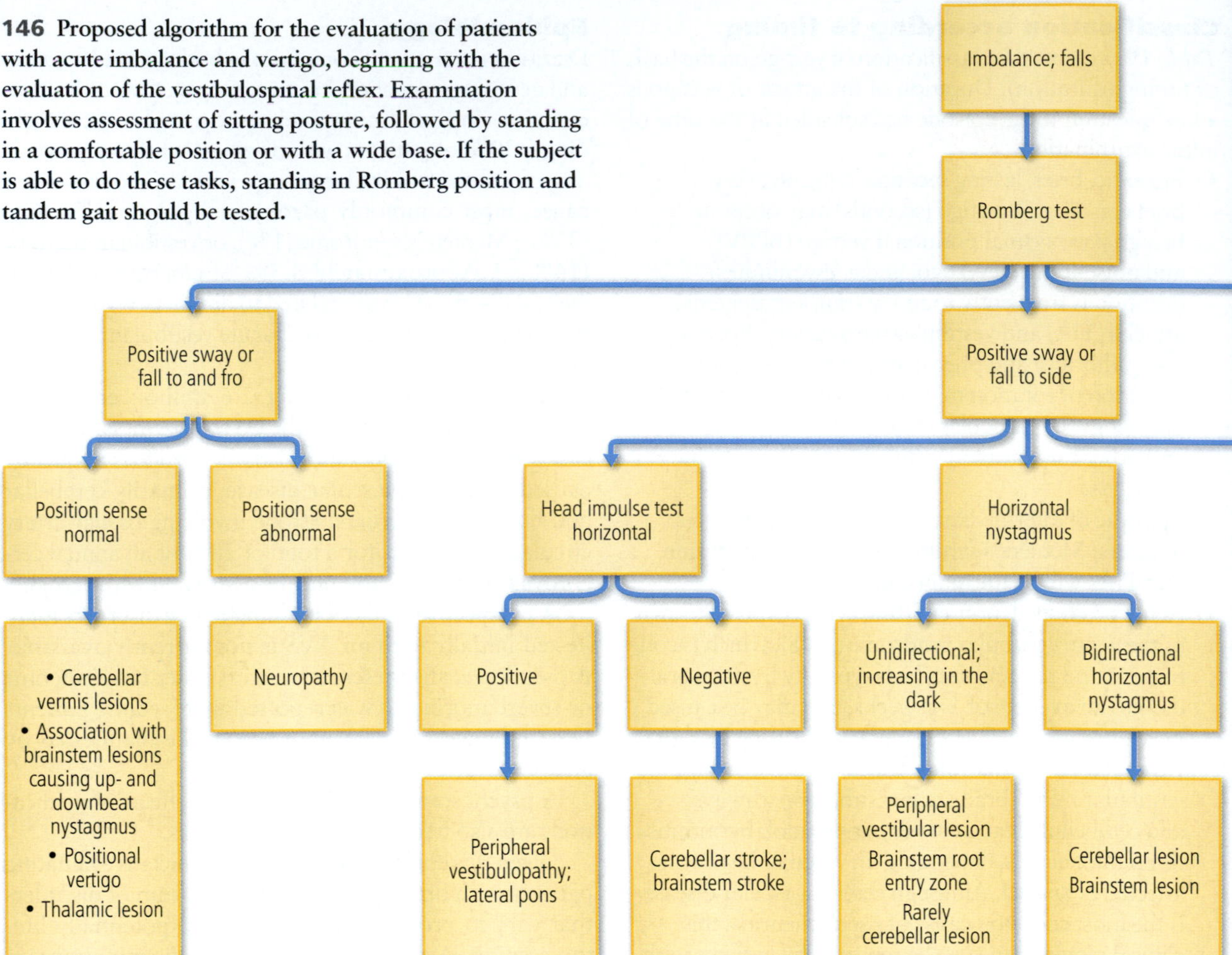

146 Proposed algorithm for the evaluation of patients with acute imbalance and vertigo, beginning with the evaluation of the vestibulospinal reflex. Examination involves assessment of sitting posture, followed by standing in a comfortable position or with a wide base. If the subject is able to do these tasks, standing in Romberg position and tandem gait should be tested.

Etiology and pathophysiology

The study of the otopathology of vertigo has been complicated by the fact that the membranous labyrinth is housed within the bony labyrinth inside the temporal bone, and the preparation of the pathology specimen for examination involves a complicated lengthy process. It is important to discuss the pathologic findings in each common form of vertigo as they are relevant to the discussion of pathogenic mechanisms.

Positional vertigo

Positional vertigo is the result of otolith displacement from the macula of the utricule and saccule into the semicircular canals (SCC), rendering the SCC gravity sensitive. Pathologic observations have been more recently confirmed by surgical findings[7]. BPPV is often idiopathic, but trauma and vestibular neuritis are possible causes.

Ménière's syndrome

This syndrome is associated with marked swelling and distention of the cochlea, the SCC, the utricle and saccule, and the endolymphatic canal. This pathologic picture is known as endolymphatic hydrops. This condition may be associated with a history of infection, trauma, or other disorders. In many instances a specific cause cannot be established.

Vestibular neuritis

Few pathologic studies have shown Wallerian degeneration of the superior vestibular nerve which is not frequently affected. A recent study showed that anatomic factors may explain increased superior vestibular nerve susceptibility to inflammation[8]; there are data to suggest that latent herpes simplex virus (HSV-1) may be responsible in several instances of vestibular neuritis.

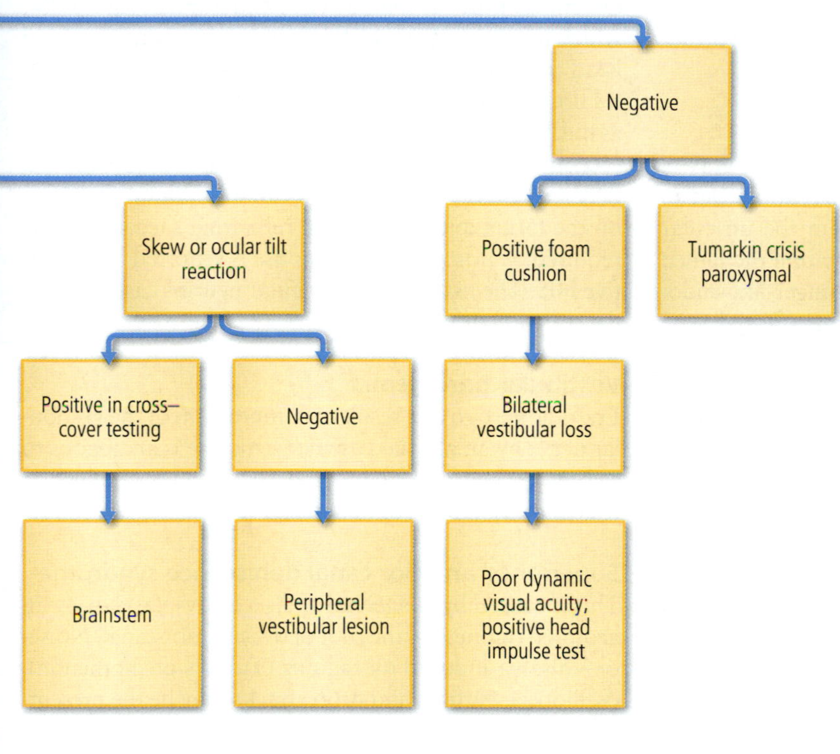

147 Arterial supply to the inner ear. In most individuals the arterial supply is provided by branches of the anterior inferior cerebellar artery (AICA). The internal auditory artery arises from AICA and has three major branches: (1) the anterior vestibular artery which irrigates the horizontal and superior semicircular canals (SCCs) and the utricule; (2) the cochlear artery which irrigates the cochlea; and (3) the posterior vestibular artery which provides arterial supply to the saccule and posterior SCC. *After Baloh and Hamagyi, 1996.*

Vascular disorders of inner ear

It is important to delineate the structures innervated by the superior vestibular nerve and their vascular supply, which include the anterior and lateral SCC and the utricule, with only minor fiber supply to the saccule. The vascular supply is provided by the anterior vestibular artery, a branch of the internal auditory artery which originates from the anterior inferior cerebellar artery (AICA). The inferior vestibular nerve innervates the posterior SCC and the majority of the saccule (**147**) and is supplied by the posterior vestibular artery. The cochlea has its own vascular supply. In a few patients with atherosclerotic disease of the vertebrobasilar system, pathologic evidence of ischemic infarction of the labyrinth and cochlea has been demonstrated[9]. Anterior vestibular artery strokes can be associated with sparing of the posterior SCC and ischemic debris from the infarcted utricule can fall into the posterior SCC and cause positional vertigo (classic BPPV). Pathologic evidence of simultaneous infarction of the labyrinth and the lateral brainstem has been previously reported[9].

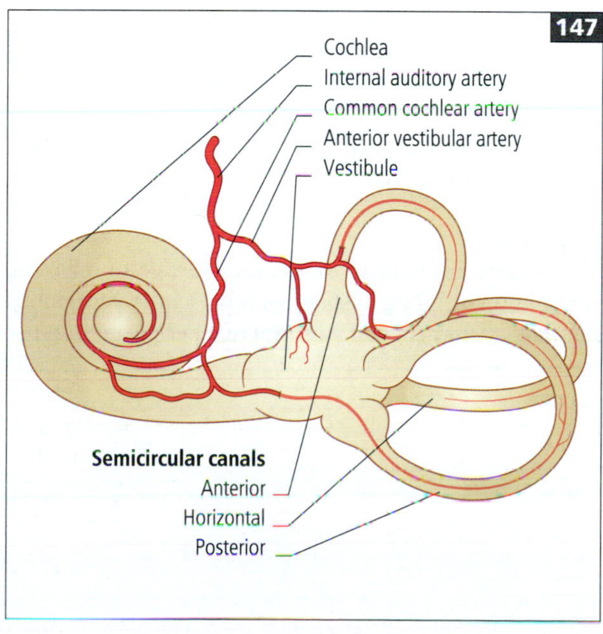

Vascular disorders of central vestibular pathways and cerebellum

Pathologic studies in pseudoneuritis cases have shown cerebellar strokes. Vertigo is also a frequent component of Wallenberg's syndrome. Systemic and infectious vasculitis can affect the blood supply to the labyrinth or brainstem.

The pathophysiology of the most common vertigo types will be discussed (other causes can be found in texts dedicated to the topic, listed in the References and Further reading).

BPPV

Movement of the head or the body in relation to gravity in BPPV causes the expected motion sensation, but in addition the ectopic otolith debris from the utricular matrix (canaliths), that is free floating within the lumen of the membranous canal, triggers a plunger-like endolymph flow surge with excitation of the affected SCC cupula. The provocative Dix–Hallpike maneuver is the best method to detect BPPV; paroxysmal vertigo and nystagmus develop in a patient who is typically comfortable in the sitting position without nystagmus prior to testing. After reaching the supine head hanging position with a delay of few seconds, an intense spinning sensation occurs with pronounced transient nystagmus. The most commonly affected SCC is the posterior canal followed by the horizontal SCC; the anterior canal is very infrequently affected primarily due to anatomic factors. Knowledge of this pathophysiologic BPPV mechanism led to the design of successful repositioning maneuvers currently used in practice, with the potential for cure or prolonged remission.

Ménière's syndrome

Ménière's syndrome is asociated with a pathologic picture described as endolymphatic hydrops. Distention of endolymph-containing membranes in the engorged inner ear structures, in particular, the SCC, the cochlea, or the saccule/utricule, causes rupture and acute vertigo, nystagmus, and hearing loss.

Migraine

The precise mechanism that causes vertigo in migraine is not known. When nystagmus is present in vertiginous migraine, it may suggest a central or a peripheral origin.

Vestibular neuritis

The acute unilateral loss of vestibular afferent input results in a typical alteration of the vestibulospinal reflex (VSR): the subject veers in an ipsilesional direction (sitting or standing). In addition, the unilateral loss of the VOR causes a contralesional, unidirectional, horizontal (h) nystagmus (fast phase) that increases in the dark. By convention, the jerk nystagmus is always named by the direction of the fast phase. The head impulse sign (HIS), which tests the integrity of the VOR in response to rapid head acceleration, is decreased or absent. To test the h-HIS, the subject is instructed to fixate on a central target as the head is rapidly accelerated by the examiner from an eccentric position to center or vice versa. As a result of a deficient VOR signal, the eyes cannot maintain fixation on the target and a corrective refixating saccade is thus required. A normal VOR response is reported as a negative HIS. The majority of vestibular neuritis cases involve the superior vestibular nerve.

Vestibular paroxysmia

Episodic vertigo as a result of compression of the vestibular nerve by an arterial vascular structure is analogous to a common neurovascular compression syndrome such as trigeminal neuralgia or hemifacial spasm.

Superior or anterior canal dehiscence syndrome

This is caused by congenital aplasia or dysplasia or by an acquired thinning of the roof of the superior canal. Noise- or Valsalva-induced nystagmus (Tullio's phenomenon), oscillopsia, vertigo, and drop attacks may be the presenting symptoms.

Bilateral simultaneous vestibular loss

This syndrome may be frequently caused by direct drug toxicity with irreversible damage to inner hair cells in the labyrinth. In current clinical practice, gentamicin ranks at the top of the list of drug toxicities. Hearing is usually spared.

Clinical features and diagnosis

Symptoms

Based on the pathophysiology of the different causes of vertigo, it is paramount to determine the duration and triggers to arrive at a correct diagnosis. Although at times patients are very precise in their description, more often than not the description is vague. Associated symptoms may include hearing impairment, tinnitus, nausea, vomiting and profuse sweating, inability to maintain sitting or standing balance or to do tandem gait, falls, oscillopsia, diplopia and, at times with central lesions, other neurologic symptoms.

Bedside vestibular signs

The physical findings vary with the specific type of vertigo pathophysiology; the basic evaluation involves an analyis of the VSR, VOR, and the otolith–ocular reflexes in addition to a complete neurologic evaluation. VSR is evaluated by the subject's ability to sit unaided and to stand first with a wide base and subsequently in Romberg position with the eyes open and closed. Following posture testing if normal, regular gait, tandem gait, and the Fukuda step tests are assessed. The direction of fall during these postural tests may be ipsi- or contralesional, depending on localization. Figure 146 proposes an algorithm for the evaluation of patients with vestibular syndromes, beginning with abnormal posture testing.

Tips

- *Testing the VSR is very helpful as an initial step in the evaluation of vestibular disorders.*
- *The direction of fall may be ipsi- or contralesional, consequently it does not lateralize the lesion localization.*

Vestibulo and otolith–ocular reflexes

In addition to the vestibulospinal assessment, the authors found three clinical signs to be very sensitive in the clinical evaluation of AVS patients, and proposed the acronym HINTS: HI: head impulse; NT: nystagmus type; and S: skew, which provide significant sensitivity/specificity. The VOR integrity is tested with the HIS; a negative (normal) HIS in an AVS patient suggests a central vestibular lesion while a positive (abnormal) HIS localizes to peripheral vestibular lesions. However, the latter tests may infrequently be positive in vestibular root entry zone lesions involving the lateral pons.

Tips

- *The HIS is the single most important bedside test in the evaluation of acute vestibular syndrome patients.*
- *In the acute setting, a normal HIS points to central lesion localization.*

Nystagmus type assessment

Spontaneous fixation and eccentric lateral and vertical gaze nystagmus is tested first in light and subsequently in dark, using either Frenzel or video-goggles, and the nystagmus type provides localizing information. Whereas unidirectional, horizontal nystagmus suggests vestibular periphery lesions, horizontal, direction-changing nystagmus points to central pathology. Vertical and primarily torsional nystagmus also point to central vestibular lesions. Subtle nystagmus may be identified by direct ophthalmoscopy, in which the examiner visualizes the optic nerve head and requests the patient to occlude the fellow eye with the palm of the hand. This technique allows detection of small amplitude nystagmus. The apparent direction of movement of the optic nerve head is opposite to the actual movement of the eye because the optic nerve head is behind the axis of rotation of the globe.

Tips

- *The evaluation of nystagmus direction (fast phases) in primary gaze is a useful tool in the classification of vestibular disorders.*
- *Vertical nystagmus is almost always due to a central lesion or an altered central mechanism. Evaluation of horizontal nystagmus must be performed in combination with the HIS results; the combined information provides high sensitivity and specificity.*

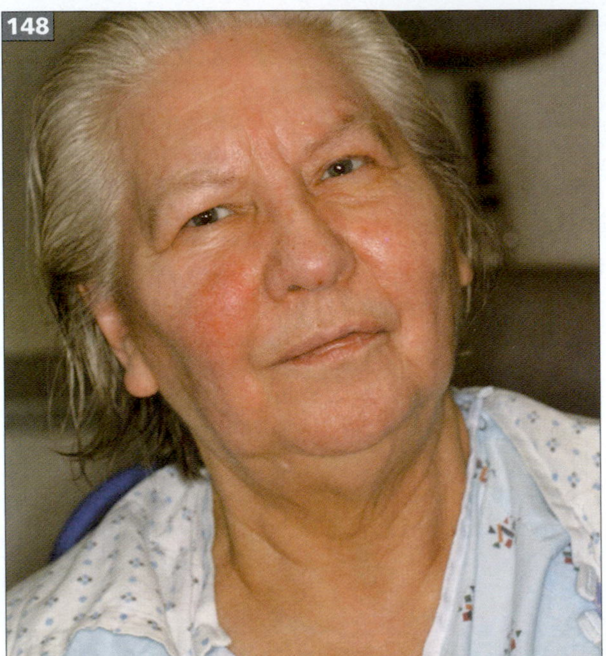

Skew deviation

Skew deviation, defined as a vertical misalignment of the eyes in primary position, is tested by asking the patient to fixate on a target while the examiner performs cross-cover testing to identify latent vertical misalignment. This sign is the result of an acute unilateral deficiency of the otolith-ocular reflex. Skew deviation detected by cross-cover test is uncommon with peripheral lesions. The Maddox rod may detect minute vertical ocular misalignment but it is generally not needed in the AVS patient as the cross-cover test provides a safe index of sensitivity/specificity in the localization question. In some cases, there is a spontaneous head tilt: ocular tilt reaction (OTR) which also suggests central vestibular localization. Skew deviation and head tilt correlate well with measures of the subjective visual vertical (SVV) and ocular torsion detected by fundoscopy, which are additional helpful tests of otolith function (**148, 149**).

Tips

- *Instruct the patient to look at a central fixation target located about 1 meter (3 feet) away and perform a cross-cover test.*
- *Any vertical refixation movement observed during this maneuver is abnormal.*
- *One eye would be higher: hypertropia, and one lower: hypotropia.*
- *Skew deviation and vertical extraocular muscle weakness may be responsible.*
- *The rest of the examination and clinical context will be the best method to interpret the results.*

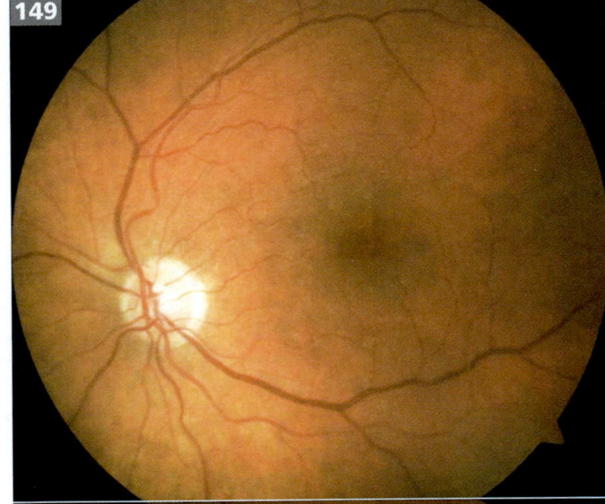

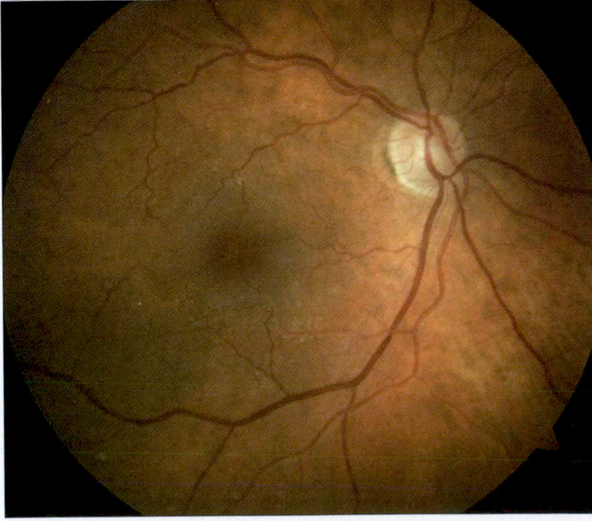

148, 149 Ocular fundoscopy from a 70-year-old patient with an acute vestibular syndrome. Observe conjugate ocular torsion to the right. The patient sitting up on an examining chair is asked to fixate on a central target and the position of the fixating eye is photographed. Normally the macula is only slightly below the optic nerve head. Additional findings included inability to sit at the bedside without support due to right lateropulsion. She had a right ocular tilt reaction (OTR). (148) Right head tilt, skew deviation, and conjugate ocular torsion. In this case the head tilt and the conjugate ocular deviation toward the right shoulder are shown. (149) Observe how the right eye (upper image) is excyclotorted and the left incyclotorted (lower image). Cross-cover test (not shown) identified the third component of the triad: skew deviation; the right eye was hypotropic. The HIS was normal. On the basis of the examination, a central vestibular pathway lesion was suspected and imaging ordered.

Horizontal head impulse test

Horizontal head impulse test (HIT) is used to evaluate the integrity of the horizontal VOR and is positive in acute peripheral vestibular syndromes, including the vestibular root entry. To test the HIT, the subject fixates on a central target as the head is rapidly accelerated in the horizontal plane. An acute vestibular lesion fails to activate the expected ocular response directed opposite to the head movement, and a refixation saccade is thus required to maintain fixation. Bedside visual acuity test (VA) is used to test an impaired VOR. Baseline VA at near is recorded and then the head is actively moved horizontally back and forth. Deterioration of two or more VA lines suggests impairment of the VOR. This test is sensitive in bilateral, peripheral vestibular loss.

Testing using fixation suppression

In long-standing vertigo cases with variable degrees of vestibular compensation, several diagnostic tests are used to detect 'latent' vestibulopathies. It is recommended to perform these tests with fixation suppression (Frenzel or video-goggles); head shaking, Valsalva maneuver, hyperventilation, vibratory stimulation of the mastoid, and the Dix–Hallpike maneuver are routinely utilized. In latent vestibulopathy cases positional nystagmus may be found; unlike BPPV, the nystagmus observed is not associated with vertigo and is not fatigable. After visualization of the tympanum, and with the patient wearing video- or Frenzel goggles, the ocular response to tragal pressure, sound stimulation, and gentle positive pressure applied with an otoscope guided manual cuff within the external auditory canal may trigger nystagmus.

Tips

- *The nystgamus elicitation techniques may be useful when primary gaze nystagmus is not present.*
- *They are performed usually with the use of Frenzel or video-goggles to suppress the potential inhibitory effect of visual fixation.*

Additional vestibular laboratory testing

Caloric and rotational testing in these circumstances may detect diagnostic abnormalities. Patients with bilateral, simultaneous vestibular loss typically do not have nystagmus and display a bilaterally positive HIS in the horizontal and vertical planes. Noise can induce vertigo and oscillopsia (Tullio's phenomenon), and the audiometer or a referee whistle can be used to test this sign.

Additional bedside evaluation

Hearing can be tested with finger rubbing, and the traditional Weber and Rinne signs should also be tested. A detailed cranial nerve and cerebellar examination is also indicated. Neurovascular evaluation searching for pulse symmetry, auscultation for arterial bruits and orthostatic blood pressure changes, and clinical evaluation of cardiac function is particularly relevant in this group of patients. The possibility of a psychiatric etiology (panic reaction), hyperventilation, and so on should be explored in patients with prominent symptoms and lack of objective pathologic findings.

Peripheral *vs.* central localization

Paroxysmal positional vertigo

BPPV is the most most common cause of vertigo, and comprises brief episodes of vertigo prompted by head extension, lying down, or turning in bed. There is a brief latency of ~30 seconds, and vertigo does not last more than 30 seconds. Symptoms fatigue with repeat maneuvers.

Typical BPPV affects the posterior SCC. The patients do not have symptoms while sitting comfortably upright and their examination shows no evidence of nystagmus. The Dix–Hallpike maneuver results in both vigorous nystagmus and intense vertigo when the subject is brought briskly from a sitting position with the head laterally turned to one side to a final position 45° below the horizontal. An upbeat, torsional nystagmus directed toward the dependent ear is the most common response (posterior semicircular canalolithiasis), and the nystagmus subsides ~30 seconds later. When the patient returns to sitting the nystagmus changes direction.

Horizontal SCC canalolithiasis causes horizontal nystagmus and develops as the patient reaches either a supine position or turns the head laterally while supine, and the horizontal nystagmus beats either to the side of head turn (canalolithiasis: geotropic) or away (cupulolithiasis: ageotropic). The neurologic examination is normal in these patients. There is a recent report of ageotropic, h-nystagmus associated with nodulus lesion of the cerebellum.

Central paroxysmal positional vertigo is uncommon and should be considered in cases with positional downbeat nystagmus. In addition, the neurologic examination is expected to be abnormal. This type of nystagmus may also be seen in patients with anterior canal BPPV and is fairly uncommon.

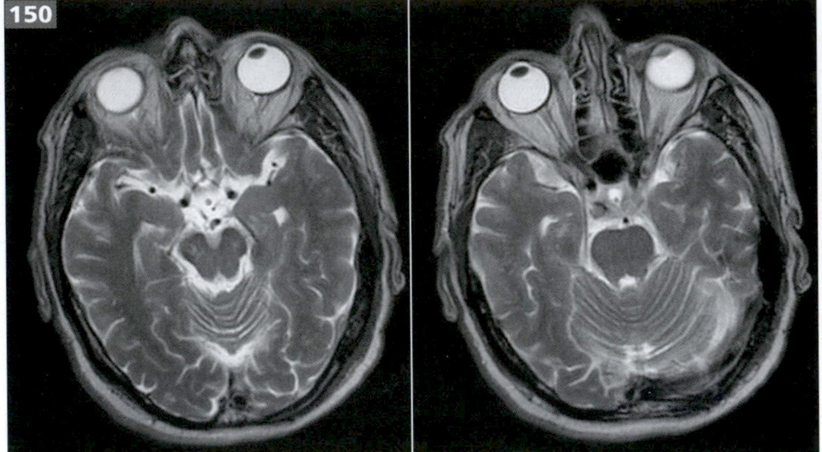

150 Axial T2-weighted MRI of the orbit. The MRI was obtained in the same patient as in 148, shortly after examination. Observe a mild head turn and conjugate horizontal ocular deviation to the right. She had right ocular lateropulsion in the sitting upright posture and left beating, unidirectional nystagmus.

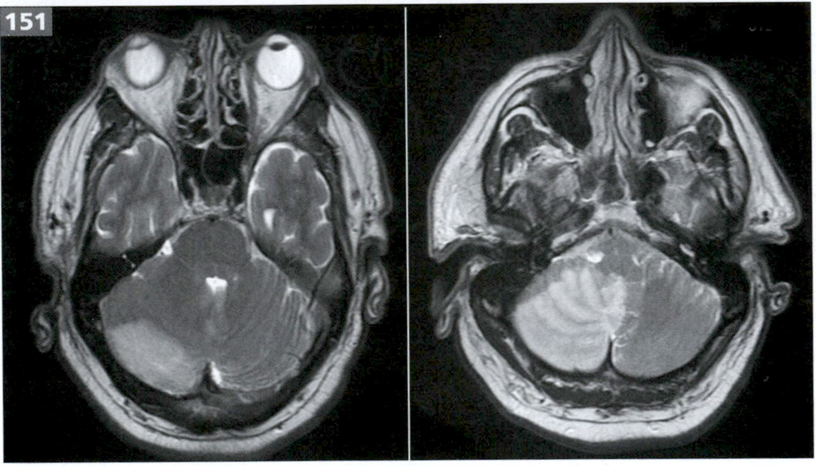

151 Axial FLAIR MRI of the brain obtained in the same patient as 148. It shows an extensive hyperintense, ischemic lesion in the right lateral inferior cerebellar hemisphere. DWI (not shown) demonstrated diffusion restriction, indicating acute infarction.

Constant, unremitting vertigo

The early clinical differentiation between a peripheral lesion with good prognosis and a central lesion with potentially poor prognosis (pseudolabyrinthitis or pseudoneuritis) is critical for the proper triage. The aforementioned acronym, HINTS, defined as a clinical triad that includes: head impulse response (HI), the nystagmus direction (N), and testing skew (TS) allows this differentiation with good sensitivity and specificity.

Central vestibular lesions

A normal (negative) HIS, horizontal, direction-changing nystagmus, skew deviation, or a full OTR indicate central localization (**148–151**), and an ischemic stroke is the most common cause. However, on occasion, MS (**152, 153**) may be responsible. Likewise, vertical or purely torsional nystagmus, and the combination of ophthalmoplegia and nystagmus, point to central localization. Patients with severe truncal ataxia, unable to sit unaided, have central vestibular pathway lesions.

In a recent series, this finding was present in ~30% of cases. Long tract abnormalities may be seen in a similar percentage of cases.

Tip

▶ *The acronym HINTS: HI Head Impulse, N: Nystagmus direction, and TS: Testing Skew provide results suggestive of INFARCT as follows: IN: Impulse Negative, FA: Fast phase alternating, and RCT: Refixation on cross-cover test.*

Peripheral vestibular lesions

Peripheral vestibular (PV) lesions in vestibular neuritis or labyrinthitis are associated with unidirectional, contralesional, horizontal nystagmus, which is typically suppressed by fixation, increases in the dark, does not change direction in different gaze positions, and increases in the horizontal gaze direction of the fast phase (Alexander's law). In addition, a positive HIS is present and overt skew deviation detected with cross-cover testing is distinctly uncommon. An abnormal HIS, however, may be seen with intra-axial lesions in the lateral pons, involving the vestibular root entry zone. In such cases, direction-changing nystagmus, skew, and the OTR triad should be tested for correct localization. In a typical Ménière's attack there is often a buildup of baseline tinnitus, hearing deterioration, and aural fullness prior to the episode of vertigo. The direction of the nystagmus cannot be used for localization as it depends on the stage of the attack and can be contralesional (paretic) in the early attack phase or ipsilesional (recovery) in the late attack phase. Symptoms subside typically within hours.

Differential diagnosis

- Lightheadness or syncope.
- Cardiac brady- or tachyarrhythmia.
- Vasovagal attacks.
- Hyperventilation and anxiety.
- Orthostatic hypotension.
- Hypovolemia; anemia.
- Migraine.
- Complex partial seizures.
- Episodic ataxia (episodes of vertigo and ataxia, several phenotypes).
- Vestibular paroxysmia (head movement related vertigo lasting longer than BPPV).
- Superior canal dehiscence syndrome (Valsalva- and noise-induced vertigo).
- Perilymphatic fistula (Valsalva-induced vertigo/ barotraumas).

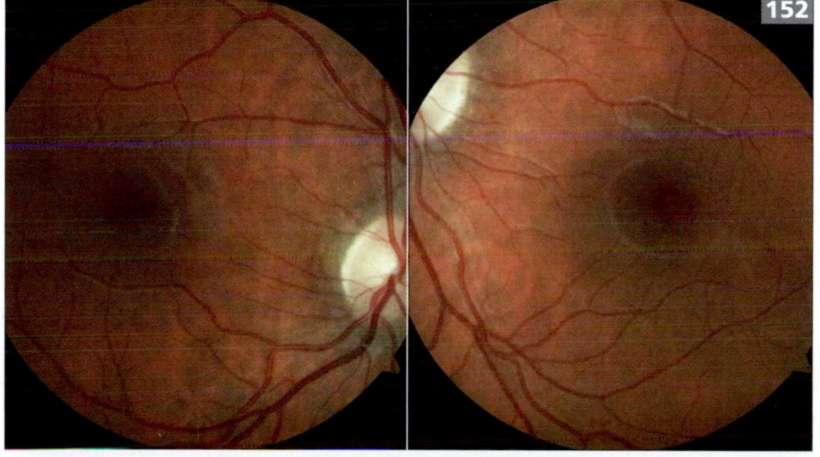

152 Ocular fundoscopy. Observe conjugate deviation of the eyes to the left in an 18-year-old, previously healthy female with an acute vestibular syndrome. On examination, she had an inability to sit without support, due to left lateropulsion; she had a left ocular tilt reaction with a hypotropic left eye, direction-changing horizontal nystagmus in lateral gaze, and a negative head impulse sign. On the basis of this examination, a central lesion in the left lateral brainstem or the cerebellum was suspected and imaging was obtained.

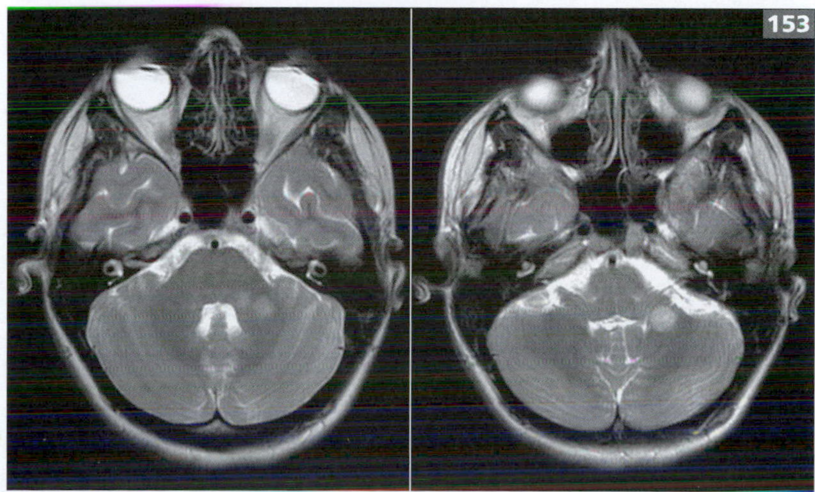

153 T2 axial MRI of the brain. Observe one round lesion of increased signal intensity in the left lateral pontomedullary junction, and two in the lateral pons (middle cerebellar peduncle) which enhanced modestly with contrast (not shown). In addition, periventricular and juxtacortical lesions suggestive of demyelinization were present. A diagnosis of multiple sclerosis was made on follow-up.

Investigations

- Patients with BPPV and an otherwise normal examination do not require further investigation.
- Patients with Ménière's syndrome require periodic audiometry and other audiologic testing (echocochleography), and a vestibular function reserve test to provide a baseline (video-nystagmography, VNG).
- Audiometry should be performed in patients with vestibulopathy, as the presence and pattern of hearing loss will be helpful in making the correct diagnosis.
- VNG with caloric testing and rotational chair stimulation should be entertained when quantitative information is needed in cases with otherwise nonspecific findings. It is very helpful in patients with bilateral vestibular ototoxicity, in combined central/peripheral lesions, and in central lesions in which quantitative oculomotor tests could detect subtle deficiencies.
- Tests of otolith–ocular function are frequently abnormal in patients with vertigo. Cross-cover testing to detect skew deviation, ocular fundus photography, and measures of the SVV may all be helpful in localization. The use of a Maddox rod to detect a subtle skew increases sensitivity, but does not add greater specificity in differentiating peripheral *vs.* central localization. The authors generally discourage use of the Maddox rod in this clinical setting.
- A brain magnetic resonance imaging (MRI) should be ordered in AVS patients in whom the HINTS triad suggests a central lesion. This recommendation also applies to initially stroke-negative brain MRI patients who may need a second scan to demonstrate the stroke when there is high suspicion of this disorder. MRI/magnetic resonance angiography (MRA) studies should also be performed in vestibular paroxysmia cases.
- The Dix–Hallpike maneuver begins with the patient sitting on a stretcher, the head is tipped back and rotated 45° to one side prior to moving the patient quickly to a supine position, so that the head is below the horizontal (~45°). It has been traditionally taught that the head is positioned over the edge of the stretcher, but the edge of a pillow may function as well, and in acute cases, goggles are not needed. In chronic BPPV cases the use of video- or Frenzel goggles is helpful to block fixation suppression and to increase the chance of observing nystagmus.
- Peripheral vestibular schwannomas are not a frequent cause of vertigo, and their initial presentation is more frequently nonspecific imbalance. Progressive unilateral hearing loss is a consistent initial presentation and VNG usually detects vestibular loss. MRI may detect occasionally asymptomatic, small intracanalicular schwannomas.
- Patients with suspected perilymphatic fistulas, superior canal dehiscence, and other causes of inner ear pathology will need thin section, high-resolution computed tomography (CT) of the temporal bone (**154**).

154 **Coronal high resolution CT scan of the right and left temporal bone, obtained in a patient with intermittent oscillopsia when physically active, with Valsalva-induced conjugate ocular torsion, conductive hearing loss, and low threshold vestibular evoked potentials. Bilateral thinning of the superior semicircular canal (SCC) roof is present (arrow) (right > left). The patient underwent surgery with repair of the dehiscence and clinical improvement.**

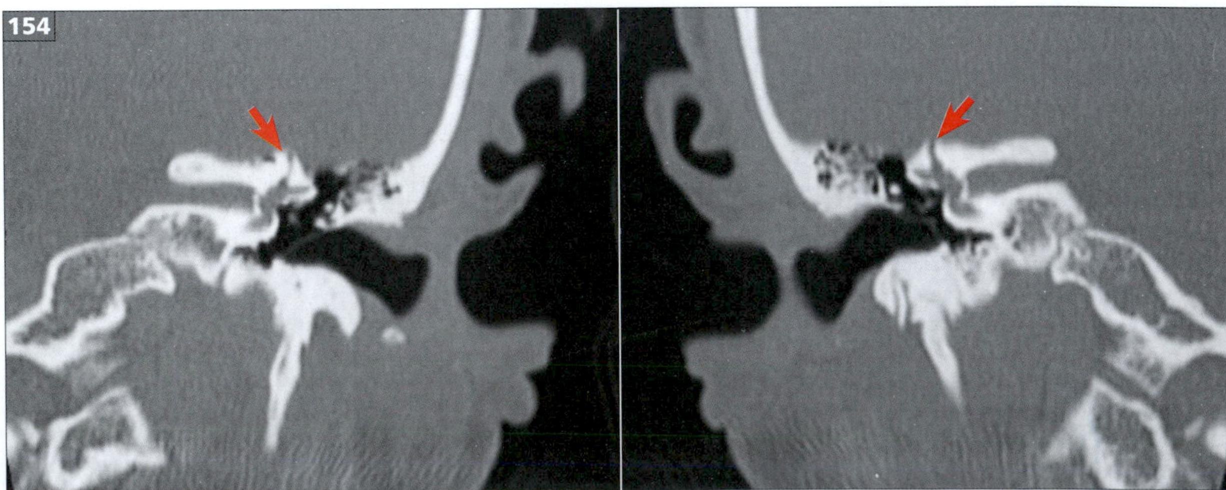

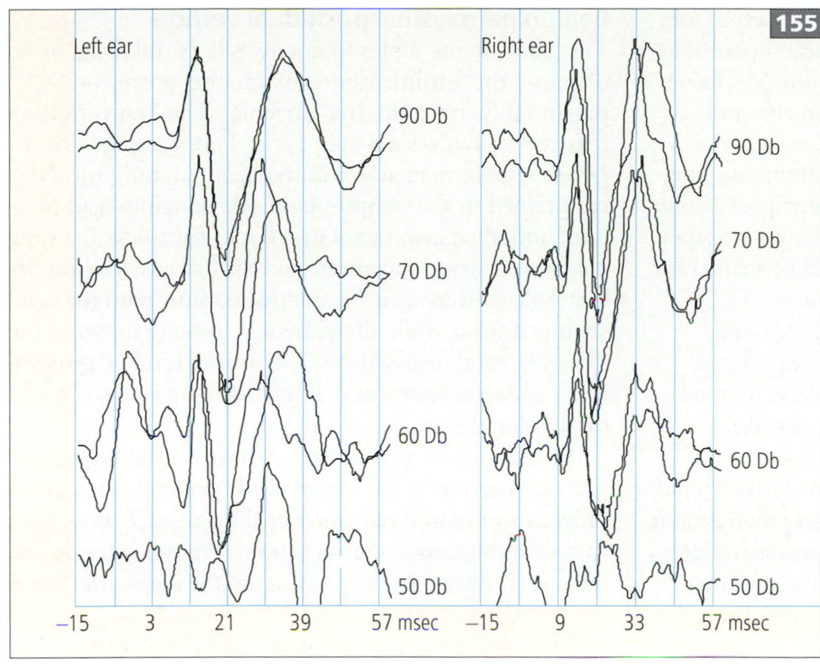

155 **Vestibular evoked potentials (VEMPs), obtained in a patient with bilateral superior canal dehiscence syndrome, show low threshold responses bilaterally. Low intensity (70 Db), 500 Hz tone bursts yielded robust responses that are normally found only with high intensity 90 Db stimuli. These findings are suggestive of superior semicircular canal (Minor's syndrome) in this clinical setting.**

- Brainstem auditory evoked potentials may be helpful in suspected central lesions. Vestibular myogenic evoked potentials (VEMPs) test the integrity of the sacculocollic reflex which is mediated by the inferior vestibular nerve. In superior vestibular neuritis, the VEMP is spared (**155**) and is absent in inferior vestibular neuritis[10].
- Otorrhinolaryngologic (ear, nose, and throat [ENT]) evaluation must be included in any patient with vertigo and associated hearing loss, prolonged history of vertigo, tinnitus, and aural fullness, signs of suppurative middle ear disease, post-traumatic vertigo, and in suspected lesions in the skull base or nasopharynx.
- Efforts to examine the patient during an attack may provide diagnostic localization and lateralization information, as this is particularly important to distinguish peripheral *vs*. central localization and, in the case of Ménière's syndrome, to rule out the possibility of bilateral involvement.

Tips

- *The evaluation of asymptomatic patients with episodes of vestibular symptoms is no different than for the patient with TIAs, epilepsy, and so on.*
- *Every effort to see the patient while symptomatic may prove valuable; flexible availability for examination when acutely symptomatic may offer a final diagnosis.*

Treatment

Reassure the patient that although the symptoms are severe, the underlying cause is not!

- BPPV involving the posterior SCC is treated successfully with canal repositioning maneuvers. This treatment has received consensus status from the American Academy of Otorhinolaringology and the American Academy of Neurology[11]. Horizontal SCC canalolithiasis can also be treated without major difficulty. Cupulolithiasis, however, may be challenging despite proposed reported positioning strategies.
- Surgery is rarely a required option for treatment resistant cases.
- In general, prolonged bending or extending the head may lead to posterior SCC BPPV recurrence. In patients with consistent BPPV recurrences, it is possible to instruct them to perform self treatment successfully.
- BPPV related to horizontal canal is treated according to the direction of the nystagmus: geotropic by turning the head in the direction of the unaffected ear and continue a 360° log roll maneuver; ageotropic is more difficult; in principle, one would want to convert the nystagmus to the geotropic variant or to use prolonged posture strategy. The subject lies on the side of the unaffected ear for several hours.

- Vestibular suppressant drugs should be reserved for the treatment of acute vertigo that is accompanied by severe autonomic or vegetative symptom. Meclizine, transdermal scopolamine, prochlorperazine and other phenothiazines, ondazentron, as well as benzodiazepines, are useful options to minimize the severity of the nausea, vomiting, and vertigo. Chronic treatment with these drugs should be avoided as they are not helpful, cause unwanted side-effects, and may delay the process of vestibular adaptation.
- Betahistine (H1 agonist and H3 antagonist) may improve the microcirculation in the inner ear and promote endolymph absorption. It has been found valuable in the treatment of Ménière's disease.
- Physical therapy is critical as it may enhance the process of adaptation. Customized vestibular rehabilitation programs are often more effective than generic techniques. Exercise routines are designed to induce the symptoms, and by a process of habituation are able to promote central compensation and thereby reduce persistent symptoms.
- Urgent ENT evaluation should be entertained in cases of suspected infection (suppurative otitis), Valsalva-related vertigo suggestive of a perilymphatic fistula, and neoplasms.
- Migraine prevention may be helpful.
- Carbamazepine may be helpful in the treatment of vestibular paroxysmia.

Ménière's disease

- Medical management is the first option (salt restriction and diuretic therapy are the major treatment modalities).
- In Europe, betahistine, a vasodilator, has been used successfully[12].
- Surgery is an option for cases that do not respond to medical management. Currently, local gentamicin ablation via a series of injections in the middle ear cavity has been found to be very effective. Usually only one injection is needed in 53% of cases, and eventual control is achieved in 75% of persons. Endolymphatic sac decompression is less commonly performed, and labyrinthectomy or vestibular nerve section is reserved for cases that do not respond to intraural gentamicin.
- Avoid sedatives and vestibular suppressant drugs on a chronic basis.

Benign paroxysmal positional vertigo

The goal of the Epley maneuver is to relocate or to disperse the otolith debris from the posterior SCC, presumably back to the utricule. The repositioning maneuver involves a 5-step cycle: 1) Beginning with the Dix–Hallpike maneuver; 2) the head laterally turned is maintained in the symptomatic side hanging-head position, until the paroxysmal nystagmus subsides; 3) a slow head turn toward the unaffected ear follows; 4) shoulder then rolls also toward the unaffected side, with the head slightly angled while the patient is looking down at the floor (the total turn is about 270° from the initial symptomatic canal position); and 5) the final step is to sit up and tip the chin down.

Practitioners recommend repeating the maneuver until nystagmus is not observed. In general, the author only tests once and re-examines the patient 1 week later to confirm success. As an anecdotal recommendation, the patient is advised to sleep sitting up the night after canal repositioning.

Even though one performance of the Epley maneuver is often successful, elderly patients may require more than one canal repositioning maneuver. Spontaneous remissions are common in young people. Recurrence may be associated with specific activities (the beauty shop, prolonged bending, and so on). Maneuvers for treatment of the horizontal SCC variant include the log rolling maneuver (360°) turn in the direction opposite to the affected canal (the affected SCC is identified by the patient's report of vertigo intensity as the head turns to trigger position while supine). A surgical procedure to plug and effectively paralyze the SCC is rarely recommended.

Tips

▶ *The success rate of a single Epley maneuver in young patients is >90%.*

▶ *These patients do not need a neurologic work-up and should be treated at once.*

▶ *Occupational and recreational activities may play a role in eventual recurrence.*

Prognosis

Sudden unilateral peripheral vestibular loss recovers after a few days, even if there is persistent loss of function. The resolution of the disabling symptoms occurs as a result of equilibration of the tonus in brainstem vestibular nuclei via central nervous system compensatory mechanisms. During this recovery period, the spontaneous symptoms resolve but the impaired response to rapid head acceleration remains and may be a permanent legacy of peripheral vestibular loss. Similar adaptation mechanisms are activated in central vestibular lesions and may be as effective.

Young BPPV patients may improve even without particle repositioning maneuvers. Older patients face frequent recurrences which may be triggered by certain activities such as attending the beauty shop, the dentist, prolonged work overhead, exercise activities, and so on.

Patients with Ménière's syndrome may have long remissions with medical treatment but may have repeat attacks and may need intervention to modify the clinical course. Vestibular schwannomas are increasingly being treated with gamma knife irradiation. Perilymphatic fistulas and symptomatic superior canal dehiscence syndrome will continue to be symptomatic unless surgically corrected.

SPECIFIC SYNDROMES

VESTIBULAR NEURITIS AND LABYRINTHITIS

Definition and epidemiology

Vestibular neuritis refers to the acute unilateral loss of vestibular function. If it coexists with acute loss of hearing, it is referred to as labyrinthitis.

- Incidence: An annual incidence of 150,000 new cases of vestibular neuritis is estimated in the US[4].

Etiology

A reactivation of HSV-1 is a likely cause. HSV-type 1 deoxyribonucleic acid has been found in vestibular ganglia and nuclei at autopsy of nonclinically symptomatic patients. A clear vascular etiology has been rarely documented. Herpes zoster virus (HZV) is also a possible cause.

Clinical features

- Acute vertigo with nausea, vomitin,g and motion intolerance.
- Truncal imbalance with ipsilesional direction of fall.
- Unidirectional, horizontal, conjugate, contralesional nystagmus that increases in the dark is observed; at times, a torsional component may be present.
- The horizontal HIS is positive and skew deviation is rare.
- If HINTS suggests a central localization: pseudoneuritis or pseudolabyrinthitis, MRI of the brain is obtained. If there is a high clinical index of suspicion of stroke, a second MRI of the brain should be ordered, even if a recent MRI scan done early after the stroke onset is negative.

Treatment

If the patient is seen early after onset, therapy with methylprednisolone has been reported effective in a randomized, double-blind trial. Vestibular suppressants often help the associated symptoms. In such a study, therapy with acyclovir was not superior to placebo.

Prognosis

Vestibular neuritis gradually improves, the unsteadiness and nystagmus resolve, but the HIS often remains abnormal. The neuritis is only rarely bilateral. The key issue here is to perform a detailed physical examination to rule out pseudoneuritis, looking for signs of brainstem or cerebellar stroke which could be a risk for further neurologic deterioration.

MÉNIÈRE'S SYNDROME

Definition and epidemiology

Ménière's syndrome is characterized by recurrent episodes of vertigo with spontaneous recovery, typically within hours. In addition, the patients have fluctuating hearing loss, usually in the low frequencies; however, over time there is a possibility of deafness. Tinnitus is frequent and typically increases with the attacks of vertigo. Aural fullness is also reported during an attack.

About 200 cases/100,000 occur[13]. Incidence may vary in different geographic locations. It is most frequent in the fifth decade.

Etiology

The pathology of Ménière's is endolymphatic hydrops and is the result of diverse etiologies but is often idiopathic. An increase in the volume of the endolymphatic fluid in the SCC and utricule/saccule occurs attributed to acoustic trauma, congenital inner ear abnormalities, and vascular disorders associated with arterial hypertension and diabetes.

Clinical features

- Vertigo attacks lasting hours and associated with nausea and vomiting.
- Horizontal torsional nystagmus that can beat away or toward the affected ear, depending on the stage of the attack.
- Hearing loss, tinnitus, and aural fullness during the attack.
- Drop attacks: patients with Ménière's syndrome may suffer from drop attacks (otolithic crisis), also known as 'Tumarkin crisis'. Typically, they fall to the ground without warning, leading frequently to significant injury. Tumarkin crisis may be an indication for intraural gentamicin therapy and in some cases vestibular neurectomy.
- Only rarely bilateral (20%).

Investigations

As an examination during the attack may provide information that otherwise may be unknown, patients should be encouraged to contact the examiner during an acute attack. Waiting for a routine appointment may not yield diagnostic information, and evaluation in an emergency setting may lead to unnecessary testing, often missing diagnostic findings.

Differential diagnosis

- Post-traumatic vertigo.
- BPPV (Ménière's patients can suffer BPPV episodes that are treated and respond to standard canal repositioning maneuvers).
- TIAs and vertebrobasilar insufficiency.
- Vestibular paroxysmia (isolated brief vertigo).
- Migraine-associated vertigo.
- Complex partial seizures (tornado epilepsy).
- Cogan and Susac's syndromes.

Treatment

- Acute episodes: vestibular suppressants (meclizine, diazepam, prochlorperazine, transdermal scopolamine) to address the autonomic symptoms. In some cases, parenteral hydration may be needed.
- Chronic management: therapy with diuretics and salt restriction. Betahistine at a dose of 48 mg tid for ~12 months may induce significant amelioration of the symptoms.
- Medical labyrinthectomy using aminoglycoside drugs given intratympanically offer san excellent alternative for patients with recurrent attacks not responding to diuretic therapy.
- Surgical labyrinthectomy or vestibular neurectomy can be offered to cases not responding to aural aminoglycosides, but only in strictly unilateral cases.

ACUTE INNER EAR ISCHEMIA

Definition and epidemiology

The actual incidence of this syndrome is unknown but it should be suspected among older patients with stroke risk factors, or younger patients that may have vasculitis. There are isolated reports of either unilateral deafness or pseudolabyrinthitis as a result of inner ear ischemia in patients with vertebrobasilar insufficiency or vertebral artery dissection[9,14]. Among AVS patients with vascular risk factors, the brain MRI often shows signs of vascular ischemic gliosis making the possibility of a vascular etiology a plausible consideration.

Clinical features

Patients with an acute ischemic event of the labyrinth, the cochlea, or both, may experience acute onset of deafness, a unilateral AVS, or both (pseudolabyrinthitis).

Differential diagnosis

- Labyrinthitis.
- Migrainous vertigo.
- Nonspecific vestibulopathy.
- Vestibular neuritis.
- Initial stage of Ménière's syndrome.

Investigations

- MRA.
- Computed tomographic angiography (CTA).
- Catheter angiography (if above choices are not available).

Treatment

- Antiplatelet aggregation agents.
- Management of vascular risk factors.
- In selected instances, short- or long-term anticoagulation may be a consideration.

MIGRAINOUS VERTIGO

Definition and epidemiology

Episodes of vertigo often preceding or coinciding with the onset of headache. These episodes may also be isolated, but the patient provides a history characteristic for migraine. Migraine is a frequent cause of vertigo, but the actual incidence and prevalence are unknown.

Clinical features

- Episodes of vertigo associated with either peripheral or central vestibular findings.
- Headache in association with the majority of the vertigo episodes.
- Headache features are consistent with the diagnosis of migraine, using the International Headache Society criteria: hemicranias, photophobia, and other auras[15]. In the past, some of these cases were probably included among basilar artery migraine cases.
- Children with benign vertigo of childhood have evolved to a classic migraine syndrome as teenagers and adults.

Tips

▸ *Migraine-associated vertigo is frequent.*
▸ *The neurologic findings may suggest a central or peripheral lesion localization and at times unsteadiness and nausea may be the only features.*
▸ *The patients must have a solid history of migraine, according to International Headache Society criteria.*
▸ *Episodic vomiting of childhood may be a forerunner of adult migraine.*

Treatment

- Migraine prophylactic agents such as propanolol may be useful and topiramate was found effective in a few studies[16].
- Vestibular suppressant drugs may be effective during the acute attack.
- Management of the associated headache with triptan could be considered, but it has not been studied.

VESTIBULAR PAROXYSMIA

Definition and epidemiology

Episodes of vertigo caused by neurovascular compression, usually of the AICA or one of its branches. The incidence or prevalence of this entity is unknown, but it probably accounts for many cases of otherwise unexplained vestibulopathy. In clinics following large numbers of patients, it may account for up to 4% of cases[17].

Clinical features

- Episodes of vertigo and imbalance are brief, lasting from seconds to a few minutes.
- Vertigo may be prompted by different positional changes, but unlike BPPV they are not consistently related to the plane of stimulation of a particular SSC.
- Less frequently a pressure feeling or numbness in the ear and decreased hearing may be reported.

Diagnosis

- Evidence of neurovascular compression with high resolution MR imaging (constructive interference in steady-state magnetic resonance, CISS).
- Exclusion of other diagnostic possibilities. A gold standard is not yet available.

Treatment

- Favorable response to treatment with carbamazepine and other antiepileptic dugs has been reported[18].
- In selective treatment-resistance cases, the possibility of vascular loop decompression could be a last resource option, as consistent benefit has not been proven.

SUPERIOR CANAL DEHISCENCE SYNDROME (MINOR'S SYNDROME)

Definition and epidemiology

The absence or thinning of the roof of the superior SCC creates a heightened response to sound and to inner ear pressure changes that leads to episodic noise-induced vertigo and oscillopsia, conductive hearing loss, and awareness and of one's own voice (autophony) with occasional oscillopsia (see **154**).

No data are presently available as to the possible incidence of this syndrome, which was described about a decade ago. Radiographic thinning of the roof of the superior SCC is not necessarily associated with clinical symptoms.

Clinical features

- Conductive hearing loss.
  - Combined conductive hearing loss and low threshold VEMP in a patient with symptoms suggestive of SCC dehiscence are indications to obtain high resolution CT scan of the temporal bone.
- Noise-induced vertigo associated with nystagmus or conjugate ocular torsion.
- Valsalva- and cough-related oscillopsia, nystagmus, and, less frequently, drop attacks.

Diagnosis

- Conductive hearing loss in one or both ears.
  - Bone conduction stimuli typically yield better hearing than air conduction stimuli.
- Noise-induced conjugate ocular torsion or oscillopsia.
- Valsalva- or cough-induced vertigo, nystagmus, or oscillopsia.
- Vestibular evoked potentials easily obtained at low intensity stimulation (see **155**).
- Radiographic evidence of superior SCC dehiscence in high resolution CT scan of the temporal bone (see **154**).

Treatment

Symptoms respond to surgical repair of the dehiscent superior SCC roof, usually a combined neurotologist–neurosurgery procedure.

BILATERAL SIMULTANEOUS VESTIBULAR LOSS

Definition and epidemiology

Loss of inner cells in the vestibular labyrinth. In general, hearing is mildly impaired or totally spared. Drug ototoxicity is the most common cause, but systemic illness and bilateral Ménière's may be responsible.

This is an infrequent syndrome. In a large balance referral center in Germany, 255 cases were registered among 6000 patients (4%)[19].

Clinical features

- Severe imbalance initially with positive Romberg test with the eyes closed. Over time it improves, but will remain always positive if the patient is tested on a foam cushion.
- No evidence of nystagmus is present despite severe imbalance.
- Poor dynamic visual acuity.
- Positive HIS in the horizontal and vertical SCC planes.

Diagnosis

- Exposure to ototoxic medications or systemic illness as a cause should be investigated.
- Bilateral caloric and rotational testing show poor or absent VOR response with evidence of phase lead and decreased gain of rotational nystagmus.
- Audiometry may be normal or minimally impaired.

Treatment

Use of aminoglycosides should be restricted, but if they are indispensable, they must be given in one daily dose with monitoring of blood levels. The combined effect of gentamicin and furosemide should be avoided. Physical therapy may improve the patient over time, as some degree of vestibular adaptation may occur.

REFERENCES

1 Baloh RW, Halmagyi MG (1996). *Disorders of the Vestibular System*. Oxford University Press, New York, Oxford.

2 Neuhauser HK, Radtke A, Von Brevern M, Lezius F, Feldman M, Lempert T (2008). Burden of dizziness and vertigo in the community. *Arch Intern Med* **168**: 2118–2124.

3 Kerber K, Meurer WJ, West BT, Fendrick MA (2006). Dizziness presentations in US Emergency Departments 1995–2004. *Acad Emerg Med* **15**:1–7.

4 Newman Toker DE, Hsiang H, Camargo C, Pelletier AJ, Butchy GT, Edlow J (2008). Spectrum of dizziness visits to US Emergency Departments: cross sectional analysis from a nationally representative sample. *Mayo Clin Proc* **83**:765–775.

5 Tarnnutzer AA, Berkowitz AL, Robinson KA, Hsieh Y-H (2011). Does my dizzy patient have a stroke? A systematic review of bedside diagnosis in acute vestibular syndrome. *CMAJ* **183**:571–591. PMCID: PMC3114934.

6 Savitz SI, Caplan LR, Edlow JA (2008). Pitfalls in the diagnosis of cerebellar infarction. *Acad Emerg Med* **14**:63–68.

7 Schucknedt HE (1969). Cupulolithiasis. *Arch Otolaryngol* **90**:765–778.

8 Goebel J, O'Mara W, Gianoli G (2001). Anatomic considerations in vestibular neuritis. *Otol Neurotol* **22**:512–518.

9 Kim JS, Lopez I, Di Patre PL, Liu F, Ishiyama A, Baloh RW (1999). Internal auditory artery infarction. Clinicopathologic correlation. *Neurology* **52**:40–45.

10 Halmagyi MG, Aw ST, Karlberg IS, Curthoys IS, Todd MJ (2002). Inferior vestibular neuritis. Neurobiology of eye movements. From molecules to behavior. *Ann NY Acad Sci* **956**:306–313.

11 Fife TD, Iverson DJ, Lempert T, *et al*., Quality Standards Subcommittee, American Academy of Neurology (2008). Practice parameter: therapies for benign paroxysmal positional vertigo (an evidence-based report of the Quality Standards Subcommittee of the American Academy of Neurology). *Neurology* **70**(22):2067–2074.

12 James AL, Burton MJ (2001). Betahistine for Meniere's disease or syndrome. *Cochrane Database Syst Rev* **1**:CD001873.

13 Arenberg IK, Balkany TJ, Goldman G, Pillsbury RC 3rd (1980). The incidence and prevalence of Meniere's disease – a statistical analysis of limits. *Otolaryngol Clin NA* **13**(5:697–601.

14 Kim JS, Lee H (2009). Inner ear dysfunction due to vertebrobasilar ischemic stroke. *Sem Neurol* **29**:534–540.

15 Olesen J, Lipton RB (1994). Migraine classification and diagnosis. International headache Society for the Diagnosis of Migraine. *Neurology* **44**:(6 suppl 4):S6–10.

16 Carmona S, Settecase N (2005). Use of topiramate (Topamax) in a subgroup of migraine-vertigo patients with auditory symptoms. *Ann NY Acad Sci* **1039**:517–520.

17 Janetta PJ (1975). Neurovascular cross-compression in patients with hyperactive dysfunction symptoms of the eighth cranial nerve. *Surg Forum* **26**:467–469.

18 Hufner K, Barresi D, Glaser M, *et al.* (2008). Vestibular paroxysmia. *Neurology* **71**:1006–1014.

19 Zingler VC, Cnyrim C, Jahn K, *et al.* (2007). Causative factors and epidemiology of bilateral vestibulopathy in 255 patients. *Ann Neurol* **61**:524-532.

Further reading

Definition and classification according to timing

Amarenco P, Hauw JJ (1990). Cerebellar infarction in the territory of the anterior and inferior cerebellar artery. A clinicopathological study of 20 cases. *Brain* **113**:139–155.

Black FO, Shupert CL, Peterka RJ, Nashner LM (1989). Effects of unilateral loss of vestibular function following hemilabyrinthectomy. *Ann Otol Rhinol, Laryngol* **98**:884–889.

Brandt T, Daroff RB (1980). The multisensory physiological and pathologic vertigo syndromes. *Ann Neurol* **7**:195–203.

Caplan LR (2008). Funny turns. They do mean something. *Arch Neurol* **65**:601–602.

Cnyrim CD, Newman-Toker DE, Karch C, Brandt T, Strupp M (2008). Bedside differentiation of vestibular neuritis from central 'vestibular pseudoneuritis'. *J Neurol, Neurosurg, Psychiatry* **79**: 458–460.

Duncan GW, Parker SW, Miller Fisher C (1995). Acute cerebellar infarction in the PICA territory. *Arch Neurol* **32**:364–368.

Fetter M, Zee DS (1988). Recovery from unilateral labyrinthectomy in rhesus monkeys. *J Neurophysiol* **59**:370–393.

Furman JM, Case SP (1999). Benign paroxysmal positional vertigo. *N Engl J Med* **341**:1590–1596.

Hotson, JR, Baloh RW (1998). Acute vestibular syndrome. *N Engl J Med* **339**:680–685.

Lee H, Sohn SI, ChoYW, *et al.* (2006). Cerebellar infarction presenting isolated vertigo: frequency and vascular topographic patterns. *Neurology* **67**:1178–1183.

Newman-Toker DE, Kattah JC, Alvernia JE, Wang DZ (2008). Normal head Impulse Test differentiates acute cerebellar stroke from vestibular neuritis. *Neurology* **70**:2378–2385.

Precht W, Shimazu H, Markham CH (1966). A mechanism of central compensation of vestibular function following hemilabyrinthectomy. *J Neurophysiol* **29**:996–1010.

Epidemiology

Newman-Toker DE, Camargo CA, Hsiang Hsieh Y, Pelletier AJ, Edlow JA (2009). Disconnect between charted vestibular diagnosis and emergency department management decisions: a cross-sectional analysis from a nationally representative sample. *Acad Emerg Med* **16**:970–977.

Newman-Toker DE, Cannon LM, Stofferhan ME, Rothman RE, Hsiang-HsiehY, Zee DS (2007). Imprecision in patient reports of dizziness symptoms quality: a cross-sectional study conducted in an acute care setting. *Mayo Clinic Proc* **82**:1329–1340.

Pathophysiology and pathology

Adams RD (1943). Occlusion of the anterior inferior cerebellar artery. *Arch Neurol Psychiatry* **49**:765–770.

Baloh RW, Lopez I, Ishiyama A, Wackym PA (1996). Vestibular neuritis: clinicopathologic correlation. *Otolaryngol Head Neck Surg* **114**:586–592.

Dix MR, Hallpike CS (1952). The pathology, symptomatology and diagnosis of certain common disorders of the vestibular system. *Proc R Soc Med* **45**:341–354.

Fetter M, Dichgans J (1996). Vestibular neuritis spares the inferior division of the vestibular nerve. *Brain* **118**:755–763.

Fife T (2009). Migraine associated vertigo: a common but difficult-to-define disorder. *Pract Neurol* **9**:27–33.

Hallpike CS, Cairns H (1938). Observations in the pathology of Meniere's syndrome. *J Laryngol, Otol* **53**:625–654.

Halmagyi MG, Curthoys IS (1988). A clinical sign of canal paresis. *Arch Neurol* **45**:737–739.

Kerber K, Brown DL, Lisbeth LD, Smith MA, Morgerstern LB (2006). Stroke among patients with dizziness, vertigo and imbalance in the emergency department. A population-based study. *Stroke* **37**:2484–2487.

Kim JS, Lee JH, Choi CG (1998). Patterns of lateral medullary infarction: vascular lesion – magnetic resonance correlation of 34 cases; *Stroke* **29**:645–652.

Schuknecht HF, Kitamura K (1981). Vestibular neuronitis. *Ann Otol, Rhinol, Laryngol* **78** (Suppl):1–19.

Theil D, Arbusow V, Derfuss T, *et al.* (2001). Prevalence of HSV-1 Lat in human trigeminal, geniculate, and vestibular ganglia and its implication for cranial nerve syndromes. *Brain Pathol* **11**:408–413.

Clinical features and diagnosis

Boatman DF, Miglioretti DL, Eberwein C, Alldoost M, Reich SG (2007). How accurate are bedside hearing tests? *Neurology* **68**:1311–1314.

Brandt T, Dieterich M (1993). Skew deviation with ocular torsion: a vestibular brainstem sign of topographic diagnostic value. *Ann Neurol* **33**:528–534.

Brandt T, Dieterich M (1994). Vestibular syndromes in the roll plane: topographic diagnosis from brainstem to cortex. *Ann Neurol* **36**:337–347.

Hain TC (2007). Head shaking nystagmus and new technology. *Neurology* **68**:1333–1334.

Halmagyi GM, Gresty MA, Gibson WP (1979). Ocular tilt reaction with peripheral vestibular lesions. *Ann Neurol* **6**:80–83.

Kattah JC, Talkad A, Wang DZ, Hsieh YH, Newman-Toker DE (2009). HINTS to diagnose stroke in the acute vestibular syndrome. Three-step bedside oculomotor examination more sensitive than early diffusion-weighted imaging. *Stroke* **40**:3504–3510.

Keane JR (1975). Ocular skew deviation. Analysis of 100 cases. *Arch Neurol* **32**:185–190.

Kim HA, Hong JH, Lee H, *et al.* (2008). Otolith dysfunction in vestibular neuritis. Recovery pattern and a predictor of symptom recovery. *Neurology* **70**:449–453.

Leigh JR, Zee DS (2006). *The Neurology of Eye Movements*. Oxford University Press, Oxford, Chapter 2, pp. 20–108.

Zee DS (1978). Ophthalmoscopy in the examination of patients with vestibular disorders. *Ann Neurol* 3(4):373–374.

Interpretation of signs and symptoms; peripheral *vs.* central

Asprella-Libonatti G (2008). Pseudo-spontaneous nystagmus: a new sign to diagnose the affected side in lateral semicircular canal benign paroxysmal positional vertigo. *Acta Otorhinolaryngol* **28**:73–78.

Baloh RW, Honrubia V, Jacobson K (1987). Benign positional vertigo. *Neurology* **37**:371–378.

Baloh RW, Yue Q, Jacobson KM, Honrubia V (1994). Persistent direction-changing positional nystagmus. Another variant of benign positional nystagmus. *Neurology* **45**:1297–1300.

Bertholon P, Brosntein A, Davies R, Rudge P, Thilo K (2002). Positional downbeating nystagmus in 50 patients: cerebellar disorders and possible anterior canalithiasis. *J Neurol, Neurosurg, Psychiatry* 72:366–372.

Bisdorff AR, Debatisse D (2001). Localizing signs in positional vertigo due to lateral canal cupulolithiasis. *Neurology* **57**:1085–1088.

Casani A, Giovanni V, Bruno F, Luigi (1997). Positional vertigo and ageotropic bidirectional nystagmus. *Laryngoscope* **107**:807–813.

Kattah JC, Kolsky MP, Luessenhop A (1994). Positional vertigo and the cerebellar vermis. *Neurology* **34**:527–529.

Nam J, Kim S, Huh Y, Kim JS (2009). Ageotropic central positional nystagmus in nodular infarction. *Neurology* **73**:1163.

Von Brevern M, Clarke AH, Lempert T (2001). Continuous vertigo and spontaneous nystagmus due to canalolithiasis of the horizontal canal. *Neurology* **56**:684–686.

Investigations

Cheng WC, Young YH, Chih-Hsiu W (2000). Vestibular neuritis; three dimensional videonystagmography and vestibular evoked myogenic otential results. *Acta Otolaryngol* **120**:845–848.

Colebatch JG, Halmagyi MG, Skuse NF (1994). Myogenic potentials induced by a click-evoked vestibulocollic reflex. *J Neurol, Neurosurg, Psychiatry* **57**:190–197.

Ho SY, Kveton JF (2002). Acoustic neuroma: assessment and management. *Otolaryngol Clinics North Am* **35**:1–8.

Treatment and prognosis

Baloh RW, Yue Q, Jacobson KM, Honrubia V (1995). Persistent, direction-changing positional nystagmus. *Neurology* **45**:1297–1301.

Brandt T, Dieterich M (2000). Perceived vertical and lateropulsion: clinical syndromes, localization and prognosis. *Neurorehabil Neural Repair* **14**:1–20.

Brandt T, Zwergal A, Strupp M (2009). Medical treatment of vestibular disorders. *Expert Opin Pharmacother* **10**:1537–1548.

Kondziolka D, Lunsford D, Mclaughlin MR, Flickinger J (1998). Long term outcomes after radiosurgery for acoustic neuromas. *New Engl J Med* **339**:1426–1433.

Palla A, Straumann D, Bronstein AM (2008). Vestibular neuritis, vertigo and high acceleration vestibulo-ocular reflex. *New Engl J Neurol* **255**:1479–1482.

Paroxysmal positional vertigo

Appiani GC, Catania G, Gagliardi M (2001). A liberatory maneuver for the treatment of horizontal paroxysmal positional vertigo. *Otol Neurotol* **22**:66–69.

Boleas-Aguirre MS, Perez N, Batuecas-Caletrio A (2009). Bedside therapeutic experiences with horizontal canal benign paroxysmal positional vertigo. *Acta Otolaryngol* **129**:1217–1221.

Epley J (1992). The canal repositioning procedure: for treatment of benign paroxysmal positional vertigo. *Otolaryngol Head Neck Surg* **107**:399–404.

Furman JM, Hain TC (2004). 'Do try this at home'. Self treatment of BPPV. *Neurology* **63**:8–9.

Tanimoto H, Kiyoshi D, Katata K, Nibu K (2005). Self treatment for benign paroxysmal positional vertigo of the posterior semicircular canal. *Neurology* **65**:1299–1300.

Vestibular neuritis

Lindsay JR, Hemenway WG (1956). Postural vertigo due to unilateral partial loss of vestibular function. *Ann Otol, Rhinol, Laryngol* **65**:692–706.

Strupp M, Zingler VC, Arbusow V, *et al.* (2004). Methylprednisolone, valacyclovir, or the combination for vestibular neuritis. *New Engl J Med* **351**:354–361.

Walker MF (2009). Treatment of vestibular neuritis. *Curr Treat Option Neurol* **11**:41–45.

Ménière's disease and Tumarkin crisis

Baloh RW, Jacobson K, Winder T (1990). Drop attacks with Meniere's syndrome. *Ann Neurol* **28**:384–387.

Black FL, Effron MZ, Burns DS (1982). Diagnosis and management of drop attacks of vestibular origin: Tumarkin otolothitic crisis. *J Otolaryngol* **90**:256–262.

Branstberg K, Ishiyama A, Baloh RW (2005). Drop attacks secondary to superior canal dehiscence syndrome. *Neurology* **64**:2126–2128.

Lange G, Maurer J, Mann W (2004). Long-term results after long term interval therapy with intratympanic gentamicin for Meniere's disease. *Laryngoscope* **114**:102–105.

Acute inner ear ischemia

Kim SJ, Lee H (2009). Inner ear dysfunction due to vertebrobasilar ischemic stroke. *Sem Neurol* **29**:534–540.

Lee H, Baloh RW (2004). Sudden deafness in vertebrobasilar ischemia: clinical features, vascular topographic patterns and long term outcome. *J Neurolog Sci* **228**: 99–104.

Lee H, Ha Y, Baloh RW (2003). Sudden bilateral simultaneous deafness with vertigo as a sole manifestation of vertebrobasilar insufficiency. *J Neurol, Neurosurg, Psychiatry* **74**:539–541.

Norrving B, Magnusson M, Holtas S (1995). Isolated acute vertigo in the elderly; vestibular or vascular disease. *Acta Neurol Scand* **5**:9143-9148.

Yamasoba T, Kikuchi S, Higo R (2001). Deafness associated with vertebrobasilar insufficiency. *J Neurolog Sci* **187**:64–75.

Migrainous vertigo

Batson G (2004). Benign paroxysmal vertigo of childhood. A review of the literature. *J Otorhinolaryngol Related Special* **9**:31–34.

Neuhaser H, Von Brevern LM, Arnold G, Lempert T (2001). The interrelations of migraine, vertigo and migrainous vertigo. *Neurology* **56**:436–441.

Vestibular paroxysmia

Janetta PJ (1984). Disabling positional vertigo. *New Engl J Med* **310**:1700–1705.

McCabe BF, Harker LA (1983). Vascular loop as a cause of vertigo. *Ann Otol, Rhinol, Laryngol* **92**:542–543.

Superior canal dehiscence syndrome

Baloh RW (2004). Superior semicircular canal dehiscence syndrome. Leaks and squeaks can make you dizzy. *Neurology* **62**:684–685.

Brantberg K, Ishiyamma A, Baloh RW (2005). Drop attacks secondary to superior canal dehiscence syndrome. *Neurology* **64**:2126–2128.

Cremer PD, Minor LB, Carey JP, Della Santina CC (2000). Eye movements in patients with superior canal dehiscence syndrome align with the abnormal canal. *Neurology* **55**:1833–1841.

Hain TC, Cherchi M (2008). Pulse synchronous pendular nystagmus in unilateral superior canal dehiscence. *Neurology* **70**:1217–1218.

Halmagyi MG, Aw ST, McGarvie LA, *et al.* (2003). Superior semicircular canal dehiscence simulating otosclerosis. *J Laryngol Otol* **117**:553–557.

Minor LB, Solomon D, Zinreich JS, Zee DS (1998). Sound-and/or pressure induced vertigo due to bone dehiscence of the superior semicircular canal. *Arch Otolaryngol Head Neck Surg* **124**:249–258.

Piton J, Negrevergne M, Portmann D (2008). Dehiscence du canal semi-circulaire supérieur: Approche et classification scanographiques. *Rev Laryngol Otol Rhinol* **129**:17–26.

Welgampola MS, Oluwaseum AM, Minor L, Carey JP (2007). Vestibular-evoked potential thresholds normalize on plugging. *Neurology* **70**:464–472.

Bilateral vestibular loss

Waterston JA, Halmagyi M (1998). Unilateral vestibulotoxicity due to gentamicin therapy. *Acta Otolaryngol* **188**:474–478.

HYPERKINETIC MOVEMENT DISORDERS

Annu Aggarwal, Victor Fung, PhilipThompson

INTRODUCTION

Hyperkinetic movement disorders are classified according to the phenomenology of the movements into the following categories:

- *Dystonia*: sustained twisting repetitive movements and posturing.
- *Tremor*: rhythmic, sinusoidal oscillation.
- *Athetosis* ('without fixed position'): slow writhing of distal limbs and fingers.
- *Chorea*: random flowing movements from one body part to another.
- *Myoclonus*: brief, abrupt shock-like jerking movements.
- *Tics*: repetitive simple or complex movements, suppressed by an effort of will.
- *Stereotypies*: complex coordinated motor behaviours repeated at the expense of other activities.

The distribution of movements is classified as:

- *Focal*: involving a single body part.
- *Segmental*: involving two contiguous regions of the body.
- *Multifocal*: involving two or more noncontiguous regions of the body.
- *Generalized*: involving leg(s), trunk, and any other body part.
- *Hemi*: one side of the body.

More than one type of movement disorder may be present. The predominant movement disorder on clinical examination determines the category and syndromic classification.

Etiologic classification and differential diagnosis

After consideration of the type of movement disorder, age of onset, pattern of inheritance if familial, history of onset and evolution, and associated neurological or systemic signs:

Primary

- Movement disorder is the only symptom or sign.
- No other neurologic signs or evidence of systemic disease.
- No radiologic abnormality.
- Includes sporadic and genetic causes (e.g. primary dystonia, essential tremor).

Secondary

- Movement disorder due to identifiable neurologic insult, structural lesion, or part of another (underlying) neurologic disease or disorder, and often accompanied by other neurologic signs:
  - Head trauma, 'cerebral palsy'.
  - Infection, immune.
  - Hereditary, metabolic, degenerative.
  - Systemic disease.
  - Vascular, tumor (hemimovement disorder).
  - Psychogenic.

Tip

▶ *The phenomenology of the predominant involuntary movement determines the syndromic diagnosis of the movement disorder. Other clinical information and investigation is then used to refine the differential diagnosis and arrive at an etiologic or pathologic diagnosis.*

DYSTONIA

Definition

Dystonia is a syndrome of sustained muscle contractions causing twisting and repetitive movements or abnormal postures of the affected body part(s). Dystonia can be inherited with variable penetrance or sporadic (primary dystonia), or secondary to brain diseases (secondary or symptomatic dystonia). Primary and secondary dystonia have a range of clinical expressions[1,2]. Important clinical characteristics of dystonia (**156**) include:

- Dystonia typically occurs during voluntary movement (action dystonia) and is a mobile (rather than fixed) movement disorder with repetitive (patterned) dystonic movements superimposed on the abnormal postures.
- Abnormal twisted postures are caused by prolonged cocontraction of agonist and antagonist muscle groups during movement.
- Often there is contraction throughout the limb with overflow of muscle contraction to those muscles not normally involved in the task.
- Tremor and jerky (myoclonic) movements are common accompaniments.
- Dystonic postures, tremor, and jerky movements of the upper limbs may be most pronounced in certain postures such as semi-pronation of forearms, shoulders abducted with fingers under nose.
- Dystonia can be task specific ('occupational cramps').
- Sensory tricks (*geste antagoniste*) relieve dystonia by touching a body part.

Tip

▶ *Always observe the patient performing the movement that is reported as causing difficulty, looking for tremor and dystonic posturing. Ask whether certain gestures or postures (sensory tricks or geste antagoniste) relieve the difficulty.*

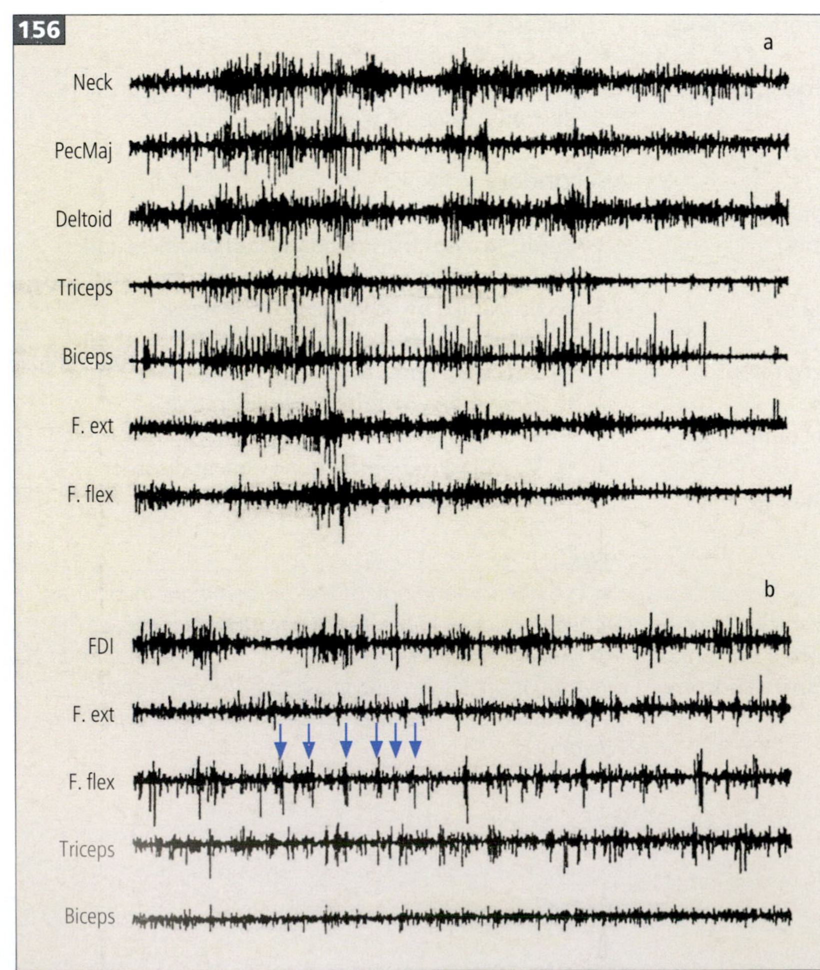

156 Surface EMGs of dystonic muscle activity in two patients with primary dystonia. (a) Long bursts of muscle activity in a patient with arm and neck dystonia with cocontraction of antagonist muscles of the arm; (b) bursts of tremor activity (arrows) punctuate the forearm extensor (F. ext) and flexor (F. flex) muscle activity in a patient with writer's cramp. *From Berardelli et al. [1998]. Brain 121:1195–1212. Reproduced with kind permission of the author and publisher.*

Epidemiology

Prevalence of 395 (per million) (may be an underestimate as diagnosis is often missed or delayed).

- Primary generalized dystonia – 34/million.
- Primary focal dystonia – 300/million:
  - Torticollis – 100/million.
  - Cranial – 80/million: oromandibular, blepharospasm, laryngeal.
  - Writer's cramp – 70/million.
  - Spasmodic dysphonia – 50/million.
- Secondary or symptomatic dystonia – 61/million.

Pathophysiology

Reduced inhibitory activity has been demonstrated at cortical, brainstem, and spinal cord levels, leading to excessive muscle activation causing cocontraction and overflow. Cortical sensorimotor maps are less well defined and motor cortical plasticity is enhanced. Together these abnormalities result in reduced precision during voluntary activation of motor pathways. Genetic factors appear to be important determinants of these physiological changes. For example, repetitive action may influence cortical plasticity in susceptible individuals leading to the development of focal dystonia and occupational 'cramps'[3].

Classification

- Age of onset:
  - Early onset: <26 years.
  - Late onset: >26 years.
- Distribution:
  - Focal: dystonia involves a single body part:
    - Cranial (blepharospasm, oromandibular, laryngeal [spasmodic dysphonia]), cervical (torticollis).
    - Upper limb, hand: writer's cramp, musician's, other occupational dystonias.
    - Axial (back, trunk): causing scoliosis, lordosis, kyphosis.
  - Segmental: dystonia involves two contiguous regions of the body.
  - Multifocal: dystonia involves two noncontiguous regions of the body.
  - Generalized: dystonia involves leg, trunk, and any other body region.
  - Hemidystonia: dystonia restricted to one side of the body.

Tip

▶ *Age of onset and distribution of dystonia are important clues to the etiology of dystonia.*

Etiology

The etiology of dystonia is classified into primary and secondary causes. In primary dystonia the only symptom or sign of neurologic involvement is dystonia. Primary dystonia is further divided into generalized young (childhood) onset dystonia, dystonia (torsion dystonia), and focal adult-onset dystonia. A valuable starting point in the assessment of dystonia is brain imaging with magnetic resonance imaging (MRI) which is normal in primary dystonia and abnormal in many examples of secondary dystonia. The list of conditions causing secondary dystonia is extensive and includes structural lesions of the basal ganglia and thalamus producing hemidystonia and many conditions that cause 'holes in the basal ganglia'. The latter are often associated with widespread brain injury of which dystonia is one of a number of manifestations that include other movement disorders, such as an akinetic rigid syndrome with prominent bulbar involvement, upper motor neuron signs, ataxia, seizures, visual failure, cognitive decline, and neuropathy. These additional features provide clues to the diagnosis and guide investigation in individual cases.

Primary dystonia

- Early onset primary (DYT1) torsion dystonia (generalized).
- Adult-onset primary dystonia (focal).

Secondary dystonia

- Inherited (genetic) dystonia with other signs:
  - Myoclonus dystonia (DYT11).
  - Dopa responsive dystonia (DYT5).
  - Dystonia–parkinsonism syndromes:
    - X-linked dystonia–parkinsonism (Lubag) (DYT3), *TAF1* gene mutation.
    - Rapid onset dystonia–parkinsonism (DYT12), *ATP1A3* gene mutation.
  - Dystonia deafness.
  - Paroxysmal dystonia.
- Focal lesions (usually basal ganglia–thalamus), hemidystonia:
  - Trauma.
  - Stroke.
  - Arteriovenous malformation (AVM).
  - Neoplasm.
  - Abscess.
- Perinatal:
  - Kernicterus.
  - 'Cerebral palsy'.

- Infective:
  - Viral encephalitis (especially Japanese B).
  - Subacute sclerosing panencephalitis (SSPE).
- Immune:
  - Systemic lupus erythematosus.
  - Antiphospholipid antibody syndrome.
  - Limbic encephalitis.
  - Anti-*N*-methyl-D-aspartate (NMDA) receptor antibody-related encephalitis.
  - Post-infectious.
  - Hemolytic uremic syndrome.
  - Demyelination.
- Toxins:
  - Manganese (ephedrone).
  - Carbon monoxide, carbon disulfide.
  - Wasp-sting encephalopathy.
- Neurodegenerations:
  - Parkinson's disease (PD).
  - Huntington's disease (HD).
  - Spinocerebellar ataxia (SCA2, 3, 17).
  - Dentatorubropallidoluysian atrophy (DRPLA).
  - Corticobasal syndrome (CBS).
  - Progressive supranuclear palsy (PSP).
  - Multiple system atrophy (MSA).
- Drug induced: acute and tardive dystonia.
- Metal disorders:
  - Wilson's disease (WD).
  - Neurodegeneration with brain iron accumulation (NBIA):
    - Pantothenate kinase associated neurodegeneration (PKAN).
    - Hypoprebetalipoproteinemia, acanthocytes, retinitis pigmentosa, pallidal degeneration (HARP).
    - Neuroaxonal dystrophy (NAD).
    - Neuroferritinopathy (NF).
    - Aceruloplasminemia (Aca).
- Metabolic:
  - Mitochondrial diseases:
    - Leigh syndrome (LS).
    - Familial striatal lucencies with Lebers optic atrophy.
  - Leukodystrophies:
    - Metachromatic leukodystrophy (MLD).
    - Pelizeaus Merzbacher disease (PMzD).
    - Krabbe's disease (KD).
  - Lysosomal storage diseases:
    - Gangliosidosis (GM1, GM2).
    - Neuronal ceroid lipofuscinosis (NCL).
    - Niemann–Pick type C (dystonic lipidosis) (NPC).
  - Organic amino aciduria (O-AA):
    - Glutaric aciduria, methylmalonic aciduria.
    - Homocystinuria.
  - Lesch Nyhan syndrome (LNS).
  - Glucose transporter type 1 deficiency (Glut 1).
- Neuroacanthocytosis (NAc).
- Ataxia telangiectasia (AT).
- Neuronal intranuclear inclusion disease (NIID).

Clinical assessment

Classify dystonia based on age of onset, distribution; differentiate primary from secondary dystonia.

History

- Age of onset.
- Evolution of symptoms.
- Distribution: body parts affected.
- Task and position specificity.
- Sensory tricks improve symptoms (geste antagoniste).
- Other relieving factors:
  - Leg dystonia present on walking forwards not backwards.
  - Oromandibular, laryngeal dystonia improving during singing.
- Diurnal variation: e.g. dopa responsive dystonia (DYT5).
- Precipitating factor: drugs, occupation.
- Family history: false negative if poorly penetrant disorder, e.g. DYT1; ask for missing relatives and unusual deaths.

Clues to secondary dystonia

- Abnormal birth or perinatal history.
- Delayed developmental motor milestones.
- Exposure to drugs (e.g. dopamine receptor blockers).
- Progressive symptoms.
- Early bulbar involvement (dysarthria, dysphagia).
- Dystonia at rest.
- Unusual distribution by age:
  - <25 years: focal or generalized with head, neck involvement.
  - 25–45 years: generalized.
  - >45 years: generalized or focal dystonia involving legs.
- Hemidystonia.
- Other neurologic signs (see examination below).
- Abnormal brain imaging.

Examination

- Observe the patient at rest, arm outstretched, supinated, semi-pronated, both shoulders extended, elbows flexed, and fingers outstretched under nose; look for twisted postures, alternating, or jerky movements (**157**).
- Observe handwriting and other skilled movements:
  - Look for abnormal grip, excessive grip pressure.
  - Arm, shoulder, and head posture while writing.
- Examine while walking (without shoes):
  - Look for toe, foot, and leg dystonia (**158**).
  - Observe trunk posture, arm swing, shoulder lift, torticollis.
- Examine for other neurologic signs:
  - Cognitive decline.
  - Visual failure – fundoscopy:
    - Pigmentary retinopathy: NBIA/ PKAN.
    - Retinopathy – optic atrophy: NCL.
    - Optic atrophy cherry-red spot: GM1, GM2.
    - Optic atrophy: familial striatal lucencies with Lebers optic atrophy, MLD, KD.
  - Abnormal ocular movements: HD, AT, NPC, PSP, SCA, O-AA.
  - Bulbar involvement (dysarthria, dysphagia): HD, WD, NBIA, NAc, LNS, AA, DYT3.
  - Parkinsonism: PD, PSP, MSA, CBS, HD, WD, NBIA, SCA, DYT3, DYT12.
  - Myoclonus: DRPLA, NCL, WD.
  - Cerebellar ataxia: MSA, WD, SCA, DRPLA, NAc, AT.
  - Pyramidal (upper motor neuron) signs: MSA, SCA, NBIA, WD, MLD.
  - Neuropathy: MLD, KD, AT.
  - Self-mutilation: LNS, NAc.
- Systemic examination:
  - Organomegaly, cataracts in storage diseases.
  - Kayser–Fleischer rings: WD.

Tip

▶ *Observation of voluntary and involuntary movement (walking, sitting, standing) begins when the patient walks into the clinic and continues throughout the interview and formal neurologic examination. Attention is paid to particular movements as indicated by the history (such as difficulty writing and other tasks).*

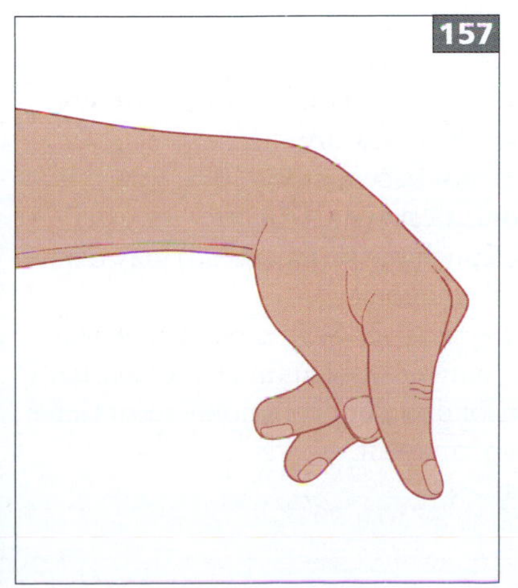

157 Dystonic posturing of the hand in symptomatic hemidystonia.

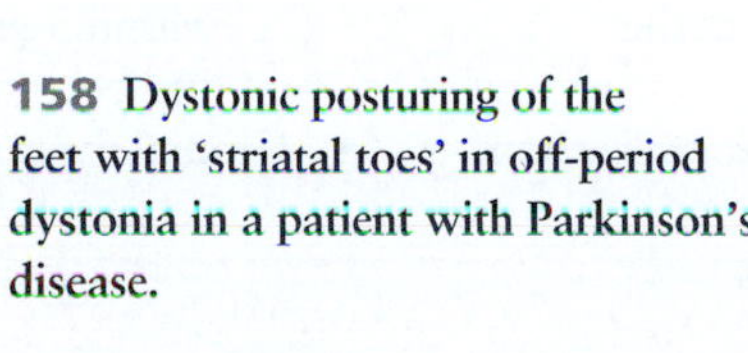

158 Dystonic posturing of the feet with 'striatal toes' in off-period dystonia in a patient with Parkinson's disease.

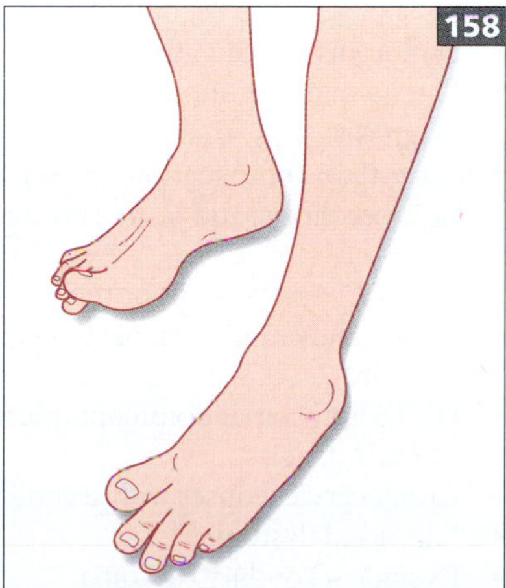

159 Spasmodic torticollis: note the hypertrophied left sternomastoid muscle.

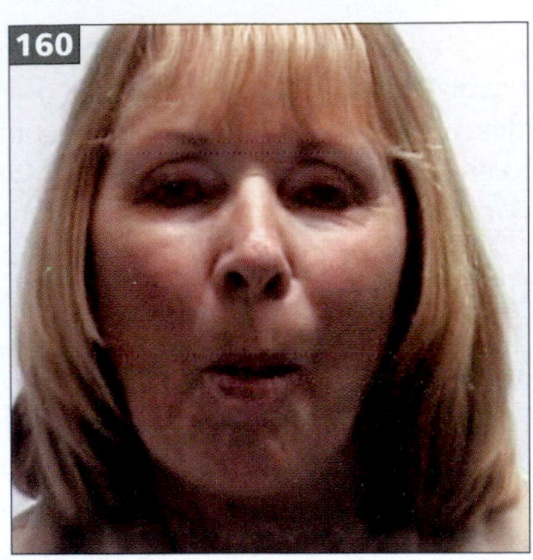

160 Oromandibular dystonia: spasm of jaw and facial (especially lower) muscles.

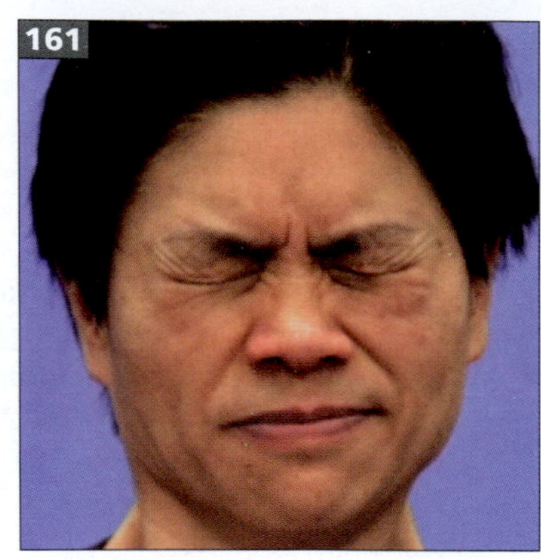

161 Blepharospasm: spasm of eye closure. Lower facial movements are also present in some cases.

Clinical features

Primary dystonia

Young-onset primary (torsion) dystonia:

- DYT1 mutations (chromosome 9) account for the majority of cases.
- Autosomal dominant inheritance with 30% penetrance.
- 70% of gene carriers have no signs of dystonia.
- If a gene carrier is asymptomatic by 25 years, they are unlikely to develop dystonia.
- Occurs in all ethnic groups but high prevalence in Ashkenazi Jews.
- Onset in first two decades (between 3 and 26 years).
- Dystonia starts in the limbs:
  - Presentation of leg action dystonia when running is common.
  - Arm or other limbs are also usually affected at onset.
- Cranial and bulbar dystonia is rare (<15%).
- In some patients dystonia remains focal (25%) or segmental (10%).
- 65% progress to become generalized over 5–10 years.
- Symptoms plateau after initial progression.
- Later worsening should prompt re-evaluation of diagnosis.
- Long-term complications include spondylosis, kyphoscoliosis, and nerve entrapment.

Non-DYT1 young-onset primary dystonia:

- Bulbar and cranial dystonia are more common than in DYT1.
- DYT6 autosomal dominant (mutation in the *THAP1* gene).
- Craniocervical onset with secondary generalization.
- Laryngeal dystonia.
- Exclude secondary dystonia.

Adult-onset primary dystonia:

- Dystonia remains focal.
- Cervical (torticollis) >cranial >upper limb.
- Familial examples, especially craniocervical dystonia – many genetic loci.
- Cervical dystonia (spasmodic torticollis) (**159**):
  - Onset 40–55 years.
  - Women are more commonly affected than men.
  - Family history in 10%.
  - Commonest focal dystonia.
  - Starts with neck discomfort, pulling sensation.
  - Limitation neck movement (neck pain is common).
  - Torticollis, laterocollis are more common than retrocollis.
  - Combination torticollis–laterocollis–retrocollis is common.
  - Consider tardive (drug-induced) dystonia when retrocollis is dominant.
  - Head tremor, dystonic jerky head movements occur in 30%.
  - Dystonic jerky head movements or head tremor may be the dominant feature.
  - Upper limb tremor occurs in 25–50%.
  - Cranial dystonia occurs in 20%.
  - Sensory trick (touching the face, head) may relieve dystonia (geste antagoniste).
  - Symptoms progress over 1–5 years, then plateau.
  - Spontaneous remissions occur in 10–20% usually within 3 years of onset but commonly recurs later and becomes permanent.
- Cranial dystonia.

- Oromandibular dystonia (**160**):
  - Onset in middle age.
  - Women are more commonly affected than men.
  - Masticatory – jaw closing >jaw opening.
  - Facial grimacing 30% (including platysma).
  - Pharyngeal, lingual, and cervical muscles may be affected.
  - Initially triggered by eating, speaking.
  - Common manifestation of tardive dystonia.
- Blepharospasm (**161**):
  - Onset at 60–70 years.
  - Women are more commonly affected than men.
  - Family history in 10%.
  - Orbicularis oculi spasm including pretarsal component.
  - Eyelid motility disorders (levator inhibition) may be combined.
  - Worse when reading, watching television, or in bright sunlight.
  - Intense spasm results in functional blindness.
  - Preceding complaints of gritty discomfort in eyes are common.
  - 70% have oromandibular dystonia (Meige syndrome).
  - 22% have cervical dystonia.
  - Spontaneous remission occurs in 10% during the first 5 years.
- Laryngeal dystonia (spasmodic dysphonia):
  - Onset 30–40 years.
  - Women are more commonly affected (60–80%).
  - Family history in 12%.
  - Vocal cord adductor dystonia (85%): voice interrupted by glottal stops (adductor spasm); varying pitch; strained 'strangled' speech.
  - Vocal cord abductor dystonia (15%): effortful whispering 'breathy' voice:
    - 30% have voice tremor.
    - 20% have segmental cranial dystonia.
- Focal limb dystonia:
  - Onset occurs at 25–35 years.
  - Men are affected more than women.
  - Usually sporadic, rarely familial (DYT1, DYT 5).
  - Upper limb:
    - Commonest is task specific dystonia, usually manifests as writer's cramp, or 'occupational cramps' in musicians, typists, golfers ('yips').
    - Dystonia is usually not severe but can be disabling and threaten the profession.
    - 'Simple' writer's cramp is dystonia only when writing, not other tasks.
    - 'Complex' writer's cramp is dystonia during many manual tasks.
    - Clinical expression of focal upper limb, hand dystonia (**162, 163**) includes: pen gripped with excessive force; pen pressed into the writing surface with excessive force; flexion or extension of wrist and fingers interfering with pen control; dystonic elevation of elbow and arm (overflow); difficulty starting to move ('freezing'); action tremor; postural tremor of affected limb in 50%; mirror dystonia of opposite hand during writing.
    - Trick maneuvers – changing grip or grip size of pen may improve pen control.
    - Remission is rare.
  - 30% of patients who learn to write with the opposite hand develop dystonia in that hand.

Tip

▶ *Adult-onset leg dystonia is almost always secondary to neurodegenerative disorders or structural (including vascular) lesions.*

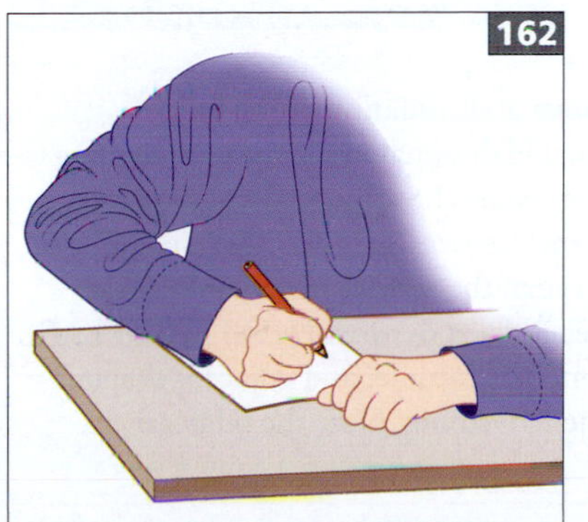

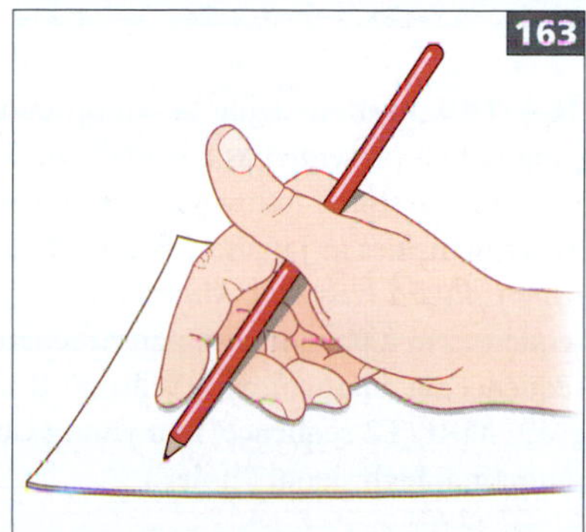

162, 163 Dystonic posturing in writer's cramp. (162) The pen is gripped tightly and pressed onto the page with excessive force. Note hyperextension of the wrist and overflow of dystonic contraction throughout the arm resulting in elevation of the elbow and shoulder; (163) extensor spasms in the thumb and index finger cause difficulty maintaining control of the pen and an inability to initiate writing.

Investigations

Young-onset primary dystonia

- DYT1 gene testing (where available).
- Screen for WD:
  - Serum ceruloplasmin.
  - 24-hour urine copper.
  - Slit lamp for Kayser–Fleischer rings.
- Brain MRI.
- Trial of levodopa.

Focal dystonia

- None where clear history and no other signs in adult.
- Investigate when signs suggest secondary dystonia.
- Laterocollis or fixed painful cervical dystonia especially in an infant or young child:
  - Cervical MRI or computed tomography (CT) to rule out atlantoaxial dislocation.
  - Sandifer syndrome (gastroesophageal reflux – hiatus hernia) in an infant.
- In others consider:
  - WD – in young adults.
  - Brain MRI.

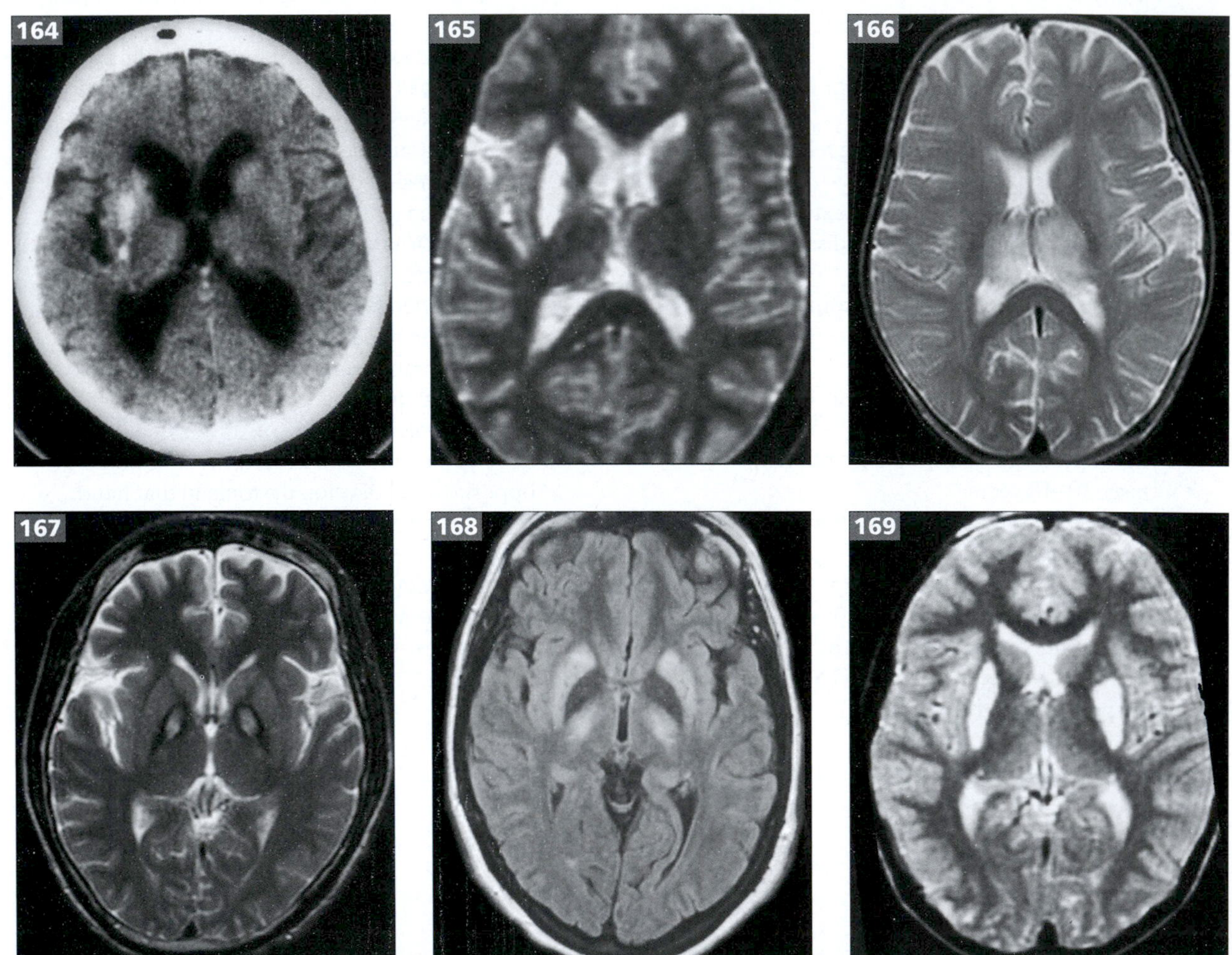

164–169 Brain imaging in symptomatic dystonia. (164) CT showing an arteriovenous malformation of the basal ganglia that presented as a hemidystonia; (165) MRI (T2 sequence) showing putaminal high signal in a patient presenting with hemidystonia following an unidentified acute infective illness; (166) MRI (T2 sequence) showing bilateral thalamic hyperintensities in Japanese B encephalitis with acute onset dystonia and parkinsonism. (*Courtesy of Dr. Darshana Sanghvi, King Edward Hospital, Mumbai*); (167) bilateral high signal in the globus pallidus ('eye of the tiger' sign) on MRI (T2 sequence) in a patient with pantothenate kinase-associated neurodegeneration and generalized dystonia; (168) MRI (FLAIR sequence) in a patient with Wilson's disease illustrating high signal in the putamen, internal capsule, and adjacent thalamus; (169) MRI (T2 sequence) in a young woman with Leigh syndrome presenting with hemidystonia. Note the bilateral putaminal high signal ('holes').

Secondary dystonia

- Brain MRI (**164–169**):
  - Focal lesions (especially basal ganglia, thalamus).
  - 'Holes' in basal ganglia:
    - Infective, toxic, anoxia, trauma, LS, O-AA.
    - Basal ganglia iron deposition, 'eye of the tiger', PKAN (NBIA).
    - Midbrain, striatal T2 hyperintensities (copper deposition): WD.
  - Pallidal T1 hyperintensities (manganese deposition): WD, acquired liver cirrhosis.
  - White matter signal changes: MLD, KD, PMzD, O-AA, WD.
  - Caudate atrophy: HD.
- Blood:
  - Acanthocytes: NAc, NBIA.
  - Serum ceruloplasmin: low in WD, absent in Aca (NBIA).
  - Serum ferritin: NF, Aca (NBIA).
  - Plasma amino acids, hyperammonemia, acidosis, hypoglycemia: O-AA.
  - White cell enzymes:
    - Betagalactosidase: GM1.
    - Aryl sulfatase A: MLD.
  - Alpha-feto protein, immunoglobulins: AT.
- Urine:
  - 24-hour copper excretion: WD.
  - Organic and amino acid: O-AA.
- Slit lamp for Kayser–Fleischer rings, liver biopsy: WD.
- Nerve conduction for peripheral neuropathy: MLD, KD, AT.
- Genetic tests:
  - HD, DRPLA, SCA 1,2, 3, 5, 7, 17.
  - NBIA: *PANK2*, *PLA2G6*, and others (see below).
  - NPC, AT.
  - DYT3, DYT12.

Tip

▶ *Brain MRI is the preferred imaging modality to visualize the basal ganglia and should include sequences to image iron and calcium.*

Selected inherited (genetic) dystonia syndromes with other neurologic signs

Dopa-responsive dystonia (Segawa's disease – DYT5)

- Rare.
- Autosomal dominant (5–10% of inherited childhood dystonia) reduced penetrance.
- Mutations of the *GTP1* gene (on chromosome 14q) which encodes guanosine triphosphate cyclohydrolase 1 (GTP-CH1), the rate-limiting enzyme in the synthesis of tetrahydrobiopterin (THB) that is essential for conversion of phenylalanine to tyrosine, as the rate-limiting step of dopamine synthesis.
- Onset is at any age; dystonia is more dominant in juvenile presentation, parkinsonism is more dominant in adult presentation.
- Females >males (4:1).
- Present with gait disturbance due to lower limb dystonia.
- Diurnal variation – worse in the evening.
- Brisk tendon reflexes, parkinsonism, postural tremor.
- Variations in presentation are common:
  - Focal arm dystonia in young adult mimicking writer's cramp.
  - Gait disturbance, upper motor signs mimicking cerebral palsy/hereditary spastic paraplegia.
  - Hypotonia, proximal weakness, floppy infant.
  - Poor feeding in infancy.
  - Oculogyric crises.
  - Paroxysmal dyskinesia
  - Late onset parkinsonism with resting tremor.
- Differential diagnosis:
  - Other enzyme defects in the THB–dopamine pathway: autosomal recessive dystonia parkinsonism with partial response to levodopa.
  - Young-onset Parkinson's disease.
  - Dopamine transporter (DaT) single photon emission tomography (SPECT) scan may help to differentiate.
- Diagnosis:
  - Genetic tests are not widely available.
  - Indirect tests: phenylalanine loading test, cerebrospinal fluid (CSF) pterin analysis
  - Dramatic and sustained response to small doses of levodopa.
- All patients with young-onset dystonia should have a trial of levodopa.

Tip

▶ *Always consider DRD in the differential diagnosis of a young presentation of dystonia and undertake a 3-month trial of levodopa.*

Myoclonus dystonia (DYT11)

- Autosomal dominant inheritance (mutations in epsilon sarcoglycan gene).
- Childhood-onset.
- Nonprogressive – severity is determined by the genetic mutation.
- Dystonia affecting cervical and upper limbs.
- Myoclonic jerks of upper body, neck, and upper limbs.
- Commonest identified cause of 'jerky' children.
- Alcohol relieves symptoms.
- Also known as essential myoclonus, 'myoclonic dystonia with lightning jerks'.

X-linked dystonia–parkinsonism (Lubag) (DYT3)

- Men from Panay Island in the Philippines are affected.
- Parkinsonism, dystonia.
- Bulbar dysfunction prominent.

Rapid onset dystonia–parkinsonism (DYT12)

- Autosomal dominant (mutation in the *ATP1A3* gene) – rare.
- Onset in teens to early adult life.
- Onset over hours to weeks then stabilizes (may fluctuate).
- Dystonia, parkinsonism.
- Cranial, bulbar, and upper limbs most affected.

Dystonia-deafness (Mohr–Tranebjaerg) syndrome

- X-linked.
- Onset first to sixth decades with peak in second to third decades.
- Severe congenital or infantile onset, sensorineural deafness precedes dystonia.
- Associated visual failure (optic neuropathy or cortical), dementia.
- Rarely expresses in female carriers without profound deafness.

Paroxysmal dyskinesias

A group of rare conditions broadly classified on clinical grounds into three main types based on duration of attacks and triggers. Molecular and genetic advances are generally confirming these phenotypes and enlarging the spectrum of associated features. The differential diagnosis includes secondary paroxysmal movement disorders[4].

Paroxysmal kinesigenic dystonia (choreoathetosis) (DYT10)

- Autosomal dominant inheritance, mutations in *PRRT2* gene[5].
- Childhood onset.
- Brief (seconds, minutes) attacks of dystonia or chorea.
- Precipitated by sudden movement.
- Several attacks per day.
- Consciousness is preserved.
- Frequency of attacks decreases with age.
- May have infantile convulsions and choreoathetosis ('ICCA').
- Treatment: anticonvulsants (carbamazepine).

Paroxysmal nonkinesigenic dyskinesia (dystonic choreoathetosis) (DYT8)

- Autosomal dominant inheritance, mutations in myofibrillogenesis regulator 1 gene.
- Onset: infancy to early childhood.
- Attacks last minutes to hours.
- Precipitated by stress, fatigue, chocolate, alcohol.
- Unilateral, bilateral dystonia or choreoathetosis.
- Frequency of attacks variable: 4/day to 2/year.
- Treatment: benzodiazepines (clonazepam).

Paroxysmal exercise-induced dystonia (DYT18)

- Autosomal dominant – sporadic, mutations in *GLUT1* gene in many[6].
- Onset: childhood or young adult.
- Precipitated by prolonged exercise (minutes to hours; typically walking).
- Duration of attacks is 5–30 minutes.
- Lower limbs mainly involved, may spread.
- Associated with epilepsy in some families (especially infantile absence seizures).
- Paroxysmal choreoathetosis with episodic ataxia and spasticity (DYT9) also due to *GLUT1* gene mutations, i.e. DYT9 and DYT18 are allelic.

Differential diagnosis of paroxysmal dyskinesias

- Epilepsy (especially frontal lobe).
- Focal structural brain lesions.
- Tonic spasms of multiple sclerosis.
- Hypocalcemic tetany (hypoparathyroidism).
- Hypoglycemia.
- Cerebral ischemia.
- Exercise-induced dystonia of lower limbs: DRD, young-onset PD.
- Episodic ataxia.
- Hartnup disease.
- Alternating hemiplegia of childhood (infants).
- Psychogenic – probably the commonest cause of sporadic paroxysmal movement disorders.

Selected secondary dystonias

Wilson's disease (WD)

- Autosomal recessive inheritance.
- Mutations of *ATP7B* gene on chromosome 13q; numerous mutations (genetic testing is available only on a research basis).
- Excessive copper accumulation.
- Onset: first two decades.

Clinical features

- First decade (~40%):
  - Hepatic – jaundice, cirrhosis, acute (fulminant) liver failure.
  - Hemolytic anemia.
- Second decade (~40%):
  - Primarily neurologic symptoms (silent cirrhosis).
  - Movement disorders: dystonia, parkinsonism, chorea, myoclonus.
  - Rubral (midbrain) tremor: 'wing beating', rest, postural, intention tremor.
  - Bulbar symptoms early and prominent.
  - Psychiatric (psychosis, depression).
  - Cognitive decline.
  - Osseomuscular symptoms: arthritis, proximal weakness.
  - Renal tubular acidosis.

Diagnosis

Diagnosis involves a combination of neurologic features and tests:

- Kayser–Fleischer rings (**170**).
- Low serum ceruloplasmin.
- High 24-hour urinary copper.
- Brain MRI (see **168**):
  - T2 hyperintense lesions of basal ganglia, midbrain, cerebellum.
  - T2 white matter signal hyperintensities (pseudosclerotic form).

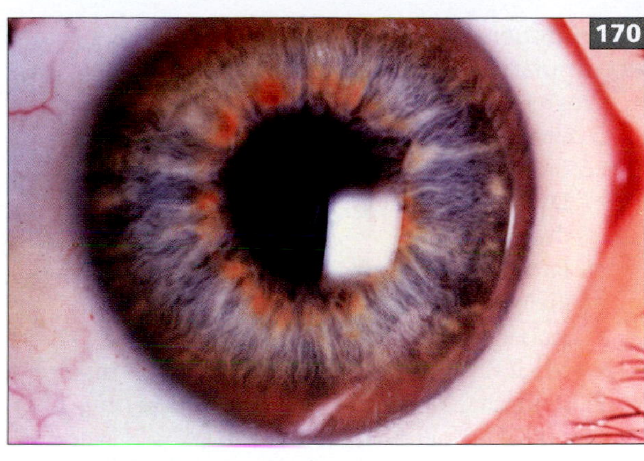

170 Kayser–Fleischer ring: peripheral copper deposition in Descemet's membrane, visible as a brown discoloration over the cornea.

- Unexplained liver disease on blood tests and ultrasound.
- WD should be considered in all patients <30 years with dystonia.
- All siblings need to be screened.

Treatment

- Untreated WD is fatal.
- Treatment can reverse even severe neurological disability.
- Treatment needs to be continued lifelong.
- Copper chelation: pencillamine, trientene.
- Reduce copper absorption using zinc.
- Liver transplant is curative:
  - Indications: intolerance/sensitivity to chelating therapy.
  - Fulminant liver failure.
- Symptomatic treatment for dystonia, neuropsychiatric behavioral problems.

Tip

► *WD is treatable and should always be considered in a young person presenting with a movement disorder.*

Neurodegeneration with brain iron accumulation (NBIA)

- Progressive iron accumulation in basal ganglia and cerebellum, with variable clinical manifestations according to age of onset[7]:
  - Dystonia (bulbar especially with dysarthria, dysphagia).
  - Parkinsonism, rigidity, spasticity.
  - Pigmentary retinopathy, optic atrophy.
  - Ataxia, cognitive decline.
  - MRI: various patterns of brain iron deposition.
- Pantothenate kinase-associated neurodegeneration (PKAN): autosomal recessive, *PANK2* gene mutation; spasticity, dystonia (especially bulbar), ocular motor abnormalities, cognitive decline; MRI – iron deposition in globus pallidus with cavitation ('eye of the tiger' sign) (see **167**).
- Hypoprebetalipoproteinemia, acanthocytes, retinitis pigmentosa, pallidal degeneration (HARP): autosomal recessive, *PANK2* gene mutation; MRI 'eye of the tiger' sign.
- Neuroaxonal dystrophy (NAD):
  - Autosomal recessive, *PLA2G6* (gene mutation).
  - MRI: iron deposition in globus pallidus, substantia nigra, cerebellum, cerebral atrophy, white matter changes.
- Neuroferritinopathy:
  - Autosomal dominant.
  - *FTL* gene mutation.
  - Age of onset 20–50.
  - Chorea (50%), cranial dystonia, orofacial dyskinesia.
  - Parkinsonism, rigidity.
  - Gait disturbance (leg dystonia).
  - Frontostriatal cognitive disturbance (late).
  - MRI: basal ganglia, dentate iron deposition and cavitation in later stage.
- Aceruloplasminemia:
  - Autosomal recessive mutation in ceruloplasmin gene (*CP*) encoding the protein ceruloplasmin.
  - Ceruloplasmin absent, elevated ferritin.
  - Age of onset variable over a wide range.
  - Diabetes, retinopathy.
  - Cognitive impairment, cranial dyskinesia, dysarthria.
  - Ataxia, chorea, parkinsonism.
  - Absent serum ceruloplasmin.
  - MRI: widespread iron deposition in basal ganglia, thalamus, red nucleus, and dentate nuclei.

Treatment

General approach:

- All young-onset primary and primary limb dystonia (<25 years) should receive a trial of levodopa–carbidopa.
- Botulinum toxin is the treatment of choice for cranial, cervical, and laryngeal dystonia.
- Secondary dystonia should be managed with specific treatment for the underlying cause and medical management as for young-onset dystonia.

Symptomatic treatment can be medical or surgical:

- Anticholinergics (trihexiphenidyl):
  - Increasing doses (1 mg/week) as tolerated, up to 50 mg/day.
  - Adverse effects: dry mouth, blurred vision, urinary retention, confusion, amnesia, constipation, weight loss, chorea. Adverse effects are common in adults, these drugs are better tolerated in children.
- Benzodiazepines (clonazepam, diazepam): caution – risk of tolerance, addiction.
- Dopamine depletion (tetrabenazine): 12.5 mg /day – increase to 25–50mg tid: adverse effects are common – parkinsonism, depression.
- Dopamine receptor antagonists (haloperidol, risperidone): adverse effects are common: parkinsonism, akathisia.
- Baclofen: (gradual increase in dose up to 100 mg/day): adverse effects include confusion, sedation, nausea.

Tip

▶ *Drugs should be not be discontinued suddenly.*

- Botulinum toxin:
  - Injected in small doses into dystonic muscle(s).
  - Effect begins within 7–10 days.
  - Most effective in cranial and cervical dystonia (in 80–90%).
  - Duration of effect lasts for about 3 months when terminal sprouting restores muscle end-plate neurotransmission.
  - Up to 5% of initial responders subsequently do not respond, due to changes in the pattern of dystonia or development of antibodies to botulinum toxin.
  - Antibody formation is associated with frequent ('booster') injections and high doses.
  - Electromyographic (EMG) guidance is helpful in laryngeal, limb, and complicated cervical dystonia.

Surgical treatments include:
- Deep brain stimulation: globus pallidus internus (GPi).
- Particularly helpful in primary and drug-induced dystonia.
- Increasing evidence for efficacy in refractory focal dystonia.
- Studies are underway for the effect in secondary dystonia.

Physiotherapy and occupational therapy is also used, and specific treatments for any underlying cause (WD, DRD [DYT5]).

Status dystonicus
- Acute and severe exacerbation of pre-existing dystonia.
- Bulbar and respiratory symptoms are common.
- Potentially life-threatening neurologic emergency.
- Precipitants: infection, drug change.
- Complications: rhabdomyolysis, renal and respiratory failure.
- Treatment is primarily supportive in intensive care unit settings, with benzodiazepines, anticholinergics, and GPi deep brain stimulation.

CHOREA

Definition

Chorea (Greek: dance) refers to irregular, random, unpredictable involuntary movements flowing from one body part to another. Clinical expression ranges from restlessness or fidgeting to ballistic movements involving proximal muscles (ballism – 'to throw'). Chorea interrupts voluntary movements and postures, resulting in variation in grip strength ('milkmaid's' grip), a dancing gait, and the inability to maintain eye closure or tongue protrusion ('jack in the box' tongue). Motor 'impersistence' may be evident as the failure to maintain postures such as outstretched arms. Chorea is usually generalized, but may be focal or unilateral (hemichorea, hemiballism).

Tip

▸ *Chorea may be mistaken for fidgeting or restlessness.*

Pathophysiology

Caused by lesions or degeneration of neurons in the circuits linking the putamen, external segment of the globus pallidus, subthalamic nucleus, and GPi. Unilateral structural lesions produce hemichorea or hemiballism.

Etiology

Inherited

- Benign hereditary chorea (BHC).
- Huntington's disease (HD).
- Huntington's disease-like syndromes (HDL); rare:
  - HDL1 prion disease.
  - HDL2 junctophillin-3 gene mutations.
  - HDL3 chromosome 4p15.3 mutations.
  - HDL4 SCA 17.
  - SCA 1,2,3.
- Freidriech's ataxia (FA).
- DRPLA.
- Oculomotor apraxia with ataxia I and II (OAA)
- NAc.
- AT.
- Neurometabolic diseases:
  - LNS.
  - O-AA.
  - Mitochondrial diseases.
- Metal disorders:
  - WD.
  - NBIA (NF).

Acquired

- Drugs:
  - Dopamine receptor blockers (antipsychotics, antiemetics).
  - Lithium.
  - Levodopa.
  - Anticholinergics.
  - Central nervous system (CNS) stimulants (amphetamines, cocaine).
  - Phenytoin.
  - Calcium channel blockers.
- Hormonal chorea:
  - Hormone replacement therapy.
  - Pregnancy (chorea gravidarum).
  - Oral contraceptives: rare; rule out recrudescence Sydenham's chorea, antiphospholipid syndrome (APS).

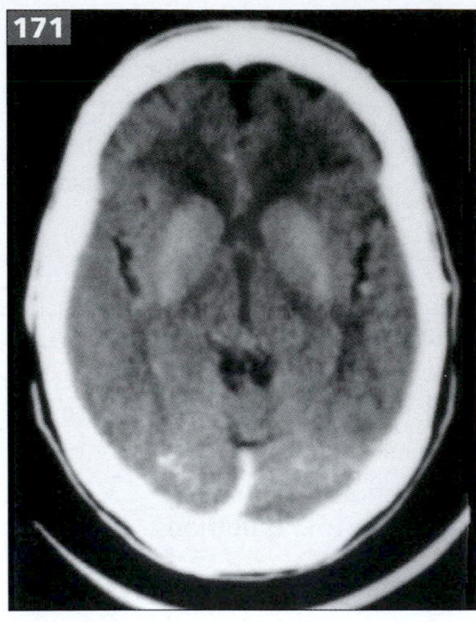

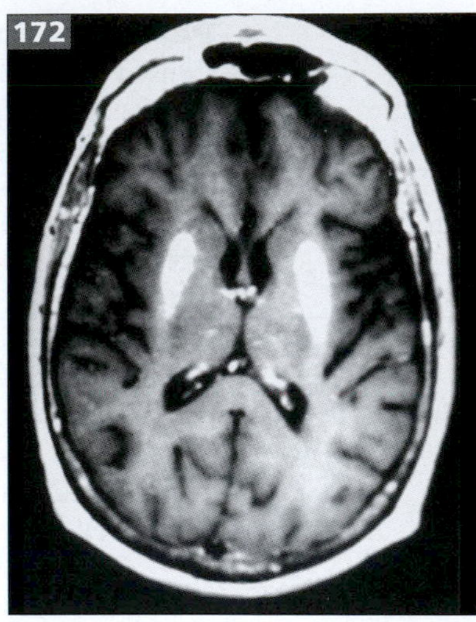

171, 172 Plain CT of the brain (171) and unenhanced T1 MRI (172) in a patient with hyperglycemia and hemorrhagic striatal infarction, presenting as severe generalized chorea. *Courtesy of Professor Kapil Sethi, University of Georgia Medical School, Augusta.*

- Immune-mediated:
  - Sydenham's chorea (SC).
  - Systemic lupus erythematosus (SLE).
  - APS.
  - Behçet's disease.
  - Celiac disease.
- Metabolic:
  - Hyperglycemic chorea (**171, 172**).
  - Osmotic demyelination (extrapontine myelinolysis).
  - Hypocalcemia, hypoparathyroidism.
  - Thyrotoxicosis.
  - Hepatocerebral degeneration (HCD)
- Infective:
  - Human immunodeficiency virus (HIV).
  - Variant Creutzfeldt–Jacob disease (vCJD).
  - Tuberculosis.
  - SSPE.
- Toxins:
  - Cerebral anoxia.
  - Carbon monoxide, carbon disulfide.
- Perinatal injury:
  - Cerebral palsy.
  - Kernicterus (neonatal hyperbilirubinemia).
- Structural lesions involving basal ganglia, subthalamic nucleus:
  - Vascular:
    - Stroke.
    - Vasculitis.
    - Polycythemia rubra vera.
    - Essential thrombocythemia.
    - Post-cardiac bypass (post-pump syndrome).
  - Tumor.
  - Demyelination.
  - Abscess.

Clinical assessment

History

- Age of onset:
  - Children and adolescents: BHC, kernicterus, LNS, AT, AA, mitochondrial diseases, SC, WD.
  - Adult: HD, HDL syndromes, NAc, SLE, APS, Behçet's disease, celiac disease, thyrotoxicosis.
  - Any age: drug-induced, structural lesions.
- Family history.
- Past history:
  - Recurrent miscarriage, migraine, thrombosis (APS).
  - Drug exposure: dopamine antagonists (including antiemetics, drugs for vertigo), anticonvulsants, stimulants.

Physical examination

- Examination with arms relaxed, arms outstretched; during eye closure; tongue protrusion; and sustained grip.
- Mental activity, voluntary movement, and walking exacerbate chorea.
- Examination while performing arithmetic or reciting months of the year backwards.
- Chorea:
  - Unpredictable, fleeting, flowing, irregular, purposeless movements.
  - Movements can be brisk, slow, or jerky.
  - Proximal and distal limbs involved.
  - Present at rest (patient appears fidgety, restless).
  - Chorea is present during voluntary movement:
    - Incorporated into 'quasipurposeful' movements.
    - Interrupts postures and movement – impersistence.
  - Dysarthria.
  - Gait unsteady, lurching, halting, with superimposed chorea.

- Distribution:
  - Generalized (HD, SC, drug-induced).
  - Orobuccolingual dyskinesia: NAc, NF, tardive dyskinesia.
  - Eyebrow raising: HD.
  - Hemichorea (structural lesion of subthalamic nucleus and connections).
- Other neurologic features:
  - Dementia: HD, CD, SCA 17, HCD.
  - Depression/behavioral, affective or psychotic disorder: HD, WD, SC, NAc.
  - Dystonia, tics, stereotypies: NAc, NF, HD, WD.
  - Abnormal eye movements: HD, NAc, AT, SCA.
  - Kayser–Fleischer rings/sunflower cataracts: WD.
  - Athetosis: kernicterus, 'cerebral palsy'.
  - Ataxia: SCA1, 2, 3, 17; vCJD, AT, NAc, FA.
  - Depressed tendon reflexes, neuropathy: FA, NAc.
- Systemic abnormalities:
  - Rash, arthropathy: SLE.
  - Cardiac signs: SC.

Differential diagnosis

- Other dyskinesias.
- See introduction.
- Orofacial dyskinesias (tardive, idiopathic): orobuccolingual predominance.

Investigations

Depends on the age of onset and distribution[8,9].

- Brain imaging: MRI (**171, 172**).
- Blood tests:
  - Blood sugar, electrolytes, hemoglobin.
  - Thyroid function tests.
  - Autoantibodies for SLE, APS, celiac disease.,
  - Antistreptolysin O and anti-DNAase B titers (SC).
  - Serum creatine kinase, acanthocytes (NAc).
- Electrocardiogram (ECG), 2D echocardiogram for cardiac involvement (SC).
- Serum ceruloplasmin, 24-hour urinary copper, examine for Kayser–Fleischer rings: WD.
- Genetic testing: HD, HDL syndromes, DRPLA, and other hereditary causes.

Treatment

Identify and treat the specific cause and symptoms.

- In severe chorea dopamine depletion (tetrabenazine) or dopamine receptor antagonists control movements and relieve exhaustion.
- In mild chorea dopamine depletion may actually cause a deterioration in motor function by inducing parkinsonism, especially in HD.
- Adverse effects of dopamine blockers: akathisia, depression, parkinsonism.
- Immune chorea: prednisolone, immune therapies for SLE, APS, SC.

Prognosis

Depends on the cause: hemichorea and hemiballismus due to stroke usually resolve within a few weeks or months.

Special conditions

Huntington's disease

HD is the commonest cause of inherited chorea. It is autosomal dominant, with expanded CAG triplet repeats in the huntingtin (*HTT*) gene (chromosome 4). A larger number of repeats correlates with earlier onset and severe disease. HD usual onset is in the fourth decade.

Clinical features

- Chorea: generalized with prominent upper facial chorea and bulbar features.
- Behavioral and cognitive problems:
  - Frontostriatal cognitive–behavioral syndrome ('subcortical dementia'): dysexecutive syndrome (impaired attention, concentration, problem solving, planning, organization, reasoning, decision making); lack of insight, disinhibition, impulse control disorder.
  - Apathy may precede chorea.
- Mood disorder – depression.
- Gait disturbance.
- Eye movement abnormalities: slow hypometric saccades, gaze impersistence, difficulty initiating saccades.
- Dystonia–parkinsonism in late stages.
- Note unusual presentations:
  - Young-onset (Westphal variant) parkinsonism, myoclonus, seizures (rare), tics.
  - Frontal – cognitive.
  - Psychiatric.
  - Behavioral.

Diagnosis

Genetic testing, MRI (caudate atrophy).

Treatment

Symptomatic.

Tip

▶ *Genetic counseling of the patient and family members is an important part of the management of HD and should be considered before undertaking testing.*

Sydenham's (rheumatic) chorea (St Vitus dance) (SC)

SC is endemic in Africa, Asia, and South America.

- Females = males pre-pubertal, females >males post-pubertal.
- Age onset: 10–16 years.
- Autoimmune: presents weeks to months after acute Group A streptococcal throat infection or following rheumatic fever.

Clinical features

- Chorea: generalized but may be hemichorea. Severity is variable from mild fidgeting to severe.
- Marked motor impersistence may give impression of paralysis ('chorea mollis').
- Tics, dystonia.
- Anxiety, obsessive compulsive behaviors, irritability.

Diagnosis

- Antistreptococcal antibodies.
- History of throat infection.
- Arthritis.
- Carditis (Jones criteria for rheumatic fever).

Treatment

- Penicillin prophylaxis until age 21 to prevent recurrent rheumatic fever.
- Symptomatic treatment of chorea (valproate or carbamazepine can be effective).
- Immunotherapy: steroids, immunoglobulin, plasma exchange in refractory cases.

Prognosis

- Remission occurs in the majority in 6 months.
- Relapse – persisting chorea occurs in 20–50%.

Neuroacanthocytosis

- Chorea, tics, stereotypies.
- Eating (lingual) dystonia.
- Neuropathy.
- Frontostriatal cognitive and behavioral syndromes.
- Thick fresh blood smear for acanthocytes.
- Mild elevation creatine kinase.

TREMOR

Definition

A rhythmic, sinusoidal (oscillatory), periodic (repetitive) movement. Apart from essential and dystonic tremor, virtually all causes of tremor are symptomatic of an underlying neurologic or systemic disorder (including drug side-effects).

Classification is by:

- Distribution – according to the body part affected.
- Pattern of occurrence: rest, postural, action or kinetic, intention, task specific.
- Tremor frequency (but there is considerable overlap).
- Cause.

Pathophysiology

Oscillation within olivo–cerebello–rubro–olivary and cerebello–thalamo–cortical pathways[10].

Functional imaging in essential tremor reveals increased olivary glucose metabolism, increased blood flow in cerebellum and red nucleus (bilaterally), and in contralateral globus pallidus, thalamus, and sensorimotor cortex. Lesions of ipsilateral cerebellum and contralateral ventral intermedius nucleus of the thalamus reduce or abolish tremor.

In essential tremor central oscillators interact with peripheral reflex loops to amplify tremor. In essential tremor it is thought the cerebellum introduces an error in the timing of muscle bursts during voluntary movement and repeated corrective movements lead to tremor. Parkinsonian resting tremor appears to result from abnormal synchronicity of basal ganglia and thalamic neuronal activity.

Variants

Essential tremor (ET)

Definition

- Postural, action or kinetic tremor (absent at rest) of upper limbs.
- Not associated with other neurologic signs.

Epidemiology:

- Commonest adult-onset movement disorder.
- Prevalence increases with age; point prevalence 300/100,000 (estimates vary widely).
- Age of onset: bimodal, young adults and 40–60 years. M=F.

Pathology

- No characteristic pathologic or biochemical findings.

Etiology

- Hereditary: autosomal dominant inheritance (50% of patients).
- Responsible gene(s) are unknown.
- Sporadic: probably the same entity as hereditary ET.

Clinical features

- Postural and kinetic tremor of fingers, hands, and forearms when held outstretched, during specific fine motor tasks (usually visually guided), and in certain arm positions ('position-specific postural tremor').
- Frequency 4–9 Hz (**173**).
- Bilateral, may be asymmetric.
- Amplitude may fluctuate (increased by emotional stress).
- Long history of tremor (>5 years) increasing in severity with age.
- Improved by alcohol in 50% of cases[11].
- Other sites affected: head (30–40%), voice (15–20%), legs (15%), jaw, face (< 5%), trunk rare.
- No other neurologic signs.

Cerebellar tremor

- Coarse 3–5 Hz tremor of upper limbs:
  - Postural tremor.
  - Action and kinetic (during movement) tremor.
  - Characteristic 'intention' tremor.
  - Amplitude increases on approaching target during goal-directed movement (under visual guidance).
- Head and trunk tremor: titubation – 'to and fro' nodding or 'yes-yes' tremor.
- May be incapacitating, poorly responsive to treatment.

Midbrain (rubral or Holmes) tremor

- Coarse 2–2.5 Hz upper limb tremor.
- Rest, postural, action, and intention tremor.
- Marked exacerbation during movement and in certain postures ('wing-beating' tremor).
- Caused by midbrain lesions affecting superior cerebellar peduncle involving cerebellothalamic projections, central tegmental tract (cerebellar–rubro–olivary pathway), and nigrostriatal tracts.
- Typically seen in multiple sclerosis, head trauma, WD.
- Other signs of midbrain damage may be present.

Parkinsonian tremor

- Rest tremor in upper limb, fingers, and hand:
  - 'Pill rolling' 5 Hz.
  - Usually asymmetric or even unilateral.
  - Abolished by movement but reappears in new posture (re-emergent tremor).
  - Leg, tongue, jaw, and lip tremor may occur.
  - Exacerbated by emotional stress.
  - Central oscillator – peripheral reflex mechanisms do not influence tremor.
  - Variable response to antiparkinsonian therapies.
- Postural, action upper limb tremor:
  - Frequency 6–8 Hz.
  - Related to cog-wheel rigidity (similar frequency).

Tip

▶ *Rest tremor is typical of PD, but may be seen in midbrain disease and rarely in other neurodegenerations. Rest tremor can also occur in dystonic tremor syndromes. Postural tremor may be an early sign of PD.*

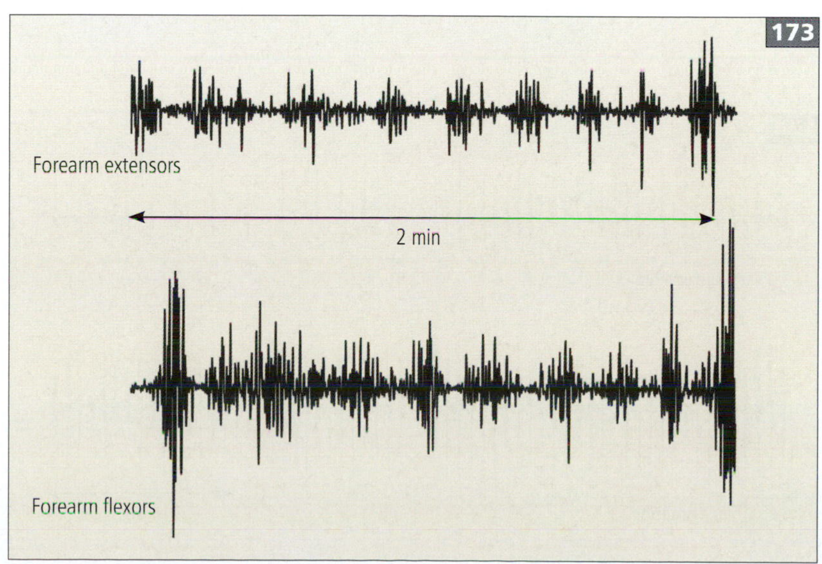

173 Surface EMGs from forearm muscles, showing typical alternating pattern of antagonist muscle activation in a 4.5 Hz postural tremor due to essential tremor.

Enhanced physiologic tremor (EPT)

Clinical features and diagnosis

- Rapid 8–12 Hz small amplitude, fine postural and kinetic tremor.
- Typically affects upper limbs and hands.
- Can be difficult to distinguish EPT from early stages of hereditary ET in a young person.

Etiology

- Exaggerated physiologic response: anxiety, fright, fatigue, strenuous exertion.
- Drugs:
  - Adrenergic drugs, amphetamines.
  - Amiodarone.
  - Antipsychotic drugs.
  - Caffeine.
  - Cimetidine.
  - Corticosteroids.
  - Cyclosporine A.
  - Lithium.
  - Oral hypoglycemics.
  - Serotonin reuptake inhibitors.
  - Sodium valproate.
  - Theophylline.
  - Thyroxine.
  - Tricyclic antidepressants.
  - Drug withdrawal: alcohol, barbiturates, benzodiazepines, opiates.
- Metabolic:
  - Metabolic encephalopathies.
  - Hypoglycemia.
  - Pheochromocytoma.
  - Thyrotoxicosis.
- Toxins:
  - Mercury.
  - 1-methyl-4-phenyl-1,2,3,6-tetrahydropyridine (MPTP).

Management

- Directed to correction of the underlying illness or cessation of relevant drugs.
- If EPT becomes symptomatic or socially embarrassing, propranolol may be helpful.

Primary orthostatic tremor

- High frequency (14–16 Hz) tremor of legs and trunk when standing still.
- Proximal arm tremor in some cases and when supporting body weight.
- Bilaterally synchronous.
- Patients complain of unsteadiness when standing still (not tremor).
- Tremor may easier to feel than to see because of high frequency.
- Confirm by EMG of leg muscles (**174**).
- Variable response to clonazepam, gabapentin, primidone, valproate, occasionally dopaminergic medications.

Dystonic tremor

Asymmetric postural, kinetic, and rarely rest tremor. Many cases of upper limb tremor previously diagnosed as ET have subtle dystonia and differentiation can be difficult. It occurs in association with focal dystonia (e.g. head tremor in torticollis, hand tremor in writers'cramp, voice tremor in laryngeal dystonia) or generalized dystonia (trunk).

Tremor is the principal feature in some cases of torticollis (tremulous torticollis) and upper limb dystonic tremor, with exacerbation in certain postures. Dystonia is subtle or overshadowed by tremor in such cases. Tremor is of variable amplitude and frequency 2–6 Hz.

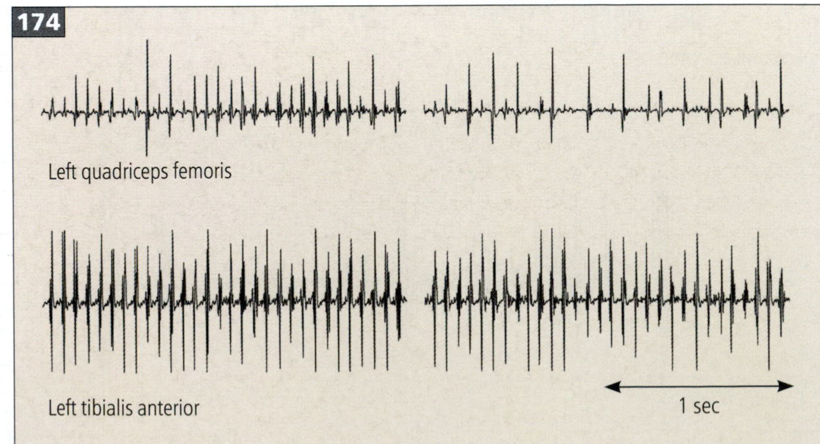

174 Surface EMGs in patient with orthostatic tremor showing characteristic 16 Hz tremor in both quadriceps femoris and tibialis anterior. Note the halving of tremor frequency in quadriceps; this correlates with an increase in the sensation of unsteadiness that is typical of this condition.

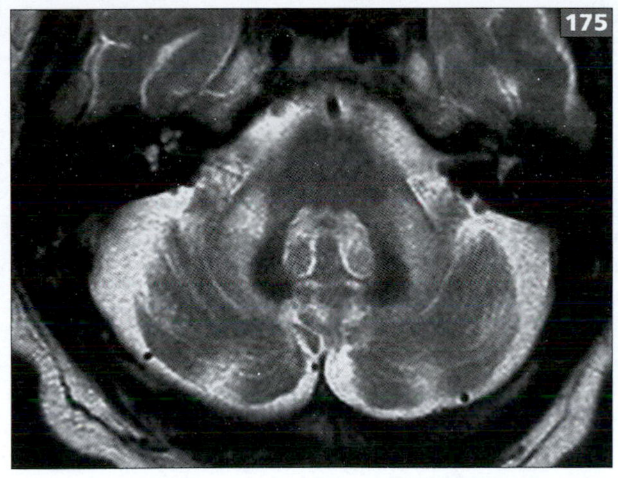

175 **MRI (FLAIR) of posterior fossa in a man with fragile X tremor ataxia syndrome. Note the characteristic high signal areas in the middle cerebellar peduncles.**

Isolated focal tremor

- Head, face, jaw, tongue, voice, trunk, upper limbs.
- Frequency 4–8 Hz.
- May be manifestation of dystonic tremor.
- Often only subtle dystonia.
- NB: focal tremor is not seen in ET pedigrees.

Isolated position-specific or task-specific tremors

- Kinetic tremor during specific tasks (6 Hz).
- Upper limbs: occupational tremors (musicians, sportsmen), primary writing tremor.
- Head and lips: musicians (e.g. wind instruments).
- Characteristics and appearance of ET but task specificity of dystonia.
- May respond to anticholinergics.

Neuropathic tremor

- Postural, kinetic tremor, upper limb more than legs:
  - Coarse flapping (alternating muscle bursts) (3–6 Hz).
  - Typically demyelinating neuropathy (IgM paraproteinemia, chronic relapsing inflammatory demyelinating neuropathy).
  - Signs of neuropathy (muscle wasting weakness, areflexia, sensory loss).
- Postural tremor upper limbs:
  - Small amplitude cocontracting (6–8 Hz).
  - Due to denervation, weakness, fatigue, synchronous motor unit discharge.
  - Amplified physiologic tremor during muscle fatigue.
  - Seen in axonal neuropathies, spinal muscular atrophy.

Fragile X tremor ataxia syndrome

- In carriers of premutation alleles (55–200 CGG repeats) of the fragile X (*FMR1*) gene.
- Males >50 years, rarer and milder in females.
- Postural, action, intention, rest tremor (3–5 Hz).
- Mimics severe ET.
- Parkinsonism, ataxia, frontal cognitive signs.
- MRI of middle cerebellar peduncle shows T2 hyperintensities (**175**).

Symptomatic palatal tremor (myoclonus)

- Regular, continuous, rhythmic (1–3 per second) contraction of soft palate.
- Generated by contractions of levator veli palatini (innervated by the facial nerve); other facial innervated muscles may be involved.
- Patients can develop a progressive cerebellar syndrome.
- Movements persist during sleep.
- Caused by lesion of the dentato–rubro–olivary pathway (Guillain–Mollaret triangle).
- Onset is several months after lesion (vascular, inflammatory, traumatic).
- Associated with pseudohypertrophy of the ipsilateral olivary nucleus (visible on MRI).

Essential palatal tremor (myoclonus)

- Regular, continuous, rhythmic (1–3 per second) contraction of soft palate.
- Generated by contractions of the tensor veli palatini (innervated by the trigeminal nerve).
- Patients present with the complaint of self-audible clicking due to tensor veli palatini contractions causing opening and closing of the Eustachian tube.
- Movements stop during sleep.
- No olivary hypertrophy.
- Many cases are now thought to be psychogenic.

Psychogenic tremor

- Variable tremor frequency.
- Entrainment (tremor adopts the frequency of rhythmic voluntary movement).
- Distractibility (tremor disrupted or attenuated by another motor task).
- Unusual and inconsistent behavioral characteristics.
- Sudden onset and spontaneous remissions.
- Psychiatric factors (somatization, secondary gain, litigation, or compensation pending).

Treatment

Not all patients require treatment. Propranolol and primidone have been shown in controlled trials to improve ET amplitude in two-thirds of cases.

- Propranolol 10–40 mg every morning or bd (up to about 240–320 mg/day).
- Metoprolol 25 mg bd to 50 mg tid.

About one-half of patients experience a reduction in tremor amplitude of up to 50%. The effect is greatest on postural limb tremor. However, not all patients are helped and the tremor is seldom abolished. Adverse effects and relative contraindications for propranolol include heart failure, bradycardia, hypotension, and asthma. The mechanism of action of propranolol is thought to be blockade of peripheral skeletal muscle β2 receptors. Selective β1 blockade is less effective than propranolol.

Primidone 62.5–750 mg daily can be given if propranolol is ineffective or contraindicated. It may be as effective as beta blockers but adverse effects are common. Care is required when introducing primidone because of acute nausea, sedation, and unsteadiness, which may warrant stopping the drug. A low starting dose minimizes adverse effects, particularly if taken in the evening before retiring. There may be no added benefit to increasing the daily dose beyond 250 mg.

Other drugs that may be helpful but also have adverse effects include gabapentin, topiramate, benzodiazepines, and acetazolamide. Patients with alcohol responsive tremors may find judicious use of alcohol helpful before social engagements. Botulinum toxin may reduce dystonic head tremor but is less effective in upper limb tremor.

Stereotactic thalamic surgery targeting the ventral intermediate nucleus of the thalamus is effective in relieving severe tremor refractory to medical therapies in 70–80% of patients. Deep brain stimulation has fewer side-effects than ablative thalamotomy, and produces greater functional improvement. Bilateral thalamic stimulation may have a lower complication rate than bilateral thalamotomy. Dysarthria and aphonia complicate up to 20–25% of bilateral thalamic lesions (or stimulators). Speech improves when one stimulator is switched off.

Prognosis

ET is slowly progressive and tremor becomes disabling in a few patients with age.

Other neurologic impairments do not occur in ET. Prognosis depends on the cause in other cases.

MYOCLONUS

Definition

Brief, shock-like, abrupt jerky movements caused by short bursts of muscle activity (positive myoclonus) or brief cessation in muscle contraction leading to a sudden lapse in limb posture (negative myoclonus or asterixis). Myoclonus in most cases is a symptom of an underlying neurologic disease or an encephalopathy.

Classification is by:

- Distribution.
- Pattern of occurrence:
  - Timing: usually irregular, may appear rhythmic if occurring in runs.
  - Spontaneous myoclonus – at rest.
  - Action myoclonus – during voluntary movement.
  - Reflex myoclonus – stimulus sensitive, e.g. sound, visual, somatosensory (touch, muscle stretch).

Tip

▶ *Repetitive action myoclonus may be mistaken for tremor, and intention myoclonus may be difficult to distinguish from intention tremor in cerebellar disease.*

Physiologic classification based on anatomic site of origin

Cortical myoclonus

- Distal, small amplitude, repetitive.
- Often focal.
- Stimulus sensitive reflex (somatosensory), spontaneous, action[12].
- Short duration bursts of muscle activity (<100 msec).
- 'Giant' cortical somatosensory evoked potentials.
- Cortical electroencephalogram (EEG) spike discharges precede myoclonus.
- Intracortical–interhemispheric spread of myoclonic activity[13].
- Causes: progressive myoclonic epilepsies, progressive myoclonic ataxias, post-hypoxic action myoclonus, epilepsia partialis continua in focal cortical lesions, myoclonus in Alzheimer's disease.

Subcortical myoclonus

- Proximal, large amplitude.
- Action myoclonus.
- Not stimulus sensitive.
- Precise site of origin not known.
- Causes: myoclonus dystonia, CJD.

Brainstem myoclonus

- Proximal – upper body, neck, proximal arms (bilateral), and trunk[13].
- Stimulus sensitive: sound, taps to upper body, face, chin, nose in hyperekplexia; limb taps in reticular reflex myoclonus.
- May have exaggerated auditory startle response.
- Characteristic pattern of muscle recruitment and spread: 'up' brainstem and 'down' spinal cord.
- May be associated with tonic spasms and falls.
- Causes: hyperekplexia (Startle disease, symptomatic forms in brainstem lesions), reticular reflex myoclonus (post-anoxic).

Spinal myoclonus

- Spinal segmental:
  - Repetitive, rhythmic jerking of affected body segment.
  - Persists in sleep.
  - Not stimulus sensitive.
  - Associated with signs of myeloradiculopathy.
  - Causes: spinal lesions.
- Propriospinal:
  - Axial–trunkal, especially abdominal muscles.
  - Trunk flexion (rarely extension).
  - Position specific (when the patient lies down).
  - Mediated by slowly conducting propriospinal fibers.
  - Spinal cord lesion may be found.
  - Many patients have a psychogenic etiology.

Peripheral myoclonus

- Rare.
- Focal lesions of peripheral nerves associated with rhythmic jerking in sensory motor supply of affected nerve.
- Central mechanisms probably involved in most cases.

Etiology

Physiological myoclonus (healthy individuals)

- Jerks when falling asleep (hypnagogic) or waking (hypnopompic).
- Nocturnal myoclonus (periodic movements of sleep).
- Hiccough (singultus).
- Benign infantile myoclonus with feeding/sleep:
  - Small amplitutude generalized myoclonus.
  - Resolves in 6–12 months.

Myoclonus dystonia (DYT11)

- Hereditary (autosomal dominant) myoclonus dystonia.
- 50% have mutations in the epsilon sarcoglycan gene.
- Sporadic.
- See under dystonia (previously called essential myoclonus).

Epileptic myoclonus (seizures accompanied by myoclonus)

- Fragments of epilepsy:
  - Epilepsia partialis continua.
  - Photosensitive myoclonus.
  - Myoclonic absence in petit mal.
- Childhood myoclonic epilepsy:
  - Infantile spasms.
  - Myoclonic astatic epilepsy (Lennox–Gastaut).
  - Juvenile myoclonic epilepsy (of Janz).

Symptomatic myoclonus (in progressive or static encephalopathy)

Progressive myoclonic epilepsy

- Early onset epilepsy, cognitive decline and dementia:
  - Lafora body disease.
  - Neuronal ceroid lipofuscinosis.
  - Sialidosis (cherry-red spot syndrome) (**176**).
  - GM2 gangliosidosis.
- Familial cortical myoclonic epilepsy.

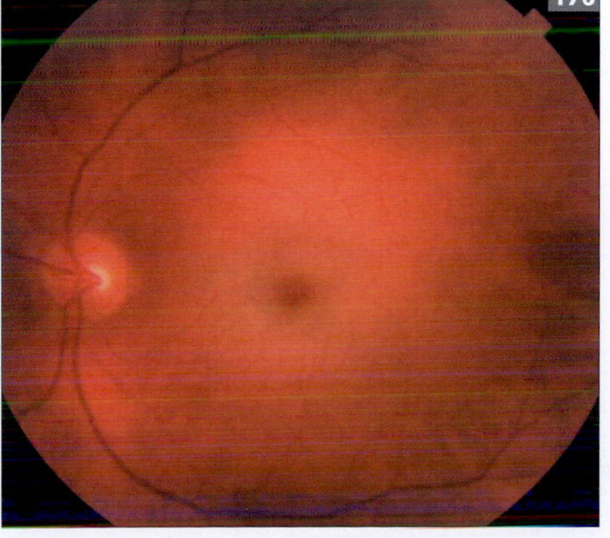

176 A macula cherry-red spot in a young man with myoclonus and ataxia due to sialidosis (neuraminidase deficiency). *Courtesy of Professor Carolyn Sue, Royal North Shore Hospital, Sydney.*

Progressive myoclonic ataxia (Ramsay Hunt syndrome)

Later onset myoclonus, ataxia with less cognitive decline.

- Common causes:
  - Post-anoxic myoclonus.
  - Myoclonic epilepsy with ragged red fibers (MERRF).
  - Baltic myoclonus (Unverricht–Lundborg disease).
  - Spinocerebellar degenerations.
- Uncommon causes:
  - Lafora body disease.
  - NCL.
  - Sialidosis (cherry-red spot syndrome).
  - DRPLA.
  - Celiac disease.
  - GM2 gangliosidosis.
  - Multiple system atrophy.
  - Action myoclonus renal failure syndrome.

Generalized multifocal myoclonus with encephalopathy

- Metabolic:
  - Liver failure, renal failure, dialysis syndrome, respiratory failure.
  - Hyperthyroidism.
  - Hyponatremia, hypoglycemia, nonketotic hyperglycemia.
  - Acute cerebral anoxia.
- Drugs and toxins:
  - Lithium.
  - Tricyclics, monoamine oxidase (MAO) inhibitors, serotonin reuptake inhibitors.
  - Narcotics.
  - Anticonvulsants.
  - Antiarrhythmics, calcium channel blockers.
  - Antibiotics (quinolones, penicillin).
  - Anesthetics.
  - Contrast media.
  - Heavy metals (bismuth).
  - Drug withdrawal.
- Infectious or post-infectious:
  - SSPE.
  - Arbovirus encephalitis.
  - Herpes simplex encephalitis.
  - Human T-lymphotropic virus I.
  - Whipple's disease.
  - Post-infectious encephalopathy.
- Focal cerebral injury:
  - Vascular, traumatic, cortical injury (epilepsia partialis continua).
  - Cortical neoplasm.
  - Thalamic lesion (asterixis).
- Paraneoplastic and autoimmune encephalopathies:
  - Limbic encephalitis:
    - Anti-NMDA receptor antibody encephalitis.
    - Voltage gated potassium channel antibody encephalitis.
    - Antiglycine receptor-associated encephalitis.
    - Antibodies to glutamic acid decarboxylase (GAD).
  - Hashimoto's encephalopathy (antithyroid autoantibodies – antithyroglobulin or antithyroperoxidase).
  - Paraneoplastic cerebellar degeneration.
  - Opsoclonus–myoclonus syndrome.

Neurodegenerations

- Dementia with myoclonus:
  - CJD.
  - Alzheimer's disease.
  - Dementia with Lewy bodies.
  - Frontotemporal dementia.
  - Motor syndromes with myoclonus.
  - Multiple system atrophy.
  - Corticobasal degeneration.
  - HD.
  - AT.
  - DRPLA.
  - Primary and secondary dystonia.

Startle syndromes

- Anxiety.
- Hereditary: hyperekplexia.
- Sporadic: brainstem injury/lesion.
- Tourette's syndrome (TS).
- Culture specific: Latah, Jumping Frenchmen of Maine, Myriachit.

Other

- Minipolymyoclonus (see below).
- Palatal myoclonus (see palatal tremor).
- Psychogenic myoclonus (see below).

Clinical assessment

The differential diagnosis of myoclonus is extensive. Careful history and examination to identify associated symptoms and signs is essential for diagnosis.

History

- Age of onset.
- Evolution of symptoms: onset and progression.
- Distribution: body parts affected.
- Precipitating factor: injury, drug or toxin exposure, occupation.
- Family history.
- Birth, perinatal history, and developmental delay.
- Other neurologic symptoms, e.g. seizures, ataxia, dystonia, dementia.
- Systemic features: organ failure.

Examination

- Observe the patient at rest with arms relaxed.
- Arm outstretched, finger–nose, during various tasks (action myoclonus).
- Negative myoclonus (asterixis) seen as lapses in sustained postures.
- While walking (bouncing gait, gait ataxia).
- Distribution (focal, generalized), rhythmicity, and amplitude of jerks.
- Stimulus sensitivity: light touch or gently flicking fingers (reflex myoclonus); loud noise or tap nose (brainstem myoclonus, hyperekplexia).
- Examine for other neurologic signs.
- Systemic examination.

Investigations

Investigations including electrophysiological tests help to define the site of origin of myoclonus, formulate a differential diagnosis, and guide further investigation.

Basic tests

- Electrolytes, glucose, renal, hepatic function, drug, toxin screen.
- MRI brain, spine.

Electrophysiologic tests

- EEG:
  - Polyspike and wave discharges suggest cortical origin of myoclonus.
  - Slowing of background rhythms suggest an underlying encephalopathy.
  - Back-averaging EEG prior to jerks: cortical myoclonus is characterized by cortical discharges preceding the myoclonus (177).
- Cortical somatosensory evoked potentials (SSEP): giant SSEPs in cortical myoclonus (177).
- Measurement of C reflexes in upper limb muscles following median nerve stimulation (177).

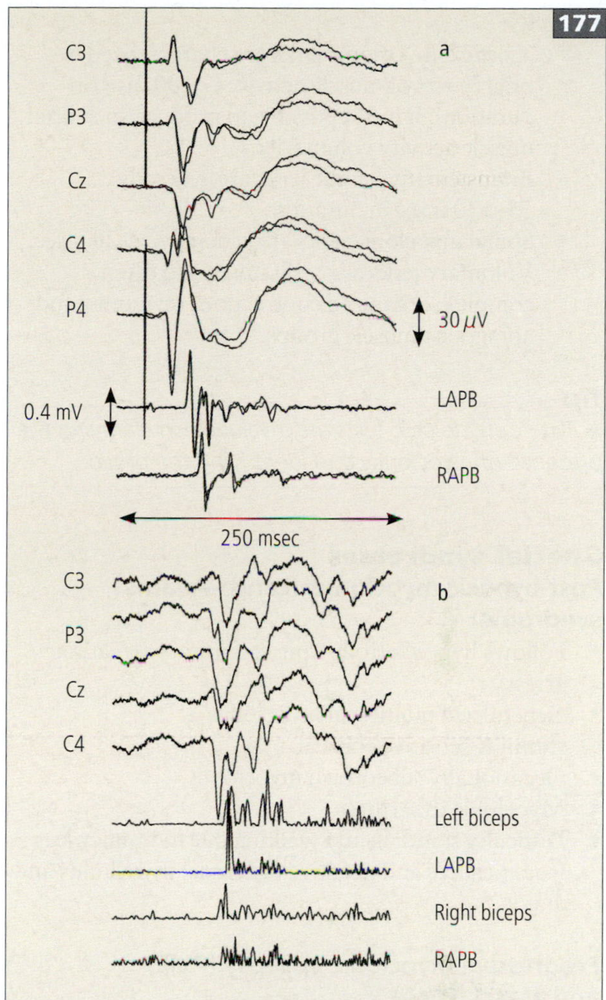

177 Somatosensory evoked potentials (SSEP) and back-averaged EEG in cortical reflex and action myoclonus due to sialidosis or the 'cherry-red spot' syndrome. (a) A giant SSEP over the right sensorimotor cortex (P4) after stimulation of the left median nerve at the wrist. A large reflex myoclonic response ('C' reflex) in the left abductor pollicis brevis (APB) muscle appears about 50 msec after the median nerve stimulus and 20 msec after the positive (downward) deflection of the enlarged SSEP. A similar response is seen in the right APB after interhemispheric spread of the SSEP activates the left sensorimotor cortex. Note the reflex myoclonic responses are repetitive; (b) backaveraged EEG recorded prior to action myoclonus in the left APB. A positive spike wave is seen over the right sensorimotor cortex (P4) preceding the left arm myoclonus. Repetitive cortical discharges are also evident along with interhemispheric spread of the discharges to the left cerebral hemisphere, but the averaged right APB responses are blurred by jitter in the timing of right limb myoclonus (the recording was triggered in relation to myoclonus in the left APB).

- EMG:
  - Cortical myoclonic jerks are characterized by brief bursts of muscle activity (<100 msec in duration). It is not possible to produce such brief muscle activity voluntarily.
  - Brainstem myoclonic jerks are generally 75–120 msec in duration.
  - Spinal myoclonic jerks are generally >120 msec.
  - Voluntary jerks are >120 msec and often complex, organized contractions of agonist and antagonist muscle groups.

Tip

▶ *Electrophysiologic tests are invaluable in clarifying the presence of myoclonus and identifying the origin.*

Special syndromes

Post-hypoxic myoclonus (Lance–Adams syndrome)

- Follows hypoxia (following respiratory or cardiac arrest).
- Generalized multifocal myoclonus – stimulus-sensitive cortical.
- Occasionally subcortical myoclonus.
- Myoclonic dysarthria.
- Difficulty standing and walking due to bouncy legs from positive and negative (asterixis) myoclonus and ataxia.

Progressive myoclonic epilepsy (PME) and ataxia (PMA)

These have different clinical profiles caused by rare inherited metabolic encephalopathies. In PME epilepsy predominates, with an earlier onset of cognitive decline and dementia. In PMA the onset may be later, myoclonus and ataxia predominate.

Startle syndromes

The auditory startle response is a normal brainstem reflex characterized by closure of the eyes, flexion of the neck, trunk, arms, and variable lower limb manifestations. The response normally habituates quickly on repetitive stimulation. In pathologic startle syndromes the response is exaggerated and does not habituate normally.

- Hereditary hyperekplexia:
  - Autosomal dominant mutations in glycine receptor gene.
  - Numerous genetic mutations are described.
  - Generalized myoclonic jerk, particularly affecting the upper body.
  - Followed by limb stiffening – patients fall if standing.
  - Does not habituate.
  - Treatment: clonazepam, valproate.
- Cultural startle syndromes: neuropsychiatric disorders characterized by exaggerated startle, echolalia, echopraxia, and automatic obedience. These were originally described in remote communities of Canadian lumberjacks as 'Jumping Frenchmen of Maine'. Persists in Malay women (Latah) and numerous other societies. Similar behaviors may be seen in TS. Pathophysiology appears different from hyperekplexia.

Opsoclonus–myoclonus syndrome

- Childhood (usually <3 years) myoclonic encephalopathy with ataxia: 'dancing eyes–dancing feet syndrome'.
- Paraneoplastic (neuroblastoma) in 50%.
- Post-infectious.
- Dramatic response to corticosteroids.
- Similar clinical picture occurs in adult paraneoplastic cerebellar degeneration.

Minipolymyoclonus

- Small amplitude trembling and twitching of outstretched fingers.
- Originally used in the context of movements produced by large motor units following denervation and reinnervation in spinal muscular atrophy (also called 'contraction pseudotremor of chronic denervation'). Subsequently used in the context of progressive epileptic encephalopathies.

Treatment

Myoclonus may be mild and not require treatment. In the case of metabolic disturbances, myoclonus may resolve with correction of the specific cause, or removal of the offending toxin or drugs. It can be entirely reversible. Polytherapy is often required to control action myoclonus:

- Valproate: adverse effects include sedation, weight gain, hair loss, tremor, polycystic ovarian syndrome in women, and hepatotoxicity. Women of child bearing age should be counseled about increased risk of fetal malformation if taken during pregnancy. Valproate is contraindicated in mitochondrial cytopathies.
- Levetiracetam: adverse effects include sedation (less than valproate), fatigue, dizziness, and behavioral change.
- Clonazepam (benzodiazepine): adverse effects include sedation, depression, fatigue, and habituation.
- Piracetam: adverse effects include sedation, diarrhea, weight gain, depression. It is the drug of choice in post-anoxic action myoclonus.

Treatment depends on the origin of myoclonus.

- Cortical myoclonus:
  - Polytherapy required in severe action myoclonus.
  - Valproate, clonazepam, piracetam/levetiracetam, zonisamide.
  - Sedation, ataxia limit the dose.
  - Gait disturbance (positive and negative myoclonus of the legs) is resistant to treatment.
- Cortical–subcortical myoclonus in primary generalized epilepsies:
  - Valproate.
  - Lamotrigine.
  - Ethosuximide, levetiracetam, clonazepam.
- Subcortical myoclonus:
  - Essential myoclonus/dystonia–myoclonus (DYT11).
  - Anticonvulsants are generally not useful.
  - Alcohol relieves symptoms but is not useful as regular treatment.
  - Clonazepam may help.
  - Pallidal deep brain stimulation is probably effective.
- Brainstem myoclonus: clonazepam, valproate.
- Spinal myoclonus: treatment is difficult – there is partial response to clonazepam but the benefit from adding other anticonvulsants is unpredictable.

Prognosis

The prognosis depends on the cause. Myoclonus due to metabolic causes usually resolves with treatment of the underlying cause.

TICS

Definition

Tics are brisk repetitive movements or vocalizations. Motor tics typically appear in the face, neck, and upper body. Tics are preceded by a premonitory sensation or an urge, often localized to a body part, that is relieved after the tic. A characteristic feature is that tics can be suppressed by an effort of will. This occurs at the expense of a rising inner tension, discomfort, or anxiety related to the premonitory sensation and inner urge. Releasing the tics relieves this mounting inner sensation. Tics increase during boredom, stress, and anxiety and may occur in response to external stimuli. Paradoxically tics also increase when the patient is alone or unobserved. Tics diminish during sleep and activities requiring concentration. Primary tic disorders are the commonest expression[14].

Classification

- Phenomenology:
  - Motor tics:
    - Simple (one discrete movement): eye blinking, eyebrow raising, pouting, facial grimacing, head jerks, shoulder shrugs.
    - Slow sinuous 'dystonic' tics of shoulder, neck.
    - Complex (sequence of movements): head shaking, arm movements, jumping, touching.
  - Vocal (phonic) tics:
    - Simple (rudimentary sounds): grunting, coughing, sniffing.
    - Complex: words/parts of words.
- Age of onset:
  - Childhood onset.
  - Adult onset (rare – suggests symptomatic or a secondary cause).

Tip

▶ *Tics are common in childhood but unusual in adult life when they are more often secondary.*

Etiology

Primary

- Simple transient tics of childhood:
  - Simple tics (motor or vocal).
  - Persist for <1 year.
  - Common (~10% school-age children).
- Chronic tics of childhood:
  - Motor or vocal lasting >1 year.
  - TS.

Secondary

- Degenerative/neurometabolic diseases:
  - HD.
  - WD.
  - NBIA.
  - Rett syndrome.
  - Lesch–Nyhan syndrome.
  - NAc.
- Neurogenetic developmental disorders:
  - Down's syndrome.
  - Klinefelter syndrome.
  - Fragile X.
  - Autism spectrum disorders.
  - Mental retardation syndromes.
- Structural lesions: basal ganglia lesions.
- Infections: SC.
- Toxic: carbon monoxide poisoning.
- Drugs: cocaine, opioids, amphetamines, anticonvulsants, neuroleptics, antidepressants, lithium.

Clinical assessment

General approach

- Classify tics: onset, type, distribution, possible etiology.
- Differentiate tics from other movement disorders, obsessions, and compulsions.

History

- Age of onset.
- Distribution: body parts affected.
- Evolution of symptoms: motor and vocal tics (interview family members also).
- Associated psychiatric symptoms: obsessions, compulsions, attention deficit hyperactivity disorder (ADHD).
- Family history.
- Clues to secondary causes of tics – other neurologic symptoms:
  - Abnormal birth/perinatal history.
  - Developmental delay.
  - Exposure to drugs, e.g. dopamine receptor blockers.
  - Infections.
  - Cognitive decline.
  - Seizures.

Examination

- Observe the patient during the interview and at rest.
- Stress exacerbates tics, e.g. when performing 'serial sevens' or reciting months of the year backwards.
- Other neurologic symptoms/signs:
  - Other movement disorders (HD, WD, SC).
  - Self mutilation, neuropathy (LNS, NAc).
- Systemic examination, e.g. organomegaly, cataracts, Kayser–Fleischer rings.

Special syndromes

Tourette's syndrome (TS)

Gilles de la Tourette described the childhood onset of chronic tics and psychiatric disorder in 1885.

Epidemiology

- Prevalence is ~1% of the population <18 years and 0.3–0.5% in adults.
- Symptoms resolve in many with age.
- Men > women (4:1).

Pathophysiology

- Familial disorder with variable expression but mode of transmission and gene defect are not known.
- Hypothesis of abnormality in corticostriatal–thalamocortical pathways causes tics and psychiatric comorbidities.

Clinical features

- Multiple motor and vocal tics present before 18 years of age.
- Onset – simple motor tics from age 5 to 18 years, initially of the face and neck spreading to shoulder, trunk, and limbs. Vocal tics emerge 1–2 years later.
- Typical waxing and waning over time.
- Exacerbations (several weeks) interspersed with relative remission.
- Tics decrease over time after adolescence.
- Tics may be mild or severe, leading to social isolation and conflict.

Associated features

- Echopraxia, echolalia, palilalia are common.
- Copropraxia, coprolalia (rare, <10%).
- Self-injurious behaviors (poking eye, biting, slapping, punching).
- Psychiatric disturbance are common:
  - Obsessional compulsive behaviors (ordering, checking, symmetry).
  - Rituals.
  - Depression.
  - ADHD.

Investigations

- Where indicated, rule out secondary causes.

Treatment

Education and counseling of the patient and family is essential. It is important to determine if there are educational and social concerns and whether these relate to the tics or associated neuropsychiatric behaviors. Psychologic support of the affected child or adolescent includes reassurance and encouragement to continue normal activities, social relationships, and schooling.

An explanation of the symptoms to teachers and arranging special schooling needs if necessary is often helpful if there are learning difficulties. The presence of tics is not necessarily an indication for pharmacologic treatment. Neuropsychiatric symptoms may require separate consideration and different treatments. Pharmacologic treatment is symptomatic and depends on the severity of symptoms. There is only evidence of efficacy for the use of major tranquillizers in reducing tic severity despite the numerous drug and behavioral treatments available. The cognitive side-effects of dopamine receptor blockade should be explained as these might have a deleterious effect on alertness in the classroom and movement in general. If it is considered necessary to commence treatment this should only be continued for a limited period of time, since fluctuation in the severity of symptoms with remissions is a characteristic feature of TS, and to minimize side-effects and the risks of long-term exposure to these drugs.

Pharmacologic treatment of tics and TS tics includes:

- Clonidine: tics and ADHD.
- Tetrabenazine: tics.
- Dopamine receptor antagonists: tics.
- Selective serotonin reuptake inhibitors (SSRIs), clomipramine: obsessive compulsive disorder and depression.
- Methyphenidate: ADHD, but may worsen tics.
- Anterior cingulotomy; thalamic deep brain stimulation is undergoing evaluation in refractory cases.
- Cognitive behavioral therapy.

STEREOTYPIES

Definition and classification

Stereotypic motor behaviors are coordinated patterns of complex movements that are repeated continually without purpose or function at the expense of other activities. Stereotypies occur in the setting of discomfort, boredom, anxiety and fear, or pleasure. Distraction or shifting the focus of attention typically interrupts stereotypies. As attention drifts, the stereotypies recur. Stereotypies may shift from one body part to another and change character. Stereotypies are particularly common in sensory deprivation, exemplified by the repetitive purposeless activities of animals in captivity.

Primary

- Common type: two-thirds of normal infants and 30% of children exhibit thumb sucking, nail biting, hair twirling, head nodding, body rocking, head banging, bruxism.
- *Note:* rhythmic head movements may be observed in normal children.
- Complex motor: hand flapping, waving, fluttering fingers in front of face, or finger writhing may be seen in 3–4 % normal preschool children[15].

Secondary

- Autistic disorders:
  - Infantile autism.
  - Asperger syndrome.
- Rett syndrome: bilateral hand wringing, hair pulling, bruxism.
- Mental retardation syndromes.
- Metabolic disorders of the CNS: LNS.
- NAc.
- Drug induced: CNS stimulants, neuroleptics.
- Infections: encephalitis.
- Trauma.
- Psychiatric disorders: catatonia, schizophrenia, obsessive compulsive disorder.
- Dementia: frontotemporal dementia (FTD), Alzheimer's disease.

Pathophysiology

Pathophysiology is unknown. Studies in patients with FTD show may be related to frontostriatal dysfunction.

Clinical features

Stereotypies may be simple (hand tapping, hand flapping, waving, opening and closing hands, head nodding, body rocking, pacing) or complex/ritualistic, e.g. spitting into one's hands and rubbing it into one's hair. They can be injurious, for example repetitive head banging, face slapping; self-mutilating, for example eye poking, biting hands, lips, or other body parts. Stereotypies are suppressed by sensory stimulation/distraction. Patients are typically unaware and unconcerned about stereotypies.

Differential diagnosis

- Mannerisms: the idiosyncratic embellishments of an individual superimposed on normal purposeful movements or activities.
- Habits: repetitive purposeless movements such as foot tapping, finger drumming, head scratching, manipulating spectacles or pens in normal adults. There is conscious awareness and control of the repetitive motor routines that typically are seen during meetings or lectures.
- Obsessive–compulsive behaviors: recurrent complex stereotypic behaviors or thoughts, of which there is a conscious awareness; ritualistic compulsive checking, cleaning, touching and arranging objects are accompanied by a sense of intrusion and knowledge of the futility of the action even though this cannot be resisted.
- Complex motor tics: associated with premonitory sensations or the urge to move (unlike stereotypies).
- Stimming: movements associated with repetitive self-stimulation.

Treatment

Patients are usually not bothered by or are unaware of stereotypies, though carers and family members are often very concerned about them. Treatment involves cognitive behavioral therapy.

DYSKINESIAS

Definition

Generic term used to describe hyperkinetic movement disorders. The term is used where combinations of movements occur as in spontaneous focal dyskinesias and drug-induced dyskinesias, including levodopa-induced dyskinesias.

All hyperkinetic movement disorders may occasionally affect a body part in isolation and present as a focal dyskinesia. In some cases focal dyskinesias are not readily classifiable as one of the major categories of hyperkinetic movement disorders because the movements are irregular, repetitive, alternating, jerky, and variable in occurrence or appearance[16]. Most cases occur spontaneously without identifiable underlying structural pathology, and are to be distinguished from tardive or drug-induced dyskinesias listed below.

Drug-induced dyskinesias

Acute dystonic reactions

- Follow rapidly after drug administration.
- Are uncommon.
- Affect children and adolescents more than adults.
- Occur within a few hours (or less often days) after one or more doses of a phenothiazine (e.g. prochlorperazine, chlorpromazine), butyrophenone (e.g. haloperidol), metoclopramide, antihistamines, tetrabenazine.
- Dystonia of head and neck muscles causes neck retraction, oculogyric crisis, opisthotonos, trismus, tongue protrusion, torticollis, dysphagia.
- Can be painful and frightening.
- Resolves in 1–2 hours or following an intravenous anticholinergic drug.
- A family history of dystonia may be present.
- A second exposure to the offending drug may be well tolerated.

Tardive dyskinesias

- Occur gradually after months or years of drug administration.
- Typically are seen with antipsychotic drugs (dopamine receptor blockers).
- Withdrawal emergent dyskinesia develops on stopping a neuroleptic.
- Thought to be less of a problem with newer atypical neuroleptics[17].
- Occur in ~15–30% patients treated with neuro leptics (5%/year).
- Choreiform orobuccolingual movements predominate.
- Patients are often not aware of movements.
- Movements are suppressible by voluntary effort.
- Risk factors:
  - Age >50 especially females.
  - Coexisting neurologic or medical disease.
  - Dose and class of neuroleptic.
  - Duration of drug exposure.
  - Anticholinergic exposure.
- ~40–50% improve after drug withdrawal.

Tardive dystonia

- Less common than tardive dyskinesia.
- Cranial, cervical (retrocollis), axial (trunk extension) dystonia.
- Remission <20% after drug withdrawal.
- Commonly associated with:
  - Akathisia, parkinsonism, tics, stereotypies.
  - Breathing noises, sniffing.

Treatment

- Stop the offending drug:
  - Remission rates are variable.
  - Beware of relapse in psychiatric condition.
  - Transient deterioration in movements may follow cessation.
  - Stop anticholinergics in tardive dyskinesia.
- Symptomatic treatment depending on type of movement disorder:
- Tetrabenazine (for dyskinesias).
- Anticholinergics for tardive dystonia.
- Botulinum toxin (for craniocervical tardive dystonia).
- Deep brain stimulation (for tardive dystonia).
- Propranolol (for akathisia).

Tip

► *Anticholinergic drugs do not prevent tardive dyskinesia and may exacerbate established choreiform dyskinesias.*

Levodopa-induced dyskinesias in Parkinson's disease

- Choreic peak dose dyskinesias.
- Dystonic off period of diphasic dyskinesias.

DRUG-INDUCED MOVEMENT DISORDERS

NEUROLEPTIC MALIGNANT SYNDROME

Definition

Neuroleptic malignant syndrome (NMS) is a potentially life-threatening condition characterized by fever, severe muscle rigidity, autonomic instability, and changes in mental state induced by abrupt blockade of CNS dopaminergic transmission[18].

Epidemiology and etiology

- Incidence: 0.01–0.02% of persons on antipsychotics.
- Neuroleptic antipsychotic drugs (typical and atypical).
- Other drugs (non-neuroleptic):
  - Metoclopramide, prochlorperazine, droperidol, promethazine.
  - Tricyclic antidepressants, carbamazepine.
- Abrupt withdrawal of dopaminergic medications, amantadine.
- Dopamine depleting agents in HD.

Risk factors

- Previous episodes (30% develop NMS on rechallenge).
- Dehydration.
- Agitation.
- Rapid rate and parenteral route of neuroleptic administration.
- Pre-existing organic brain disease or psychiatric illness, particularly if taking lithium.

Pathophysiology

Profound decrease of central dopaminergic function leads to rigidity and tremor. Sustained muscle contraction causing rigidity results in increased heat production amplified by altered hypothalamic and autonomic thermoregulation, causing fever and rhabdomyolysis.

Clinical assessment

Rapid onset, usually within a few days of starting treatment with a dopamine receptor antagonist, but sometimes after stopping treatment. Variable combinations of the following features:

- Fluctuating level of consciousness and alertness.
- Confusion, agitation, restlessness (often precedes rigidity and fever).
- Akinetic mutism.
- Generalized muscle rigidity, tremor, dyskinesia.
- Autonomic dysfunction (hypertension, hypotension).
- Tachycardia, tachypnea.
- Hyperthermia (fever, diaphoresis).
- Dehydration.
- Oculogyric crises, gaze paresis infrequently.
- Extensor plantar responses may be present.

Differential diagnosis

- CNS disorders:
  - Infection (viral encephalitis, HIV, post-infectious encephalomyelitis).
  - Trauma.
  - Seizures.
  - Acute dystonic reaction.
- Systemic disorders:
  - Infection (septicemia, tetanus, rabies).
  - Metabolic encephalopathy.
  - Endocrinopathy (thyrotoxicosis, pheochromocytoma).
  - Autoimmune disease (SLE, polymyositis).
  - Heatstroke (history of physical exertion, no diaphoresis or rigidity).
- Drugs/toxins:
  - Toxins (carbon monoxide, phenols, strychnine).
  - Food-related allergic reactions.
  - Drug withdrawal: salicylates, dopamine inhibitors and antagonists, stimulants, MAO inhibitors, anesthetic agents, alcohol, sedatives.
  - Substance abuse: cocaine, amphetamines.
  - Central anticholinergic syndrome: fever, dry skin, confusion. Differentiated from NMS by peripheral signs of atropine poisoning (dry mouth, mydriasis, bowel paresis, urinary retention) and absence of rigidity.
  - Malignant hyperthermia: inherited mutation of the ryanodine receptor (CACNA1S) and other myopathies. Exposure to volatile anesthetics or depolarizing agents (succinyl choline) triggers persistent muscle contraction, muscle rigidity, rhabdomyolysis, hyperpyrexia, and metabolic acidosis.
  - Serotonin syndrome: see below.
  - Catatonia: see below.

Investigations

- Elevated creatine kinase (but may be normal).
- Leucocytosis.
- Myoglobinuria.
- Hypoxia, respiratory and metabolic acidosis.
- Renal function tests.
- Urine, blood, CSF examination, cultures to exclude infection.

Treatment

- General:
  - Early recognition.
  - Discontinue the offending antipsychotic drugs.
  - Restart dopaminergic drugs (if discontinued).
  - Transfer to intensive care unit:
    - Hydration, cooling.
    - Ventilatory assistance if required.
    - Rhabdomyolysis: alkanization of urine, renal replacement therapy.
- Specific:
  - Benzodiazepines: midazolam 1–10 mg/hour, diazepam 30 mg/day, lorazepam 3 mg/day.
  - Dopamine agonists, levodopa/carbidopa.
  - Dantrolene.
  - Electroconvulsive therapy may be successful in refractory cases.

Prognosis

The syndrome lasts 7–10 days in uncomplicated cases receiving oral neuroleptics, recovering spontaneously without the need for specific drugs. A longer course is seen with depot neuroleptics. Mortality has declined with early recognition and metabolic support, but medical complications (respiratory, cardiac, renal) occur in up to 40%. Contractures may develop, and residual cerebellar damage may occur as a sequel to hyperpyrexia.

The need for antipsychotics should be reviewed, as there is recurrence in 30% with rechallenge. If antipsychotics are clinically indicated, medication should be restarted in small doses, and titrated slowly. Atypical antipsychotics should be used.

Prevention

- A careful history of prior antipsychotic use and previous complications.
- Clear indications for antipsychotic use.
- Increases in dose should be made judiciously based on symptom response.

SEROTONIN SYNDROME

Definition

A potentially life-threatening disorder resulting from excessive stimulation of central and peripheral serotonin receptors by therapeutic or recreational drugs, often taken in combination[19].

Etiology

- Drugs associated with the serotonin syndrome:
  - SSRIs.
  - Tricyclic antidepressants.
  - MAO inhibitors.
  - Lithium.
  - Anticonvulsants: valproate.
  - Analgesics: meperidine, fentanyl, tramadol, pentazocine.
  - Antiemetics: ondansetron, metoclopramide.
  - Antimigraine drugs: sumatriptan.
  - Bariatric medications: sibutramine.
  - Antibiotics: linezolide, ritonavir.
  - Cough, cold remedies: dextromethorphan.
  - Amphetamines, cocaine, lysergic acid diethylamide (LSD).
  - Herbal products: tryptophan, St. John's wort, ginseng.
- Drug combinations associated with serotonin syndrome:
  - Phenelzine and meperidine.
  - Tranylcypromine and imipramine.
  - Phenelzine and SSRIs.
  - Paroxetine and buspirone.
  - Linezolide and citalopram.
  - Moclobemide and SSRIs.
  - Tramadol, venlafaxine, and mirtazapine.

Clinical features

Variable combinations of:

- Fluctuating confusion, restless agitation, akinetic mutism.
- Tremor, myoclonus.
- Rigidity, hyper-reflexia, clonus.
- Autonomic hyperactivity: tachycardia, diaphoresis, fever, flushed facies.
- Diarrhea.

Investigations

- Elevated creatine kinase.
- Raised transaminases.
- Leukocytosis.

Diagnosis

- Clinical suspicion.
- Note overlap with signs of NMS and catatonia.
- Serotonergic drug use.
- Rule out infections and other causes of hyperthermia.

Treatment

- Stop drug(s) – may resolve rapidly after cessation of offending drugs.
- Benzodiazepines (lorazepam).
- Propranolol, bromocriptine, dantrolene are contraindicated.

CATATONIA

Definition

A fluctuating syndrome of abnormal motor and cognitive behavior, typically accompanying psychiatric disorders such as schizophrenia, severe depression, and mania but also encountered in severe medical illness such as head injury, systemic and CNS infection, toxic, metabolic, and immune encephalopathies[20].

Clinical features

Variable combinations of:

- Mood disorder.
- Prodrome of hyperactivity, restless agitation, distractibility.
- Delirium, stupor, staring, withdrawn.
- Akinetic mutism, unresponsive, inertia.
- Abnormal posturing, waxy flexibility, catalepsy, rigidity.
- Automatic obedience, echophenomena, utilization behavior.
- Stereotypies – repetitive purposeless movements.
- Autonomic dysfunction: fever, diaphoresis, tachycardia.

Investigations

- Normal or elevated creatine kinase.
- Other investigations normal in the absence of medical illness.

Diagnosis

- Clinical suspicion.
- Note overlap with NMS.
- Rule out infections, toxic, metabolic, immune encephalopathies.

Treatment

- Supportive therapy.
- Benzodiazepines (diazepam, lorazepam) – often dramatic response.
- Electroconvulsive therapy in refractive cases.
- High mortality if unrecognized.
- May deteriorate with neuroleptic administration.

PSYCHOGENIC MOVEMENT DISORDERS

Epidemiology and etiology

Psychogenic movement disorders account for 2% of all movement disorders and up to 20% of cases seen at specialist movement disorder clinics[21].

Clinical assessment

History

- Sudden onset and rapid progression.
- Waxing and waning.
- Paroxysmal events.
- Multiple neurologic and somatic complaints.
- Past psychiatric illness.
- Identifiable stressor(s).
- Family member with similar neurologic illness.
- Self-inflicted injuries.

Examination

- Pattern of movements[22]:
  - Shaking, jerking, fixed dystonic posturing, bizarre gait.
  - Often mixture of movement types.
  - Exaggerated slowness and effort.
- Accompanying signs often suggest conversion disorder or somatization:
  - 'Nonorganic' weakness, sensory loss.
  - Nonepileptic pseudoseizures.
  - Convergence spasm.
  - Unintelligible speech.
- Alleviation – or improvement of movements with distraction, suggestion, or placebo.
- Exacerbation by suggestion/examination.
- Deficits not congruent with known neurologic disease.
- Unexplained variation in examination findings.
- Disability out of proportion to examination findings.
- Voluntary rhythmic movements (e.g. making circles with feet, opening and closing hands) entrain or disrupt psychogenic movement disorders.
- Restraint of the affected limb: may intensify the movements.

Treatment

- Careful discussion of the diagnosis.
- Reassure the patient that treatment is available.
- Analysis and treatment of triggers.
- Physiotherapy.
- Patient and family counseling.
- Psychiatric consultation.

REFERENCES

1 Geyer HL, Bressman SB (2006). The diagnosis of dystonia. *Lancet Neurol* 5:780–790.
2 Ozelius LJ, Lubarr N, Bressman SB (2011). Milestones in dystonia. *Mov Disord* **26**:1106–1126.
3 Berardelli A, Rothwell JC, Hallett M, Thompson PD, Manfredi M, Marsden CD (1998). The pathophysiology of primary dystonia. *Brain* **121**:1195–1212.
4 Bruno MK, Hallett M, Gwinn-Hardy K *et al.* (2004). Clinical evaluation of idiopathic paroxysmal dyskinesias: new diagnostic criteria. *Neurology* **63**:2280–2287.
5 Wang JL, Cao L, Li XH, *et al.* (2011). Identification of PRRT as the causative gene in paroxysmal kinesigenic dyskinesias. *Brain* **134**:3493–3501.
6 Pons R, Collins A, Rotstein M, Engelstadt K, De Vivo DC (2010). The spectrum of movement disorders in Glut-1 deficiency. *Mov Disord* **25**:275–281.
7 Gregory A, Polster BJ, Hayflick SJ (2009). Clinical and genetic delineation of neurodegeneration with brain iron accumulation. *J Med Genet* **46**:73–80.
8 Cardoso F (2004). Chorea: non genetic causes. *Curr Opin Neurol* **17**:433–436.
9 Schneider SA, Walker RH, Bhatia KP (2007). The Huntington's disease-like syndromes: what to consider in patients with a negative Huntington's disease gene test. *Nat Clin Pract Neurol* **3**:517–525.
10 Elble R, Deuschl G (2011). Milestones in tremor research. *Mov Disord* **26**: 1096–1105.
11 Bain PG, Findley LJ, Thompson PD, *et al.* (1994). A study of hereditary essential tremor. *Brain* **117**:805–824.
12 Obeso JA, Rothwell JC, Marsden CD (1985). The spectrum of cortical myoclonus. From focal reflex jerks to spontaneous motor epilepsy. *Brain* **108**:193–224.
13 Brown P, Day BL, Rothwell JC, Thompson PD, Marsden CD (1991). Intrahemispheric and interhemispheric spread of cerebral cortical myoclonic activity and its relevance to epilepsy. *Brain* **114**: 2333–2351.
14 Jankovic J, Kurlan R (2011). Tourette syndrome: evolving concepts. *Mov Disord* **26**:1149–1156.
15 Singer HS (2011). Stereotypic movement disorders. In: WJ Weiner, E Tolosa (eds). *Handbook of Clinical Neurology, Volume 100 (3rd Series). Hyperkinetic Movement Disorders*. Elsevier. Chapter 45, pp. 631–639.
16 Aggarwal A, Thompson PD (2011). Unusual focal dyskinesias. In: WJ Weiner, E Tolosa (eds). *Handbook of Clinical Neurology, Volume 100 (3rd Series). Hyperkinetic Movement Disorders*. Elsevier. Chapter 44, pp. 617–628.
17 Tarsy D, Baldessarini RJ (2006). Epidemiology of tardive dyskinesia: is risk declining with modern antipsychotics? *Mov Disord* **16**:589–598..
18 Factor SA (2005). Neuroleptic malignant syndrome. In: SA Factor, AE Lang, WJ Weiner (eds). *Drug Induced Movement Disorders*, 2nd edn. Blackwell Futura. Ch 9, pp. 174–212.
19 Boyer EW, Shannon M (2005). The serotonin syndrome. *N Engl J Med* **352**:1112–1120.
20 Fink M, Taylor MA (2009). The catatonia syndrome. *Arch Gen Psychiatry* **66**:1173–1177.
21 Lang AE (2011). Phenomenology of psychogenic movement disorders. In: M Hallett, AE Lang, J Jankovic, *et al.* (eds). *Psychogenic Movement Disorders and other Conversion Disorders*. Cambridge University Press, Cambridge. Ch 2, pp. 6–13.
22 Brown P, Thompson PD (2001). Electrophysiological aids to the diagnosis of psychogenic jerks, spasms, and tremor. *Mov Disord* **16**:595–599.

Further reading

Brown P, Rothwell JC, Thompson PD, Britton TC, Day BL, Marsden CD (1991). The hyperekplexias and their relationship to the normal startle reflex. *Brain* **114**: 1903–1928.

Kimber TE, Thompson PD (2011). Senile chorea. In: WJ Weiner, E Tolosa (eds). *Handbook of Clinical Neurology Volume 100 (3rd Series). Hyperkinetic Movement Disorders*. Elsevier. Ch 13, pp. 213–217.

DEVELOPMENTAL DISEASES OF THE NERVOUS SYSTEM

James H. Tonsgard

INTRODUCTION

This chapter is divided into two sections: (1) Developmental malformations of the nervous system, and (2) Neurocutaneous disorders. Many of the neurocutaneous disorders could easily be considered in a discussion of tumors of the nervous system. However, several of the disorders show significant developmental abnormalities that justify their inclusion in this chapter. Furthermore, as discussed below, the nervous system emerges from the ectoderm of the primitive embryo from which the skin, as well as portions of the skull and face, also develops. As a consequence, germline or early somatic mutations of the ectoderm may produce defects in both the skin and nervous system resulting in neurocutaneous disorders.

EMBRYONIC DEVELOPMENT OF THE NERVOUS SYSTEM

In order to understand the diseases in this section it is essential to have at least some familiarity with developmental biology. By the end of the second week of gestation, the embryonic disc contains the three basic tissue types: mesoderm, ectoderm, and endoderm. Neuronal precursor cells develop from the ectoderm on the dorsal surface along the anterior-posterior axis of the disc. As these cells proliferate, they form a neural plate which indents, forming a groove with ridges or folds on either side (**178a**). As the folds fuse in the midline to form the neural tube, the neural tube separates from the ectoderm. The neural tube forms by day 23 (**178b**). Cells at the margins of the folds separate from the neural tube and form the neural crest, the precursor of both the autonomic and peripheral nervous systems. Closure of the anterior end of the neural tube occurs by day 24 and the posterior end by day 29. Closure of the neural tube is a

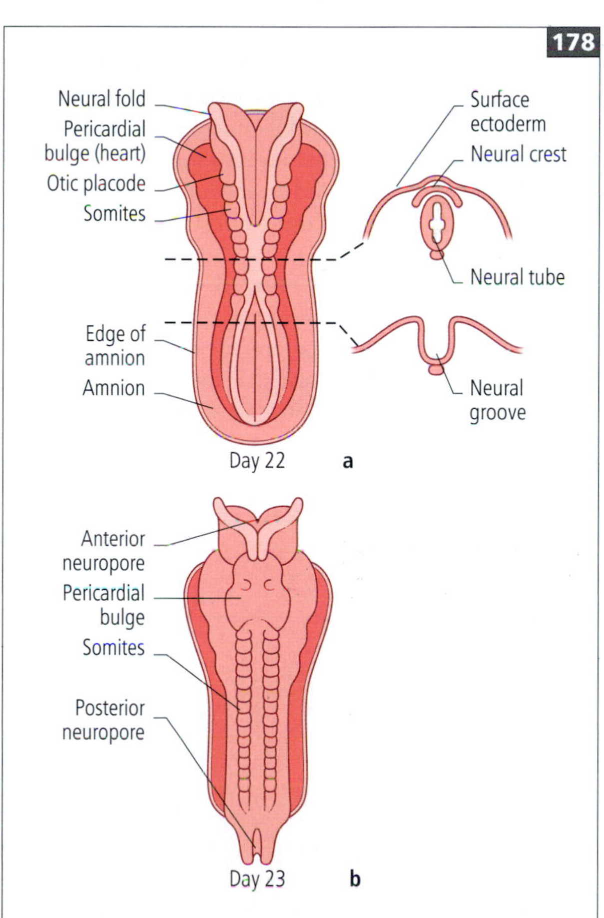

178 Development of the nervous system and closure of the neural tube. (a) Dorsal and transverse section through the embryo at day 22 at the start of closure of the neural tube; (b) dorsal view at day 23, with closure of the anterior neuropore beginning, while the posterior neuropore remains open. *Adapted with permission of Sinauer Associates, Gilbert SF, Developmental Biology, 6th edn.*

continuous process that proceeds from between two and five different sites along the anterior–posterior axis (**179**).

Induction of the nervous system is regulated by genes controlling dorsal–ventral longitudinal organization and genes affecting the anterior–posterior axis, creating transverse divisions or segments. Patterning of the dorsal–ventral axis results in four longitudinal domains of the central nervous system (CNS). Patterning along the anterior–posterior axis results in segmentation of the CNS into the forebrain, midbrain, hindbrain, and spinal cord (**180**). The rostral end of the neural tube undergoes extensive changes, forming three dilatations or segments: the prosencephalon or forebrain, the mesencephalon or midbrain, and the rhombencephalon or hindbrain. The prosencephalon divides transversely to form the telencephalon and diencephalon. Lateral division or cleavage of the telencephalon produces two paired structures which become the cerebral hemispheres. The rhombencephalon eventually divides into the metencephalon which becomes the pons and cerebellum and the myelencephalon which becomes the medulla (**180**)[1].

Formation of the cerebral cortex

Formation of the mature nervous system is dependent on the induction or formation of precursor cells, followed by the proliferation and maturation of cells within periventricular germinal centers and finally, migration to their intended sites. A cross-section of the developing brain shows that it is initially organized into an outer pial (preplate) or marginal zone (MZ) and inner ventricular zone (VZ) (**181a**). Stem cells proliferate and differentiate into immature neurons and glial precursors within the VZ and subventricular zone (SVZ). Starting in the seventh fetal week, neuroblasts in the VZ migrate upward to form a subpial preplate zone (PP). Subsequently, neurons migrate into the PP (**181c1**). These neurons divide, with some forming the superficial molecular layer or MZ (layer I) and others moving to the deep subplate. Thereafter, waves of neurons pass through the subplate, successively forming layers VI, V, IV, III, and II in an inside-out pattern, with the last neurons moving into layer II (**181b/c3**).

The majority of primitive neurons migrate radially or upward along glial fibers that extend from the VZ to the outer molecular layer. However, some neurons move tangentially or laterally within the VZ and SVZ, and intermediate zone (the future white matter). Radial and tangential movements are determined by characteristics of the radial glial fibers as well as a number of molecules (BLBP, ErbB4 receptor, and Notch receptors). The molecules that contribute to movement include cytoskeletal proteins (filamin A, doublecortin, Lis 1, ARFGEF2), signaling molecules (reelin), molecules modulating glycosylation that provide stop signals, neurotransmitters, neural cell adhesion molecules, and growth factors. Toxins such as alcohol and cocaine may also affect this process. Migration of neurons primarily occurs between the 12th and 24th fetal weeks.

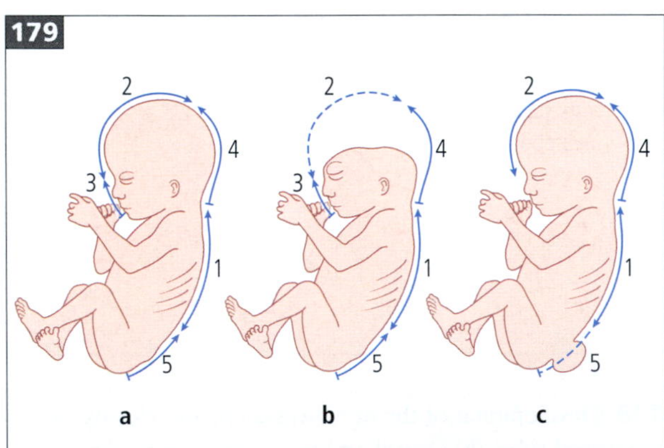

179 Closure of the neural tube. (a) Normal fetus with the putative sites of neural closure numbered with arrows showing the direction of closure; the number of closure sites is debated. (b) Anencephaly caused by failure of fusion of the anterior neuropore. (c) Spina bifida caused by failure of closure of the posterior neuropore. *Adapted with permission of Sinauer Associates, Gilbert SF, Developmental Biology, 6th edn.*

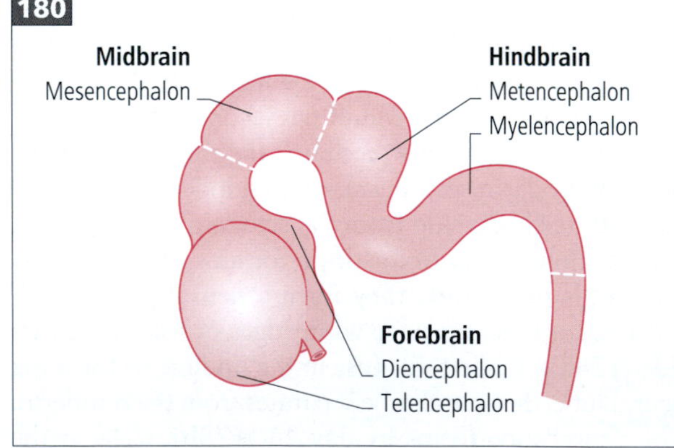

180 The early embryonic brain is divided into three segments: forebrain, midbrain, and hindbrain. Cleavage of the telencephalon of the forebrain produces two paired structures that become the cerebral hemispheres. The metencephalon becomes the pons and cerebellum, while the myelencephalon becomes the medulla.

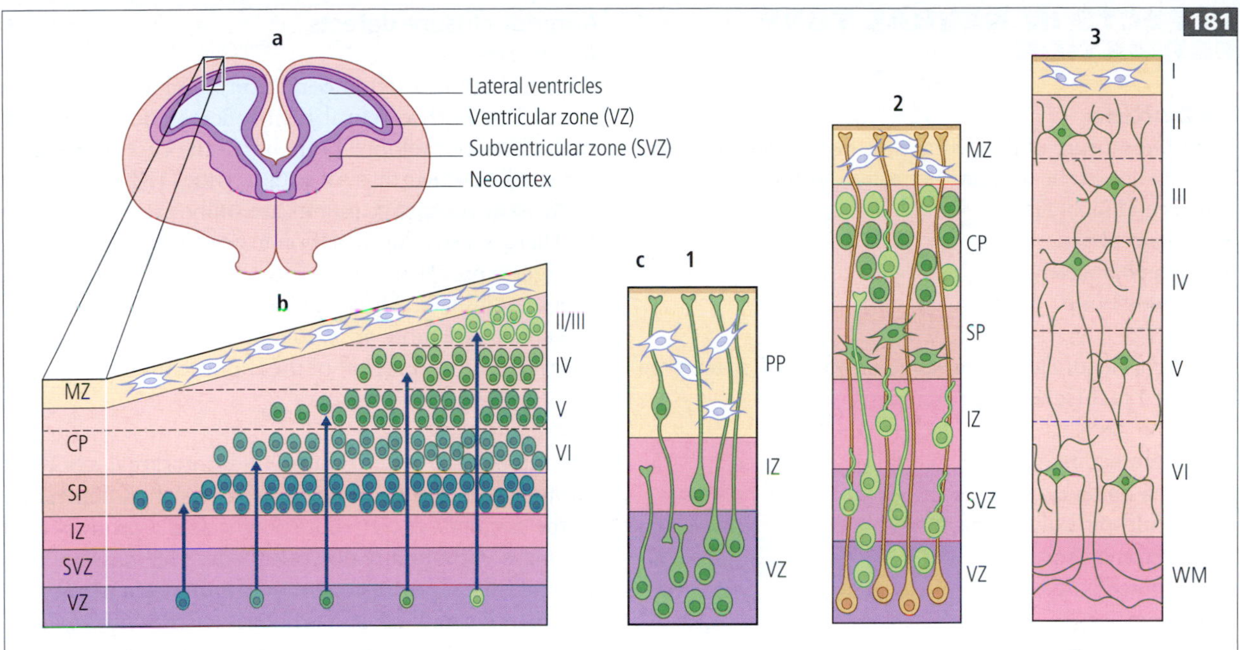

181 Development of the cortex. (a) An axial section of the immature brain. (b) Successive waves of neuron migration beginning with the deepest cortical layers. (c) 1: The first immature neurons migrate from the ventricular zone (VZ) through the intermediate zone (IZ), to form the preplate (PP). 2: Subsequently migrating neurons (green), moving along radial glial fibers (brown), split the PP into the marginal zone (MZ) and the subplate (SP) and begin to form the cortical plate (CP). The MZ contains Cajal–Retzius cells (white) which control the position of the migrating neurons. 3: The mature CP has six defined layers (I–VI), while the MZ, SP, and VZ have disappeared and the IZ has become white matter (WM).

Neurons within the subplate are transient and proliferate between 22 to 34 weeks gestation, form synaptic connections between the deep nuclei of the brain and the cortex, and express regulatory protein receptors, neurotransmitter receptors, and growth factor receptors. Cells that remain within the VZ become the ependyma lining the ventricles. The relatively cell-free area between the cortical plate and the VZ becomes the white matter (WM) of the mature brain. Myelination is under the control of the glial elements and occurs during the first 2 years of post-natal life and beyond[2].

Thus, the development of the brain can be understood as a complicated series of processes that includes induction, fusion, bending, proliferation, patterning, segmentation, cleavage, differentiation, migration, mitotic arrest, and finally myelination. Blood vessel formation and vascular proliferation are also of critical importance.

DEVELOPMENTAL MALFORMATIONS OF THE NERVOUS SYSTEM

Malformations of the nervous system may be caused by defects in development, broadly classified into:

- Failure of neural tube closure.
- Abnormal segmentation and sulci formation.
- Abnormal proliferation and migration of neuronal cells and precursors.
- Agenesis–hypoplasia.

The causes of errors in this series of processes include:

- Single gene defects as well as multiple gene mutations.
- Trauma.
- Teratogens such as hypoxia, hypothermia, chemical toxins, drugs, infections, radiation, maternal diabetes, and maternally produced toxins (as in phenylketonuria). The effects of toxins are dependent on:
  - Route of administration.
  - Dosage.
  - Timing.
  - Genetic and teratogenic factors may sometimes be combined.

For the purposes of this chapter, the malformations are divided into:

- Defects in neural tube formation.
- Defects of mid- and hindbrain development.
- Defects of forebrain and cerebral development.

DEFECTS IN NEURAL TUBE FORMATION

Definition

Defective closure of the neural tube (dysraphism). Defective closure of the anterior neuropore is termed **cranioschisis** and includes:

- Anencephaly.
- Encephalocele.
- Meningocele.

Defective closure along the spine or posterior neuropore is termed **rachischisis** and includes:

- Meningocele.
- Myelomeningocele (spina bifida).
- Spina bifida occulta.
- Occult spinal dysraphism.
- Diastomatomyelia.
- Tethered cord.

Epidemiology

The incidence varies widely in different populations. In the United States, neural tube defects (NTDs) occur in 1 out of every 1000 pregnancies. The recurrence risk in siblings is 2–5%, representing as much as a 50-fold increased risk over the general population. Defects in closure of the cranium are more frequent than closure defects of the spine. The mildest defect, spina bifida occulta, occurs in 5% of the normal population.

Etiology and pathophysiology

Defects in folding, fusion, or closure of the neural tube occur between days 20 and 29 of gestation. Defects involve a variable portion of the dorsal midline structures of the primitive neural tube including its covering of meninges, bone, and skin. Defects can occur anywhere along the neural axis.

Closure of the neural tube is believed to proceed from between two and five sites along the neural tube. This may explain why defects can occur, for example, in the cervical region in a patient without affecting closure more caudally. Both genetic and environmental factors are known to play a role in NTDs. NTDs are associated with a number of genetic syndromes and chromosomal abnormalities, but no one single gene has been implicated as a causative agent.

Several of the genes involved in folate-dependent pathways have been implicated in NTDs, although the exact mechanism is unknown. Some mothers with NTDs during pregnancy appear to have autoantibodies to folate receptors. Folate supplementation is thought to bypass competitive blocking autoantibodies.

NTDs can also be induced by toxins such as retinoic acid and valproic acid.

Anterior closure defects

Anencephaly

Anencephaly is a lethal condition in which there is an absence of both cerebral hemispheres and the cranial vault. The undeveloped brain lies in the base of the skull as a small vascular mass of neural tissue (**182**).

- Most anencephalic infants are stillborn.
- There is a striking variation in prevalence with the highest prevalence in the UK and Ireland, and the lowest in Asia, Africa, and South America.
- Females are more affected than males.
- It is the most frequent of the cranioschises.

Cranial meningocele

Cephalocele is a herniation of intracranial contents through a defect in the skull. It is classified depending on the contents. A cranial meningocele is a protrusion of meninges without any nervous tissue. The mass appears as a fluid-filled protrusion covered either by a membrane or skin in the midline, and is not associated with any neurologic deficit. Meningoceles may occur anywhere along the neuroaxis.

Encephalocele

Encephalocele is a herniation of intracranial contents including brain and meninges. It is a round mass protruding from the skull, most commonly in the occipital area (**183**). Frontal encephaloceles are much less common, but are more frequent in the Asian population. The amount of herniated neural tissue in the defect is variable, and in part determines severity of the deficits.

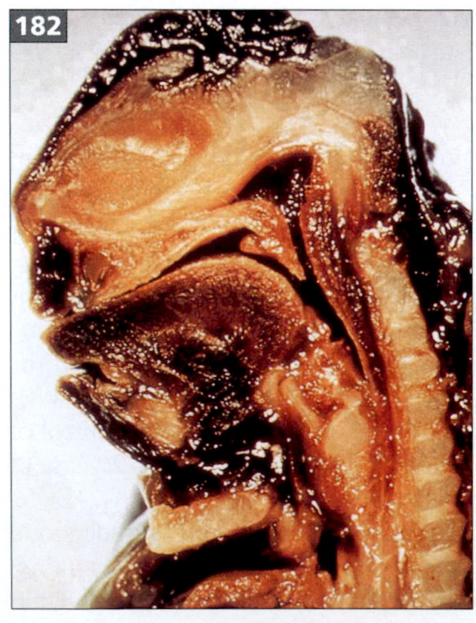

182 Sagittal section of a pathologic specimen of a dead fetus with anencephaly, showing absence of the cranial vault and its contents.

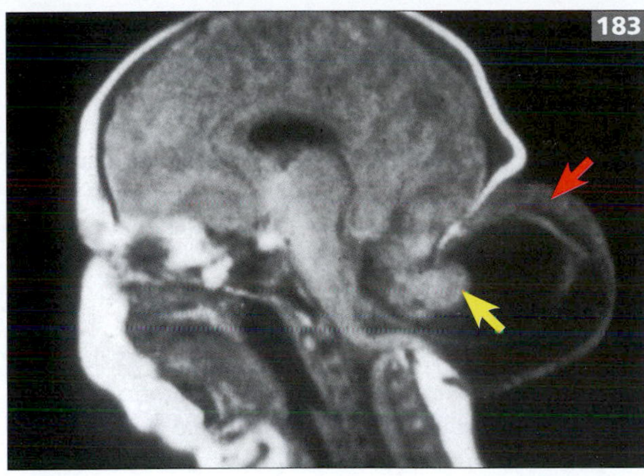

183 Encephalocele. Sagittal T1-weighted MRI of the brain, showing a defect in the suboccipital area in a patient with a Chiari III malformation, and herniation of hypoplastic cerebellar tissue (yellow arrow) and meninges (red arrow) through the bony defect.

Tip

▶ *Encephaloceles are defects in the skull, commonly associated with Dandy–Walker and Klippel–Feil syndromes, Arnold–Chiari malformation, porenecephaly, agenesis of the corpus callosum, cleft palate, and several chromosomal disorders. These associations affect outcome.*

Spinal and posterior closure defects

Meningocele

Meningocele is a protrusion of meninges without accompanying neural tissue. It is evenly distributed along the spinal axis and may go undetected. Meningoceles that are covered by normal skin are unlikely to be associated with other defects. Meningoceles in cranial and upper cervical spine can be associated with aqueductal stenosis, Arnold–Chiari malformations, and hydromyelia (**183**).

Meningomyelocele

Meningomyelocele is a cystic protrusion in the midline that involves spinal cord, nerve roots, meninges, vertebral bodies, and skin. Meninges and spinal cord or roots protrude through the defect in the neural arch as a dural sac containing spinal cord or roots closely applied to the body of the sac (**184**). Meningomyeloceles are commonly associated with hydrocephalus due to an accompanying Arnold–Chiari malformation (**185**) (see Hindbrain Defects p. 215). Aqueductal stenosis is a less common cause of hydrocephalus in meningomyeloceles. Characteristics of meningomyelocele include:

- The lumbosacral area is the most common location.
- Thoracic defects are less frequent and associated with more complications.
- The lumbosacral and thoracic defects account for 90% of meningomyeloceles.
- When the cervical spinal cord is involved, two distinct types of abnormalities are seen: a myelocystocele herniating posteriorly into a meningocele (**185**) and a meningocele without an underlying cord defect.

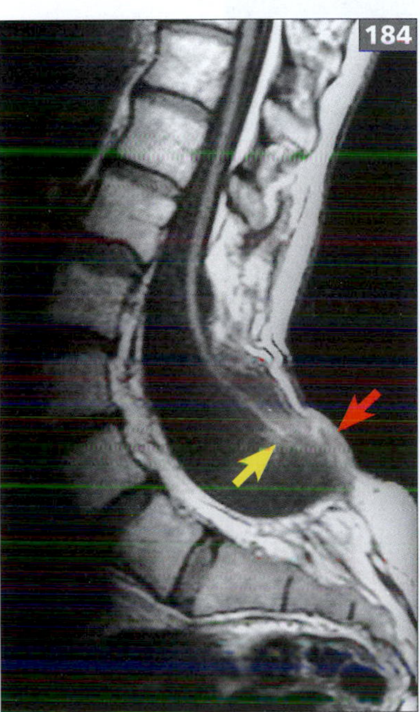

184 Sagittal T1-weighted MRI of the lumbosacral spine, showing a lumbosacral meningomyelocele (red arrow) and narrowing of the elongated lumbar cord with cord tethering (yellow arrow).

185 Chiari II malformation. T1-weighted MRI midline sagittal view of the brain and upper cervical cord, showing elongated brainstem with downward displacement of the cerebellum and obliteration of the fourth ventricle (arrows).

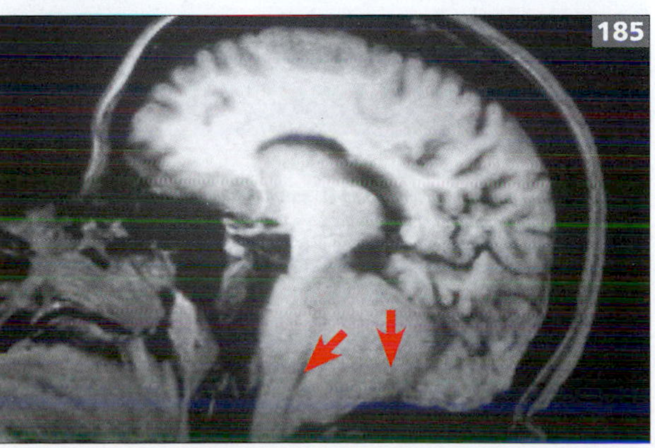

Spina bifida occulta

Spina bifida occulta is an incomplete closure of the vertebral arch. It commonly involves the lamina of L5 and S1. The incidence is about 5% of the population. When there is any associated neurologic dysfunction, it is referred to as an occult spinal dysraphism.

Occult spinal dysraphism

An occult spinal dysraphism is spina bifida occulta associated with:

- Fibrous bands causing distortion of the cord.
- Intraspinal lipoma.
- Dermoid or epidermoid cyst.
- Fibrolipoma, subcutaneous lipoma.
- Diastomatomyelia.
- Commonly results in the tethered cord syndrome.

Diastomatomyelia

Diastomatomyelia is a midline longitudinal division of the spinal cord due to a septum (**186, 187**). The septum is made of bone, cartilage, or fibrous tissue attached posteriorly to the vertebrae or dura and may extend for as many as 10 spinal segments (thoracic or lumbar). The division of the cord may be complete, each half with its own dural sac and nerve roots. This longitudinal fissuring and doubling of the cord is referred to as diplomyelia. Diastomatomyelia is usually associated with a hairy patch, dimple hemangioma, lipoma, or teratoma overlying the defect (**188**).

Clinical features

Anterior closure defects

Anencephaly

Anencephaly is incompatible with life; most fetuses are stillborn. Some infants survive for several days and demonstrate responses to stimuli that are purely spinal reflexes. Neuroendocrine defects are frequent due to pituitary hypoplasia.

Cranial encephalocele

Small frontal encephaloceles protruding into the nasal cavity may cause no neurologic signs; trauma to frontal defects may result in cerebrospinal fluid (CSF) rhinorrhea or infection. Occipital encephaloceles are associated with mental retardation, seizures, motor dysfunction, and visual defects. The degree of disability depends both on the amount of neural tissue in the encephalocele and the other conditions associated with the defect.

Posterior closure defects

Meningocele

A meningocele in the thoracic or lumbar cord that is covered by skin is unlikely to be associated with any deficits. Cervical meningoceles are associated with hydrocephalus, and severe motor deficits due to the associated defects mentioned above (see Pathology).

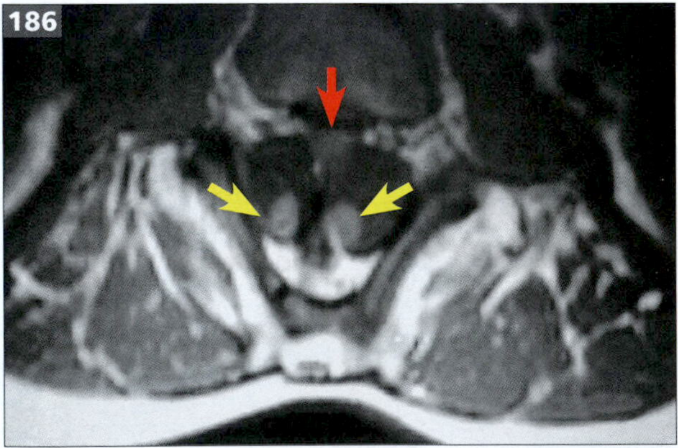

186 Diastomatomyelia. T1-weighted axial MRI of the lumbar spine, showing the neural tissue (yellow arrows) passing around the bony bar (red arrow) with a misshapen vertebral body.

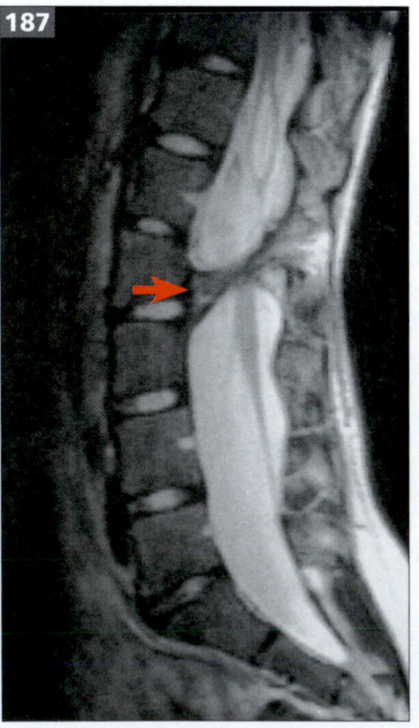

187 Diastomatomyelia. T2-weighted MRI, midline sagittal view , showing a bony bar (arrow) across the center of the spinal canal.

Meningomyelocele

The location determines the type and severity of complications; lumbosacral defects are the most common, and thoracic and cervical lesions tend to be more complicated. Characteristics include:

- Variable weakness of the legs.
- Loss of bowel and bladder control.
- Sensory defects that can result in skin ulceration.
- Deep tendon reflexes are absent.
- Dislocation of the hips may occur.
- Hydrocephalus is common.
- Infection may complicate closure of the defect or treatment of the hydrocephalus.
- Growth of child stretches the spinal cord causing a tethered cord syndrome.

Spina bifida occulta

This is not associated with any clinical deficits, and is often associated with changes in the overlying skin, such as hyperpigmentation, hair, discoloration, dimple, or dermal sinus (**188, 189**).

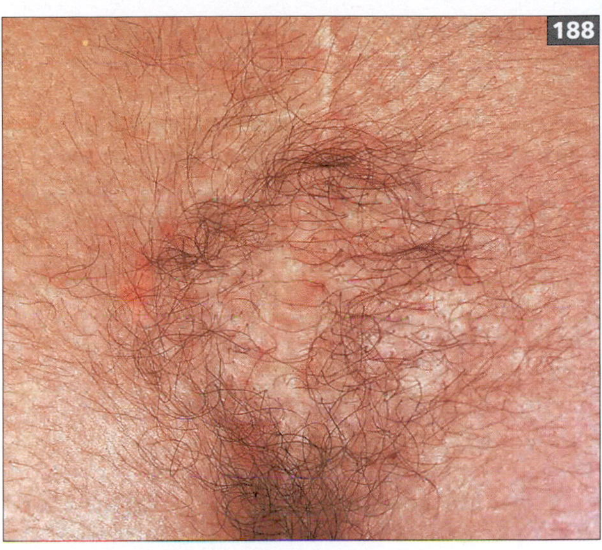

188 Photograph of the lower back of a patient with spina bifida occulta, showing a tuft of hair over the site of the spinal defect and a vertical surgical scar.

Occult spinal dysraphism

This is associated with clinical deficits; the degree of deficits is variable and sometimes severe:

- Absent Achilles tendon reflexes.
- Incontinence, sensory loss in the feet or legs.
- Gait abnormalities.
- Static deficits and progressive dysfunction can be seen with growth.
- Sometimes the defect goes unnoticed until late childhood when increase in height results in stretching of the cord.
- A common presentation is the tethered cord syndrome.

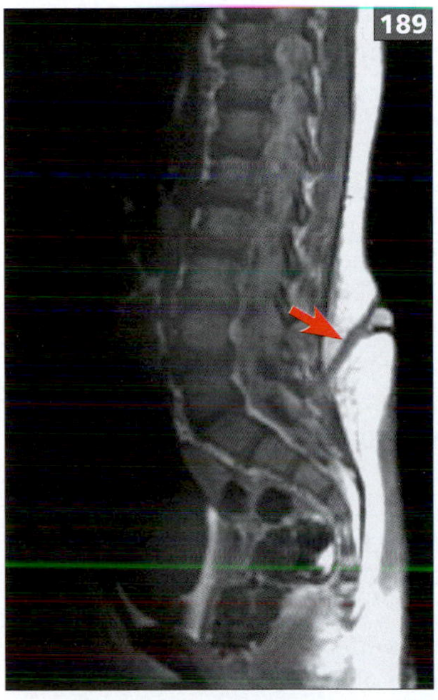

189 Sagittal post-contrast T1 MRI of lumbar spine, showing a dermal sinus tract extending from the skin to the sacral canal (arrow) with associated intraspinal infection.

Diastomatomyelia

This is always associated with clinical symptoms, including:

- Commonly accompanied by progressive scoliosis.
- Overlying cutaneous abnormality.
- Tethered cord syndrome.

Tethered cord syndrome

This is due to adhesion of the conus medullaris to one of the lower lumbar vertebrae. The conus fails to ascend within the spinal canal/dural sac as the child increases in height. Causes include intradural fibrous adhesions, diastomatomyelia, intradural lipoma, dermal sinus tract, tight filum terminale. Onset of symptoms occurs in late childhood or later, including:

- Progressive sensorimotor deficits in the legs or feet (most patients).
- Severe pain in the perineum, gluteal region, or legs (common).
- Midline cutaneous lesions (many but not all patients).
- Bowel and bladder dysfunction (frequent).
- Upper motor neuron signs coexist with symptoms of conus dysfunction (rare).

Investigations

Cranial encephalocele

- Magnetic resonance imaging (MRI) of the brain defines the amount of neural tissue contained in the defect and shows other associated defects such as agenesis of the corpus callosum, Dandy–Walker malformation, and Arnold–Chiari malformation.
- Plain spine X-rays to look for a Klippel–Feil defect.
- Chromosome studies for chromosomal abnormalities, genetic diseases or syndromes.

Spinal defects

(Including meningocele, meningomyelocele, spina bifida occulta, occult spinal dysraphisms, and diastomatomyelia.)

- X-rays of the spine delineate the vertebral abnormalities: failure of fusion of one or more vertebral arches, hemivertebrae, block vertebrae, or a bony spur.
- MRI of the spine is essential to delineate these defects.
- Ultrasound is useful to investigate sacral dimples or dermal sinus tract and can demonstrate intradural lipomas as well as low-lying conus in infants.
- Urodynamic studies are helpful in patients with tethered cord syndrome.

Diagnosis

Pre-natal diagnosis

Enhanced birth defect screen or AFP3/AFP4, measuring alpha fetoprotein, dimeric inhibin A, beta human chorionic gonadotropin, and unconjugated estradiol, is commonly used at 15–20 weeks of gestation to evaluate the potential for NTDs and chromosomal anomalies. Based on the results of this screening, pregnant women may be referred for amniocentesis. Maternal gene *MTHFR* 677T is a risk factor for meningomyelocele.

Tips

▶ *Elevated levels of amniotic fluid alpha fetoprotein and acetyl cholinesterase are found in patients with open NTDs.*

▶ *Pre-natal ultrasound is effective in diagnosing the NTDs with the exception of the occult dysraphisms.*

Post-natal diagnosis

Ultrasound, plain X-rays, and MRI as discussed above.

Treatment

Prevention

Because of the markedly increased risk for recurrence of NTDs in subsequent pregnancies, mothers of children with NTDs should receive appropriate genetic counseling and screening.

Tips

▶ *Folic acid supplementation of at least 4 mg/day reduces the risk of NTDs by as much as 70%.*

▶ *Folic acid is a water soluble B vitamin that is essential for cell function, division, and differentiation*[3].

Pre-natal treatment

Intrauterine repair of myelomeningocele may reduce the incidence of Arnold–Chiari malformations and hydrocephalus in some patients prior to 20 weeks gestation, although there are significant maternal and fetal risks[4].

Post-natal treatment

- Prompt closure of meningomyeloceles reduces the risk of infection and improves subsequent function.
- Ventriculoperitoneal shunting is required for patients with hydrocephalus.
- Patients with loss of sphincter control require a daily regimen of catheterization and bowel emptying.
- Patients with meningomyeloceles should have a coordinated multi-disciplinary team to deal with urologic, orthopedic, neurologic, and neurosurgical complications.
- Treatment of tethered cord depends on the cause. Surgical intervention is required in patients with progressive deficits, severe pain, or progressive scoliosis.

Prognosis

Anterior closure defects

- Anencephaly is a universally lethal condition.
- Occipital encephaloceles are associated with mental retardation, seizures, variable motor dysfunction, and frequent visual impairment.

Spinal and posterior closure defects

- Meningoceles and spina bifida occulta are not associated with any neurologic sequelae.
- Meningomyelocele:
  - Overall, long-term mortality rate has improved and approaches zero in recent series for sacral and lumbar lesions. Outcome is largely dependent on the need for ventriculoperitoneal shunting.
  - 65% require ventricular peritoneal shunting.
  - 50% are ambulatory and 50% attend regular school and achieve at an age-appropriate level.
  - Patients do face a lifetime of disability with potential motor problems, shunt infections and shunt failures, and chronic urinary catherization.
- Occult spinal dysraphisms, diastomatomyelia, and tethered cord syndrome have a variable response to surgical intervention:
  - Pain is relieved or improved in almost all patients.
  - Motor function is improved in 25–80%.
  - Bowel and bladder function improves in 16–67%.
  - Scoliosis is improved or stabilized in 43–67%[5].

DEFECTS IN HINDBRAIN DEVELOPMENT

Definition

Arnold–Chiari malformations are the most common of the defects involving the lower hindbrain or medulla. The central feature of all of the Chiari malformations is downward displacement of the cerebellar tonsils and brainstem through the foramen magnum:

- In Chiari Type II the medulla can actually be doubled over alongside the cervical cord.
- Chiari Type III is associated with a cervical encephalocele and meningocele.
- Chiari Type IV consists of cerebellar hypoplasia and should be reclassified as a separate cerebellar malformation (see below).
- Dandy–Walker syndrome is the best known of the defects affecting the cerebellum. In this syndrome there is hypoplasia of the cerebellar vermis and cystic dilatation of the fourth ventricle.
- Cerebellar vermis hypoplasia is hypoplasia of the cerebellar vermis without a posterior fossa cyst.
- Malformations associated with the 'molar tooth' sign, including Joubert syndrome, are a group of malformations affecting the midbrain.

Tips

▶ *Chiari type I malformation consists of downward displacement of the cerebellar tonsil and brainstem in isolation.*

▶ *Chiari Type II consists of elongation of the medulla, often associated with kinking or folding of the medulla and it is invariably associated with a meningomyelocele.*

Epidemiology

Arnold–Chiari malformations are the most common. The exact incidence of the type I malformations is unknown, but it is a common incidental finding. It is frequently discovered in late childhood or adolescence. Chiari type II malformations are by definition associated with meningomyelocele and apparent at birth.

The Dandy–Walker malformation is primarily a sporadic condition. The incidence varies widely: 1 in 5000 to 1 in 50,000 live births. The Dandy–Walker malformation has been reported in association with a number of chromosomal anomalies.

Cerebellar vermis hypoplasia is a rare disorder that is X-linked in some patients and apparent in infancy. Joubert syndrome is a rare autosomal recessive disorder due to a defect in chromosome 9q34 that is apparent in infancy.

Etiology and pathogenesis

Development of the posterior fossa is a complicated process that begins after neural tube closure and after the brain has divided into three primary structures: the prosencephalon, mesencephalon, and rhombencephalon. The pons, cerebellum, and medulla are derived from the rhombencephalon: the cerebellum is derived from the most rostral portion of the hindbrain, the pons from the next portion of the hindbrain or metencephalon, and the medulla from the lower portion of the hindbrain or myelencephalon. Only the midbrain is derived from the mesencephalon.

A number of genes have been identified in the subdivision, bending, and patterning process that forms the structures of the mid- and hindbrains. The first parts of the cerebellum develop between 6 and 7 weeks gestation. The cerebellar vermis is fully developed by 4 months gestation, and the cerebellar hemispheres develop between 5 and 7 months of fetal life. However, the cerebellum is not fully developed until 20 months of life[6].

Arnold–Chiari malformations

Type I

- Elongation of the medulla.
- Downward displacement of the medulla and cerebellar tonsils through the foramen magnum (**190**).
- Hydromyelia and syringomyelia occur in 30–70% of patients. This is a cystic dilatation of the central canal of the spinal cord that can be progressive and extend for several vertebral segments (**191**). Syringobulbia, i.e. fluid within the brainstem, is also sometimes seen (**192**).

Type II

- Medulla is elongated and sometimes folded, causing thinning of the upper cervical cord and upward displacement of cervical roots (**193**).
- Vascular injury to the medulla may also occur.
- The pons is often thin.
- Aqueductal stenosis or compression of outflow of the fourth ventricle causes hydrocephalus.
- Hydromyelia and syringomyelia of the cervical cord also occur.
- Meningomyelocele is invariably associated.
- Increased gyri, heterotopias of the brain, and Klippel–Feil syndrome can be associated with Type II malformation.

Type III

- Cerebellar herniation.
- High cervical or occipital–cervical meningomyelocele.
- Open, dystrophic posterior fossa.

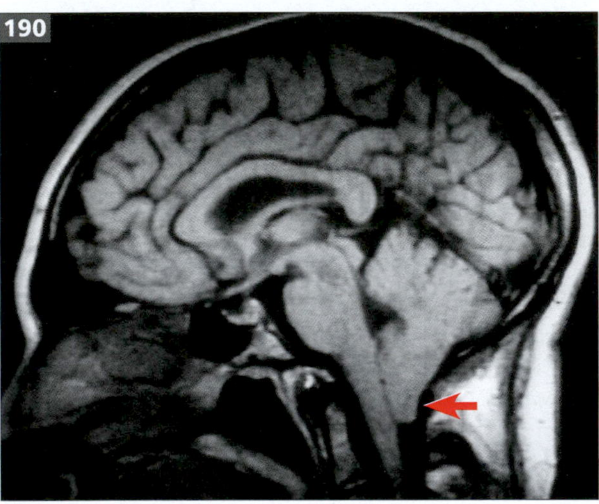

190 Chiari I malformation. Midline sagittal T1-weighted MRI, showing displacement of the cerebellar tonsils (arrow).

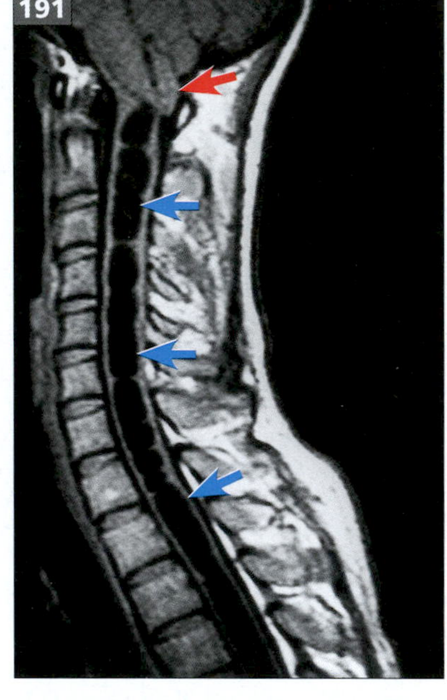

191 Syringomyelia. Sagittal T1-weighted MRI of the cervical spine showing displacement of cerebellar tonsils (red arrow) and a large bead-like syrinx (blue arrows) extending into the thoracic cord.

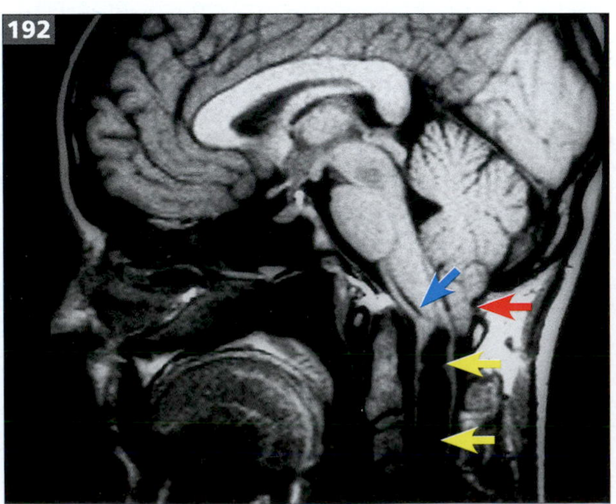

192 Syringomyelia and syringobulbia. T1-weighted sagittal MRI of the brain and brainstem and upper cervical cord, showing herniated cerebellar tonsils (red arrow), cervical syrinx (yellow arrows), and syringobulbia (blue arrow) extending to the level of the pontomedullary junction.

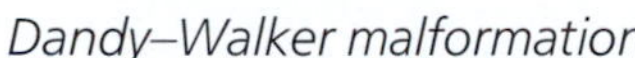

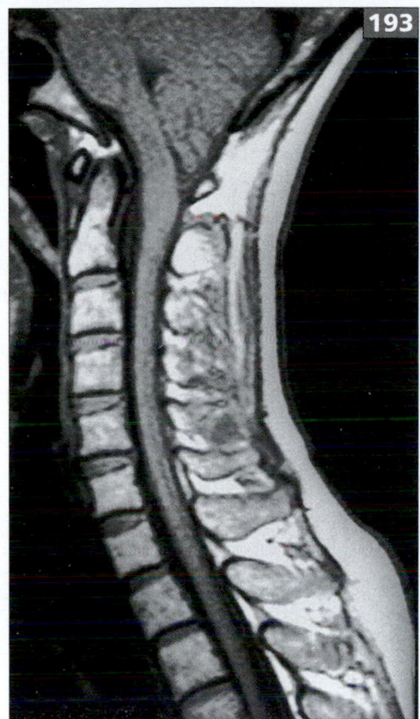

193 Chiari II malformation. Sagittal T1-weighted MRI of brainstem and cervical cord, showing elongation of the medulla, with downward displacement of the medulla and cerebellar tonsils.

Dandy–Walker malformation

- Posterior fossa is enlarged.
- Tentorium and lateral sinuses are displaced upward.
- Cerebellar vermis is hypoplastic or absent and upwardly displaced.
- Cerebellar hemispheres are simplified and displaced upward.
- Fourth ventricle is deformed by a large ependymal lined cyst that extends into the spinal canal (**194**).
- Third and lateral ventricles are usually enlarged and hydrocephalus is frequently present.
- Associated other defects include: agenesis of the corpus callosum, a variety of cortical malformations, aqueductal stenosis, Klippel–Feil syndrome, and a variety of somatic malformations[7].

Cerebellar vermis hypoplasia

- The vermis is small but in a normal position relative to the brainstem.
- There is a retrocerebellar fluid collection, not a cyst, which does communicate with the fourth ventricle.

Joubert syndrome

- There is an abnormally deep interpeduncular fossa.
- Hypoplasia of the vermis.
- Elongated superior cerebellar peduncles.
- Fourth ventricle is also enlarged so that axial views of the midbrain have a 'molar tooth' appearance (**195**).

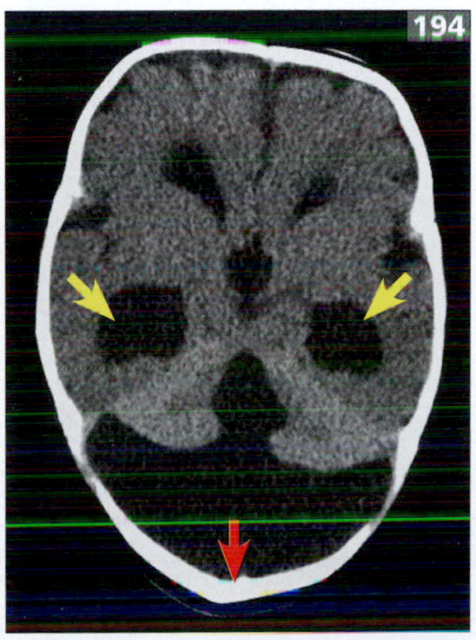

194 Dandy–Walker malformation. CT of the brain, showing absence of the midline cerebellar vermis and a large posterior fossa cyst communicating with the fourth ventricle (red arrow) and dilated lateral ventricles (yellow arrows).

195 Joubert syndrome. Axial FLAIR MRI of the brainstem shows distortion of the fourth ventricle (red arrow) and prominent, elongated superior cerebellar peduncles (yellow arrows) forming a 'molar tooth' sign.

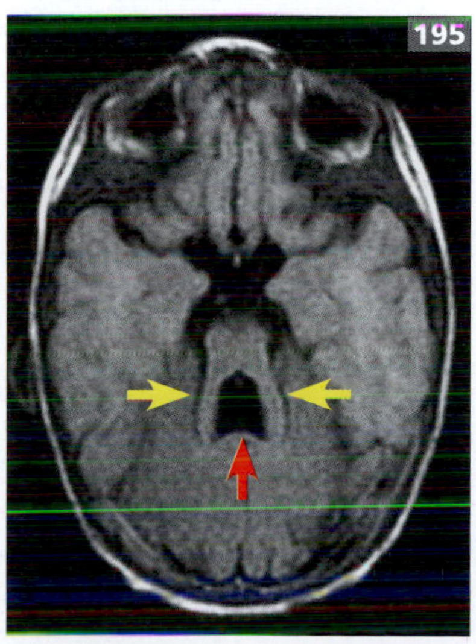

Clinical features

Arnold–Chiari malformations

Type I

- May be noted incidentally on MRI imaging and remain asymptomatic.
- Symptoms may appear in late childhood or adolescence.
- Headaches, neck pain, ataxia, and problems with gag or swallowing; sometimes headache will be worse with coughing or the Valsalva maneuver.
- Ataxia, nystagmus (particularly downbeat nystagmus), extensor plantar responses, posterior column signs, and scoliosis can be seen.

Type II

- Meningomyelocele.
- Hydrocephalus.

Type III

- Cervical meningomyelocele.
- Not usually compatible with life.

Dandy–Walker malformation

- Presentation is in infancy.
- Large head, back of the head is large and flattened.
- Hypotonia, and developmental delay.
- Hydrocephalus often brings these children to clinical attention.
- Nystagmus, apnea, and seizures are frequent.
- Rarely patients die suddenly from uncal herniation.
- Mental impairment is frequent, but as many as 50% have normal intelligence.

Cerebellar vermis hypoplasia

- Similar presentation to the Dandy–Walker malformation.
- X-linked form appears to be associated with severe mental retardation, seizures, choreoathetosis and spasticity, and coarse facial features.

Joubert syndrome

- Hypotonia, developmental delay.
- Nystagmus or oculomotor apraxia.
- Apnea, and seizures.
- Wide spectrum of severity, with some patients severely retarded.
- Somatic defects including retinal dystrophy, coloboma, renal disease, and hepatic fibrosis.

Investigations

Arnold–Chiari malformations

- MRI of the brain.
- MRI of the spine is essential to look for a syrinx of the cord as well as to assess the meningomyelocele that accompanies Type II and Type III.
- Dynamic CSF flow studies can be useful in assessment of the adequacy of posterior fossa CSF flow around the cerebellar tonsils.
- Plain X-rays are helpful in diagnosing associated vertebral anomalies.

Dandy–Walker syndrome and cerebellar vermis hypoplasia

- MRI of the brain is essential in diagnosing and evaluating these syndromes.
- MRI of the brain is also important in identifying other potentially associated brain abnormalities.
- Chromosome testing is valuable in cerebellar hypoplasia.

Joubert syndrome

- MRI of the brain.
- Visual assessment including electroretinography (ERG) is recommended.
- Chromosome testing.
- Sleep study is important because of the frequency of apnea.
- Imaging of the kidneys because of kidney dysplasia in some patients.
- A variety of genetic mutations have been found.

Diagnosis

Diagnosis is made by MRI of the brain. Chiari malformation is pathologic if the tip of the cerebellar tonsils is more than 5 mm below the foramen magnum after the first decade of life. Prior to that, the tonsils may need to be more than 6 mm below the foramen magnum. Dandy–Walker syndrome is diagnosed by the presence of all of the features on MRI. Joubert syndrome and other midbrain malformations are readily recognized by the presence of the 'molar tooth' sign on MRI.

Treatment

Arnold– Chiari malformations

Type I

- Intervention is not without controversy, because patients may be found to have the MRI finding incidentally.
- It is important not to intervene unless the patient is symptomatic.
- Some symptoms such as headache, neck pain, incontinence, or difficulties with coordination are nonspecific and may not respond to treatment.

Tips

▶ *Surgical decompression of the posterior fossa should only be done in patients who have a cervical cord syrinx and progressive or intractable symptomatology.*

▶ *Intervention is not based on the degree of displacement of the tonsils.*

Type II

- The majority have hydrocephalus and require a ventriculoperitoneal shunt.
- *In utero* repair of the meningomyelocele may reduce the incidence of hydrocephalus, but is not without risks.

Dandy–Walker syndrome

- Shunting procedure to treat the accompanying hydrocephalus.
- When the posterior fossa cyst clearly communicates with the ventricles, a cystoperitoneal shunt may be sufficient. It is not uncommon, however, for patients to have both a ventriculoperitoneal shunt and a shunt of the cyst.
- Management of seizures.
- Intellectual assessments.

Joubert syndrome

- Patients may require respiratory support.
- Feeding difficulties related to poor oral motor coordination may require a gastrostomy tube.
- Seizures require treatment but are usually not severe problems.
- Vision, kidney, and liver function must be assessed regularly because of associated complications.

Prognosis

Arnold–Chiari malformations

Type I

Surgical decompression is not without complications including pseudomeningocele, CSF leaks, meningitis, and a cerebellar slump in which the enlargement of the foramen magnum is too generous. Some patients also appear to have an inflammatory reaction to certain types of patches used for the duraplasty to close the posterior fossa. Results of decompression vary in different series with 45–86% of patients with Type I Chiari and syrinx showing objective signs of improvement.

Type II

See discussion of meningomyelocele.

Type III

This defect is usually associated with death within the first year of life.

Dandy–Walker syndrome

- Compatible with a fairly normal life span.
- Seizures are usually not extremely difficult to treat.
- Patients may require revisions of their ventricular and cyst shunts.
- Rarely, patients die unexpectedly from uncal or tonsilar herniation.

Joubert syndrome

There is substantial variability in the severity of the condition. The vast majority of patients survive the neonatal period and show improvement in breathing, motor function, and feeding over time.

DEFECTS IN FOREBRAIN AND CEREBRAL DEVELOPMENT

Definition

A large number of defects in the formation of the cerebral hemispheres have been identified. These defects are organized according to the developmental processes involved:

1. Disorders of prosencephalic or forebrain development, which are largely defects in cleavage: holoprosencephaly (HPE), agenesis of the corpus callosum, and septo-optic dysplasia (SOD).
2. Disorders of neuronal proliferation: primary microcephaly.
3. Disorders of neuronal migration: periventricular heterotopia, lissencephaly 1, Aristaless-related homeobox (ARX) spectrum disorders, and subcortical band heterotopia.
4. Disorders of cortical organization: polymicrogyria and schizencephaly.

DISORDERS OF PROSENCEPHALIC DEVELOPMENT

Epidemiology

Disorders of prosencephalic or forebrain cleavage that survive to delivery are uncommon (1 in 10,000–15,000 live births), but the incidence is higher in spontaneous abortions where it may occur in 1 in 250. It can be a recessive, autosomal dominant, or sex-linked condition.

The sex ratio in alobar HPE is 3:1, female: male. There is no sex predilection for the lobar form. The incidence of agenesis of the corpus callosum and hypoplasia of the corpus callosum is 1.8 per 10,000 live births, and of SOD is 1 in 10,000 live births.

Etiology and pathophysiology

Holoprosencephaly

Holoprosencephaly (HPE) is a defect in which there is impaired midline cleavage of the embryonic forebrain. Classically there is a failure to divide sagittally into cerebral hemispheres, transversely into telencephalon and diencephalon, and horizontally into olfactory tracts and bulbs. Less severe forms have been identified so that it is customary to further divide these defects into alobar, semilobar, and lobar holoprosencephaly.

An identifiable genetic causes represent 15–20% of cases, both monogenetic and chromosomal. Teratogens such as hyperglycemia (diabetes mellitus), alcohol, and retinoic acid are implicated in some cases.

Alobar holoprosencephaly

- Small single ventricle without an interhemispheric fissure (**196**).
- Thalami are undivided.
- Corpus callosum and the olfactory tracts and bulb are absent.

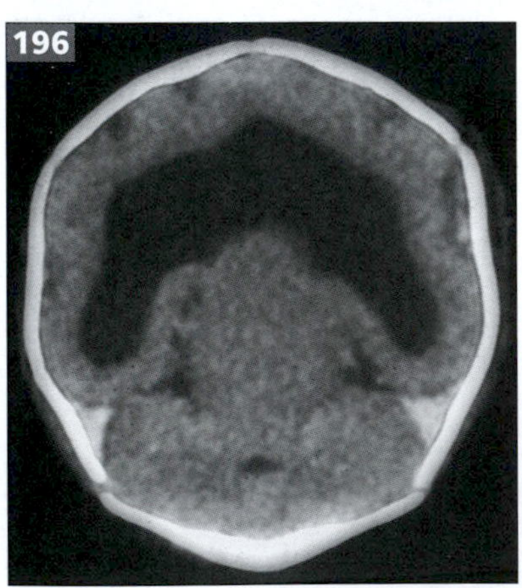

196 Alobar holoprosencephaly. CT of the brain, showing a single ventricle, absence of the corpus callosum and smooth simplified cortex with fused thalami.

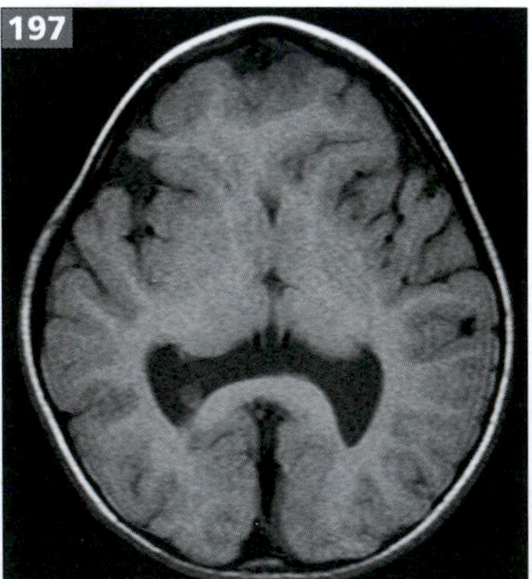

197 Semilobar holoprosencephaly. Axial T1-weighted MRI of the brain shows persistent fusion of the frontal lobes, with partial segmentation of the temporal and occipital lobes, and the posterior horns of the lateral ventricles.

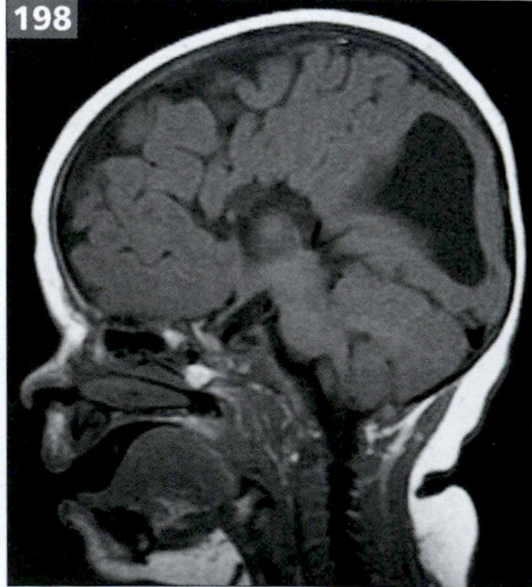

198 Agenesis of the corpus callosum. Sagittal T1-weighted MRI of the brain, with absence of the corpus callosum and partial visualization of posterior horn of the lateral ventricle.

Semilobar holoprosencephaly
- Rudimentary cerebral hemispheres are present (**197**).
- Interhemispheric fissure is incomplete.
- Corpus callosum is largely undeveloped.
- Olfactory tracts and bulbs are either absent or hypoplastic.

Lobar holoprosencephaly
- Cerebral hemispheres are well formed
- Interhemispheric fissure is incomplete.
- Corpus callosum is usually absent or incomplete.
- Thalami are not completely separated.
- Olfactory bulbs and tracts are absent or hypoplastic.

Agenesis of the corpus callosum

Agenesis of the corpus callosum is often part of the HPE spectrum (**198**). The corpus callosum has four parts (from front to back): rostrum, genu, body, and splenium. Formation starts with the genu and then progresses front to rear. If development is incomplete, the posterior portion is absent.
- Seen in a variety of chromosomal disorders and genetic syndromes.
- Autosomal recessive as well as X-linked inheritance has been demonstrated.
- In some cases, advanced maternal age may be a contributing variable.

Septo-optic dysplasia

A heterogeneous group of disorders with midline brain abnormalities:
- Hypoplasia or absence of the septum pellucidum and corpus callosum.
- Optic nerve hypoplasia.
- Pituitary/hypothalamic dysfunction.

There are two separate groups of SOD patients: one group exhibits a high incidence of cortical malformations, and the second group appears to be within the HPE spectrum. Mutation in the HESX gene has been implicated in some patients, but a genetic cause cannot be identified in most.

Clinical features

Holoprosencephaly

Alobar HPE

There is a variable number of severe facial dysmorphic features including: cyclopia, nasal proboscis, hypotelorism, single nostril nose, absence of olfactory tracts and bulbs, median cleft lip, hypognathia, single maxillary incisor, pituitary hypoplasia or even absence, and iris coloboma (**199**).

Amentia is a feature, sometimes with response to sensory stimuli and social smiling. Other defects include meningomyelocele, Dandy–Walker malformation, and heart, skeletal, and gastrointestinal (GI) defects.

Semilobar and lobar HPE

These include facial dysmorphism: ocular hypo- or hypertelorism, flat nose, cleft lip, iris coloboma. Pituitary abnormalities including diabetes insipidus are commonly found.

Agenesis of the corpus callosum
- This is an extremely heterogeneous group, with association with at least 50 congenital syndromes (including Aicardi syndrome), chromosomal disorders, and metabolic diseases[8].
- High incidence of cardiac, musculoskeletal, genitourinary, and GI defects.
- >50% have other malformations of the CNS.
- Mental impairment and seizures are frequent.

Septo-optic dysplasia

SOD are a heterogeneous group of patients. Visual defects, including nystagmus, diminished acuity, and color blindness are found in all patients, also microophthalmia and coloboma of the iris or retina. Pituitary abnormalities occur in 62%, including diabetes insipidus. Mental retardation, spastic quadriplegia, and seizures are also present.

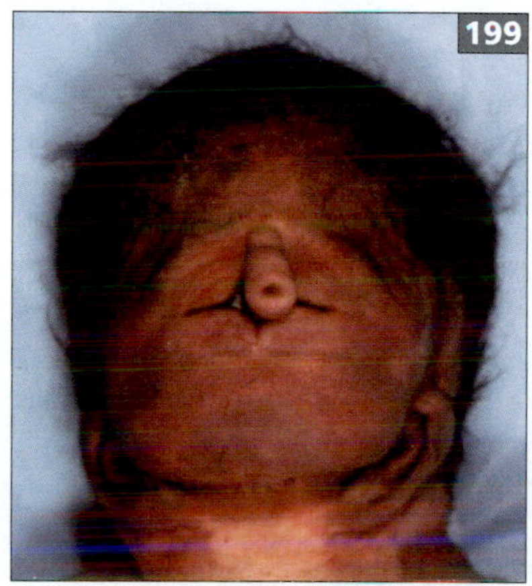

199 Autopsy photograph of a patient with alobar holoprosencephaly showing severe facial dysmorphisms including a small head, single nasal proboscis, and cyclopia.

Investigations

- MRI of the brain.
- Plain skeletal X-rays.
- Tests of electrolytes and endocrine and pituitary function.
- Echocardiogram and renal ultrasound.
- Patients with seizures require electroencephalography (EEG) to characterize their seizure type.
- Chromosomal testing as well as specific gene testing.

Diagnosis

Diagnosis is made by MR imaging of the brain.

Treatment

Treatment depends on the associated defects. These patients require a coordinated multidisciplinary team to treat their various problems.

Because of the association with pituitary defects, particularly diabetes insipidus, careful monitoring of serum electrolytes and fluid intake is essential. Appropriate nutritional support usually requires placement of a gastrostomy tube. Patients with seizures require seizure medicines.

Patients with cleft lip and palate require repair if they survive beyond the first 6 months of life. Because the spectrum of severity can be quite wide, the decision to repair any cardiac defects depends on the individual patient.

Prognosis

The spectrum of severity is quite wide, but life expectancy in most of these patients is reduced. Alobar HPE is probably not compatible with life beyond infancy. Patients with milder defects may survive into childhood or beyond and deserve appropriate and careful support.

DISORDERS OF NEURONAL PROLIFERATION (PRIMARY MICROCEPHALY)

Definition and epidemiology

Primary microcephaly (MCPH) is a congenital reduction in brain size (at least 4 SD below age and sex means), in the absence of other gross structural abnormalities both within and outside the brain.

MCPH is an autosomal dominant disorder. The incidence varies in different ethnic groups from 1 in 10,000 in northern Pakistan to 1 in 2 million in Scotland.

Etiology and pathophysiology

MCPH appears to be a primary disorder of neurogenic mitosis in which there are reduced numbers of neurons. Eight genetic loci have been found and five of the genes identified. All of the MCPH proteins appear to be ubiquitous and localize to the centrosome for at least part of the cell cycle.

Normal head measurements have been documented up to 20 weeks gestation. Head growth declines subsequently. After birth, the head size is 4–12 SD below the mean. Thereafter, the degree of MCPH remains unchanged. Pathology shows:

- Simplification of the cortical gyral pattern and reduction in brain volume.
- Slight reduction in white matter volume.
- The architecture of the brain is normal, with no evidence of any migrational defect.

Clinical features

- Mental retardation, but the degree of mental retardation is only mild to moderate.
- Motor milestones are slightly delayed and speech is significantly delayed, but most children learn to talk.
- Height and weight are usually normal.
- Seizures are reported in some patients.
- No spasticity or cognitive decline is present.

Investigations

MRI of the brain to look at the structure, computed tomography (CT) scan of the brain to look for calcification, eye examination to rule out congenital infection, TORCH titers to rule out congenital infection.

Tips

▶ *MCPH or primary microcephaly must be distinguished from other genetic and nongenetic causes of microcephaly such as congenital infection, fetal alcohol syndrome, fetal irradiation, cocaine exposure, and Rubinstein Taybi syndrome.*

▶ *The head size in MCPH is at least 4 SD below the mean, and the brain otherwise appears to be normal.*

Treatment

These patients usually do not require specific treatment.

Prognosis

Patients with MCPH tend to be happy children with reasonable motor coordination. They can be taught daily living skills and may have some ability to read and write. Life expectancy is normal.

DISORDERS OF NEURONAL MIGRATION

A number of defects in neuronal migration have been identified. A complete review is beyond the scope of this chapter; here, four defects will be discussed. One of these defects, subcortical band heterotopia, shares a genetic basis with lissencephaly 1[9].

Definition

Periventricular nodular heterotopia

Ectopic neurons occur, located along the wall of the lateral ventricles, often bilaterally (**200**). Heterotopias also may occur as a single lesion adjacent to the ventricle or in the superficial white matter.

Lissencephaly 1

In classical lissencephaly or type 1 lissencephaly, the brain is nearly devoid of gyri and the cortical mantle is thickened (pachygyria) (**201**). The brain therefore has a smooth surface due to the absence or near absence of gyri. Microscopically, the brain lacks the normal six-layered structure of the cortex. A variety of disorders are associated with this appearance.

ARX spectrum disorders

These result in X-linked mental retardation in males, due to a defect in radial and tangential migration of gamma aminobutyric acid (GABA)ergic neurons and early cholinergic neurons.

Subcortical band heterotopia

Heterotopic neurons form a thick band of gray matter that may be circumferential or more limited to either the fontal or occipital poles (**202**). Heterotopic neurons are positioned midway between the outer molecular layer and the deep ventricular zone.

Epidemiology

Periventricular nodular heterotopia

- Autosomal recessive and an X-linked dominant form are described.
- X-linked form is lethal in males.
- A number of syndromes are included (e.g. frontal, frontoparietal, perisylvian, parasagittal, and generalized heterotopia syndromes).
- Genetic disorders are now described with heterotopias.

Lissencephaly 1

This is an autosomal dominant disorder, with three clinical phenotypes:

- Miller-Dieker phenotype is due to a large deletion of the *LIS1* gene and neighboring genes.
- Isolated lissencephaly is due to a small deletion or mutation in the *LIS1* gene.
- X-linked with abnormal genitalia (XLAG) is due to a mutation in the *ARX* homeobox gene.

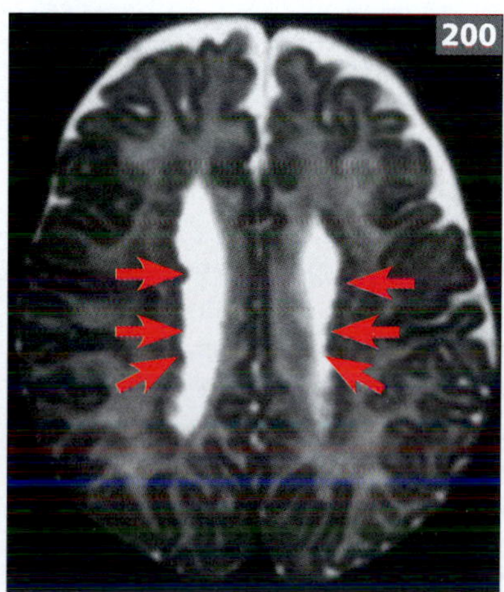

200 Periventricular nodular heterotopia. T2-weighted axial MRI of the brain, showing gray matter ependymal nodules along the ventricular surface (arrows).

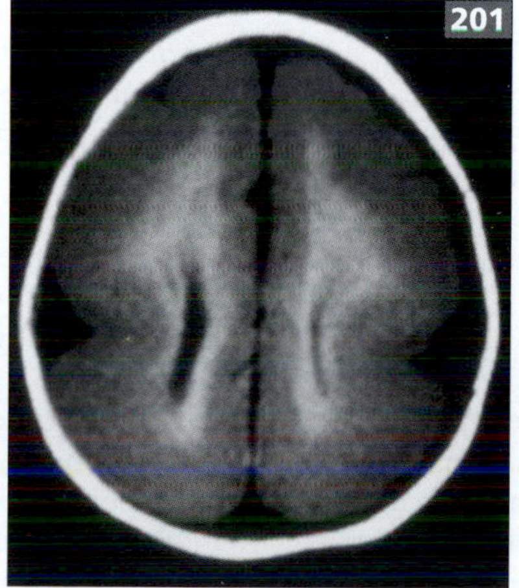

201 Lissencephaly. Axial T1-weighted MRI of the brain, showing a thickened cortical mantle with few gyri.

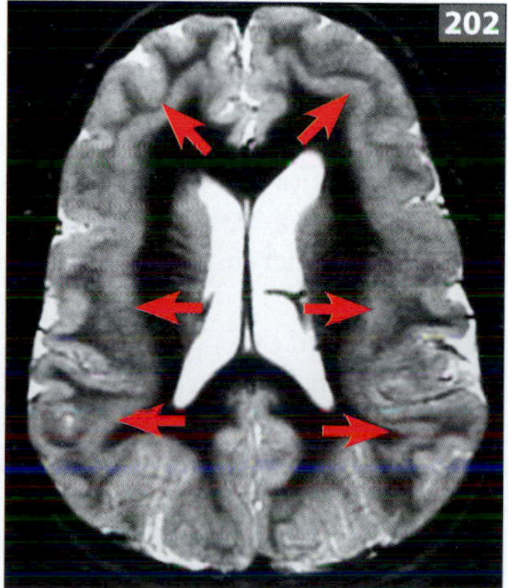

202 Subcortical band heterotopia. Axial inversion recovery MRI of the brain, showing a circumferential band of gray matter (arrows) between the cortex and the ventricular surface.

Most Lis1 mutations are *de novo*, with a low risk of recurrence. However, some parents have a balanced translocation involving the Lis1 gene with a higher risk of recurrence. Patients with lissencephaly may also have a mutation in the *DCX* gene or in the *TUBA1A* gene. The *DCX* gene is located on the X chromosome; a mutation in one of the X chromosomes in females results in subcortical band heterotopia (discussed below), whereas males inheriting the *DCX* mutation have classical lissencephaly. *TUBA1A* mutations are autosomal dominant disorders. Three-quarters of the patients with classical lissencephaly have a mutation either in the *LIS1* gene or the *DCX* gene.

ARX spectrum disorders

These occur in as many as 7% of families with X-linked mental retardation. Female carriers may have some changes.

Subcortical band heterotopia

Predominantly females with a mutation in the *DCX* gene located on the X chromosome (see discussion of lissencephaly above).

Etiology and pathophysiology

Periventricular nodular heterotopia

Females with the X-linked form appear to have a somatic mosaic phenotype due to random X chromosome inactivation.

- Neurons that express the mutant X chromosome fail to migrate.
- All X-linked and most sporadic cases have a mutation in the filamin 1 gene which encodes an actin-binding protein which is essential for neuronal migration.
- A second gene, *ARFGEF2*, has been shown to be defective in some patients.

Pathology shows:

- Rounded nodules of neurons that are often confluent are found along the walls of the lateral ventricles.
- The number and size of nodules vary.
- Cortex is otherwise normal in appearance.

Lissencephaly 1

The lissencephaly genes Lis1, DCX, and TUBA1A encode proteins closely related to microtubules. A network of microtubules is critical to neuronal migration. Migrating neurons extend processes along a framework of radial glia. The centrosome and nucleus of the neurons are pulled along the process. Microtubules are essential to the movement of the centrosome and nucleus, thereby controlling neuronal migration.

Pathology shows:

- The cortex is smooth and gyri are either absent or severely reduced.
- The cortical mantle is thickened.
- Microscopically, there is a four-layered cortex. The fourth layer is a broad band of disorganized neurons and the white matter may contain neuronal heterotopia.

ARX spectrum disorders

A wide variety of phenotypes are seen; some patients have no visible malformations, while the most severely affected patients have lissencephaly, hydranencephaly, and agenesis of the corpus callosum.

A mutation, deletion, insertion, or duplication in the *ARX* gene that is involved in ventral telencephalic morphogenesis, migration of GABAergic neuron progenitors, and early cholinergic neurons. There is a polyalanine tract insertion. Severity increases with the length of the polyalanine tract insertion.

Subcortical band heterotopia

Mutation in the *DCX* gene (see discussion of lissencephaly above). Pathology shows:

- Bands of gray matter in the white matter are present between the cortex and the lateral ventricles.
- The cortex is fairly normal in appearance, except for rather shallow sulci.

Clinical features

Periventricular nodular heterotopia

- The spectrum of severity is quite wide and to some degree correlates with the extent of the heterotopia.
- Most patients have seizures which often come to attention in adolescence.
- Seizures vary from mild to severe and intractable.
- Cognitive impairment can be mild.
- No motor impairment is present.

Lissencephaly 1

Patients with the Miller–Dieker phenotype have a dysmorphic appearance that includes a prominent forehead, bitemporal hollowing, short nose, protuberant upper lip, and small jaw. Other associated anomalies are present, such as omphalocele and cardiac defects. Isolated lissencephaly patients are without dysmorphic features. All lissencephaly patients have profound mental retardation, motor impairment, and seizures. The seizures are usually severe and intractable, with onset in infancy.

ARX spectrum disorders

At least 10 different clinical phenotypes have been described. The cardinal feature is X-linked intellectual disability that is usually severe. Patients are usually divided into the nonmalformation group and the malformation group.

Nonmalformation patients have intractable epilepsy (often starting as infantile spasms), dystonic movements, and dysarthria or failure to speak. Some patients show marked difficulty with use of their hands. Malformation patients have profound mental retardation, intractable epilepsy, and a variety of brain abnormalities including agenesis of the corpus callosum, lissencephaly, and even hydranencephaly. Patients with lissencephaly may also have ambiguous genitalia.

Subcortical band heterotopia

The clinical course can be similar to lissencephaly 1, but the severity can be mild in some patients. There are no dysmorphic features.

Investigations and diagnosis

- MRI of the brain is diagnostic.
- EEG is useful in characterizing seizures.
- Chromosomal and genetic studies to exclude other conditions associated with lissencephaly.

Treatment

Treatment is symptomatic. Patients with periventricular nodular heterotopia may only require treatment for seizures. Patients with subcortical band heterotopia may also only require treatment of seizures, although some may need additional support. Patients with lissencephaly 1 are more severely affected and usually require:

- Gastrostomy tubes and nutritional support.
- Physical and occupational therapy.
- Surgical treatment of seizures may be useful in patients with focal heterotopias.

Prognosis

Prognosis is defined by the severity of seizures. Patients with periventicular nodular heterotopia tend to have a milder course. Patients with lissencephaly, *ARX* spectrum, and subcortical band heterotopia have a more severe clinical course with intractable seizures and significant motor and cognitive impairment which contribute to a reduced life expectancy.

DISORDERS OF CORTICAL ORGANIZATION

The defects in this section are characterized by excessive migration of neurons, differentiating them from conditions such as periventricular nodular heterotopia, where some neurons fail to migrate from the ventricular zone. Thus, the defect seems to be a failure to arrest normal neuronal migration.

Definition

Polymicrogyria

Excessive numbers of small prominent convolutions are present, giving the brain a lumpy appearance. Two major varieties of polymicrogyria are described: layered (with a four-layered cortex), and nonlayered (often associated with heterotopias). Polymicrogyria can be diffuse or focal.

Schizencephaly

Unilateral or bilateral clefts in the brain are present that extend to the ventricles. Clefts result in communication between the ventricle and the subarachnoid space. The cleft is lined with polymicrogyric cortex (**203**).

Epidemiology

Polymicrogyria

- Seen in association with other brain malformations such as heterotopia.
- Six distinct syndromes are seen (two of the most common will be discussed).

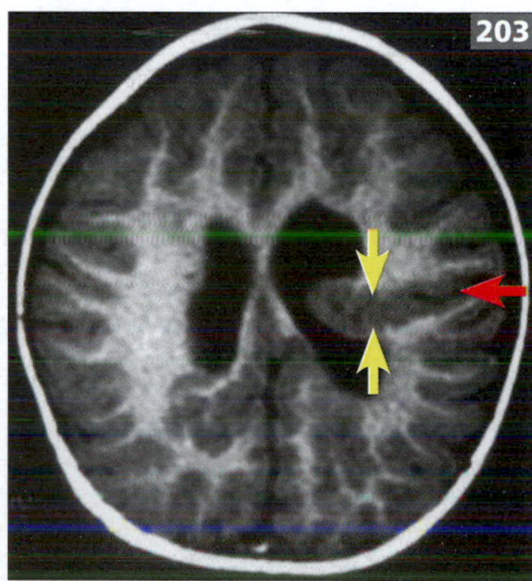

203 Schizencephaly. Axial T1-weighted MRI of the brain, showing a cleft (red arrow) extending from the ventricle to the surface of the cortex. The cleft is lined with polymicrogyric cortex (yellow arrows).

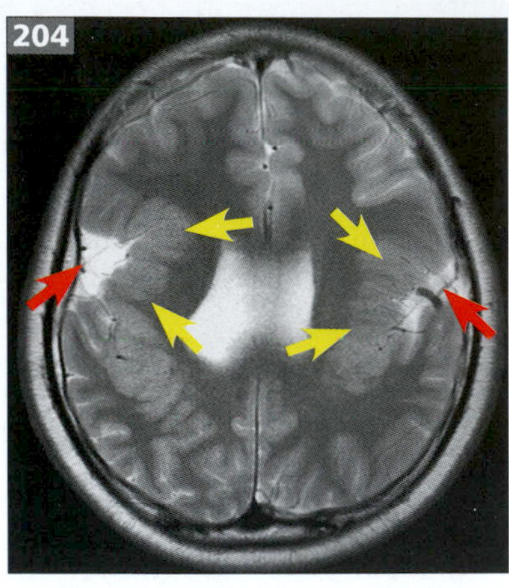

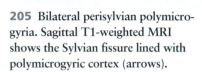

204 Bilateral perisylvian polymicrogyria. T2-weighted axial MRI of brain, showing deep Sylvian fissures (red arrows) lined with polymicrogyric cortex (yellow arrows).

205 Bilateral perisylvian polymicrogyria. Sagittal T1-weighted MRI shows the Sylvian fissure lined with polymicrogyric cortex (arrows).

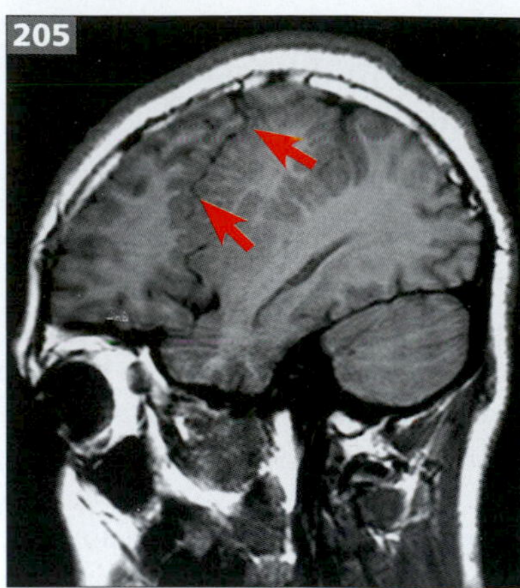

Bilateral perisylvian polymicrogyria
Variable inheritance patterns, including autosomal recessive and dominant and X-linked dominant and recessive (204, 205).

Bilateral frontal polymicrogyria
Primarily a sporadic condition, although there is one report of autosomal recessive inheritance. Both conditions are uncommon but the true incidence is unknown.

Schizencephaly
This is a rare condition, predominantly sporadic although at least one familial case is reported.

Tips

- *Schizencephaly must be distinguished from porencephaly.*
- *In porencephaly, an ischemic injury results in destruction of tissue between the lateral ventricle and the surface of the brain resulting in an open channel, while in schizencephaly there is a deep cleft that communicates with the lateral ventricle and is lined with cortex; this lining is the key distinguishing feature.*
- *The clinical features and prognosis of the two conditions are quite different, with schizencephaly having a much more severe outcome.*

Etiology and pathophysiology

Polymicrogyria
Genetic loci have been identified in some patients. Toxins including hypoxia, congenital infection, and carbon monoxide poisoning have also been implicated.

Excessive numbers of small convolutions with shallow and enlarged sulci are present. Cortical folding is irregular due to packing of the microgyri. Histologically, there are two types: layered, which shows a four-layered cortex with a layer of laminar necrosis; and nonlayered, in which the molecular layer is continuous and does not follow the profile of the convolutions and the neurons have a radial distribution without a laminar organization.

Schizencephaly
Familial cases may have mutations in the *EMX2* gene that is implicated in patterning of the developing forebrain. Toxins are suggested to be the predominant cause. Pathology shows a deep cleft, either unilateral or bilateral, extending the full thickness of the brain. The walls of the cleft are usually widely separated, and the clefts are commonly in the perisylvian area.The cortex lining the clefts is polymicrogyric.

Clinical features

Polymicrogyria
Clinical manifestations depend in part on the extent of the abnormality. Virtually all patients have seizures. Patients with bilateral perisylvian polymicrogyria typically have impairment of oral motor function and dysarthria. Most have mental retardation and some have severe generalized motor dysfunction, but severity varies widely. Patients with bilateral frontal polymicrogyria have developmental delay and seizures.

Schizencephaly
- Microcephaly.
- Intractable seizures.
- Severe intellectual and motor impairment, cortical blindness.

Investigations and diagnosis

- Diagnosis is made on the basis of MRI of the brain.
- EEG is useful in characterizing seizures.
- Since polymicrogyria can be found in other conditions, those need to be excluded.

Treatment

Treatment is symptomatic. Seizures are the main complication of these disorders which requires treatment. Severely impaired children require gastrostomy and nutritional supplementation.

Prognosis

Prognosis is determined in part by the severity of the seizures and degree of motor impairment. It is variable in polymicrogyria. In schizencephaly the impairments are invariably severe and life span is shortened.

NEUROCUTANEOUS DISORDERS

The neurocutaneous disorders present a very different spectrum of problems compared to the malformations of the nervous system. However, there are areas of overlap. Many malformations of the nervous system involve poor regulation of cell division and proliferation, which is also an essential problem in the neurocutaneous disorders. Moreover, several of the neurocutaneous disorders, particularly tuberous sclerosis, neurofibromatosis type 1 (NF-1), incontinentia pigmenti, hypomelanosis of Ito, the linear sebaceous nevus syndrome, and Lhermitte–Duclos disease are associated with brain lesions caused by abnormal neuronal migration or organization.

Activation of mTOR pathway

The neurocutaneous disorders are a heterogeneous group that, at first glance, has little in common other than involvement of both skin and brain. The association of skin and nervous system defects can be understood at least in part because both are derived from the embryonic ectoderm. However, as we develop a greater molecular understanding of these conditions, it is apparent that most of the neurocutaneous disorders involve activation of the signaling components, both upstream and downstream of the protein kinase mammalian target of rapamycin (mTOR) (**206**). Upstream of mTOR, the key signaling molecules are p21 Ras GTPase, Raf, Mek, Erk, the lipid kinase PI3K, the Akt kinase,TSC1/TSC2, and the GTPase Rheb. Downstream are the pathways for angiogenesis, protein translation, gene amplification, and cell cycling. Defects in these signaling molecules and pathways are the basis for tuberous sclerosis, NF-1, Proteus syndrome, Cowden syndrome, Lhermitte–Duclos, and von Hippel–Lindau disease[10].

Tip

▶ *All of the neurocutaneous disorders are progressive, implying: individual complications may worsen over time; complications are age specific, with different complications occurring at different times.*

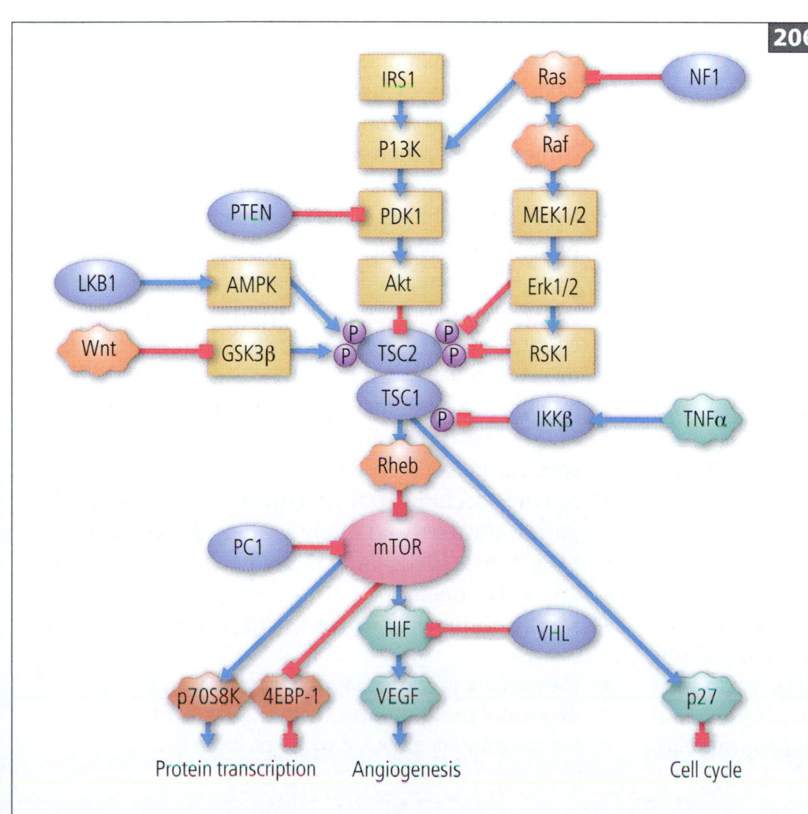

206 The mammalian rapamycin target (mTOR) signaling pathway, showing key signaling molecules upstream of mTOR including Ras, the lipid kinase PI3K, the AKt kinase, and the GTPase Rheb, which are all known to be deregulated in different human cancers. Mutations in the mTOR component genes, *TSC1, TSC2, LKB1, PTEN, VHL, NF1, PKD1* (*PC1*), and *IKK*, result in the development of tuberous sclerosis, Peutz–Jeghers syndrome, Cowden syndrome, Bannayan–Riley–Ruvalcaba syndrome, Lhermitte–Duclos disease, Proteus syndrome, von Hippel–Lindau disease, neurofibromatosis type 1, polycystic kidney disease, and incontinentia pigmenti, respectively. Activation of the PI3K–Akt pathway and increased vascular endothelial growth factor (VEGF) receptors are implicated in neurofibromatosis 2. HIF: hypoxia-inducible factor; TNF: tumor necrosis factor.

NEUROFIBROMATOSIS TYPE 1

Definition and epidemiology

NF-1 is a common autosomal dominant disorder, presenting with hyperpigmented macules of the skin (café-au-lait spots). There is multi-system involvement including frequent learning problems, bony abnormalities, eye abnormalities (optic gliomas and iris Lisch nodules), and an increased risk of cancer. Tumours of the peripheral nerves (cutaneous or dermal neurofibromas) and tumors of nerve trunks and roots (plexiform neurofibromas) occur.

The incidence of NF-1 is 1 in 2500 to 3000 live births. NF-1 is an autosomal dominant disorder that equally affects males and females. It is reported in all racial and ethnic groups, although it may occur less frequently in people of Middle Eastern descent. Manifestations of NF-1 are often apparent at birth and become more apparent in the first several years of life. One-half of all cases are spontaneous mutations.

Etiology and pathogenesis

NF-1 is due to a defect in a gene on chromosome 17q that encodes the protein neurofibromin, a Ras guanosine triphosphate (GTP)ase activating protein (Ras GAP). Neurofibromin stimulates the hydrolysis of GTP bound to p21 Ras, converting it to the inactive state. Active Ras stimulates cell growth and proliferation and is part of the mTOR signaling pathway. Neurofibromin expression is ubiquitous but is particularly prominent in the nervous system. NF1 is a disorder of poorly regulated cell growth and proliferation, i.e. increased growth and proliferation, thought to be secondary to excessive stimulation of Ras[11].

The cardinal pathologic feature is a *neurofibroma* which is a tumor of the nerve consisting of a proliferation of Schwann cells, fibroblasts, mast cells, blood vessels, and extracellular matrix with nerve fibers running through the tumor mass. Neurofibromas can occur along small nerve fibers, spinal roots, plexi, nerve trunks, and autonomic nerves. Dermal neurofibromas are well circumscribed tumors in the skin. Plexiform neurofibromas are similar, but contain more extracellular matrix and sometimes appear in grape-like clusters distorting large nerves. Plexiform neurofibromas may be well circumscribed or highly invasive and infiltrative.

Clinical features

The clinical features are highly variable even within the same pedigree, and virtually any organ system can be affected. There are a large number of potential complications, but some are quite rare. The complications of NF-1 are age specific, which helps greatly in assessing and counseling patients. The major complications/features are listed below.

Skin

- Café-au-lait spots are hyperpigmented macules that must be at least 0.5 cm in children and ≥1.5 cm in adults and are found in virtually all patients (**207**).
- Freckling,small hyperpigmented macules in areas protected from the sun such as the groin or axilla.
- Cutaneous or dermal neurofibromas: start as small, raised, soft papules or sometimes as purplish depressible macules along small nerve fibers and can enlarge over time to become pedunculated or even pendular (**207**). Cutaneous neurofibromas occur in late teenage or adult years in virtually all patients, but the number varies tremendously in different patients.
- Plexiform neurofibromas sometimes involve the skin, underlying muscle, and nerve and often involve large nerves or the sympathetic chains (**208–210**). They are congenital. Including very small ones, they are found in 50% of patients. Large plexiform neurofibromas occur in <20%[12].

Brain

- High intensity signals seen on MRI in the basal ganglia, thalamus, pons, and cerebellum, are commonly called unidentified bright obects (UBOs) that are prominent in some children and tend to disappear in adult years (**211**).
- Grade I astrocytomas in the cortex, white matter, optic tracts, hypothalamus, and brainstem are found in 3–15% of patients and may regress over time. They are rarely symptomatic (**211**).
- Grade III and IV gliomas are an uncommon complication primarily of young adults. The most common location is in the cerebellum.
- Learning problems occur in as many as 60% of patients and include specific learning disabilities as well as attention deficit hyperactivity disorder (ADHD) and other executive function problems. Mental retardation is uncommon and occurs in no more than 6% but there can be a general lowering of intelligence quotient (IQ), albeit within the normal range. There are some patients who have autistic spectrum disorder.
- Seizures occur in 10% of patients and are usually partial complex and rarely are difficult to control.
- Headaches, particularly migraines, occur in at least 15% of patients.
- Stroke occurs in less than 1% of patients (see vascular disease).
- Dysarthria is common in early childhood and improves with therapy.

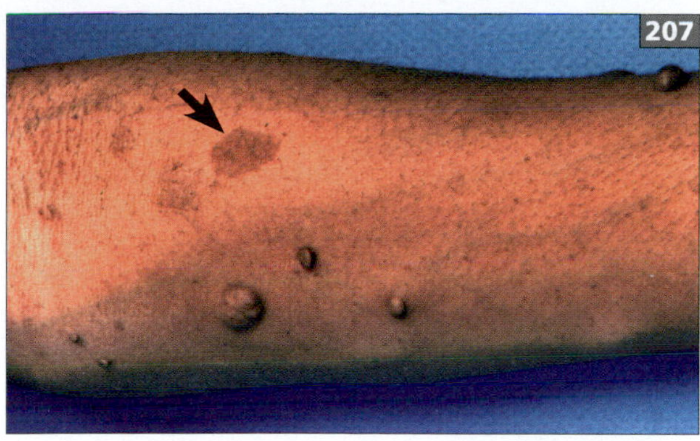

207 Café-au-lait spot (arrow) and several pedunculated dermal neurofibromas on the forearm of a patient with neurofibromatosis type 1.

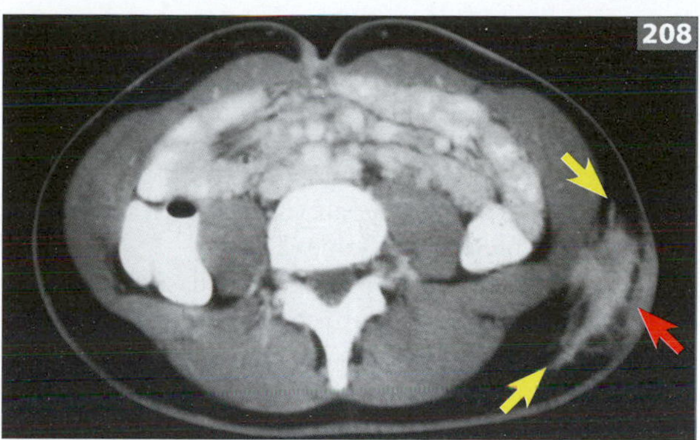

208 Superficial plexiform neurofibroma. CT of the abdomen showing an area of increased signal on the left side of the patient's flank in the subcutaneous fat with some thickening of the skin (red arrow). The plexiform neurofibroma has thin 'fingers' that extend to the limit of the abdominal musculature (yellow arrows).

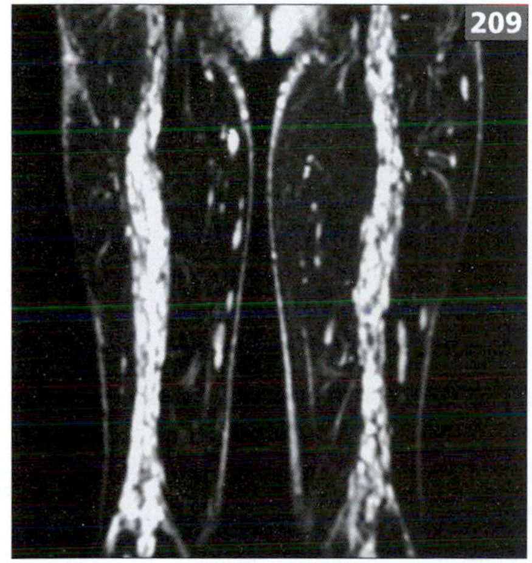

209 MRI of the proximal legs, showing nodular clusters of plexiform neurofibromas along the length of both sciatic nerves, with a number of isolated intramuscular and cutaneous neurofibromas that are visualized by increased signal intensity.

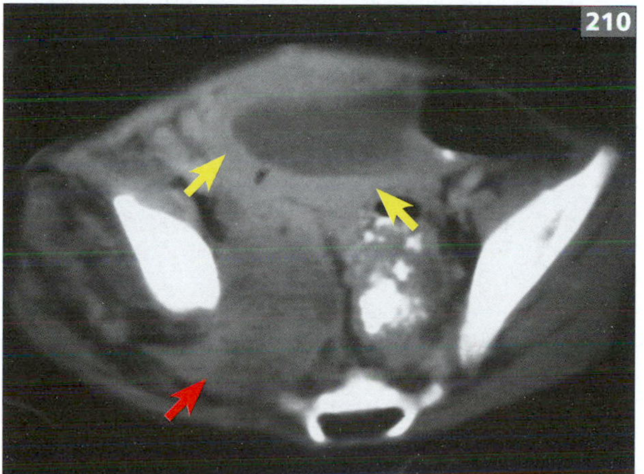

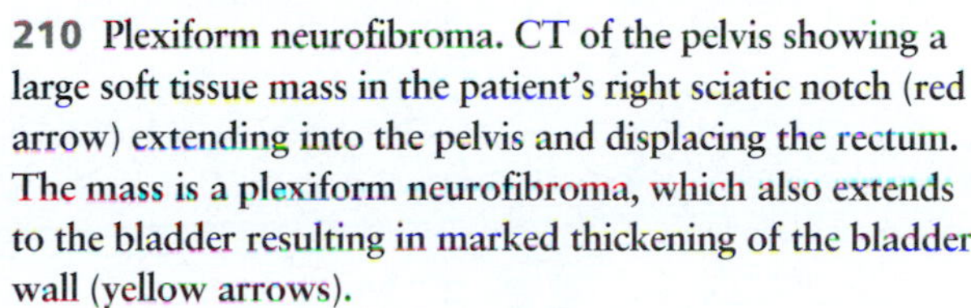

210 Plexiform neurofibroma. CT of the pelvis showing a large soft tissue mass in the patient's right sciatic notch (red arrow) extending into the pelvis and displacing the rectum. The mass is a plexiform neurofibroma, which also extends to the bladder resulting in marked thickening of the bladder wall (yellow arrows).

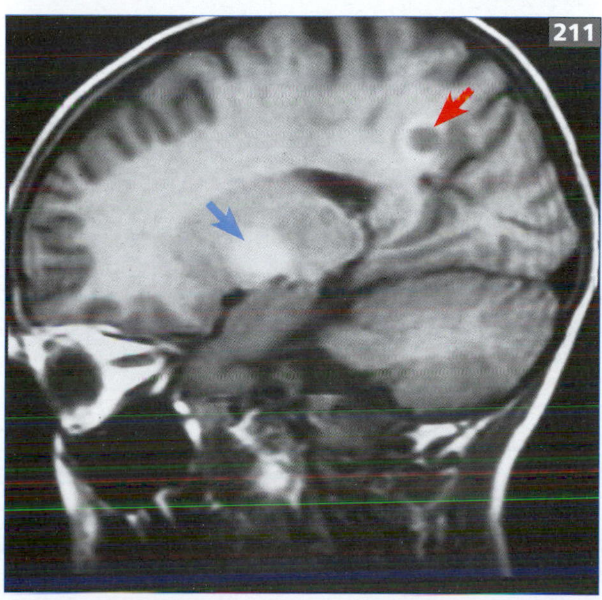

211 Grade I glioma and unidentified bright object (UBO) in neurofibromatosis type 1. Sagittal T1-weighted MRI of brain, showing a target-like grade I glioma (red arrow) and an area of increased signal in the basal ganglia (blue arrow) commonly called a UBO.

Eye

- Optic gliomas are grade I astrocytomas found in 15% of patients, with onset typically between 18 months and 8 years of age. These are generally nonprogressive lesions and do not cause visual problems, but in 20%, they grow and impair vision, even leading to functional blindness in some (**212**)[13].
- Iris Lisch nodules are hyperpgimented, slightly raised macules on the iris that appear in early teenage to young adult years and are not associated with any visual disturbance. In brown-eyed patients, Lisch nodules appear hypopigmented. They are found in 85–90% of adults (**213**).

Cardiovascular

- Hypertension in infants and children is usually attributable to renal artery stenosis and can be difficult to control in some patients. Hypertension in young adults may be caused by pheochromocytoma which is found in approximately 1% of adults.
- Vascular disease occurs in 3% of patients and includes renal artery stenosis (commonly involving the aorta, femoral artery, renal artery and its branches, and sometimes the superior mesenteric artery). The carotid arteries may also be involved with complete occlusion either unilaterally or bilaterally with a moyamoya pattern and stroke (**214, 215**). Vascular malformations occasionally occur, which can rupture causing massive hemorrhage.
- Pulmonic stenosis is seen in as many as 15%.

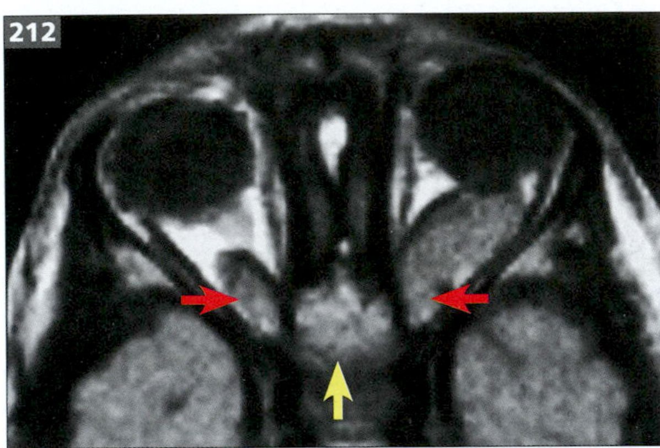

212 Optic glioma. Axial T1-weighted MRI of the brain through the orbits, showing markedly enlarged optic nerves bilaterally (red arrows) as well as an enlarged optic chiasm (yellow arrow).

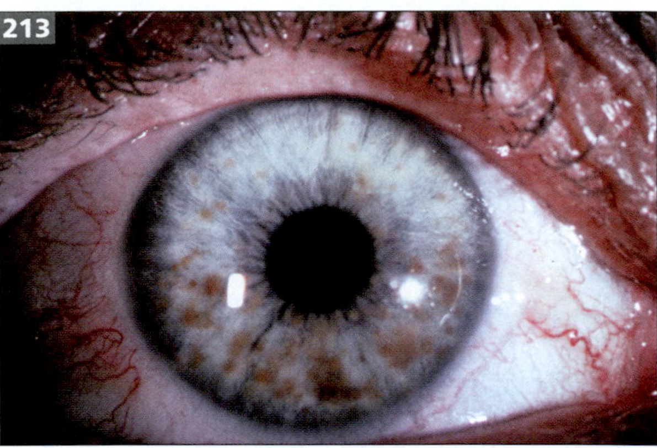

213 Lisch nodules. Photograph of the eye of a patient with neurofibromatosis type 1 showing a large number of reddish brown spots predominantly in the lower pole of the iris.

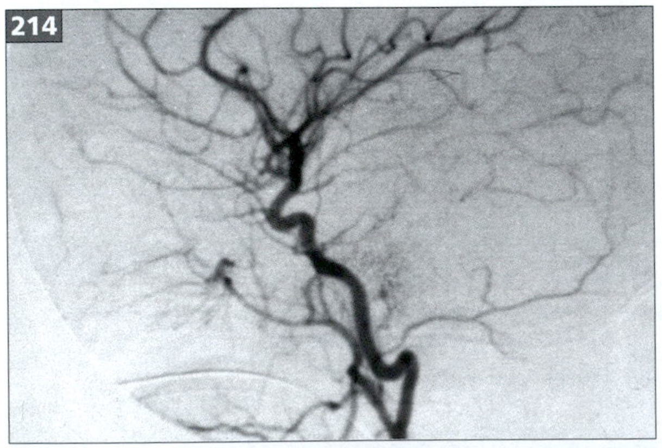

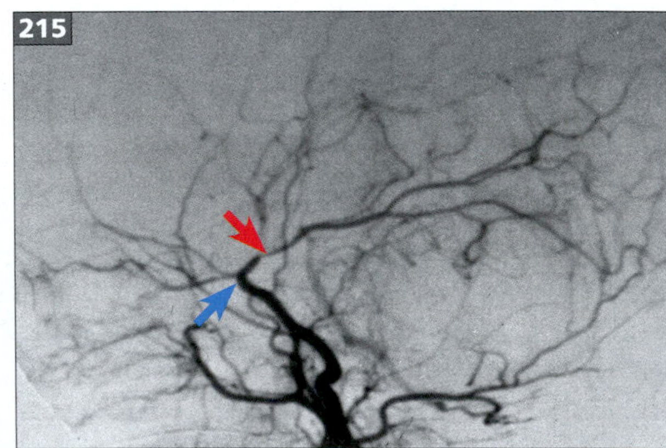

214, 215 Vascular disease in neurofibromatosis type 1. (214) Normal angiogram of the left internal carotid artery. (215) Angiogram of the right internal carotid artery of the same patient, showing an abrupt occlusion (red arrow) with absence of the anterior cerebral artery (blue arrow) and middle cerebral artery branches, with retrograde filling of the posterior cerebral artery.

Skeletal/orthopedic

- Hypotonia and problems with fine and gross motor co-ordination occur in 60% of patients.
- Significant scoliosis occurs in at least 3%, with milder scoliosis in as many as an additional 10%. There are at least four clinical presentations:
  - A severe, rapidly progressive, so-called dystrophic type (**216**) that presents between 3 and 5 years of age.
  - Secondary to erosion and instability of vertebrae from paraspinal plexiform neurofibromas or dural ectasias, that frequently manifests in adolescence or adult years.
  - Benign scoliosis of teenage years.
  - Subtle scoliosis that rarely becomes clinically significant and may only be seen on spine films.
- Dystrophic abnormalities of long bones, particularly the tibia and fibula, occur in 1–3% (**217**). This is usually detectable at birth and leads to bowing and fracture. A progressive reabsorption of bone, primarily the sphenoid wing of the orbit, but sometimes the mandible, occurs in <1% of patients and is usually apparent in childhood (**218**).
- Decreased bone density occurs in some patients.

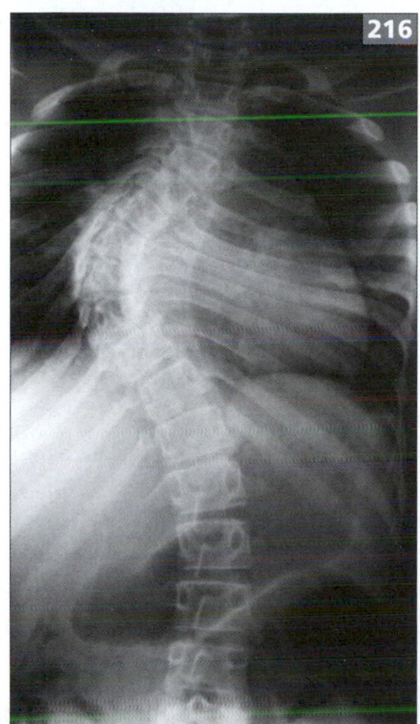

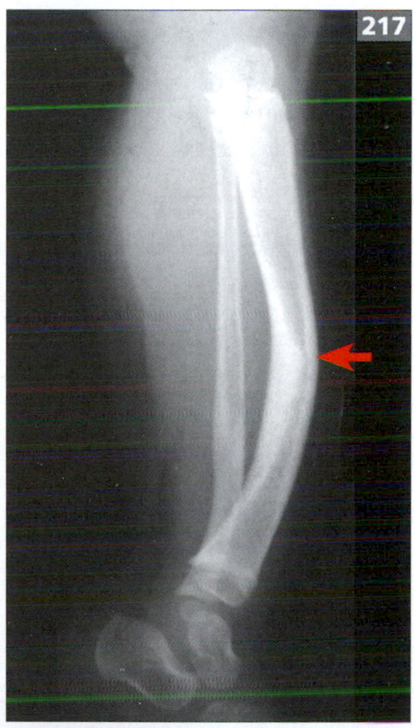

216 Anterior–posterior chest X-ray, showing marked scoliosis characteristic of the dystrophic scoliosis seen in neurofibromatosis type 1.

217 Lateral view X-ray of the tibia and fibula, showing anterior bowing and narrowing of the intramedullary canal (red arrow).

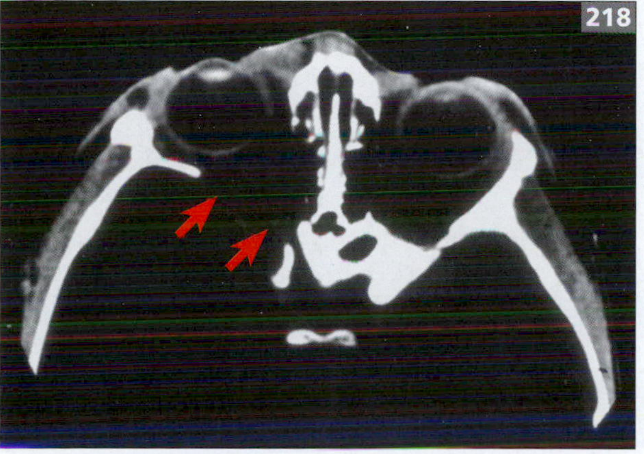

218 Bone windows of CT of the orbits, showing absence of a portion of the back of the orbit on the right (arrows) due to hypoplasia of the sphenoid wing.

Endocrine/growth

- Pheochromocytoma occurs in <1%.
- Thyroid tumors are seen in <1%.
- Precocious puberty may occur in patients with optic gliomas.
- Macrocephaly and short stature are common.
- Spinal cord, nerve roots, nerve trunks, and autonomic nervous system are affected. Plexiform neurofibromas commonly involve the dorsal roots of the spine, as well as nerve trunks and plexi and the sympathetic chains. Some form of plexiform neurofibroma occurs in 50% of patients. Common locations are the sympathetic chain in the neck, the dorsal roots, the pelvic or sacral plexus, the sciatic and femoral nerves, and the brachial plexus.
- Spinal compression can result from dumb-bell-shaped growth of paraspinal plexiform neurofibromas, particularly in the high cervical spinal cord (**219, 220**).
- Dural ectasias occur in the thoracic and sacral cord in <1% of patients. This appears to be a defect in the formation of the dura, which, while intact, can be quite large and associated with pain.

Malignancies

There is an increased risk of true malignancy of approximately 3% over the general population. Between 6 and 10% of patients develop malignant peripheral nerve sheath tumors which are highly malignant tumors that develop within plexiform neurofibromas, usually between the ages of 15 and 50 years (**221**). Uncommon types of cancer, such as pheochromocytoma and thyroid cancer, occur with increased frequency, as do malignant brain tumors, although all of the tumor types are infrequent. There may be an increased incidence of breast cancer in women[14].

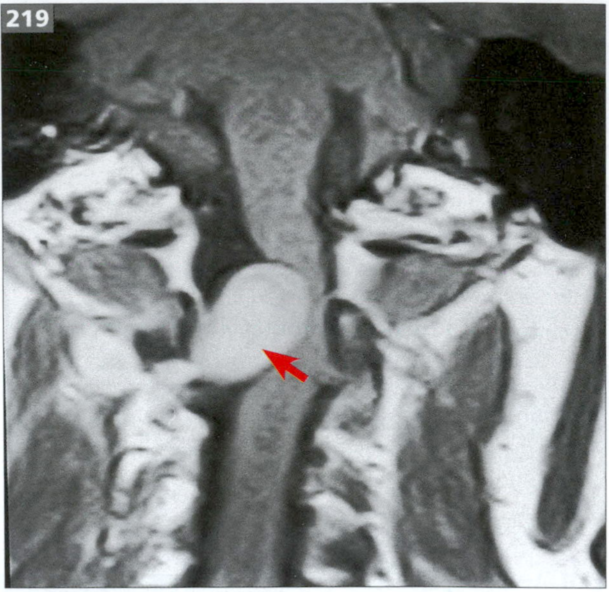

219 Cervical cord compression. Coronal T1-weighted image of the cervical spine after gadolinium, showing a dumbbell-shaped paraspinal plexiform neurofibroma (arrow) extending into the dural space and compressing the spinal cord at C2.

220 Cervical cord compression. Axial T1-weighted image of the cervical spine after gadolinium, showing a paraspinal plexiform neurofibroma extending through the neural foramen (red arrows), displacing the spinal cord at C2.

221 Malignant peripheral nerve sheath tumor. Axial CT view of the abdomen, showing a large heterogeneous paraspinal mass (arrows) in the lumbar area. The mass is a plexiform neurofibroma. Only a small portion of the tumor immediately adjacent to the lumbar spine showed a high-grade malignancy.

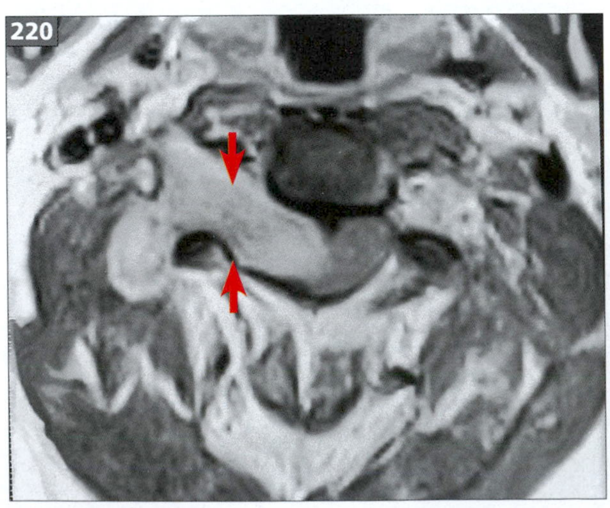

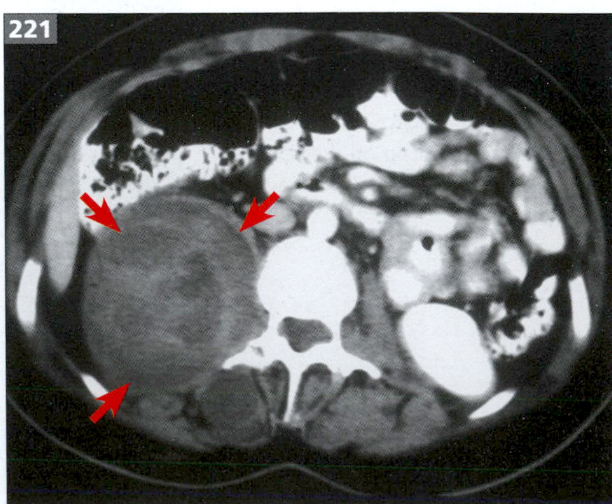

Investigations

Investigations are largely for symptomatic patients. Routine imaging for screening purposes is not recommended because many lesions remain asymptomatic, and if an asymptomatic abnormality is discovered, it is not clear how often imaging would need to be done. Following lesions of uncertain significance can lead to substantial anxiety.

Brain

The intellectual development of patients with NF-1 should be monitored carefully. Formal developmental or neuropsychological testing is important if there is a suggestion of developmental delay or school problems. Imaging of the brain is not recommended unless patients are symptomatic. Seizures can sometimes be subtle. If there are staring episodes or sleep disturbances, a 24-hour EEG is recommended.

Eye

Regular annual eye examinations to measure acuity and the appearance of the optic nerve are recommended in all patients between the ages of 18 months and 10 years. Significant deterioration in acuity needs to be assessed by MRI.

Cardiovascular

Hypertension in children requires a CT angiogram of the kidneys. Since patients with renal artery stenosis also have cerebral vascular disease, a brain MR angiogram (MRA) may also be warranted. Young adults with hypertension should be screened for pheochromocytoma with a test for blood catecholamines.

Skeletal/orthopedic

If there is any suggestion of bowing of the long bones, particularly the tibia, within the first year of life, plain X-rays will reveal a pseudarthrosis. Any evidence of spinal curvature should also be investigated by X-ray. Muscle or skeletal pain is an unusual complaint and should be investigated, preferably with MRI. Disturbances in gait or paresthesias may indicate spinal cord compression and should be evaluated by spine MRI.

Diagnosis

The diagnosis of NF-1 can usually be made clinically, and frequently at birth. Since café-au-lait spots and freckling may increase or appear over time, the diagnosis is sometimes delayed until 5–6 years of age. The diagnosis of NF-1 requires at least two of the following:

- Six or more café-au-lait spots that are ≥0.5 cm in diameter in pre-pubertal patients, or ≥1.5 cm in diameter in post-pubertal patients.
- Freckling in the axilla or groin area.
- Two or more cutaneous neurofibromas.
- One plexiform neurofibroma.
- Two or more iris Lisch nodules.
- An optic glioma.
- Characteristic bony lesions: sphenoid wing hypoplasia, dystrophic scoliosis, or a pseudarthrosis.
- A first-degree relative with NF-1.

The diagnosis can be confirmed by genetic testing with at least 95% accuracy. Genetic testing can also identify patients with mosaicisms, large deletions, and some mutations that can help to predict the clinical course.

Treatment

Treatment is symptomatic at the present time. However, it is important to institute a regular regime of annual examinations to detect complications. Since the complications are age specific, it is possible to focus on different problems at different ages[15].

- Birth and infancy:
  - Check long bones.
  - Look for externally visible plexiform neurofibromas.
  - Monitor developmental milestones.
- Early childhood:
  - Monitor language and developmental milestones.
  - Check spine for scoliosis.
  - Annual eye examination.
  - Check blood pressure.
- Childhood:
  - Monitor learning, attention span, and socialization.
  - Annual eye examination.
  - Check spine for scoliosis.
- Teenage years:
  - Monitor learning and socialization.
  - Check for cutaneous neurofibromas.
- Adults:
  - Check for hypertension.
  - Check for cutaneous neurofibromas.
  - Investigate any cause of pain.
  - Genetic counseling/family planning.
  - Surgical removal of visible and stigmatizing cutaneous tumors is appropriate. Careful debulking or even complete removal of plexiform neurofibromas is possible in some patients.
  - Speech therapy, neuropsychological testing, physical and occupational therapy, tutoring, and help with learning disabilities are all important parts of care.

Prognosis

The majority of patients can lead normal and productive lives. NF-1 is associated with a mildly shortened life span because of the incidence of malignancy in young adults. Large numbers of cutaneous neurofibromas or large visible plexiform neurofibromas may seriously affect function and socialization in a small percentage of patients.

Large plexiform neurofibromas will sometimes produce pain. A larger problem is recognizing and effectively treating learning problems.

NEUROFIBROMATOSIS TYPE 2

Definition and epidemiology

NF-2 is a genetic disorder characterized by multiple CNS tumors. The hallmark is VIIIth nerve tumors (vestibular schwannoma), usually bilateral. Tumors of spinal roots, spinal cord, brainstem as well as meningeal-derived tumors are frequent.

Incidence is 1 in 25,000 live births. NF-2 is an autosomal dominant disorder that affects males and females equally. It occurs in all racial and ethnic groups. One-half of all cases are spontaneous mutations, and approximately one-third of nonfamilial cases are due to somatic mosaicisms.

Etiology and pathogenesis

NF-2 is due to a defect in chromosome 22q encoding the protein merlin, which is one of a group of proteins that links actin to cell-surface glycoproteins that control growth and cell remodeling. It acts as a tumor suppressor and regulator of Schwann and meningeal cells, with the highest level of expression in Schwann cells, meningeal cells, peripheral nerves, and the lens. Loss of merlin causes cell proliferation and tumor formation. The exact mechanism is unknown but activation of the P13kinase–AKT pathway is implicated. Merlin is one of the ezra, radixin, moesin (ERM) cytoskeleton proteins.

Schwannoma

- Nodular tumor surrounded by a fibrous capsule consisting of epineurium and some nerve fibers. The tumors are predominantly of Schwann cells with alternating patterns of cellularity.
- Virtually never malignant.
- Usually extrinsic to the nerve and separate from the majority of the axons; when small nerves are involved, the tumor frequently engulfs the nerve, making separation from the nerve difficult.
- Vestibular schwannomas can sometimes be quite large, displacing and compressing the pons, with resulting contralateral motor weakness and cerebellar dysfunction (222).
- Prominent vascular endothelial growth factor (VEGF) receptors on tumors provides an opportunity for treatment using antibodies to VEGF receptors[16].

Meningiomas

- Arise from arachnoid cells of the leptomeninges.
- Predominantly fibrous, but meningothelial tumors also occur.
- Common locations include the orbital ridge, cerebellar pontine angle, interhemispheric fissure, and skull base (223).
- Frequently large, compressing adjacent brain; typically multiple.
- Meningioma en plaque occurs in some patients late in their disease.

Ependymomas, and hamartomas

- Found in as many as one-third of NF-2 patients.
- The most common site for ependymomas is the brainstem or cervical cord and can be associated with syrinx formation (224).
- Hamartomas of the brain are frequent; they are a mixture of Schwann cells, glia, and meningeal cells.

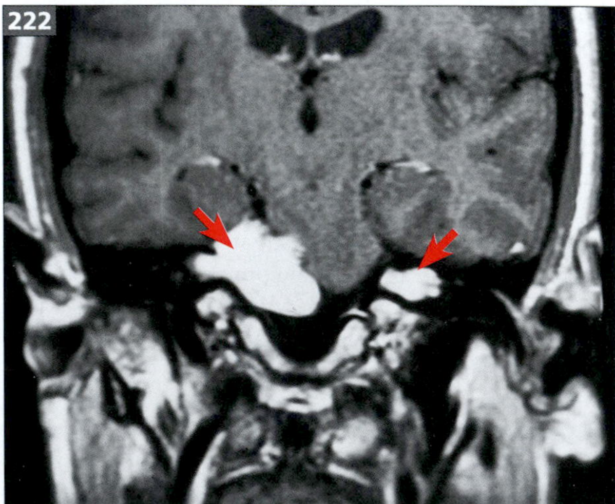

222 Bilateral vestibular schwannomas. Coronal T1-weighted MRI with gadolinium enhancement in a patient with neurofibromatosis type 2, showing bilateral enhancing vestibular nerve tumors (arrows) compressing and displacing the pons.

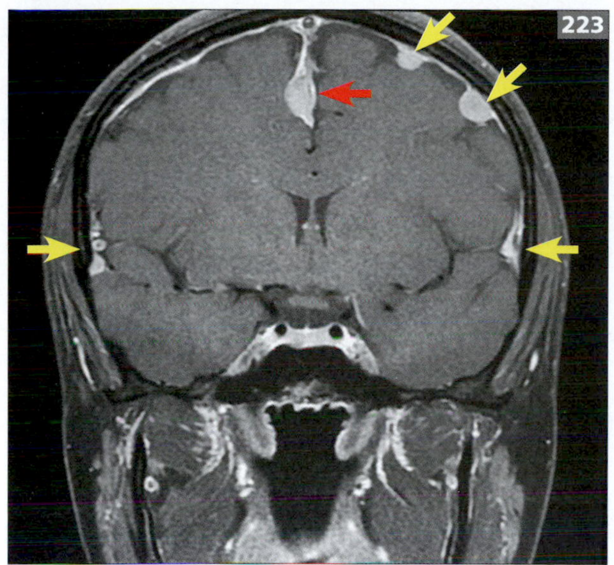

223 Multiple meningiomas. Coronal T1-weighted MRI with gadolinium enhancement, showing a meningioma in the interhemispheric fissure (red arrow) as well as multiple enhancing meningiomas (yellow arrows) attached to the dura in a patient with neurofibromatosis type 2.

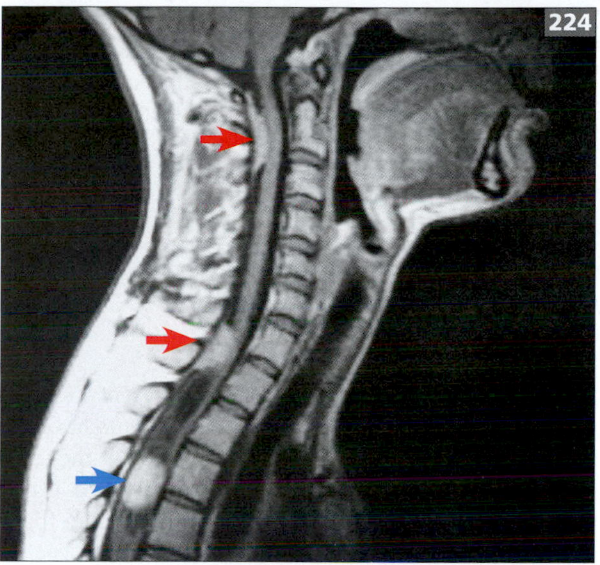

224 Spinal cord lesions in neurofibromatosis type 2. Sagittal T1-weighted MRI of the cervical and thoracic spinal cord with gadolinium enhancement, showing two enhancing extramedullary tumors which are meningiomas (red arrows) and an enhancing intramedullary cervical-cord astrocytoma (blue arrow) with syrinx (beginning at T1).

Clinical features

The mean age of onset is 19 years. Presentation is usually attributable to an VIIIth nerve tumor with hearing loss, often unilateral. Tinnitus, dizziness, and loss of balance are also frequent.

Motor dysfunction typically occurs later in the course. In children, the presentation is quite different with symptoms related to a tumor of the brain, brainstem, or spinal cord. Cataracts, strabismus, and facial weakness can also be presenting signs in children.

NF-2 is a relentlessly progressive disorder but the pace of the progression is quite variable. Some patients have prolonged periods of stability or quiescence.

Hearing loss and vestibular complaints

Hearing loss is progressive and initially unilateral. Because most patients have bilateral vestibular tumors, complete deafness is inevitable. Vertigo as well as tinnitus is common and sometimes debilitating.

Facial weakness

Facial weakness is a frequent iatrogenic complication due to injury of the VIIth nerve after surgery on vestibular nerve tumors. VIIth nerve palsies result in dryness of the eye and potential corneal injury.

Motor impairment

Meningiomas compress adjacent brain and depending on location produce motor dysfunction and corticospinal or cerebellar signs. Ependymoma of the spinal cord will sometimes produce motor weakness and sensory complaints referable to the spinal cord. Extradural meningiomas and schwannomas are commonly found along the spinal cord and are also a source of pain and weakness. Ependymomas commonly affect the lower brainstem and will sometimes produce cranial nerve palsies and motor weakness. Peripheral motor neuropathy is an uncommon association.

Eye

Subcapsular, posterior cataracts occur in most patients. They do not necessarily impair vision. Orbital ridge meningiomas produce proptosis and visual impairment. Retinal hamartomas are common and may affect peripheral vision in some patients.

Strabismus or limitation in eye movement is common due to schwannomas of the VIth or IIIrd cranial nerve. Corneal injury is common because of VIIth nerve injury and Vth nerve schwannomas.

Sensory complaints

Parathesias, or less commonly, sensory loss, occur as a result of paraspinal tumors or syrinx formation associated with an ependymoma. Pain in a dermatome distribution may occur due to a schwannoma of a spinal root or a spinal cord meningioma.

Seizures

Seizures are common and may be attributable to cortical meningiomas as well as hamartoma.

Skin

Dermal or subcutaneous tumors are present in most patients but are usually subtle. Most patients have no more than a few skin tumors. Histologically they are often a mixture of neurofibroma and schwannoma. Café-au-lait spots may be present, but never more than four, unlike NF-1.

Investigations

MRI of the brain with contrast enhancement is used. Both meningiomas and schwannomas enhance with contrast, making small tumors more easily identifiable. Internal auditory canal views are often essential to detect small vestibular schwannomas. MRI of the brain should probably be done annually in most NF-2 patients. MRI of the entire spinal cord with contrast can be done less frequently, usually every 2 years. Annual audiograms should be performed to monitor hearing.

Diagnosis

The diagnosis can usually be made clinically. Genetic testing is now available that is accurate in at least 90% of patients with germline mutations and typical NF-2. Genetic testing can also be performed on tumor tissue in questionable or unusual cases.

One-third of patients with no family history have somatic mosaicisms. These patients can be more difficult to diagnose and can require blood testing as well as tumor cytogenetics. Mosaicisms are the most likely cause of atypical NF-2 cases, i.e. patients with a single vestibular schwannoma or patients with unilateral disease.

The diagnosis can be made clinically if there is:

- Bilateral vestibular schwannoma *or*
- First-degree relative with NF-2 and unilateral vestibular schwannoma or any two of: meningioma, schwannoma, glioma, *or*
- Unilateral vestibular schwannoma and any two of: meningioma, schwannoma, glioma, neurofibroma, posterior subcapsular cataract, *or*
- Multiple meningiomas (two or more) and unilateral schwannoma or any two of: schwannoma, glioma, neurofibroma, cataract.

Tip

▶ *The Manchester (modified NIH) diagnostic criteria for NF-2 are probably the most reliable[17].*

NF-2 must sometimes be distinguished from schwannomatosis and meningiomatosis. The former is characterized by the presence of multiple schwannomas. There are no other tumor types or vestibular schwannomas in this disease. Recent studies have shown that a substantial percentage of patients with familial schwannomatosis and a small percentage of patients with sporadic schwannomatosis actually have NF-2. Distinguishing these two diseases requires genetic testing of the blood as well as of tumor samples.

Meningiomatosis is characterized by multiple meningiomas without any other tumor type. Most, but not all, of these patients have NF-2.

Treatment

Treatment is largely symptomatic and not without controversy. Physicians must remember that intervention has potential consequences/complications.

Vestibular tumors

Resection of vestibular tumors in NF-2 is often more difficult than treatment of sporadic vestibular schwannomas because the tumors can be multifocal and recur. Resection of vestibular tumors can be complicated by hearing loss and facial weakness. The treatment approach is to some extent dictated by the size of the vestibular schwannomas. Fractionated radiotherapy is used in some centers. A recent study suggests that chemotherapy directed at VEGF expression may significantly reduce the size of large inoperable vestibular tumors and improve hearing.

Meningiomas

While meningiomas are benign tumors, it is difficult to resect them completely. Often the best course is to observe tumors and operate only when symptomatic. The development of appropriate chemotherapy offers the best long-term hope.

Ependymomas

These are usually indolent intradural spinal cord tumors in NF-2. They almost never show evidence of malignancy and can often be observed without surgical intervention.

Cataracts and eyes

Cataracts usually do not require removal. Poor eyelid closure due to VIIth nerve injury can be surgically facilitated. Frequent eye drops help with dryness.

Hearing loss
Cochlear implantation has shown some benefit in NF-2 patients and may influence the surgical approach on vestibular tumors. Signing is an important skill for patients and families to develop because of inevitable hearing loss.

Genetic counseling
The risk of NF-2 for each pregnancy is 50%. The risk is less in mosaics. Assessment of children of patients is important, because many patients with NF-2 are diagnosed after they have already had children.

Prognosis
NF-2 is a severe progressive disorder that results in shortened life span. However, the spectrum of severity can be quite wide and the tumors in NF-2 are often quite indolent. Age of onset and number of tumors are helpful predictors of outcome: early onset and multiple brain and spinal tumors are associated with poorer prognosis. Nevertheless, as molecular understanding of this disease improves, chemotherapeutic approaches may provide substantial help.

TUBEROUS SCLEROSIS

Definition and epidemiology
Tuberous sclerosis complex (TSC) is a progressive disease characterized by hypopigmented macules of the skin, migrational errors of the brain, seizures, and hamartomas of multiple organ systems, including skin, kidney, brain, lungs, and heart.

- Prevalence: 1 in 6800 to 1 in 17 300 children.
- Age of onset is usually infancy.
- TSC is an autosomal dominant disorder, with males and females equally affected.
- High spontaneous mutation rate, with only 40% familial cases.

Etiology and pathogenesis
TSC is due to inactivation of either the *TSC1* gene on chromosome 9q or the *TSC2* gene on chromosome 16p, encoding the proteins hamartin and tuberin, respectively. These proteins are abundantly expressed in brain, as well as other tissue, and function as a heterodimeric signalling complex. Expression is prominent in the embryo and is important in brain development and cellular organization. Hamartin may interact with the ERM proteins (see NF-2) and regulate cytoskeleton-mediated processes, while tuberin appears to be a GTPase activating (GAP protein, see NF-1). The hamartin/tuberin complex is an important negative regulator of mTOR[18].

TSC affects all tissues, including the lymphatic system, with the possible exceptions of the peripheral nervous system, skeletal muscle, and pineal gland.

Brain
The brain is normal in size, but may show areas of broadening and firmness on the surface referred to as cortical tubers (225). The number of tubers varies in different patients. The cut surface reveals a lack of demarcation of cortex from white matter. The tubers are composed of interlacing rows of fibrous astrocytes. The normal layered architecture of the cerebral cortex is diffusely disturbed in the tubers, with increased glial cells, atypical large neurons, and giant glial cells and disruption of the normal radial architecture (226).

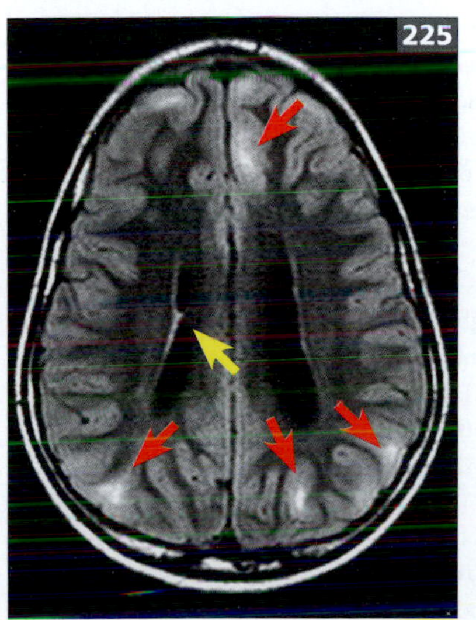

225 Cortical tubers. Axial FLAIR MRI of the brain, showing areas of increased signal within the cortex (red arrows) as well as slight swelling of those gyri. There are also subependymal nodules (yellow arrow) on the ventricular surface.

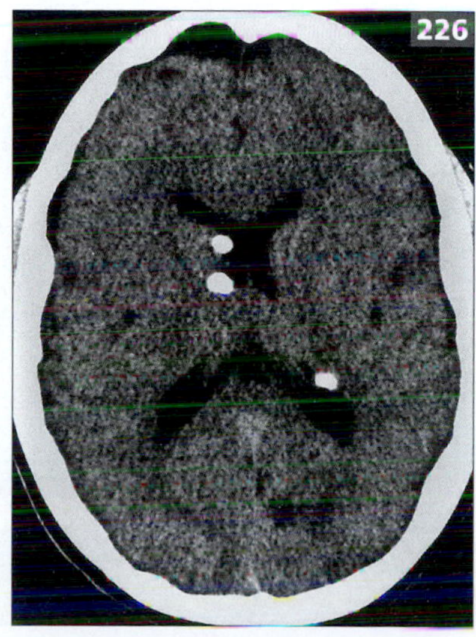

226 CT noncontrast scan of the brain, showing bright, calcified subependymal nodules bilaterally on the ventricular surface in tuberous sclerosis.

The surface of the lateral ventricles may be encrusted with subependymal nodules made of glial cells, blood vessels, and abnormal neurons, which tend to calcify (227). Some subependymal nodules have the potential to increase in size, transforming into subependymal giant cell tumors (SEGAs) which can obstruct the foramina of Monro, causing hydrocephalus in 10% of patients (228).

Kidney

Angiomyolipomas (AMLs), found in 80% of patients, are tumor-like masses in the kidneys, consisting of sheets of disorganized smooth muscle, fat, and foam cells, and large thick-walled blood vessels. They vary in size, measuring as much as 20 cm (8 in) in diameter. They are typically multiple and bilateral, bulging from the surface of the kidney or compressing and distorting the renal pelvis.

Renal cysts vary in size from millimeters to several centimeters in diameter, and occur throughout the parenchyma in 20% of patients. The cysts are lined with hyperplastic epithelium (229).

Heart

Rhabdomyomas are found in 50% of children and are thought to represent hamartomas of myocytes. They vary in size from millimeters to several centimeters and are most commonly found in the ventricles. They may be entirely intramural or protrude from the cardiac surface. They may obstruct valvular function or impinge on the cardiac conduction system.

Lungs

Lymphangiomyomatosis occurs in 1% of patients, almost exclusively females. The lungs are enlarged and heavy and the normal structure is replaced by innumerable cysts.

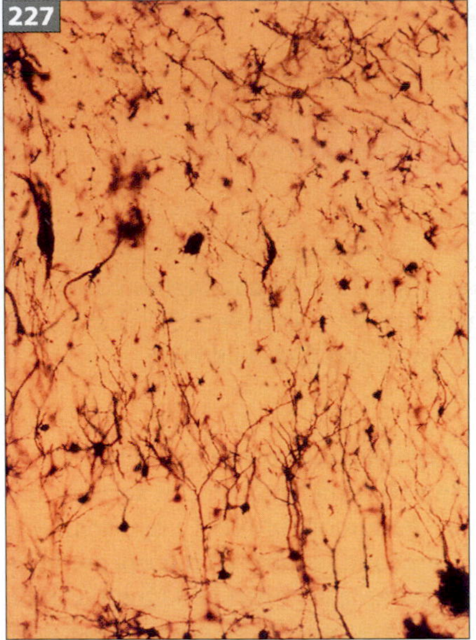

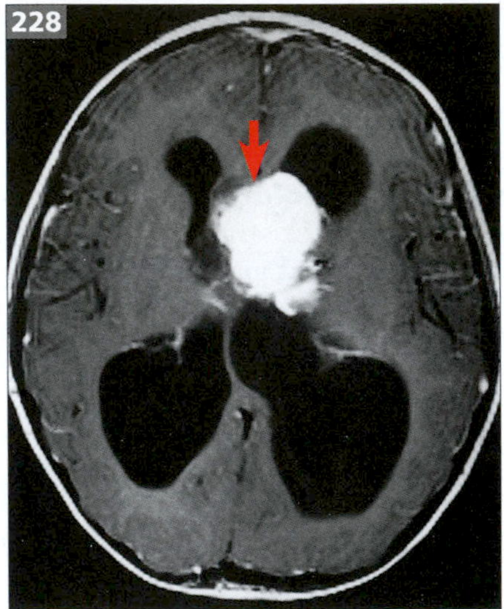

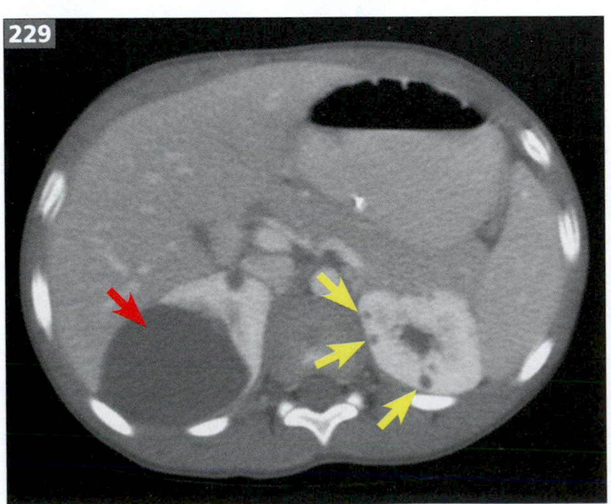

227 Golgi–Cox staining of the lower border of a cortical tuber in tuberous sclerosis, showing relatively normal, radially oriented pyramidal cells in the lower third of the section, with small, primitive, multipolar neurons above, and a complete absence of layered cortex, lacking radial orientation.

228 Axial T1-weighted MRI with gadolinium enhancement, showing an enhancing subependymal giant cell astrocytoma (SEGA) at the foramen of Monro (arrow), with obstruction of the foramen and resulting enlarged lateral ventricles (hydrocephalus).

229 Renal cysts. CT of the abdomen, showing a large cyst of the right kidney (red arrow) with several smaller cysts (yellow arrows) in both kidneys.

Clinical features

TSC is a highly variable condition even within the same pedigree. Patients may range from severe mental retardation with intractable seizures to mild, unnoticed disease. Typically diagnosis is made in infancy, due to the appearance of seizures or developmental delay, but mild cases may not be appreciated until adult years. Mutations in the *TSC1* gene are associated with a milder phenotype. The complications of TSC, like the other neurocutaneous disorders, are age specific.

Brain

Seizures occur in 92% of patients, usually starting in infancy or early childhood. Virtually all seizure types occur. Infantile spasms are the presenting sign in 70%. TSC is the cause of 25% of all infantile spasms. Seizures are often difficult to control. Patients with seizures and mental retardation are more likely to have higher numbers of cortical tubers.

IQ is normal in 55.5%. Profound mental retardation with IQ <21 is found in 30%. Moderate to severe retardation is found in the vast majority of patients who present with infantile spasms. Autistic spectrum disorder occurs in a significant number of patients. Behavioral difficulties are common and can be severe.

Hydrocephalus is due to enlargement of SEGAs in childhood (mean age of onset is 9 years), and is found in 10%.

Skin

Hypomelanotic macules are present in 61–97% of cases of TSC. They vary from a few millimeters to several centimeters in size and have an oval, ash-leaf shape. They are present at birth, but may be difficult to see in light-skinned individuals. They are readily seen with a Wood's lamp.

Adenoma sebaceum are small, red-pink, flat- topped skin lesions with a smooth, glistening surface, a few millimeters in size, that are distributed in a butterfly-like pattern on the face. They appear in mid to late childhood in 70% of patients. Fibrous plaques are a similar lesion, usually appearing in late childhood or adult years in 19%. Both of these lesions are angiofibromas, characterized by hyperplasia of connective and vascular tissue (**230**).

Shagreen patches are thick, slightly elevated, flesh-colored macules, most often seen in the lumbosacral region. They are plaques of subepidermal fibrosis. Ungual fibromas are angiofibromas of the nail bed that appear in late adolescence (**231**).

Kidney

Complications such as hypertension, renal failure, and hemorrhage are all due to the progressive enlargement of angiomyolipomas and are the second most common cause of morbidity and mortality in TSC. Lesions greater than 4 cm (1.6 in) in diameter are likely to become symptomatic and require frequent monitoring and possible intervention. These are complications of adult years. Hemorrhage in these tumors can be life threatening. Tumors respond at least transiently to mTOR inhibitors.

230 Adenoma sebaceum. Photograph of the face of a patient with tuberous sclerosis, showing diffuse severe angiofibromas of the cheeks, chin, forehead, and nasolabial folds.

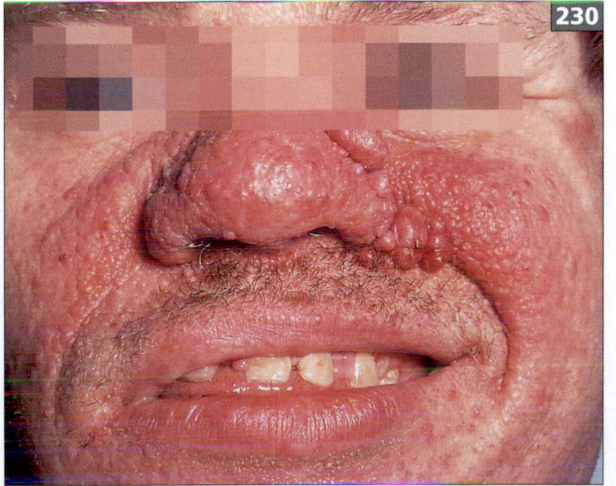

231 Ungual fibromas. Photograph of the toes of a patient with tuberous sclerosis, showing multiple angiofibromas growing out of the nail bed, with a small superficial hemorrhage.

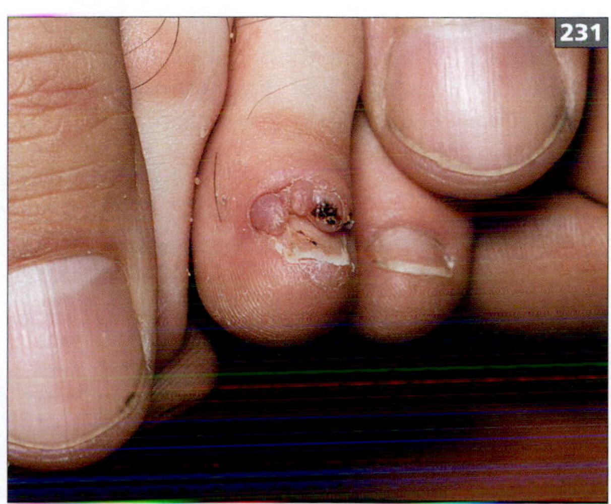

Heart

Complications such as congestive heart failure and arrhythmias are due to rhabdomyomas. These are apparent in the fetus on ultrasound. They are present in 30–50% of patients and are only symptomatic in a small percentage of patients within the first few months of life. Thereafter, the tumors tend to regress and remain asymptomatic.

Lungs

Dyspnea, pneumothorax, hemoptysis, chest pain, and cough occur in as many as 26% of women, due to lymphangiomyomatosis. This is a progressive disorder that occurs exclusively in adults with presentation between 30 and 35 years of age. It is found almost entirely in women with TSC.

Eye

Retinal hamartomas occur in 40–50% of patients. They are congenital and appear to be nonprogressive. They may impair vision in some patients but for the vast majority of patients they are asymptomatic.

Investigations

CT of the brain demonstrates subependymal nodules because of their tendency to calcify and is a useful diagnostic test in the first year of life. Thereafter, CT can be used to follow SEGAs which can cause hydrocephalus. Ultrasound and CT are useful for detecting and measuring angiomyolipomas and cysts. MRI of the brain demonstrates the cortical tubers and white matter changes.

Echocardiography demonstrates the cardiac rhabdomyomas which are apparent even *in utero*.

EEG is essential in the characterization and treatment of seizures. Regular chest X-ray shows pulmonary changes in adults. Genetic testing is available to confirm the diagnosis and determine whether the defect is in *TSC1* or *TSC2*.

Diagnosis

Genetic testing is available which can identify mutations in 85–90% of patients. The diagnosis can usually be made clinically by the presence of two major or one major and two minor criteria:

- Major criteria: facial angiofibroma, ungula fibroma, shagreen patch, hypopigmented spots, cortical tuber, subependymal nodule, SEGA, retinal hamartoma, cardiac rhabdomyoma, renal angiomyolipoma, lymphangiomyomatosis.
- Minor criteria: dental enamel pits, hamartomatous rectal polyps, gingival fibroma, confetti skin lesions, multiple renal cysts.

Treatment

Treatment is essentially symptomatic, and much of the treatment is focused on the neurologic complications.

Seizures need to be aggressively managed. Seizures are often difficult to control and may require consideration of more invasive treatments such as a vagal nerve stimulator, epilepsy surgery, or vigabatrin, a seizure medication that can be associated with constriction of visual fields but is often quite effective in TSC. mTOR inhibitors may also be helpful in seizure control.

Hydrocephalus may require ventriculoperitoneal shunting. Hydrocephalus in TSC is caused by SEGAs. Recent trials of mTOR inhibitors indicate that as many as 77% of patients demonstrate a response of 30% or more tumor shrinkage. This suggests that hydrocephalus and SEGAs may ultimately effectively be treated with chemotherapy. Educational support and behavior management are important issues.

Cardiac manifestations rarely require intervention and should be managed conservatively. Kidney lesions are monitored closely and ablation of enlarging angiomyolipomas needs to be discussed. mTOR inhibitors also appear to be of benefit in some patients with angiomyolipomas. Pulmonary function needs to be followed in adults with lymphangiomyomatosis.

Prognosis

TSC is a progressive disorder with a shortened life span. However, because of the marked variability of expression, a significant percentage of patients may lead normal lives. Chemotherapy offers considerable hope.

STURGE–WEBER SYNDROME

Definition and epidemiology

Sturge–Weber syndrome (SW) is a neurocutaneous disorder characterized by a clinical triad of:

- A facial capillary cutaneous angioma (port wine stain) of the face; this is usually unilateral and in the distribution of the ophthalmic division of the trigeminal nerve, but sometimes is bilateral.
- Abnormal blood vessels of the meninges (leptomeningeal angioma), usually ipsilateral to the skin lesion.
- Abnormal blood vessels in the eye leading to glaucoma.

However, the syndrome is defined by the leptomeningeal angioma. Not all patients have the other features.

The incidence of SW is 1 in 50,000 live births. It is a sporadic condition that affects males and females equally. A congenital abnormality, the facial angioma, is apparent at birth, but not all babies with facial angiomas have SW. The risk of SW in children with a facial angioma is 8%.

Etiology and pathogenesis

While the cause of SW is unknown, a developmental abnormality of the embryonic vascular plexus in the cephalic mesenchyme adjacent to the telencephalic vesicle is postulated. Genetic studies of families with capillary malformations suggest at least one candidate gene, RASA1. It is hypothesized that there is abnormal regulation of blood vessels and extracellular matrix expression that produce tortuous abnormal blood vessels in the leptomeninges, with sluggish blood flow that results in progressive ischemia to the underlying cortex[19].

Leptomeninges appear thickened and discolored by the angioma. Calcification of the meningeal arteries and cortical and subcortical veins underlying the angioma is present, as is laminar necrosis of the cortex (232). Neuronal loss and gliosis occur, with progression of the condition and recurrent thrombi due to venous stasis. There is progressive ischemia and atrophy of the underlying cortex.

Leptomeningeal angioma and cortical injury is more common in the occipital pole of the brain, but can involve the entire hemisphere. Involvement of both hemispheres is uncommon but occurs.

Clinical features

Skin

Cutaneous angioma on one side of the face and scalp is present, usually involving the first (ophthalmic) division of the trigeminal nerve. The angioma is a deep red color (port wine stain) that is present at birth, and may be flat or slightly raised (233).

Eye

Glaucoma occurs in 30–70% of patients, with a bimodal occurrence, with the majority developing glaucoma in infancy and the remainder developing it in childhood or adult years. The mechanism is not clear. Hemianopsia is common due to ischemic brain injury.

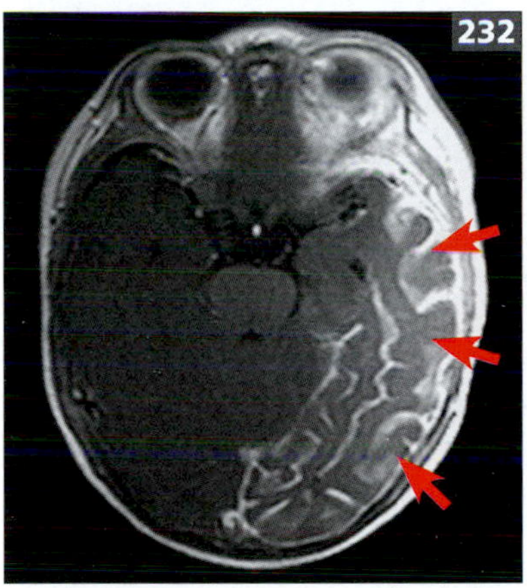

232 Sturge–Weber meningeal angioma. Post-contrast axial MRI of the brain, showing enhancement of temporal, parietal, and occipital gyri (arrows) in the left hemisphere, with some left cortical atrophy.

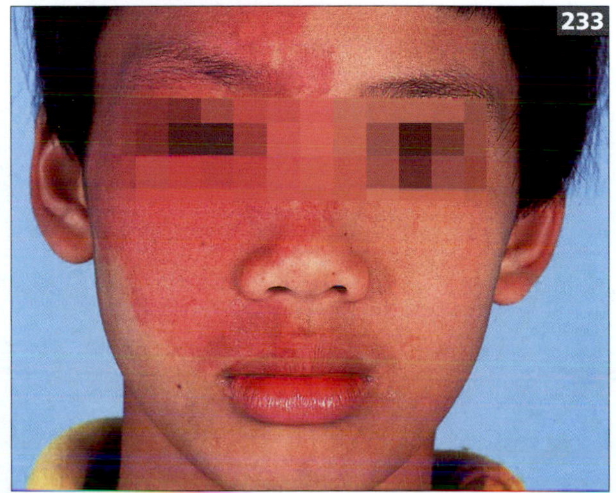

233 A patient with a reddish cutaneous capillary angioma on one side of the face, involving the first and second divisions of the trigeminal nerve.

Brain

Seizures, either partial or generalized, occur in 75–90%, usually begin in infancy or early childhood, and are the first neurologic symptom. Seizures can be intractable in 50%. Developmental delay is commonly appreciated after initially normal milestones in approximately two-thirds of patients. Mental retardation is present in 50%.

Hemiparesis and hemiatrophy of the contralateral extremities are present in the majority of patients. Recurrent transient focal deficits occur, usually hemiparesis or visual deficits, that last for hours or days. Headaches occur in 30–45%.

Patients with bilateral disease are much more likely to have severe problems. The pace of problems seems to decrease after childhood, and adults with SW can be remarkably stable.

Investigations

MRI with enhancement demonstrates the vascular malformation. This can usually be seen within the first year of life, but may not be easily visible initially. Fluid- attenuated inversion recovery (FLAIR) sequences in the MRI, as well as MR venography, may be useful. CT demonstrates calcification of the underlying cortex relatively early, usually within the first 2 years of life.

Positron emission tomography (PET) imaging may be useful in demonstrating decreased metabolism in the affected areas. EEG, particularly prolonged recordings, are essential in characterizing seizures and detecting subtle subclinical activity.

Diagnosis

The diagnosis is usually straightforward in patients with all three characteristic features: facial angioma, leptomeningeal angioma, and the presence of glaucoma. However, in the first few months of life, the leptomeningeal angioma may be hard to detect and glaucoma can have a later onset. Additionally, not all patients have all three features. Some may only have the leptomeningeal angioma, so that repeat imaging of patients with recurrent focal seizures in infancy is important.

Treatment

Aggressive control of seizures is needed. Radiologic studies suggest that seizures are associated with ischemic injury to the cortex underlying the leptomeningeal angioma because of abnormal regulation of blood flow in these vessels. This leads to laminar necrosis. The goal is to minimize seizures. Epilepsy surgery should be discussed in some patients with intractable seizures. This is controversial, because of the variable clinical course.

Antithrombotic therapy is recommended, such as daily aspirin. Glaucoma should be treated (with beta blockers, carbonic anhydrase inhibitors, or trabeculectomy). Educational assessment is useful to identify learning difficulties and provide appropriate support. The most severely affected patients are those with bilateral disease who are not good surgical candidates. Laser treatment of the face is effective in eliminating the facial angioma and usually begins in the second to third year of life.

Prognosis

Prognosis varies widely because the extent of the leptomeningeal angioma can vary significantly. The pace of the clinical course of SW seems to be faster in early childhood and often stabilizes thereafter. SW can present difficult problems and devastating complications in some patients; however, in others the course is much milder.

Patients with seizure disorders can be seizure-free for many years with minimal deficits. In some patients, while intractable, seizures can also be quite mild and relatively infrequent. Half of patients graduate from secondary/high school and a significant percentage live independently.

HEREDITARY HEMORRHAGIC TELANGIECTASIA (OSLER–RENDU–WEBER SYNDROME)

Definition and epidemiology

Hereditary hemorrhagic telangiectasia (HHT) is an autosomal dominant disorder characterized by multiple telangiectases involving the skin, mucous membranes, viscera (particularly the GI [nose, pharynx, gut] and genitourinary tracts), and occasionally the nervous system. HHT is often complicated by ateriovenous malformations (AVMs) in the brain, lung, GI tract, and liver.

Prevalence of HHT is variable: 1 in 1331 in Netherlands Antilles to 1 in 39,000 in northern England. A world-wide prevalence of 1 in 5000 is postulated. While telangiectasias appear in childhood, the manifestations are primarily in adults. Males and females are equally affected.

Etiology and pathophysiology

HHT has an autosomal dominant inheritance. Linkage analysis indicates five genes, three of which have been identified: endoglin or *ENG* (HHT type 1), activin receptor-like kinase or *ALK1/ACVRL* (HHT type 2), and Smad 4 (HHT in association with juvenile polyposis). Additional genes are predicted on chromosome 5 (HHT3), and chromosome 7 (HHT4).

The genes for HHT encode proteins that modulate transforming growth factor (TGF)-β superfamily signaling in vascular endothelial cells. Mutations lead to the development of fragile telangiectatic vessels and AVMs. TGF-β modulates several processes of endothelial cells, including migration, proliferation, and adhesion, and the composition and organization of the extracellular matrix. More than 80% of patients are accounted for by mutations in *ENG* or *ACVRL*[20].

The fundamental lesion is probably a dysplasia of the vessel wall. Bleeding is due to the mechanical fragility of the vessel. Pulmonary and hepatic AVMs create a right-to-left shunt that may lead to cerebral hypoxia and polycythemia, and may allow the passage of emboli (thrombotic, septic) from the systemic venous circulation or right heart to the brain causing stroke and cerebral abscess.

Telangiectases range from small, focal dilatations of post-capillary venules to large, markedly dilated and convoluted venules which extend through the entire dermis, have excessive layers of smooth muscle without elastic fibers, and often connect directly to dilated arterioles. Telangiectases are commonly found in skin, face, nares, tongue, oral mucosa, conjunctiva, trunk, and GI tract (**234**, **235**).

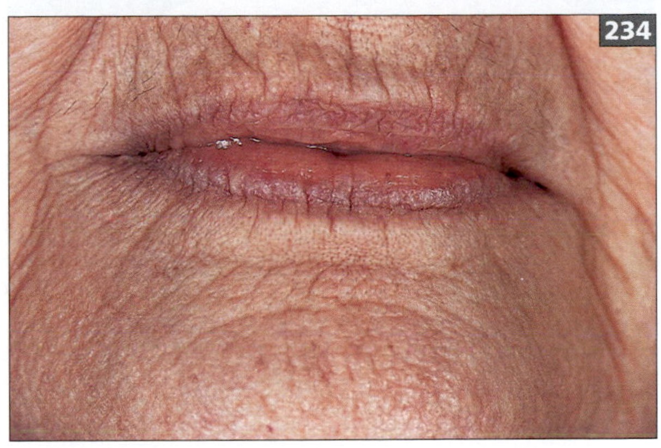

234 Photograph of a patient with hereditary hemorrhagic telangiectasia, showing multiple small telangiectases of the upper and lower lips.

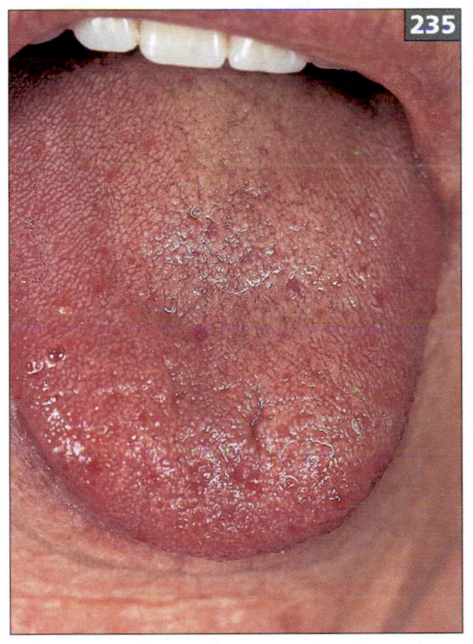

235 Photograph of the tongue of a patient with hereditary hemorrhagic telangiectasia, showing multiple small red telangiectases of the tongue.

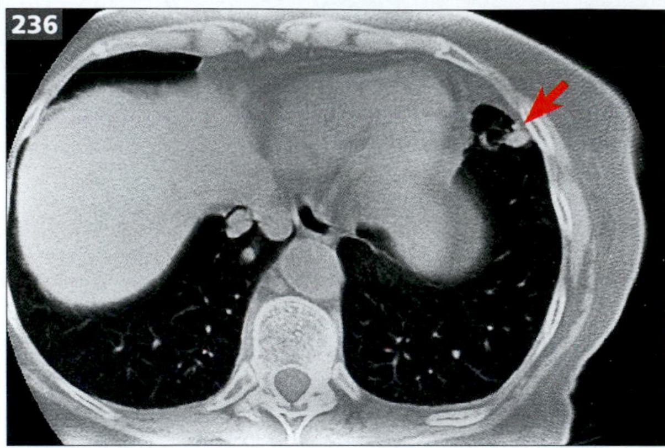

236 Axial CT of the chest showing a pulmonary arteriovenous malformation in the left lower lobe (arrow).

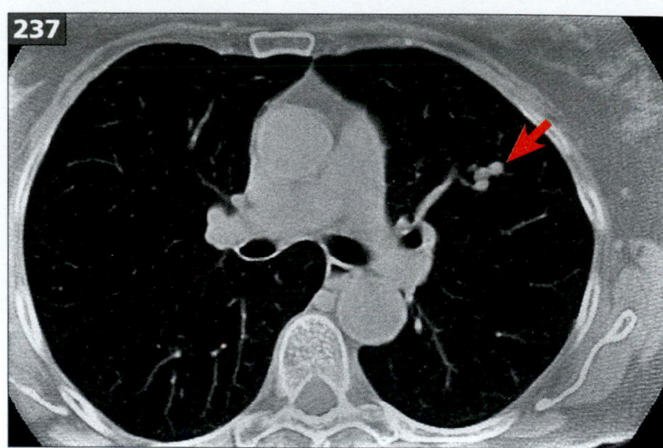

237 Axial CT of the chest showing a pulmonary arteriovenous malformation in the left anterior mid zone (arrow) of the left lung.

AVMs form a direct connection between arteries and veins, without capillaries. They are found in the brain (5–10%), spinal cord, lungs (5–15%), particularly lower lobes, and GI tract including liver (**236, 237**).

Clinical features

HHT is highly variable, even within the same pedigree. Spontaneous and recurrent nosebleeds are the most common and earliest manifestation, often in early childhood. Pulmonary and cerebral AVMs may be more common in HHT1, whereas hepatic vascular malformations may be more common in HHT2, but these differences are not substantial enough to influence screening. A rare form of HHT linked to a defect in the SMAD4 gene is associated with juvenile polyposis.

Telangiectases

These are bright red or violaceous, ranging in size from that of a pinhead to >3 mm. They blanch under pressure and have a tendency to bleed (**234, 235**). They are widely distributed, apparent on face, tongue, oral mucosa, and trunk. Telangiectases first appear during childhood, enlarge during adolescence, and may assume spidery forms, resembling the cutaneous telangiectases seen with liver cirrhosis, in late adult life.

Other features

- Severe iron deficiency anemia.
- Severe or recurrent bleeding:
  - Epistaxis (often in childhood) is a severe recurring problem.
  - Upper or lower GI and liver hemorrhage (in later adult years).
  - Hematuria.
- Sudden focal neurologic dysfunction:
  - Stroke syndrome due to intracranial hemorrhage or arterial obstruction by paradoxical embolism or thrombus or an intracranial AVM.
  - Spinal cord hemorrhage or infarction.
- Progressive focal neurologic dysfunction:
  - Enlargement of the intracranial or intraspinal vascular lesions.
  - Brain abscess due to septic emboli to brain via pulmonary fistulae.
  - Seizures.
- Pulmonary AVMs causing:
  - Dyspnea, fatigue, cyanosis, polycythemia, clubbing, chest bruit.
  - Pulmonary hypertension.
  - Pulmonary infection/abscess.
- Liver vascular malformations leading to:
  - High output heart failure.
  - Portal hypertension.
  - Jaundice.
  - Portosystemic encephalopathy.
- Pregnancy: there is an increased risk of hemorrhage during pregnancy.

Investigations

- Blood tests:
  - Full blood count.
  - Genetic testing.
- Brain AVM:
  - CT and CT angiography.
  - MRI of brain, MRA also can be helpful. Screening is somewhat controversial because most cerebral AVMs will never bleed; however, when they do, the consequences can be severe.
- Pulmonary AVM:
  - High resolution helical CT and contrast echocardiography are effective screening tools.
  - Pulmonary angiography.
- GI AVM, telangiectases, angiodysplasias:
  - Endoscopy.
  - Angiography.
- CT for liver lesion.

Diagnosis

Diagnosis is clinical. Any two of the following are suspicious for HHT and three are felt to be diagnostic:

- Recurrent and severe spontaneous epistaxis.
- Telangiectases elsewhere than in the nasal mucosa.
- Visceral involvement.
- First-degree relative with HHT (the disease is found in heterozygotes, but penetrance may be incomplete).

Genetic testing is available for the three identified gene defects.

Treatment

Telangiectases

- Nasal:
  - Humidification.
  - Packing of the nose is probably best done with lubricated deflatable packing.
  - Topical application to the nasal mucosa of VEGF inhibitor can be helpful.
  - Transfusion.
  - Estrogen therapy.
  - Septal dermoplasty.
  - Laser ablation.
  - Cautery eradicates a bleeding lesion, but satellite ones tend to form. The success of different treatments appears to correlate with the type of lesion causing the bleeding. Laser treatments may work best with isolated lesions, whereas dermoplasty may be better for more diffuse lesions[21].
- Skin:
  - Topical agents: oxidized cellulose applied to lesion.
  - Laser ablation.

AVMs

- Pulmonary:
  - Embolization is effective and safe.
  - Asymptomatic lesions should be embolized.
  - Ligation of arterial supply.
  - Antibacterial prophylaxis at the time of dental or surgical procedures.
- CNS:
  - Neurovascular surgery.
  - Stereotactic radiosurgery.
- GI:
  - Transfusion.
  - Photocoagulation.
  - Estrogen–progesterone therapy.
  - Repeated endoscopy for GI bleeding is not recommended.

Liver

Liver problems can be quite severe and hepatic artery embolization should be avoided. Patients should be considered for liver transplantation.

Pregnancy

Risks of hemorrhage during pregnancy should be discussed.

Prognosis

Prognostic variability is marked in HHT. Older studies indicated that the mortality approaches 50%. However, with genetic testing it has become apparent that the spectrum of severity is wide with some patients only having recurrent nosebleeds. Early diagnosis, detection of lesions, and monitoring have significantly improved the outlook.

LINEAR NEVUS SEBACEOUS SYNDROME

Definition and epidemiology

Linear nevus sebaceous syndrome (LNSS) involves hypertrophic sebaceous gland nevus on the face or scalp, with mental retardation and seizures.

Incidence of LNSS is unclear. The epidermal nevus syndrome, which includes a wide variety of conditions many of which are asymptomatic except for the nevus, is reported to occur in as many as 1 in 1000 live births. The incidence of LNSS is certainly lower, and in the author's experience quite rare. Males and females are equally affected.

Etiology and pathogenesis

LNSS is postulated to be a somatic mosaic disorder involving a lethal autosomal dominant gene. A cutaneous lesion in a linear distribution is found on the face or scalp characterized by papillomatous epidermal hyperplasia and an excessive number of sebaceous glands.

Clinical features

Sebaceous nevus

This appears as waxy nodules with granular pitted surface on the face or scalp (**238**). It becomes hairy, hyperplastic, and darker in adolescence. Tumor formation, including malignancy, can occur in adult years.

Brain

- Seizures occur in 75%: partial or partial complex, often intractable.
- Mental retardation in 61%.
- Migrational errors: heterotopia, pachygyria, agenesis of corpus callosum, hemimegalencephaly.
- Large hemicranium.
- Motor dysfunction including hemiplegia.

Eye

Eye abnormalities occur in 59–68%:

- Coloboma.
- Strabismus.
- Cataract.
- Optic nerve hypoplasia.

Skeletal

Skeletal abnormalities occur in 68%:

- Fibrous dysplasia of the skull.
- Scoliosis.
- Unilateral hypoplasia of a variety of bony structures.

Investigations

- MRI of the brain to look for migrational errors.
- Careful eye examination.
- EEG to characterize seizures.

Diagnosis

Diagnosis is based on the clinical triad of facial/scalp nevus, seizures, and mental retardation.

Treatment

Treatment is symptomatic. Seizures can be intractable and difficult to control. Because there is some potential for malignant transformation of the nevus in adult years, some thought should be given to removal of the nevus.

Prognosis

While there are apparently patients with the nevus alone that are asymptomatic, patient with the full triad are severely impaired and as a result, have a shortened life span.

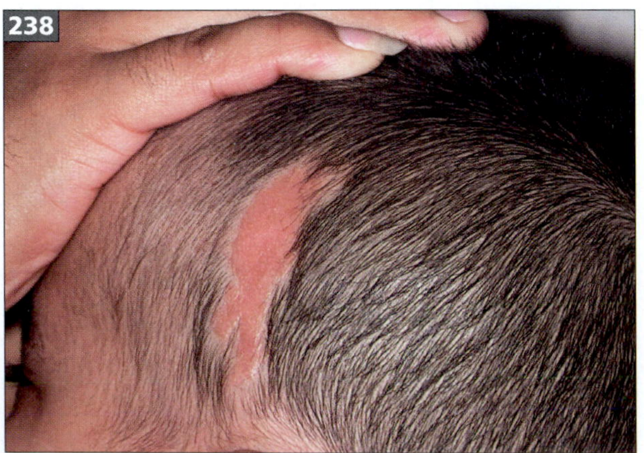

238 Linear sebaceous nevus. Photograph of the head of a child, showing a raised, waxy, colored lesion.

COWDEN'S SYNDROME AND LHERMITTE–DUCLOS DISEASE

Definition and epidemiology

Cowden's syndrome (CS) is an autosomal dominant disorder characterized by hamartomatous neoplasms of the skin, mucosa, GI tract, bones, CNS, eyes, and genitourinary tract. The neurologic manifestation is Lhermitte–Duclos disease (LD) which is a hamartomatous overgrowth of cerebellar ganglion cells.

- Rare autosomal dominant disorder.
- Predominantly found in Caucasians.
- Females are more commonly affected (60%).
- Symptoms are not usually apparent until early adult years.

Etiology and pathogenesis

CS is caused by a mutation in chromosome 10q in the *PTEN* tumor suppressor gene. *PTEN* is a phosphatase that negatively regulates signal transduction in the PI3K/AKT pathway. Inactivation of *PTEN* stimulates AKT and promotes cell growth through stimulation of the mTOR pathway. It is felt that LD represents a hypertrophic process superimposed on a developmental malformation of the cerebellum[22].

LD is a dysplastic enlargement of the cerebellar cortex. The folia appear thickened and distorted. The granular layer is thickened because of hypertrophy of the granular cells. The molecular layer is also thickened because of hyperplasia and hypertrophy of the myelinated fibers extending from the abnormal granular cells. Purkinje cells are reduced in number. The dysplasia is not well demarcated from the normal cerebellum.

Clinical features

Brain (LD abnormality)

- Ataxia.
- Increased intracranial pressure.
- Cranial nerve palsies.
- Macrocephaly in 50–80%.
- Mental retardation in 10%.

Skin and oral mucosa

- Trichilemmoma.
- Acral keratosis and palmar and plantar keratosis.
- Oral mucosal papillomas.

Cancer and tumors

- Breast cancer.
- Thyroid cancer, especially follicular thyroid cancer and goiter.
- Genitourinary tumors or malformations (endometrial cancer, renal cell carcinoma, uterine fibroids).
- Nonadenomatous polyps of the GI tract.

Investigations

- MRI of brain shows enhancing masses of the cerebellum with a laminated pattern.
- Semi-annual mammograms after age 30 years.
- Endoscopy of the GI tract every 3–5 years.
- Thyroid scans regularly.

Diagnosis

Clinical diagnosis is made by the presence of one pathognomonic criterion or one major criterion, usually with a minor criterion:

- Pathognomonic criteria:
  - Mucocutaneous lesions.
  - Trichilemmomas, facial.
  - Acral keratoses.
  - Papillomatous papules.
  - Mucosal lesions.
- Major criteria:
  - Breast carcinoma.
  - Thyroid carcinoma, nonmedullary.
  - Macrocephaly.
  - LD.
  - Endometrial cancer.
- Minor criteria:
  - Other thyroid lesions.
  - Mental retardation.
  - GI hamartomas.
  - Fibrocystic disease of the breast.
  - Lipomas.
  - Fibromas.
  - Genitourinary tumors.

Treatment

Treatment is largely surgical and symptomatic. There is considerable interest in the use of mTOR inhibitors.

Prognosis

The lifetime risk of breast cancer is 25–50%. The risk of thyroid cancer is 10%. Surgical excision of cerebellar lesions is frequently associated with recurrence.

VON HIPPEL–LINDAU DISEASE

Definition

Von Hippel–Lindau disease (VHL) is an uncommon autosomal dominant disorder characterized by multiple benign and malignant vascular tumors of the CNS, eye, kidneys, adrenal glands, pancreas, and reproductive adnexal organs (epididymis, fallopian tubes).

Etiology and pathogenesis

VHL is discussed in detail in Chapter 13, Tumors of the nervous system. However, it is mentioned here because it is a neurocutaneous disorder and because its etiology and pathogenesis are related to stimulation of the mTOR signaling pathway, which is implicated in most of the other neurocutaneous disorders discussed in this chapter. The vHL gene is located on chromosome 3p and encodes a protein which acts as a tumor suppressor gene. The protein forms a complex with other proteins, including elongin B and C, and Cullin 2, to form a VCB–CUL2 complex. The complex determines ubiquitin-dependent proteolysis of large cellular proteins. When normal oxygen levels are present, the complex binds to the alpha subunits of hypoxia-inducible factor (HIF) 1 and 2 for degradation of proteins. If VHL protein is absent, HIF stimulates angiogenesis which is critical in some tumor formation[23].

INCONTINENTIA PIGMENTI

Definition and epidemiology

Incontinentia pigmenti is a rare X-linked disorder primarily affecting skin, brain, and eyes. It is characterized by a swirled pattern of hyperpigmentation, with a history of preceding vesicles in the newborn.

- Rare disorder, primarily noted in Caucasians.
- Primarily affects females, though some males have been reported.
- X-linked disorder that is generally felt to be lethal *in utero* in males.
- At least one-half of cases are familial.

Etiology and pathogenesis

Incontinentia pigmenti is believed to be due to mutations in the *NEMO/IKKγ* gene on chromosome Xq28. This gene encodes a transcription factor that regulates the expression of multiple genes, including cytokines, chemokines, and cell adhesion molecules. A deficiency of this transcription factor facilitates apoptosis induced by tumor necrosis factor (TNF) and other cytokines. The disease seems to involve a complicated process of cell death and increases in multiple cytokines that produce an inflammatory response in the epidermis associated with both systemic and local eosinophilia.

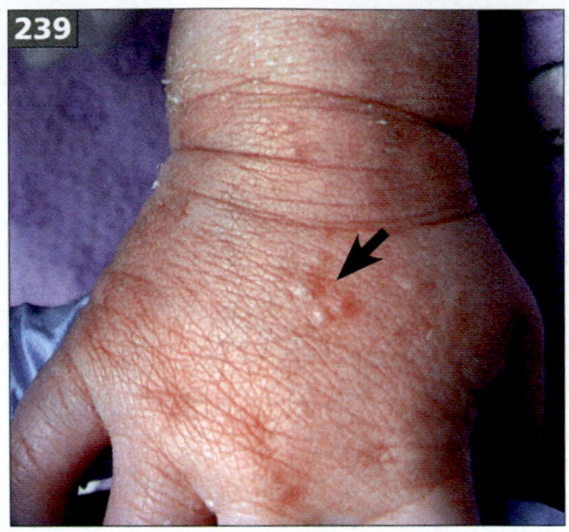

239 **Incontinentia pigmenti. Photograph of the hand of a newborn, showing vesicles (arrow) with an erythematous base.**

There are four clinical stages to this disease[24], with the following pathological features:

1. The epidermis and dermis show a spongy inflammation with massive eosinophilia with vesiculation.
2. There is epidermal hyperplasia and hyperkeratosis with papillomas and persistent eosinophilic inflammation.
3. Melanin is found in melanophages in the dermis, leading to the concept that the epidermis is incontinent of melanin.
4. The epidermis is atrophic, with loss of sweat glands, and melanocytes are reduced in number.

Clinical features

Skin

The four clinical stages are as follows:

1. Vesicular or inflammatory stage is present in 90% within the first 2 weeks of life, characterized by erythema and superficial vesicles distributed in a linear fashion, most commonly on the trunk or extremities (**239**). This is sometimes confused with herpes zoster. The blisters clear by 4 months of age.
2. The verrucous stage occurs in 70%, usually between 2 and 6 weeks of age, and consists of dry papules and plaques, which may or may not be in the same area as the vesicles (**240**). These are usually found on the extremities and clear by 6 months of age.
3. The third stage is whorls or streaks of brown or gray hyperpigmentation (**241**). These are found on the trunk and extremities and may not be in the same areas as the previous lesions. This stage usually begins between 12 and 26 weeks of age and persists for several years or decades.
4. The final stage is patches of atrophic, hairless, hypopigmented skin, predominantly on the extremities, that begins in teenage years.

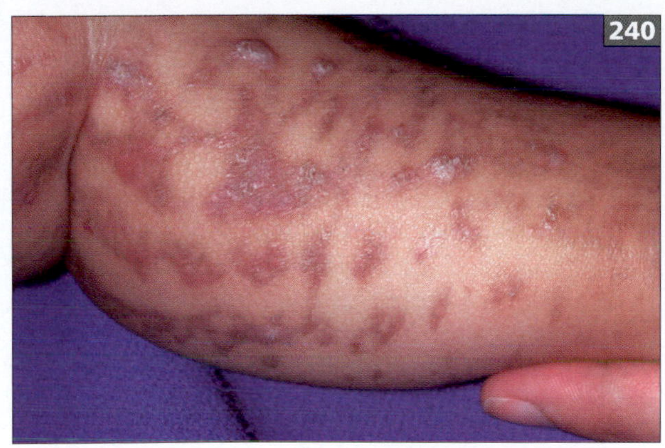

240 Incontinentia pigmenti. The inner aspect of the leg of a 7-week-old baby, demonstrating crusted nodules of the early verrucous stage and hyperpigmented streaks.

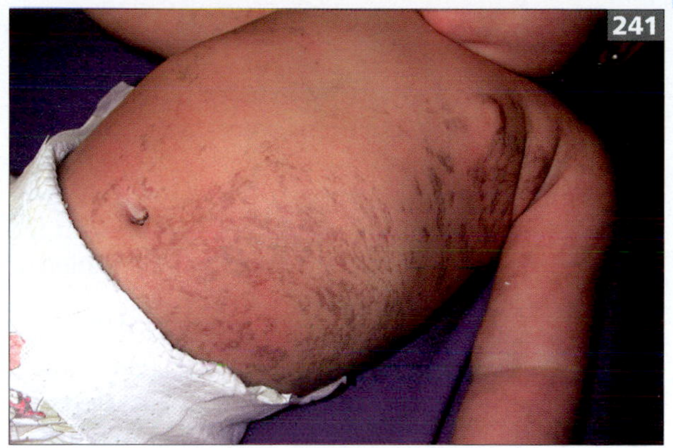

241 The abdomen of a 9-month-old child, showing the third stage of incontinentia pigmenti, with whorls and streaks of grayish-brown hyperpigmentation.

Brain

- Seizures in 13% including infantile spasms.
- Spastic paralysis in 11%.
- Microcephaly in 5%.
- Developmental delay and mental retardation in some.

Eye

- Strabismus in 18%.
- Optic nerve atrophy in 4%.
- Retinal lesions (vaso-occlusive events, hypopigmentation, fibrovascular proliferation, retinal detachment).

Other organ involvement

- Alopecia.
- Nail dystrophy.
- Dental abnormalities in 80%.

Investigations

- Skin biopsy to document the pathology.
- Genetic testing for *NEMO/IKKγ* gene mutations.
- Peripheral white blood cell count looking for leukocytosis and eosinophilia.
- Eye examination.
- Brain MRI.

Diagnosis

In patients *without* a family history of incontinentia pigmenti, one major criterion is required:

- Typical neonatal rash with erythema, vesicles, and eosinophilia.
- Typical hyperpigmentation, mainly on the trunk following the lines of Blaschko, fading in adolescence.
- Linear atrophic, hairless lesions.

In patients *with* a family history of incontinentia pigmenti, the presence of one criterion:

- Suggestive history of typical rash.
- Vertex alopecia.
- Dental anomalies.
- Retinal disease.
- Multiple male miscarriages.

Treatment

Treatment of incontinentia pigmenti is largely symptomatic. The skin lesions usually do not cause major problems. The vesicular stage may need to be treated with sterile dressings. Genetic counseling can be offered.

Prognosis

The prognosis is generally good, although there is a group of patients with seizures, motor impairment, and mental retardation.

HYPOMELANOSIS OF ITO

Definition and epidemiology

Hypomelanosis of Ito is a rare disorder characterized by large areas of hypopigmentation in irregular streaks or whorls on the trunk and extremities, following the lines of Blaschko and appearing within the first year of life (**242**). There is absence of any history of inflammation or blisters preceding the pigmentary changes.

Hypomelanosis of Ito is a sporadic disorder. The incidence is unclear, varying from rare to 1 in 10,000 children. It is more easily detected in patients with increased skin pigmentation (Japanese, Hispanic, African-American), but it is unclear whether this represents a racial predilection. It is more frequent in females (2:1 female to male), and is apparent within the first year of life.

Etiology and pathogenesis

Hypomelanosis of Ito is believed to be due to a somatic cell mosaicism. A variety of chromosomal abnormalities have been implicated including trisomy 18, triplody, and tetrasomy 12p, but the majority seem to involve the X chromosome. It is hypothesized that the chromosomal anomalies disrupt expression or function of pigmentary genes. Pigmentary genes control a variety of processes, including melanoblast migration from the neural crest in fetal life. Alternatively, some investigators feel that hypomelanosis of Ito is due to functional disomy of the chromosome Xp.

The histopathology shows abnormal melanocytes that are also reduced in number, with absent or reduced dendrites.

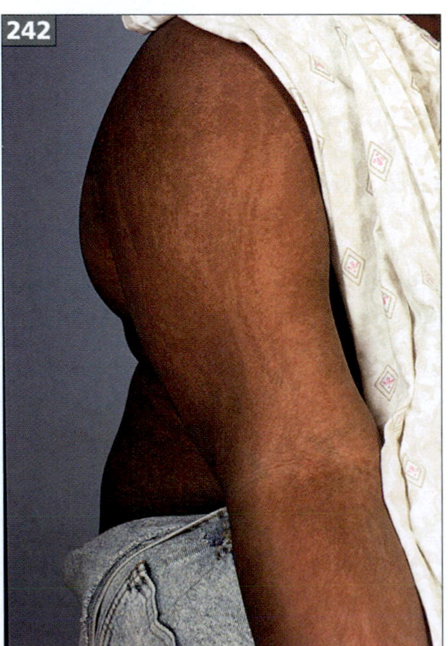

242 Hypomelanosis of Ito. Photograph of the arm, showing extensive lacy and whorl-like depigmentation.

Clinical features

Skin

- Extensive areas of the extremities and trunk with irregular streaks or whorls or lacy patterns of hypopigmentation that follow the lines of Blaschko (**242**).
- Appears in first year of life without preceding history of vesicles or scarring.

Noncutaneous abnormalities

- Occur in 75–94%.
- Brain:
  - Mental retardation in 60%.
  - Borderline IQ in 15%.
  - Seizures.
- Other organs: a wide variety of defects in eyes, bones, and teeth.

Investigations

- MRI of the brain is indicated in patients with mental retardation.
- Chromosome studies.
- Eye examination.

Diagnosis

Diagnosis of hypomelanosis of Ito is based on skin findings and a history that the skin findings appeared within the first year of life and were not preceded by either vesicles or warty lesions or scarring.

Treatment

The skin lesion does not require treatment. Treatment of other problems is symptomatic.

Prognosis

The high frequency of mental retardation and seizures indicates a high risk of disability.

REFERENCES

1 Stiles J, Jernigan TL (2010). The basics of brain development. *Neuropsychol Rev* **20**:327–348.

2 Spalice A, Parisi P, Nicita F, Pizzerdi G, Bel Balzo F, Ianneti P (2009). Neuronal migration disorders: clinical, neuroradiologic and genetic aspects. *Acta Paediatr* **98**:421–433.

3 De Marco P, Merello E, Mascelli S, Capra V (2006). Current perspectives on the genetic causes of neural tube defects. *Neurogenetics* 7:201–221.

4 Danzer E, Johnson MP, Adzick NS (2012). Fetal surgery for myelomeningocele: progress and perspective. *Dev Med Child Neurol* **54**:8–14.

5 Bowman RM, Boshnjaku V, McLone DG (2009). The changing incidence of myelomeningocele and its impact on pediatric neurosurgery: a review from the Children's Memorial Hospital. *Childs Nerv Syst* **25**:801–806.

6 Parisi MA, Dobyns WB (2003). Human malformations of the midbrain and hindbrain: review and proposed classification scheme. *Mol Genet Metab* **80**:36–53.

7 Golden JA, Rorke LB, Bruce DA (1987). Dandy–Walker syndrome and associated anomalies. *Pediatr Neurosci* **13**:38–44.

8 Volpe P, Campobasso G, De Robertis V, Rembouskos G (2009). Disorders of prosencephalic development. *Prenat Diagn* **29**:340–354.

9 Guerrini R, Dobyns WB, Barkovich AJ (2007). Abnormal development of the human cerebral cortex: genetics, functional consequences, and treatment options. *Trends Neurosci* **31**:154–162.

10 Rosner M, Hanneder M, Siegel N, Valli A, Fuchs C, Hengstschlager M (2008). The mTOR pathway and its role in human genetics. *Mutat Res* **659**:284–292.

11 Williams VC, Lucas J, Babcock MA, Gutmann DH, Korf B, Maria BL (2009). Neurofibromatosis type 1 revisited. *Pediatrics* **123**:124–133.

12 Mautner VF, Asuagbor FA, Dombi E, *et al.* (2008). Assessment of benign tumor burden by whole-body MRI in patients with neurofibromatosis 1. *Neuro Oncol* **10**:593–598.

13 Listernick R, Ferner RE, Liu GT, Gutmann DH (2007) Optic pathway gliomas in neurofibromatosis-1: controversies and recommendations. *Ann Neurol* **61**:189–198.

14 Evans DGR, Baser ME, McGaughran J, Sharif S, Howard E, Moran A (2002). Malignant peripheral nerve sheath tumors in neurofibromatosis 1. *J Med Genet* **39**:311–314.

15 Tonsgard JH (2006). Clinical manifestations and management of neurofibromatosis type 1. *Semin Pediatr Neurol* **13**:2–7.

16 Plotkin SR, Stemmer-Rachaminov AO, Barker FG II, *et al.* (2009). Hearing improvement after bevacizumab in patients with neurofibromatosis type 2. *N Engl J Med* **361**:358–367.

17 Evans DGR, Baser ME, O'Reilly B, *et al.* (2005). Consensus Statement: Management of the patient and family with neurofibromatosis 2: a consensus conference statement. *Br J Neurosurg* **19**:5–12.

18 Kohrman MH (2012). Emerging treatments in the management of tuberous sclerosis complex. *Pediatr Neurol* **46**:267–275.

19 Comi AM (2006). Advances in Sturge–Weber syndrome. *Curr Opin Neurol* **19**:124–128.

20 Govani FS, Shovlin CL (2009). Hereditary hemorrhagic telangiectasia: a clinical and scientific review. *Eur J Hum Genet* **17**:860–871.

21 Mahoney EJ, Shapshay SM (2006). New classification of nasal vasculature patterns in hereditary hemorrhagic telangiectasia. *Am J Rhinol* **20**:87–90.

22 Abel TW, Baker SJ, Fraser MM, *et al.* (2005). Lhermitte–Duclos disease: a report of 31 cases with immunohistochemical analysis of the PTEN/AKT/mTOR pathway. *J Neuropathol Exp Neurol* **64**:341–349.

23 Lonser RR, Glenn GM, Walther M, *et al.* (2003). von Hippel–Lindau disease. *Lancet* **361**:2059–2067.

24 Berlin AL, Paller AS, Chan LS (2002). Incontinentia pigmenti: a review and update on the molecular basis of pathophysiology. *J Am Acad Dermatol* **47**:169–187.

Further reading

Malformations of the nervous system

Barkovich AJ, Guerrini R, Kuzniecky RI, Jackson GD, Dobyns WB (2012). A developmental and genetic classification for malformations of cortical development: update 2012. *Brain* **135**:1348–1369.

Defects in neural tube formation

Bassuk AG, KibarZ (2009). Genetic basis of neural tube defects. *Semin Pediatr Neurol* **16**:101–110.

Dias MS, Skaggs DL (2005). Neurosurgical management of myelomeningocele (Spina Bifida). *Pediatr Rev* **26**:50–60.

Lew SM, Kothbauer KF (2007). Tethered cord syndrome: an updated review. *Pediatr Neurosurg* **43**:236–248.

Shaer CM, Chescheir N, Schulkin J (2007). Myelomeningocele: a review of the epidemiology, genetics, risk factors for conception, prenatal diagnosis, and prognosis of affected individuals. *Obstet Gynecol Surv* **62**:471–479.

Defects in hindbrain development

Tubbs RS, Lyerly MJ, Loukas M, Shoja MM, Oakes WJ (2007). The pediatric Chiari malformation: a review. *Childs Nerv Syst* **23**:1239–1250.

Vaillant C, Monard D (2009). SHH pathway and cerebellar development. *Cerebellum* 8:291–301.

Malformations of the forebrain and cerebral development

Altaba AR, Palma V, Dahmane N (2002). Hedgehog-GLI signaling and the growth of the brain. *Nature Rev Neurosci* **3**:24–33.

Cohen MM (2006). Holoprosencephaly: clinical, anatomic, and molecular dimensions. *Birth Defects Res Clin Mol Teratol* **76**:658–673.

Polizzi A, Pavone P, Iannetti P, Manfre L, Ruggieri M (2006). Septo-optic dysplasia complex: a heterogeneous malformation syndrome. *Pediatr Neurol* **34**:66–71.

Roessler E, Muenke M (1998). Holoprosencephaly: a paradigm for the complex genetics of brain development. *J Inher Metab Dis* **21**:481–497.

Defects of neuronal proliferation

Abuelo D (2007). Microcephaly syndromes. *Semin Pediatr Neurol* **14**:118–127.

Disorders of neuronal migration

Guerrini R, Marini C (2006). Genetic malformations of cortical development. *Exp Brain Res* **173**:322–333.

Shoubridge C, Fullston T, Gecz J (2010). ARX spectrum disorders: making inroads into the molecular pathology. *Hum Mutat* **31**:889–900.

Spalice A, Parisi P, Nicita F, Pizzerdi G, Bel Balzo F, Ianneti P (2009). Neuronal migration disorders: clinical, neuroradiologic and genetic aspects. *Acta Paediatr* **98**:421–433.

mTOR pathway

Gipson TT, Johnston MV (2012). Plasticity and mTOR: towards restoration of impaired synaptic plasticity in mTOR-related neurogenetic disorders. *Neural Plast* 486402 Epub 2012 Apr 30.

Neurofibromatosis

Mautner VF, Tatagiba M, Lindenau M, *et al.* (1995). Spinal tumors in patients with neurofibromatosis type 2: MR imaging study of frequency, multiplicity, and variety. *Am J Roentgenol* **165**:951–955.

North K, Joy P, Yuille D, Cocks N, Hutchins P (1995). Cognitive function and academic performance in children with neurofibromatosis type 1. *Dev Med Child Neurol* **37**:427–436.

Tonsgard JH, Kwak SM, Short MP, Dachman AH (1998). CT imaging in adults with neurofibromatosis-1: frequent asymptomatic plexiform lesions. *Neurology* **50**:1755–1760.

Tuberous sclerosis

Ess KC (2006). The neurobiology of tuberous sclerosis complex. *Semin Pediatr Neurol* **13**:37–42.

Holmes GL, Stafstrom CE, the Tuberous Sclerosis Study Group (2007). Tuberous sclerosis complex and epilepsy: recent developments and future challenges. *Epilepsia* **48**:617–630.

Huttenlocher PR, Heydemann PT (1984). Fine structure of cortical tubers in tuberous sclerosis: a Golgi study. *Ann Neurol* **16**:595–602.

Koenig MK, Butler IJ, Northrup H (2008). Regression of subependymal giant cell astrocytoma with rapamycin in tuberous sclerosis complex. *J Child Neurol* **23**:1238–1239.

Napolioni V, Moavero R, Curatolo P (2009). Recent advances in neurobiology of tuberous sclerosis complex. *Brain Develop* **31**:104–113.

Rosser T, Panigraphy A, McClintock W (2006). The diverse clinical manifestations of tuberous sclerosis complex: a review. *Semin Pediatr Neurol* **13**:27–36.

Sturge–Weber syndrome

Lo W, Marchuk DA, Ball KL, *et al.* (2011). Updates and future horizons on the understanding, diagnosis, and treatment of Sturge-Weber syndrome brain involvement. *Dev Med Child Neurol* **54**:214–223.

Thomas-Sohl KA, Vaslow DF, Maria BL (2004). Sturge Weber syndrome: a review. *Pediatr Neurol* **30**:303–310.

Hereditary hemorrhagic telangiectasia

Faughnan ME, Palda VA, Garcia-Tsao G, *et al.* (2011). International guidelines for the diagnosis and management of hereditary haemorrhagic telangiectasia. *J Med Genet* **48**:73–87.

Linear nevus sebaceous syndrome

van de Warrenburg BPC, van Gulik S, Renier WO, Lammens M, Doelman JC (1998). The linear naevus sebaceous syndrome. *Clin Neurol Neurosurg* **100**:126–132.

Cowden's syndrome

Boonpipattanapong T, Phuenpathom N, Mitranun W (2005). Cowden's syndrome and Lhermitte-Duclos disease. *Br J Neurosurg* **19**:361–365.

Von Hippel–Lindau disease

Greer SN, Metcalf JL, Wang Y, Ohh M (2012). The updated biology of hypoxia-inducible factor. *EMBO J* **31**:2448–2460.

Hypomelanosis of Ito

Fritz B, Kuster W, Orstavik KH, Naumova A, Spranger J, Rehder H (1998). Pigmentary mosaicism in hypomelanosis of Ito: Further evidence for functional disomy Xp. *Hum Genet* **103**:441–449.

Taibjee SM, Bennett DC, Moss C (2004). Abnormal pigmentation in hypomelanosis of Ito and pigmentary mosaicism: the role of the pigmentary genes. *Br J Dermatol* **151**:269–282.

HEREDITARY AND METABOLIC DISEASES OF THE CENTRAL NERVOUS SYSTEM IN ADULTS

Alma R. Bicknese

INTRODUCTION

The first step to identifying metabolic or inherited degenerative disease in an adult is to recognize that it could exist. Many view this disease class as only occurring in childhood, so diagnosis is often delayed. The adult patterns are generally slower in onset and do not have the classic appearance of their pediatric manifestations. Adult presentations require recognition of subtle findings or disease patterns that vary from more common adult degenerative neurologic disorders.

Inquire about family history, but be aware that many adults do not know or cannot accurately recall family history. Motor symptoms such as ataxia, dystonia, or spasticity may be the initial presentation, but cognitive decline and psychiatric disturbance often precede onset of neurologic symptoms. When suspicious of an inherited or metabolic disorder in the early stages, neuropsychiatric evaluation may be helpful in detecting early brain dysfunction.

Early symptoms of degenerative diseases

Personality changes and behavior disturbances are often the first symptoms of disease. Irritability, shortened attention span, and poor memory are often overlooked or blamed on stressful events. Cognitive decline and mental regression may be seen in some inherited metabolic diseases (*Table 20*); these may not be obvious until work performance is impacted. Inability to perform demanding tasks such as book keeping or supervision may lead to poor evaluations or job loss months or years before seeking medical advice.

It may be difficult to distinguish common psychiatric diseases such as depression from early degeneration and the clinician should be alert for atypical presentations or subtle neurologic findings pointing to a degenerative disease. A neuropsychologist may be able to help differentiate psychological from degenerative symptomatology.

TABLE 20 **DISORDERS ASSOCIATED WITH DEMENTIA**

Adrenoleukodystrophy
CADASIL
Ceroid lipofuscinosis
FXTAS
Huntington's disease
Krabbe's disease
Lafora body disease
Metachromatic leukodystrophy
Mitochondrial disorders
Niemann–Pick Type C
Sandhoff disease

CADASIL: cerebral autosomal dominant arteriopathy with subcortical infarcts and leukoencephalopathy; FXTAS: fragile X-associated tremor/ataxia syndrome.

In later stages, agitation, violent behavior, and impulsive acts may occur and lead to social or legal conflicts. Conversely, symptoms more typical of depression may occur such as withdrawal, indifference, or being abnormally quiet[1,2].

Tip

▶ *The best resource for specific genetic disease information is GeneReviews, an NIH online textbook that is peer reviewed, can be referenced, and is updated at least every 3 years. Go to: http://www.ncbi.nlm.nih.gov/sites/GeneTests and click on the GeneReview link.*

TABLE 21 **DISORDERS ASSOCIATED WITH PSYCHIATRIC SYMPTOMS**

CADASIL
Ceroid lipofuscinosis
FXTAS
G_{M2} gangliosidosis
Homocystinuria
Huntington's disease
Metachromatic leukodystrophy
Niemann–Pick Type C
PKAN
Porphyria
Sandhoff disease
Wilson's disease

CADASIL: cerebral autosomal dominant arteriopathy with subcortical infarcts and leukoencephalopathy; FXTAS: fragile X-associated tremor/ataxia syndrome; PKAN: pantothenate kinase-associated neurodegeneration.

TABLE 22 **DISEASES ASSOCIATED WITH EXTRA-PYRAMIDAL SIGNS OR GAIT DISTURBANCE**

Adrenoleukodystrophy
Ceroid lipofuscinosis
FXTAS
G_{M2} gangliosidosis
Homocystinuria
Huntington's disease
Krabbe's disease
Lafora body disease
Metachromatic leukodystrophy
Mitochondrial disorders
Niemann–Pick Type C
PKAN
Sandhoff disease
Wilson's disease

FXTAS: fragile X-associated tremor/ataxia syndrome; PKAN: pantothenate kinase-associated neurodegeneration.

TABLE 23 **DISORDERS WITH CHARACTERISTIC MRI FINDINGS**

Disorder	**Finding**
Adrenoleukodystrophy	Occipital white matter changes with contrast uptake at margins (early)
CADASIL	White matter changes in anterior temporal horns (early) Subcortical lacunar infarcts
FXTAS	White matter changes in superior cerebellar peduncle
G_{M2} gangliosidosis	Cerebellar atrophy
Huntington's disease	Severe atrophy of the caudate and putamen
Lafora body disease	MR spectroscopy
Mitochondrial disorders	Symmetric basal ganglia lesions, infarcts that do not follow vascular pattern
PKAN	'Eye of the tiger' sign
Wilson's disease	'Face of the panda' sign, increased T2 signal in caudate and putamen

CADASIL: cerebral autosomal dominant arteriopathy with subcortical infarcts and leukoencephalopathy; FXTAS: fragile X-associated tremor/ataxia syndrome; PKAN: pantothenate kinase-associated neurodegeneration.

Psychiatric symptoms

When a previously psychologically healthy individual either begins exhibiting atypical psychiatric symptoms, or if presentation is outside of the usual age of onset for disorders such as schizophrenia or bipolar disorder, one should consider the possibility of an inherited metabolic disease (*Table 21*). Metabolic diseases may initially present with a psychotic break, agitated depression, or even a delusional or hallucinational syndrome.

Some metabolic diseases may fluctuate and have repeated psychotic or delusional episodes. Neurologic findings such as tremor, decreased facial movement, or bradykinesia can be side-effects of psychiatric medications, making interpretation of examination difficult.

The most important evidence for a metabolic disorder is the recognition of subtle neurologic signs that may be signs of a brain disorder:

- Speech disorders including dysarthria, changes in quality of speech, and new onset stuttering.
- Ocular changes including progressive loss of vision or disorders of eye movements. Consultation with a neuro-ophthalmologist may be helpful to detect early findings.
- Exaggerated *or* absent deep tendon reflexes.
- Progressive spasticity or Babinski signs.
- New onset extrapyramidal symptoms or tremor (*Table 22*).
- Seizures or abnormal slowing on electroencephalogram (EEG).
- Abnormal magnetic resonance imaging (MRI) findings (*Table 23*).

METABOLIC AND DEGENERATIVE DISEASES IN ADULTS

HUNTINGTON'S DISEASE

Definition and etiology

Huntington's disease (HD) is an autosomal dominant disorder with very high penetrance with rare *de novo* mutations. Over 90% of cases can be confirmed by family history. It is caused by instability (expansion) of the CAG repeat in exon 1 mapped to chromosome 4q16, and encodes the protein 'huntingtin', whose function is unknown[3] (**243**). Prevalence is about 7:100, 000 in Western European populations, but pockets of higher incidence occur, and prevalence is probably much lower in Asia and Africa.

Age onset is late childhood to eighth decade, with a mean onset at 35–40 years. Males and females are equally affected.

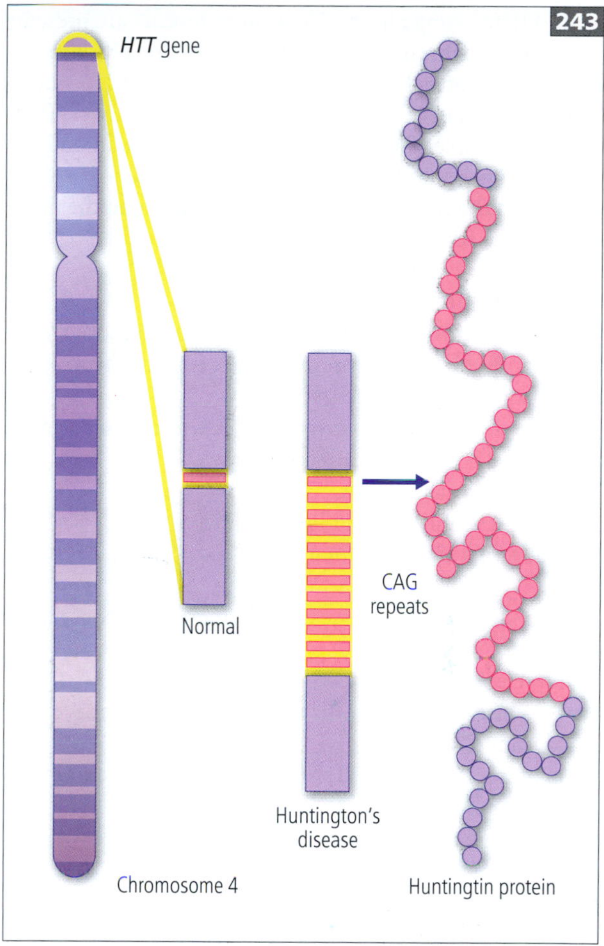

243 The *HTT* gene is located on the short (p) arm of chromosome 4 at p16.3, and codes for the huntingtin protein. The mutation that gives rise to Huntington's disease causes excessive repetition of the CAG nucleotide triplet. A normal gene contains less than 26 CAG repeats, but the mutated allele may contain up to 250 repeats, leading to the production of an abnormally long, toxic version of the protein.

The number of CAG repeats can increase from one generation to the next; this occurs during gametogenesis, particularly during spermatogenesis (paternal inheritance). This phenomenon (called anticipation) makes the symptoms become apparent at an earlier age in successive generations. Normal alleles: have 26 or fewer repeats; intermediate alleles: have 27–35 repeats. An individual is not at risk for themselves, but is at risk of having an affected child.

In HD-causing alleles, 36 or more repeats are present; in reduced penetrance, 36–39 repeats are present. An individual is at risk for HD, but may not develop symptoms. Full penetrance HD-causing alleles have 40 or more repeats, leading to severe neuronal loss, initially in the striatum (putamen and caudate nucleus) and subsequently in the cerebral cortex (**244**). In general, the more repeats, the earlier disease onset.

Clinical features

About one-third of patients will first be diagnosed with primary psychiatric symptoms, the rest with neurologic symptoms. Early changes include:

- Mild motor decline with clumsiness and slowed gait.
- Irritability, anxiety, or agitation.
- Apathy or depression.
- Subtle eye movement abnormalities.
- Delusions and hallucinations.

As the disease progresses, movement disorders predominate:

- Dystonia and chorea.
- Parkinsonian symptoms including mask-like face and hypophonic speech.
- Gait may be slow and stiff, or a staggering gait reminiscent of intoxication.
- Dysphagia and weight loss may occur.
- Tremor may be prominent.
- Depression and suicidal ideation are common.

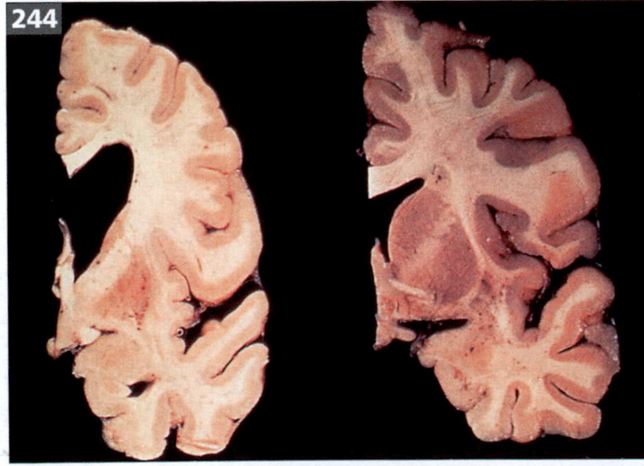

244 Coronal section through the frontal lobe of one cerebral hemisphere from a patient with advanced Huntington's disease (left), showing severe atrophy of the caudate nucleus and frontal lobe, with dilatation of the frontal horn of the lateral ventricle of the brain, compared with a normal brain (right).

In later stages:

- Rigidity, severe bradykinesia.
- Dysphagia, inability to swallow and severe weight loss.
- Seizures.
- In the end, the patient cannot walk or speak.

Diagnosis

MRI shows atrophy of the caudate and putamen, sometimes before symptom onset.

Tip

▶ *Warning! Do not test asymptomatic relatives or children! This disease has variable course and a positive test can be devastating for a young person. Refer to a genetics counselor, who will provide pre- and post-test support.*

Treatment

Treatment is symptomatic:

- Baclofen and diltiazem may be helpful for rigidity.
- Haloperidol or atypical antipsychotics may help chorea.
- Levodopa should be used cautiously for parkinsonian symptoms as it may significantly worsen chorea.
- Valproate is useful for myoclonus.

A number of rare diseases may present like HD, and should be considered when the genetic test is negative or without family history.

Chorea – acanthocytosis

- Autosomal recessive.
- Early appearance is similar to HD including psychiatric symptoms.
- Acanthocytes are present in 5–50% of the red cell population.
- Caused by mutations in the *VPS13A* gene, which produces a protein called chorein.
- Self-mutilation is common.

Huntington's disease-like 1 (HDL1)

- Prion disease with symptom overlap with HD.
- Autosomal dominant inheritance.
- Mutation in the prion protein gene *PRNP* on chromosome 20p.

Huntington's disease-like 2 (HDL2)

- Clinically indistinguishable from HD.
- May be exclusive to individuals of African descent.
- CTG/CAG repeat expansion in the *JPH3* gene.

Tip

▶ *Don't know when or how to order a specific genetic test? GeneTests is a National Institutes for Health (NIH) sponsored on-line resource that lists laboratories around the world offering a specific test. Go to: http://www.ncbi.nlm.nih.gov/sites/GeneTests and click on the laboratory link.*

CEREBRAL AUTOSOMAL DOMINANT ARTERIOPATHY WITH SUBCORTICAL INFARCTS AND LEUKOENCEPHALOPATHY (CADASIL)

Definition and etiology

Cerebral autosomal dominant arteriopathy with subcortical infarcts and leukoencephalopathy (CADASIL) is autosomal dominant with high penetrance. Within the same family and same mutation, variable patterns of disease are noted. CADASIL is caused by mutations to the *NOTCH3* gene. *NOTCH3* affects the function and survival of vascular smooth muscle cells. Dysfunction leads to apoptosis, leading to small vessel vasculopathy and eventually strokes (*Table 24*). Most strokes are 'lacunar' and involve one modality, but recurrent strokes lead to increasing dysfunction. World-wide prevalence is unknown (1:50,000 in Scotland). Penetrance is probably 100%, but expression or severity varies widely.

Age of onset is young adulthood until the sixth decade. Males and females are equally affected.

Clinical features

Significant symptoms include:

- Migraine with aura: average age of onset 26, occurs in 40% of patients.
- Cognitive defects: average age of onset 35, occurs in 60% of patients:
  - Slowly progressive with acute exacerbations with strokes.
  - Verbal cues and executive functions are first involved.
- Strokes: average age of onset 46, with range 19–67years:
  - Individual strokes involve small vessels: 'lacunar' pattern.
  - As strokes recur, frontal lobe symptoms with pseudobulbar palsy, gait disturbance, and urinary incontinence are seen.
  - May be wheelchair bound by early 60s.
- Psychiatric disorders: average age onset 35, occur in 30% of patients:
  - Depression and personality changes predominate, which can be the presenting finding.

TABLE 24 **DISORDERS ASSOCIATED WITH STROKE**

CADASIL
Fabry's disease
Homocystinuria
Mitochondrial disorders

CADASIL: cerebral autosomal dominant arteriopathy with subcortical infarcts and leukoencephalopathy.

- Epilepsy occurs in about 10% of patients, usually around stroke onset.
- Reversible acute encephalopathy has been reported, which can be severe and result in death.

Diagnosis

MRI findings depend on age and severity of disease:

- Progressive white matter lesions are seen:
  - Age 20–30 years: white matter hyperintensities in anterior temporal horns, with nonspecific periventricular and external capsule changes.
  - Age 30–death: slow increase in hyperintensities in other brain areas, that may go on to involve the entire white matter.
- Subcortical lacunar lesions in the gray/white junction are common, may appear early, and are specific for CADASIL.
- MRI findings consistent with microbleeds can occur, primarily in the thalamus.
- Diagnosis is by *NOTCH3* molecular genetic analysis, which detects at least 90% of mutations. Most mutations are in exons 2 through 6 and 11. If negative, proceed to complete sequencing.
- If needed, electron microscopy of skin biopsies will demonstrate electron-dense (osmiophilic) granules in the media of arterioles.

Treatment

Treatment is symptomatic, with advice to avoid certain risks: smoking increases the progression of the disease, and the use of contrast or performing standard angiography in CADASIL should be avoided as it may provoke stroke.

FRAGILE X-ASSOCIATED TREMOR/ATAXIA SYNDROME (FXTAS)

Definition and etiology

Fragile X-associated tremor/ataxia syndrome (FXTAS) is an X-linked disorder produced by instability and abnormal methylation of the *FMR1* gene, which in turn is caused by an increased number of CGG trinucleotide repeats (**245**). Some families show anticipation, where the disease worsens between generations.

The number of repeats determines the severity: 50–200 repeats (premutation) produces FXTAS; >200 repeats (mutation) produces a more severe childhood disorder (fragile X syndrome). FXTAS primarily affects males, with some affected females. Women and girls can rarely have either fragile X or FXTAS, and may have premature ovarian failure.

Prevalence: 1:250 women and 1:800 men have the premutation. Penetrance varies depending on age and sex:

- Male premutation carriers are at highest risk:
  - Age 50–59: 17%.
  - Age 60–69: 38%.
  - Age 70–79: 47%.
  - Age ≥ 79: 75%.
- The overall estimated prevalence is about 1:3000 males.
- Female penetrance is not as well understood but prevalence is estimated at 1:5200.

Clinical features

Symptoms may begin as young as early 50s, but can be delayed a decade or more. Major criteria include:

- Intention tremor.
- Progressive ataxia.

Minor criteria include:

- Parkinsonian symptoms.
- Cognitive decline:
  - Short-term memory disorder.
  - Executive function deficits.
- Personality changes with volatile mood – anger outbursts, inappropriate or impulsive actions.
- Peripheral neuropathy – sensory or autonomic.
- Females may have the same symptoms as males, but usually less severe. In addition they may have:
  - Fibromyalgia.
  - Hypothyroidism.
  - Epilepsy.

245 The *FMR1* gene is located on long (q) arm of the X-chromosome at q27.3. Mutation of the gene causes excessive repetition of the CGG nucleotide triplet, from 30 repeats in normal functional alleles, to over 200 in mutated alleles. This leads to abnormal methylation and decreased production or absence of the *FMR1* gene's protein product, FMRP. A CGG sequence in the *FMR1* gene which is repeated between 55 and 200 times is described as a premutation and can lead to adult onset FXTAS. Repeats greater than 200 lead to Fragile X syndrome in boys.

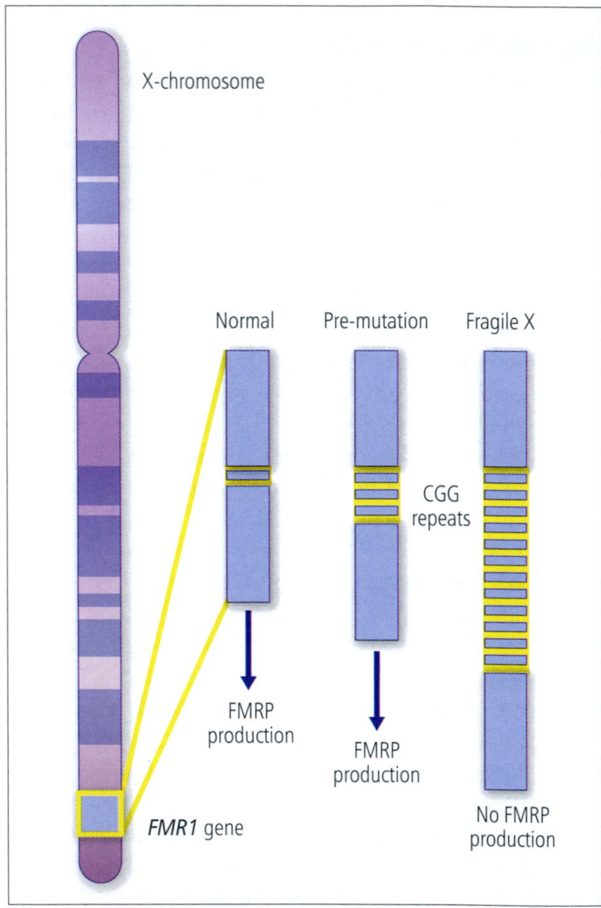

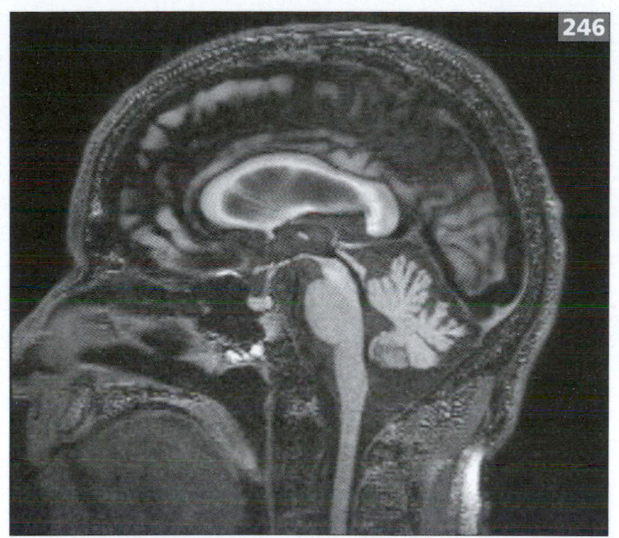

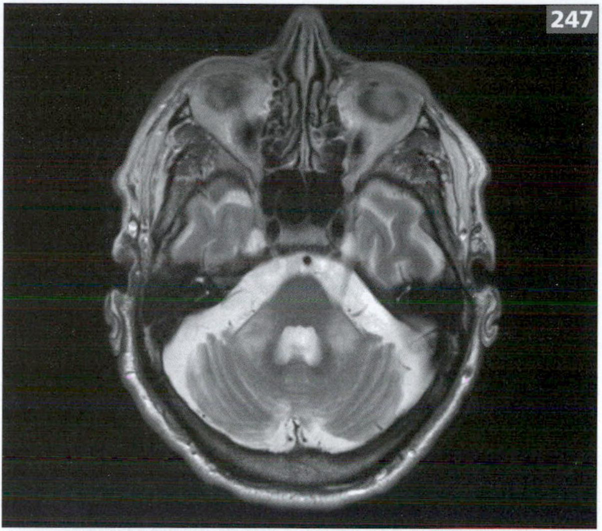

246, 247 FXTAS imaging. Sagittal (243) and axial (244) MRI images show characteristic increased signal in the cerebellar peduncles and pons. The sagittal image also demonstrates increased signal in the corpus callosum, along with generalized cerebral atrophy.

Diagnosis

MRI shows major and minor criteria:

- Major criteria: white matter lesions in the middle cerebellar peduncles and/or brainstem (246, 247).
- Minor criteria: lesions in cerebral white matter or generalized atrophy.

Diagnosis requires the presence of a premutation along with MRI and physical findings.

- **Definitive diagnosis** requires the presence of the premutation AND both one major MRI and two major neurologic signs.
- **Probable diagnosis** requires the presence of the premutation and EITHER one major MRI finding or two major neurologic findings.
- **Possible diagnosis** requires the premutation AND both one minor MRI finding AND one major neurologic finding.

Mutations in the *FMR1* gene can affect multiple generations in the same family in different ways. The grandfather and mother may have the premutation, while her son may have fragile X syndrome. Once fragile X is diagnosed, grandparents, aunts, uncles, siblings and cousins are at risk for carrying the premutation and developing FXTAS. Testing of family members should be done in conjunction with a genetic counselor who will review testing options, the probability of having the disorder if the premutation is present, and recurrence risk with additional pregnancies.

X-LINKED ADRENOLEUKODYSTROPHY

Definition and etiology

X-linked adrenoleukodystrophy (ALD) is an X-linked peroxisomal disorder with progressive central nervous system (CNS) demyelination and adrenal failure due to accumulation of saturated, very long chain fatty acids (VLCFAs). ALD is caused by mutations in the *ABCD1* gene (ATP-binding cassette, subfamily D [ALD], member 1) located on the long arm of the X chromosome. *ABCD1* encodes for adrenoleukodystrophy protein (ALDP); this combines with another protein to form a membrane transporter within peroxisomal membranes. Without this transporter, VLCFA cannot be metabolized and accumulates in brain and adrenal cells.

Prevalence in hemizygotes (affected males) is 1:20,000 and in hemizygote and heterozygote (carrier) females is 1:16,800. The age onset and clinical manifestations can vary within the same family.

Clinical features

- Childhood cerebral form: 30% of patients – onset usually 4–8 years: rapidly progressive.
- Adrenomyeloneuropathy (AMN): 40–45% cases (*Table 25*):
  - Onset mid-20s to middle age.
  - Slowly progressive spastic paraparesis without upper limb involvement.
  - Impaired vibration and position sense.

TABLE 25 **DISORDERS ASSOCIATED WITH NEUROPATHY**

Adrenoleukodystrophy
Fabry's disease
FXTAS
G_{M2} gangliosidosis
Homocystinuria
Krabbe's disease
Metachromatic leukodystrophy
Mitochondrial disorders
Porphyria
Sandhoff disease

FXTAS: fragile X-associated tremor/ataxia syndrome.

  - Urinary and sexual dysfunction.
  - Mild peripheral nerve involvement – slowing of sensory and motor conduction velocities.
  - Hypogonadism is common.
  - Mild cognitive decline.
  - Adrenal insufficiency can occur after onset of paraparesis.
- Addison disease only: 10%:
  - Onset 2 years to adulthood, usually around age 7.
  - Most develop AMN by middle age.
- Atypical presentations seen in 5–10% of affected males:
  - Headache, increased intracranial pressure, focal neurologic defects – usually presents prior to age 10, rarely in adults.
  - Adult onset progressive dementia, behavior disturbance, and paralysis.
  - Progressive ataxia in child or adult.
  - Neurogenic bladder and bowel abnormalities or impotence without other neurologic or endocrine disorders.
  - Some with the gene will remain asymptomatic.
- Females: about 20% of carriers develop milder symptoms after age 35, and about 20% of carrier females develop spastic paraparesis in middle age.

Diagnosis and investigations

ADL should be suspected in young or middle-aged adult males with progressive lower limb spasticity, sensory changes, bladder and bowel abnormalities or impotence, and in all males with primary adrenal failure. ADL should also be considered in middle-aged and older females with progressive lower limb spasticity and sensory changes with or without bladder and bowel abnormalities.

MRI of the brain usually shows a characteristic pattern of symmetric hyperintense T2 signal in the parieto-occipital region with contrast enhancement at the advancing margin (**248**). White matter changes progress from posterior to anterior, with all white matter eventually involved. MRI may be normal in females and mildly affected males.

Laboratory evaluation for elevated VLCFA is the preferred first diagnostic test, and is positive in 100% of males and about 80% of females. The *ABCD1* gene can be tested:

- Sequencing is positive for 99% of males and 93% of females.
- Duplication/deletion testing will diagnose 6% of females.

Treatment

Treatment is supportive. Patients should be monitored for, and treated for, adrenal insufficiency. Adrenocorticotropic hormone (ACTH) levels will rise. Other treatments such as Lorenzo's oil have not been studied in adults.

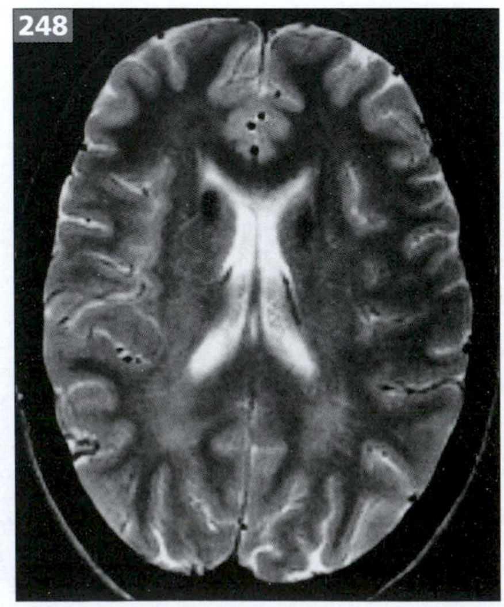

248 Adrenoleukodystrophy. T2W axial MRI showing diffuse bilateral increased signal, mainly in the parieto-occipital white matter. The more anterior white matter is also beginning to look affected.

PANTOTHENATE KINASE-ASSOCIATED NEURODEGENERATION (PKAN)

Definition and etiology

Pantothenate kinase-associated neurodegeneration (PKAN) was formerly known as Hallervorden–Spatz syndrome. PKAN is an autosomal recessive disorder caused by mutations in the *PANK2* gene. *PANK2* codes for pantothenate kinase 2, which participates in the synthesis of coenzyme A and in the phosphorylation of pantothenate (vitamin B5), N-pantothenoyl-cysteine, and pantetheine. Without pantothenate kinase 2, cysteine and cysteine-containing compounds collect in the basal ganglia, causing chelation of iron in the globus pallidus, and oxidative cell death. Males and females are equally affected.

Disease frequency is unknown, but is estimated at 3:1,000,000. Onset is early childhood until adulthood (75% prior to age 10, 25% late teens until the third decade).

Clinical features

Neurologic disability with extrapyramidal symptoms is the key feature in PKAN. Psychiatric symptoms can be the initial presentation in adults but motor impairment is inevitable.

- Extrapyramidal dysfunction:
  - Dystonia.
  - Rigidity.
  - Choreoathetosis.
  - Parkinsonian features and dysarthria can be prominent in late-onset PKAN.
- Corticospinal dysfunction:
  - Spasticity.
  - Hyper-reflexia.
  - Babinski sign.
- Psychiatric symptoms:
  - Cognitive decline – similar to frototemporal dementia.
  - Personality changes.
  - Impulsivity.
  - Emotional lability – violent outbursts.
  - Depression.
  - Psychosis.
- Retinal degeneration or optic atrophy occur in two-thirds of cases.

HARP (hypoprebetalipoproteinemia, acanthocytosis, retinitis pigmentosa, and pallidal degeneration) is now considered a variant of PKAN.

Diagnosis

Diagnosis is by MRI, which shows iron deposition in basal ganglia. Abnormalities are restricted to the globus pallidus and substantia nigra, producing the 'eye of the tiger' abnormality on T2-weighted imaging (**249**). This eventually develops in virtually all patients. Hypointensity of the dentate nuclei in T2 sequencing is sometimes seen. *PANK2* gene analysis should be performed when MRI findings are present.

Treatment

Survival with progressive disability is usually 10 years, but 30 years has been reported. No treatments to prevent disease progression are available.

- L-dopa may be effective in early cases.
- Spasticity can be modulated by baclofen, trihexyphenidyl, and intramuscular botulinum toxin.
- Supplementation with pantothenate, coenzyme Q, and other antioxidants has been attempted, but is not proven to be effective.

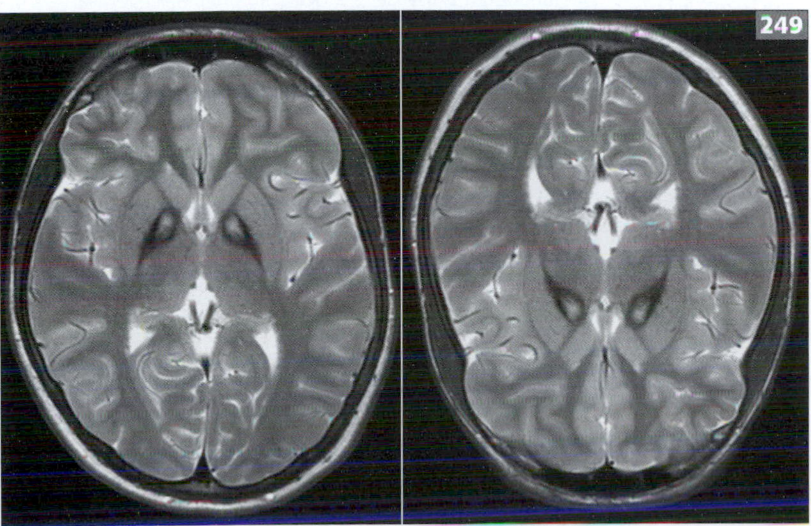

249 T2-weighted MRI showing iron deposition in the pallidus and substantia nigra in pantothenate kinase-associated neurodegeneration mutations (left). When the axial image is rotated, an 'eye of the tiger' abnormality is seen (right). *Courtesy of the Children's Hospital and Research Center Oakland.*

INHERITED DISEASES WITH PROMINENT VISCERAL AND NEUROLOGIC FINDINGS

WILSON'S DISEASE (WD)

Wilson's disease (WD) (familial hepatolenticular degeneration) is an autosomal recessive disease that causes heavy copper deposition in liver, cornea, kidneys, and CNS. The gene is located on chromosome 13q14.3 and codes for a copper transporting P-type protein ATP7B. This results in low serum ceruloplasmin and high serum and urine copper. Normal variations in another gene, the prion protein gene (*PRNP*), can modify the course of WD[4].

Prevalence: 1:30,000 (30 per million) are affected; 1:100 individuals in the general population have one copy of the WD gene. Age of onset is 8 to >50 years, and males and females are equally affected.

Clinical features

WD may present with primarily liver or CNS findings.

Liver disease

Isolated liver findings are common in childhood, but may be subtle or overlooked. Hepatic cirrhosis precedes neurologic dysfunction.

CNS findings

CNS findings are common in WD, and become increasingly common after age 12 years.

Copper deposits in the Descemet's membrane (Kayser–Fleischer rings) are universally present when there is CNS disease, and are detected by slit lamp examination (**250**, *Table 26*).

Behavioral and cognitive changes are common and are the first manifestation in about 20% of cases. These changes often precede extrapyramidal symptoms. Patients show loss of emotional control, and difficulty in conforming to societal norms is usual. Intellectual decline is present but may be masked by bizarre behavior. WD may be misdiagnosed as schizophrenia or other psychiatric disorders, which delays treatment, worsening the outcome.

Extrapyramidal symptoms have two major and often dissociated findings:

- Rigidity: Wilsonian form has faciolinguopharyngeal rigidity with facial masking, dysarthria, and dysphagia. Rigidity progresses and can involve the trunk and limbs.
- Tremor (Westphal–Strumpell form) may initially be in one limb.

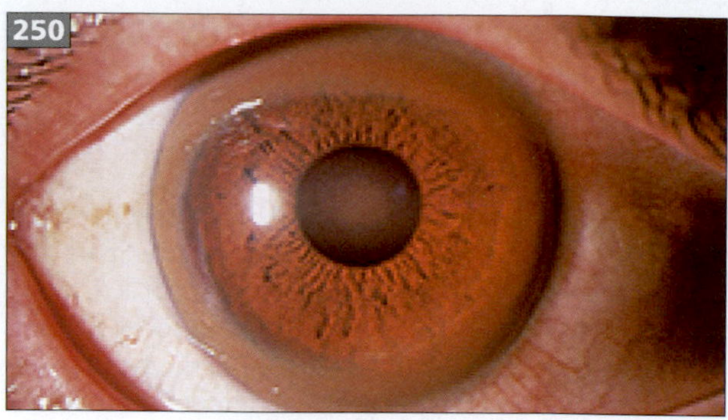

250 Kayser–Fleischer ring: a 1–3 mm thick brown ring (but may be other colors) of sulfur–copper complexes at the corneal margin.

As symptoms progress, the face becomes mask-like and there may be a forced grin. Speech and swallowing become more difficult and may be lost. Parkinsonian symptoms worsen, and a gross and irregular tremor develops, which is worse with arms outstretched (rubral tremor). Dyskinesia or chorea may be prominent in some patients.

TABLE 26 **DISORDERS WITH EYE FINDINGS**

Disorder	Finding
Fabry's disease	Cornea verticillata, focal dilation retinal arteries (slit lamp)
G_{M2} gangliosidosis	Oculomotor apraxia
Homocystinuria: CBS	Downward ectopia lentis
Homocystinuria: MTHFR	Oculomotor apraxia
Huntington's disease	Oculomotor apraxia (vertical more than lateral)
Mitochondrial disorders: Leigh syndrome, Leber optic atrophy, PEO	Retinitis pigmentosa Optic atrophy External ophthalmoplegia
Niemann–Pick disease	Early – abnormal saccades Late – supranuclear palsy
PKAN	Retinal degeneration, optic atrophy
Wilson's disease	Kayser–Fleischer rings (slit lamp)

CBS: cystathionine β-synthase deficiency;
MTHFR: methylenetetrahydrofolate reductase;
PEO: progressive external ophthalmoplegia;
PKAN: pantothenate kinase-associated neurodegeneration.

Diagnosis and investigations

Laboratory investigation should include:

- Serum ceruloplasmin and total copper: false-positives and false-negatives have occurred, and cannot be relied on to diagnose or exclude disease.
- 24-hour urinary copper secretion – if low, repeat with penicillamine to increase secretion.
- Slit lamp examination for Kayser–Fleischer rings – universally present with CNS disease.
- Liver biopsy is the 'gold standard'.
- Genetic analysis is available. Genetic testing is not always positive and should *not* be used to rule out WD. Most cases are caused by two mutations:
  - H1069Q is the mutation found in populations of European origin. It accounts for 35–45% of WD in a mixed European population.
  - R778L is the mutation found in Asian populations, accounting for approximately 57% of WD in a mixed Asian population.

MRI finding include:

- T1-weighted images show increased signal intensity in globus pallidus and midbrain.
- T2-weighted images can show increased signal intensity in caudate and putamen. Some show high signal with central dark signal intensity. In some the thalamus and globus pallidus is affected (251).
- The 'face of the Panda' is sometimes seen on T2 imaging of the midbrain. Extensive hyperintensity of the midbrain with relative sparing of red nucleus and superior colliculus reminds some of a panda's markings (252).

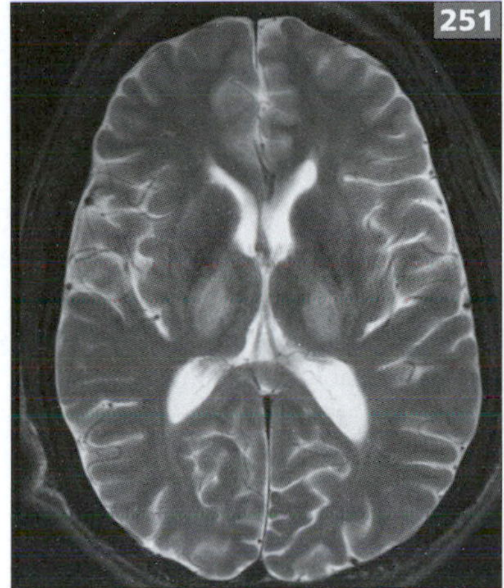

251 Wilson's disease. T2-weighted MRI image shows hyperintense signal in the bilateral thalami, and subtle hyperintense signal in the putamen. *Courtesy of Dr. Paramdeep Singh.*

Treatment

Copper chelating agents that increase urinary excretion of copper are the first-line treatment for WD. Penicillamine was introduced in 1956 and remains the standard treatment, but other agents are available in select cases.

Dietary modification includes avoidance of food high in copper (meat, shellfish, chocolate, mushrooms, dried beans and peas) and increasing consumption of food high in antioxidants. Antioxidant supplements such as Vitamin E may be of use.

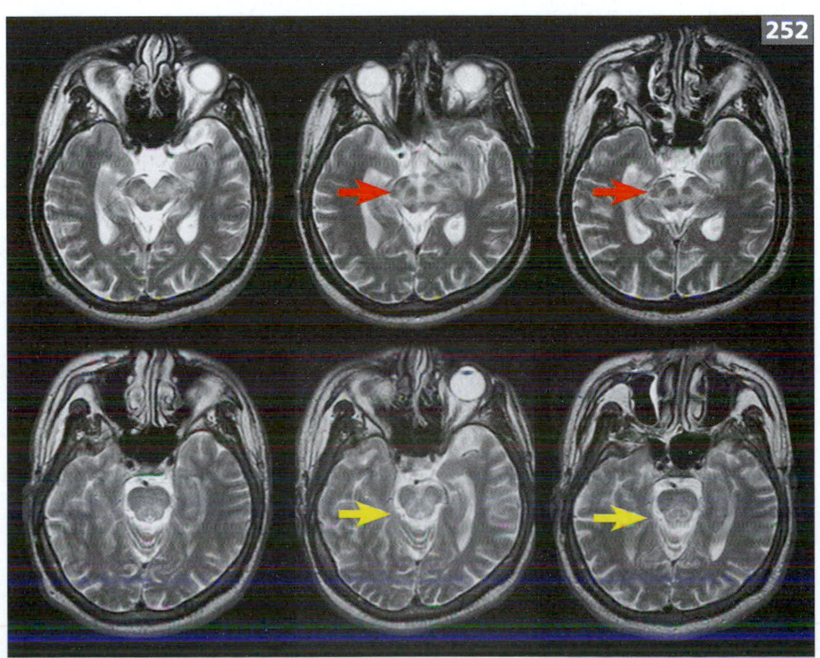

252 Wilson's disease. Copper deposition leads to a characteristic MRI brainstem 'panda' image. Red arrows point to the 'face of the giant panda' seen in the midbrain. There is hyperintense signal surrounding normal red nuclei. The yellow arrows point to the 'panda cub' in the pons. *Courtesy of Dr. David S Liebeskind.*

ACUTE INTERMITTENT PORPHYRIA

Definition and etiology

Porphyrias are disorders caused by the deficiency of enzymes that participate in the synthesis of heme, which lead to the accumulation of intermediaries called porphyrins. Acute intermittent porphyria (AIP) is an autosomal dominant disorder with variable penetrance. Many patients remain asymptomatic throughout life. It is caused by a porphobilinogen deaminase deficiency; this enzyme catalyzes the conversion of porphobilinogen to hydroxymethylbilane. Without it, porphyrin precursors, porphobilinogen and δ-aminolevulinic acid accumulate.

Prevalence is 1–5:100,000, and is higher in those with a Swedish background. Onset is post-puberty, between ages 18 and 40. AIP usually remits by age 40 unless a major provocation occurs. Males are affected less frequently than females.

TABLE 27 **DISEASES ASSOCIATED WITH AN ACUTE NEUROLOGIC DECLINE**

CADASIL
Fabry's disease
Homocystinuria
Mitochondrial disorders
Porphyria
Decompensation in well-controlled childhood metabolic disorders during illness

CADASIL: cerebral autosomal dominant arteriopathy with subcortical infarcts and leukoencephalopathy.

Clinical features

Patients have episodes of acute decompensation or attacks provoked by metabolic stress, fasting, or a large number of drugs (*Table 27*). Phenobarbital, other antiepileptics, and estrogens are frequently involved, but a large number of common drugs may provoke an attack.

Attacks consist of a triad of abdominal pain, psychiatric/CNS symptoms, and peripheral neuropathies. Symptom severity can vary from mild abdominal pain to significant neuropathy or psychiatric disease.

- Brain dysfunction varies in severity:
  - Depression and insomnia are common.
  - May be mistaken for bipolar disorder.
  - Restlessness, crying, confusion, violent behavior, hallucinations, and psychosis may occur.
  - Mental status changes, cortical blindness, seizures, or coma may occur.
  - CNS dysfunction and abdominal pain usually occur together.
- Predominantly motor polyneuropathy:
  - Distal weakness of fingers and wrist extensors is common – wrist drop is classic.
  - Can be severe and generalized with involvement of respiratory musculature leading to respiratory failure.
  - May be confused with Guillain–Barré syndrome.
  - Sensory and autonomic dysfunction may occur.
  - Cranial nerves VII and X are vulnerable, and may cause dangerous dysphagia.
- Abdominal pain is severe, continuous, and lasts several days.

Diagnosis and investigations

Diagnosis is by demonstrating increased urinary porphobilinogen secretion. A 12–24-hour urine collection is best. Porphobilinogen is not included in most 24-hour urine porphyrin screens and may need to be ordered individually. Nearly all patients will have elevated porphobilinogen between attacks. Measurement of porphobilinogen deaminase activity is of little value, as 10% of AIP patients have normal assays, and most patients with deficiency never become symptomatic. MRI is usually normal.

Treatment

The treatment goal is to decrease heme synthesis and thus porphyrin precursors. Most patients should be admitted during attacks because of pain and risk of respiratory depression from peripheral neuropathy.

- High doses of glucose can inhibit heme synthesis and be used for mild attacks.
- Severe attacks can be treated with hematin at a dose of 4 mg/kg/day for 4 days.
- Pain should be treated with narcotics.
- Seizures can be treated with either levetiracetam or gabapentin. However, most classic antiepileptics provoke attacks.

DISORDERS OF AMINO ACID METABOLISM

Introduction

The common end-point of this class of metabolic disorders is the specific abnormal levels of urine and blood amino acids. Symptoms may fluctuate depending on metabolic stress or dietary intake. Most present in childhood, but homocystinuria may not manifest until adult life. Of note, adults who were diagnosed with childhood aminoaciduria may manifest symptoms under conditions of metabolic stress.

HOMOCYSTINURIA

Definition

Disorders in methionine metabolism lead to the accumulation of homocysteine and its metabolites. There are three separate enzymes of interest in the methionine pathway; mutations in each may cause homocystinuria. Homocysteinemia is a variant when only blood has elevated homocysteine levels.

Each enzyme has a specific cofactor/vitamin that affects its metabolism. The pathway starts at methionine, which is converted to homocysteine and then to cysteine. This portion is called the transulfuration pathway. Conversion of homocysteine back to methionine is by the remethylation pathway. A minor alternative pathway uses betaine as a methyl donor (**253**).

Methionine metabolism is affected by environmental factors and comorbidities including oral contraceptives, methotrexate treatment, high-protein diet, folate deficiency, and smoking. Common comorbidities that may provoke crises include hypothyroidism, renal failure, and malignancies. All forms of homocystinuria are autosomal recessive.

Cystathionine ß-synthase deficiency

Definition and etiology

Cystathionine β-synthase deficiency (CBS) is the classic and most severe form of homocystinuria. CBS can be differentiated from other forms of homocystinuria by elevated methionine levels.

- Subtypes:
  - Vitamin B6 responsive.
  - Vitamin B6 unresponsive.
- Prevalence: 1:100,000.
- Age of onset: wide variability from infancy to middle age.

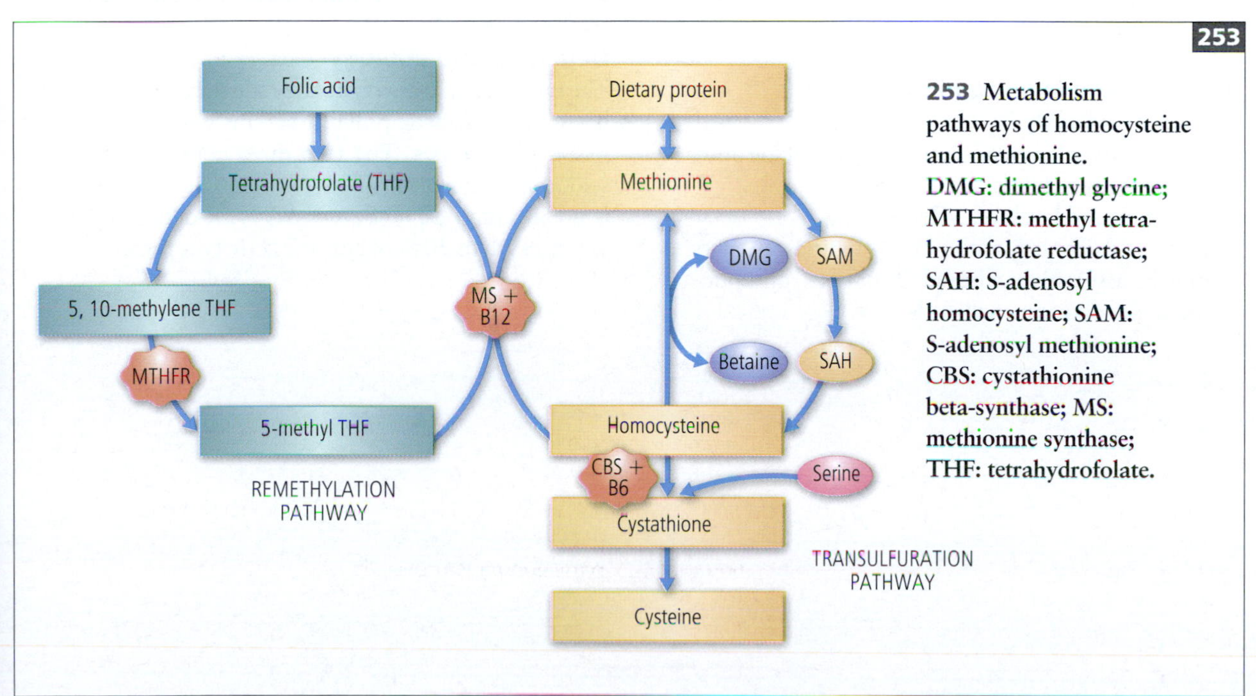

253 Metabolism pathways of homocysteine and methionine. DMG: dimethyl glycine; MTHFR: methyl tetrahydrofolate reductase; SAH: S-adenosyl homocysteine; SAM: S-adenosyl methionine; CBS: cystathionine beta-synthase; MS: methionine synthase; THF: tetrahydrofolate.

Clinical features

Symptoms can be severe or mild. Up to one-third of patients present with a thromboembolic event in adult life. Signs and symptoms may include one or all of the following:

- Developmental delay/intellectual disability:
  - Mean intelligence quotient (IQ) for B6-responsive subtype: 79.
  - Mean IQ for B6-unresponsive subtype: 57.
  - IQ ranges from severe retardation to above average (130+).
- Downward ectopia lentis and/or severe myopia: lens dislocation typically occurs before age 10.
- Skeletal abnormalities:
  - Marfanoid appearance (excessive height, long limbs).
  - Osteoporosis.
  - Scoliosis, high-arched palate, pes cavus, pectus excavatum, or pectus carinatum, can also occur.
- Thromboembolism:
  - Deep venous thrombosis.
  - Stroke.
  - Myocardial infarction.
- Psychiatric problems:
  - Personality disorders.
  - Anxiety.
  - Depression.
  - Psychotic episodes.
- Dystonia.
- Seizures.
- Skin findings:
  - Malar flush.
  - Hypopigmentation.
  - Livedo reticularis.

Diagnosis and investigations

- Amino acid analysis:
  - Elevated plasma and urine homocysteine and methionine levels.
  - Decreased levels of cysteine.
- Enzyme activity: cystathionine β-synthase activity may be assessed in cultured fibroblasts, amniotic fluid, and chorionic villi cells.
- Genetic testing:
  - *CBS* is the only gene linked to classic homocystinuria.
  - Two most common mutations are CBS I278T and G307S, and account for about one-half of cases in the United States.
  - Targeted mutation analysis: sequence analysis will detect about 95% of cases.
- Pyridoxine (B6) challenge: should be performed on all patients. Baseline homocysteine levels are obtained, and then 100 mg B6 is given. A 30% reduction is considered positive; if no effect, escalating doses of B6 are given up to 500 mg.

Carriers

Carriers are usually symptom free, although there are concerns of increased thromboembolic events when under physiologic stress. Homocysteine levels are usually normal. Diagnosis is usually by gene analysis.

Treatment

In pyridoxine-responsive individuals, life-long supplementation is necessary. Patients should undertake a protein-restricted diet, and infants should be on a methionine-restricted diet.

Betaine treatment (6–9 g/day) promotes an alternative remethylation pathway. It is useful for B6-unresponsive patients, or when diet manipulation is unsuccessful. B12 (intramuscular injections) and folate (5 mg/day) are also used.

Methylenetetrahydrofolate reductase deficiency

Definition and etiology

The methylenetetrahydrofolate reductase (*MTHFR*) gene has multiple genetic polymorphisms which produce different phenotypes. The two most common mutations seldom produce neurologic problems as enzyme activity is greater than 20%. Severe *MTHFR* deficiency is seen when less than 20% of enzyme activity is present.

C677T polymorphism

The *MTHFR* nucleotide at position 677 has two possibilities, C (cytosine) or T (thymine). The 677T allele produces a thermolabile enzyme with reduced activity. Individuals with two copies of 677C have a 'wild type' genotype. 677CT heterotypes are nearly normal; 677TT have mild hyperhomocysteinemia. Folate supplementation is recommended.

Prevalence: about 10% of the North American population is homozygous for T. In periods of stress or with a low-folate diet, homocysteine levels may rise. 677TT adults are at increased risk of cardiovascular events in heart and brain. 677TT women have a higher risk of infants with spina bifida and pre-eclampsia. Studies have linked 677TT to increased risk of schizophrenia, decreased bone mass, leukemia, and colon cancer. Gene testing for this variant is widely available.

1298C polymorphism

The *MTHFR* nucleotide at position 1298 has two possibilities, A (adenine) or C (cytosine). 1298AA is normal wild type. This mutation produces no significant effect by itself, but in compound heterozygotes (one copy of 677T and one copy of 1298C) appear to have higher homocysteine levels than 677TT homotypes.

Compound heterozygote woman have increased risk of infants with spina bifida and pre-eclampsia.

Severe MTHFR deficiency

Over 30 separate mutations have been reported to produce severe *MTHFR* deficiency. The age of onset and severity appear correlated to enzyme activity. Symptoms may begin at birth, but may present into the sixth decade. Exacerbations may be triggered by illness. Severe *MTHFR* is associated with low or low normal methionine levels.

Clinical features

Infantile and early childhood form:

- First 3 months:
  - Hypotonia.
  - Lethargy or coma.
  - Brain atrophy with white matter changes.
- 3 months–10 years:
  - Microcephaly.
  - Severe developmental delay.
  - Epilepsy.
  - White matter changes on brain MRI.

Childhood and adult forms may have similar neurologic complications. Some adults will have developmental issues and microcephaly, but many appear relatively asymptomatic until presentation.

- Mixed upper motor neuron findings – hypo- or hypertonia.
- Extrapyramidal findings:
  - Dystonia.
  - Chorea.
- Abnormal eye movements.
- Acute paraplegia – subacute combined degeneration of the cord.
- Thromboembolism:
  - Cerebral sinus thrombosis.
  - Stroke.
  - Myocardial infarction.
- Psychiatric problems are more common in adults:
  - Personality disorders.
  - Anxiety.
  - Depression.
  - Psychotic episodes.
- Mental status changes:
  - Confusion.
  - Coma.
- Polyneuropathy.

Diagnosis and investigations

- MRI:
  - Diffuse white matter changes.
  - Atrophy common.
- Diagnosis is based on elevated urine and serum homocysteine:
  - Low methionine.
  - Low folate.
- Gene testing is available in a few laboratories, but many mutations are not identified.

Treatment

Betaine is the mainstay of treatment, to activate the alternative pathway. Most treatment uses a cocktail of cofactors and products of alternative pathways, including:

- Folate.
- Cobalamine.
- Carnitine.
- Pyridoxine.
- Methyltetrahydrofolate.
- Riboflavin.

However, a cocktail in isolation is usually ineffective.

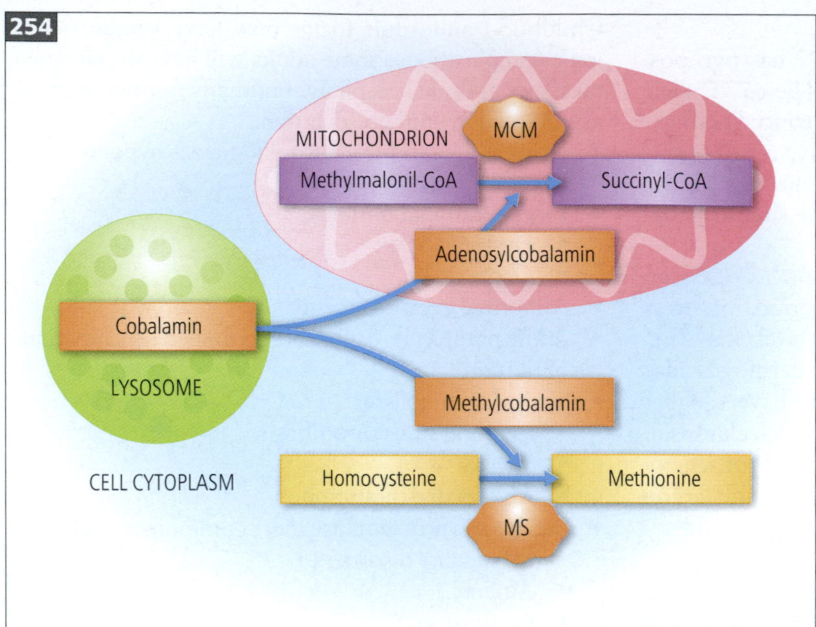

254 Summarized diagram of the pathways utilizing cobalamin. MCM (methylmalonyl-CoA mutase) deficiency causes methylmalonic aciduria, and MS (methionine synthase) deficiency causes hyperhomocysteinemia. Disorders affecting the early steps of cobalamin metabolism may cause a combined MCM/MS deficiency, characterized by hyperhomocysteinemia and/or homocystinuria combined with methylmalonic aciduria.

Disorders of cobalamin (vitamin B12) metabolism

Definition and etiology

Vitamin B12, also known as cobalamin, is a cofactor for two enzymes, methylmalonyl-CoA mutase (*MUT* gene) and methionine synthase (methionine synthase reductase [*MTR*] gene). Disorders of cobalamin metabolism may affect one or both enzymes (**254**).

- Methylmalonyl-CoA mutase (MCM) enzyme dysfunction:
  - Vitamin B12 dependent.
  - *MUT* gene mutation.
  - Causes methylmalonic aciduria.
- Methionine synthase (MS) enzyme dysfunction:
  - Vitamin B12 dependent.
  - *MTR* gene mutation, rarely associated with dysfunction of the enzyme that regenerates MS.
  - Causes hyperhomocysteinemia and/or homocystinuria.
- Combined MCM/MS deficiency:
  - Cobalamin is released from the lysosomes and requires several biochemical modifications before it can be utilized by MCM and MS.
  - Defects in the early steps of the cobalamin metabolism result in deficient activity of both enzymes.
  - Characterized by hyperhomocysteinemia and/or homocystinuria combined with methylmalonic aciduria.
  - There are five genes involved in isolated MS and MS/MCM function function, and all are autosomal recessive.

Males and females are equally affected, and the disease frequency is unknown. Disease onset is from infancy to middle age.

Clinical features

Combined MS/MCM dysfunction

There is a wide variation in age of onset. Infancy is the most common age of presentation. Infants are small and often have acidosis and megaloblastic anemia. Seizures are common. Some develop hemolytic uremic syndrome.

Childhood presentation is nonspecific with microcephaly, cytopenia/megaloblastic anemia, hypotonia, and often symptoms of progressive neurologic dysfunction and seizures.

Adults may present with acute crisis, or a chronic decline. Acute presentations will have confusion or mental status changes. Most acute presentations are triggered by a metabolic stressor and are associated with megaloblastic anemia. Chronic presentations are insidious, with:

- Early progressive cognitive decline.
- Nonspecific white matter changes on MRI.
- Myelopathy with cystic changes in spinal cord.
- Microangiopathic renal syndrome may occur.

Megaloblastic anemia is common, but not universal. *MUT/MTR* mutations will have elevated methylmalonic acid and homocysteine. Most will have elevations in both blood and urine, but a minority may have elevation only in blood.

Isolated MS dysfunction

This is less common, and has a wide variation in onset. Infancy is the most common presentation with severe failure to thrive and megaloblastic anemia. Hypotonia, seizures and developmental delay or decline occur. Adult presentation varies widely:

- Weakness.
- Megaloblastic anemia.
- Psychosis and mental status changes.
- Significant thrombophilia.
- Hemolytic uremic syndrome.
- Optic nerve atrophy.

Diagnosis and investigations

Diagnosis is based on initial laboratory tests, which include:

- Urine organic acid analysis.
- Plasma amino acid analysis.
- Vitamin B12 level, to rule out deficiency.
- Total and free carnitine, and fractionated acyl carnitines.

Genetic testing is available for all five genes, although not all mutations can be detected.

Treatment

Acute attacks include:

- Correction of base deficits.
- Calorie supplementation using dextrose.
- Protein restriction.
- Vitamin B12 supplementation with hydroxycobalamin at 1 mg/day. NB. Do not use the cyanocobalamin form of B12.

Preventative treatment includes hydroxycobalamin injections every 1–3 days. Supplemental treatments are usually given but have little evidence of clinical efficacy. They include carnitine, betaine, pyridoxine, folate, and methionine. Protein restriction is not needed unless there is an acute crisis.

INCLUSION BODY DISORDERS

Introduction

Intracellular inclusion bodies are the hallmark of this group of diseases. In the past, tissue histology was needed for diagnosis, but several genes have been identified and can often be used for diagnosis. Myoclonus is a prominent symptom for this class of disorders.

LAFORA BODY DISEASE

Definition and etiology

Lafora body disease is an autosomal recessive disorder involving one of two genes: *EPM2A* or *NHLRC1* (*EPM2B*). *EPM2A* codes for a protein 'laforin' of unknown function, while the product of the *NHLRC1* gene is unknown. Males and females are equally affected. Prevalence is unknown. It is rare in most populations, but several regions of Europe, the Middle East, North America, and Africa have higher frequencies. Onset is in mid teens into early adulthood, but it can present as young as age 6 and as old as the third decade.

Clinical features

Early findings include:

- Epilepsy: myoclonic epilepsy prevails, but most have a mixed pattern including absence, visual seizures, and tonic–clonic seizures (*Table 28*). It may be initially mistaken for juvenile myoclonic epilepsy. The epilepsy rapidly becomes intractable.
- Migraine-like headaches.
- Cognitive decline.
- Depression and apathy.

Late findings include:

- Dysarthria and ataxia.
- Prominent visual hallucinations.
- Agitation.
- Increasing dementia leading to vegetative state.
- Intractable epilepsy.
- Nonepileptic myoclonus.

TABLE 28 **DISORDERS ASSOCIATED WITH PROMINENT SEIZURES**

Disorder
Ceroid lipofuscinosis
Lafora body disease
Metachromatic leukodystrophy
Mitochondrial disorders
Niemann–Pick Type C
Huntington's disease (late)

Diagnosis and investigations

- MRI is initially normal. MR spectroscopy shows reduced *N*-acetylaspartate (NAA)/creatine ratio in frontal and occipital cortex, basal ganglia, and cerebellum.
- Visual evoked potentials show abnormally high voltage.
- Diagnosis: mutations are sometimes not detected, requiring skin biopsy to detect Lafora bodies.

Tip

▶ *A negative gene test does not rule out inclusion body diseases. If the clinical findings are highly suspicious follow a negative gene test with a biopsy.*

Treatment

No specific treatment exists. Supportive care, management of epilepsy, and myoclonus must be addressed. Most patients die within 10 years of diagnosis.

ADULT NEURONAL CEROID LIPOFUSCINOSES

Definition and etiology

Adult neuronal ceroid lipofuscinoses (ANCL) (Kuf's disease) is a progressive degenerative disease. It is usually an autosomal recessive disorder, but may be dominant in some families. Inclusion bodies develop within the cytoplasm of white blood cells and neurons and can be seen with electron microscopy (EM).

Ceroid lipofuscinoses can occur from infancy to adulthood. Phenotypes are described by age of onset. Genetics is complicated as although eight genes have been identified, they are not specific to phenotype or always to inclusion body type. The five genes most associated with ANCL are *CTSD*, *PPT*, *CLN3*, *CLN5*, and *CLN4*. Males and females are equally affected. Disease onset is usually in the third decade, but can be from the second to sixth decades.

Clinical features

There are two major clinical phenotypes:

- Type A: progressive myoclonic epilepsy with associated:
  - Dementia.
  - Ataxia.
  - Late pyramidal and extrapyramidal signs.
  - Seizures are often uncontrollable.
- Type B: behavior abnormalities and dementia, with associated:
  - Motor dysfunction.
  - Ataxia.
  - Extrapyramidal signs.
  - Bulbar (brainstem) signs.
- Pre-senile form (over age 50) usually have type B symptoms.

Diagnosis and investigations

Three genes code for lysosomal enzymes, and have biochemical assays:

- Palmitoyl-protein thioesterase 1, encoded by the gene *PPT1*.
- Tripeptidyl-peptidase 1, encoded by the gene *TPP1*.
- Cathepsin D, encoded by the gene *CTSD*.

Inclusion bodies subtypes include:

- Granular osmophilic deposits (GROD). Associated genes are *PPT1*, *CTSD*, and *CLN8*. Autosomal dominant ANCL usually has GROD and has not been linked to a specific gene.
- Curvilinear profiles (CV). Associated genes are *CLN8*, *MFSD8* (major facilitator superfamily domain-8), *CLN6*, and *TPP1*.
- Fingerprint profiles (FP). Associated genes are *CLN3*, *CLN5*, *CLN6*, and *MFSD8*.
- Mixed type inclusions (GROD, CV, FP).

Tip

▶ *Talk to your pathology laboratory before ordering EM on white blood cells. This requires special processing and often needs time to arrange.*

Adult diagnosis is primarily by EM histology to identify inclusion bodies. White blood cells usually have characteristic inclusion bodies, so biopsies are not normally required. However, biopsies are taken of neuron dense tissues such as conjunctiva, skin, or rectal mucosa. Three different tissues should be negative to rule out inclusion body disease. If characteristic inclusion bodies are present, assay *PPT1*, *TPP1* and *CTSD* enzyme activity. If negative, gene sequencing is available, but this is often negative.

Treatment

Treatment is symptomatic. Epilepsy can be worsened by carbamazepine and lamotrigine and these drugs should be avoided. Usual survival is about 10 years from diagnosis.

LATE-ONSET LYSOSOMAL STORAGE DISEASES

Introduction

Hereditary metabolic encephalopathies are most common in early childhood, but can present at any point in life, and in adults have a slower and more diffuse effect on the nervous system. Because these diseases have diverse symptoms and progression, classic pediatric disease patterns should not be relied on for diagnosis. As most are recessive, a family history is usually lacking. Even when family history is present, there can be significant variation in age of onset and severity, masking recognition in older individuals.

LATE-ONSET G_{M2} GANGLIOSIDOSIS

Definition and etiology

This is a group of autosomal recessive disorders caused by mutations in at least one of three genes: *HEXA*, *HEXB*, and *GM2A*. Deficiency in one gene product prevents catabolism of G_{M2} gangliosides and other molecules with terminal N-acetyl hexosamines, leading to accumulation of these sphingolipids inside lysosomes and eventual cell death (255).

- Hexosaminidase A is a heterodimer composed of an α subunit and a β subunit. The α subunit is encoded by the *HEXA* gene while the β subunit is encoded by the *HEXB* gene.
- Hexosaminidase B is a homodimer composed of two β subunits.

Tay–Sachs disease may be caused by either:

- *HEXA* gene mutations which lead to a decrease activity of hexosaminidase A, or
- G_{M2} activator gene mutation (*GM2A*); this encodes for the hexosaminidase A cofactor. Deficiencies result in infantile Tay–Sachs disease.

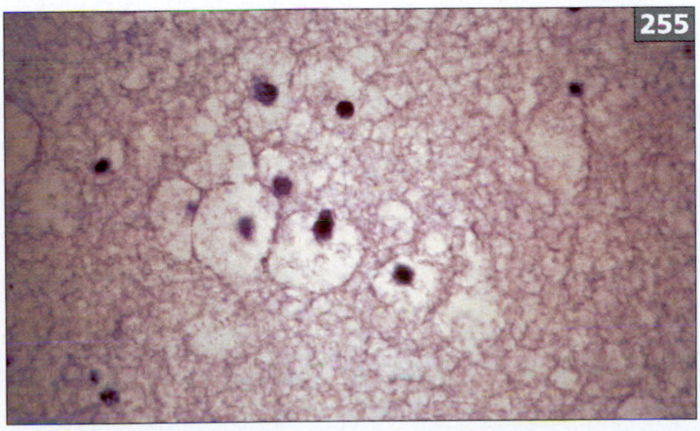

255 Distension of nerve cells with glycolipids.

Sandhoff disease is caused by *HEXB* gene mutations which lead to decreased activity of both hexosaminidase A and hexosaminidase B.

Tay–Sachs disease

Definition and etiology

Gene frequency depends on the population. For *HEXA*, the carrier rate is 1:25–30 in Ashkenazi Jews, 1 per 2500–3600 prior to carrier screening. The carrier rate for Louisiana Cajun, French Canadian, and Pennsylvania Dutch populations is 1:50. The carrier rate for most populations is 1:250–1:300. Prevalence is 1 per 309,000 live births. For *GM2A*, the gene frequency is unknown.

Males and females are equally affected. Onet is from infancy to middle age.

Clinical features

Unlike the better known infantile and late adolescent variants, chronic G_{M2} gangliosidosis has variable onset and slow progression, with some surviving into their eighth decade. Most are *HEXA* compound heterozygotes with less than 10% enzyme activity.

Up to 60% have psychiatric disturbances, which may precede neurologic symptoms. These can be mild to severe. Up to 30% present with schizophrenia or atypical psychosis, with agitation, delusions, hallucinations, and paranoia. Recurrent depression is common. This should *not* be treated with classic antidepressants that deplete hexosaminidase A activity. Dementia is usually not prominent.

Neurologic symptoms include cerebellar tremor, pyramidal signs, and lower motor neuron findings:

- Diffuse cerebellar atrophy is an early finding, even with minimal symptoms.
- Lower motor neuron disease with early proximal and late distal weakness.
- Sensory involvement is late or absent.
- Dysarthria.
- Oculomotor apraxia.
- Dystonia or choreiform movements.

Diagnosis and investigations

Biochemical assay of HEXA activity is the preferred diagnostic test for the general population. Up to 50% have negative genetic testing. If biochemical assay is positive, then deoxyribonucleic acid (DNA) testing should be performed. Pseudodeficiency with decreased activity can occur. DNA testing can differentiate pseudodeficiency from disease alleles. DNA analysis may be preferred in high-risk populations with known mutations; Ashkenazi Jews have 98% detection with either DNA analysis or biochemical assay.

Sandhoff disease: G_{M2} gangliosidosis Type II

Definition and etiology

Sandhoff disease is a *HEXB* mutation. Gene frequency depends on the population; 1 per 500 Jewish persons is a heterozygous unaffected carrier. Frequency is unknown for other populations, but most recognized cases are NOT in Jewish persons. Males and females are equally affected. Onset is from infancy to middle age.

Clinical features

Unlike the better known infantile and juvenile forms, adult Sandhoff disease usually presents as motor neuron disease. Dementia, psychiatric symptoms, and extrapyramidal symptoms have been reported but appear rare.

LATE-ONSET METACHROMATIC LEUKODYSTROPHY

Definition and etiology

Late-onset metachromatic leukodystrophy (MLD) is an autosomal recessive disease involving the lysosomal enzyme arylsulfatase A (ARSA), preventing degradation of sulfated glycolipids with a secondary buildup of metachromatic granules resulting in widespread demylination. It is caused by a mutation in the *ARSA* gene. Disease frequency is 1:40,000, with males and females equally affected. Onset is early infancy to middle age, with 50–60% of patients with late infantile MLD, 20–30% of patients with juvenile MLD, and 15–20% of patients with adult MLD. Age at onset is similar in affected family members.

Clinical features

Adult MLD frequently begins with psychiatric symptoms or cognitive decline:

- Decreased work or school performance.
- Personality changes:
  - Drug or alcohol use.
  - Emotional lability.
- Progressive memory loss.
- Atypical psychosis.
- Seizures.

Motor abnormalities may appear later, but can be the presenting symptom, with ataxia, dystonia, and choreoathetosis. Peripheral neuropathy can be prominent but is NOT universal in adult MLD and cannot be used to exclude diagnosis. Neuropathy is, however, prominent in infantile MLD.

TABLE 29 **DISEASES THAT CAN BE ASSOCIATED WITH NONSPECIFIC CORTICAL WHITE MATTER CHANGES**

Adrenoleukodystrophy (late)
CADASIL (late)
FXTAS (late)
Homocystinuria
Krabbe's disease
Metachromatic leukodystrophy
Mitochondrial disorders

CADASIL: cerebral autosomal dominant arteriopathy with subcortical infarcts and leukoencephalopathy; FXTAS: fragile X-associated tremor/ataxia syndrome.

Diagnosis and investigations

- Elevated cerebrospinal fluid (CSF) protein is often present but NOT universally in adult MLD. It is prominent in infantile MLD.
- MRI shows white matter changes (*Table 29*): periventricular white matter with initial posterior involvement with gradual rostral to caudal progression; anterior lesions may occur in adult MLD, cerebral atrophy is expected in chronic cases.
- ARSA enzyme deficiency is the preferred initial test. It occurs in 10% of normal controls, and ARSA enzyme pseudodeficiency can occur in otherwise healthy individuals with enzyme activity of 5–20% of normal.
- *ARSA* gene testing confirmation is required to rule out pseudodeficiency, as there are specific alleles on genetic testing. *ARSA* gene testing may be negative in some affected individuals, so should not be the first test.

Most patients survive for 5–10 years, but fulminate courses with short survival have been described.

FABRY'S DISEASE

Definition and etiology

Fabry's disease is an X-linked lysosomal enzyme disorder of α-galactosidase, resulting in accumulation of glycosphingolipids with α-galactosyl moieties. The inability to process these glycosphingolipids results in their buildup in multiple organs. Most of the early, prominent symptoms are the result of accumulation in the blood vessels and the peripheral and central autonomic nervous system, although all tissues are affected. As the disease progresses, accumulation in kidneys and heart will lead to organ failure. Progressive arterial accumulations result in infarction. Fabry's disease usually affects males (1:60,000) but about 30% of female carriers have some disease involvement. This is usually mild, but some cases have severe disease due to nonrandom X chromosome inactivation. Onset is late childhood (usual) into middle age.

Clinical features

Early symptoms

- Pain:
  - Attacks of severe pain and parasthesias in fingers and toes (acroparasthesia).
  - Late childhood onset is common, but adult onset has been reported.
  - Attacks last days to weeks.
  - Precipitated by physiological stress, such as fever, exercise, and dehydration.
  - Lancinating or burning pain, often severe.
  - Parasthesias usually occur with pain.
  - Joint swelling and elevated erythrocyte sedimentation rate (ESR) are common, and may lead to misdiagnosis of rheumatologic disease.
  - Pain responds to anticonvulsants.
- Skin lesions:
  - Typically are small, red flat or slightly raised telangiectases called angiokeratoma.
  - Usually around the umbilicus and thighs (bathing-trunk distribution).
- Eye findings:
  - Focal dilation of retinal arteries.
  - Corneal opacities – curved or straight lines radiating out from the center of the cornea (cornea verticillata), best seen with a slit lamp.
- Tinnitus and vertigo.
- High frequency hearing loss, occasionally progresses rapidly to deafness.

Late symptoms

- Progressive renal failure.
- Stroke: thromboembolic events leading to focal findings:
  - Usually occurs in young adult life.
  - Predilection for the basilar system, but any vessel may be involved.
- Cardiac:
  - Valvulopathy (mitral valve insufficiency).
  - Cardiac arrhythmia.
  - Coronary artery disease.
  - Cardiomyopathy – may present in isolation in adults; left ventricular hypertrophy is common.

Mild cases presenting in adulthood may not have classic findings of acroparasthesia, pain, and angiokeratoma. Here, patients may have:

- Peripheral neuropathy.
- Unexplained cardiomyopathy.
- Cerebrovascular events before age 40.
- Most will have corneal findings on slit lamp examination.

Diagnosis and investigations

- α-Galactosidase activity:
  - Males have nondetectable activity.
  - Affected females have variable activity (nondetectable up to normal range).
- α-*GAL* gene sequencing.
- Biopsy will show linear deposits; seldom used as a primary diagnostic method, but can be used in unusual cases, such as in isolated cardiomyopathy.

Treatment

- Enzyme replacement therapy is commercially available in North America and Europe, using IV treatments usually monthly for life.
- Aspirin or other antiplatelet treatment for stroke prevention.
- Pain attacks usually respond to anticonvulsants such as phenytoin, carbamazepine, and gabapentin.

Prior to enzyme replacement therapy, most affected males became increasingly debilitated from recurrent stroke and progressive heart and renal failure. Current survival is improved, but long-term outcome studies are lacking.

LATE-ONSET KRABBE'S DISEASE

Definition and etiology

This is an autosomal recessive disease caused by a mutation of the *GALC* gene which encodes for galactocerebrosidase (GALC). The deficiency of this lysosomal enzyme leads to the accumulation of several sphingolipids, including galactosylceramide and psychosine, which result in oligodendrocyte death and demyelination. Disease frequency is 1:100,000, and 1:150 carriers. Males and females are equally affected. Onset is in infancy (90%) to the fifth decade (10% juvenile to adult).

Clinical features

Adult presentations vary widely even in the same family. For instance, some may maintain normal intellect and have primarily motor findings. Symptoms may include:

- Intellectual decline.
- Progressive spasticity.
- Peripheral neuropathy of motor and sensory nerves – burning parasthesias, visual loss and optic atrophy.

Diagnosis and investigations

MRI typically shows atrophy and abnormal signal in cerebral white matter, with demylination in brainstem and cerebellum. At least one adult had abnormality restricted to the pyramidal tract and optic radiations. MR spectroscopy may show elevated myoinositol-containing and choline-containing compounds, with decreased N-aspartylaspartate in affected white matter areas.

Nerve conduction studies usually show motor neuropathy, but a few reported normal in adult onset disease. CSF protein is usually elevated. GALC enzyme assay is the preferred first evaluation:

- Usually less than 5% of normal.
- Patients with 8–20% activity may be normal or symptomatic.

GALC gene testing is available. Most adult-onset cases have 809G>A mutation, detected by sequence analysis. Individual states within the USA have introduced newborn screening for *GALC* deficiency. The frequent occurrence of decreased *GALC* activity with no neurologic symptoms has been documented. It is unclear if these children will later develop the disease, or if asymptomatic cases exist.

NIEMANN–PICK TYPE C

Definition and etiology

Niemann–Pick Type C (NPC) is an atypical autosomal recessive lysosomal storage disease caused by one of two genes: *NPC1* (98% of families) or *NPC2* (2% of families). The exact function of the NPC1 and NPC2 protein is unknown, but deficits cause accumulation of unesterified cholesterol in perinuclear vesicles. Males and females are equally affected. Disease frequency is at least 1:120,000, but is most likely underestimated. There is a higher incidence in native Hispanic families in the American southwest and Acadians of Nova Scotia. Onset is infants to adults. *Note*: Age of onset usually, but not always, is consistent within families. Infantile cases may have family members with late onset.

Clinical features

- Infantile: present at birth with splenomegaly, hepatic and/or pulmonary disease.
- Late infantile: splenomegaly, hypotonia, progression to supernuclear palsy, developmental arrest or regression.
- Juvenile: clumsiness, progressing to ataxia, supranuclear gaze palsy, progressive intellectual regression, variable splenomegaly.
- Adults: may present with either motor or psychiatric findings. Onset occurs from teens up to the sixth decade. Splenomegaly occurs in about 50%.

Psychiatric presentation occurs in about 30%. Neurologic findings may be absent on presentation, but will develop later:

- Psychosis or schizophrenia:
  - Can be acute or insidious.
  - Paranoid delusions.
  - Auditory or visual hallucinations.
  - Symptoms may fluctuate.
- Major depression:
  - Social withdrawal.
  - Disturbed behavior.
  - Aggressiveness or agitation.

Bipolar disorder, transient isolated visual hallucinations or obsessive compulsive disorder have been reported.

Neurologic symptoms vary. The most characteristic neurologic finding is vertical supranuclear gaze palsy (VSGP), occurring in about 75%. Other findings may include:

- Cerebellar ataxia.
- Dysarthria.
- Dementia – mild to severe.
- Movement disorders:
  - Dystonia.
  - Parkinsonism.
  - Chorea.
- Progressive spasticity.
- Epilepsy.
- Cataplexy.

Diagnosis and investigations

- Neuro-ophthalmology evaluation is important; abnormal saccadic eye movements are usually the first neurologic sign. VSGP occurs first, followed by lateral gaze.
- Splenomegaly is present in about 50% of cases.
- MRI is normal until late in disease. Late findings include:
  - Atrophy of cerebellar vermis.
  - Thinning of corpus callosum.
  - Mild generalized cortical atrophy.

Definitive diagnosis requires cultured fibroblasts. These accumulate unesterified cholesterol in lysosomes. Sequencing of *NPC1* and *NPC2* is available, but is not recommended for primary diagnosis. It is performed for prognosis and recurrence risk. The clinical course varies, with many patients surviving for 10 or more years.

MITOCHONDRIAL DISORDERS

Introduction

Mitochondrial disorders are a heterogeneous group of disorders whose primary deficit is failure of energy production due to alteration in mitochondrial enzyme function. Mitochondria are passed from mother to child via the fertilized egg, so that all mitochondria are maternally inherited[5].

Mitochondria contain their own DNA (mtDNA) which codes for most proteins within the mitochondria. There is a high mutation rate for mtDNA, which influences inheritance and disease presentation. There are hundreds of mitochondria in each cell, and each mitochondrion may have one or two mtDNA copies. Random partition of mitochondria occur as cells divide (heteroplasmy), which can lead to different proportions of normal or abnormal mitochondria from cell to cell, and organ to organ. There is a threshold of expression: phenotypic expression occurs when the proportion of abnormal mtDNA reaches a critical level.

Tip

▶ *Available mitochondrial genetic tests have increased rapidly over the last decade. Several laboratories offer complete sequencing of the mitochondrial genome and/or tests of known nuclear DNA mutations. Expect rapid advances in understanding and genetic testing to occur. Information can become rapidly outdated.*

A significant number of mitochondrial proteins are encoded in the nuclear DNA (nDNA), and are transported into the mitochondria. Disease may be caused by either nDNA or mtDNA mutations. Inheritance in nDNA mutations is NOT maternal. Most nDNA mitochondrial diseases present in childhood.

There is no one identifying feature of mitochondrial disease. Patients may have one or more symptoms that can occur at any time in life. Mitochondrial disease should be suspected when a neurologic presentation is atypical or may have more than one of the following findings:

- Encephalopathy.
- Seizures.
- Early-onset or atypical late-onset dementia.
- Myoclonus.
- Movement disorders – dystonia, dyskinesias, chorea.
- Complicated migraine.
- Stroke.
- Unexplained white matter changes (multiple sclerosis-like).
- Neuropathy.
- Cardiac conduction defects or cardiomyopathy.
- Hearing deficits.

- Disorders of extraocular muscles – ptosis, acquired strabismus, or ophthalmoplegia.
- Diabetes.
- Renal tubular disease.
- Visual loss (retinitis pigmentosa).
- Lactic acidosis.

MRI findings suggestive of mitochondrial disease include:
- Symmetric basal ganglia or brainstem lesions.
- Symmetric increased T2 intensity in white matter:
  - Generalized.
  - Primarily occipital or frontal.
- Cerebral atrophy.
- Cerebellar atrophy.

DISEASES OF MITOCHONDRIAL DNA

Definition and etiology

There are multiple mitochondrial syndromes that have stereotypic presentations and clinical course. Specific mtDNA mutations are often associated with these syndromes, but it must be remembered that the same mutation may be associated with more than one syndrome. For instance, a mutation most commonly associated with NARP may be found in a patient with a primary myopathy or encephalopathy. Evaluation includes serum lactic acid, and, if negative, either MR spectroscopy or CSF analysis of lactate. Mutations may be identified in with blood cells, but a muscle biopsy is often needed to detect mutations.

Mitochondrial encephalomyopathy with lactic acidosis and stroke-like episodes (MELAS)

- Onset at any age.
- Stroke-like events causing subacute focal brain dysfunction.
- Seizures and/or migraine headaches.
- Lactic acidosis:
  - Secondary hyperalaninemia.
  - Both may be normal between crisis.

MRI findings include diffusion-weighted imaging-positive lesions that are not hypointense on apparent diffusion coefficient. They do not follow vascular territory, and have a predilection for the posterior circulation.

Frequently seen clinical findings include retinitis pigmentosa, cerebellar ataxia, myopathy, cardiomyopathy, and diabetes.

Mitochondrial encephalopathy with ragged red fibers

- Myoclonus
- Epileptic seizures: myoclonic epilepsy, generalized seizures, or focal seizures.
- Cerebellar ataxia.
- Mitochondrial myopathy with ragged red fibers.

Frequently seen clinical findings include:
- Dementia.
- Optic neuropathy.
- Deafness.
- Corticospinal tract degeneration.
- Peripheral neuropathy.
- Myopathy.
- Proximal renal tubule dysfunction.
- Cardiomyopathy.
- Lactic academia with secondary hyperalaninema.

Neurogenic weakness with ataxia and retinitis pigmentosa (NARP)

MT-ATP6 is the only gene associated with NARP. Not all clinical cases have a detectable deletion. Clinical findings include:
- Proximal muscle weakness.
- Sensory neuropathy.
- Ataxia.
- Retinal pigmentary degeneration.

Frequently associated clinical findings include:
- Primary intellectual disability.
- Dementia.
- Epileptic seizures.

Leber hereditary optic neuropathy (LHON)

- Subacute painless bilateral vision loss.
- Males: females 4:1.
- Median age onset 24 years.

Frequently associated clinical findings include dystonia and cardiac pre-excitation syndromes.

Subacute necrotizing encephalomyelopathy

Definition and etiology

Subacute necrotizing encephalomyelopathy (Leigh syndrome) can be produced by nDNA and mtDNA mutations of genes encoding for enzymes involved in energy production, such as mitochondrial respiratory chain complexes I, II, III, IV, and V, and components of the pyruvate dehydrogenase complex. Leigh syndrome is therefore more than one disease with similar phenotypes.

- Two-thirds of pediatric cases are nDNA mutations.
- Most identified adult disease is secondary to mtDNA mutations, but a few cases have been linked to nDNA genes *SURF1* and *COQ*.
- An X-linked form has been described; this is caused by a mutation of the *PDHA1* gene which encodes for a component of the pyruvate dehydrogenase complex.

Prevalence is probably 1:40,000, with males and females equally affected.

Clinical features

Key features are symmetric necrotizing lesions of the basal ganglia, thalamus and diencephalon, and brainstem, seen on MRI or autopsy. Cerebellum and spinal cord gray matter may also be involved, but cortex is seldom involved. Leigh syndrome may result in respiratory failure and death. Symptoms may fluctuate with apparent remissions and exacerbations, and include:

- Ataxia.
- Movement disorders – dystonia, chorea.
- Nystagmus, ophthalmoparesis.
- Dysphagia.
- Peripheral neuropathy.
- Myopathy.
- Cardiomyopathy.
- Optic atrophy.
- Seizures.
- Slowly progressive dementia.

Treatment

Treatment is primarily symptomatic, with frequent monitoring of respiratory function, swallowing, and cardiac function. Supplementation with coenzyme Q, riboflavin, and thiamine has been attempted (*Table 30*). A high-fat diet may be effective with mutations in complex I.

TABLE 30 **VITAMINS, SUPPLEMENTS, AND MEDICATIONS USED IN MITOCHONDRIAL DISEASES**

Supplement	Daily dose	Comments
Coenzyme Q10	5–15 mg/kg divided doses	Variable absorption, maximum benefit may take months
L-carnitine	30–100 mg/kg divided doses	May cause diarrhea if started quickly
Thiamine (vitamin B1)	100–800 mg	
Riboflavin (vitamin B2)	400 mg	
Niacinamide (vitamin B3)	100–500 mg	Avoid niacin form
Folate	1–10 mg	
Vitamin E	400–1200 IU divided	May interfere with coenzyme Q10 absorption
Selenium	25–50 μg	
Lipoic acid	200–600 mg divided	
DURING CRISIS OR STRESS		
Prednisone	5–60 mg	Withdrawal may cause relapse
Creatine	100 mg/kg/day divided	Up to 7 g
STROKE WITH MELAS SYNDROME		
L-arginine	0.5 g/kg given IV in first hours, then 0.15–0.3 g/kg oral divided	Two papers support use

MELAS: mitochondrial encephalomyopathy, lactic acidosis, and stroke-like episodes.

Mitochondrial deletion syndromes

Definition and etiology

These involve larger deletions of mtDNA. If inherited, they derive from the mother. Mitochondrial deletion syndromes more often arise *de novo* and the mother and siblings are not affected. There are three overlapping phenotypes, Kearns–Sayre and Pearson syndromes, and progressive external ophthalmoplegia (PEO).

Kearns–Sayre syndrome

- Must have triad of symptoms:
  - Onset before age 20.
  - Pigmentary retinopathy.
  - PEO.

In addition, patients must have one of the following:

- Cardiac conduction block.
- CSF protein greater than 1 g/l (100 mg/dl).
- Cerebellar ataxia.

Patients may also have hearing loss, depression, dementia, weakness, or an endocrine deficiency such as diabetes mellitus, hypoparathyroidism, or growth hormone deficiency.

Patients require frequent monitoring for cardiac and endocrine dysfunction. Most die before age 30.

Pearson syndrome

- Sideroblastic anemia.
- Exocrine pancreas dysfunction.
- Usually fatal in infancy.

PEO

- Age at onset: childhood to middle age.
- Ptosis.
- Paralysis of extraocular muscles.
- Mild to severe proximal limb weakness.
- If there are more components of Kearns–Sayre syndrome, then it is referred to as PEO plus (PEO+).
- Most have a normal life-span.
- Children may inherit from an affected mother.

Treatment

Treatment of mtDNA deletion syndromes is primarily supportive. Some Kearns–Sayre syndrome patients have low CSF folinic acid and require supplementation. Supplementation with coenzyme Q, L-carnitine, and B vitamins is usual, as these are presumed to improve enzyme function, but there have been no controlled trials.

REFERENCES

1 Sedel F, Baumann N, Turpin JC, Lyon-Caen O, Saudubray JM, Cohen D (2007). Psychiatric manifestations revealing inborn errors of metabolism in adolescents and adults. *J Inherit Metab Dis* 30(5):631–641.

2 Pagon RA, Bird TD, Dolan CR, Stephens K, Adam MP (eds). *GeneReviews* (Internet). University of Washington, Seattle; 1993-. Available from: http://www.ncbi.nlm.nih.gov/books/NBK1116/

3 Lyon G, Kolodny EH, Pastores GM (2006). Childhood and adolescent hereditary metabolic disorders. In: *Neurology of Hereditary Metabolic Diseases in Children*, 3rd edn. Mcgraw Hill Professional, New York.

4 Sedel F, Lyon-Caen O, Saudubray JM (2007). Therapy insight: inborn errors of metabolism in adult neurology – a clinical approach focused on treatable diseases. *Nat Clin Pract Neurol* 3(5):279–290.

5 Cohen BH, Gold DR (2001). Mitochondrial cytopathology in adults: What we know so far. *Cleveland Clinic J Med* 68(7):625–642.

TRAUMA OF THE BRAIN AND SPINAL CORD

James L. Stone, Prasad S. S.V. Vannemreddy

INTRODUCTION

Traumatic brain injury (TBI) is a major public health problem affecting more than 1.4 million people per year in the United States and the leading cause of death in those under 45 years of age. Resultant direct and indirect medical costs are approximated at $60 billion per year.

About 500,000 patients require hospital treatment for TBI every year in the United States, representing 200–300 patients per 100,000 population. Eighty percent of TBI patients have a mild injury and the remaining 20% a moderate (10–15%) or severe TBI (5%).

In recent decades improvements in pre-hospital care, especially airway management, triage to a Level 1 trauma center, prompt computed tomographic (CT) imaging, removal of significant intracranial hemorrhagic collections, and avoidance of secondary insults (hypotension, hypoxemia) has reduced severe TBI mortality to about 30%. This has occurred without an increase in those severely disabled or vegetative.

Guidelines for the management of severe TBI have been widely adopted in the United States and updated in 2007[1]. Management of increased intracranial pressure (ICP) remains a challenge in severe TBI, and noninvasive neurophysiologic monitoring of moderate and mild TBI is a realistic goal. Following spinal injuries, timely realignment, decompression, and internal fixation are routinely performed, but spinal cord injury often remains irreversible or only shows minimal improvement with corticosteroid treatment.

TABLE 31 **GLASGOW COMA SCALE (GCS) SCORE**

Eye opening	**Score** (1–4)
Spontaneous	4
To voice	3
To pain	2
None	1
Verbal response	**Score** (1–5)
Oriented	5
Confused, disoriented	4
Inappropriate words	3
Incomprehensible sounds	2
None	1
Best motor response	**Score** (1–6)
Obeys	6
Localizes	5
Withdraws (flexion)	4
Abnormal flexion posturing	3
Extension posturing	2
None	1
Total	(3–15)

HEAD INJURY

Definition and etiology

Despite intensive treatment disability or death occurs in the majority of patients with severe coma-producing TBI, and physical and neuropsychologic disabilities are frequent in those with moderate and mild injuries.

The Glasgow Coma Scale (GCS) is widely used to quantify severity of injury (*Table 31*). Patients who open their eyes spontaneously, follow commands, and are fully oriented score all 15 points. Patients who do not open their eyes spontaneously or to stimuli, and cannot verbalize or move any extremities have the lowest score of 3. The patient's best responses are taken. A comatose patient is referred to as a severe TBI and defined as having a GCS score equal or less than 8, a moderate injury is usually lethargic and has a GCS of 9–12, and mild injury has less alteration in consciousness and a GCS of 13–15.

Severe TBI carries an overall mortality of about 30%. Approximately 10–20% of moderate injuries will deteriorate into coma, with serious morbidity or death in just under 10%. Additionally the severe and moderate injuries yield large numbers of disabled survivors (20–30%).

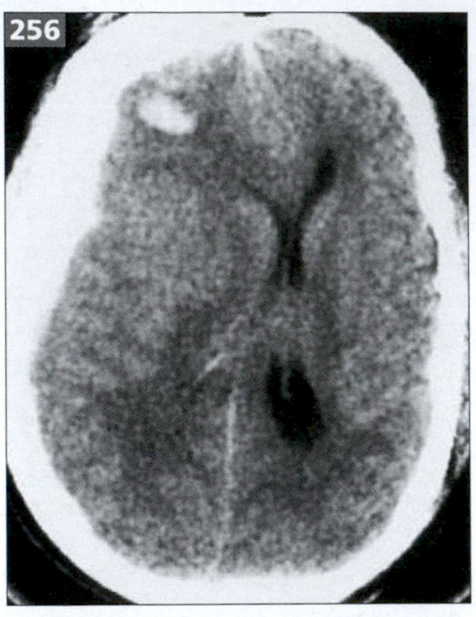

256 CT scan showing acute subdural hemorrhage with underlying parenchymal injury. Note the displacement of ventricles and midline shift.

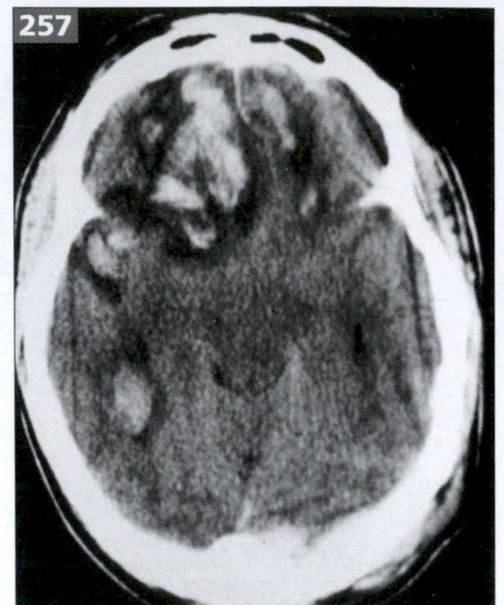

257 CT scan showing large delayed-onset hemorrhagic contusion evident 2–3 days after injury with adjacent areas of contusion and significant mass effect.

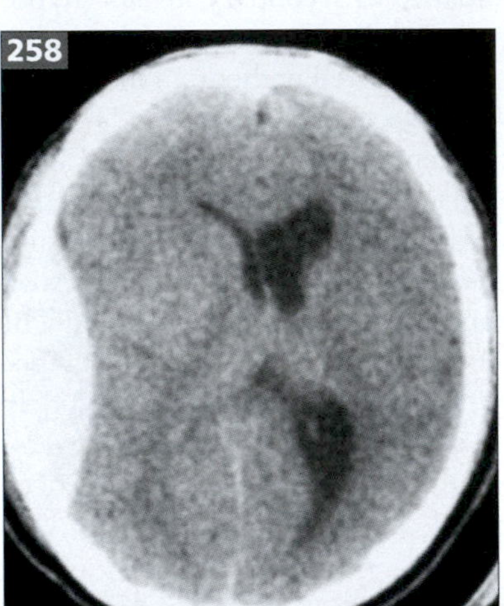

258 CT scan showing the typical lens-shaped acute extradural hematoma (EDH) of the parietal region. Note the associated midline shift. EDH is associated with the best prognosis among all the intracranial hemorrhages (traumatic or otherwise) when evacuated at an appropriate time.

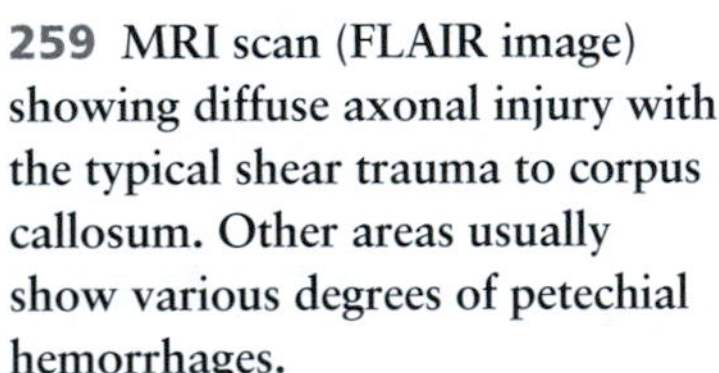

259 MRI scan (FLAIR image) showing diffuse axonal injury with the typical shear trauma to corpus callosum. Other areas usually show various degrees of petechial hemorrhages.

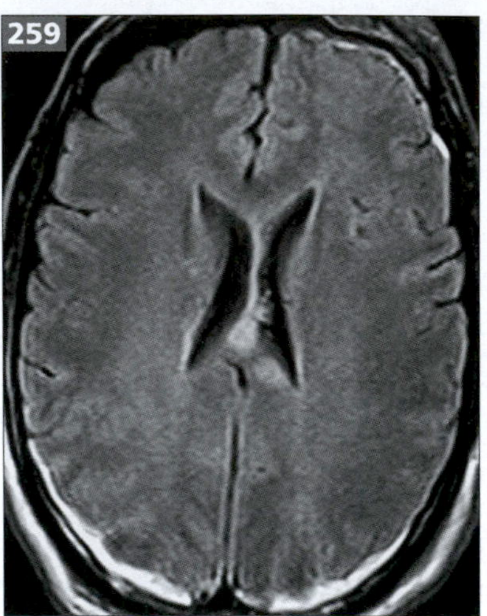

In the United States, of the approximately 400,000 patients admitted awake and alert each year following a mild TBI, about 1.5% or 6000 will deteriorate and die. Extreme caution is necessary in that any patient with a GCS of 13, an abnormal CT brain scan, skull fracture or skull puncture has a risk similar to that of moderate injuries and should not be considered a mild head injury.

In terms of prognosis after severe TBI, motor score is most valuable, and, when combined with patient age and pupillary response, the motor score is as reliable as the complete GCS score[2].

Etiology and clinical features

Head injuries may be classified as closed (blunt) or open (penetrating). A closed head injury, with or without fracture but intact dura, usually results from vehicular injury, blunt assault, or fall. Open injury is associated with dural penetration due to a gunshot or stab wound, compound depressed skull fracture from an angulated object, or basal skull fracture with cerebrospinal (CSF) leakage.

Focal brain injuries, often precipitated by translational or linear acceleration–deceleration phenomena, result from inertial movements of the brain within the skull that may tear venous or small arterial structures resulting in subdural hemorrhage (**256**). The basifrontal and temporal lobes may strike the rough skull base, resulting in frontal and temporal contusions and cortical lacerations associated with local brain swelling. Focal skull injuries include depressed, linear, and basal skull fractures, or sutural diastases.

Tip

► *A chronic subdural hematoma can mimic stroke, either a cerebrovascular accident (CVA) or a transient ischemic attack (TIA), and sometimes a tumor (when papilledema is present).*

Focal lesions may be coup (directly under the impact site) or contrecoup (distant diametrically opposed to the impact). Significant parenchymal contusional hemorrhages, either primary or delayed in onset, may require surgical removal (**257**). Extradural (epidural) hematomas (EDH) result from a focal impact almost always associated with a nearby skull fracture and stripping of the dura from the inner table of the skull (**258**). The hematoma forms a lens shape as blood fills into this space and causes further stripping of the dura from the skull. A lucid interval may be present; however, clinical deterioration can be rapid. Underlying brain damage is usually more severe with an acute subdural hematoma (mortality >50%) rather than an EDH. The mortality of acute EDH continues to decrease in recent decades as outcome is largely related to triage and timely decompression by craniotomy.

Posterior fossa skull fractures and hematomas are particularly dangerous due to the proximity of the brainstem and result from impacts to the back of the head. The presence of any skull fracture must be taken seriously in any patient and increases the likelihood of a significant acute or delayed intracranial hematoma by a factor of about 400 in a conscious patient and a factor of 20 in a comatose patient.

A diffuse axonal injury (DAI) to the brain consists of scattered shearing of white matter axons, histologically appearing days after injury as swollen retraction balls of axoplasm. Their distribution is centripetal and magnitude related to the force of injury. Extension of these white matter shearing lesions, from sites of relative tethering such as the corpus callosum down into the brainstem, is believed to represent an increasing degree of injury related to rotational or angular acceleration–deceleration of the skull and brain. Hemorrhages into the deeper gray matter or ventricles also often signify DAI (**259**). The severity of injury in a primate model correlates with a clinical continuum from simple cerebral concussion to prolonged traumatic unconsciousness. Experimental evidence suggests that the axonal injury may not be complete at onset, but progresses in the hours after injury. This raises the hope of partial reversal by pharmacologic means if such agents could be identified.

Head injury as a result of blunt assault or fall results more often in focal injuries such as cerebral contusions and subdural hematomas, whereas vehicular injuries more often result in diffuse head injuries. Severe focal, diffuse, or penetrating injuries such as gunshot wounds are often associated with brain swelling and increased ICP. A 'blast injury' force as seen in proximity to a discharging explosive device may result in concussion or prolonged unconsciousness even without skull penetration by fragments or shrapnel. High intensity shock waves consisting of advancing wave-fronts are believed to cause secondary complex interference patterns, which may result in diffuse physiologic or actual mechanical tissue disruption[3]. This mechanism may result in neuropsychologic deficits and post-traumatic stress disorders (PTSD).

Diagnosis and investigations

An adequate airway, usually by endotracheal intubation, must be promptly established in combative or struggling patients. This includes all severe (GCS 8 or less), possibly some moderately (GCS 9–12) head injured patients, those with respiratory distress, or a borderline patient with any significant intracranial abnormality of CT scan of the brain. Attention to airway, ventilation, and circulatory stability is necessary before adequate diagnosis and treatment can be carried out.

Tip

▶ *The ABC of emergency resuscitation is: Airway, Breathing, and Circulation.*

Secondary insults may occur minutes, hours, or days after injury and compound the primary brain injury in about 30% of severe injuries. These insults include hypotension (systolic blood pressure <90 mmHg), hypoxia (PO_2 <60 mmHg), carbon dioxide retention (PCO_2 >45 mmHg) and anemia (hematocrit <30%), all known to worsen brain swelling, ICP, morbidity, and mortality. Hyperglycemia and hyperthermia are to be avoided. Injury to visceral organs, or long bone fractures, may contribute to blood loss hypovolemia, hypotension, and increased morbidity.

The patient's level of consciousness may be depressed secondary to hypotension, and abdominal/pelvic ultrasound or diagnostic peritoneal lavage take priority over a CT scan of the head in this circumstance.

Other diagnoses may be present such as intoxication, anoxic insult, metabolic encephalopathy, post-ictal state, or status epilepticus. Nonconvulsive status epilepticus may occur and require prolonged electroencephalogram monitoring to capture and monitor adequately.

Following respiratory and circulatory stabilization, rapid neurologic assessment is performed including the GCS and pupillary light responses. It is not always possible to examine the patient before muscle paralyzing agents or sedation with hypnotics such as propofol, or benzodiazepines have been given. Unilateral pupil enlargement (midposition 4–5 mm or dilated >5 mm) in an obtunded patient, with or without fixation to light, is highly localized and indicative of ipsilateral tentorial herniation unless proved otherwise.

Cerebellar, lower cranial nerve, or precipitous respiratory abnormalities (tonsillar herniation) may be found with posterior fossa injuries.

Doll's eye maneuver or cold calorics with head elevation should only be performed if the status of the cervical spine and tympanic membranes can be determined. Patients must be stimulated and the best responses recorded, such as: follows commands, responds to voice, light pain, moderate pain, or deep pain. Asymmetries, decorticate or decerebrate responses, flaccid no extremity response, DTRs, and plantar responses are recorded. Sensory examination is only possible in awake, cooperative patients. Trauma patients are usually kept in a rigid collar, despite normal cervical spine studies, until the neck can be cleared clinically or ligament injury ruled out with magnetic resonance imaging (MRI).

Concern is given to CSF leakage from the nose (rhinorrhea) indicative of cribriform or anterior fossa fracture, or ear (otorrhea) suggestive of temporal bone fracture. Antibiotic administration is controversial, but a spinal drain is often indicated when leaks persist after several days.

Rigidity of the neck may indicate a cervical spine fracture (present in about 5–8% of severe TBI, and 10–15% of severe facial fractures), occipital fracture, or tonsillar herniation.

Patients with a concussion or mild head injury who present for medical attention should at least receive plain skull X-rays, and any patient with a GCS score less than 15, focal neurologic signs, headache, vomiting, skull fracture, or significant scalp swelling should receive a plain CT scan of the head. Further treatment will usually depend upon the CT scan results.

MRI brain scans are usually unnecessary and inconvenient in the earlier stages of TBI diagnosis and treatment. In the subacute phase, characteristic MRI findings can often establish a suspected diagnosis of DAI.

Treatment

In the early resuscitation phase, elevated ICP or transtentorial–uncal herniation is suggested by clinical findings such as anisocoria or pupillary dilatation, motor posturing, or progressive level of consciousness deterioration not attributed to extracranial factors. Emergency treatment of suspected herniation or elevated ICP consists of intubation and hyperventilation, and rapid intravenous administration of mannitol (i.e. 1 g/kg) or hypertonic saline solution (variable concentrations given) as the patient is emergently sent for a CT brain scan.

Patients are brought promptly to surgery for significant subdural or epidural hematomas (usually equal or greater than 1 cm) or parenchymal contusions (equal or greater than 30 ml in the temporal or posterior fossa), and/or a midline shift of 0.5 cm or greater. Similarly, compound depressed skull fractures exceeding the thickness of the skull and penetrating injuries may require acute or subacute surgery.

Post-traumatic subarachnoid hemorrhage in the basal cisterns, fissures, cortical sulci, or on the tentorium are a frequent finding in all forms of TBI, but uncommonly associated with vasospasm and specific treatment is not required. Patients with nonsurgical lesions on an initial CT scan require a repeat CT scan, often as early as 4–6 hours later, to detect enlarging or evolving lesions such as hemorrhagic cerebral contusions.

Subsequent observation in the intensive care unit and placement of an ICP monitor is recommended according to US guidelines updated in 2007 for patients with:

- A GCS score of 8 or less, with an abnormal but nonsurgical CT scan, *or*
- A normal scan with two or three of the following: age over 40, motor posturing, or systolic blood pressure <90 mmHg.

Head elevation is routinely in the range of 30°. ICP monitoring with a ventricular catheter is preferred in that ventricular CSF drainage may be used as a first choice to control elevated ICP (>20 mmHg) before resorting to mannitol (0.25–0.50 g/kg), hyperventilation (PCO_2 30–35 mmHg), or second-tier therapies such as barbiturate coma, hypothermia, or decompressive hemicraniectomy for edema.

ICP management may be augmented by cerebral perfusion pressure (CPP = mean arterial blood pressure minus ICP) management. The CPP is ideally maintained between 50 and 60 mmHg, in that CPP >70 mmHg has been associated with adult respiratory distress syndrome (ARDS).

Patients who maintain elevated ICP (>20 mmHg) require follow-up CT brain scans for enlarging or evolving lesions, including hydrocephalus. Other helpful invasive cerebral monitoring modalities include brain tissue oxygen content, pH, lactate, and temperature monitoring. Cerebral blood flow with estimations of hyperemia or ischemic desaturation as well as cerebral metabolic rate of oxygen consumption can be obtained with a jugular bulb venous catheter.

ICP monitors are generally discontinued after ICP has normalized for 24–48 hours. Those patients who have required ventricular drainage for 5–10 days may develop hydrocephalus and require a shunting procedure.

Tip

▶ *Hemicraniectomy is an option in the acute or subacute period to control refractory increases in ICP.*

Anticonvulsants are continued post-injury in patients having a seizure, but only for 1 week in those without significant cortical or hemispherical lesions considered at risk of a seizure.

CONCUSSION

Definition and etiology

Concussion is a frequently encountered form of mild head injury and the most common form of head injury in athletic injuries. The term cerebral concussion has been used interchangeably with mild TBI. Approximately 250,000 concussions occur yearly in the US in football alone.

Classic cerebral concussion was defined as a loss of consciousness (LOC), usually brief, and associated with retrograde and post-traumatic (anterograde) amnesia. By such definition, full consciousness is regained by 24 hours, and the condition may be accompanied by abnormal microscopic neuronal changes. In recent decades cerebral concussion has come to be defined as a physiologic dysfunction secondary to a minor head injury without associated pathologic changes in the brain.

A cerebral concussion is often a consequence of sudden angular acceleration–deceleration head motions that usually accompany, but may be independent of, impact to the head. Helmets greatly absorb impacts to the head, have virtually eliminated skull fracture, significantly reduce focal impact brain injury, but cannot eliminate concussion.

A five- to tenfold increase in extracellular potassium concentration lasting 3–5 minutes is associated with a concussion producing loss of consciousness, resulting in nerve action potential failure and LOC. Excitatory amino acids such as glutamate are believed to open gated channels resulting in the ionic flux. Occasionally the process requires several seconds or longer, allowing some purposeful action before collapse.

Clinical features

With cerebral concussion, confusion is more frequently found than LOC, clearly indicating a problem of cerebral processing, affecting orientation, higher thought processes, and memory. There may be disturbances of vision, unsteadiness, vacant stare, a foggy state, delayed responses, slurred speech, and emotional outbursts. Symptoms of headache, especially with exertion and dizziness, are common, and nausea and vomiting may occur. Simple concussion is completely reversible and unless repetitive, is not believed to be associated with neurological sequelae.

In order to categorize, study, and treat concussion several classification schemes have been devised, such as the American Academy of Neurology Practice Parameter Grading System For Concussion. Grading the severity of concussion has been helpful in both treating athletic injuries and prognostication regarding the safe return to sporting activity. Athletes should not return to contact sports while significant residual symptoms persist.

Repeated concussions can result in cumulative cytoarchitectual and gross structural brain damage, usually manifesting as increasing severity and duration of symptoms with successive concussions. In recent years, professional athletes from several contact sports were forced to retire due to repeated concussions. Some suffer from problems such as headaches, slurred speech, visual problems, depression, or dementia. Adolescents, high school or college students who experience multiple concussions are strongly encouraged to discontinue contact sports[4].

A rare and controversial issue is the second impact syndrome (SIS). This involves the athlete who suffers a concussion and returns to the contact sport (minutes to weeks later) to experience a second head injury before recovery from the earlier concussion. This may result in death or severe disability from malignant brain swelling. It is believed that the first concussion caused a focal or diffuse abnormality in cerebral vascular regulation leading to excessive blood congestion, and a second injury occurred before this congestion has recovered. The SIS has been reported in high school age as well as adult contact sport athletes, highlighting the risks of persistent signs and symptoms in the return to contact sports.

Neuropsychologic testing appears to be effective in obtaining useful data on the short-term and long-term effects of concussion and mild TBI, and is useful to those involved in decisions involving athletes. Brief but concise neuropsychologic tests batteries, administered to the contact sport athlete before the season begins, and similar testing after a concussion, is sensitive to document the absence of a lingering effects before return to play.

Conditions that may mimic recurrent concussion symptoms in the contact sport athlete include a previously asymptomatic or undiagnosed Chiari malformation, basilar invagination, hydrocephalus, arachnoid cyst, or migraine headaches.

SPINAL CORD INJURY

Definition and etiology

Spinal stability is the ability of the spinal column to limit displacement of its segments under physiological loads, so as to prevent damage or irritation of the neural structures, and to prevent irreversible deformity or pain due to structural changes. Biomechanical instability refers to the ability of spine to resist forces in experimental settings or controlled environment ex vivo.

Acute spinal cord injury (SCI) is a devastating injury affecting many young, productive individuals with a male preponderance. The average age is 37.6 years which has increased over the last four decades, likely due to increased longevity and associated accidental falls.

The most common cause for acute SCI is a motor vehicle accident in industrialized countries, falls, and pedestrian injuries. Gunshot SCI is unfortunately common in the US and exceeds the number of sport injuries, which have been reduced due to protective and preventive measures. SCI is expensive to the person, family, and the nation.

An average 15,000 people sustain SCI per year in the US, and a young individual with high cervical SCI will incur medical costs in the range of $740,000 the first year and $135,000 each year of survival[5]. About 400,000 people are living with the effects of SCI in the US.

Complete SCI

These injuries produce a complete paraplegia or a complete tetraplegia. Loss of motor and/or sensory function for more than three segments below the level of injury is termed complete SCI. Only about 3% of injuries with complete SCI at the initial physician examination may regain some function within 24 hours.

Complete paraplegia is permanent loss of motor and nerve function at T1 level or below, with loss of sensation and movement in the legs, bladder, bowel, and perineum. Arms and hands retain normal function. Some people may retain partial trunk movement.

Complete tetraplegia is characterized by loss of hand and arm movement as well. Some may require an artificial ventilator to support respiratory function. Partial hand and arm movements may by retained in some.

Incomplete SCI

These are far more common than complete SCI and the patients retain some sensory and motor function below the level of injury. This is determined after the period of spinal shock has subsided, which is usually 6–8 weeks post-injury.

- Anterior cord syndrome: an incomplete SCI characterized by damage to the anterior part of the spinal cord, resulting in impaired temperature, touch, and pain sensations below the level of injury.
- Central cord syndrome: characterized by damage of the central part of the spinal cord, with loss of function in upper extremities predominantly and some variable weakness in the lower limbs. The hands may be maximally involved and sensory loss minimal.
- Posterior cord syndrome: this results in impaired coordination due to damage to the posterior columns of the spinal cord.
- Brown–Sequard syndrome: usually found secondary to a stab wound and results in damage to one-half of the spinal cord or hemisection, resulting in impaired loss of movement but preserved sensation on one side of the body and preserved motor function with sensory loss on the other half of the body. Incomplete Brown–Sequard may be found in some anterior cord syndromes.
- Conus medullaris syndrome: this results from injury to the sacral portions of the spinal cord resulting in saddle anesthesia, loss of bladder/bowel function, with weakness of lower extremities. Recall that the spinal cord usually terminates at the L1 level.
- Cauda equine syndrome: characterized by injury to the nerves located below the L1 region of the spine, resulting in partial or complete loss of sensation. In some cases, these nerve roots can regenerate and recover function.

Tip

▶ *Incomplete injuries have the best chances for recovery. Avoiding a second injury during transfers is all the more important.*

Clinical features

The American Spinal Injury Association (ASIA) provides a scoring system and a scale for measuring the disability. Both the score and scale are extensively used in clinical and research settings (*Table 32*). The clinical picture is a result of the level of injury, mechanism, and severity

In a severe injury with spinal shock, all reflexes below the lesion are lost, including the bulbocavernous, cremasteric, and abdominal reflexes, with motor as well as sensory deficits accompanied by hyporeflexia. Gradually the reflexes may return, and deep tendon reflexes become brisk. A complete and flaccid paralysis becomes spastic over a period of time.

In a high cervical lesion, respiratory compromise because of phrenic nerve denervation and diaphragm paralysis is seen. Sphincter tone is lost and sacral functions are compromised.

Spinal shock results in hypotension and bradycardia due to loss of sympathetic tone (contrary to the hypovolemic shock more commonly seen in trauma, with hypotension and tachycardia). Spinal shock can be due to a mixed expression of loss of sympathetic tone, loss of muscle tone due to paralysis, and blood loss.

Chronic SCI findings vary again depending upon the initial presentation, respiratory support, immobilization, urinary dysfunction, urinary tract infection, pulmonary problems, and decubitus ulcers. These are also the usual causes of death.

Tip

▶ *A central cervical spinal cord injury is difficult to evaluate during an acute phase especially with obtunded sensorium. Degenerative changes in the cervical spinal cord must make the clinical picture very suspect.*

TABLE 32 **CLASSIFICATION OF SPINAL CORD INJURY** (AMERICAN SPINAL INJURY ASSOCIATION)

A. Complete
No sensory or motor function preserved in the lowest sacral segments (S4–5).

B. Sensory incomplete
Sensory but no motor function preserved below the neurologic level including the sacral segments S4–5.

C. Motor incomplete
Motor function is preserved below the neurologic level, and more than half of the key muscles below the neurologic level have a muscle grade less than 3; there must be some sparing of sensory and/or motor function in the segments S4–5.

D. Motor complete
Motor function is preserved below the neurologic level, and more than half of the key muscles below the neurologic level have a muscle grade above or equal to 3. There must be some sparing of sensory and/or motor function below S4–5.

E. Normal
Sensory and motor functions are normal. Patient may have abnormalities on reflex examination.

Diagnosis and investigations

Like in any acute trauma condition, cardiorespiratory function takes priority and the patient has to be stabilized initially. All trauma patients, especially the unconscious, are considered as spinal injured, unless proven otherwise. Stabilization procedures have to keep this in mind, especially intubation in a high cervical spinal cord injury or transfers in an unstable cervical and/or thoracic spine trauma. Effective treatment of hypotension is essential to maintain perfusion to the spinal cord, with or without spinal shock.

A complete neurologic examination has to follow careful history-taking, eliciting the mechanics of injury. It is important to ask if the patient had been able to walk after the injury or paralysis was sudden and complete. A delay implies instability issues or developing hematoma in the canal. Not uncommonly, patients with an incomplete SCI or cervical fracture without SCI will describe a several minute period, immediately after injury, of inability to move their extremities.

Sensory and motor examination provides the injury level to the spinal cord while sphincter examination is essential for the sacral functions. Physical examination of the spine can provide details about the surface landmarks and gross displacements of spinal segments.

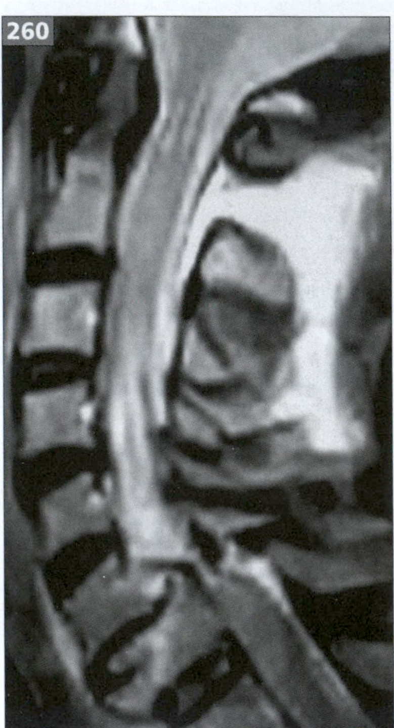

260 MRI (T2 image) showing the fracture dislocation of the cervical spine which is usually associated with complete spinal cord injury.

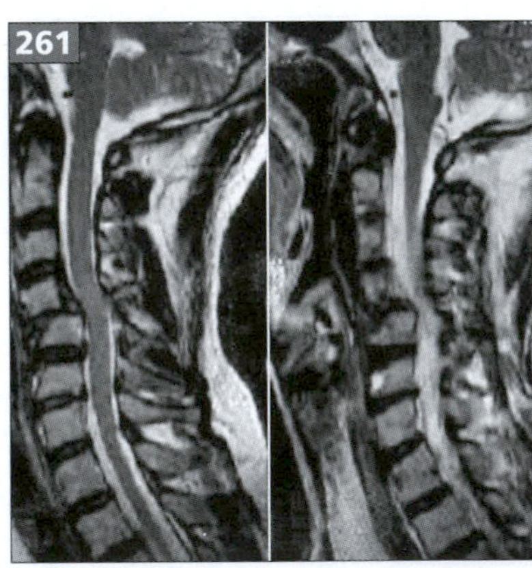

261 A displaced cervical spine at C4 and C5, mostly ligamentous injury. A subluxation usually has incomplete SCI. (MRI-T2 sequence.)

Imaging

Cervical, thoracic, and lumbosacral plain films are usually routinely obtained. Radiographs and high resolution CT/MRI scans provide information regarding the nature and mechanics of the spinal cord injury. While in some cases SCI exists without radiological abnormality (SCIWORA), the usual patient has fractures, fracture dislocations (**260**), or instability due to ligamentous injury sometimes seen as subluxation (**261**).

MRI is excellent in providing the succinct details of spinal cord status and has prognostic significance. A long segment spinal cord edema usually has a bad prognosis as does a hemorrhage into the cord substance with contusion. In awake patients with or without polytrauma, clearance of the cervical spine is usually provided following dynamic X-rays, CT scans, or MRI scans.

A CT with dynamic flexion/extension views and a MRI with or without X-rays may be indicated in unconscious patients within 48 hours to clear the patient. High resolution CT of spine with reconstructions provides greater detail regarding the body and ligamentous instability in the obtunded patient. Both CT and MRI help in the diagnosis of ligamentous instability which may not be obvious in the resting position of the spine in an unconscious patient.

Tip

► *SCI exists without radiological abnormality and radiological abnormality can exist without SCI. Thus both clinical and radiological examinations are crucial.*

Treatment

Both complete and incomplete SCI require acute and chronic management protocols. Acute care includes stabilization of cardiorespiratory function, management of spinal shock, and immobilization of the unstable spinal injury. Spinal shock with hypotension and bradycardia requires aggressive treatment using pressors in order to maintain normal perfusion to the damaged neural tissue. Secondary damage due to ischemia must be prevented by normalization of blood pressure.

High-dose methyl prednisolone treatment is offered as an option according to the guidelines provided by both the American Association and Congress of Neurological Surgeons. According to the reviewer, the evidence suggested 'harmful side-effects are more consistent than any suggestion of clinical benefits'. A total of 639 manuscript titles and abstracts on corticosteroids and human SCI published between 1966 and 2001 were included in the study. There is no convincing evidence to support that methyl prednisolone administration within 8 hours of acute cervical SCI improved neurological recovery. A significant increase in severe medical complications was noted when the administration continued for 24 hours.

Surgical treatment

Following external immobilization during the emergency care and clinicoradiologic evaluations, indications for internal fixation of the spinal column are assessed. Diagnostics and implant technology have improved tremendously over the past decade, and newer internal surgical stabilization techniques have been introduced. The goals of surgical intervention in acute SCI are stabilization of spinal column and decompression of spinal cord.

The timing of such intervention is unclear and several prospective studies are being conducted. Early surgery is, however, indicated in cases of incomplete SCI, since decompression would facilitate the recovery of the neural structures. In complete SCI such an emergency procedure may not produce the desired outcome, while operative stress on an unstable patient could be counter-productive.

A stable patient is considered for surgical intervention which could be anterior, posterior, or combined. This decision is based upon the location of compressive elements and the instability, along with the degree of instability. In several instances the surgeon may make a selection based on the familiarity of an approach and condition of the patient.

Indications for emergency surgery (applicable to the incomplete lesions of spinal cord):

- Progression of neurologic deficits.
- Complete subarachnoid block radiographically (MRI or myelography).
- Myelogram, CT, or MRI showing bone fragments or soft tissue elements in the spinal canal producing spinal cord compression.
- Compression of an important nerve root requiring decompression.
- Penetrating trauma or compound spinal injury.
- Nonreducible fracture displacement due to locked facets producing spinal cord compression.
- Acute anterior spinal cord syndrome secondary to disc herniation or fracture/dislocation.

Cervical spine

Preoperative traction is helpful in achieving closed reduction of the displaced segments. In a seriously ill patient with medical contraindications, a reducible injury may be externally immobilized in a halo traction device (**262, 263**): for a reducible C1–2 injury, halo immobilization is useful in patients over 60 years of age, and a type III odontoid fracture that traverses the body of C2 vertebra heals very well.

A ruptured transverse ligament with atlantoaxial dislocation (AAD) with a displacement of more than 6 mm is preferably treated with internal fixation by transarticular screws and posterior C1–2 fusion.

Most unstable spine injuries below C2 are treated by anterior decompression and internal fixation by screw–plate systems. A single level injury may need bone graft and plate fixation, while a burst fracture may require more extensive decompression and fusion techniques including posterior stabilization.

Posterior lateral mass screw–plate/rod fixation has been used extensively for long segment fixation.

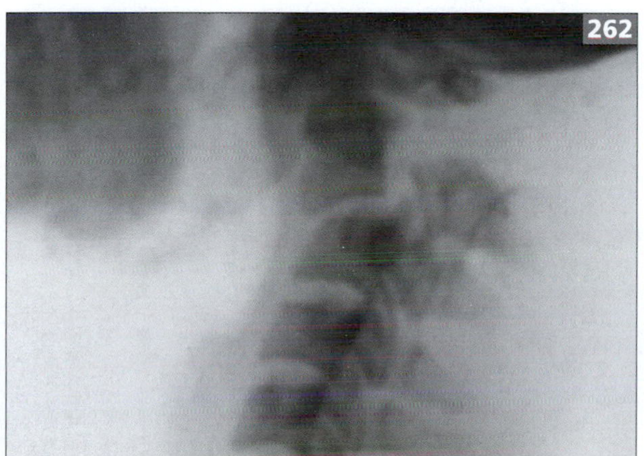

262 Radiograph showing hangman's fracture with severe displacement of fracture segments at C2–3.

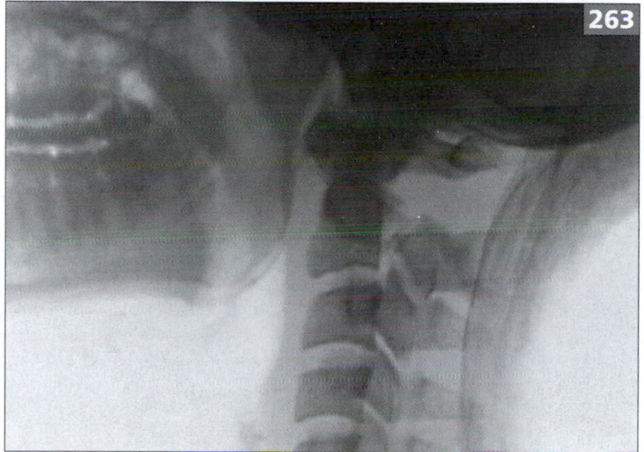

263 The hangman's fracture in 262 was reduced using cervical traction. This injury can heal in a Halo external immobilization or surgical internal fixation. Note the posterior gap between C1 and C2 due to bilateral fracture of C2 pedicles.

Thoracic and thoracolumbar spine

As the thoracic, thoracolumbar, and lumbar spine injuries are the more common injuries, several advancements in hardware technology have expanded the indications for stabilization. The surgical route can be anterior, posterior, or in some cases circumferential.

Surgical treatment with internal fixation of upper thoracic spine is more complicated since suitable hardware is not easily available and the cervicothoracic junction is difficult to approach from the front. A posterior long segment rod fixation through laminar or pedicle hooks is useful in some instances.

Anterolateral approach via a thoracotomy for the mid-thoracic spine is practiced to place an anterior plate with bone-packed cages filling the intervetebral spaces.

Chronic SCI

Rehabilitation and disability management through physiotherapy and occupational therapy improves the outcome of these patients, especially those with incomplete SCI. Complete injuries require management of airway, pulmonary complications, decubitus ulcers, and complications resulting from immobility.

Bladder and bowel care requires attention and patients are taught to accommodate changes in life-style to prevent further complications. Long-standing SCI can lead to a variety of pain syndromes, autonomic dysreflexia, syringomyelia, and spasticity that need specialized treatments.

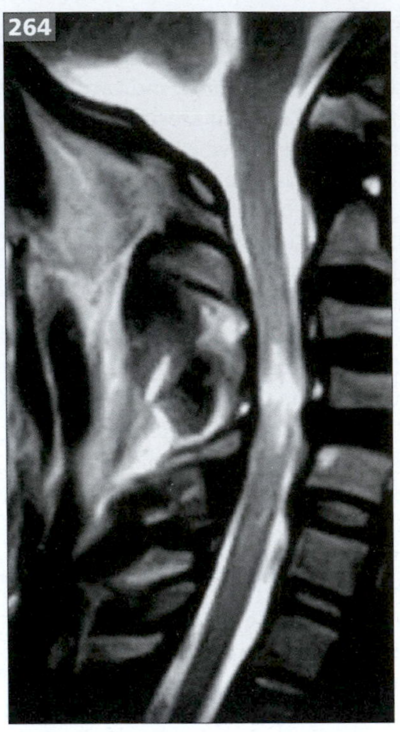

264 MRI (T2) scan showing spinal cord edema at C4 and C5, a frequent indicator of poor prognosis.

Prognosis

An incomplete SCI has a potential for good recovery and the advances in technology along with the paramedical support systems have yielded encouraging results. However, despite these advances acute SCI has mortality of up to 20%. Mortality is higher with acute complete or severe incomplete cervical SCI, where respiratory paralysis sets in early. In the subacute phase, ARDS or gastric bleeding may be encountered. Among those with incomplete SCI, the central cord syndrome and Brown–Sequard syndrome, many regain independent mobility by the end of the first year. Anterior cervical cord syndrome usually has a poorer recovery. C4–C5 edema is a frequent indicator for a poor prognosis (**264**).

Complete SCI is not reversible. A complete SCI without improvement after 72 hours is very unlikely to show functional recovery and only one-third of complete cervical SCI requiring ventilator support survive 5 years.

REFERENCES

1 Brain Trauma Foundation *et al.* (2007). Guidelines for the management of severe traumatic brain injury. *J Neurotrauma* **24** (Suppl 1):S1–S87.

2 Valadka AB, Andrews BT (2005). *Neurotrauma. Evidence-Based Answers to Common Questions*. Thieme, New York.

3 Taber KH, Warden DL, Hurley RA (2006). Blast related traumatic brain injury: what is known ? *J Neuropsychiatry Clin Neurosci* **18**:141–145.

4 Kelly JP, Rosenberg JH (1997). Diagnosis and management of concussion in sports. *Neurology* **48**:575–580.

5 National Spinal Cord Injury Statistical Center (2005). Spinal cord injury: facts and figures at a glance. *J Spinal Cord Med* **28**:379.

Further reading

American Spinal Injury Association (2002). *Standards for Neurological Classification of Spinal Cord Injury* (rev. 2000). ASIA, Chicago.

Bailes JE, Day AL (2001). *Neurological Sports Medicine: A Guide for Physicians and Athletic Trainers*. American Assoc Neurological Surgeons, Rolling Meadows, IL.

Bhattacharjee Y (2008). Shell shock revisited: solving the puzzle of blast trauma. *Science* **319**:406–408.

Fantus RJ, Stone JL (2008). Watch your head. *Bull Am Coll Surg* **93**:48–49.

Gennarelli TA (1993). Cerebral concussion and diffuse brain injuries. In: Cooper PR (ed). *Head Injury*. Williams & Wilkins, Baltimore, pp. 137–158.

Hadley MN, Walters BC, Grabb PA, *et al.* (2002). Guidelines for the management of acute cervical spine and spinal cord injuries. *Clin Neurosurg* **49**:407.

Jallo, Loftus CM (2009). *Neurotrauma and Critical Care of the Brain*. Thieme, New York.

Jordan BD, Tsairis P, Warren RT (1998). *Sports Neurology*, 2nd edn. Lippincott-Raven, Philadelphia.

Maroon JC, Lovell MR, Norwig J, Podell K, Powell JW, Hartl R (2000). Cerebral concussion in athletes: evaluation and neuropsychological testing. *Neurosurgery* **47**:659–672.

McKinley W, Santos K, Meade M, Brooke K (2007). Incidence and outcomes of spinal cord injury syndromes. *J Spinal Cord Med* **30**:215.

(No authors listed) (1997). Practice Parameter: The management of concussion in sports (summary statement). Report of the Quality Standards Subcommittee. *Neurology* **48**:581–585.

Prasad VS, Schwartz A, Bhutani R, Sharkey PW, Schwartz ML (1999). Characteristics of injuries to the cervical spine and spinal cord in polytrauma patient population: experience from a regional trauma unit. *Spinal Cord* **37**:560–568.

Spinal cord injury statistics. www.brainandspinalcord.org

Stone JL (1993). *Head Injury and Its Complications*. PMA Publishers, Costa Mesa, CA.

Winn HR (ed) (2004). *Youmans Neurological Surgery*, 5th edn. Vol **4**: Trauma. WB Saunders, Philadelphia.

STROKE AND TRANSIENT ISCHEMIC ATTACKS OF THE BRAIN AND EYE

Graeme J. Hankey

INTRODUCTION

Definition

Stroke

Stroke is traditionally defined as a clinical syndrome characterized by an acute loss of focal brain function with symptoms lasting more than 24 hours or leading to (earlier) death, and which is thought to be due to inadequate blood supply to a part of the brain (ischemic stroke) or spontaneous hemorrhage into a part of the brain (primary intracerebral hemorrhage) or over the surface of the brain (subarachnoid hemorrhage).

The American Stroke Association now advocates a definition of stroke that incorporates the findings of brain imaging so that stroke is defined as an episode of focal neurologic (brain, retina, spinal cord) dysfunction (even if less than 24 hours in duration) in which the autopsy, computed tomography (CT) brain scan, or magnetic resonance imaging (MRI) brain scan shows features consistent with focal brain infarction (**265–267**) or hemorrhage (**268–271**, next page).

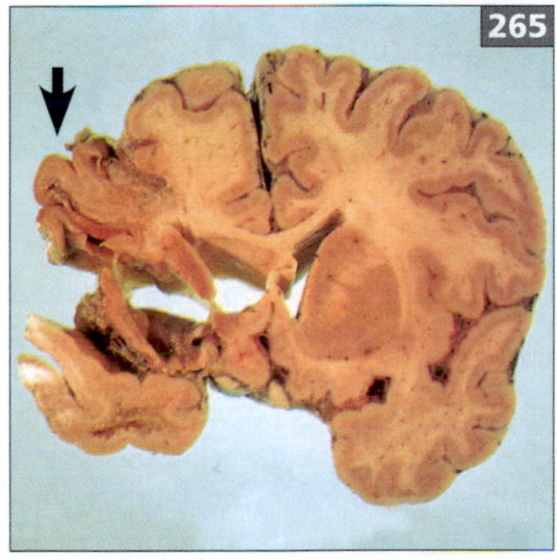

265 Brain, coronal section, showing necrosis of the right parietal and temporal lobes, basal ganglia, and internal capsule (arrow) due to an old infarct in the right middle cerebral artery territory, causing a total anterior circulation syndrome. *Courtesy of Professor BA Kakulas, Department of Neuropathology, Royal Perth Hospital.*

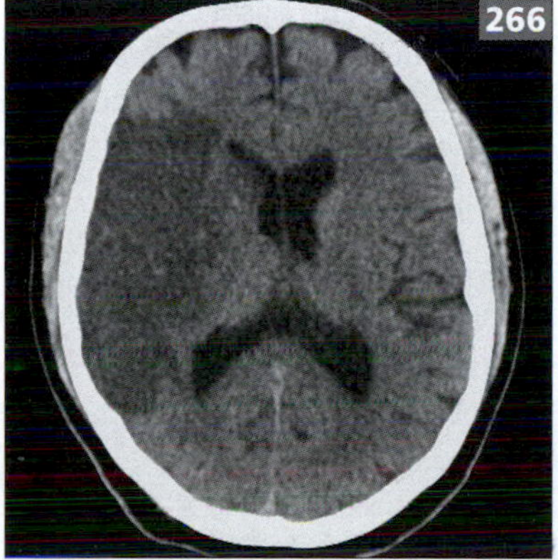

266 Plain CT brain scan showing a focal region of low density, consistent with infarction, in the right frontal, temporal, and parietal lobes in the territory of supply of the right middle cerebral artery.

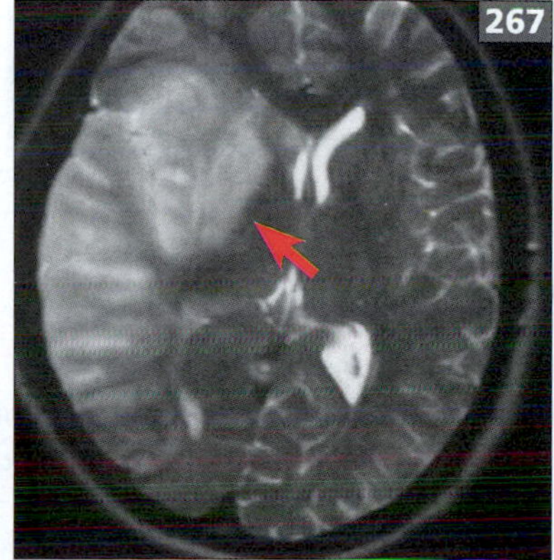

267 T2W axial MRI of an infarct in the right hemisphere (arrow), obtained at 12 hours after symptom onset, in a patient with a left hemiparesis, visual–spatial–perceptual dysfunction, and a left homonymous hemianopia (a total anterior circulation syndrome). Note the altered signal in gray and white matter and the mass effect.

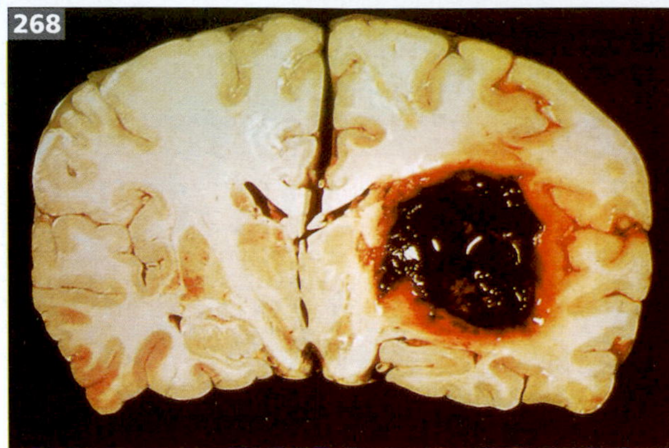

268 Brain, coronal section, showing a fresh putaminal hemorrhage in a patient with severe hypertensive small vessel disease. *Courtesy of Professor BA Kakulas, Department of Neuropathology, Royal Perth Hospital.*

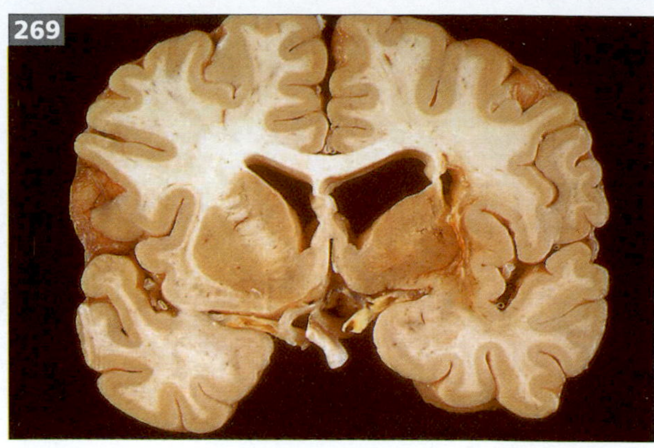

269 Brain, coronal section, showing an old putaminal hemorrhage as a slit-like cavity, with surrounding brown hemosiderin pigmentation. *Courtesy of Professor BA Kakulas, Department of Neuropathology, Royal Perth Hospital.*

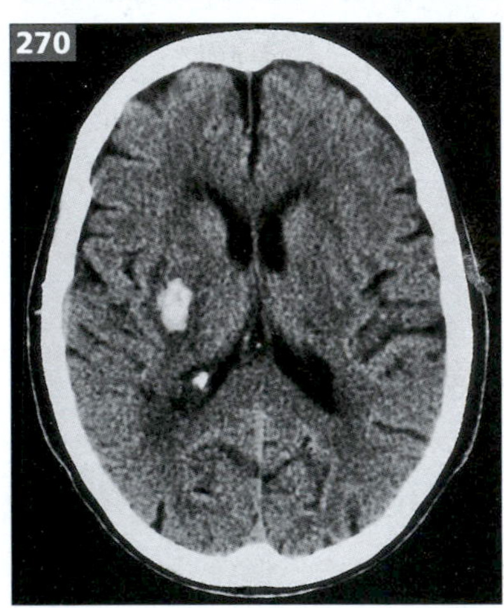

270 Plain (non-contrast) cranial CT scan on the day of stroke onset, showing a homogeneous area of high attenuation, representing an acute hematoma, in the right posterior putamen. The surrounding rim of low density is mild brain edema.

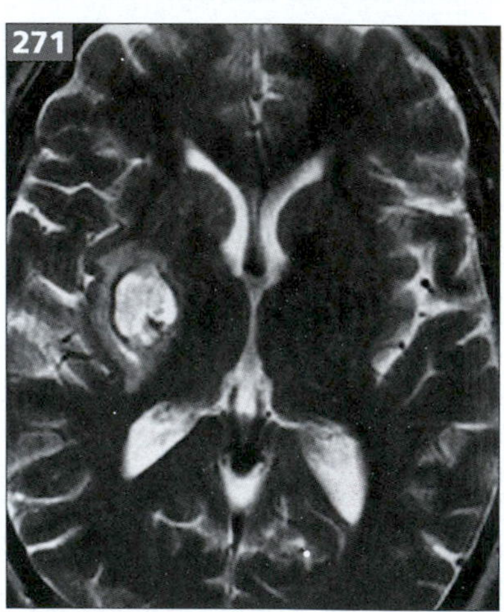

271 T2W MRI showing a right basal ganglia (putamen) hemorrhage 10 days after stroke. Note the increased (bright) signal centrally (methemoglobin) and the dark low signal encircling this, due to hemosiderin.

Transient ischemic attack of the brain or eye

A transient ischemic attack of the brain or eye (TIA) is traditionally defined as a clinical syndrome characterized by an acute loss of focal cerebral or monocular function with *symptoms* lasting less than 24 hours (in practice most last less than 1 hour) and which is thought to be due to inadequate blood supply to a part of the brain or eye.

The American Stroke Association now advocates a definition of TIA that incorporates the findings of MRI brain imaging so that TIA is defined as a transient episode of neurologic dysfunction caused by focal brain, spinal cord, or retinal ischemia, without imaging evidence of acute focal brain infarction – i.e. the MRI diffusion-weighted imaging (DWI) brain scan shows no features of acute focal brain infarction (272, 273). The rationale for this new definition is that: a) the classic 24-hour definition is misleading because many patients with transient (<24-hour) events actually have associated cerebral infarction; b) the 24-hour time limit for transiently symptomatic cerebral ischemia is arbitrary (having more to do with the earth's rotation than biology) and not reflective of the typical duration of these events; and c) disease definitions in clinical medicine, including those for ischemic injuries, are most useful when tissue based. The main argument against the new definition is that it requires brain imaging that will vary depending on the availability of imaging resources, and many patients may not be able to undergo MR brain imaging because of contraindications or claustrophobia. As a consequence, stroke and TIA incidence rates will differ depending on whether and when detailed imaging studies are performed.

Tip

► *Although bright, high signal-intensity lesions ('light bulbs') on DWI and low apparent diffusion coefficient (ADC) values have a high sensitivity (about 90%) and specificity (about 90%) for the diagnosis of acute focal cerebral ischemia, the same findings have been reported in other diverse conditions such as focal brain hemorrhage, abscess, and tumor (i.e. they are not 100% specific).*

The overlap between stroke and TIA, and the concept of an acute stroke syndrome ('brain attack' or 'unstable brain ischemia')

There is a continuum from TIA to ischemic stroke in terms of duration of symptoms rather than an arbitrary cut-off at 24 hours between TIA (<24 hours) and stroke (>24 hours). Patients with TIA and mild ischemic stroke share a similar age and sex distribution, prevalence of vascular risk factors, and long-term prognosis for serious vascular events. Thus, from the point of view of pathogenesis and treatment (secondary prevention), there seems no need to distinguish TIA from ischemic stroke, and indeed many trials of secondary prevention have included patients with TIA and nondisabling, mild ischemic stroke because they are essentially the same condition. However, there are at least four situations in which it may be important to distinguish TIA from minor ischemic stroke: 1) when formulating a differential diagnosis in clinical practice, the differential diagnosis of focal neurologic symptoms lasting minutes (e.g. epileptic seizures, migraine) is somewhat different from that of attacks lasting several hours to days (e.g. demyelination, intracranial tumor, intracerebral hemorrhage); 2) when conducting epidemiologic studies of cerebrovascular disease consistency of diagnostic criteria is essential for comparing results over time and in different regions. Further, complete case ascertainment in incidence and prevalence studies is much less likely for TIA than stroke since patients who experience brief attacks are more likely to ignore or forget them, and are less likely to report them to a doctor than patients who suffer more prolonged or disabling events; 3) when conducting case–control studies, there is less change in 'acute phase' blood factors related to thrombosis and tissue infarction, and there is, by definition, no survival bias, among TIA patients compared with stroke patients; 4) when assessing case-mix in individual units and audits of rehabilitation needs and management, distinguishing TIA from minor stroke may be relevant.

A potential problem in the era of increasingly rapid assessment and treatment of patients with acute cerebrovascular disease is if, and how, to use the above time-based definitions of TIA and stroke in patients who are being seen, and in some cases treated with potentially dangerous interventions (e.g. thrombolysis, thrombectomy), within a few hours of the onset of symptoms. For example, if a hemiparetic patient is assessed 1 hour after the onset of symptoms, one question is whether this attack will recover and turn out to be a TIA, or not recover and become a stroke? There is no certain way of knowing, unless the patient is already recovering, but the longer the duration of symptoms of focal neurologic dysfunction the more likely the deficit will persist and the greater the risk of subsequent early stroke. For patients whose symptoms have resolved within 24 hours of onset, they can be diagnosed retrospectively as having had a TIA (by the traditional definition). However, for those who are being assessed within 24 hours of symptoms onset and their focal neurologic symptoms are still present, with or without relevant physical signs, it is appropriate to describe the acute presentation of focal cerebral ischemia by a term such as a 'brain attack' or 'acute stroke syndrome' or 'unstable brain ischemia'.

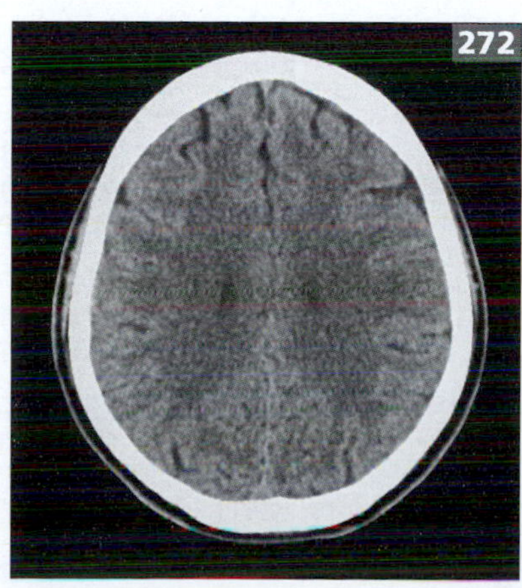

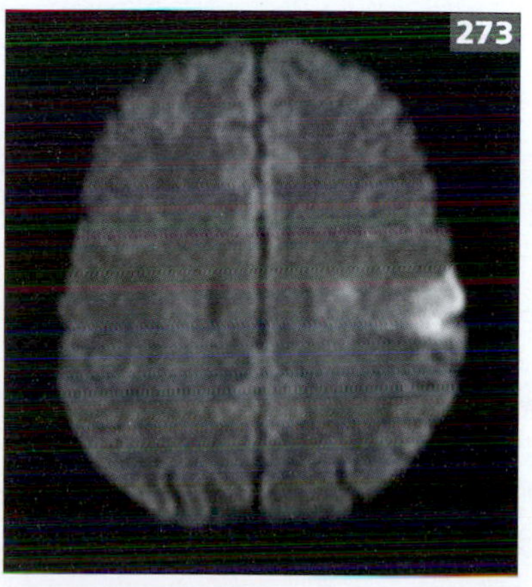

272 Normal plain CT brain scan (left) in a patient with sudden onset right arm weakness that resolved within 1 hour.

273 Magnetic resonance (MR) diffusion weighted image (DWI) (left) showing restricted diffuction, consistent with left posterior frontal ischemia.This would be classified as a TIA by the traditional definition but as an ischemic stroke by the American Stroke Association definition.

This emphasizes the need to exclude rapidly other differential diagnoses of TIA and stroke (e.g. hypoglycemia, brain tumor), establish the pathologic and etiologic subtype of the stroke and risk of recurrent stroke, and intervene with appropriate treatments that may include reperfusion therapy for focal brain ischemia, maintenance of physiological homeostasis, prevention of complications of stroke, early prevention of recurrent stroke and other serious vascular events, and early rehabilitation. 'Time is brain' in this setting.

The anachronistic term 'cerebrovascular accident (CVA)' should be abandoned because it misleadingly implies that stroke is a chance event (accident) and that little can be done.

EPIDEMIOLOGY

Incidence

The incidence of all cerebrovascular events in the community of Oxfordshire, UK between 2002 and 2004 was 3.36 (95% confidence interval [CI]: 3.14–3.58) per 1000 population per year (*Table 33*)[1]. This is higher than the incidence of all coronary vascular events (3.13, 95% CI: 2.93–3.35 per 1000 population per year).

The incidence of first-ever (incident) cerebrovascular events was 2.27 (95% CI: 2.09–2.45) per 1000 per year, indicating that most cerebrovascular events (about two-thirds) are first-ever events. Most (in Oxfordshire at least) were also ischemic in nature, causing ischemic stroke (incidence 2.01, 95% CI: 1.85–2.19 per 1000 per year) or transient ischemic attacks (incidence 1.1, 95% CI: 0.98–1.23 per 1000 per year).

Global incidence

Throughout the world, about 16 million people experience a first-ever stroke each year. Of these, about 9.6 million (60%) arise in low or middle-income countries[2].

Between 1970 and 2008, the incidence of stroke in high-income countries fell by 42%, from 163 (95% CI: 98–227) per 100,000 person years in 1970 to 94 (72–116) per 100,000 person years in 2008 (p for trend = 0.004)[3]. This equates to a fall of about 1.0% per year. This significant decline in stroke incidence in high-income countries coincided with a significant increase in treatments and decline in prevalence of causal risk factors.

In contrast, the incidence of stroke in low- and middle-income countries increased by more than 100%, from 52 (95% CI: 33–71) per 100,000 person years in 1970 to 117 (95% CI: 79–156) per 100,000 person years in 2008 (p for trend <0.0001)[3]. This equates to an increase of about 5.6% per year. The significant increase in stroke incidence in low- and middle-income countries has coincided with increasing exposure of the population to raised blood pressure, smoking, physical inactivity, and diets that are low in fruit and vegetables but high in salt and fat, as well as an increasing average age.

TABLE 33 **ANNUAL RATES* OF ACUTE CEREBROVASCULAR EVENTS IN THE OXFORD VASCULAR STUDY (OXVASC) POPULATION OF OXFORDSHIRE, UK, 2002–2004**

Cerebrovascular events	Men	Women	Total
All cerebrovascular events			
All	2.99 (2.71–3.29)	3.75 (3.43–4.1)	3.36 (3.14–3.58)
Incident	1.96 (1.73–2.2)	2.6 (2.33–2.89)	2.27 (2.09–2.45)
Ischemic stroke			
All	1.87 (1.65–2.11)	2.17 (1.92–2.43)	2.01 (1.85–2.19)
Incident	1.36 (1.17–1.56)	1.47 (1.27–1.69)	1.41 (1.27–1.56)
Intracerebral hemorrhage			
All	0.18 (0.11–0.26)	0.12 (0.07–0.2)	0.15 (0.11–0.2)
Incident	0.13 (0.08–0.2)	0.12 (0.07–0.2)	0.12 (0.09–0.17)
Subarachnoid hemorrhage			
All	0.05 (0.02–0.1)	0.15 (0.09–0.23)	0.1 (0.07–0.14)
Incident	0.03 (0.01–0.07)	0.12 (0.07–0.2)	0.07 (0.04–0.11)
Transient ischemic attack			
All	0.89 (0.74–1.06)	1.31 (1.13–1.52)	1.1 (0.98–1.23)
Incident	0.45 (0.34–0.57)	0.89 (0.74–1.07)	0.66 (0.57–0.77)

* 95% confidence intervals

Prevalence

Stroke is the most prevalent neurologic disorder under the age of 85 years. There is estimated to be about 62 million survivors of stroke world-wide. The age- and sex-adjusted prevalence of stroke has been estimated between 14.7 per 1000 and 17.5 (95% CI: 17.0–18.0) per 1000 in northern England[4].

Case fatality

Case fatality within 30 days of stroke is about 10–15% but increases steeply with age to about 30% in individuals older than 85 years.

A recent systematic review of 35 population-based studies in 18 high-income countries of the early (21 day to 1 month) case fatality of stroke from 1970 to 2008 showed only a nonstatistically significant trend toward a mild decline in early case fatality after stroke in the past 35 years, indicating that recent advances in acute treatments for stroke have not translated into significant declines in early case fatality.

Mortality

The average age-adjusted stroke mortality is about 50–100 per 100,000 people per year in developed countries. However, there are substantial differences among different countries, for example, from greater than 180 per 100,000 people in the Russian Federation to less than 15 per 100,000 people in Canada and Australia (**274**). These differences may reflect differences in the prevalence of genetic and environmental risk factors and differences in the management of stroke.

Global mortality

Throughout the world, about 5.7 million people die after a stroke each year[2]. Stroke therefore contributes about 10% of all deaths around the world, making it the second most common cause of death after ischemic heart disease. Of these 5.7 million deaths, 5 million (87%) arise in low- or middle-income countries. Among the 5.7 million deaths due to stroke each year, nearly 90% can be attributed to high blood pressure (54%), high blood cholesterol (13%), high blood glucose (13%), and tobacco smoking (8%). In addition, gross national income per capita is a major independent, significant predictor of age-adjusted mortality from stroke; for every US$1000 decrease in gross national income per capita, the relative risk of stroke increases by 4% (95% CI: 3–5%).

In developed countries there has been a steady reduction in mortality from stroke during the past 40 years; trends in developing countries are less certain. The most plausible explanation for the reduction in mortality in western countries is a decline in stroke incidence due to improved control of stroke risk factors (especially high blood pressure and cigarette smoking) combined with a parallel improvement in living standards.

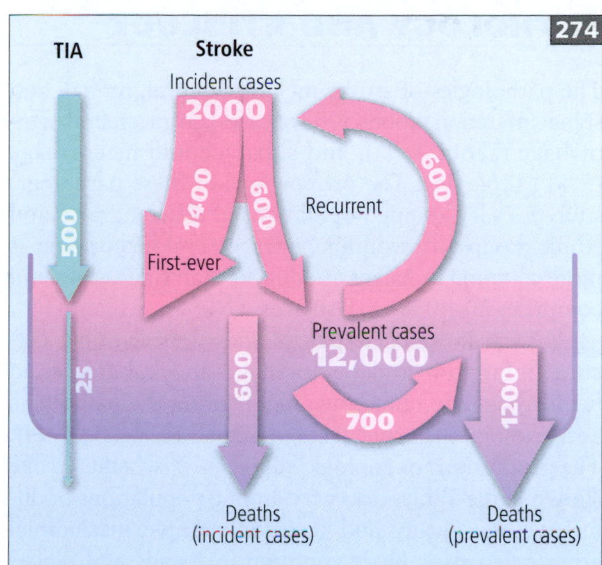

274 Epidemiology of ischemic stroke. In a population of one million people, there are about 2000 new (incident) cases of ischemic stroke each year, of which 1400 (70%) are first-ever and 600 (30%) are recurrent, who are added to a pool of at least 12,000 prevalent survivors. Of the 2000 incident cases, about 600 (30%) are likely to die during the year, and 700 (35%) remain dependent. Of the 12,000 (or more) prevalent cases, about 1200 are likely to die during the year.

Disability

Throughout the world, stroke accounts for the loss of about 51 million disability-adjusted life years (DALYs – the sum of life years lost as a result of premature death and years lived with disability adjusted for severity) each year, of which about 44 million (87%) arise in low- or middle-income countries. Stroke-related disability was the sixth most common cause of reduced DALYs in 2002.

Cost

Stroke accounts for about 2–4% of total health-care costs world-wide, and more than 4% of direct health-care costs in industrialized countries. In Germany, for example, the lifetime cost of stroke is about €40,000.

PATHOLOGY AND ETIOLOGY

The pathologies of stroke include cerebral, retinal, and spinal infarction (about 80% of cases), intracerebral hemorrhage (about 15%), and subarachnoid hemorrhage (5%) (*Table 34*). The proportions of these pathologic subtypes vary among populations of different races and ethnic groups; for example, intracerebral hemorrhage is more common in Asians and Blacks than Caucasians and comprises 20–40% of all strokes.

The cardiovascular pathologies underpinning cerebral infarction and hemorrhage and subarachnoid hemorrhage are numerous, highlighting the pathologic and etiologic heterogeneity of stroke (*Tables 34–44*). The proportions of etiologic subtypes of ischemic stroke shown in the Tables also vary among populations of different ethnic groups and ages; for example, intracranial atherosclerosis is more common in Asians and Blacks than Caucasians, and embolism from the heart is more common in the very elderly and young (due to atrial fibrillation [AF] in the elderly, and congenital and rheumatic heart disease in the young)[5].

Tip

▶ *Stroke is not a disease. It is a clinical syndrome caused by one of many possible diseases. Hence, the clinical features, prognosis, and treatments for stroke are variable.*

TABLE 34 **PATHOLOGIES OF STROKE**

Cerebral, retinal, and spinal cord infarction (ischemic stroke)	**80%**
Large artery diseases *(Table 35)*	40%
• Extracranial	25–30%
(aorta, carotid, vertebral arteries)	10–15%
• Intracranial	20%
(ICA, MCA, ACA, vertebral, basilar, PCA)	15%
Small artery diseases *(Table 36)*	<5%
Heart diseases *(Table 37)*	<1%
Blood diseases (thrombophilias) *(Table 38)*	
Cerebral venous disease *(Table 39)*	
Intracerebral hemorrhage (hemorrhagic stroke) *(Tables 40–43)*	**15%**
Subarachnoid hemorrhage *(Table 44)*	**5%**

ACA: anterior cerebral artery; ICA: internal carotid artery; MCA: middle cerebral artery; PCA: posterior cerebral artery

Cerebral infarction (ischemic stroke)

Sites of cerebral infarction:

- Wedge-shaped cortical/subcortical infarcts in the cerebral and cerebellar hemispheres (**275**): usually due to large or branch artery occlusion by *in-situ* thrombosis or embolism from a proximal source in the heart, aortic arch, or extracranial carotid and vertebral arteries.
- Elongated sickle-shaped strips of infarction of variable width from the frontal to the occipital lobes due to infarction in the border zone between the most distal parts of the anterior and middle cerebral arteries (**276**), often due to ipsilateral severe carotid occlusive disease.
- Small, deep lacunar infarcts, commonly in the internal capsule, thalamus, and ventral pons due to disease affecting the small (40–800 μm diameter) perforating arteries of the brain (**277**); i.e. the lenticulostriate perforating branches of the middle cerebral artery, the thalamoperforating branches of the proximal posterior cerebral artery, and the perforating branches of the basilar artery to the brainstem. These usually manifest as a 'lacunar' clinical syndrome and make up about 25% of ischemic strokes and TIAs.

275 Axial section of the brain at postmortem showing a large hemorrhagic cortical/subcortical infarct in the right frontal lobe due to embolic occlusion of the right anterior cerebral artery and prerolandic branch of the upper division of the right middle cerebral artery by an embolus from the origin of the right internal carotid artery.

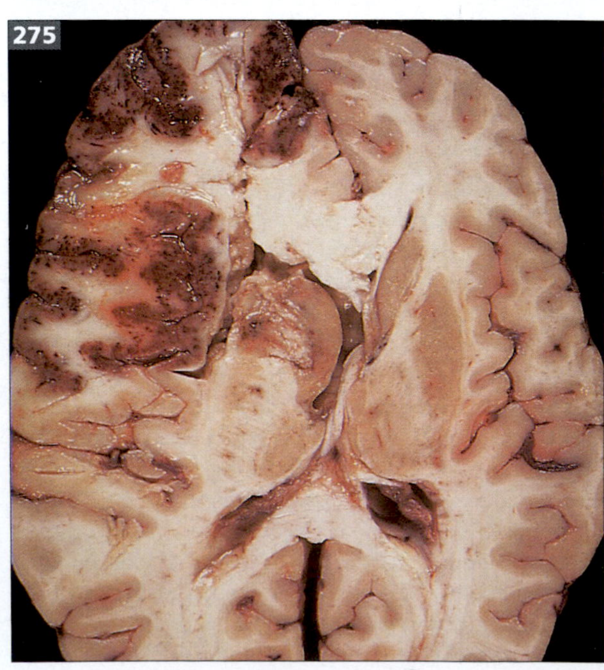

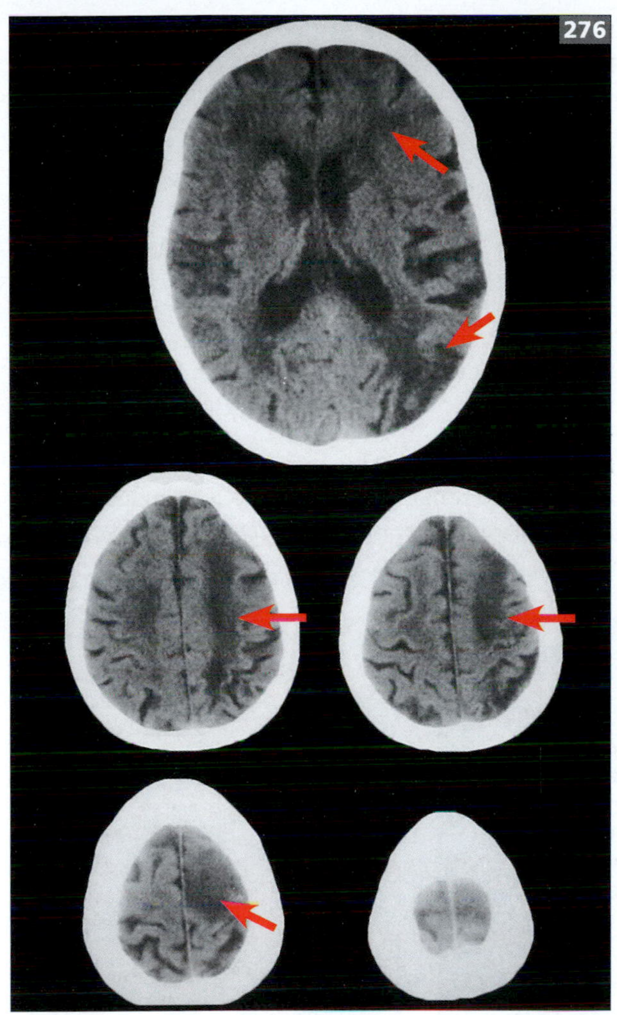

276 CT scan showing a border-zone infarct in the left cerebral hemisphere (arrows). Note the low-density area (infarct) runs along the border between the middle cerebral artery and anterior cerebral artery territory, and the border between the middle cerebral artery and posterior cerebral artery territory.

277 Brain at autopsy showing a lacunar infarct (arrow) in the internal capsule of a patient with a previous lacunar syndrome. *Courtesy Professor BA Kakulas, Department of Neuropathology, Royal Perth Hospital.*

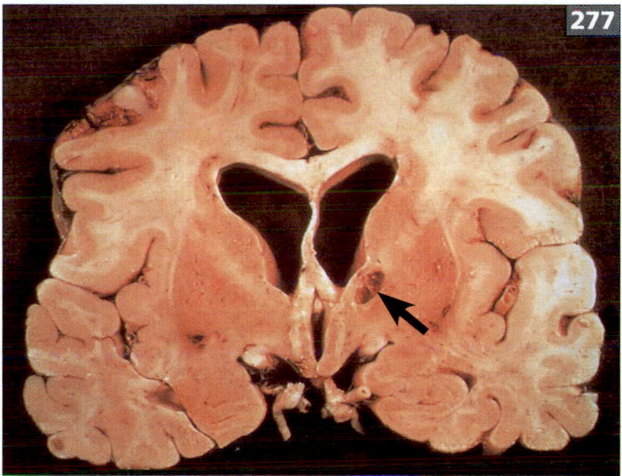

Extracranial and intracranial large artery disease

The large arteries supplying blood to the brain are the aortic arch, extracranial carotid, and vertebral arteries, and intracranial internal carotid, middle cerebral, anterior cerebral, vertebral, basilar, and posterior cerebral arteries.

The most common diseases of the large cerebrovascular arteries are atherosclerosis and dissection. Other large artery diseases are shown in *Table 35*.

Atherosclerosis

The major sites of large artery atherosclerosis are large and medium-sized arteries (e.g. aortic arch), particularly at places of arterial branching (e.g. the carotid bifurcation), tortuosity (e.g. the carotid siphon), and confluence (e.g. the basilar artery) (**278–280**, next page). Individuals with atheroma affecting one artery almost always have atheroma affecting several other arteries, either with or without clinical manifestations.

Some sites are remarkably free of atheroma (e.g. the internal carotid artery [ICA] between its origin and the siphon, and the main cerebral arteries distal to the Circle of Willis). Consequently, occlusion of a branch of the middle cerebral artery (MCA) is more likely to be due to embolism than local thrombosis on an atheromatous plaque.

The main pathologic manifestations of atherosclerosis are:

- Fatty streaks: focal accumulations of subendothelial smooth muscle cells and macrophages containing lipid (cholesterol and cholesterol ester).
- Fibrous plaque: a central core of lipid and cell debris surrounded by smooth muscle cells, collagen, elastic fibers, and proteoglycans. A band of fibrous tissue (the fibrous cap) separates the lipid core (the atheroma) from the lumen of the vessel.
- Mature atheroma has three main constituents:
  - Proliferated cells, predominantly smooth muscle cells.
  - Lipids (cholesterol-esters) and lipid-laden macrophages ('foam cells').
  - Connective tissue elements such as elastins and glycosaminoglycans.
- Complicated lesions: mature fibrous plaque with various types of degenerative changes such as calcification (due to precipitation of calcium salts in the tissues), intraplaque hemorrhage or plaque rupture, intimal ulceration or erosion, and mural thrombosis and thromboembolism (**281**).

The main cause of atherosclerosis is prolonged exposure to causal risk factors, such as high blood pressure, high blood lipids (low-density lipoprotein [LDL]-cholesterol and apoB lipoprotein), high blood glucose (diabetes), and cigarette smoking in individuals genetically predisposed to form atheroma in response to these exposures.

Hyperhomocysteinemia is an uncommon hereditary cause of atheroma, predisposing to it by injuring endothelial cells and increasing smooth muscle proliferation.

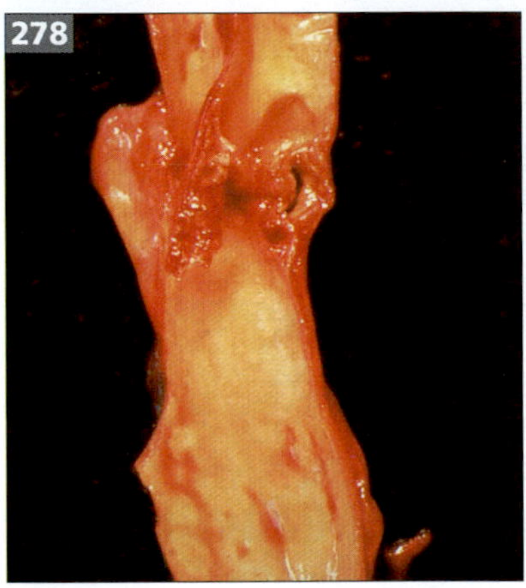

278 Longitudinal section of the common carotid artery and proximal internal carotid artery at autopsy showing atheroma of the origin of the internal carotid artery.
Reproduced with permission from Hankey GJ and Warlow CP [1994]; Transient ischaemic attacks of the brain and eye. WB Saunders.

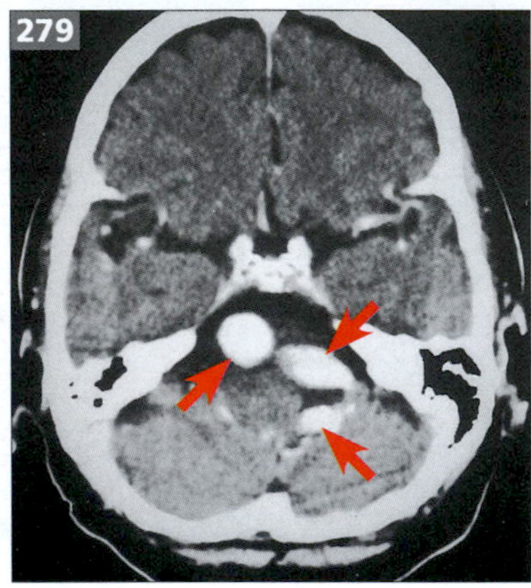

279 CT brain scan with contrast showing a very ectatic basilar artery (arrows).

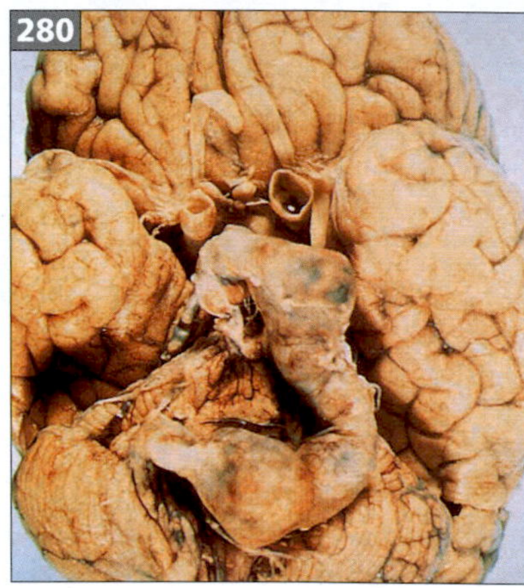

280 Photograph of the base of the brain at post-mortem showing atheromatous aneurysmal dilatation and tortuosity of the basilar artery.
Reproduced with permission from Hankey GJ and Warlow CP [1994]; Transient ischaemic attacks of the brain and eye. WB Saunders.

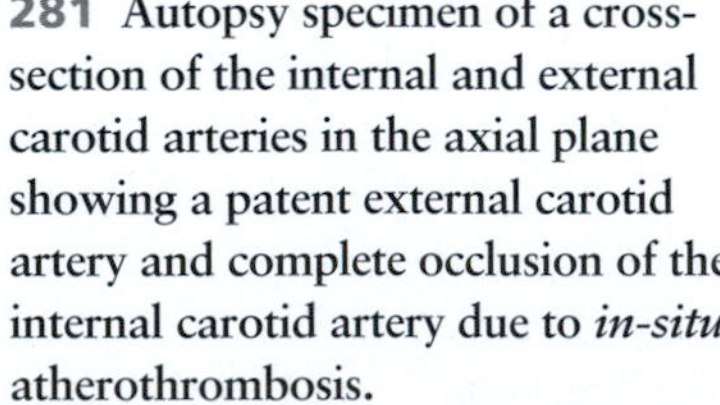

281 Autopsy specimen of a cross-section of the internal and external carotid arteries in the axial plane showing a patent external carotid artery and complete occlusion of the internal carotid artery due to *in-situ* atherothrombosis.

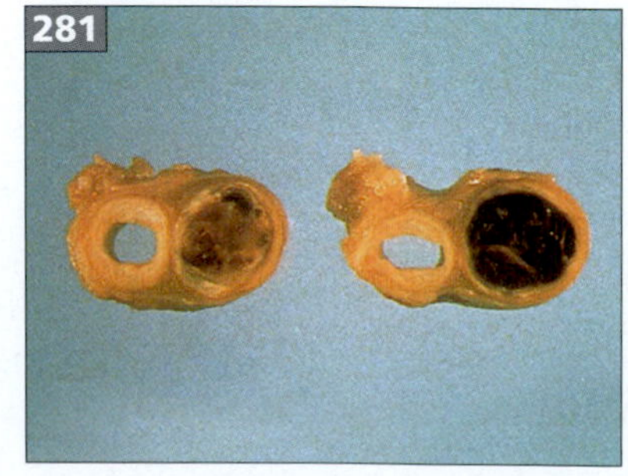

TABLE 35 **LARGE ARTERY DISEASES OF THE BRAIN**

	Causative gene/chromosome location	Inheritance pattern
Atherosclerosis		
• Hereditary: homocystinuria	Cystathione beta synthase and others Methyltetrahydrofolate reductase c677T	AR AR
• Acquired (exposure to risk factors)		
Dissection		
• Spontaneous		
• Trauma (e.g. rapid, extreme neck rotation)		
• Ehlers–Danlos syndrome type IV	Collagen type III gene (COL 3A1)	AD
• Homocystinuria	Cystathione beta synthase and others	AR
• Marfan's syndrome	FBN1 and TGF,R2 genes	AD
• Fibromuscular dysplasia		
Fabry's disease	Alpha-galactosidase A gene	XL-R
Moyamoya disease	3p24.2-26, 17q25	Polygenic or AR
Pseudoxanthoma elasticum	ATP-binding cassette subfamily C member 6 gene (ABCC6)	AR or AD
Sickle cell disease	Hemoglobin beta	AR
Neurofibromatosis 1		
Down's syndrome		
Irradiation		
Arteritis		
• Takayasu's arteritis		
• Giant cell arteritis		
• Behçet's disease		

AD: autosomal dominant; AR: autosomal recessive; FBN1: fibrillin; TGF,R2: transforming growth factor, beta receptor II; XL-R: X-linked recessive

Dissection

Dissection is the second most common type of large artery disease[6]. Dissection is characterized by a tear in the intima or media, leading to bleeding within the arterial wall, which tracks or dissects longitudinally and circumferentially between the intima and media, or media and adventitia, of the arterial wall. The dissection can tear through the intima allowing the partially coagulated intramural blood to enter the lumen of the artery.Thrombus can also form on the intimal flap or any subendothelial collagen, and later embolize to the brain. Most carotid dissections occur at the base of the skull and extend proximally (towards the bifurcation of the common carotid artery into the internal and external carotid arteries) and distally (towards the intracranial internal carotid artery (282); common carotid artery and intracranial carotid dissections are rare. Most vertebrobasilar dissections occur at the C2 level, possibly reflecting increased susceptibility to mechanical torsion and stretch at this location.

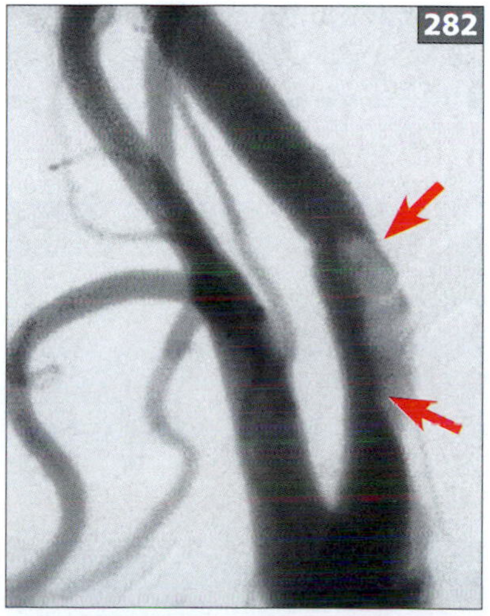

282 Intra-arterial angiogram of a localized internal carotid dissection with a small intimal flap (arrow).

Ehlers–Danlos syndrome type IV, the vascular type, results from mutations in the gene for type III procollagen. It is a rare connective tissue disorder inherited as an autosomal-dominant trait, characterized mainly by arterial dissection, intracranial aneurysm, and the spontaneous rupture of large and medium-sized arteries, and a gravid uterus or intestines. Carotid intima–media thickness is one-third lower and circumferential wall stress 40% higher than in matched controls. The higher circumferential wall stress is probably a major risk factor for the dissection and rupture of fragile arterial tissue. The fragility of the arterial wall in mice with mutations affecting type I and type III collagens has been attributed to a large decrease in the number of collagen type I fibrils in the aortic media and adventitia.

Marfan syndrome is a connective tissue disorder inherited as an autosomal-dominant trait and is characterized by abnormalities involving the skeletal, ocular, and cardiovascular systems. It results from mutations in the gene encoding fibrillin-1 (FBN1), leading to abnormalities in the assembly of elastic fibers. A clinical hallmark and the major cause of morbidity and premature death from this syndrome is aortic root dilatation and associated aortic regurgitation, dissection, and rupture. The exact mechanisms leading to dilatation are not fully understood, but steady and pulsatile stresses are probably important, leading to the mechanical fatigue and ultimate failure of abnormal elastic fibers to sustain physiological pulsatile stress. Marfan syndrome also predisposes to mitral valve prolapse and AF.

Fibromuscular dysplasia (FMD) is a group of nonatherosclerotic, noninflammatory arterial diseases that most commonly involve the carotid and renal arteries, and can be complicated by arterial dissection and intracerebral aneurysms with a risk of subarachnoid or intracerebral hemorrhage. The prevalence of cervicocranial FMD is about 2/1000. Histologic classification discriminates three main subtypes, intimal, medial, and perimedial. Intimal FMD, is characterized by irregularly arranged mesenchymal cells within a loose matrix of subendothelial connective tissue and a fragmented internal elastic lamina. The most common form, medial FMD, is characterized by a homogeneous collar of elastic tissue that presents as multiple stenoses interspersed with aneurysmal outpouchings, with a preserved internal elastic lamina. Perimedial FMD involves excessive tissue deposition at the junction of the media and adventitia. The three types are not mutually exclusive. Angiography typically shows medial FMD as multiple stenoses and a 'string-of-beads' appearance (**283, 284**). The etiology of FMD is unknown, although various hormonal and mechanical factors have been suggested. Differential diagnoses include atherosclerotic stenoses and stenoses associated with vascular Ehlers–Danlos and Williams' syndromes, and type 1 neurofibromatosis.

Fabry disease

Fabry disease is an X-linked sphingolipidosis caused by deficiency of α-galactosidase A (α-gal). The defect of this lysosomal enzyme leads to a failure in the metabolism of glycosphingolipids containing α-D-galactosyl moieties, particularly globosotriaosylceramide, which accumulate in the lysosomes of most organ cells. Progressive accumulation of globosotriaosylceramide in endothelial and vascular smooth muscle cells causes progressive stenosis and occlusion of small arterial vessels. Furthermore, the large vessels dilate, resulting in dolichoectatic changes and flow stagnation, increasing the risk of artery-to-artery embolism and vessel thrombosis[7]. These changes occur more frequently in the posterior circulation. The incidence of FD is estimated to be 1 in 117,000 live births and 1 in 40,000 men.

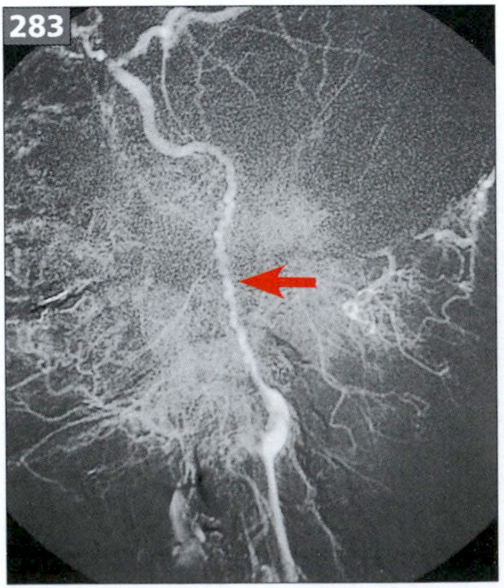

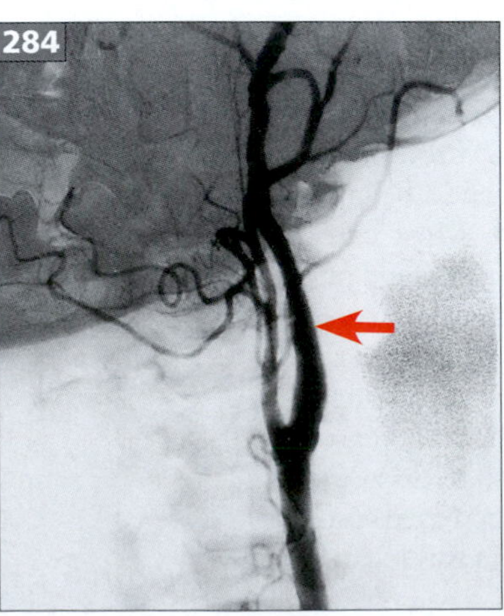

283, 284 **Intra-arterial angiograms of fibromuscular hyperplasia. Note the narrowed and beaded appearance of the internal carotid artery (arrow).**

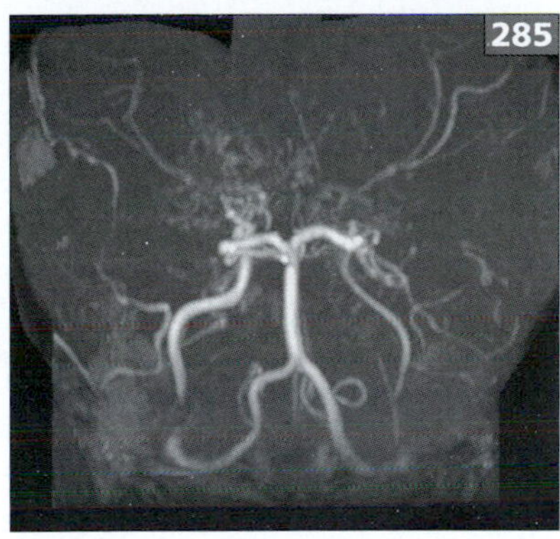

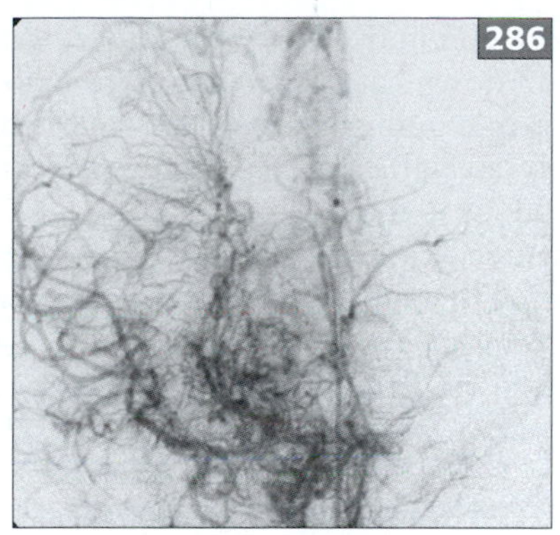

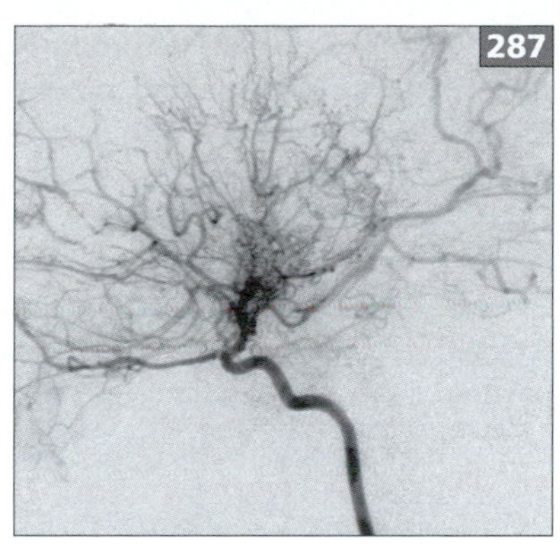

285 MR angiography, posterior–anterior view, showing stenosis of the distal intracranial internal carotid artery, extending to the proximal anterior and middle arteries, with secondary development of an extensive collateral network at the base of the brain along with the classic 'puff of smoke' appearance.

286, 287 Catheter angiogram, posterior–anterior and lateral views, in a patient with moyamoya disease, showing reduced flow in the internal, middle, and anterior cerebral arteries coupled with prominent flow voids through the basal ganglia and thalamus from moyamoya-associated collateral vessels, virtually diagnostic of moyamoya.

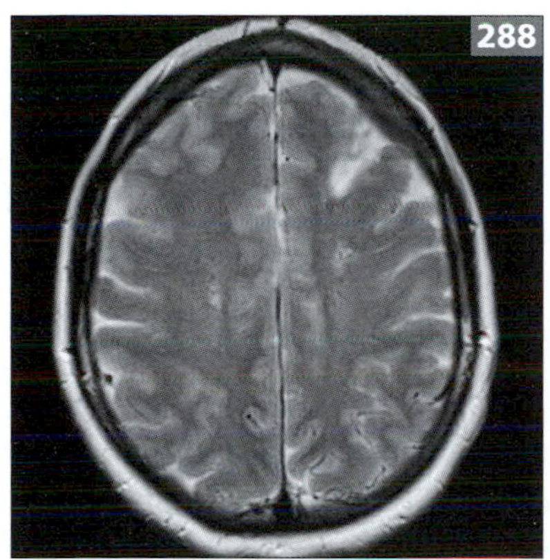

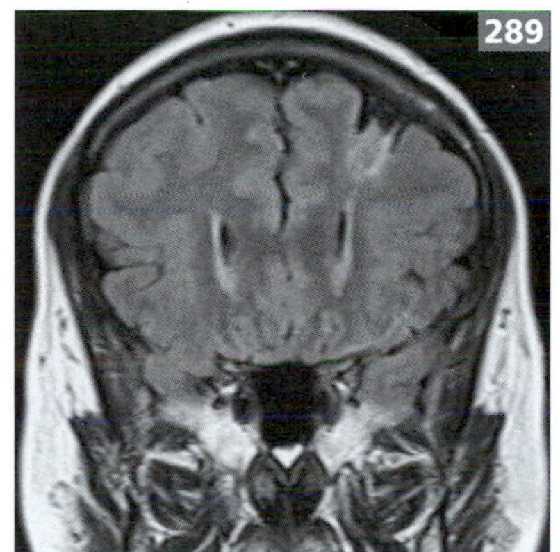

288, 289 MRI brain scan, axial (288) and coronal (289) planes, in a patient with moyamoya disease, showing an area of increased signal intensity due to old infarction and atrophy in left frontal lobe cortex, in the border zone between the territory of supply of the left anterior and middle cerebral arteries.

Moyamoya disease and syndrome

Moyamoya disease and syndrome are characterized by chronic, progressive occlusion of the terminal carotid arteries bilaterally[8]. As a consequence, numerous collateral telangiectatic vessels develop at the base of the brain which give rise to the appearance of a 'puff of smoke' on catheter angiography (285–289). Stenosis occurs in the distal internal carotid artery and often involves the proximal anterior and middle cerebral arteries. Affected vessels do not show arteriosclerotic or inflammatory changes leading to occlusion. Rather, vessel occlusion results from a combination of hyperplasia of smooth muscle cells and luminal thrombosis. The media is often attenuated, with irregular elastic lamina. Caspase-dependent apoptosis has been implicated as a contributory mechanism in the associated degradation of the arterial wall. Moyamoya-associated collaterals are generally dilated perforating arteries that are believed to be a combination of pre-existing and newly developed vessels. These collaterals show evidence of stress related to increased flow, including the combination of fragmented elastic lamina, thinned media in the vessel wall, and the presence of microaneurysms; these findings help to explain why some patients present with hemorrhage. Other moyamoya-related vessels are collapsed and their lumens thrombosed, findings that may account for the cause of ischemic symptoms.

Moyamoya disease is commonly found in individuals of Asian heritage and there is no known cause. Genetic factors appear to play a major role in moyamoya. The proportion of patients who have affected first-degree relatives is 10% in Japan. Less common associations, which may be causal, include sickle cell disease, neurofibromatosis type 1, cranial therapeutic irradiation, Down's syndrome, and rarely, congenital cardiac anomaly, renal artery stenosis, giant cervicofacial hemangiomas, and hyperthyroidism.

Pseudoxanthoma elasticum

Pseudoxanthoma elasticum (PXE) is an inherited systemic disease of connective tissue related to mutations in the *ABCC6* (ATP binding cassette subtype C number 6) gene which primarily affects the skin, retina, and cardiovascular system. It is characterized pathologically by elastic fiber mineralization and fragmentation (so called 'elastorrhexia'), large artery calcifications, and stenosis, and clinically by high heterogeneity in age of onset and the extent and severity of organ system involvement. The diagnosis relies on clinical features and the histologic demonstration of abnormal, calcified elastic fibers in the dermis through the use of special stains.

Sickle cell disease

Sickle cell disease is a multi-system disease, associated with episodes of acute illness and progressive organ damage. The arteriopathy is characterized by intimal thickening, proliferation of fibroblasts and smooth muscle cells and, eventually intraluminal thrombus formation, which is usually confined to the supraclinoid internal carotid artery and proximal portions of the middle and anterior cerebral arteries. The pathophysiology is that deoxygenation causes sickle hemoglobin (HbS) to polymerize, leading to sickled erythrocytes. Interaction of sickled erythrocytes with leukocytes and the vascular endothelium results in vaso-occlusion, which then leads to tissue infarction, hemolysis, and inflammation. Inflammation enhances expression of adhesion molecules, further increasing the tendency of sickled erythrocytes to adhere to the vascular endothelium, resulting in further endothelial activation, thrombus formation, and vascular occlusion. Reperfusion of the ischemic tissue generates free radicals and oxidative damage. The damaged erythrocytes release free hemoglobin into the plasma, which strongly bind to nitric oxide, causing functional nitric oxide deficiency and contributing to the development of the vasculopathy.

Neurofibromatosis 1

Neurofibromatosis 1 (NF-1) is an autosomal-dominant disease, with extremely variable expressivity, but most patients have café-au-lait spots, intertriginous freckling, dermal and plexiform neurofibromas, and learning disabilities, and some also develop cardiac and vascular disease. Cerebrovascular abnormalities usually result from stenoses or occlusions of the internal carotid, middle cerebral, or anterior cerebral artery. The large vessel disease is characterized histologically by Schwann cell proliferation. As a result of the stenosis, small collaterals, in the form of telangiectatic vessels, form around the area of the stenosis and appear as a 'puff of smoke' ('moyamoya') on cerebral angiography. Intracranial aneurysms and cervical arteriovenous fistulae and aneurysms may also occur in NF-1 patients, but are less common and tend to be seen in older patients.

Irradiation

The effects of external therapeutic irradiation (for malignancy) on the arterial wall have been well documented in animal and in human studies. The factors which may influence such injury include the type of radiation, number of fractions, dose, and time interval from treatment. The vascular injury induced by irradiation involves all layers of the vessel wall and is characterized by endothelial cell proliferation, medial scarring and loss of smooth muscle, and adventitial fibrosis. Irradiation may also accelerate the development of atherosclerosis.

Arteritis

Takayasu arteritis is a chronic, idiopathic, inflammatory disease that primarily affects large vessels, such as the aorta and its main branches (**290**)[9]. The clinical features usually reflect limb or organ ischemia resulting from gradual stenosis of involved arteries. Takayasu arteritis often occurs in females during their reproductive years. The differential diagnosis includes: 1) other causes of inflammatory aortitis (such as syphilis; tuberculosis; systemic lupus erythematosus [SLE]; rheumatoid arthritis; spondyloarthropathies; Buerger, Behçet, Cogan, and Kawasaki diseases; and giant cell arteritis); 2) developmental anomalies (such as Ehlers–Danlos syndrome and Marfan syndrome); and 3) other aortic abnormalities (such as neurofibromatosis, ergotism, and radiation fibrosis).

Giant cell arteritis is a panarteritis characterized by intimal proliferation and thickening, destruction of the internal elastic lamina, and infiltration of the media by mononuclear cells (predominantly T lymphocytes of the helper/inducer subset), giant cells, and occasional eosinophils with granuloma formation (**291–293**). Any medium or large artery in the body (aorta, carotid, vertebral, coronary, femoral, and so on) may be affected, but most commonly branches of the external carotid

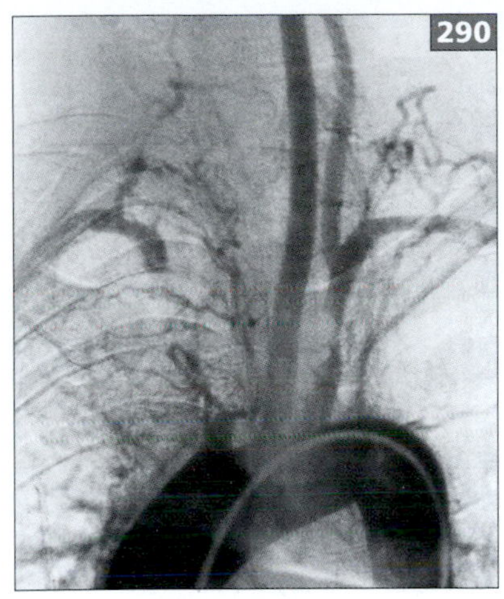

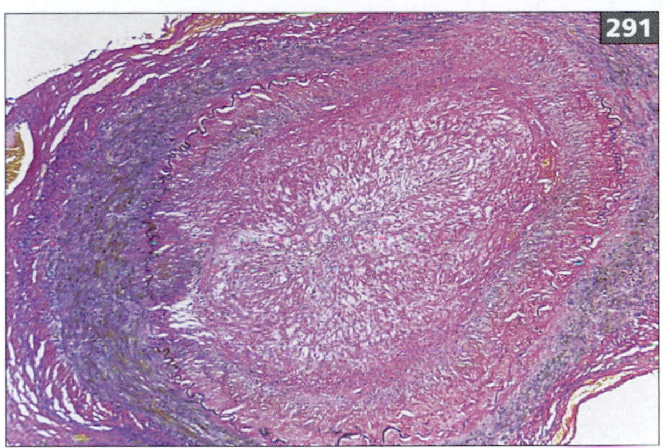

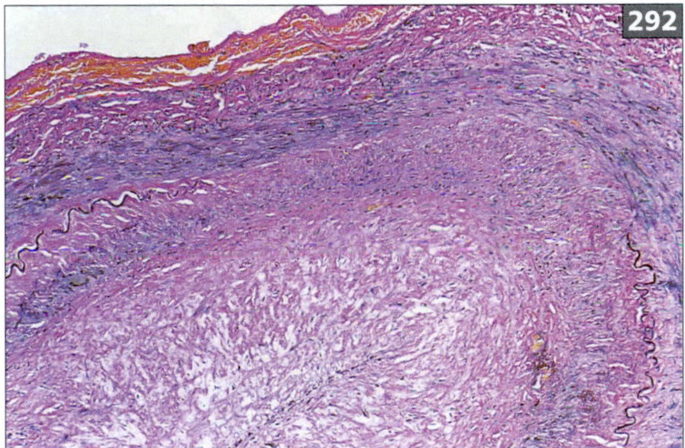

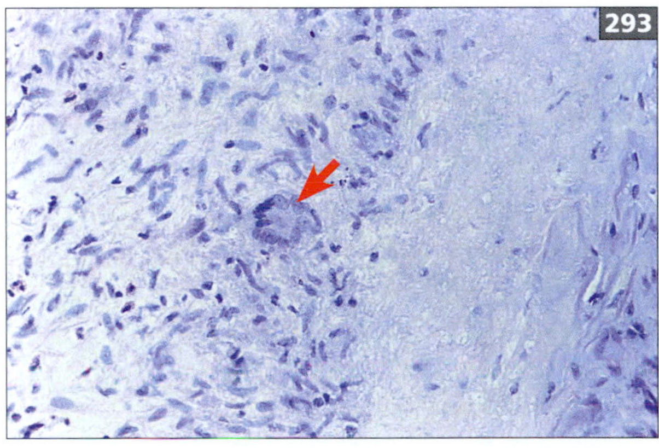

290 An arch aortogram from a patient with Takayasu's arteritis. Note the stricture of the right subclavian and occlusion of the left subclavian arteries. *Photo courtesy Dr Alan Reid, Consultant Radiologist, Royal Infirmary, Glasgow, UK.*

291 Cross-section of a temporal artery. Low-power magnification, showing that the lumen is occluded by extensive granulomatous inflammatory reaction involving the total thickness of the vessel.

292 Higher power, showing that the intimal surface is replaced by a fibroblastic proliferation, occluding the lumen, and that the sub-intimal zone has extensive fibrinoid necrosis with marked disruption of the internal elastic lamina. There is histiocytic proliferation, nodules of eosinophil cells, and occasional multinucleated giant cells. In the outer muscle and adventitial coats there is a light infiltrate of lymphocytes and plasma cells.

293 High-power section of a temporal artery biopsy of a patient with active giant cell arteritis, showing (in the centre of the field) a multinucleate giant cell with the nuclei arranged around the periphery of the cell in a horseshoe pattern (arrow).

(superficial temporal, facial, occipital arteries), ophthalmic, vertebral, and posterior ciliary arteries, as well as the aorta and its branches. These are all vessels with substantial quantities of elastin in their walls. Curiously, other vessels with lesser amounts of elastin, such as the proximal central retinal artery, and the petrous and cavernous portions of the internal carotid arteries, and their branches, may also be involved, but the cervical segment of the carotid artery is minimally involved and there is a striking lack of arteritic involvement of the intracranial arteries except in rare cases. Particularly common sites of arterial stenosis are the internal carotid artery just before dural penetration and the extracranial vertebral artery just before entering the skull.

Intracranial small vessel disease

The term small vessel disease encompasses all of the pathologic processes that affect the small vessels of the brain, including small arteries and arterioles but also capillaries and small veins[9,10].

TABLE 36 **SMALL VESSEL DISEASES OF THE BRAIN**

TYPE 1 **Arteriolosclerosis**

TYPE 2 **Cerebral amyloid angiopathy**	**Causative gene/chromosome location**	**Inheritance pattern**
• Hereditary:		
– Hereditary cerebral hemorrhage with amyloidosis of the Dutch type	Amyloid precursor protein gene	AD
– Cystatin C-related familial cerebral amyloid angiopathy	Cystatin C gene	AD
– Familial amyloid polyneuropathy	Tranthyretin gene	AD
• Sporadic		

TYPE 3 **Inherited or genetic small vessel diseases distinct from cerebral amyloid angiopathy**

	Causative gene/chromosome location	**Inheritance pattern**
• CADASIL	Notch 3 gene	AD
• CARASIL	Unknown gene	AR
• HERNS	3p21.1–p21.3	AD
• Fabry disease	Alpha-galactosidase A gene	XL-R
• MELAS	Mitochondrial DNA	Maternal
• Homocystinuria	Cystathione beta synthase and others	AR
• Pseudoxanthoma elasticum	ATP-binding cassette subfamily C member 6 gene (ABCC6)	AR or AD
• Sickle cell disease	Hemoglobin beta	AR
• Angiotensin-converting enzyme	Ins/Del	AR
• Small vessel diseases caused by COL4A1 mutations		
• Hereditary cerebroretinal vasculopathy		
• Hereditary multi-infarct dementia of the Swedish type		
• Neurofibromatosis 1		

TYPE 4 **Infectious, inflammatory, and immunologically mediated small vessel diseases (vasculitis)**

- Infectious vasculitis:
  - Bacterial: syphilis, tuberculosis, Lyme disease, *Mycoplasma pneumoniae*, *Bartonella henselae*, *Rickettsia* spp., acute bacterial meningitis
  - Fungal: aspergillosis, mucormycosis, coccidioidomycosis, candidosis
  - Viral: varicella zoster virus, HIV, hepatitis C virus, cytomegalovirus, parvovirus B19
  - Parasitic: cysticercosis
  - Infective endocarditis
- Systemic vasculitis:
  - Wegener's granulomatosis
  - Churg–Strauss syndrome
  - Behçet's disease
  - Polyarteritis nodosa
  - Henoch–Schönlein purpura
  - Kawasaki disease
  - Giant cell arteritis
  - Takayasu's arteritis
- Connective tissue diseases:
  - Systemic lupus erythematosus
  - Rheumatoid arthritis
  - Sjögren's syndrome
  - Dermatomyositis
  - Mixed connective tissue disease
- Miscellaneous:
  - Antiphospholipid antibodies syndrome
  - Sarcoidosis
  - Lymphoma (Hodgkin's and non-Hodgkin's)
  - Inflammatory bowel disease
  - Graft-versus-host disease
  - Drugs: amphetamine, cocaine, ephedrine, phenylpropanolamine
  - Primary angiitis of the CNS

TYPE 5 **Venous collagenosis**

- Collagenous thickening of the walls of veins and venules close to the lateral ventricles

TYPE 6 **Other small vessel diseases**

- Post-radiation angiopathy
- Nonamyloid microvessel degeneration in Alzheimer's disease

AD: autosomal dominant; AR: autosomal recessive; ATP: adenosine triphosphate; CADASIL: cerebral autosomal-dominant arteriopathy with subcortical infarcts and leukoencephalopathy; CARASIS: cerebral autosomal-recessive arteriopathy with subcortical infarcts and leukoencephalopathy; HERNS: hereditary endotheliopathy with retinopathy, nephropathy, and stroke; HIV: human immunodeficiency virus; MELAS: mitochondrial myopathy, encephalomyopathy, lactic acidosis; XL-R: X-linked recessive.

The difference between small arteries and arterioles is the absence of a continuous elastic lamina. Intracranial small arteries have two origins: *superficially* they stem from the subarachnoid circulation as the terminal vessels of medium-sized arteries, which originate from larger arteries; and, *deeper* at the base of the brain, they stem directly from the large arteries as arterial perforators. The two systems converge towards each other and, after having passed the cortical layers and the deep gray structures, respectively, they merge in the deepest areas of the subcortical white matter where there is a borderzone (or watershed area).

Lipohyalinosis, arteriosclerosis, vessel wall leakage, and collagen deposition in venular walls are recognized microvascular changes. Suggested pathogenetic mechanisms are ischemia/hypoxia, hypoperfusion due to altered cerebrovascular autoregulation, blood–brain barrier leakage, inflammation, degeneration, and amyloid angiopathy. An etiopathogenic classification is shown in *Table 36*[10–12].

Arteriolosclerosis

Arteriolosclerosis (or age-related and vascular risk factor-related small vessel diseases) is mainly characterized by loss of smooth muscles cells from the tunica media, deposits of fibro-hyaline material, narrowing of the lumen, and thickening of the vessel wall. Other pathologic features may include fibrinoid necrosis, lipohyalinosis, microatheroma (distal manifestation of atherosclerosis), microaneurysms (elongated and dilated vessels: saccular, lipohyalinotic, asymmetric fusiform, bleeding globe) and segmental arterial disorganization. In addition to the brain, arteriolosclerosis also affects the kidney and retina. It is strongly associated with ageing, hypertension, and diabetes.

Cerebral amyloid angiopathy

Cerebral amyloid angiopathy is a progressive accumulation of congophilic βA4 immunoreactive, amyloid protein in the walls of small-to-medium sized arteries and arterioles predominantly located in the leptomeningeal space, the cortex, and, to a lesser extent, also in the capillaries and veins. In its most severe form, the vessels become dilated and disrupted, with focal wall fragmentation and extravasation of blood and sometimes luminal occlusion. It is also a pathologic hallmark of Alzheimer's disease. It is very frequent in the elderly population (frequency increases with age: present in 50% of individuals in their 9th decade). It is associated with cerebral ischemic changes (white matter lesions and microinfarcts) and also large lobar hemorrhages (which are frequently recurrent), and MRI brain imaging evidence of multifocal microbleeds (see intracerebral hemorrhage below) (**294**).

Inherited and genetic small vessel diseases

The most prominent inherited or genetic small vessel diseases (distinct from cerebral amyloid angiopathy) are cerebral autosomal-dominant arteriopathy with subcortical infarcts and leukoencephalopthy (CADASIL) and Fabry's disease (see above). CADASIL causes a type of stroke and dementia whose key features include recurrent subcortical ischemic events and vascular dementia and which is associated with diffuse white matter abnormalities on neuroimaging (**295**, **296**)[10–12].

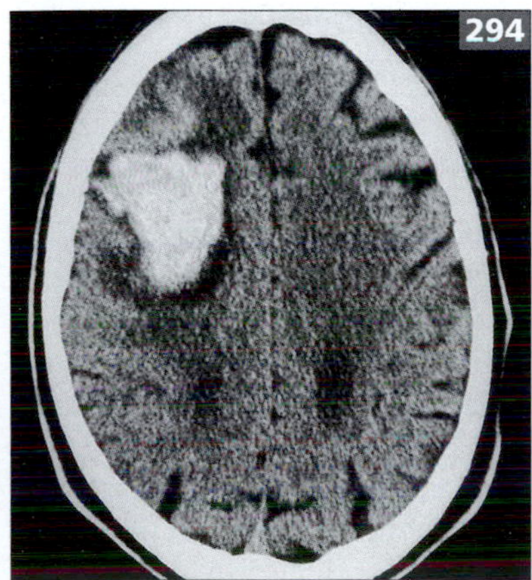

294 Noncontrast cranial CT scan showing a focal area of high density, due to recent hemorrhage, in the frontal lobe on the right due to amyloid angiopathy.

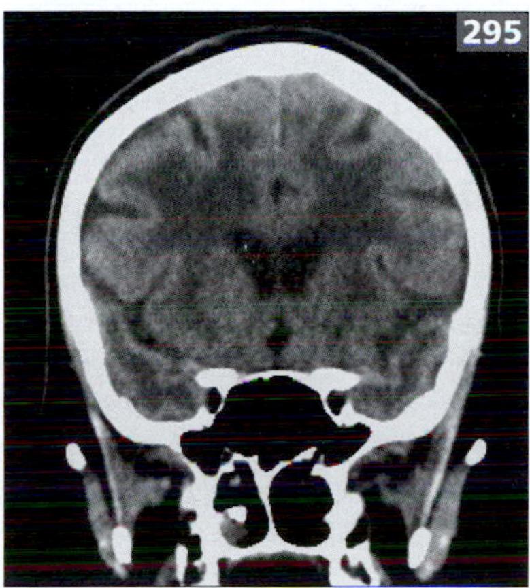

295 Plain CT brain scan, coronal plane, showing low density, consistent with infarction, in subcortical white matter of the frontal and temporal lobes due to CADASIL.

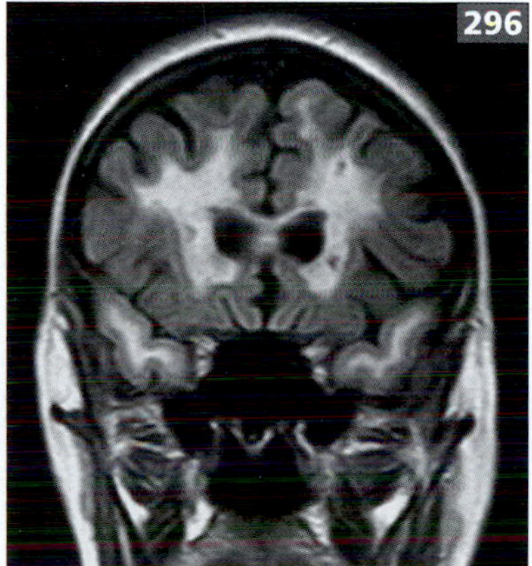

296 MRI brain scan, FLAIR sequence, coronal plane, showing high intensity, consistent with infarction, in subcortical white matter of the frontal and temporal lobes due to CADASIL.

Pathologic examination reveals multiple small, deep cerebral infarcts, a leukoencephalopathy and a non-atherosclerotic, nonamyloid angiopathy involving mainly the small cerebral arteries. The receptor of the mutant *Notch3* gene on chromosome 19 accumulates in arteries and precapillaries and causes severe alterations of vascular smooth muscle cells; electron microscopy shows granular deposits within the vascular basal lamina throughout the arterial system.

CADASIL is suggested by: 1) one or more of recurrent subcortical ischemic strokes (especially before age 60 and in the absence of vascular risk factors), migraine (especially with aura, including atypical or prolonged auras), and/or early cognitive decline or subcortical dementia; 2) bilateral, multifocal, T2/FLAIR hyperintensities in the deep white matter and periventricular white matter, with lesions involving the anterior temporal pole, external capsule, basal ganglia, and/or pons; and 3) an autosomal-dominant family history of migraine, early-onset stroke, or dementia. The clinical spectrum of CADASIL is broad, and there is a poor genotype–phenotype correlation.

Mitochondrial myopathy, encephalopathy, lactic acidosis, and strokelike episodes (MELAS) is a progressive disorder caused by mitochondrial dysfunction[7]. Almost 80% of patients with MELAS have a mitochondrial DNA (mtDNA) A-to-G transition at nucleotide 3243 of the transfer ribonucleic acid (RNA) of leucine. The prevalence of this mutation varies from about 8 to 240 per 100,000. The mtDNA mutations are maternally transmitted in a nonMendelian manner. The etiology of strokelike episodes in MELAS has not been completely explained. Patients may present with neurologic deficits that correlate with MRI DWI that show hyperintense cortical multifocal laminar lesions. The ADC suggests the presence of vasogenic edema. These lesions may not follow a defined arterial territory distribution, have a predilection for the posterior areas of the brain, and may spread progressively to other brain areas. The different hypotheses that have been proposed are that the lesions are: 1) ischemic in nature and caused by cerebral small vessel mitochondrial and vascular dysfunction; 2) due to a mitochondrial-mediated cytopathic mechanism whereby the transfer RNA of leucine mtDNA mutation decreases protein synthesis and causes oxidative phosphorylation failure, leading ultimately to adenosine triphosphate (ATP) depletion and energy failure; and 3) due to endothelial mitochondrial failure that affects the blood–brain barrier and causes a shift in extracellular ion homeostasis.

In neurofibromatosis 1, small vessel disease may arise which is characterized by mesodermal dysplasia or fibromuscular hyperplasia, abnormal proliferation of spindle cells in the wall, degeneration, healing, and subsequent muscle loss accompanied by extensive fibrosis. The process may culminate in formation of micronodular smooth muscle aggregates or nodules that arise from the vessel wall. Small vessel disease usually presents as a stenotic or occlusive lesion that lacks an obvious neural component but neural proliferation in the vessel walls may exist at different stages of disease progression.

Inflammatory and immunologically mediated small vessel diseases

Inflammatory and immunologically mediated small vessel diseases are a heterogeneous group of rare diseases characterized by the presence of inflammatory cells in the vessel walls (vasculitis)[9]. They may arise spontaneously and be isolated to the central nervous system (CNS) or arise in the context of a systemic or local infection (e.g. tuberculous basal meningitis [**297**]) or, more commonly, a systemic vasculitis (see Chapter 12 Inflammatory Disorders of the Nervous System).

Venous collagenosis

Venous collagenosis is a collagenous thickening of the walls of veins and venules closely located to the lateral ventricles, causing narrowing and sometimes occlusion of the lumen. It is associated with white matter lesions.

Other small vessel diseases

Post-radiation angiopathy is a delayed side-effect of cerebral irradiation (after months or years). It is characterized by fibrinoid necrosis and hyaline thickening of the wall of small vessels of the white matter causing narrowing of the lumen, thrombotic occlusion, and degeneration of myelin sheaths and a diffuse leukoencephalopathy.

Heart diseases

Embolism from the heart causes about one-fifth of ischemic strokes and transient ischemic attacks (**298**).

There are several heart diseases (*Table 37*) that may give rise to different types of emboli to the brain. The most substantial embolic threats are nonrheumatic and rheumatic atrial fibrillation (AF,) infective endocarditis, prosthetic heart valve, recent myocardial infarction, dilated cardiomyopathy, intracardiac tumors, and rheumatic mitral stenosis. Emboli may comprise red fibrin thrombus (AF, left ventricular aneurysm, or akinetic segment), calcium (mitral annulus calcification), micro-organisms (infective endocarditis), tumor (left atrial myxoma), prosthetic heart valves, and devices inserted to occlude patent foramen ovale (PFO).

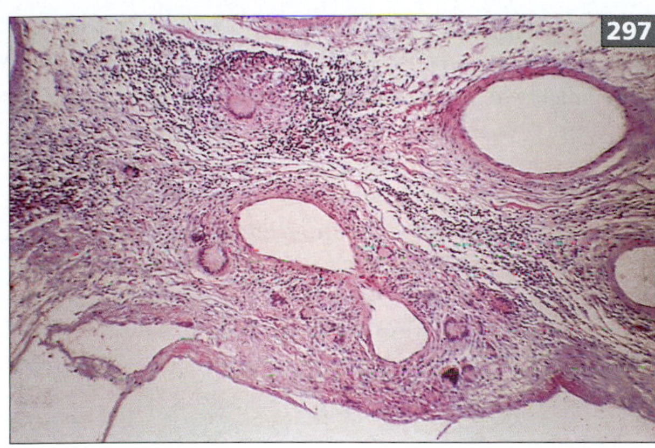

297 Histologic section of basal meninges, showing infiltration with mononuclear cells and multinucleate giant cells in a patient with infective arteritis of the CNS due to tuberculosis.

298 Illustration of the pathway a left atrial or ventricular thrombus takes as it embolizes to the brain.

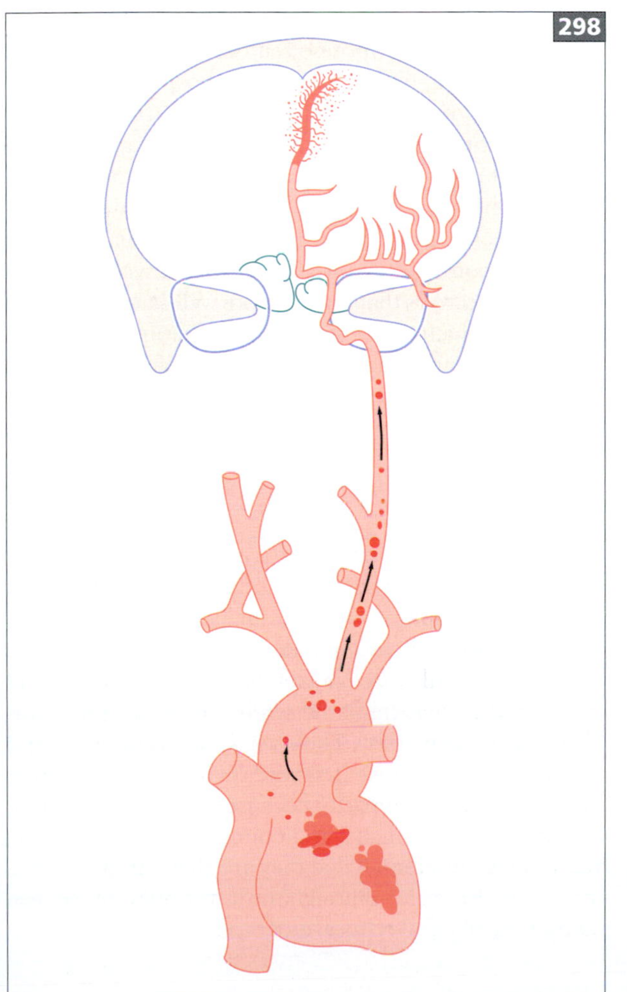

TABLE 37 **CARDIAC SOURCES OF EMBOLISM**
(in anatomical sequence)

Right to left shunt (paradoxical emboli from the venous system) via
- Patent foramen ovale
- Atrial septal defect
- Ventricular septal defect
- Pulmonary arteriovenous malformation

Left atrium
- Thrombus:
  - Atrial fibrillation/flutter*
  - Sinoatrial disease (sick sinus syndrome*)
  - Atrial septal aneurysm
- Myxoma and other tumors*

Mitral valve
- Rheumatic endocarditis (stenosis* or regurgitation)
- Infective endocarditis*
- Nonbacterial thrombotic (marantic) endocarditis*
- Bioprosthetic and mechanical heart valve*
- Papillary fibroelastoma*
- Mitral annulus calcification
- Mitral valve prolapse
- Libman–Sacks endocarditis
- Antiphospholipid syndrome

Left ventricle
- Mural thrombus:
  - Acute myocardial infarction (recent, within previous few weeks)*
  - Chronic myocardial infarction with ejection fraction <28%*
  - Symptomatic congestive heart failure with ejection fraction <30%*
  - Nonischemic dilated cardiomyopathy*
  - Mechanical 'artificial' heart*
  - Left ventricular aneurysm or akinetic segment
  - Blunt chest injury (myocardial contusion)
- Myxoma and other tumors*
- Hydatid cyst
- Primary oxalosis

Aortic valve
- Rheumatic endocarditis (stenosis* or regurgitation)
- Infective endocarditis*
- Noninfective thrombotic (marantic) endocarditis
- Bioprosthetic and mechanical heart valve*
- Libman–Sacks endocarditis
- Antiphospholipid syndrome
- Calcific stenosis/sclerosis/calcification
- Syphilis

Congenital heart disease (particularly with right to left shunt)

Cardiac manipulation/surgery/catheterization/valvuloplasty/angioplasty

*Substantial risk of embolism (>2% per year).

Atrial fibrillation

AF is the most common sustained cardiac arrhythmia[13]. It results in a loss of organized atrial contraction and is associated with stasis in the left atrial appendage (LAA), reduced LAA flow velocities, and thrombus formation. When AF is of more than 2 days' duration, atrial thrombi may be seen in up to 14% of patients on transesophageal echocardiography, ranging from 0.2 to 4.2 cm in size. Embolic strokes caused by AF are typically larger, more commonly disabling and fatal, and occur at more advanced age compared with strokes occurring in sinus rhythm. However, up to 25% of AF-associated strokes originate from alternate sources, including the left ventricle, aortic arch, extracranial arteries, and *in situ* disease of the intracranial cerebral arteries.

AF is most commonly caused by disorders that increase the pressure in the atria, such as hypertension, cardiomyopathy (ischemic, dilated, or hypertrophic) and valvular heart disease (and pulmonary embolism); disorders that cause dilatation of the atria, such as obstructive sleep apnoea and obesity; disorders that cause ischemia of the atria, such as ischemic heart disease; disorders that cause inflammation of the atria, such as pericarditis and myocarditis; disorders that genetically predispose to AF, such as familial AF; and reversible causes of AF, such as drugs (alcohol, caffeine), surgery (cardiac, pulmonary, esophageal, or general surgery), and endocrine disorders (hyperthyroidism, pheochromocytoma).

Valvular heart disease

Rheumatic valvular disease, particularly mitral, is a well-recognized cause of embolism to the brain, particularly when the patient is in AF and has thrombosis in the left atrium. Even when the patient is in sinus rhythm and there is no thrombus in the left atrium, degenerate and sometimes calcific fragments of valve can be discharged into the circulation. Infective endocarditis (see below) and intracerebral hemorrhage caused by anticoagulation are among the many other causes of stroke in these patients.

Nonrheumatic sclerosis, and particularly calcification, of the aortic and mitral valves can occasionally be a source of embolism of thrombotic or calcific material.

Uncomplicated mitral leaflet prolapse should no longer be considered a cause of embolism from the heart to the brain; there must be something additional, such as gross mitral regurgitation, AF, or infective endocarditis.

Prosthetic heart valves, particularly mechanical rather than tissue ones, are well recognized to be complicated by thrombosis, and sometimes thromboembolism or infective endocarditis. The stroke risk is similar among the different types of mechanical valve, but those in the mitral position are more prone to thrombosis than those in the aortic position. For all valves, the overall risk of embolism is about 2% per year, provided patients with mechanical valves are anticoagulated. For patients unable to comply with systemic anticoagulation and in the elderly, tissue valves include the Carpentier–Edwards and Hancock porcine heterograft valves and the Carpentier–Edwards pericardial valve; the overall results are similar to mechanical valves, being about equal at the end of 10 years. Some disagreement remains about the need for systemic anticoagulation during the first few months after insertion of a bioprosthesis, when the embolic stroke risk is highest.

Infective endocarditis

Infective endocarditis is caused by microbial infection of the endocardial surface or of prosthetic material in the heart. More than 80% of cases are caused by *Staphylococcus aureus* or by species of *Streptococcus* or *Enterococcus*. The annual incidence is 3–10 cases per 100,000.

About one-fifth of patients with infective endocarditis have an ischemic stroke or transient ischemic attack as a result of embolism of valvular vegetations (**299**, **300**). Cerebrovascular symptoms can be the presenting feature, but they more often occur in someone who is clearly unwell, perhaps already in hospital, but before the infection has been controlled. Hemorrhagic transformation of an infarct occurs in 20–40% and may be excacerbated or precipitated by unwise anticoagulation. Primarily hemorrhagic strokes – intracerebral or, rarely, subarachnoid or mixed intracerebral and subdural – are as or more commonly caused by a pyogenic vasculitis and vessel wall necrosis than by the more well-known mycotic aneurysms which can be single or multiple and most often affect the distal branches of the middle cerebral artery. These aneurysms do not always rupture and they may resolve with time.

Nonbacterial thrombotic (marantic) endocarditis

Small sterile vegetations, consisting of fibrin and platelets, appear on the cardiac valves in cachectic and debilitated patients as a result of cancer (usually adenocarcinomas) and sometimes of disseminated intravascular coagulation, burns, and septicemia. Similar vegetations are found in SLE and antiphospholipid syndrome (APS), and possibly protein C deficiency. These vegetations are friable and may embolize to cause ischemic stroke (and sometimes multifocal encephalopathy because of multiple emboli), ischemia in other organs, and pulmonary embolism. The vegetations are so small that they are all but impossible to diagnose during life, although the larger ones can be seen on transesophageal echocardiography.

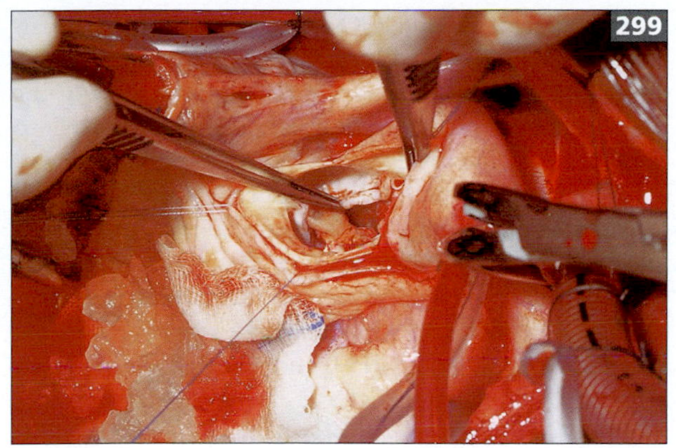

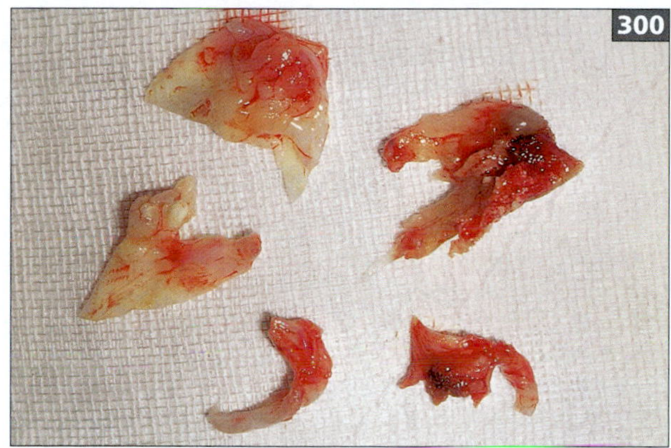

299, 300 **Vegetations consisting of platelets, fibrin, and colonizing microorganisms removed surgically from an infected heart valve.**

Left ventricular mural thrombus

Left ventricular mural thrombus, diagnosed by echocardiography, occurs within days of an acute myocardial infarction in up to 20% of patients (particularly if not treated with antithrombotic drugs), mostly in those with large anterior myocardial infarcts (**301**). However, clinically evident systemic embolism to the brain complicates less than 5% of all acute myocardial infarctions. Other causes of ischemic stroke after an acute myocardial infarction include: emboli as a result of cardiac catheterization, angioplasty, or surgery, or AF; low-flow infarction caused by systemic hypotension or cardiac arrest; and paradoxical embolism caused by deep venous thrombosis and a PFO. Causes of hemorrhagic stroke include hemorrhagic transformation of any ischemic stroke and primary intracerebral hemorrhage due to thrombolytic and antithrombotic treatments.

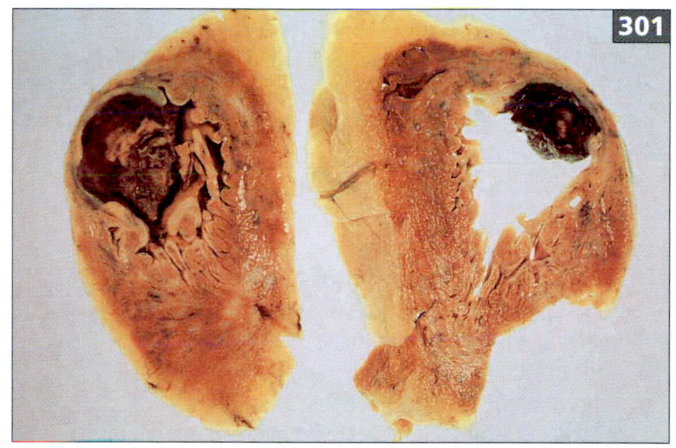

301 **Cross-section of the left ventricle, showing mural thrombus adjacent to an area of myocardial infarction.**

Intracardiac tumors

Myxomas, found in the left atrium much more often than in any other cardiac chamber, are the most common intracardiac tumor but are still extremely rare. Some are familial. Tumor or complicating thrombus may embolize to the brain, eye, and elsewhere. Myxomatous emboli cause not only focal cerebral ischemia but also fusiform and irregular aneurysmal dilatations at sites of earlier symptomatic or even asymptomatic embolic occlusions, and these can rupture to cause intracerebral or subarachnoid hemorrhage. Brain metastases have also been described. Myxomas can also cause intracardiac obstruction with shortness of breath, palpitations, and syncope. Frequently they cause constitutional problems, such as malaise, fatigue, weight loss, fever, rash, arthralgia, myalgia, anemia, raised erythrocyte sedimentation rate, and hypergammaglobulinemia.

Other, even rarer, primary and secondary cardiac tumors may embolize, such as valvular fibroelastoma.

Sinoatrial disease (sick sinus syndrome)

Sinoatrial disease (sick sinus syndrome) can be associated with intracardiac thrombus and embolism, particularly if bradycardia alternates with tachycardia or the patient is in AF.

Paradoxical embolism

Paradoxical embolism is a condition in which emboli of venous origin enter the systemic circulation by being shunted from the right to the left atrium. A PFO accounts for up to 95% of paradoxical emboli, pulmonary shunts for only 5%, and atrial septal defects (ASDs) for 1% or even less.

TABLE 38 **BLOOD DISEASES WHICH MAY CONTRIBUTE TO THE ETIOLOGY OF ISCHEMIC STROKE**

	Polymorphism	Inheritance pattern
Inherited blood coagulation disorders		
Protein C deficiency		
Protein S deficiency		
Protein Z deficiency		
Antithrombin deficiency		
Plasminogen activator inhibitor 1	Arg 506 Gly	AD
Factor V Leiden mutation	G20210A	AD
Prothrombin mutation	4G/5G	AR
Acquired blood coagulation disorders		
Antiphospholipid antibodies (anticardiolipin antibodies, lupus anticoagulant, anti-β_2-glycoprotein)		
Coagulation disorders associated with cancer		
Hyperhomocystinemia		
Disturbances of primary hemostasis:		
• High vWF		
• Low ADAMTS13		
• Disorders of fibrin formation and fibrinolysis		
• High fibrinogen		
• Impaired fibrinolysis:		
– Plasminogen activator inhibitor 4G/5G promoter polymorphism of the encoding gene		
– Increased thrombin-activatable fibrinolysis inhibitor		
Polycythemia rubra vera		
Thrombocytosis:		
• Primary thrombocytosis:		
– Essential thrombocythemia		
– Polycythemia vera		
– Idiopathic myelofibrosis		
– Chronic myeloid leukemia		
– Myelodysplasia		
– Acute leukemia		
• Secondary thrombocytosis:		
– Infection		
– Inflammation		
– Connective tissue disease		
– Iron deficiency		
– Blood loss (e.g. surgery)		
– Malignancy		
– Post-splenectomy		
– Hemolytic anemia		
Leukemia		
Sickle cell disease		

ADAMTS13: a disintegrin and metalloprotease with thrombospondin motif; vWF: von Willebrand factor.

During fetal life, the PFO is an integral part of the circulation. The collapsed lungs substantially increase the resistance in the pulmonary circulation, requiring the blood to be shunted from the right atrium directly into the left atrium and systemic circulation. After birth, resistance in pulmonary circulation declines and facilitates flow through the lungs. The pressure in the right atrium falls below that of the left atrium, the septum primum is pushed against the septum secundum, and the two generally fuse. However, in some persons, a slit-like opening persists, which is called PFO, and gives rise to (momentary) right-to-left shunts (RLSs).

PFO is found in 24% of healthy adults and 38% of patients with cryptogenic stroke. This ratio and case reports indicate that PFO and stroke are associated, probably because of paradoxical embolism. In healthy people with PFO, embolic events are not more frequent than in controls. However, once ischemic events occur, the risk of recurrence is increased.

A coexisting atrial septal aneurysm (ASA) is a substantial and probably the most important risk factor for stroke in patients with PFO[14]. An ASA not only prevents spontaneous closure of the foramen after birth but it also produces frequent openings of the PFO cleft, perhaps even with every heart beat. Other risk factors for stroke in the presence of PFO are a previous embolic ischemic event and possibly the size of the PFO, the degree of functional shunting, the presence of a Eustachian valve (EV), and a coexisting hypercoagulable state. Before birth, the EV directs oxygenated blood from the inferior vena cava towards and across the PFO into the systemic circulation. In patients with a PFO, a persisting EV is frequently encountered. By directing the blood from the inferior vena cava to the interatrial septum, a persisting EV may prevent spontaneous closure of PFO after birth and may, therefore, predispose to paradoxical embolism.

Blood coagulation diseases

Occasionally, ischemic strokes, intracranial venous thrombosis, and transient ischemic attacks complicate an underlying hematologic disorder, which itself may be quite common (such as sickle cell disease in Afro-Caribbeans) or extremely rare (such as protein S deficiency). While inherited blood coagulation disorders (e.g. deficiencies of protein C, protein S, protein Z, and antithrombin III; and mutations in genes encoding for the anticoagulant proteins and coagulation factors factor V Leiden and prothrombin G20210A) are recognized risk factors for venous thromboembolic events, there is no substantial evidence for a causal relation between most blood coagulation disorders and arterial thromboembolic events, including ischemic stroke (*Table 38*).

The strongest association is between the acquired APS and ischemic stroke. APS is defined by the presence of a medium or high titer of antiphospholipid antibodies (lupus anticoagulant, anticardiolipin antibodies, and anti-β_2-glycoprotein-1 antibodies) on at least two occasions more than 12 weeks apart in patients with recurrent thromboembolism[15]. The thrombosis is more often venous than arterial and in any sized vessel. Other features are nonspecific and include recurrent miscarriage, migraine, memory loss, confusion, visual disturbances, abdominal pain, heart valve vegetations, a characteristic rash – livideo reticularis, thrombocytopenia, hemolytic anemia, circulating lupus anticoagulant, and false-positive nonspecific serological tests for syphilis. Primary APS is not associated with any other autoimmune disease whereas the secondary form most commonly occurs in patients with SLE, but also with other autoimmune diseases. The cause of thrombosis, the prognosis for recurrent stroke, and the nature of the relationship and overlap with SLE are all uncertain.

The prevalence of APS is estimated to be 2–4% of the general population (>50% primary). However, the association between acquired APS and ischemic stroke is almost by definition and the clinical significance of isolated mildly elevated antiphospholipid antibody titers is unclear. Indeed, antiphospholipid antibodies are not specific to APS, particularly if they are not present in high titers on *repeated* testing. They can be found in some normal individuals, and also in SLE and other collagen vascular disorders, malignancy, lymphoma, paraproteinemias, human immunodeficiency virus (HIV) and other infections, patients with multiple vascular risk factors, on hemodialysis, or in the elderly, and as a result of a variety of drugs such as phenothiazines, hydralazine, phenytoin, valproate, procainamide, and quinidine.

Other possible associations with ischemic stroke include the coexistence of a hereditary prothrombotic condition with a PFO (and/or ASA), oral contraceptive use, or other cardiovascular risk factors. Increased fibrinogen and homocysteine concentrations are also associated with increased risk of ischemic stroke but whether they are causal is still debated. Disseminated intravascular coagulation (DIC) and thrombotic microangiopathies seem to cause microvascular occlusive events rather than arterial ischemic stroke. Further research is required to appreciate the role of von Willebrand factor (vWF), a disintegrin and metalloprotease with thrombospondin motif (ADAMTS13) – also known as vWF-cleaving protease (VWFCP) – a metalloprotease enzyme that cleaves vWf, and factors involved in fibrinolysis in the occurrence of ischemic stroke.

Cerebral venous thrombosis (CVT)

The main pathologic manifestations of CVT are:

- Most patients have dural sinus thrombosis with or without cortical vein involvement (**302, 303**); isolated cortical venous thrombosis is rare.
- The thrombus itself is like other venous thrombi elsewhere in the body. When it is fresh, it is a red thrombus rich in red blood cells and fibrin and poor in platelets; when it is old, it is replaced by fibrous tissue sometimes showing recanalization.
- Hemorrhagic infarction of the brain is common.

302, 303 Autopsy specimen of brain, vertex of the brain (302), and coronal section through the frontal lobes (303), showing bilateral parasagittal hemorrhagic infarction due to superior sagittal sinus thrombosis.

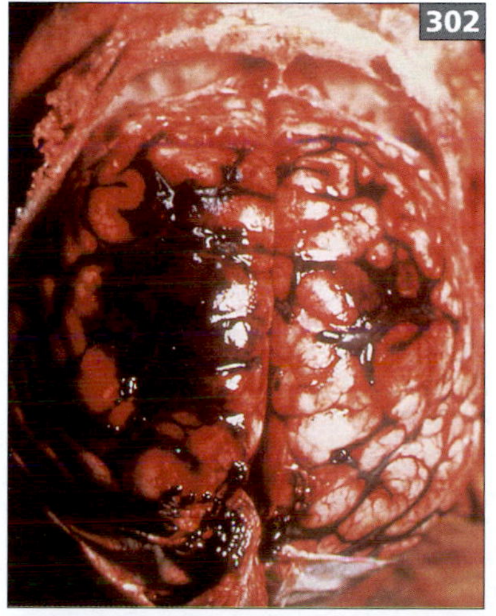

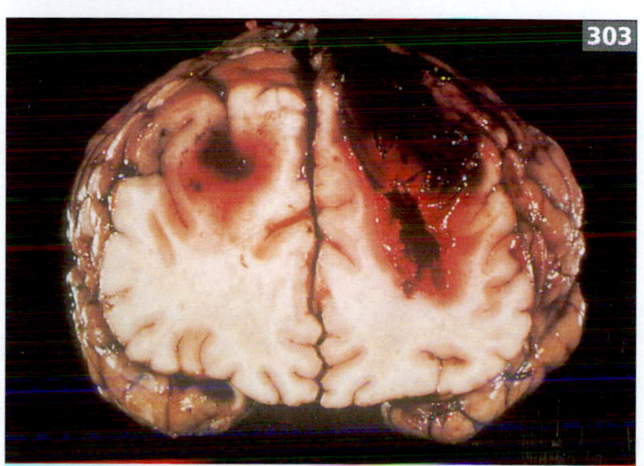

TABLE 39 **CAUSES OF CEREBRAL VEIN THROMBOSIS**

Local conditions directly affecting the veins and sinuses

NONINFECTIVE

- Head trauma (open or closed, with or without fracture)
- Intracranial surgery
- Brain infarction or hemorrhage
- Tumor invasion of dural sinuses (meningioma, metastases, glomus tumor)
- Catheterization of, and infusions into, the internal jugular veins (e.g. for parenteral nutrition)

INFECTIVE

- Direct septic trauma
- Local regional infection (scalp, sinuses, ears, mastoids, nasopharynx)
- Intracranial infection:
  - Bacterial meningitis
  - Meningovascular syphilis
  - Subdural empyema
  - Bacterial or fungal brain abscess

Systemic conditions

NONINFECTIVE

Surgery

- Any surgical procedure, with or without deep venous thrombosis

Hormonal

- Pregnancy or more commonly the puerperium
- Oral contraceptives (estrogens or progestogens)

Medical

- Severe dehdration of any cause (including angiography or myelography)
- Hyperviscosity syndrome:
  - Multiple myeloma
  - Waldenstrom's macroglobulinemia
- Hypercoagulable state:
  - Red blood cell disorders:
  - Polycythemia
  - Post-hemorrhagic anemia
  - Sickle cell disease/trait
  - Paroxysmal nocturnal hemoglobinuria
- Platelet disorders:
  - Essential thrombocythemia

Systemic noninfectve medical conditions continued

- Coagulation disorders:
  - Deficiency of antithrombin III, protein C, protein S, or circulating lupus anticoagulants
  - Activated protein C resistance (factor V Leiden gene mutation)
  - Prothrombin 20210 gene mutation
  - Disseminated intravascular coagulation
  - Heparin- or heparinoid-induced thrombocytopenia
  - Antifibrinolytic treatment
- Extracranial malignancy (non-metastatic effect):
  - Visceral carcinoma, carcinoid, lymphoma, leukemia, L-asparaginase
- Connective tissue disease:
  - Systemic lupus erythematosus
  - Wegener's granulomatosis
  - Giant cell arteritis
- Cardiac:
  - Congenital heart disease
  - Congestive heart failure
  - Pacemaker
- Gastrointestinal:
  - Inflammatory bowel disease
  - Cirrhosis
- Various others:
  - Behçet's disease
  - Sarcoidosis, uveomeningities
  - Nephrotic syndrome
  - Androgen therapy, ecstasy, dihyrdroergotamine
  - Diabetes mellitus
  - Parenteral injections
  - Hyperhomocystinemia
  - Epidural anesthesia

INFECTIVE

- Bacterial: septicemia, endocarditis, typhoid, tuberculosis
- Viral: measles, hepatitis, encephalitis, herpes, HIV, CMV
- Parasitic: malaria, trichinosis
- Fungal: aspergillosis

CMV: cytomegalovirus; HIV: human immunodeficiency virus.

Unlike arterial thrombosis, damage to the vessel wall is a causal factor in only about 10% of patients with intracranial cerebral venous thrombosis (ICVT); the underlying disease condition consists of infection, infiltration, or trauma. More important are disorders of coagulation (70%)[16]. The most common inherited coagulation defect is factor V Leiden mutation, which is found in about 20% of patients without other obvious causes. The third component of Virchow's triad of causes of thrombosis, stagnant flow, contributes no more than a few percent (associated with dehydration or with dural puncture, sometimes in combination with hyperosmolar contrast agents). In 20% of patients no contributing factors can be identified and the cause remains shrouded in mystery. Perhaps as yet undiscovered prothrombotic mutations are responsible to some extent.

Often there is no single cause but a combination of contributing factors, for example the post-partum period and protein S deficiency, pregnancy and Behçet's disease, oral contraceptives and the factor V Leiden mutation, or the same combinations with dural puncture as a third factor. The risk of ICVT in the post-partum period increases with maternal age, and with Cesarean section.

In neonates, ICVT is usually associated with acute systemic illness, such as shock or dehydration; in older children, the most frequent underlying conditions are local infection (the leading cause until the antibiotic era), coagulopathy and, more in Mediterranean countries, Behçet's disease. Causes of CVT are listed in *Table 39*.

Intracerebral hemorrhage

Intracerebral hemorrhage (ICH) accounts for 15–40% of all strokes, depending on geography and race[17].

Sites of primary intracerebral hemorrhage (irrespective of age):

- Putamen or internal capsule (**268, 269**) 30%.
- Caudate nucleus 5%.
- Entire basal ganglia region 5%.
- Lobar (**304**) 30%.
- Thalamus 15%.
- Cerebellum 10%.
- Pons or midbrain (**305**) 5%.

ICH is caused by rupture of an intracerebral artery. Predisposing factors include diseases or malformations of cerebral arteries (anatomical factors), diseases of the blood clotting system (hemostastic factors), and excessively high systemic arterial blood pressure (hemodynamic factors). Arteriovenous malformations are the most common cause of ICH in the young, degenerative small vessel disease in middle and old age, and amyloid angiopathy in old age. These and other causes of ICH, and their relative frequencies, are listed in *Table 40*.

Chronic hypertension

Chronically raised blood pressure leads to degenerative change (lipohyalinosis – fibrinoid necrosis), in small perforating arteries, most of which are found in deep regions: basal ganglia, thalamus, cerebellum, and brainstem, which ultimately leads to their rupture in the basal ganglia, cerebellum, or brainstem, or less often in the subcortical white matter. Microaneurysms occur on these vessels but are not necessarily the site of rupture.

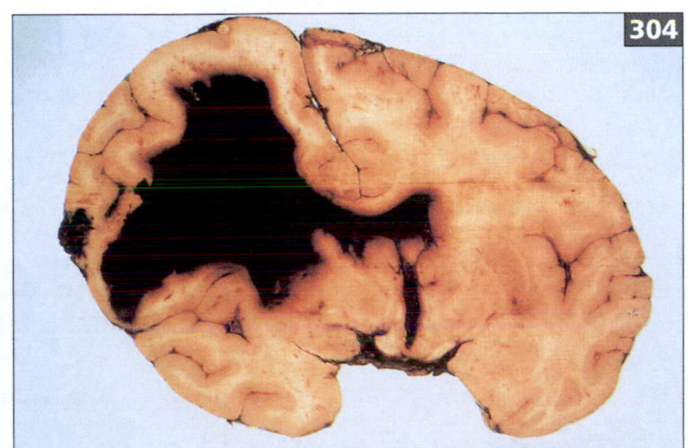

304 Brain coronal section at autopsy, showing a large lobar intracerebral hematoma that was fatal.

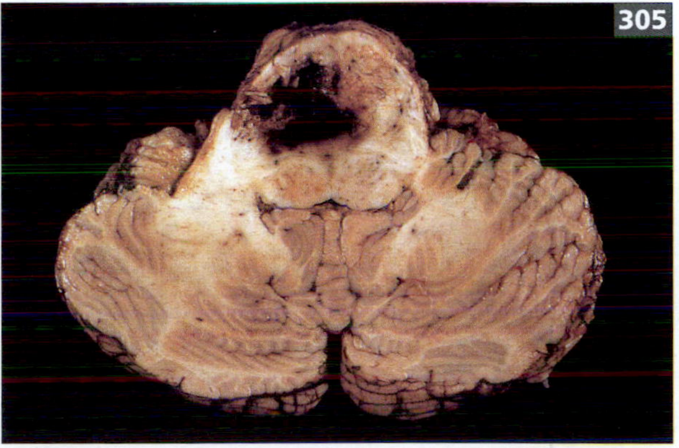

305 Autopsy specimen of a cross-section of the midpons and cerebellum in the axial plane of a patient who was 'locked-in', showing hemorrhage in the ventral pons bilaterally.

TABLE 40 **CAUSES OF INTRACEREBRAL HEMORRHAGE**

Arterial disease (anatomical factors)

- 'Complex' disease (fibrinoid necrosis) in small, penetrating vessels:
  - Most common cause in middle and old age
  - Hemorrhages often deep in putamen (40%), caudate nucleus (8%), thalamus (15%), cerebral hemispheres (lobar) (20%), cerebellum (8%) and brainstem (8%)
- Amyloid (congophilic) angiopathy:*
  - Most common cause in old age
  - Hemorrhages often in lobes of cerebral hemispheres
  - May be associated with dementia
- Vascular malformations (arteriovenous and cavernous angiomas):
  - Dural or brain
  - Most common cause in young normotensive people
  - Seizures and headaches commonly antedate hemorrhage
  - Cavernous angiomas tend to be multiple and familial

• Autosomal-dominant polycystic kidney disease	*PKD1*, *PKD2* gene	AD inheritance
• Cerebral cavernous malformations	7q21–q22, 7p13–p15, 3q25.2–q27	AD or sporadic
• Hereditary hemorrhagic telangiectasia (Osler–Weber–Rendu disease)	Endoglin and activin receptor-like kinase 1 genes	AD

- Caroticocavernous fistula
- Saccular aneurysms:
  - Cause of 1 in 13 intracerebral hemorrhages (2 in 13 <65 years old), usually in conjunction with subarachnoid hemorrhage
- Atheromatous aneurysm
- Septic arteritis and mycotic aneurysms
- Necrotizing angiitis of the CNS*
- Arterial dissection
- Intracerebral tumors:
  - Primary (glioblastoma, oligodendroglioma, medulloblastoma, hemangioblastoma)
  - Metastases (melanoma, bronchial carcinoma, renal carcinoma, choriocarcinoma, endometrial carcinoma)
- Intracranial venous thrombosis*
- CADASIL (cerebral autosomal-dominant arteriopathy with subcortical infarcts and leucoencephalopathy) (**306**)
- Moyamoya syndrome
- Occult head injury*
- Trauma
- Hemorrhagic brain infarction

Raised blood pressure (hemodynamic factors)

- Acute arterial hypertension:
  - Alcohol (also antiplatelet action, and coexistent liver disease)
  - Amphetamines (may also cause a vasculitis)
  - Cocaine and other sympathomimetic drugs
  - Monoamine oxidase A inhibitors
  - Exposure to extreme cold
  - Trigeminal nerve stimulation
  - Post carotid endarterectomy, heart transplantation, or correction of congenital heart lesions
- Chronic arterial hypertension, causing complex small vessel disease (see above)

Bleeding diathesis (hemostatic factors)*

- Anticoagulants
- Antiplatelet drugs: probably a relatively minor contributory factor
- Thrombolytic treatment
- Thrombocytopenia
- Hemophilia and other hereditary coagulation factor deficiencies (e.g. factor V)
- Leukemia
- Diffuse intravascular coagulation

*Causes of multiple hemorrhages in the brain parenchyma.

Amyloid angiopathy

Cerebral amyloid or 'congophilic angiopathy' is the most common cause of superficial ('lobar') hemorrhages in older individuals. Hemorrhages associated with amyloid angiopathy typically occur at the border of the gray and white matter of the cerebral hemispheres and are irregular (**307**, **308**). They may also rupture towards the surface and spread through the subarachnoid space. Cerebellar hemorrhages associated with amyloid angiopathy are less common. The amyloid-laden vessels may be so brittle that even mild head trauma precipitates a hemorrhage. Recurrence of hemorrhage associated with amyloid angiopathy is much more common than with 'hypertensive' small vessel disease. Recurrent hemorrhages often appear in the same region of the brain.

Cerebral amyloid angiopathy also causes diffuse demyelination of the subcortical white matter, causing intellectual deterioration. White matter changes may also result from atherosclerotic changes in the long perforators from the cerebral convexity to the white matter, which is much more common in the general population (leukoaraiosis).

Cerebral arteriovenous malformations

Cerebral arteriovenous malformations (AVMs) are tangles of dilated arteries and veins without a connecting capillary network; the intervening brain tissue is usually normal (**309**, **310**). On angiography, they are recognizable by the large feeding arteries and the rapid shunting of blood to veins that are enlarged and tortuous, often with

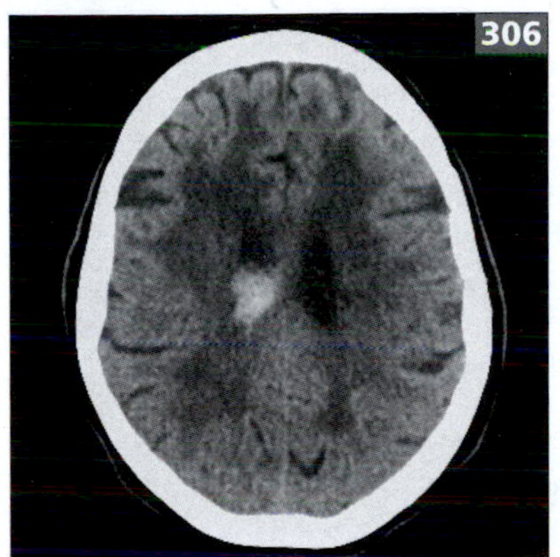

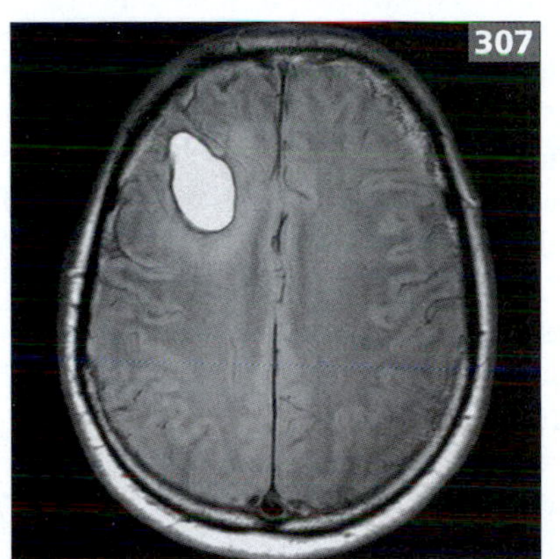

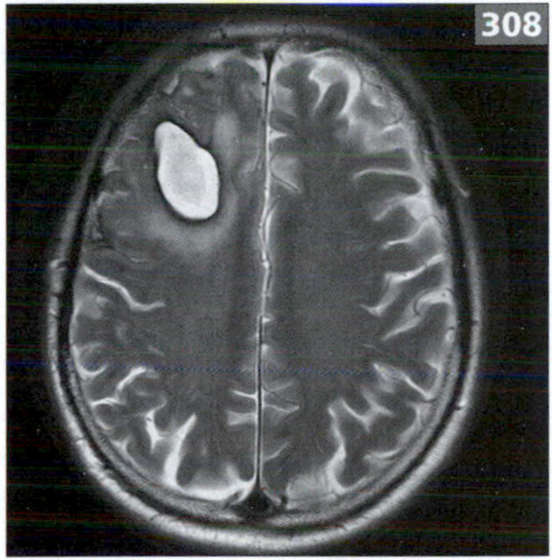

306 Plain CT brain scan, showing intracerebral hemorrhage with intraventricular extension in a patient with CADASIL. (Note the widespread subcortical ischemic leukoencephalopathy.)

307, 308 MRI brain scan, axial plane, proton density-weighted turbo spin echo clear (307) and T2* (308), showing hemorrhage in the right frontal lobe due to probable amyloid angiopathy.

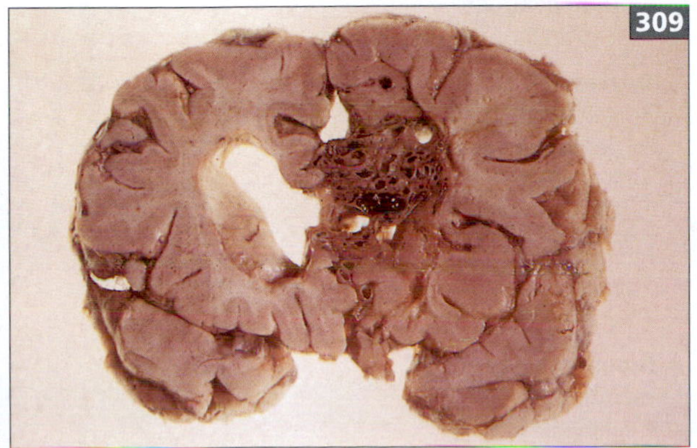

309 Brain section, coronal plane, showing a large arteriovenous malformation in the left medial frontal lobe and dilated lateral ventricles.

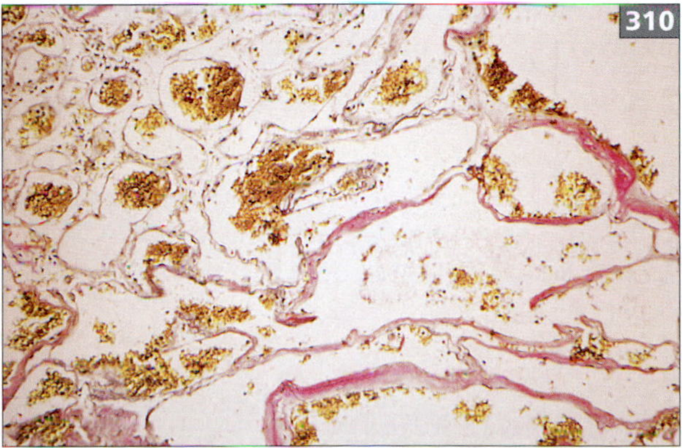

310 Histologic section of an arteriovenous malformation, showing a network of tangled, thin-walled blood vessels interposed between arteries and veins.

a central nidus of dilated vessels, between the arteries and veins. Multiple AVMs are exceptional, but their frequency is probably underestimated because a second AVM is often very small; about half the patients with multiple AVMs have hereditary hemorrhagic telangiectasia (Osler–Weber–Rendu disease). Familial occurrence of AVMs is even more exceptional.

There are saccular aneurysms on the feeding arteries or within the nidus itself in about 20% of AVMs, the aneurysms being likely sources of bleeding. AVMs in which one or more aneurysms have formed are more likely to (re)rupture: the annual risk of bleeding is as high as 7%, against the usual rate of 2–3%/year for AVMs without associated aneurysm.

Cerebral AVMS initially present with ICH in about half of patients. The next most common manifestation is epilepsy (about one-quarter), while many are asymptomatic at the time of detection. Demonstrable AVMs are the most common single cause of ICH in the young, but they account for no more than about one-third of those cases. Other causes include the use of illicit drugs such as cocaine and amphetamines, and the use of anticoagulant drugs with poorly controlled anticoagulation (i.e. international normalized ratios [INRs] above 4). The annual detection rate of AVMs is approximately 1 per 100,000 per year.

Hemorrhages from AVMs are mostly in the white matter ('lobar'), but they also occur in the deep nuclei of the cerebral hemisphere. Subarachnoid hemorrhage results if the hematoma reaches the surface of the brain, but of all hemorrhages secondary to a ruptured AVM only 4% are purely subarachnoid, without a parenchymal component. If there is no associated aneurysm on the arterial side, the site of rupture is usually on the venous side of the malformation.

Rupture of a vein might perhaps explain the often slower onset and better recovery of the clinical deficits as the result of hemorrhages from AVMs compared with ICHs from rupture of perforating arteries, or saccular aneurysms.

TABLE 41 **CAUSES OF MULTIPLE HEMORRHAGES IN THE BRAIN**

Hypertension (**311**)
Amyloid angiopathy (**312**)
Intracranial venous thrombosis
Thrombolytic and anticoagulant treatment
Metastases, especially melanoma (**313**), bronchial carcinoma, renal carcinoma, choriocarcinoma
Cerebral vasculitis
Diffuse intravascular coagulation
Hemostatic disorder
Leukemia
Eclampsia
Head trauma

TABLE 42 **CAUSES OF PRIMARY INTRAVENTRICULAR HEMORRHAGE**

Aneurysms
- Posterior inferior cerebellar artery or its choroidal branch
- Anterior inferior cerebellar artery

Arteriovenous malformations
- In the ependymal lining
- Of the choroid plexus
- Dural fistula of a cerebral venous sinus

Occlusive arterial disease
- Moyamoya syndrome: idiopathic, atherosclerotic or with associated aneurysm
- Lacunar hemorrhagic infarction

Clotting disorders
- Hemophilia

Tumors
- Pituitary adenoma or metastasis
- Ependymoma
- Meningioma
- Schwannoma

Infectious diseases
- Brain abscess
- Parasitic granuloma

Drugs
- Cocaine
- Amphetamine

Wernicke's encephalopathy (see Chapter 15)

Cavernous malformations

Cerebral cavernous malformations are small (1 mm to several cm in diameter), thin-walled vascular structures, consisting of a mulberry-like conglomerate lined by endothelium without muscular or elastic layers and with no intervening brain tissue; they are single or multiple, and occasionally calcified. Cavernous malformations are located in the hemispheric white matter or cortex in about one-half of all cases, in the posterior fossa (most often the brainstem) in one-third, and in the basal ganglia or thalamus in one-sixth. Exceptional locations include the ventricular system, where cavernous malformations may become extremely large, the pineal region, the cavernous sinus, the optic chiasm or other cranial nerves, and the spinal cord. Coexistence of spinal and cerebral cavernous malformations is not uncommon. Cavernous malformations may also occur in the skin, orbit, and almost any internal organ. The lesions are not static but often grow or shrink, and can even appear *de novo* in sporadic cases[18]. Brain radiation in children is a probable risk factor.

Infective endocarditis

Infective endocarditis is complicated by ICH in about 5% of cases. It most commonly results not from rupture of 'mycotic' aneurysms – actually bacteria as well as fungi may be involved – but as a result of acute, pyogenic necrosis of the arterial wall early in the disease, caused by virulent organisms such as *Staphylococcus aureus*. Mycotic aneurysms may develop and rupture later, during antimicrobial therapy or with less virulent bacteria, such as *Streptococcus viridans*, *S. sanguis*, *Staphylococcus epidermidis*, or *Salmonella* species.

In general, lobar hemorrhage is an exceptional first sign of endocarditis, i.e. in a patient without any history of heart disease, recent cerebral ischemia, recent malaise, fever, or loss of weight.

Antithrombotic therapy

The risk of ICH in patients on oral anticoagulants increases with the intensity of anticoagulation, but in most patients with ICH while on anticoagulants the INR values are within appropriate limits. Antiplatelet drugs are probably only a relatively minor contributory factor in the pathogenesis of ICH against a background of much more powerful determinants, most often small vessel disease. ICH after thrombolytic treatment for myocardial infarction is mostly of the lobar type, related to amyloid angiopathy in elderly patients; this complication is fatal in at least one-half of patients.

Multiple intracerebral hemorrhages

Occasionally patients present with multiple concurrent hemorrhages in the brain for which there are several causes (*Table 41*).

Primary intraventricular hemorrhage

Primary intraventricular hemorrhage is uncommon. The usual causes are shown in *Table 42*.

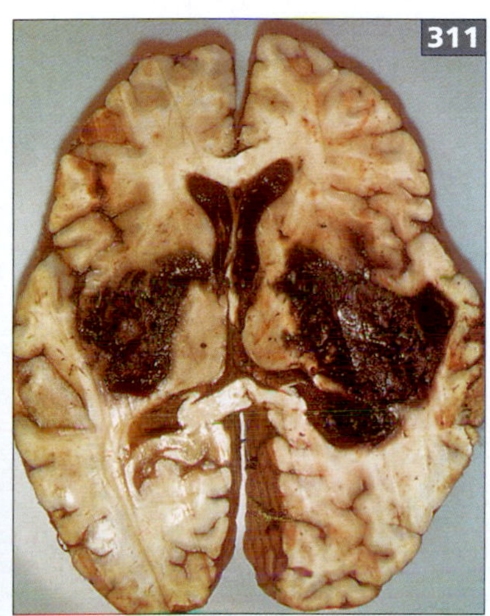

311 Axial slice of the brain at autopsy, showing bilateral basal ganglia hemorrhage with rupture into the ventricles in a patient with severe hypertension.

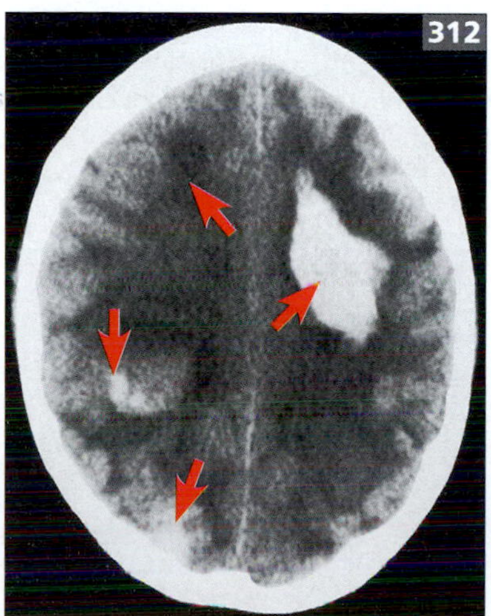

312 CT brain scan from a patient with pathologically proven amyloid angiopathy. Note multiple hemorrhages of different ages in different parts of the brain (arrows).

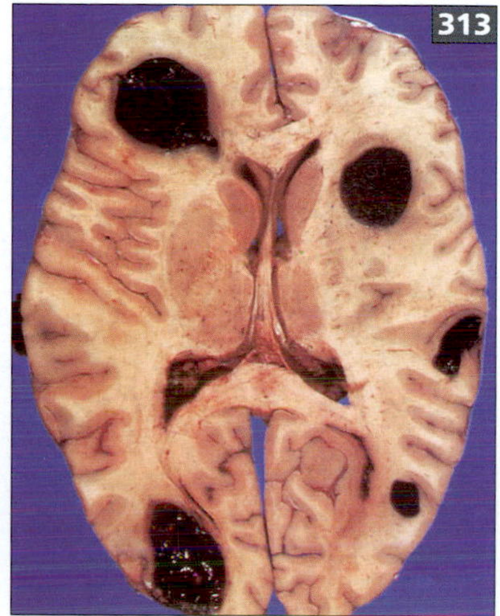

313 Axial section showing multiple areas of hemorrhage into metastases of malignant melanoma. *Courtesy of Professor BA Kakulas, Department of Neuropathology, Royal Perth Hospital, Western Australia.*

TABLE 43 **CAUSES OF SPONTANEOUS SUBDURAL HEMATOMAS**

Acute, of arterial origin • Rupture of a small pial artery, spontaneous, or in association with cocaine/amphetamine • Saccular aneurysm of major intracerebral artery • Arteriovenous malformation • Intracavernous aneurysm of the carotid artery • Aneurysm of middle meningeal artery • Moyamoya syndrome
Chronic, by rupture of a (bridging) vein • Anticoagulant or thrombolytic treatment • Coagulation defects, genetically determined or acquired • Low cerebrospinal fluid pressure, secondary to spontaneous leak from a spinal root sleeve lumbar puncture, or with unknown cause • Tension pneumocephalus • Rupture of an arachnoid cyst • Dural arteriovenous fistula • Dural metastasis • Autosomal dominant polycystic kidney disease

Subdural hemorrhage

Hemorrhage into the subdural space (**314, 315**) is not a stroke by definition but it frequently enters into the differential diagnosis of a TIA and stroke. Its causes are shown in *Table 43*.

Subarachnoid hemorrhage

Blood is present in the subarachnoid space, which may be diffuse or localized and may have extended into the brain parenchyma (**316**). The causes of subarachnoid hemorrhage are listed in *Table 44*[19].

Saccular aneurysms

Most commonly, subarachnoid blood is maximal adjacent to a ruptured saccular aneurysm at the base of the brain (**317**). Saccular aneurysms are small, thin-walled blisters protruding from the arteries of the circle of Willis or its major branches (**318**). They are located at bifurcations and branchings:

- Anterior communicating artery complex – 40%.
- Internal carotid artery – 30%:
  - Origin of the posterior communicating artery from the stem of the ICA.
  - Terminal bifurcation of the ICA, into the middle and anterior cerebral arteries.
- Middle cerebral artery: first major bifurcation (**319**) – 20%.
- Posterior circulation: tip of basilar artery – 10%.

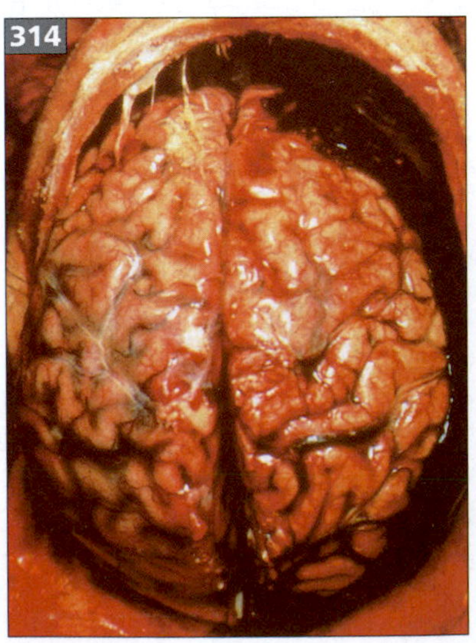

314 Autopsy specimen of a fatal subdural hematoma over the right hemisphere.

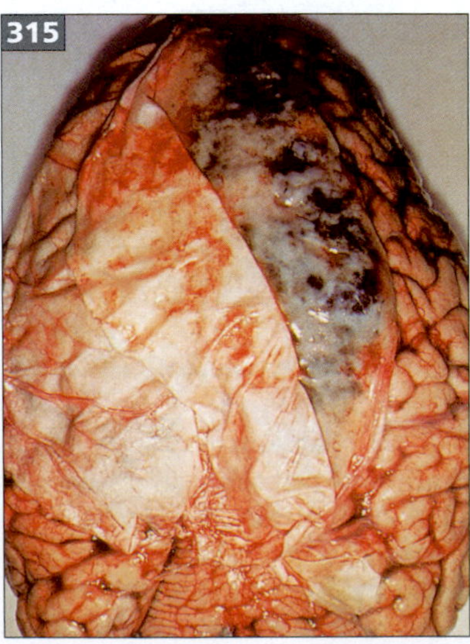

315 Autopsy specimen of a fatal subdural hematoma over the parasagittal region of one hemisphere, beneath the dura, which has been retracted.

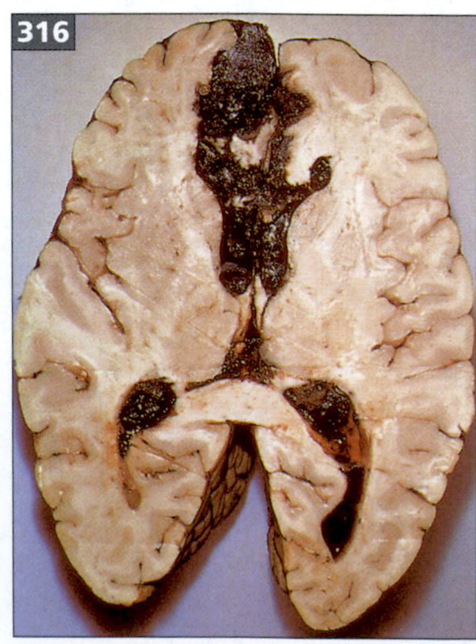

316 Section of the brain in the axial plane, showing subarachnoid hemorrhage in the anterior interhemispheric fissure and intraventricular extension of the hemorrhage due to a ruptured anterior communicating artery aneurysm. *Courtesy of Professor BA Kakulas, Department of Neuropathology, Royal Perth Hospital, Western Australia.*

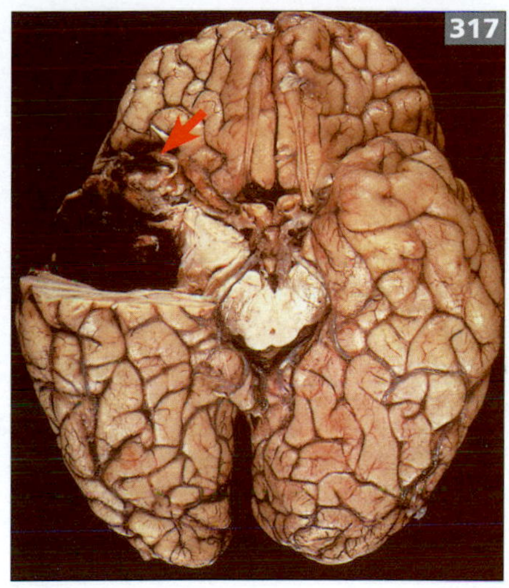

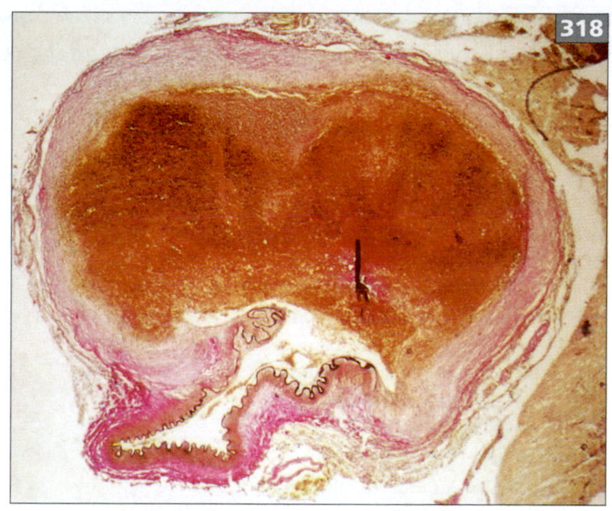

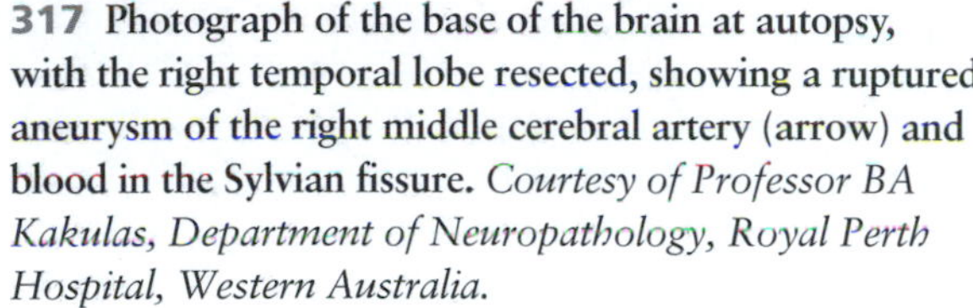

317 Photograph of the base of the brain at autopsy, with the right temporal lobe resected, showing a ruptured aneurysm of the right middle cerebral artery (arrow) and blood in the Sylvian fissure. *Courtesy of Professor BA Kakulas, Department of Neuropathology, Royal Perth Hospital, Western Australia.*

318 Section of a saccular aneurysm at the base of the brain, taken at autopsy, showing disruption of the internal elastic lamina and hemorrhage.

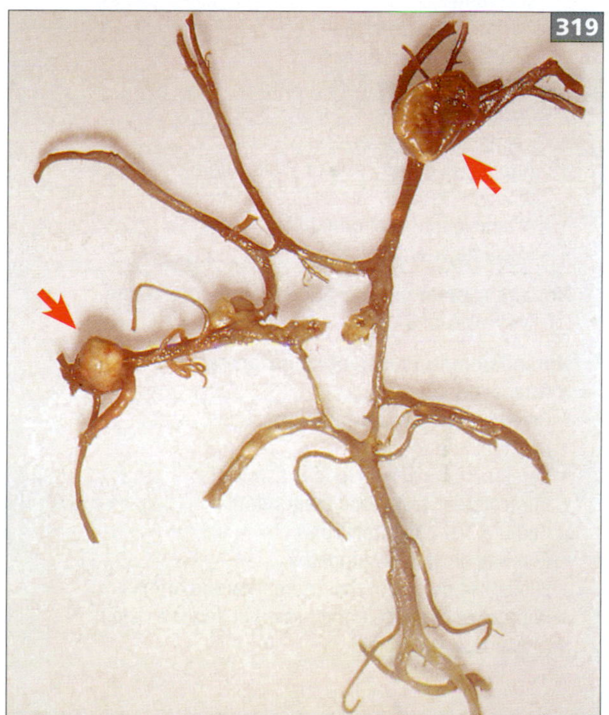

319 Dissection of the arteries on the surface of the base of the brain, showing the circle of Willis and bilateral aneurysms of the middle cerebral arteries. *Courtesy of Professor BA Kakulas, Department of Neuropathology, Royal Perth Hospital, Western Australia.*

Saccular aneurysms vary in size from 2 mm to 3 cm in diameter, with a mean of 7.5 mm. They are variable in form, round with a narrow stalk, broad-based without a stalk, or narrow cylinders. They are multiple in about 25% of cases.

Saccular aneurysms are not congenital but develop during the course of life, usually after the second decade. The formation of aneurysms is probably acquired (possibly due to hypertension, smoking, alcohol abuse, and atheroma) and due to a defect in the media and elastica of the arterial wall; perhaps focal destruction of internal elastic membrane by hemodynamic forces at the apices of the bifurcations[20]. In the exceptional case of childhood aneurysms, there is often an underlying cause such as trauma, infection, or connective tissue disorder (*Table 44*).

TABLE 44 **CAUSES OF SUBARACHNOID HEMORRHAGE (SAH)**

Ruptured saccular aneurysms
(85% of cases of SAH)
- Long-term exposure to causal risk factors (genes [family history], hypertension, smoking, alcohol)
- Disorders of connective tissue:
  – Ehlers–Danlos syndrome type IV
- Autosomal dominant polycystic kidney disease
- Infantile fibromuscular dysplasia
  – Marfan's syndrome*
  – Pseudoxanthoma elasticum*
  – α1-antitrypsin deficiency
  – Neurofibromatosis*
- Disorders of angiogenesis:
  – Hereditary hemorrhagic telangiectasia
  – Progressive hemifacial atrophy (Parry–Romberg syndrome)
- Associated hypertension:
  – Congenital heart disease
  – Coarctation of the aorta
  – Aortitis syndrome
- Local hemodynamic stress:
  – Anomalies of the circle of Willis (more common in women)
  – Arteriovenous malformations
  – Moyamoya syndrome

Nonaneurysmal perimesencephalic hemorrhage
(10% of cases of SAH)

Noninflammatory lesions of intracerebral vessels
- Arterial dissection
- Cerebral arteriovenous malformations
- Fusiform aneurysms
- Cerebral dural arteriovenous fistulae
- Intracerebral cavernous malformation
- Cerebral venous thrombosis
- Cerebral amyloid angiopathy
- Blister-like bulges of the internal carotid artery
- Rupture of circumferential artery in pontine cistern
- Moyamoya syndrome

Inflammatory lesions of cerebral arteries
- Mycotic aneurysms
- Borreliosis
- Behçet's disease
- Primary angiitis of the central nervous system
- Polyarteritis nodosa
- Churg–Strauss syndrome
- Wegener's granulomatosis

Sickle cell disease

Tumors
- Pituitary apoplexy
- Cerebral metastases of cardiac myxoma
- Malignant glioma
- Acoustic neuroma
- Cervical meningioma
- Angiolipoma
- Schwannoma of accessory nerve or spinal root
- Spinal meningeal carcinomatosis
- Melanoma of the cauda equina
- Cervical spinal cord hemangioblastoma

Drugs
- Cocaine use
- Anticoagulants

Head trauma

Superficial siderosis of the central nervous system

Vascular lesions in the spinal cord
- Saccular aneurysm of spinal artery
- Spinal arteriovenous fistula or malformation
- Cavernous malformation at spinal level

*A relationship with cerebral aneurysms has been assumed in the past but subsequently questioned for these conditions.

They are prone to rupture following an acute rise in bood pressure, such as with heavy physical exertion and sexual intercourse, but this remains to be established. The few studies which have collected data on the activities immediately preceding the onset of subarachnoid hemorrhage (SAH) have reported physical exertion preceding the hemorrhage in 2–20% of patients; sexual intercourse in 0–11%; activities with a Valsalva maneuver in 4–20%; and stress in 1–2%. Because few of these studies accounted for the usual frequency of these factors in everyday life, it is uncertain whether they actually increase the risk of aneurysm rupture or not.

Perimesencephalic hemorrhage

In 10% of cases, the center of the SAH is in the cisterns around the midbrain or ventral to the pons (perimesencephalic), usually ventral to it, but there is no other pathology; the angiogram is normal, showing no evidence of an aneurysm and the patients do not come to autopsy: they recover and go on to live a normal life. The cause of the bleeding is unknown but it is not a ruptured aneurysm. The long-term outcome is invariably excellent. Rarely, other vascular pathologies, such as arterial dissection, are identified.

RISK FACTORS

Risk factors for stroke are characteristics of an individual, or of a population, which are associated with an increased risk of stroke compared with an individual, or a population, without those characteristics.

A causal association between a risk factor and stroke is inferred by the:

- Strength of the association (high relative risk or relative odds).
- Consistency of the association in different studies and populations.
- Presence of a dose-response relationship (the more the risk factor, the higher the frequency of the disease).
- Independence from confounding factors.
- Temporal sequence with the risk factor *first* and *then* the disease, remembering that the onset of the symptoms of stroke may be years after the onset of the underlying pathology (e.g. atheroma, aneurysm etc.).
- Biological and epidemiologic plausibility.
- Effect on the incidence of stroke of experimental removal of the risk factor in randomized trials.

The importance of a risk factor is determined by causality and the absolute risk difference between those with and those without the causal risk factor. Even if the relative risk is high, the relevance will be small if the risk factor is rarely present in the population. For example, although the relative risk of stroke for patients with rheumatic AF is very high, the fact that rheumatic heart disease is now rare in developed countries means that it is still a rare cause of stroke, i.e. it 'explains' only a small proportion of strokes and so has a low attributable risk. On the other hand, a risk factor which is common and yet does not carry a particularly high relative risk (e.g. mild hypertension) will 'explain' a much higher proportion of strokes (compared with severe hypertension which is rare). Also, if the background risk of stroke in a population is very low (e.g. in young women), exposure to quite a high relative risk (e.g. by taking oral contraceptives) will not increase the absolute risk of stroke very much.

The INTERSTROKE study reported that 90% of stroke could be attributed to 10 risk factors[21], as shown in *Table 45*.

TABLE 45 **RISK FACTORS FOR ALL STROKE**

Risk factor	**Prevalence**		**Odds ratio** (99% CI)	**Population-attributable risk** (99% CI)
	Controls	**Cases**		
History of hypertension	32%	56%	2.6 (2.3–3.1)	35% (30–39%)
Regular physical activity	12%	8%	0.7 (0.5–0.9)	28% (14–48%)
Waist-to-hip ratio (T3 *vs.* T1)	33%	41%	1.6 (1.4–2.0)	26% (19–36%)
Apolipoprotein B to A1 ratio (T3 *vs.* T1)	33%	47%	1.9 (1.5–2.4)	25% (16–37%)
Current smokers	24%	36%	2.1 (1.7–2.5)	19% (15–23%)
Diet risk score (T3 *vs.* T1)	30%	35%	1.4 (1 .1–1.6)	19% (11–30%)
Cardiac causes* (AF, MI, RhVD, PVD)	5%	12%	2.4 (2.8–3.2)	7% (5–9%)
Diabetes	12%	19%	1.4 (1.1–1.7)	5% (3–9%)
Depression	14%	20%	1.4 (1.1–1.6)	5% (3–10%)
Psychosocial stress	15%	20%	1.3 (1.1–1.6)	5% (2–10%)
Alcohol intake >30 drinks/month	11%	16%	1.5 (1.2–1.9)	4% (1–14%)

3000 cases of acute first stroke (within 5 days of symptom onset) compared with 3000 controls with no history of stroke who were matched with cases for age and sex, and who were assessed in 22 countries between 2007 and 2010 in the INTERSTROKE study. (*Lancet* [2010]. **376**:112–23).

Multivariable model adjusted for age, sex and region.

*Cardiac causes includes atrial fibrillation (AF) or flutter, previous myocardial infarction (MI), rheumatic valve disease (RhVD), or prosthetic valve disease (PVD).

TABLE 46 **RISK FACTORS FOR ISCHEMIC STROKE**

Risk factor	**Prevalence**		**Odds ratio** (99% CI)	**Population-attributable risk** (99% CI)
	Controls	**Cases**		
Apolipoprotein B to A1 ratio (T3 *vs.* T1)	33%	49%	2.4 (1.9–3.1)	35% (25–46%)
History of hypertension	32%	55%	2.4 (2.0–2.8)	31% (27–37%)
Regular physical activity	12%	8%	0.7 (0.5–0.9)	29% (14–50%)
Waist-to-hip ratio (T3 *vs.* T1)	33%	43%	1.7 (1.4–2.1)	26% (18–36%)
Current smokers	24%	37%	2.3 (1.9–2.8)	21% (17–26%)
Diet risk score (T3 *vs.* T1)	30%	35%	1.3 (1.1–1.6)	17% (9–30%)
Cardiac causes* (AF, MI, RhVD, PVD)	5%	14%	2.7 (2.0–3.7)	8% (6–11%)
Diabetes	12%	21%	1.6 (1.3–2.0)	8% (5–12%)
Depression	14%	21%	1.5 (1.2–1.8)	7% (4–11%)
Psychosocial stress	15%	20%	1.3 (1.0–1.6)	5% (2–10%)
Alcohol intake >30 drinks/month	11%	16%	1.4 (1.1–1.8)	1% (0–8%)

2337 cases of acute first ischemic stroke (within 5 days of symptom onset) compared with 3000 controls with no history of stroke who were matched with cases for age and sex, and who were assessed in 22 countries between 2007 and 2010 in the INTERSTROKE study (*Lancet* [2010]. **376**:112–23).

Multivariable model adjusted for age, sex and region.

T1; T3: First (lowest) and third (highest) tertiles of distribution.

TABLE 47 **RISK FACTORS FOR HEMORRHAGIC STROKE**

Risk factor	**Prevalence**		**Odds ratio** (99% CI)	**Population-attributable risk** (99% CI)
	Controls	**Cases**		
History of hypertension	32%	60%	3.8 (3.0–4.8)	44% (37–52%)
Regular physical activity	12%	7%	0.7 (0.4–1.1)	28% (7–67%)
Waist-to-hip ratio (T3 *vs.* T1)	33%	35%	1.4 (1.02–1.9)	26% (14–43%)
Diet risk score (T3 *vs.* T1)	30%	34%	1.4 (1.01–2.0)	24% (12–43%)
Alcohol intake >30 drinks/month	11%	16%	2.0 (1.3–3.0)	15% (8–24%)
Current smokers	24%	31%	1.4 (1.1–2.0)	9% (4–20%)
Psychosocial stress	15%	19%	1.2 (0.9–1.7)	3% (1–16%)

In 663 cases of acute first hemorrhagic stroke (within 5 days of symptom onset) compared with 3000 controls with no history of stroke who were matched with cases for age and sex, and who were assessed in 22 countries between 2007 and 2010 in the INTERSTROKE study (*Lancet* 2010; **376**: 112–23).

Multivariable model adjusted for age, sex and region.

T1; T3: First (lowest) and third (highest) tertiles of distribution.

TABLE 48 **RISK FACTORS FOR SUBARACHNOID HEMORRHAGE (SAH)**

Risk factors	**Relative risk**	**(95% CI)**	**Prevalence** (%)	**PAR** (%)
Cigarette smoking	2.4	(1.8–3.4)	28	29
Systolic BP >140 mmHg	2.0	(1.5–2.7)	12	19
Alcohol >300 g/week	5.6	(1.9–16.7)	6	19
Alcohol 100–299 g/week	3.5	(1.1–11.0)	5	11
First-degree relative with SAH	6.6	(2.0–21.0)	2	11
AD polycystic kidney disease	4.4	(2.7–7.2)	0.1	0.3

AD: autosomal dominant; PAR: population-attributable risk.

Other causal risk factors for stroke include increasing age, carotid stenosis, a positive family history for stroke, and possibly poor oral hygiene, recent infection, increased plasma fibrinogen (and viscosity), increased hematocrit, and genetic variation of mitochrondrial DNA (mtDNA) sub-haplogroup K. Other markers of an increased risk of stroke include previous stroke or TIA, peripheral arterial disease, obstructive sleep apnea, microalbuminuria, and socioeconomic deprivation.

The effect of risk factors on stroke incidence is usually additive or multiplicative so that the presence of several risk factors puts an individual at particularly high risk. Consequently, clinicians are now encouraged to stratify individuals into categories of stroke risk on the basis of their risk factor profile and estimate of absolute risk of a vascular event.

Table 46 shows the risk factors for ischemic stroke, and *Table 47* shows the major risk factors for primary (nontraumatic) hemorrhagic stroke, in the INTERSTROKE study[21].

Risk factors for SAH are listed in *Table 48*. The most important modifiable risk factors are hypertension, cigarette smoking, and heavy alcohol intake[20,21]. The most important nonmodifiable risk factor is familial predisposition to SAH. At least 5%, and up to 20%, of patients with SAH have a positive family history for SAH. SAH occurs six to seven times more often in first-degree than in second-degree relatives of patients with SAH. Familial clustering does not necessarily imply a genetic predisposition to aneurysm formation, but because familial hypertension only partly explains the familial clustering of SAH, genetic factors related to aneurysm formation are likely to play a role.

SAH is also associated with heritable disorders, such as autosomal-dominant polycystic kidney disease, Ehlers–Danlos type IV, and neurofibromatosis type 1, but these account for a small minority of patients with SAH.

CLINICAL ASSESSMENT

The aim of the clinical assessment is to establish:

1. The *diagnosis* of a vascular event of the brain.
2. The anatomical *location* of the neurologic and cardiovascular lesion.
3. The underlying *cause* (pathology and etiology) of the stroke.
4. The functional *severity* of the stroke (*Table 49*).

Prognosis and *treatment* are covered in later sections of this chapter.

TABLE 49 **CLINICAL ASSESSMENT OF PATIENTS WITH SUSPECTED STROKE OR TRANSIENT ISCHEMIC ATTACK (TIA)**

1. Is this patient having a vascular event of the brain (TIA/stroke) or not?
2. Where is the stroke or TIA (anatomy)?
3. What type of stroke is it (pathology)?
4. What is the cause of the stroke or TIA (etiology)?
5. How severe is the stroke?
6. What is the prognosis for survival, free of handicap and recurrent stroke?
7. What is the treatment to optimize survival, free of handicap, and to minimize complications and recurrent stroke?

Diagnosis

Is it a stroke/TIA or a nonvascular syndrome? The characteristic clinical features of a stroke and TIA are:

- Loss of *focal* neurologic function (*Table 50*).
- Of sudden onset.
- Which is *maximal at onset*, without spread or intensification.
- Thought to be due to either *inadequate blood supply* to a part of the brain as a result of arterial thrombosis or embolism, associated with disease of the arteries, heart, or blood (ischemic stroke), or to a *hemorrhage* into a part of the brain or over the brain (hemorrhagic stroke).
- The exception is the minority of patients with SAH who present with headache but have no focal neurologic symptoms or signs; neck stiffness is not invariable and may not occur for several hours (see below).

Symptoms and signs of focal neurologic dysfunction

Focal neurologic symptoms and signs (*Table 50*) are clinical features which arise from a disturbance in an identifiable focal area of the brain: for example, unilateral weakness (corticospinal tract) or clumsiness/ataxia (cerebellum), unilateral sensory loss (spinothalamic tract), speech disorder (dominant hemisphere), and double vision (oculomotor pathways). In patients with TIA and stroke, they are caused by focal cerebral ischemia or hemorrhage.

Tip

▶ *As stroke may strike any part of the brain, eye, or spinal cord, much of (central) neurology can be learned 'stroke by stroke'.*

Nonfocal neurologic symptoms

Nonfocal neurologic symptoms are not neuroanatomically localizing (*Table 51*), and therefore should not be interpreted as being due to a TIA or stroke because they are seldom caused by focal cerebral ischemia or hemorrhage. However, neurologic symptoms are not always easy to categorize (*Table 52*); sensory and motor disturbances in a pseudo-radicular pattern (such as a wrist drop or tingling in two or three fingers) may reflect focal neurologic dysfunction, as may cognitive changes such as amnesia but these can be difficult to characterize and quantify, particularly when transient. Vertigo, confusion, and dysarthria may reflect either focal or nonfocal pathology, depending on whether other definite focal neurologic symptoms occur concurrently (e.g. diplopia) and whether they occur in the relevant milieu (e.g. sudden onset in an elderly person with a plethora of vascular risk factors).

Sudden onset

Most symptoms of stroke arise suddenly and are maximal at onset, without intensification or spread. The onset is usually so abrupt that the patient can describe exactly what they were doing at the time of onset. Occasionally, the symptoms may worsen gradually or in a step-wise fashion, but nonetheless their onset is usually sudden. If the patient cannot recall the precise onset of the symptoms, but is nevertheless quite aware of the symptoms, then the diagnosis of stroke is in doubt.

TABLE 50 **FOCAL NEUROLOGIC SYMPTOMS**

Motor symptoms
- Weakness or clumsiness of one side of the body, in whole or in part (hemiparesis)
- Simultaneous bilateral weakness (paraparesis, quadriparesis)*
- Difficulty swallowing (dysphagia)*
- Imbalance (ataxia)*

Speech/language disturbances
- Difficulty understanding or expressing spoken language (dysphasia)
- Difficulty reading (dyslexia) or writing (dysgraphia)
- Difficulty calculating (dyscalculia)
- Slurred speech (dysarthria)*

Somatosensory symptoms
- Altered feeling on one side of the body, in whole or in part (hemisensory disturbance)

Visual symptoms
- Loss of vision in one eye, in whole or in part (transient monocular blindness or amaurosis fugax)
- Loss of vision in the left or the right half or quarter of the visual field (hemianopia, quadrantanopia)
- Bilateral blindness
- Double vision (diplopia)*

Vestibular symptoms
- A spinning sensation (vertigo)*

Behavioural/cognitive symptoms
- Difficulty dressing, combing hair, cleaning teeth, and so on; geographical disorientation; difficulty copying diagrams such as a clock, flower, or intersecting cubes (visual–spatial–perceptual dysfunction).
- Forgetfulness (amnesia)*

*As an isolated symptom, this does not necessarily indicate transient focal cerebral ischemia, because there are many other potential causes.

TABLE 51 **NONFOCAL NEUROLOGIC SYMPTOMS**

Generalized weakness and/or sensory disturbance
Lightheadedness, faintness, 'dizziness'
'Blackouts' with altered or loss of consciousness or fainting, with or without impaired vision in both eyes
Incontinence of urine or feces
Confusion
Any of the following symptoms, if isolated:* • A spinning sensation (vertigo) • Ringing in the ears (tinnitus) • Difficulty swallowing (dysphagia) • Slurred speech (dysarthria) • Double vision (diplopia) • Loss of balance (ataxia)

*If these symptoms occur in combination, or with focal neurologic symptoms, they may indicate focal cerebral ischemia.

TABLE 52 **KEY FOCAL NEUROLOGIC SYMPTOMS AND SIGNS TO ELICIT FROM THE CLINICAL HISTORY**

1. **Nature:** Was the deficit of the motor, somatosensory, visual, and/or other system?
2. **Quality:** Was there a loss of function (e.g. weakness, numbness, or blindness, as is usually the case in TIA and stroke) or a gain of function (e.g. jerking, parasthesiae, visual scintillations, as is not usually the case in TIA and stroke, but in other disorders such as partial epilepsy or migraine)?
3. **Anatomical distribution:** Did the deficit involve, e.g., a part of the face, arm, or leg; or the entire face, arm, and leg?
4. **Onset:** Was the onset of symptoms sudden, stuttering, or gradual?
5. **Evolution:** Did the deficit recover, stabilize, or progress?

The onset of symptoms of stroke is seldom associated with a precipitating event. However, low flow to the brain or eye ('hemodynamic' stroke) can be precipitated by hypotensive drugs, a general anesthetic, cardiac arrest, or cardioversion, in people with severe carotid and vertebrobasilar occlusive disease, and a compromised collateral cerebral and ocular circulation[22]. Vigorous physical activity and coitus have also been associated with hemorrhagic stroke, particularly SAH. The last trimester of pregnancy and the puerperium is a time when otherwise healthy young women may be predisposed to stroke as a result of paradoxical embolism from the venous system of the legs or pelvis, intracranial hemorrhage due to eclampsia, a ruptured arteriovenous malformation, and intracranial venous sinus thrombosis.

Duration of symptoms

The duration of symptoms of TIA and ischemic stroke is a continuum (see above); the only 'relevance' of longer duration TIAs and minor ischemic stroke is that a relevant ischemic lesion is more likely to be demonstrated by brain imaging, and the risk of stroke is higher – increasing duration of focal neurologic symptoms is one of the five main predictors of early recurrent stroke, along with age, blood pressure, clinical features, and diabetes (and duration of symptoms) in the 'ABCD2' prognostic model of early stroke risk after TIA (see prognosis, below). However, some of the prognostic significance of long duration 'TIAs' may be diagnostic in origin. This is because longer duration focal neurologic attacks are more likely to be vascular in origin than short duration attacks and are therefore more likely to be accurately diagnosed as TIAs than short duration attacks which are sometimes migraines, seizures, or syncope misdiagnosed as a TIA.

Tip

► *It is not known how short a TIA can be (and still be a TIA).*

Clinical features of cerebral venous thrombosis

The clinical features of CVT consist essentially of headache, focal neurologic deficits, epileptic seizures, and impairment of consciousness, in different combinations and degrees of severity[16]. The symptoms and signs depend to some extent on which vein is affected, and to an important extent on whether the thrombotic process is limited to the dural sinus or extends to the cortical veins. The onset of the headache is usually gradual, but in up to 15% of patients it is sudden, which may initially suggest the diagnosis of a ruptured aneurysm.

Clinical features of subarachnoid hemorrhage

The key clinical feature suggestive of SAH is a sudden onset of severe, diffuse headache that peaks within minutes and usually lasts 1–2 weeks[19]. Although the suddenness of onset is the most characteristic feature, there are no features of the headache that distinguish reliably between SAH and nonhemorrhagic thunderclap headache. In general practice, headache is the only symptom in about one-third of patients with SAH.

TABLE 53 **CLINICAL SYNDROMES DETERMINED BY NEUROANATOMY AND NEUROVASCULAR ANATOMY**

Arterial territory	Area supplied	Typical syndromes if total territory involved
INTERNAL CAROTID ARTERY **Ophthalmic artery**	Retina and optic nerve	Monocular blindness or altitudinal field defect
Anterior choroidal artery	Globus pallidus (internal), internal capsule (posterior limb), choroid plexus	Contralateral hemiparesis, hemisensory loss, and homonymous hemianopia
Middle cerebral artery	Frontal lobe, parietal lobe, superior temporal lobe	Contralateral central facial weakness, hemiparesis and hemisensory loss (arm>leg), homonymous hemianopia, global aphasia (dominant hemisphere), or visual–spatial–perceptual dysfunction (nondominant hemisphere)
Medial lenticulostriate	Internal capsule	Contralateral pure motor hemiparesis
Lateral lenticulostriate	Putamen, globus pallidus (external), caudate nucleus, internal capsule, corona radiata	Contralateral hemiparesis, dysphasia (dominant hemisphere) or visual-spatial-perceptual dysfunction (non-dominant hemisphere)
Superior division of MCA	Frontal and anterior parietal lobes	Contralateral central facial weakness, hemiparesis and hemisensory loss, ipsilateral deviation of head and eyes, global or motor aphasia (dominant hemisphere)
Prerolandic branch		Contralateral face and arm weakness, motor aphasia (dominant hemisphere)
Rolandic branch		Contralateral central facial weakness, hemiparesis and hemisensory loss; dysarthria (resembling a lacunar syndrome)
Anterior parietal branch		Conduction aphasia and bilateral ideomotor apraxia
Inferior division of MCA *Posterior parietal branch* *Angular branch* *Posterior temporal branch* *Anterior temporal branch* *Temporal polar branch*	Inferior parietal and lateral temporal lobes	Homonymous hemianopia, Wernicke's aphasia, or agitated confusional state (dominant hemisphere), left visual neglect (right-sided lesion)
Anterior cerebral artery	Anterior and superior medial frontal lobe	Contralateral foot and leg weakness or hemiparesis (leg>arm), abulia, incontinence, grasp reflexes
VERTEBRAL ARTERY **Posterior inferior cerebellar artery**	Lateral medulla, inferior cerebellum	Ipsilateral Horner's syndrome, ipsilateral facial sensory loss (pain, temperature), vertigo, ipsilateral paralysis of palate and laryngeal closure (dyphagia and ineffective cough), ipsilateral ataxia of limbs, contralateral spinothalamic sensory loss in limbs; cervical radiculopathies can occur due to involvement of radicular branches of the vertebral artery

Other features with or without headache include vomiting (75%), depressed consciousness (67%), focal neurologic dysfunction (15%) (*Table 50*), intraocular subhyaloid hemorrhages (linear or flame-shaped hemorrhages in the preretinal layer, **320**) (14%), epileptic seizures (7%), delirium (1%), radicular or precordial pain (spinal SAH), severe hypertension, and electrocardiographic changes that can mimic those of acute myocardial infarction.

An epileptic seizure at the onset of the headache is a strong indicator of aneurysmal SAH. Vomiting is not a distinctive feature because about 43% of patients with nonhemorrhagic thunderclap headache also report vomiting at onset. Preceding bouts of similar headaches are also not distinctive; they are recalled by 20% of patients with aneurysmal SAH and 15% of patients with innocuous thunderclap headache. After 3–12 hours, neck stiffness may develop in conscious patients.

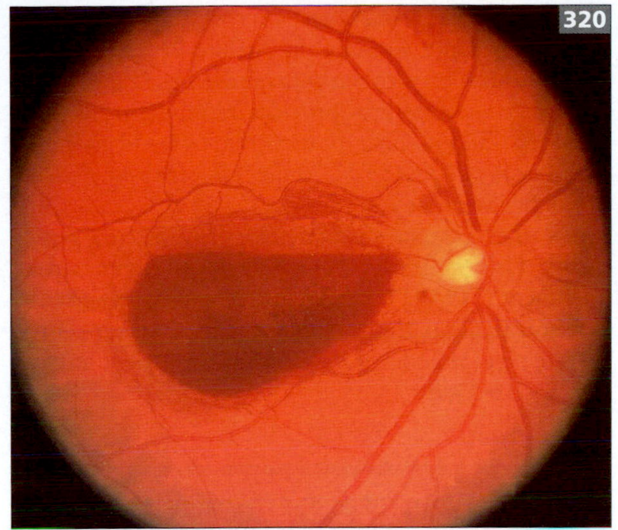

320 Ocular fundus of a patient with subhyaloid hemorrhage, appearing as sharply demarcated linear streaks of brick red-colored blood or flame-shaped hemorrhage in the preretinal layer, adjacent to the optic discs and spreading out from the optic disc. *Courtesy of the late Matthew Wade, Department of Medical Illustrations, Royal Perth Hospital, Western Australia.*

Location

Anatomical correlation

The site and extent of the brain damage caused by focal brain ischemia or hemorrhage determines the clinical features (*Table 53*).

While the answer to the first question 'Is the patient having a vascular event of the brain (TIA/stroke) or not?' often lies in the history, the answer to the next question 'Where (in the brain and vasculature) is the stroke or TIA?' is often determined by the neurologic examination. For example, eliciting a visual field defect, particularly a superior or inferior quadrantanopia, points to a lesion in the contralateral temporal or parietal lobe, respectively, and a homonymous hemianopia to a lesion in the optic tract or occipital lobe. Eliciting a cranial nerve palsy in conjunction with associated motor (corticospinal tract) and sensory (e.g. spinothalamic tract) signs usually points to a lesion in the nucleus or fascicle of the cranial nerve and adjacent long tracts within the brainstem.

However, there are limitations and caveats to the neurologic examination in acute stroke. For example, in the first few hours after a stroke, some of the normally reliable signs of a corticospinal tract (upper motor neuron) lesion, such as spasticity, brisk reflexes, cocontraction, flexor and extensor spasms in response to noxious and proprioceptive stimuli, are immature or absent.

TABLE 53 continued

Arterial territory	Area supplied	Typical syndromes if total territory involved
BASILAR ARTERY **Top of basilar artery***	Rostral midbrain, part of thalamus inferior temporal, occipital lobes	Coma or somnolence, ptosis or lid retraction, variable pupillary abnormalities, supranuclear vertical gaze paresis, ophthalmoplegia, hemiballismus, ataxia, cortical blindness
Superior cerebellar artery	Midbrain (dorso-lateral), superior cerebellar peduncle, superior cerebellum	Ipsilateral Horner's syndrome, ipsilateral limb ataxia and tremor, contralateral spinothalamic sensory loss, contralateral central facial weakness, contralateral IVth nerve palsy sometimes
Anterior inferior cerebellar artery	Base of pons, rostral medulla, rostral cerebellum, cochlea, vestibule	Ipsilateral Horner's syndrome, ipsilateral facial sensory loss (pain, temperature), ipsilateral nuclear facial and abducens palsy, ipsilateral deafness and tinnitus, vertigo, nausea, vomiting, nystagmus,ipsilateral ataxia of limbs, dysarthria
Paramedian branches	Paramedian pons	Any of the lacunar syndromes: – pure motor hemiparesis – axic hemiparesis – pure hemisensory loss – hemiparesis–hemisensory loss – internuclear ophthalmoplegia

*30% of the population have a single common arterial stem supplying the medial aspect of both thalami.

Some anatomically localizing neurologic deficits also require a cooperative and conversant patient and a willing and patient doctor to elicit them, such as:

- Alexia and agraphia (dominant hemisphere angular gyrus).
- Apraxia (dominant parietal lobe).
- Visual agnosias (nondominant parieto-occipital cortex).
- Visual and sensory inattention (nondominant parietal lobe).

Some constellations of symptoms and signs may also not suggest immediately a single focal neurologic lesion, but are indeed caused by a single lesion, such as:

- Bilateral ptosis caused by a unilateral IIIrd nerve nucleus lesion (usually ischemic).
- Lower motor neuron facial palsy with ipsilateral conjugate gaze palsy and contralateral hemiparesis (Foville's syndrome due to a low pontine lesion).
- Selective involvement of the face, hand, and foot in the cheiro–oral–pedal syndrome (thalamic or brainstem lesion).
- Weakness of one arm and the opposite leg (so-called cruciate hemiparesis) caused by a unilateral medullary pyramid lesion.
- Right hemiparesis and (sympathetic) apraxia of the left hand (left frontal–parietal lesion).

Some signs are false localizing signs. For example, a unilateral IIIrd cranial nerve and bilateral VIth cranial nerve palsies can be indirect effects of space-occupying lesions elsewhere, and thus false localizing signs of raised intracranial pressure.

Clinical classification

The Oxfordshire Community Stroke Project (OCSP) classification of stroke syndromes, based on easily observed clinical features, provides information about the anatomical and vascular location, etiology, and prognosis of the stroke (*Table 54*)[23]. About 1% of stroke patients do not fit one of these syndromes.

Another commonly used classification of stroke etiology is the Trial of Org 10172 in Acute Stroke Treatment (TOAST) criteria which aims to identify the most probable pathophysiological mechanism on the basis of clinical findings and results of investigations (see Diagnosis section).

TABLE 54 **THE OXFORDSHIRE COMMUNITY STROKE PROJECT CLASSIFICATION OF CLINICAL STROKE SYNDROMES**

Total anterior circulation syndromes (TACS):
about 20% of cases (**321–324**)

- Hemiparesis and homonymous hemianopia contralateral to the brain lesion, *and*
- *Either* dysphasia *or* visuospatial perceptual disturbance
- ± Hemisensory deficit contralateral to the brain lesion

Partial anterior circulation syndromes (PACS):
about 30% of cases (**325–327**)

- One or more of unilateral motor or sensory deficit, aphasia or visuospatial neglect (combined or not with homonymous hemianopia)
- Motor or sensory deficit may be less extensive than in lacunar syndromes (for example, hand alone)

Lacunar syndromes (LACS):
about 25% of cases (**328–333**)
Any one of the following four syndromes, involving at least two of the three areas (face, arm, leg), and involving the limb in its entirety:

- Pure motor hemiparesis, *or*
- Pure hemisensory deficit of one side of the body, *or*
- Hemisensory–motor deficit, *or*
- Ataxic hemiparesis (dysarthria, clumsy hand syndrome, or ipsilateral ataxia with crural hemiparesis)
- No visual field defect
- No new disturbance of higher cortical or brainstem function

Posterior circulation syndromes (POCS):
about 25% of cases (**334–339**)
Any one of:

- Cranial nerve impairment
- Unilateral or bilateral motor or sensory deficit
- Disorder of conjugate eye movement
- Cerebellar dysfunction
- Homonymous hemianopia
- Cortical blindness

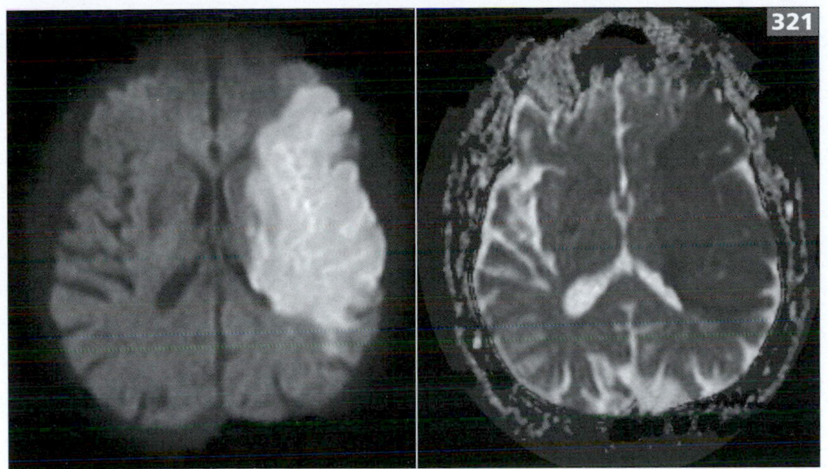

321, 322 MRI brain scan, diffusion weighted image (DWI) in the axial plane (321), in a patient with a total anterior circulation syndrome, showing restricted diffusion, due to recent infarction, in the left frontal, temporal, and parietal lobes. Magnetic resonance angiography (MRA) in the coronal plane (322) shows absent flow, due to occlusion, in the left middle cerebral artery.

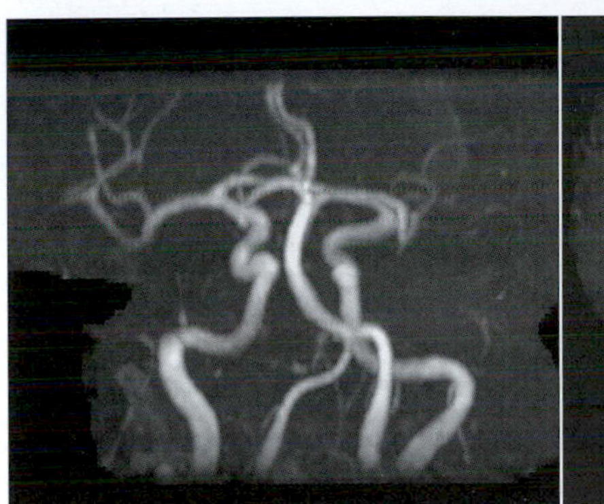

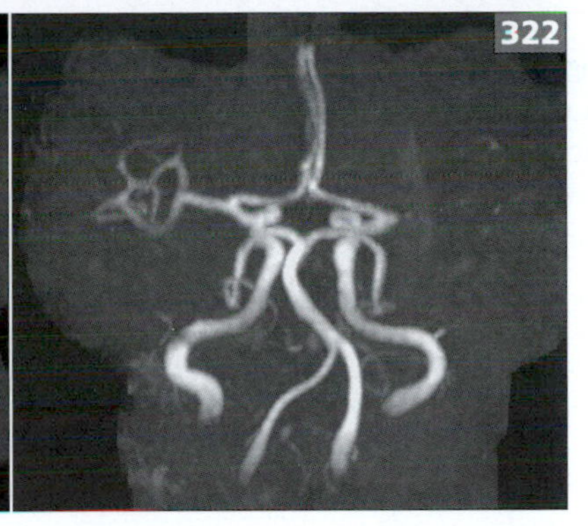

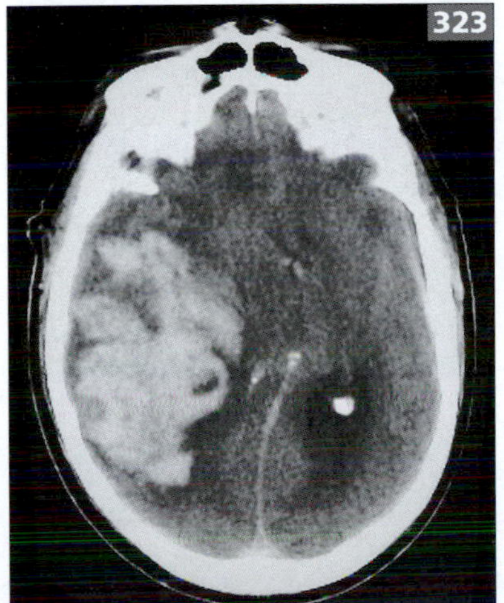

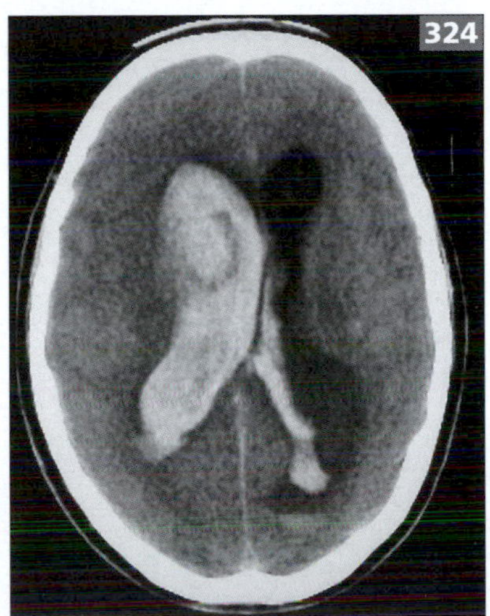

323, 324 CT brain scans of a large, recent, right temporal hemorrhage causing a total anterior circulation syndrome in a patient taking warfarin. Note the extension into the lateral ventricles.

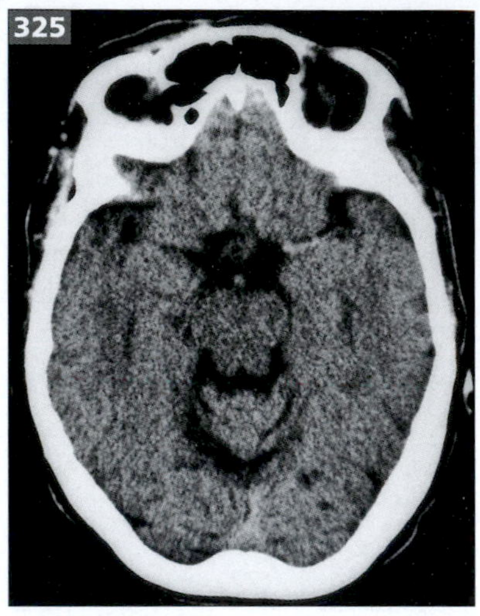

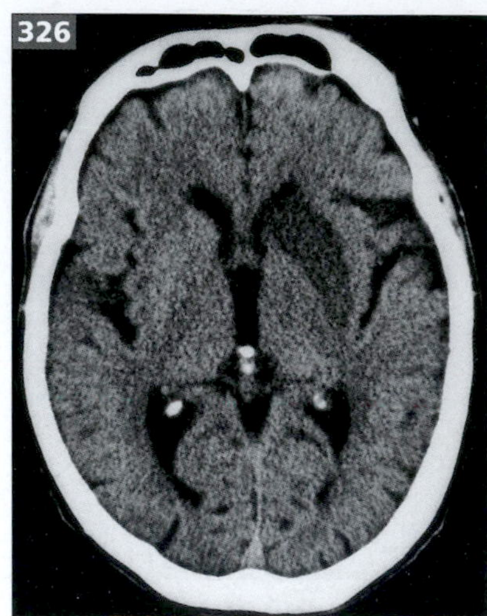

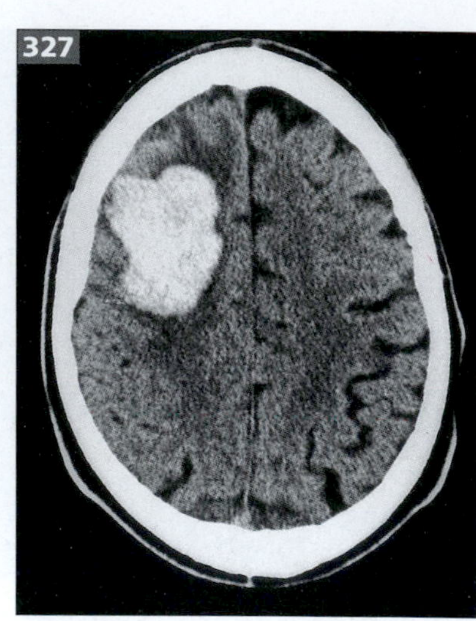

325, 326 Plain cranial CT scan, showing hyperdensity (due to blood clot) in the origin of the left middle cerebral artery (325), and left striatocapsular infarction (326) in a patient who presented with a partial anterior circulation syndrome (right hemiparesis and dysphasia/cognitive deficit).

327 Plain cranial CT scan, showing a homogeneous area of high density due to hemorrhage in the right frontal lobe of an elderly man with amyloid angiopathy and a partial anterior circulation syndrome (left hemiparesis and cognitive/visual–spatial–perceptual dysfunction).

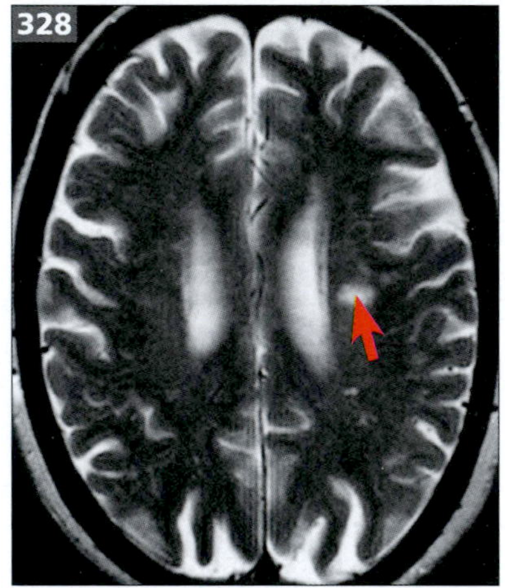

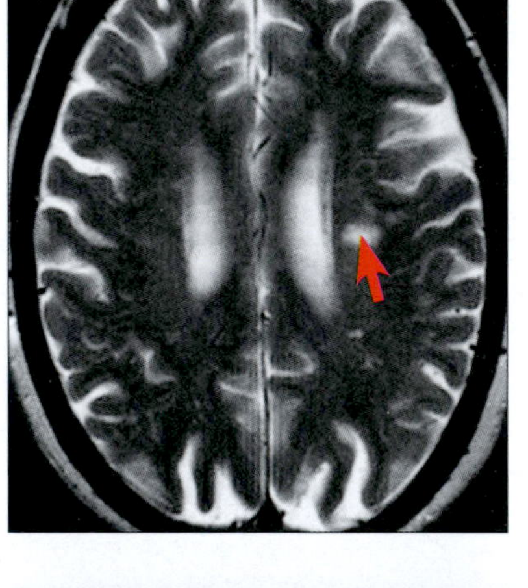

328 T2W MRI of a lacunar infarct in the centrum semiovale (arrow).

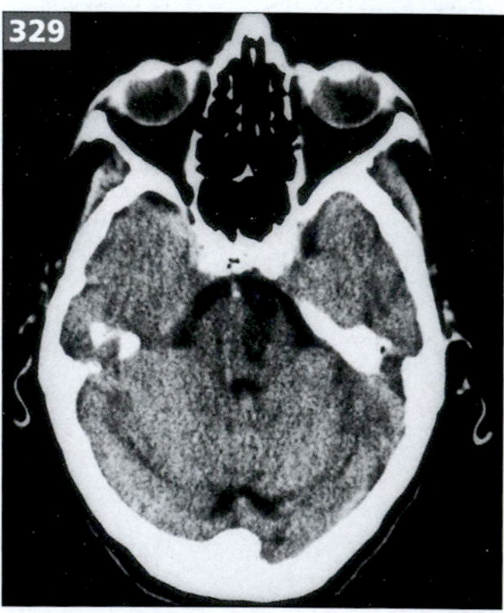

329 Plain cranial CT scan, axial plane, showing high density (whiteness) due to acute thrombus in the basilar artery and a wedge-shaped area of low density in the left paramedian pons, representing lacunar infarction due to occlusion of a paramedian branch of the basilar artery.

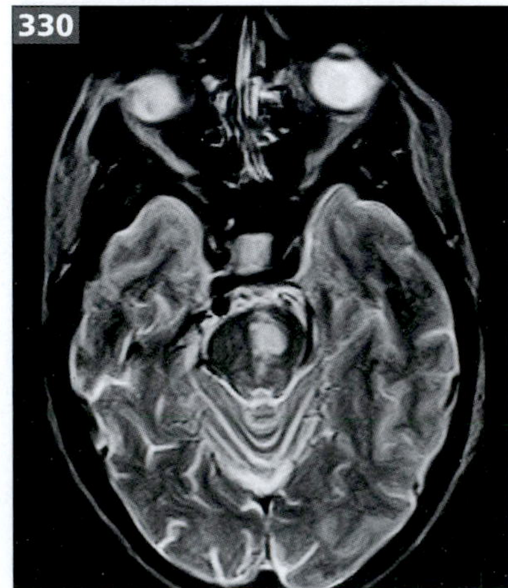

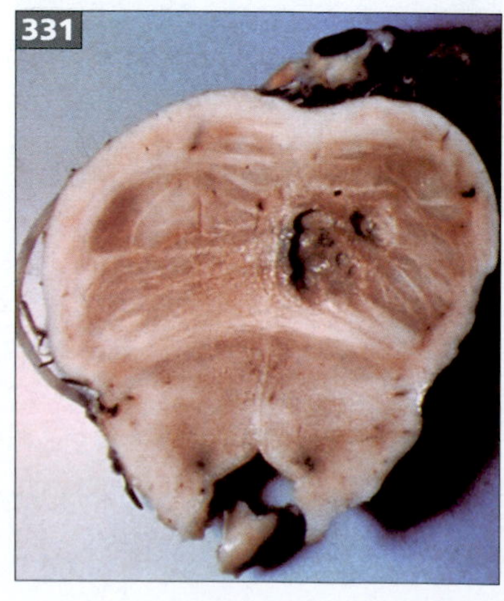

330, 331 MRI brain (330) and autopsy specimen of brainstem (331), showing an axial section through the mid-pons and floor of the fourth ventricle; there is a small area of cavitation due to organized lacunar infarction in the ventral pons on the left, resulting from occlusion of a left paramedian perforating branch of the basilar artery. The patient had an ataxic hemiparesis (lacunar syndrome).

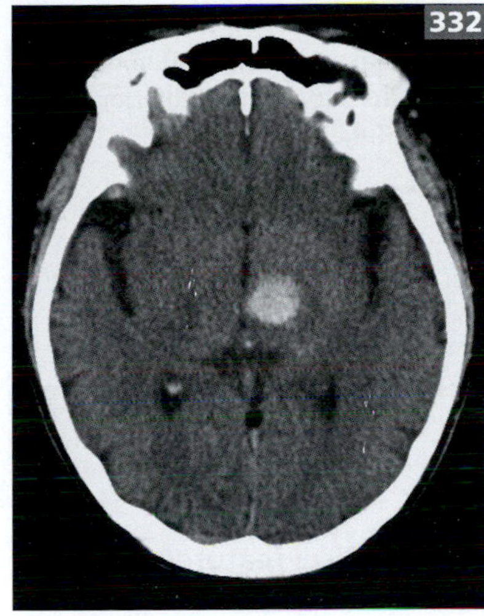

332 Plain (noncontrast) cranial CT scan on the day of stroke onset. It shows a homogeneous area of high attenuation in the left thalamus, representing an acute hematoma, causing a pure right hemisensory deficit (lacunar syndrome).

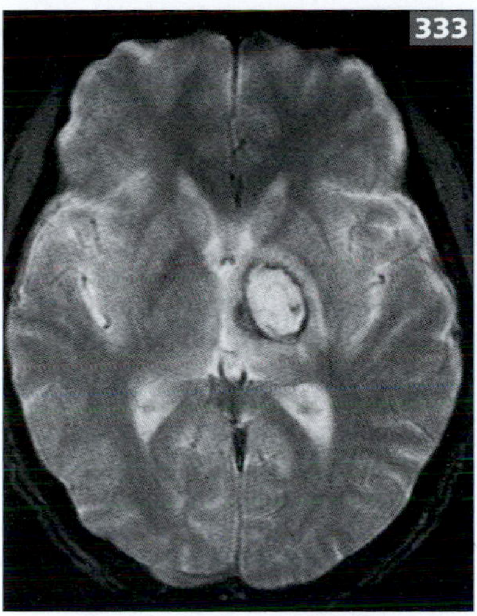

333 T2W MRI of a left thalamic hemorrhage 21 days after stroke, causing right hemisensory deficit (lacunar syndrome). Note the increased (bright) signal centrally (methemoglobin) and the dark low signal ring encircling this due to hemosiderin.

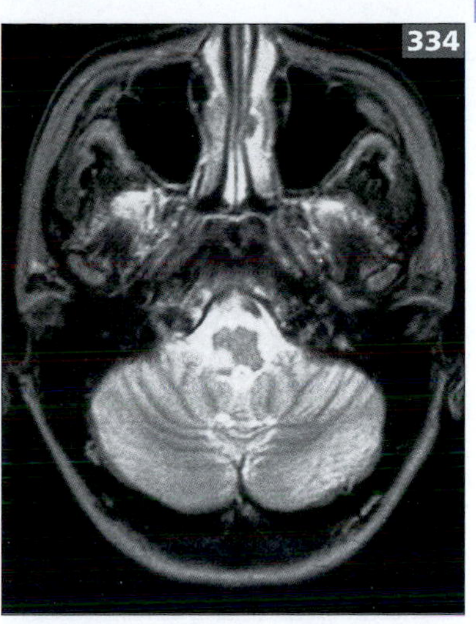

334 MRI brain scan, T2-weighted image, showing an area of high attenuation, consistent with recent infarction, in the right lateral medulla causing a posterior circulation syndrome.

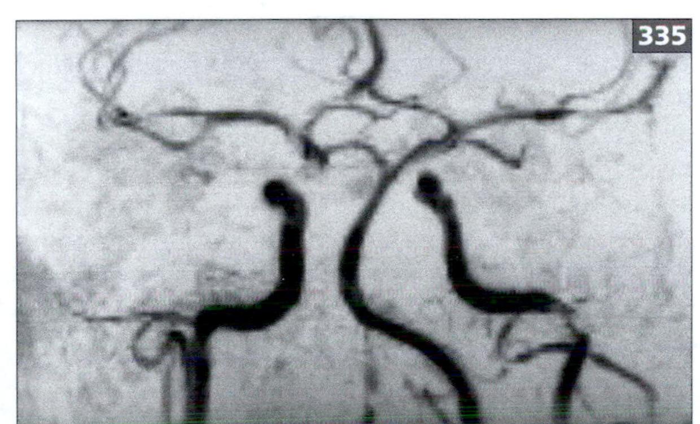

335 MRA showing patchy signal in the right vertebral artery consistent with dissection of the right vertebral artery, and absence of signal in the right posterior inferior cerebellar artery, causing right lateral medullary infarction.

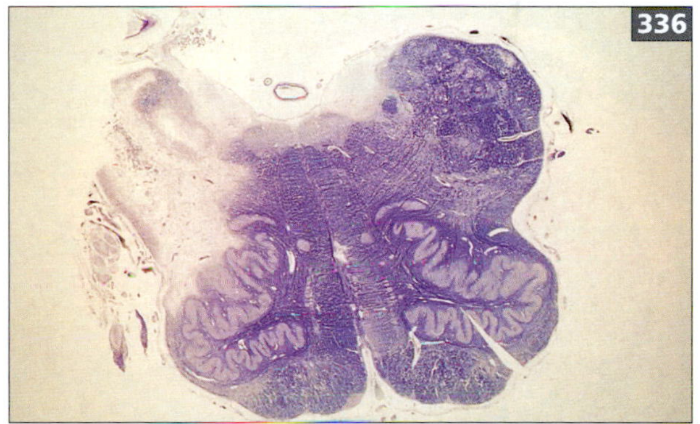

336 Autopsy specimen of brain, horizontal slice through the medulla at the level of the olives, showing pallor due to infarction in the right lateral medulla.

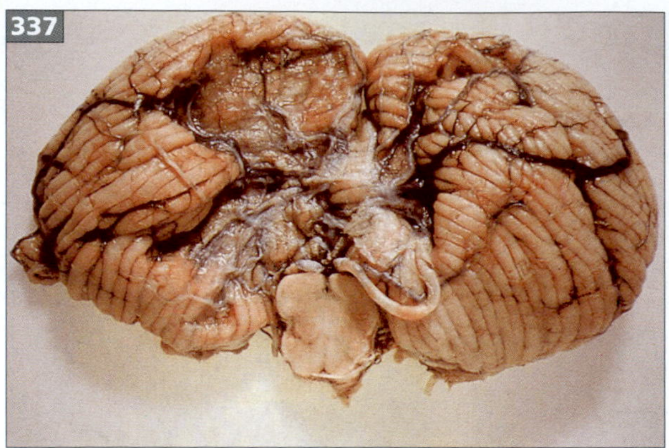

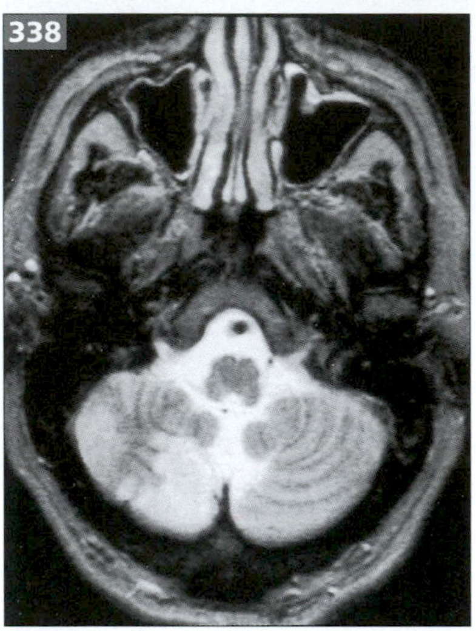

337, 338 MRI scan, T2-weighted image (337), and ventral surface of the cerebellum and medulla at autopsy (338), showing infarction in the left posterior inferior cerebellum due to occlusion of the posterior inferior cerebellar artery.

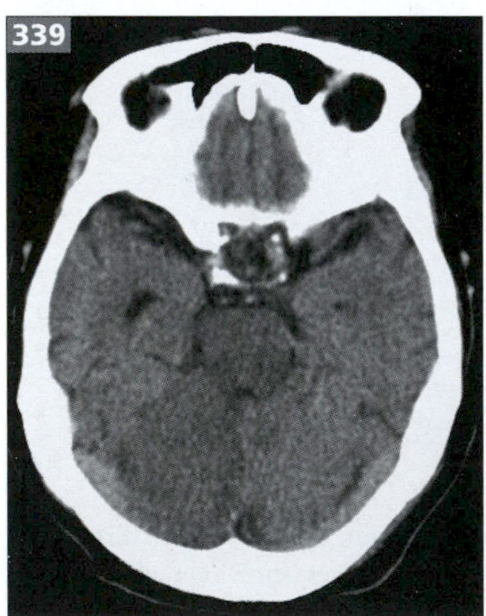

339 Plain CT brain scan showing low density, due to infarction, in the pons and right cerebellar hemisphere causing a posterior circulation syndrome characterized by depressed consciousness, quadriparesis, and sensory impairment, and left cerebellar ataxia.

Anatomically localizing clinical features of CVT

Thrombosis of the superior sagittal sinus alone leads to the syndrome of intracranial hypertension, i.e. headache and papilledema (340). Papilledema can cause transient visual obscurations and sometimes irreversible constriction of the visual fields, beginning in the inferonasal quadrants. The increased pressure of the cerebrospinal fluid (CSF) may also give rise to VIth nerve palsies, and sometimes to other cranial nerve deficits.

Involvement of *cortical veins* causes one or more areas of venous infarction, with or without hemorrhagic transformation. If the affected veins drain into the sagittal sinus, the venous infarcts are typically located near the midline in the parasagittal and parieto-occipital regions, often on both sides. In the case of the lateral sinus, the venous infarct is usually located in the posterior temporal area. If the thrombotic process extends to the petrosal sinus, the Vth or VIth cranial nerves may be affected, and with jugular vein thrombosis, the IXth to XIth cranial nerves.

Clinically, the venous infarcts present with epileptic seizures or with focal deficits, such as hemiparesis or aphasia. If unilateral weakness develops (with thrombosis originating in the superior sagittal sinus), it tends to predominate in the leg, in keeping with the parasagittal location of most venous infarcts. Obstruction of cortical veins draining into the posterior part of the superior sagittal sinus, or into the lateral sinus, will relatively often lead to hemianopia, aphasia, or a confusional state. Impairment of consciousness may result from multiple lesions in the cerebral hemispheres, or from transtentorial herniation and compression of the brainstem.

Either epilepsy or a focal deficit is a presenting feature in 10–15% of patients; during the course of the illness seizures occur in 10–60% of reported series, and focal deficits in 30–80%.

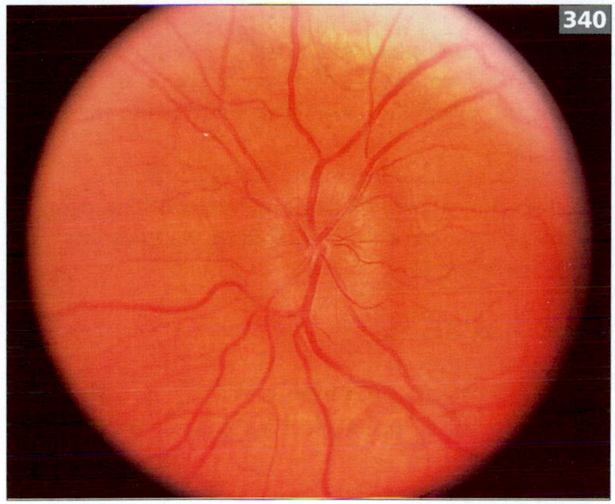

340 **Ocular fundus showing papilledema in a patient with headache due to intracranial hypertension. Note the congested swollen optic disc, loss of the physiological cup, blurred disc margins, and congested retinal veins.**

TABLE 55 **FOCAL NEUROLOGIC SIGNS FOLLOWING SUBARACHNOID HEMORRHAGE, AND THEIR LIKELY CAUSE**

Sign	Most common explanation
Hemiparesis	Large subarachnoid hemorrhage in Sylvian fissure (middle cerebral artery aneurysm)
Paraparesis	Aneurysm of anterior communicating artery, spinal arteriovenous malformation
Cerebellar ataxia, Wallenberg syndrome or both	Dissection of vertebral artery
IIIrd cranial nerve palsy	Aneurysm of internal carotid artery at the origin of posterior communicating artery; rarely aneurysm of basilar artery or superior cerebellar artery, or pituitary apoplexy
VIth cranial nerve palsy	Nonspecific rise of intracranial pressure
IXth–XIIth cranial nerve palsy	Dissection of vertebral artery
Sustained downward gaze and unreactive pupils	Acute hydrocephalus, with dilatation of the small proximal part of the Sylvian aqueduct

Note: intracerebral hemorrhages may give rise to other deficits, depending on their site.

Involvement of the *cortical veins alone*, without sinus thrombosis and its associated signs of increased CSF pressure, is rare but can present as 'stroke' and so may have been under-recognized.

Thrombosis of the *deep venous system*, including the great vein of Galen, may lead to bilateral hemorrhagic infarction of the corpus striatum, thalamus, hypothalamus, the ventral corpus callosum, the medial occipital lobe, and the upper part of the cerebellum. In these cases the clinical picture is dominated by coma and disturbance of eye movements and pupillary reflexes. Partial syndromes exist and can be survived, sometimes with surprisingly few sequelae.

Thrombosis of *cerebellar veins* leads to clinical features resembling those with arterial territory infarcts in the cerebellum (dominated by headache, vertigo, vomiting, and ataxia, sometimes followed by impaired consciousness), but with a more gradual onset.

Anatomically localizing clinical features of SAH

The neuroanatomical significance of focal neurologic signs in a patient with SAH is shown in *Table 55*.

Cause

After establishing the clinical features of stroke (*vs.* not stroke), its pathologic subtypes, and the anatomical site of the brain and vascular pathology, the next step is to seek clinical features of the underlying cause of the brain and vascular pathology[5].

Causes of ischemic stroke

Arterial disease

Large artery atherosclerosis

- Total, partial, or posterior circulation syndrome.
- Multiple risk factors for atherosclerosis (increasing age, hypertension, diabetes, smoking, hyperlipidemia).
- Family history of atherosclerotic ischemic events of the brain, heart, and limbs.
- Preceding TIAs.
- Ischemic oculopathy (341–344).
- Retinal emboli (345–347).
- Carotid, subclavian, vertebral, femoral, or renal bruits.
- Absent carotid pulses; unequal radial pulse.
- Other clinical complications of atherothrombosis: angina, past myocardial infarction, claudication, absent foot pulses.

Small artery disease

- Lacunar syndrome.
- Capsular warning syndrome.
- Vascular risk factors such as smoking, hypertension, and diabetes.
- Systemic features of arteritis.
- Family history of small vessel disease (e.g. CADASIL).

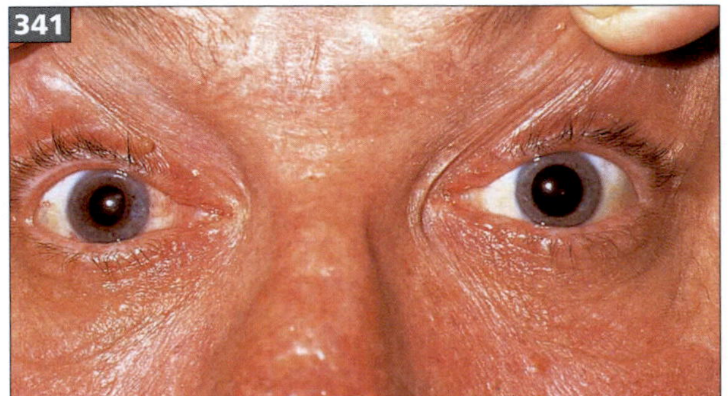

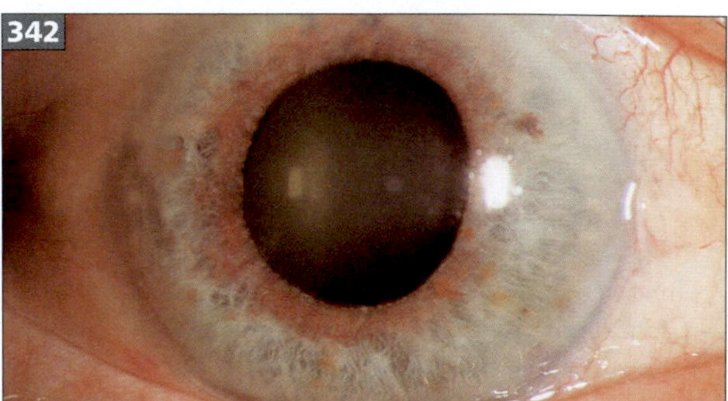

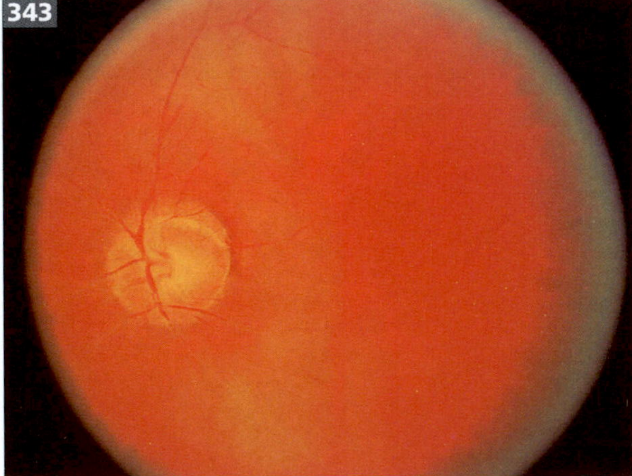

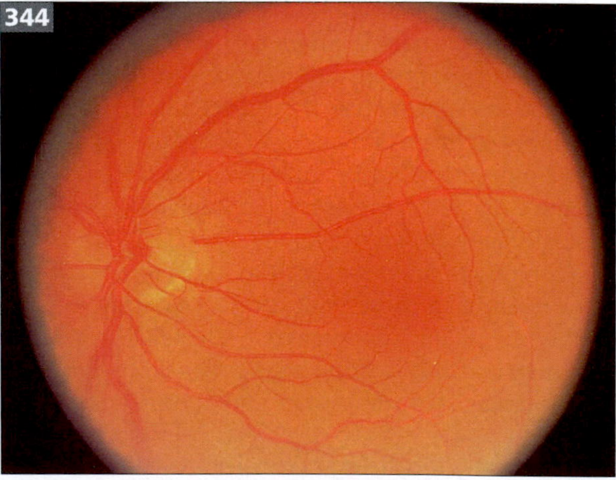

341–344 This patient's right eye is affected by ischemic oculopathy (341). Note the congested sclera, cloudy cornea, new vessel formation (neovascularization) around the limbus of the iris (rubeosis iridis) and mid-dilated pupil, which indicate chronic anterior segment ocular ischemia due to carotid occlusive disease. *Reproduced with permission from Hankey GJ and Warlow CP [1994]; Transient Ischemic Attacks of the Brain and Eye; WB Saunders, London.* (342) Close-up view of the right eye in 341, showing rubeosis iridis more clearly; (343) Fundus of the severely ischemic right eye of the same patient, showing attenuated vessels and pallor of the retina due to retinal edema caused by severe ischemia. (344) Fundus of the normal left eye of the same patient.

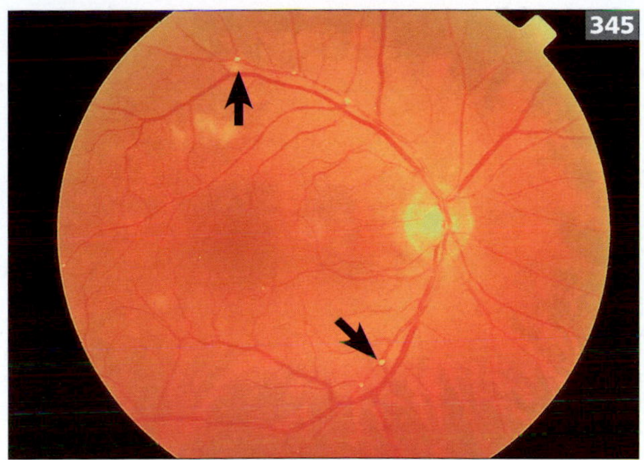

345 Fundus examination showing cholesterol emboli (arrows) as bright, orange–yellow, refractile, crystalline, glinting lipid emboli, so-called Hollenhorst cholesterol plaques. They are usually unilateral, multiple, and found at the bifurcation of retinal arterioles. They frequently arise from ulcerated atherosclerotic plaque in the ipsilateral carotid system. *Reproduced with permission from Hankey GJ and Warlow CP [1994]; Transient Ischemic Attacks of the Brain and Eye; WB Saunders, London.*

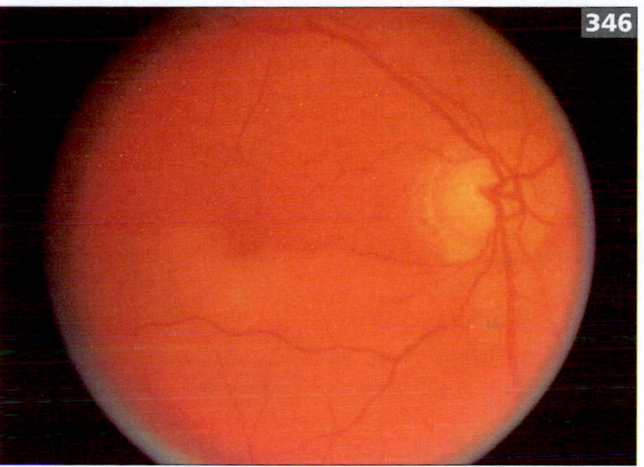

346 Ocular fundus of a patient with inferior temporal branch retinal artery occlusion showing pallor of the inferior half of the retina due to cloudy swelling of the retinal ganglion cells caused by retinal infarction.

347 Ocular fundus showing narrow arterioles and veins, pallor of the retina, and a cherry-red spot over the fovea due to accentuation of the normal fovea, which is devoid of ganglion cells, by the opalescent halo, in a patient with central retinal artery occlusion.

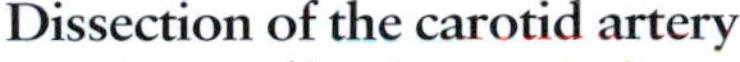

Dissection of the carotid artery

- History of head or cervical trauma (e.g. chiropractic manipulation).
- Headache, face or neck pain.
- Horner's syndrome ipsilaterally (involvement of the cervical sympathetic chain, ascending in the wall of the carotid artery) (**348**).
- Acute or delayed (up to several weeks) focal monocular or carotid territory ischemic symptoms (ipsilateral visual loss, contralateral hemisensorimotor deficit; difficulty speaking).
- Neck bruit.
- Pulsatile tinnitus.
- Dysgeusia (altered taste).
- Cranial nerve palsy (single or multiple): III–VII, IX–XII, in at least 10% of patients with extracranial internal carotid artery (ICA) dissection. The lower cranial nerves, IX–XII, lie close to the ICA below the jugular foramen in the retrostyloid and posterior retroparotid space, and may be compressed or stretched by the dissected ICA if it is expanded or aneurysmal because of the extra blood in its wall. Alternatively, the blood supply to the cranial nerves may be compromised by the dissection; the nutrient vessels to the cranial nerves are small (200–300 μm in diameter) branches of the ICA.

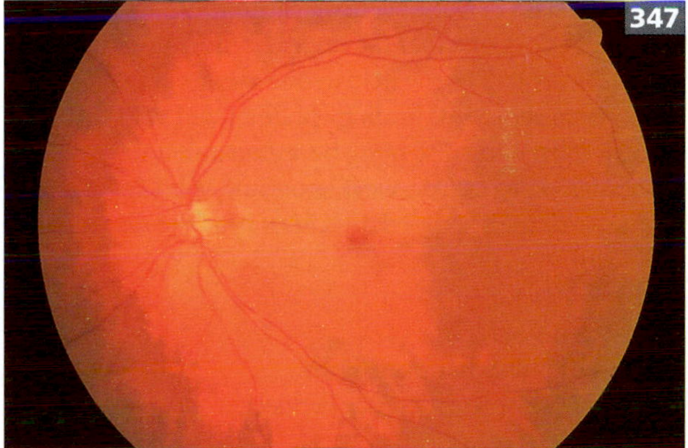

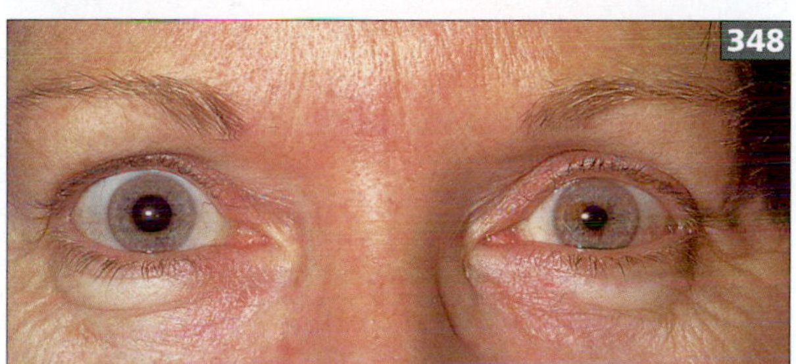

348 Horner's syndrome, due to interruption of the ascending postganglionic pupillodilator oculosympathetic fibers in the wall of the internal carotid artery by dissecting blood.

Dissection of the vertebral artery
- Pain in the neck and back of the head.
- Focal vertebrobasilar ischemic symptoms (occipital/temporal lobe, brainstem, cerebellum; most commonly features of a lateral medullary or cerebellar infarct).
- Upper limb peripheral motor deficits: bilateral distal upper limb amyotrophy.

Giant cell arteritis
- Systemic upset (fever, malaise, fatigue, anorexia, weight loss, night sweats, depression, and arthralgias).
- Myalgia (pain and stiffness in the neck, shoulders, and buttocks).
- Headache (temporal, occipital, or generalized; severe and persistent).
- Pain, swelling, thickness, redness, tenderness, and nodularity over the affected arteries, sometimes with reduced or absent pulsation (e.g. superficial temporal arteries may stand out and be tender on brushing the hair) (349).
- Pain on chewing (jaw and tongue claudication due to maxillary and lingual artery occlusion).
- Ischemic symptoms of the eye (usually sudden, painless deterioration of vision in one eye) or brain.
- Reduced visual acuity from 6/6 to no light perception.
- Visual field defects: particularly altitudinal visual field defects (loss of either the upper or more commonly the lower half of the field in one eye).
- Ophthalmoscopic findings of distended veins, a swollen optic disc (may be segmental) and, occasionally, cotton-wool spots and splinter- or flame-shaped hemorrhages at or near the disc margin (350).

Takayasu's arteritis
- Absent pulses in upper limbs.
- Blood pressure difference between arms.

CNS vasculitis (351)
- Multiple strokes.
- Encephalopathy.
- Headache.

Behçet's disease
- Recurrent oral and genital ulcers (352).
- Superficial thrombophlebitis.
- Deep venous thrombosis.

Moyamoya syndrome
- Multiple strokes.
- Hemorrhagic stroke.
- Cognitive decline.

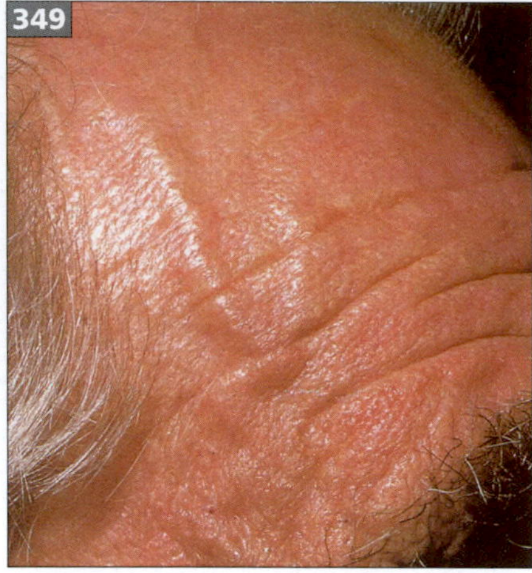

349 Lateral photograph of the forehead of a patient with giant cell arteritis, showing a visibly enlarged, tender temporal artery.

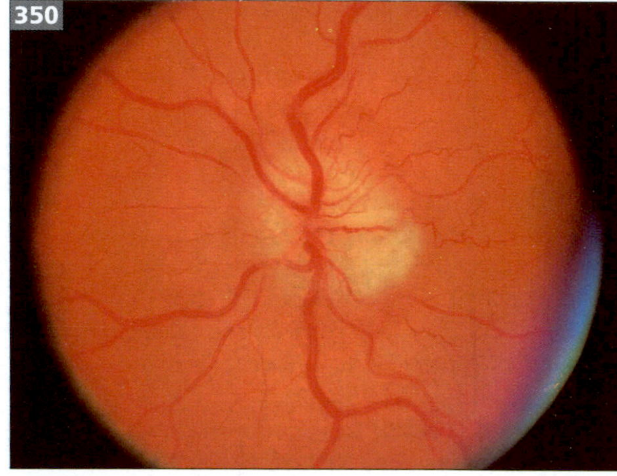

350 Fundus photograph of anterior ischemic optic neuropathy due to giant cell arteritis of the posterior ciliary artery, showing a swollen optic disc, cotton-wool spots at the disc margin, and distended veins. *Courtesy of the late Mr Matthew Wade, Department of Medical Illustrations, Royal Perth Hospital, Western Australia.*

Retinoarteriopathy and retino-cochlear-cerebral arteriopathy
- Visual loss.
- Progressive or episodic deafness.
- Abnormal fundoscopy.

Sneddon's syndrome
- Generalized livido reticularis.
- Ischemic or hemorrhagic stroke.

CADASIL
- Family history.
- Multiple strokes.
- Migraine with aura.
- Dementia.
- Psychosis.

Fabry's disease
- Skin lesions (angiokeratomas, hypohydrosis/ anhidrosis).
- Neuropathic pain.
- Acroparesthesia.
- Painful small-fiber peripheral neuropathy.
- Whorled corneal opacities (corneal verticillata).
- Corneal dystrophy.
- Cataract.
- Retinal vascular changes.
- Episodic diarrhoea, vomiting, or constipation.
- Postprandial bloating and pain, early satiety.
- Weight loss.
- Left ventricular hypertrophy, systolic or diastolic dysfunction, mitral valve insufficiency, premature coronary artery disease, arrhythmia.
- Proteinuria, lipiduria, renal tubular dysfunction (polyuria), renal failure.
- Vertebrobasilar dolicoectasia.

Hereditary angiopathy, nephropathy, aneurysm, and muscle cramps (HANAC syndrome), other COL4A1 disorders
- Small vessel disease.
- Cerebral aneurysms.
- Porencephaly.
- Retinal arterial tortuosity.
- Kidney disease.
- Muscle cramps.

Homocystinuria
- Hypopigmentation.
- Malar flush.
- Livido reticularis.
- Mental retardation.
- Developmental delay.
- Seizures.
- Personality disorder, behavioral disorder, depression.
- Skeletal abnormalities: osteoporosis, pectus excavatum or carinatum, genu valgum, scoliosis, dolicholstenomelia with marfanoid appearance (rarely, arachnodactyly).
- Ectopia lentis, myopia, glaucoma, cataracts, retinal detachment, optic atrophy.
- Foul odor of the urine.
- Pancreatitis.
- Premature atherosclerosis, thromboembolic events.

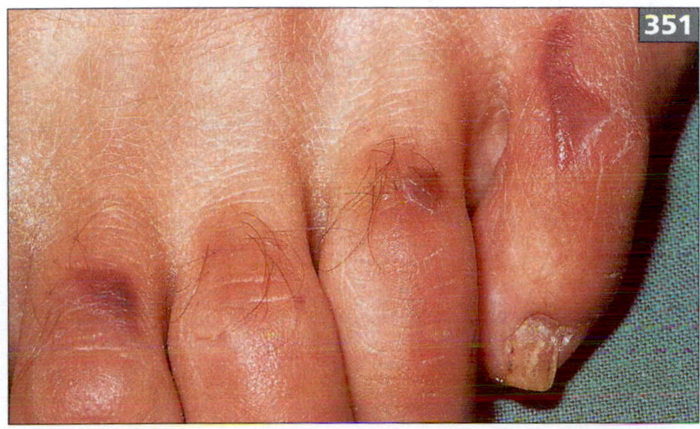

351 Vasculitic infarcts of the skin in a patient with polyarteritis nodosa.

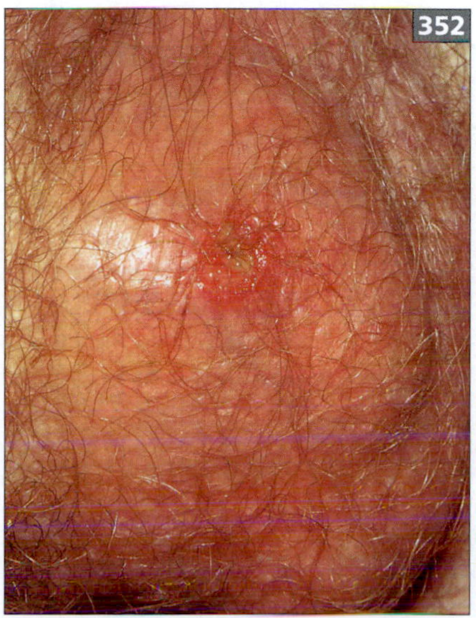

352 Genital (scrotal) ulcer in a young man with Behçet's disease.

Marfan syndrome

- Pectus carinatum or excavatum.
- Upper-to-lower-segment ratio <0.86 or arm-span-to-height ratio > 1.5.
- Scoliosis >20%.
- Ectopia lentis.
- Dilation or dissection of the ascending aorta.
- Lumbosacral dural ectasia.

Ehlers–Danlos type IV

- Easy bruising.
- Thin skin with visible veins.
- Characteristic facial features.
- Rupture of arteries, uterus, and intestines.

Pseudoxanthoma elasticum

- Skin changes (increased elasticity and yellow–orange papular lesions).
- Ocular changes (angioid streaks).
- Hypertension.

Cardiac disease

A cardiac source of embolism is suspected in patients with total, partial, or posterior circulation ischemic stroke (i.e. involving cortex); multiple infarcts in different arterial territories; and hemorrhagic transformation of the infarction, although none of these features is specific for cardiogenic embolism.

Atrial fibrillation

- Irregularly irregular pulse.
- Electrocardiogram (ECG) documentation of AF: underlying hypertensive, ischemic, or valvular heart disease or thyrotoxicosis as the cause of the AF.

Valvular heart disease

- History of rheumatic fever or prosthetic valve surgery.
- Cardiac murmur.
- PFO: Stroke during Valsalva's maneuver or after prolonged immobilization.

Infective endocarditis

- Predisposing risk factors:
  - Native valve condition (31%).
  - Invasive procedure within previous 60 days (25%).
  - Prosthetic valve (20%).
  - Presence of pacemaker (12%).
  - Congenital heart disease (10%).
  - Current intravenous drug use (9%).
  - Previous endocarditis (7%).
- Fever >38°C at some point is almost invariable (so the absence of any fever should lead to consideration of an alternative diagnosis).
- A new regurgitant cardiac murmur (almost one-half of patients).
- A regurgitant murmur across a prosthetic valve.
- Any systemic embolus (e.g. splinter hemorrhages [353], hematuria).
- Abnormal liver function tests or sepsis of unknown origin.
- Painless Janeway lesions on the palms (354) or soles, and immunologic findings such as Roth spots on fundoscopy and Osler nodes are now rare, being found in no more than 5% of cases of infective endocarditis, but they are useful if they are present and recognized.

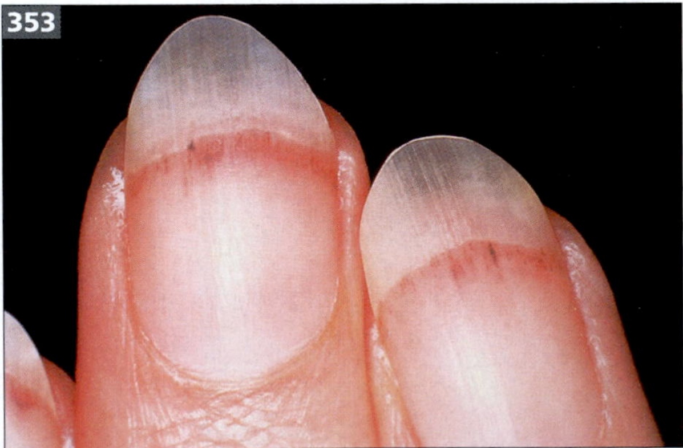

353 Linear splinter hemorrhages under the nails, which can be difficult to differentiate from traumatic lesions.

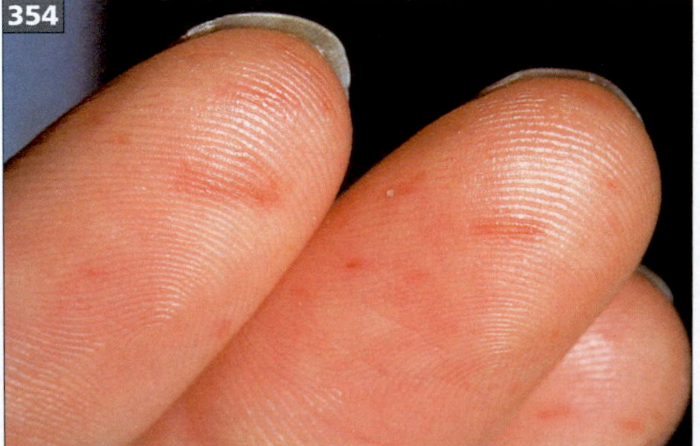

354 Pulps of the fingers showing erythematous maculopapular lesions (Janeway's spots) which were nontender.

Pulmonary disease

Pulmonary arteriovenous fistulae:

- Right-to-left shunt.
- No PFO.
- Hereditary hemorrhagic telangiectasia (Osler–Rendu–Weber disease).

Hematologic disease

Genetic thrombophilic diseases:

- Arterial and venous strokes.
- Family history.

Sickle cell disease

- African ethnic origin.
- Pain crisis.
- Bacterial infection.
- Vaso-occlusive crises.
- Pulmonary and abdominal crises.
- Anemia.
- Myelopathy.
- Seizures.

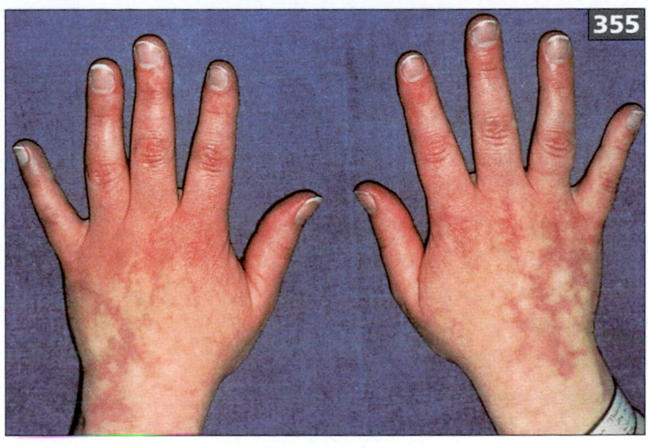

355 Livedo reticularis in a patient with antiphospholipid antibody syndrome.

Antiphospholipid syndrome

- TIA, stroke, or multifocal encephalopathy due to arterial or venous thrombosis in any size of vessel before 50 years of age.
- Unexplained deep vein thrombosis or pulmonary embolism before 50 years of age.
- Recurrent thrombosis (without evidence of inflammation in the vessel wall).
- Thrombosis at an unusual site.
- Three or more unexplained consecutive spontaneous miscarriages before the 10th week of gestation, with maternal anatomical or hormonal abnormalities excluded and paternal and maternal chromosomal causes excluded.
- Recurrent spontaneous miscarriage/fetal loss due to intrauterine death after 10 weeks gestation with normal fetal morphology documented by ultrasound or by direct examination of the fetus.
- Severe intrauterine fetal growth retardation.
- Severe or early onset pre-eclampsia.
- Pre-eclampsia with severe thrombocytopenia.
- Prematurity (one or more premature births of a morphologically normal neonate before the 34th week of gestation because of eclampsia or severe pre-eclampsia defined according to standard definitions, or recognized features of placental insufficiency).
- Cardiac valve disease (in combination with other symptoms above).
- New diagnosis of systemic lupus erythematosus.
- Migraine-like headaches.
- Livedo reticularis (355).
- Nonhealing ulceration of the ankles and skin necrosis.
- Raynaud's phenomenon.
- Unexplained persistent thrombocytopenia.

Metabolic disease

Mitochondrial encephalomyopathy, lactic acidosis, and stroke -like episodes (MELAS)

- Developmental delay.
- Short stature.
- Optic atrophy.
- Ophthalmoplegia.
- Sensorineural deafness.
- Migraine-like headache.
- Seizures.
- Episodic vomiting, gastrointestinal dysmotility.
- Diabetes.
- Cognitive decline.
- Nephropathy.
- Exercise intolerance, dilated cardiomyopathy, left ventricular hypertrophy, cardiac conduction block, pre-excitation syndrome.
- Myopathy.
- Peripheral neuropathy.
- Elevated CSF protein.

Cerebral venous thrombosis

Predisposing causes of CVT are multiple. The risk factors for venous thrombosis in general are linked classically to the Virchow triad of stasis of the blood, changes in the vessel wall, and changes in the composition of the blood. Risk factors are usually divided into acquired risks (e.g. surgery, trauma, pregnancy, puerperium, APS, cancer, exogenous hormones) and genetic risks (inherited thrombophilia) (**356–358**).

Causes of hemorrhagic stroke

Intracerebral hemorrhage

There may be a history of preceding neck trauma (arterial dissection); physical activity such as heavy exertion, defecation, lifting, sexual intercourse; administration of anticoagulant, antiplatelet or recreational drugs; ischemic stroke (hemorrhagic transformation of an infarct); puerperium (choriocarcinoma, intracranial venous thrombosis).

The past history may be noteworthy for hemophilia, hemorrhage in other sites of the body (hemostatic disorder), hypertension, cancer (particularly melanoma, bronchial or renal carcinoma), epileptic seizures (cortical AVM, tumor, amyloid angiopathy), headache (AVM), and valvular heart disease (septic embolism).

General examination may reveal petechiae or bruising (generalized hemostatic disorder); signs of malignant disease (clubbing, cutaneous melanoma, hepatosplenomegaly, lung collapse), needle marks (drug addict), hypertension and hypertensive end-organ disease (retinopathy [**359, 360**], cardiomegaly), retinal hemorrhages (**361**), or a heart murmur (infective endocarditis).

Cerebral amyloid angiopathy, related to the deposition of β-amyloid proteins in the cerebral vessels, is a leading cause of recurrent lobar hemorrhage in elderly patients. Cerebral amyloid angiopathy may present with stereotyped recurrent transient neurologic symptoms before the

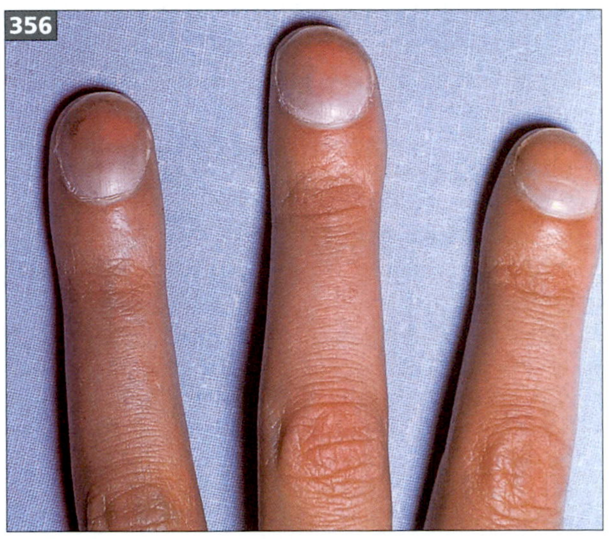

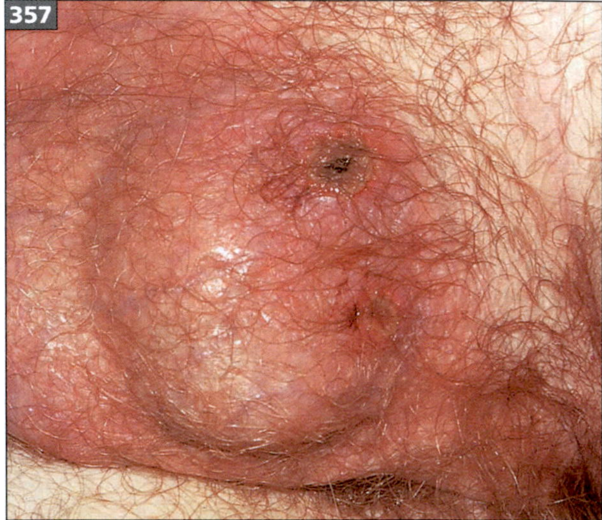

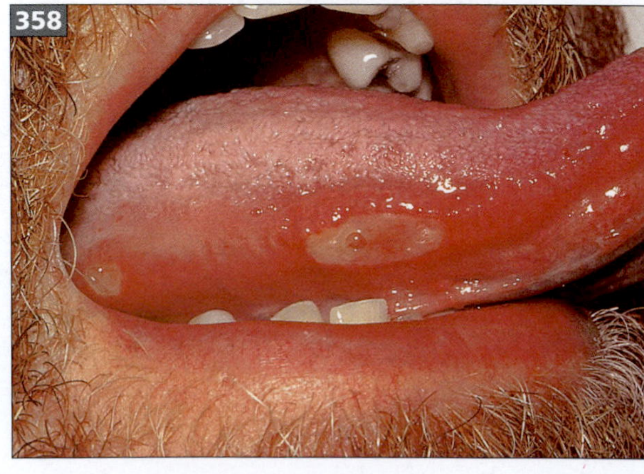

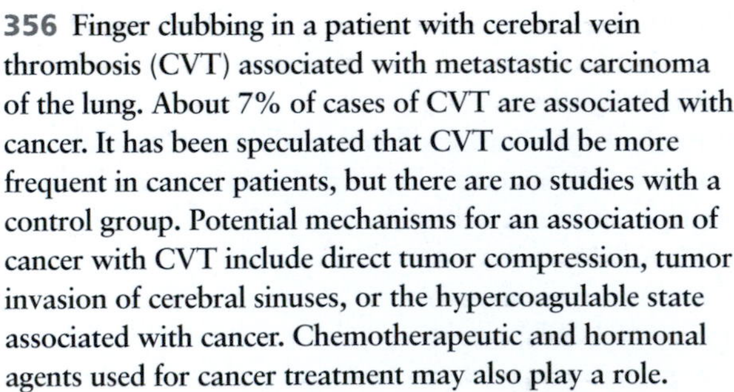

356 Finger clubbing in a patient with cerebral vein thrombosis (CVT) associated with metastastic carcinoma of the lung. About 7% of cases of CVT are associated with cancer. It has been speculated that CVT could be more frequent in cancer patients, but there are no studies with a control group. Potential mechanisms for an association of cancer with CVT include direct tumor compression, tumor invasion of cerebral sinuses, or the hypercoagulable state associated with cancer. Chemotherapeutic and hormonal agents used for cancer treatment may also play a role.

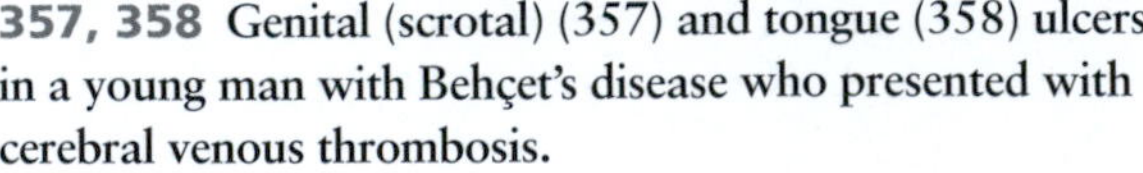

357, 358 Genital (scrotal) (357) and tongue (358) ulcers in a young man with Behçet's disease who presented with cerebral venous thrombosis.

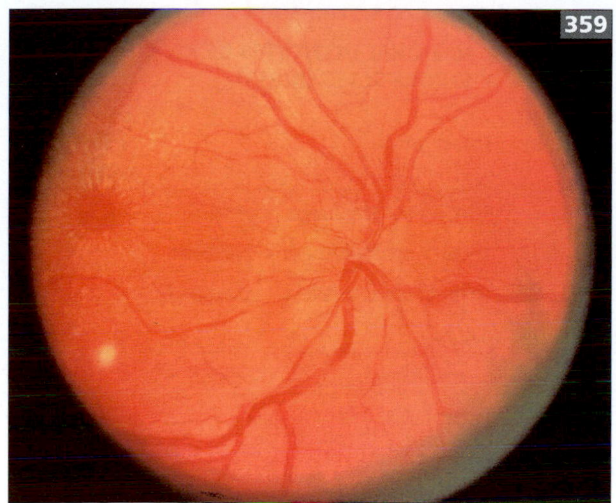

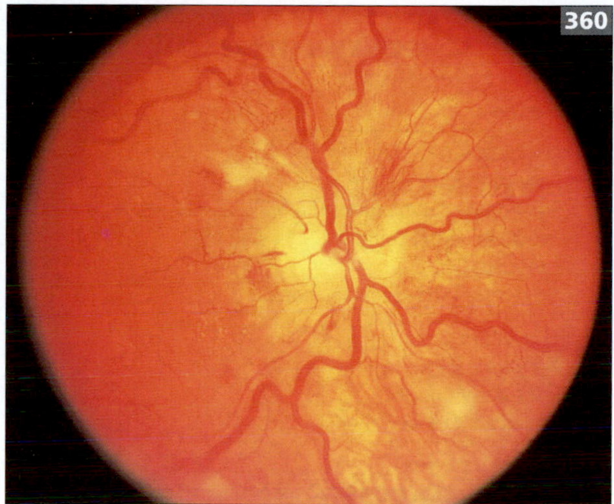

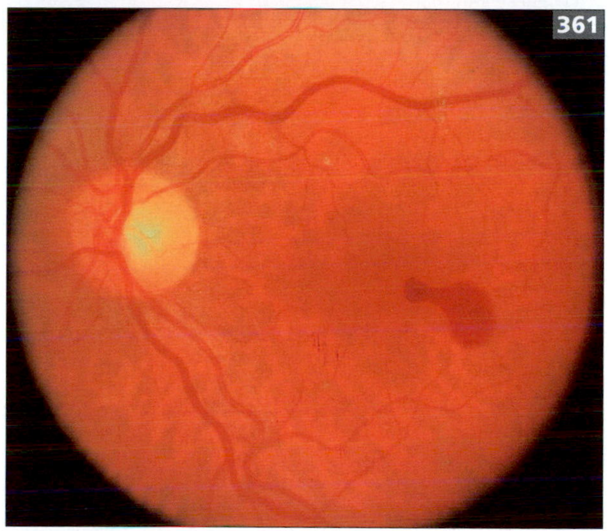

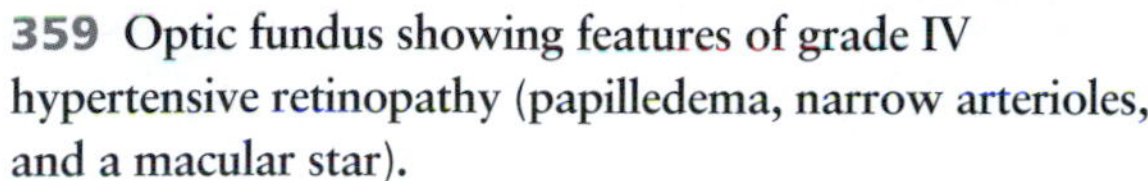

359 Optic fundus showing features of grade IV hypertensive retinopathy (papilledema, narrow arterioles, and a macular star).

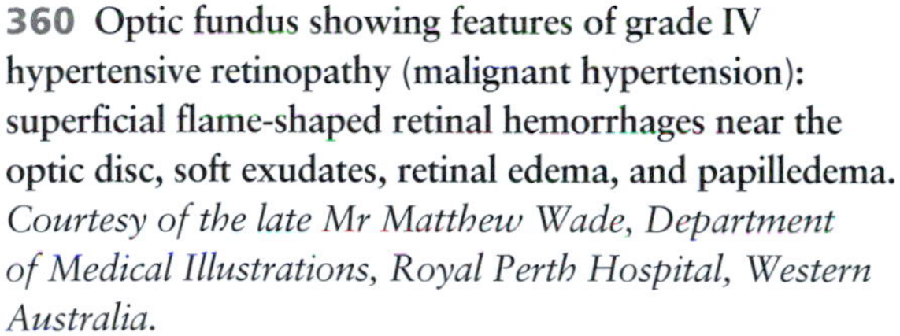

360 Optic fundus showing features of grade IV hypertensive retinopathy (malignant hypertension): superficial flame-shaped retinal hemorrhages near the optic disc, soft exudates, retinal edema, and papilledema. *Courtesy of the late Mr Matthew Wade, Department of Medical Illustrations, Royal Perth Hospital, Western Australia.*

361 Ocular fundus showing a retinal hemorrhage due to thrombocytopenia in a patient who presented with a symptomatic intracerebral hemorrhage.

onset of ICH. Clearly, this presentation of cerebral amyloid angiopathy poses a difficult challenge to clinicians because recurrent neurologic events without apparent blood on CT of the head will often lead to a progressive increase in dosages of antithrombotic medications. This can have profoundly adverse consequences in patients prone to ICH, such as those with cerebral amyloid angiopathy, and thus the MRI gradient echo sequence (see investigations, below) should be considered in patients with an appropriate clinical scenario: an older patient (>65 years) with or without a history of dementia, and possibly previous lobar hemorrhage.

Cavernous malformations in the brain are often asymptomatic – even if complicated by hemorrhage, which is mostly minute. If a cavernous malformation is symptomatic, epileptic seizures are at least as common a manifestation as hemorrhage. The third main clinical syndrome is that of a transient or permanent focal deficit corresponding to a brain region or a cranial nerve, sometimes associated with an expanding cavernous malformation. Not unexpectedly this occurs relatively often with lesions in the brainstem. The deficits usually develop in a gradual fashion but may remit, mimicking multiple sclerosis, or they may cause myoclonus of the face or palate.

Subarachnoid hemorrhage

Risk factors for aneurysm formation that may be present include cigarette smoking, hypertension, alcohol consumption, personal or family history of SAH, polycystic kidney disease, and heritable connective tissue diseases (Ehlers–Danlos syndrome type IV, pseudoxanthoma elasticum, fibromuscular dysplasia). The neurologic examination findings sometimes provide a clue to the site of the SAH and ruptured aneurysm (see *Table 55*).

TABLE 56 **SCANDINAVIAN STROKE SCALE**

Function	Score
Consciousness:	
• Fully conscious	6
• Somnolent; can be woken to full consciousness	4
• Reacts to verbal command, but is not fully conscious	2
• No reaction to verbal command	0
Eye movement:	
• No gaze palsy	4
• Gaze palsy present	2
• Conjugate eye deviation	0
Arm, motor power:*	
• Raises arm with normal strength	6
• Raises arm with reduced strength	5
• Raises arm with flexion in elbow	4
• Can move, but not against gravity	2
• Paralysis	0
Hand, motor power:*	
• Normal strength	6
• Reduced strength in full range	4
• Some movement, fingertips do not reach palm	2
• Paralysis	0
Leg, motor power:*	
• Normal strength	6
• Raises straight leg with reduced strength	5
• Raises leg with flexion of knee	4
• Can move, but not against gravity	2
• Paralysis	0
Orientation:	
• Correct for time, place, and person	6
• Two of these	4
• One of these	2
• Completely disorientated	0
Speech:	
• No aphasia	10
• Limited vocabulary or incoherent speech	6
• More than yes/no, but not longer sentences	3
• Only yes/no or less	0
Facial palsy:	
• None/dubious	2
• Present	0
Gait:	
• Walks 5 m without aids	12
• Walks with aids	9
• Walks with help of another person	6
• Sits without support	3
• Bedridden/wheelchair	0
Total	__

*Motor power is assessed only on the affected side.

TABLE 57 **NATIONAL INSTITUTES OF HEALTH STROKE SCALE (NIHSS)**

Item	Description	Points available
1a	Level of consciousness – general	3
1b	Level of consciousness – questions	2
1c	Level of consciousness – commands	2
2	Gaze	2
3	Visual fields	3
4	Facial palsy	3
5	Motor – arms	8
6	Motor – legs	8
7	Ataxia	2
8	Sensory	2
9	Language (dysphasia)	3
10	Dysarthria	2
11	Inattention (neglect)	2
Total		42

Full details available at:
(http://www.ninds.nih.gov/doctors/NIH_Stroke_Scale.pdf)

TABLE 58 **MODIFIED RANKIN SCORE**

Grade	Description
0	No symptoms at all
1	No significant disability, despite symptoms: able to carry out all usual duties and activities
2	Slight disability: unable to carry out all previous activities, but able to look after own affairs with assistance
3	Moderate disability: requiring some help but able to walk without assistance
4	Moderate to severe disability: unable to walk without assistance, and unable to attend to own bodily needs without assistance
5	Severe disability: bedridden, incontinent, and requiring constant nursing care and attention
6	Death

TABLE 59 **FIRST-LINE (ROUTINE) DIAGNOSTIC TESTS FOR SUSPECTED TIA OR STROKE**

Test	Potential indications and findings associated with TIA or stroke	Notes
CT or MRI brain scan	• Suspected TIA or stroke • Exclude nonvascular causes of focal neurologic symptoms • Distinguish ischemic and hemorrhagic stroke • May help stratify risk of hemorrhagic transformation of fresh brain infarct associated with early thrombolysis • Ascertain likely cause of the ischemic or hemorrhagic stroke from the site and size of the lesion(s)	
Full blood count	Anemia, disseminated intravascular coagulation, myeloproliferative disorders, sickle cell disease, thrombocytopenia, thrombocytosis, thrombotic thrombocytopenic purpura	
Erythrocyte sedimentation rate	Inflammatory arteriopathies (temporal arteritis, etc.), and infective endocarditis	Nonspecific but sensitive; raised in >60% of patients with infective endocarditis
Biochemistry profile (glucose, urea, electrolytes, creatinine, calcium)	Hypoglycemia, hyperglycemia, hyponatremia, hypernatremia, hypocalcemia, hypercalcemia	Hypoglycemia is the most likely of these to cause focal neurologic symptoms
Electrocardiography	Arrhythmias (e.g. atrial fibrillation/flutter), ischemia, myocardial infarction, left ventricular hypertrophy	
Urinalysis	Proteinuria, albuminuria, hematuria	Bacteremia in the elderly from urinary tract infections may produce neurologic findings

Severity

The level of consciousness can be assessed with the Glasgow Coma Scale (GCS). The GCS was originally designed to assess the neurologic severity of head injuries. Its main limitations in stroke are when there is aphasia or a motor deficit (the best motor response should then be evaluated in any nonparetic limbs). The severity of the neurologic deficit is more thoroughly assessed by the Scandinavian Stroke Scale (*Table 56*) and the National Institutes of Health Stroke Scale (NIHSS) (*Table 57*) which both measure and score neurologic impairments.

The NIHSS quantifies different categories of impairments, including consciousness. It is widely used in monitoring stroke patients and as a selection criterion for thrombolytic therapy. Although it takes only minutes, is reliable and reproducible, and can be performed by a non-neurologist, some training is still required.

The severity of the stroke can also be assessed by the Modified Rankin Scale score (mRS) which quantifies disability, and to some extent, handicap (*Table 58*). Other scores of disability and handicap include the Barthel index, functional independence measure, stroke impact scale, and SF-36.

INVESTIGATIONS

FIRST-LINE INVESTIGATIONS

The decision to investigate, and the choice of investigations, is primarily driven by the need to answer a specific clinical question relevant to the diagnosis or management of the patient. However, it is also based on the patient's symptoms, age, pre- and post-stroke condition, willingness to accept any risks, costs or inconvenience associated with the investigations, and the cost-effectiveness of the investigations.

All patients with TIA or stroke in whom active management is being considered should undergo at least the following first-line investigations (*Table 59*), even if the clinical assessment strongly suggests a common cause.

Tip

▶ *Do not presume that the results of investigations will necessarily be any more sensitive or specific than the clinical findings. Investigations contribute most to the diagnostic process when set in a proper clinical context and when they take the pre-test probability of the disorder to be diagnosed into account.*

Brain imaging (CT or MRI scan)

- The purpose of immediate imaging of the brain is to:
- Exclude nonvascular causes of the suspected TIA or stroke (e.g. tumor [362–364], subdural hematoma [365, 366]).
- Distinguish intracranial hemorrhage (367) from cerebral infarction (368). The CT must be done within about 1 week of stroke onset otherwise the CT features of acute hemorrhage (high signal intensity – whiteness) may resolve (in the same way that a bruise resolves under the skin) and all that remains are CT changes of low signal density (blackness) in the area of previous hemorrhage, that can be misinterpreted as previous infarction.
- Ascertain the location, nature and size of early ischemic changes in patients being considered for early thrombolysis, as some of these features may be associated with response to reperfusion therapy (research is ongoing).
- Ascertain the likely cause of the ischemic or hemorrhagic stroke (from the site[s] and shape of the infarct[s] or hemorrhage[s]).

CT of the head

Noncontrast CT of the head remains the first diagnostic standard for suspected transient ischemic attack or acute stroke. This is because it is widely and rapidly available, and has near perfect sensitivity for acute intracranial hemorrhage, the most important differential diagnosis to ischemic stroke. Hemorrhage in the brain is visible immediately on CT (i.e. it doesn't take a few hours to develop its characteristic white appearance), but the distinct appearance of the fresh hemorrhage changes with time, disappearing slowly in the subsequent days to weeks, depending on the size of the hemorrhage. Thereafter the hemorrhage appears as a region of low density on CT scan, which can be mistaken for an old infarct.

In acute ischemic stroke, a number of early signs have been described (e.g. density of the middle cerebral artery or one of its branches in the Sylvian fissure, obscuration of the lentiform nucleus, loss of the insular ribbon, effacement of cortical sulci, compression of the frontal horn of the lateral venticle) (369). The prognostic value of these signs (and their size) in stratifying risk of hemorrhagic transformation of the infarct, and response to thrombolytic therapy, continues to be investigated. Formalized CT scores have been developed, such as the Alberta Stroke Program Early CT Score (ASPECTS).

CT is limited however in identifying early evidence of ischemia, small areas of ischemic injury, and ischemic lesions in the posterior fossa. The sensitivity of CT in acute ischemic stroke varies, depending on the imaging features of infarction, examination time from clinical onset, study population, and other variables. Sensitivity estimates range from 12% to 92%, with an overall estimate of 40–60% for the 6-hour time window. Among patients with suspected TIA, the CT reveals alternative explanations for the transient neurologic symptoms in about 1.2% of the patients.

The presence of a normal CT brain scan therefore does not necessarily mean that the patient has not had a stroke. A patient with a clinical diagnosis of stroke, and an early CT brain scan which is either normal, or shows a relevant hypodense lesion consistent with infarction, is classified as having an ischemic stroke.

Tip

▶ *Hemorrhagic transformation of an infarct can occur very early after stroke onset and makes the infarct look just like an intracerebral hemorrhage on brain CT or MR.*

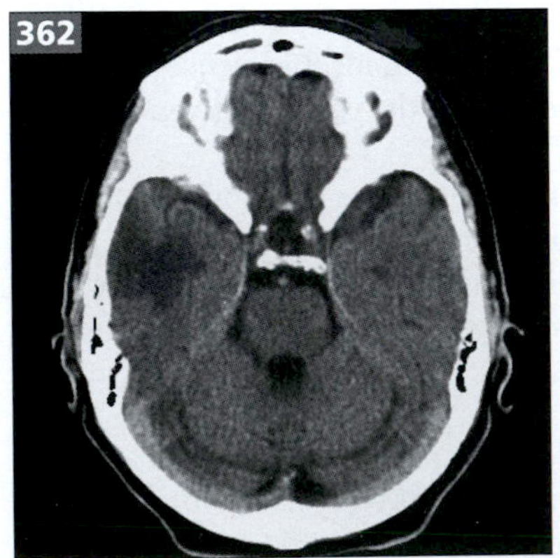

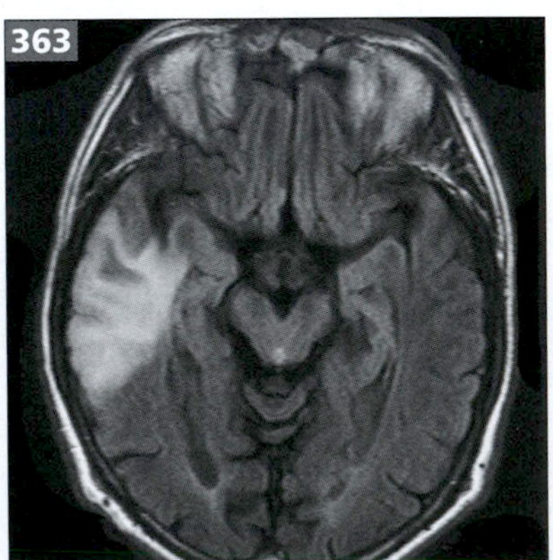

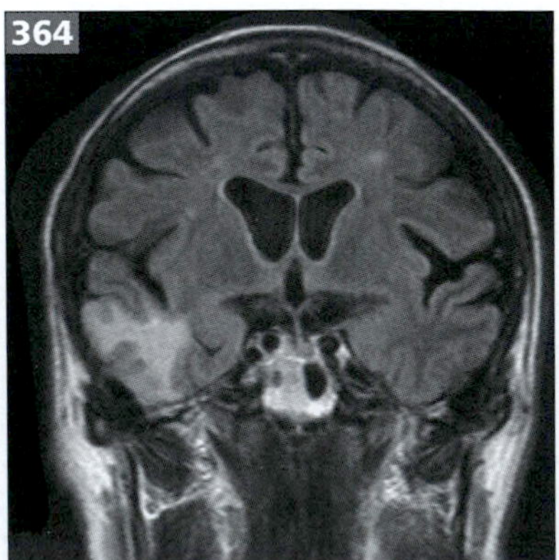

362–364 CT brain scan, axial plane, showing a low density in the right temporal lobe that was initially mistaken for infarction, but was shown histologically to be tumor; MRI brain scan axial plane (363) and coronal plane (364), showing the same lesion.

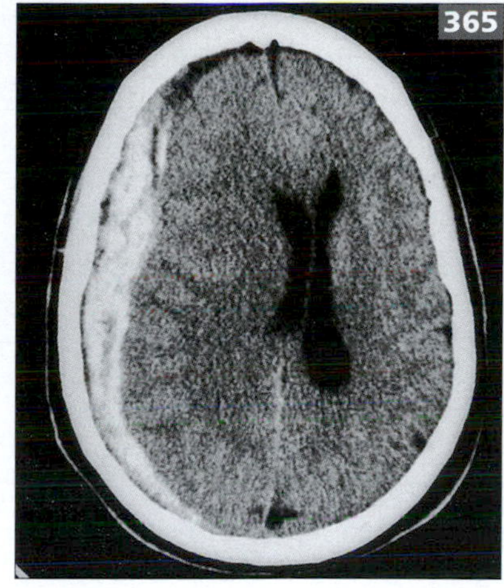

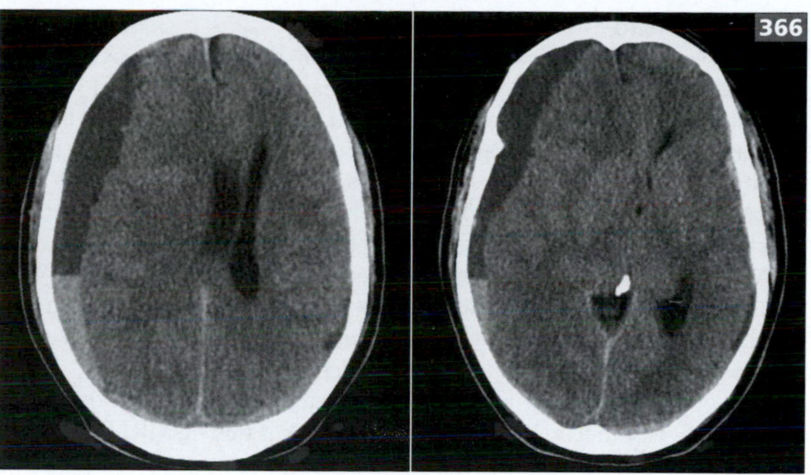

365 Plain cranial CT scan, showing a recent subdural hematoma as a high density (white) area over the right hemisphere, causing mass effect with compression of the right lateral ventricle and midline shift.

366 Bilateral acute on chronic subdural hematoma, right larger than left. Note the layer of higher density sediment posteriorly, indicating some recent hemorrhage.

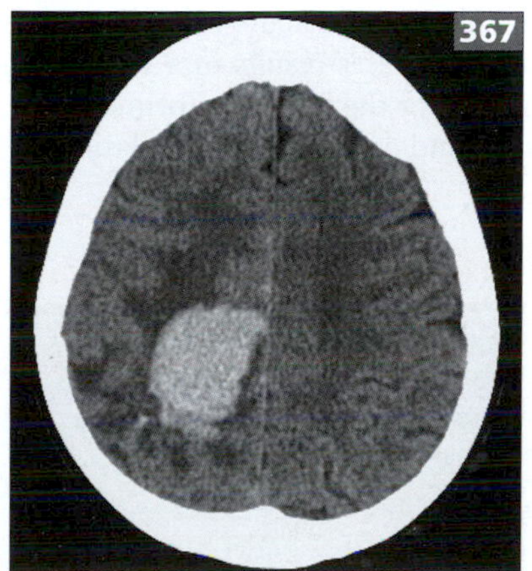

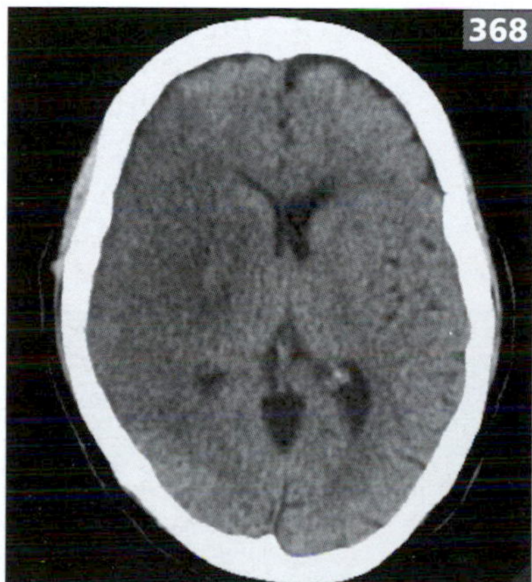

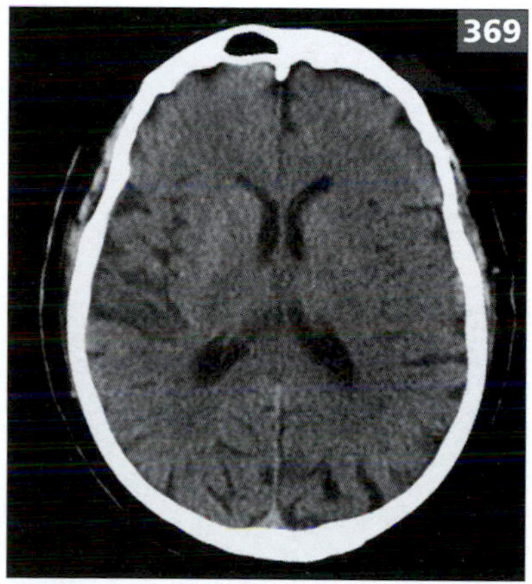

367 Plain CT brain scan, showing an area of high signal intensity, consistent with fresh hemorrhage, in the right parasagittal posterior frontal lobe.

368 Plain CT brain scan, showing an area of low signal intensity, consistent with fresh infarction, in the right frontal and temporal lobes (middle cerebral artery territory).

369 Plain CT brain scan, at 3 hours after onset of symptoms of right hemiparesis and dysphasia, showing obscuration of the left lentiform nucleus, loss of the left insular ribbon, and effacement of cortical sulci over the left hemisphere, consistent with fresh infarction, in the left frontal and temporal lobes (middle cerebral artery territory).

MRI of the head

MRI has significant advantages over CT, in that it improves sensitivity and specificity of the diagnosis of TIA and stroke, particularly acute infarction (**370**). For the diagnosis of stroke, CT brain scan has a sensitivity of about 26% (20–32%) whereas MRI brain a sensitivity of about 83% (78–88%)[24, 25]. MRI is also more effective for identifying other pathologies. For example, appropriate MRI sequences can help diagnose intracerebral hemorrhage months or even years after the event when the CT shows only a hypodense area indistinguishable from an infarct (**371**). This is because the characteristic signal changes of parenchymal hemorrhage due to hemosiderin formation persist indefinitely. The only drawback is that not all hematomas form hemosiderin during their resolution and therefore not all hematomas are discernible as such on MRI performed late after the stroke.

However, there are limitations to the widespread use of MRI, which include availability, cost, patient tolerance, and increased time needed for the evaluation. As the availability of MRI increases, it is likely that it will eventually become the standard for evaluation of patients with stroke and TIA, in developed countries at least.

Gadolinium contrast

If nonvascular pathologies are suspected, MRI should be ordered with gadolinium contrast to increase the sensitivity for blood–brain barrier breakdown, which can be seen with mass lesions or inflammatory processes. An acute brain infarct will enhance with contrast injection, beginning approximately 3 days after the injury, and may continue to enhance for many weeks. Using the information from DWI, ADC, and contrast-enhanced images will often help to determine the timing of the injury if this is not clear from the medical history.

Diffusion-weighted imaging (DWI)

MRI DWI should be considered superior to noncontrast CT scan for the diagnosis of acute ischemic stroke in patients presenting within 12 hours of symptom onset. MRI DWI measures the net movement of water in tissue due to random (Brownian) molecular motion of water[26].

Within minutes to a few hours after arterial occlusion and the onset of acute ischemia, failure of the oxygen-dependent sodium–potassium ATPase pump in cell membranes leads to a disruption in membrane ionic homeostasis and restricted diffusion of water molecules in and out of cell membranes. In acute infarction, the reduced diffuction of free water results in a reduction of the ADC in the region of the ischemia (primarily in the intracellular space) and an excess accumulation of

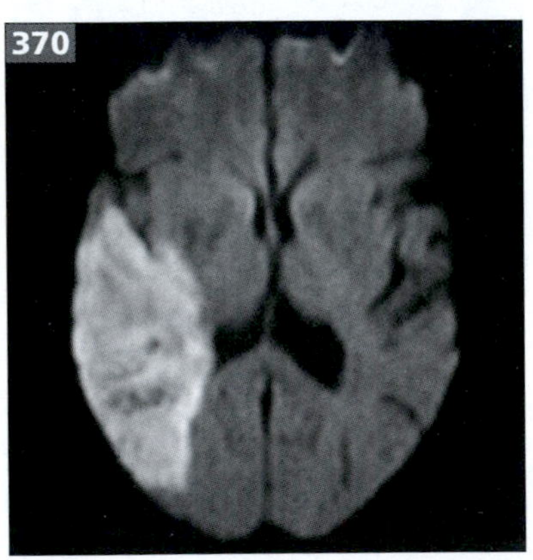

370 MRI DWI brain, axial plane, showing restricted diffusion due to cytotoxic edema caused by recent infarction in the right temporal lobe.

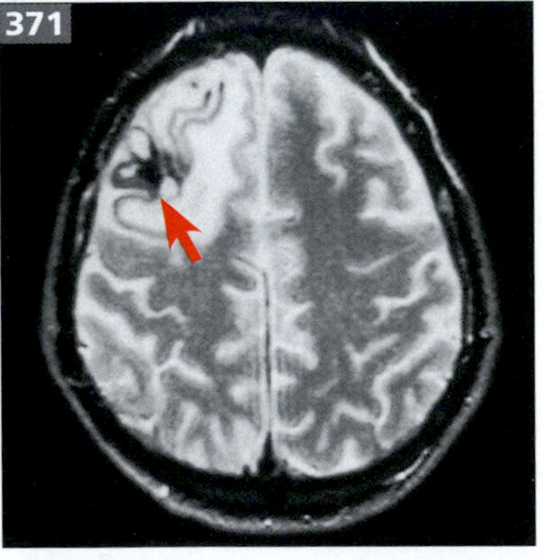

371 T2-weighted MRI of a patient 1 year after a severe head injury. The black areas in the right frontal lobe (arrow) are hemosiderin, indicating previous brain hemorrhage – in this instance traumatic. The black areas will persist indefinitely and are quite specific for hemorrhage, thus MRI can be used to identify hemorrhage a long time after the event, when CT cannot.

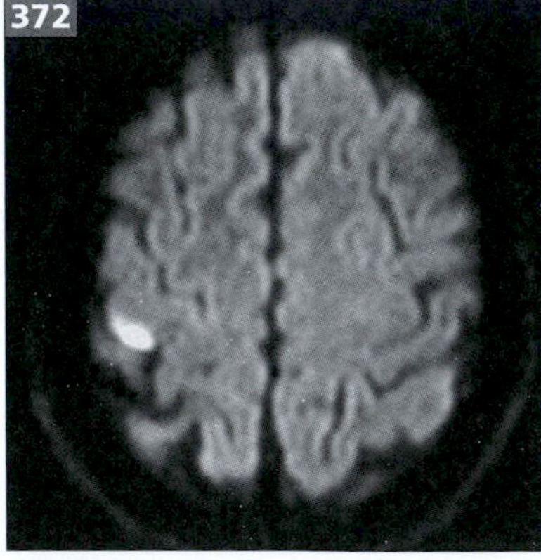

372 MRI DWI brain, axial plane, showing small area of increased signal due to restricted diffusion in the motor cortex of the right cerebral hemisphere in a patient who experienced transient left hand weakness for 1 hour.

intracellular water (cytotoxic edema). This area appears as a relative dark signal in the territory of the ischemia on the ADC map (see **321**, right) and as a bright signal on DWI, after combination with the T2 sequence (see **321**, left); i.e. the DWI sequence is created from a combination of the T2 sequence and the ADC map.

It is important to compare the DWI sequence with the ADC map to confirm acute ischemia. One important pitfall in interpretation of the DWI sequence includes 'T2 shine-through', in which a bright signal on the T2 image (from a subacute or older lesion) results in a falsely bright signal on DWI. A lack of a corresponding dark signal on the ADC confirms this artifact. Therefore, to differentiate acute from subacute or older lesions (T2 shine-through), DWI is used in conjunction with T2-weighted images and ADC maps.

Decreases in the ADC and increased signal on DWI studies are thought to represent irreversible ischemia in most instances. The sensitivity and specificity of this technique in the detection of acute ischemia are 88–100% and 86–100% respectively.

The value of the ADC decreases from within 30 minutes of acute infarction and reaches a nadir at about 3 days. As the infarct evolves, free water diffusion increases as cells lyse and release fluid into the extracellular compartment and the permeability of vessels increases. Hence the value of the ADC increases and equals that of normal brain (pseudonormalization) before becoming abnormally high. An acute infarct, which appears bright on DWI, will therefore progressively fade after 10–14 days, and diffusion will transiently pseudonormalize and then eventually become increased on the ADC image. In chronic ischemia the value of the ADC remains abnormally high owing to the largely extracellular water content, and diffusion-weighted images dark.

MRI DWI is particularly helpful in the assessment of patients with transient focal neurologic symptoms that have resolved and in whom it is uncertain whether the symptoms were really focal or not, and whether they were ischemic in nature from the patient's history alone[26] (**372**). Although a negative DWI does not exclude a TIA, a positive DWI in a clinically relevant area of the brain strongly supports the diagnosis of TIA (indeed, the diagnosis of the event then becomes a stroke, if the DWI is positive, according to the American Stroke Association criteria – see beginning of chapter).

Patients with TIA whose symptoms last longer than 1 hour or who have motor weakness or aphasia are more likely to have a positive lesion on DWI (*Table 60*). A negative MRI or DWI also does not exclude the diagnosis of stroke (*Table 61*). Among patients with minor stroke, one-third have a negative MRI and DWI, particularly among patients with less severe stroke, of younger age, female gender, and increased time from stroke onset to scan.

TABLE 60 **FREQUENCY OF DWI ABNORMALITY IN PATIENTS WITH TRANSIENT NEUROLOGIC EPISODES OF DIFFERENT DURATIONS**

Duration of symptoms (hr)	**DWI hyperintensity** (%)
0–1	33.6
1–2	29.5
2–3	39.5
3–6	30.0
6–12	51.1
12–18	50.0
18–24	49.5

Pooled data from 10 MRI studies enrolling 818 patients.

TABLE 61 **CAUSES OF AN INACCURATE MRI DWI DIAGNOSIS OF TIA**

False-positive DWI diagnosis of TIA (at least 10%)
- Nonischemic cause of DWI hyperintensity (e.g. seizure focus, brain abscess, herpes simplex encephalitis, brain trauma, and rarely brain tumors [but usually due to T2 shine-through])
- Neurologically asymptomatic cause of DWI hyperintensity
- Chronic, persistent cause of DWI hyperintensity (i.e. old lesion)

False-negative DWI diagnosis of TIA (at least 10%)
- Very early imaging after onset of ischemia (i.e. too early)
- Short-duration TIA (insufficient time to cause early ischemic changes on DWI)
- Penumbral ischemia (ischemia is sufficient to cause neurologic symptoms but insufficient to cause failure of the sodium–potassium ATPase pump in the neuronal cell membranes)
- Ischemic region too small to image
- Ischemic region too difficult to image (e.g. in brainstem)
- Confounding background lesion(s)
- Late imaging after onset of ischemia (e.g. >2 weeks after resolution of symptoms)

ATP: adenosine triphosphate.

Baseline DWI volume may also be useful in predicting baseline clinical stroke severity and final lesion volume in anterior-circulation stroke syndromes.

Perfusion-weighted imaging

Perfusion-weighted imaging (PWI) allows the measurement of capillary perfusion. The method most commonly used in clinical practice and research is the dynamic susceptibility contrast-enhanced technique, in which paramagnetic contrast agent is injected as an IV bolus and the signal change is tracked by susceptibility-weighted, T2*-weighted magnetic resonance (MR) sequences.

Relative cerebrovascular hemodynamic measures reflecting cerebral blood volume, mean transit time, time to peak, and cerebral blood flow (CBF) can be derived from the MR signal intensity-over-time curve in a semi-quantitative fashion. Parameter maps display the area of critically reduced perfusion.

There is insufficient evidence to support or refute the value of PWI in diagnosing acute ischemic stroke. However, it is hypothesized that patients with a larger perfusion than diffusion deficit on MRI (e.g. a PWI:DWI ratio >1.2) may be those with a surviving ischemic penumbra who are likely to benefit from early reperfusion therapy. Ongoing clinical trials are examining this hypothesis.

Gradient echo T2-weighted susceptibility images

The gradient echo T2-weighted susceptibility images can also be a helpful sequence in defining the cause of focal neurologic symptoms. This sequence has been demonstrated to have sensitivity equivalent to that of CT for acute hemorrhage and is more sensitive for previous hemorrhage (373–377).

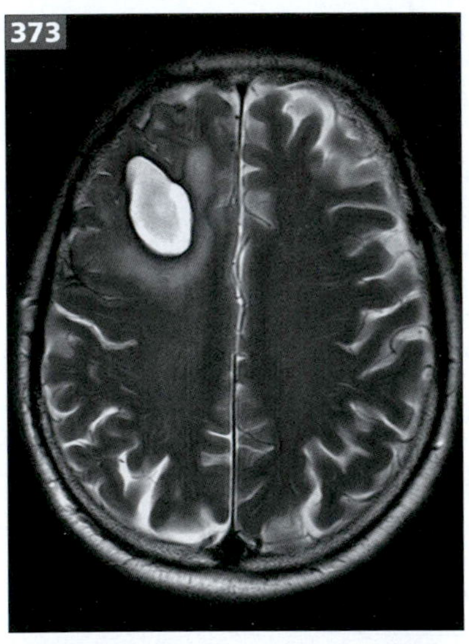

373–374 MRI brain, axial plane, gradient echo T2-weighted susceptibility images showing acute hemorrhage in the right anterior frontal lobe.

375–376 MRI brain, axial plane, gradient echo T2-weighted susceptibility images showing acute hemorrhage in the right posterior frontal lobe.

377 MRI brain, axial plane, gradient echo T2-weighted susceptibility images showing previous small hemorrhages in the right posterior parietal lobe.

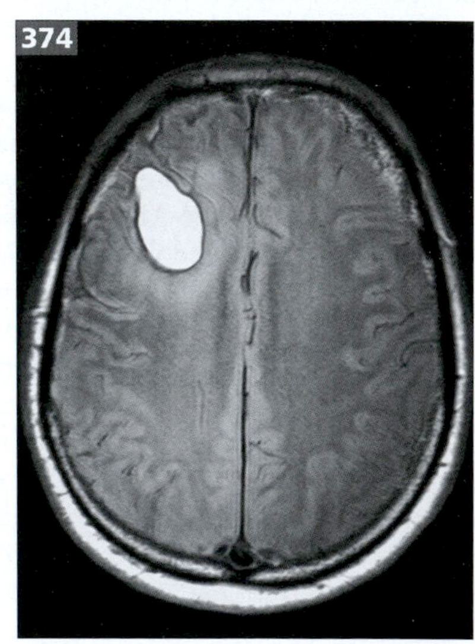

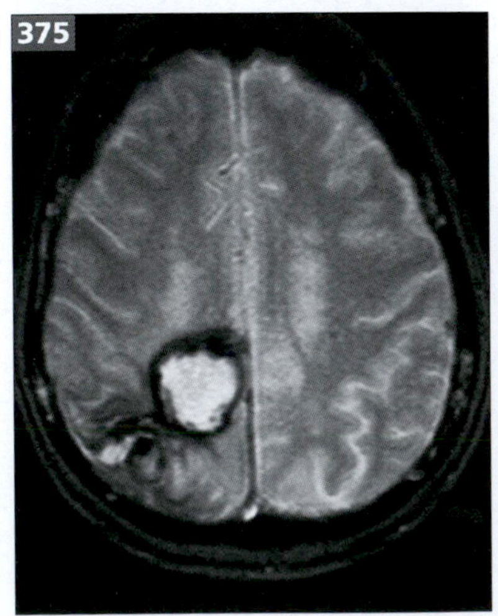

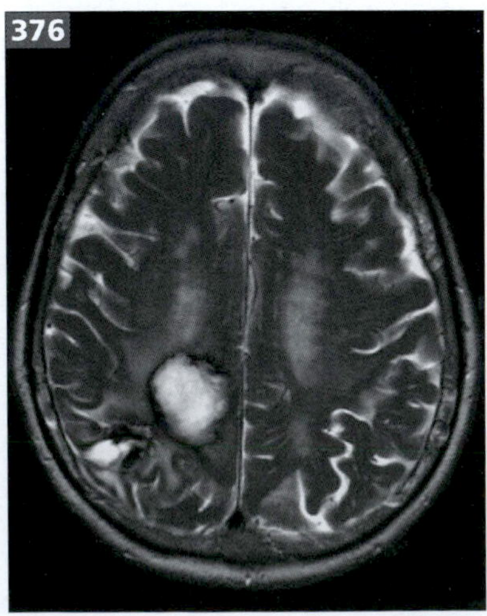

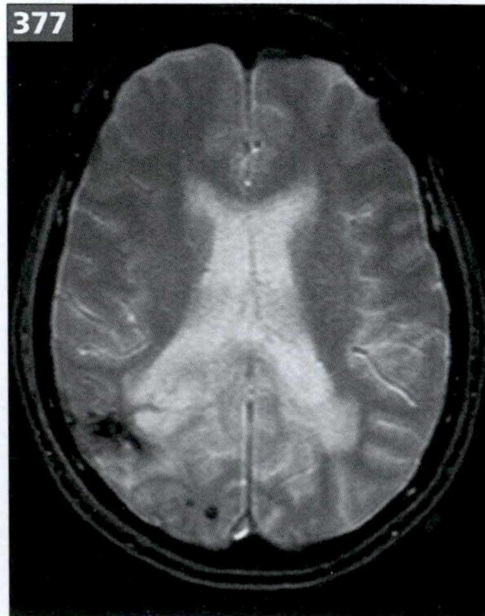

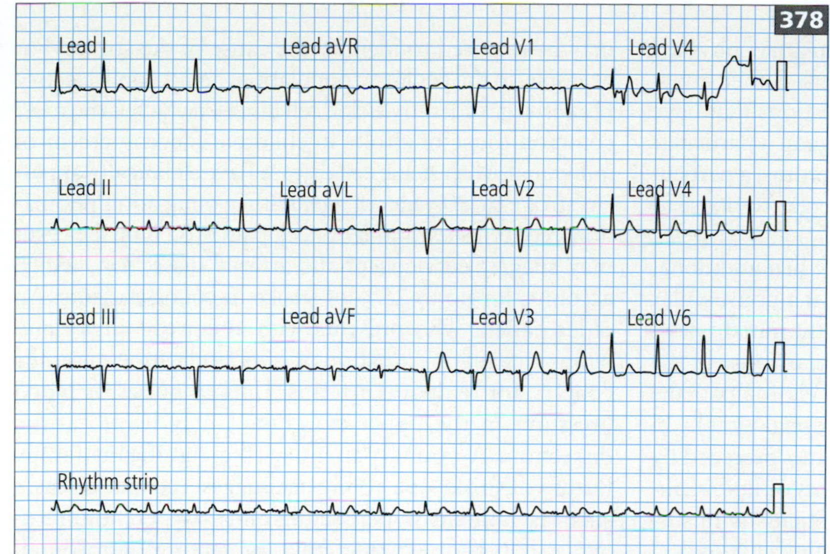

378 Electrocardiograph showing atrial fibrillation.

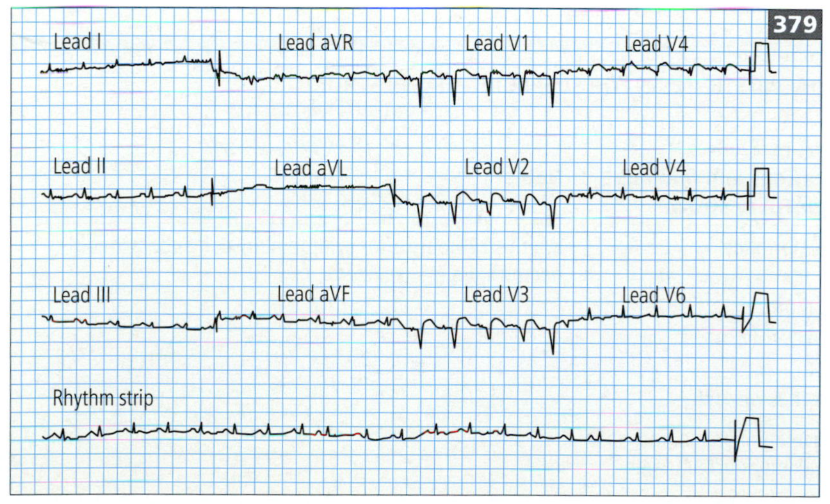

379 Electrocardiograph of a patient with a recent acute anteroseptal myocardial infarction, showing sinus tachycardia, and Q waves and ST segment elevation in leads V1–V3.

Electrocardiography

All patients with suspected TIA or stroke should undergo ECG, as it may reveal AF (378) or flutter, evidence of previous, recent, or ongoing myocardial ischemia (379), and evidence of left ventricular hypertrophy. The American Stroke Association also recommends checking cardiac enzyme levels in all patients with acute ischemic stroke.

SECOND-LINE INVESTIGATIONS

After assessing the patient's medical history, physical examination, and first-line investigations, futher investigation may be required to address questions that have arisen from the initial assessment and suggest a particular nonvascular cause of the neurologic symptoms, a particular cause of the TIA or stroke, or a particular response to therapy or prognosis.

Table 62 presents various scenarios when additional testing may be considered. For example, if a nonvascular cause of the symptoms is suggested from the initial assessment, tests that may identify a nonvascular cause of the symptoms include serum ammonia levels for patients with hepatic encephalopathy; electroencephalography in patients with transient altered mental status preceded by positive phenomena, such as flashing lights or limb shaking; and arterial blood gas levels for patients with suspected hypercarbia or significant unexplained hypoxia.

For patients in whom the diagnosis of stroke and its pathologic subtype is established, further investigations may be required to identify the cause of the stroke. For example, in the pediatric population, hemoglobin electrophoresis may identify sickle cell disease, which is the most common cause of stroke in children. Eleven percent of individuals with sickle cell disease have a clinically apparent stroke by 20 years of age. In the young adult population, recent neck trauma or neck pain preceding the event may suggest cervicocephalic arterial dissection, which accounts for up to 25% of stroke in young patients. An older patient who presents with amaurosis fugax and temporal pain on palpation or jaw claudication raises the concern for temporal arteritis. Uneven pulses or blood pressures in the upper extremities may herald aortic dissection. A young patient with a significant family history of stroke at a young age suggests genetic diseases such as familial hypercoagulability, hypercholesterolemia, hyperhomocysteinemia, or cerebral autosomal-dominant arteriopathy with subcortical infarcts and leukoencephalopathy. In patients with a history of recurrent

TABLE 62 **SECOND-LINE (OPTIONAL) DIAGNOSTIC TESTS FOR SUSPECTED TIA OR STROKE** *(selected indications)*

Test	Potential indications and findings associated with TIA or stroke	Notes
Cerebrospinal fluid evaluation	Subarachnoid hemorrhage	Wait 6–12 hours after symptom onset if subarachnoid hemorrhage is suspected
	CNS and systemic infection	
	Multiple sclerosis	
	Primary CNS or other vasculitis	
Coagulation profile: prothrombin time, aPTT, international normalized ratio	Indicated if intracerebral or subarachnoid hemorrhage or taking anticoagulants	
	May also identify a hypercoagulable state such as lupus anticoagulant (prolonged aPTT)	
	Useful to establish baseline before anticoagulation or thrombolysis	
Fasting cholesterol/lipid and glucose concentrations	Hyperlipidemic and diabetic states	Important for risk factor identification in patients with ischemic stroke or TIA
Duplex carotid and vertebral ultrasonography	For patients with embolic carotid and vertebrobasilar territory ischemic events	Carotid ultrasound is a good screening technique for imaging the carotid bifurcation and measuring blood velocities, but it has limited ability to image the extracranial vasculature proximal or distal to the bifurcation
	Atherosclerotic stenosis/occlusion, dissection as possible causes of symptoms	The use of carotid ultrasound as the sole test may lead to erroneous determination of the degree of stenosis, which may have implications in terms of medical and surgical therapy

idiopathic stroke/transient ischemic attack or those with other previous thromboembolic events (deep venous thrombosis or pulmonary embolism), an evaluation for a hypercoagulable state is prudent once the primary evaluation is performed. A reasonable hypercoagulable evaluation for arterial thrombosis includes anticardiolipin antibodies, lupus anticoagulant, and β_2 glycoprotein I antibodies. If a PFO is identified and no other mechanism of TIA or stroke is apparent, additional studies to identify venous hypercoagulable conditions, including protein C or S deficiency, factor V Leiden, prothrombin gene mutation, antithrombin III deficiency, and elevated homocysteine concentration, may be performed and a source ascertained (e.g ultrasound of the leg and pelvic veins). Once the condition is identified, a hematologist should be consulted for preventive strategies.

In patients with CVT, routine blood studies should be performed, including a complete blood count, chemistry panel, prothrombin time, and activated partial thromboplastin time. A normal D-dimer level according to a sensitive immunoassay or rapid enzyme-linked immunosorbent assay (ELISA) may be considered to help identify patients with low probability of CVT. If there is a strong clinical suspicion of CVT, a normal D-dimer level should not preclude further evaluation. Screening for potential prothrombotic conditions that may predispose a person to CVT (e.g. use of contraceptives, underlying inflammatory disease, infectious process) is recommended in the initial clinical assessment. Testing for prothrombotic conditions, including protein C, protein S, antithrombin deficiency, APS, prothrombin G20210A mutation, and factor V Leiden, can be beneficial for the management of patients with CVT. Testing for protein C, protein S, and antithrombin deficiency is generally indicated 2–4 weeks after completion of anticoagulation. There is a very limited value of testing in the acute setting or in patients taking warfarin.

TABLE 62 continued

Test	Potential indications and findings associated with TIA or stroke	Notes
Transcranial Doppler ultrasonography (TCD)	Ongoing emboli detection, intracranial stenoses, right-to-left shunting	TCD is useful for monitoring the development of vasospasm in large vessels at the base of the brain and for determining major occlusive disease in those arteries, although CTA, MRA, and DSA are more accurate for occlusive/stenotic lesions. TCD is also useful for monitoring large brain vessels in patients with sickle cell disease
Magnetic resonance angiography (MRA)	Identify large vessel atherosclerotic stenosis, occlusion or dissection, vascular malformation or aneurysm	Contrast-enhanced (CE) MRA appears to be more sensitive and specific, and more accurate, than Doppler ultrasound alone for imaging the extracranial vasculature. However, it may overestimate degree of arterial stenosis Consequently, the addition of CE-MRA to the ultrasound evaluation still results in a misassignment to the surgical group in 17% of cases
		Cervical magnetization transfer MRI, with fat suppression and axial fat-saturated T1 images, is most sensitive for dissection
Computed tomographic angiography (CTA)	Identify large vessel stenosis/occlusion, dissection, or vascular malformation or aneurysm	Risks associated with radiation and contrast exposure. May underestimate degree of arterial stenosis. CTA is equal to, or better than, DSA for large aneurysms

TABLE 62 continued

Test	**Potential indications and findings associated with TIA or stroke**	**Notes**
Intra-arterial cerebral angiography (intra-arterial digital subtraction angiography [DSA])	Primary CNS and other medium and large vessel vasculitis, nonatherosclerotic arteriopathies (e.g. moyamoya syndrome); arteriovenous malformations; aneurysms May also be useful in patients with doubtful or contradictory findings with other vascular imaging techniques (ultrasound, MR or CT angiography)	Intra-arterial DSA remains the optimal technique for imaging the cerebral vasculature, particularly when making decisions about invasive therapies. In addition to providing information about a specific vascular lesion, DSA can provide valuable information about collateral flow, perfusion status, and other occult vascular lesions that may affect patient management. However, DSA is associated with a risk, albeit small (<1%), of serious complications, such as stroke or death
Abdominal and renal angiography	Polyarteritis nodosa	
Radiography of the chest	Cardiomegaly (large left atrial or ventricular size); aortic dissection; hilar lymphadenopathy (sarcoid)	Routinely recommended, but low yield
Transthoracic echocardiography	Indicated if embolic TIA or ischemic stroke, particularly if no other likely source, and if abnormal heart clinically, on ECG or on chest X-ray Findings include valve lesions, global or segmental left ventricular dysfunction, patent foramen ovale in young patients, spontaneous echo contrast, intracardiac tumors, and vegetations (endocarditis)	Images anterior/ventral portion of the heart (e.g. left ventricle) better than posterior portion of the heart (left atrium and appendage, ascending aorta and arch)
Transesophageal echocardiography	Cryptogenic stroke in young patients, aortic atheromatous disease, infective endocarditis. More sensitive than transthoracic echocardiography for cardiac sources of embolism, particularly in left atrium, interatrial septum, heart valves and aortic arch	Transesophageal echocardiography is the best imaging modality for infective endocarditis, particularly if prosthetic material is present Specificity for detecting vegetations, abscesses, or other evidence of infective endocarditis can approach 100% Serial studies should be performed if the initial diagnosis of endocarditis remains in doubt
Antinuclear antibodies, anti-dsDNA, ENAs, complement, ANCA, rheumatoid factor	Systemic lupus erythematosus, other connective tissue diseases, Wegener's granulomatosis, Churg–Strauss syndrome	A positive rheumatoid factor is potentially useful as a minor criterion for infective endocarditis
Lupus anticoagulant, anticardiolipin, and anti-β_2-glycoprotein antibodies	Antiphospholipid syndrome (cerebral ischemia in combination with deep venous thrombosis, recurrent miscarriage, livedo reticularis, cardiac valvular vegetations, thrombocytopenia and migraine)	The lupus anticoagulant assay detects immunoglobulins that cause prolonged clotting times *in vitro*, but are associated with thrombosis *in vivo* A positive lupus anticoagulant or high anticardiolipin antibody titre should be repeated 12 weeks later to meet the diagnostic criteria for the antiphospholipid syndrome, which are a) lupus anticoagulant, b) medium or high titre (>40 IgG or IgM phospholipid units [1 unit is 1 μg of antibody], or >99th centile) of IgG or IgM anticardiolipin antibody, or c) anti-β_2-glycoprotein I antibody in serum or plasma on two or more occasions, at least 12 weeks apart, measured by standardized enzyme-linked immunosorbent assay (ELISA)

TABLE 62 continued

Test	**Potential indications and findings associated with TIA or stroke**	**Notes**
Factor V Leiden, prothrombin gene G20210A mutations	Cerebral or deep venous thrombosis; specific mutations	Risk factors for cerebral, pelvic, and leg vein thromboses
Mitochondrial DNA (MELAS)	Ischemic stroke in a young person; arterial dissection; specific mutations	
NOTCH3 (CADASIL)		
GLA (Fabry's disease)		
CBS and others (homocystinuria)		
FBN1 (Marfan syndrome)		
COL3A1 (Ehlers–Danlos type IV)		
ABCC6 (Pseudoxanthoma elasticum)		
HBB (sickle cell disease)		
Hemoglobin electrophoresis; peripheral blood smear	Indicated if suspected sickle cell disease: patients of African origin or descent, pain crisis, anemia	
Antithrombin III, protein C, S, and Z deficiency	Cerebral or deep venous thrombosis; specific deficiencies	Antithrombin III and protein S and C evaluations should be undertaken after the acute phase. They are lowered by oral anticoagulants; antithrombin III concentrations are also lowered by nonfractionated heparin. Abnormally low concentrations in the acute phase, or in anticoagulated patients, should be confirmed 6 weeks later or when oral anticoagulants are stopped
Fibrinogen, D-dimer, Factor VIII, von Willebrand factor, plasminogen activator inhibitor-1, endogenous tissue plasminogen activator activity	Possible hematologic risk factors for ischemic stroke, TIA and cerebral venous thrombosis	
Alpha-galactosidase A activity	Fabry's disease	
High sensitivity C-reactive protein	Infective endocarditis, arteritis	Raised in over 60% of patients with infective endocarditis. Its role as a predictor of future risk of ischemic events is still being determined
Serum titres for syphilis, *Borrelia*, herpes zoster virus, hepatitis B and C virus, and HIV infection	Infective arteritis; specific infections	Prevalent infections and work-up may vary according to region
Blood cultures	Infective endocarditis	Positive blood cultures for *S. aureus*, *Streptococcus*, or *Enterococcus* species, or other serology and cardiac imaging (echocardiography) are the mainstays of definitive diagnosis

TABLE 62 continued

Test	Potential indications and findings associated with TIA or stroke	Notes
Cryoglobulins	Hepatitis C virus, other cryoglobulinemias	
Pathergy test	Behçet's disease	
Pregnancy test	Pregnancy changes levels of many clotting factors	Risk is greatest in the third trimester or immediately postpartum
Serum and urine drug toxicology concentrations	Suspected toxic encephalopathy; suspected infective endocarditis due to IV drug use; suspected toxic cause of stroke (e.g. amphetamines, cocaine, alcohol); therapeutic levels of prescribed drugs (phenytoin, etc.) and toxic levels of drugs of abuse	
Cardiac enzyme levels	Myocardial ischemia	Recent or ongoing myocardial infarction is a risk factor for cardioembolism
Serum ammonia level	Hepatic encephalopathy	
Plasma homocysteine and methionine concentrations	Hyperhomocystinemia	Risk factor for venous thrombosis, acute coronary syndrome, and stroke
Thyroid function test	Atrial fibrillation; cognitive impairment; hypothyroidism/hyperthyroidism	
Vitamin B12 level	Cognitive impairment; deficiency produces neurologic symptoms (paresthesias, ataxia, confusion)	
Electroencephalogram (EEG)	Unilateral slow wave activity, nonconvulsive or convulsive status epilepticus	
Ophthalmologic examination	Arteriopathies: genetic, inflammatory, infectious, retinocerebral	
	Retinopathies: hypertensive, diabetic, ischemic, hemorrhagic, Roth's spots	
	Subarachnoid hemorrhage (subhyaloid hemorrhages)	
Skin biopsy	CADASIL	
Muscle biopsy	MELAS	
Aortic positron emission tomography	Takayasu's arteritis	
Temporal artery biopsy	Giant cell arteritis	
Brain and meningeal biopsy	Primary CNS vasculitis	

ANCA: antineutrophil cytoplasmic antibody; aPTT: activated partial thromboplastin time; CADASIL: cerebral autosomal-dominant arteriopathy with subcortical infarcts and leukoencephalopthy; dsDNA: double-stranded deoxyribonucleic acid; ENA: extractable nuclear antigen; IG: immunoglobulin; MELAS: mitochondrial encephalomyopathy, lactic acidosis, and stroke-like episodes; MRI: magnetic resonance imaging.

Vascular imaging

Ultrasound

Extracranial ultrasound

Carotid and vertebral artery duplex studies consist of two elements: a B-mode evaluation that obtains an ultrasonographic image of the carotid artery and a Doppler mode evaluation that assesses the velocity and direction of blood flow within the artery.

Doppler measures that have been correlated with angiographic stenosis include ICA peak systolic velocity (PSV) and end-diastolic velocity, as well as ratios of ICA PSV and common carotid artery PSV[27]. The combination of a PSV >130 cm/s and an end-diastolic velocity >100 cm/s defines a stenosis of 70–99%. Other criteria for the diagnosis of a stenosis of 70–99% are an ICA PSV/common carotid artery PSV ratio >4.0; and a combination of PSV >210 cm/s, end-diastolic velocity >70 cm/s, ICA PSV/common carotid artery PSV ratio >3.0, and ICA end-diastolic velocity/common carotid artery end-diastolic velocity ratio >3.3 (*Table 63*).

Figures **380–382** display an example of a stenosis in the proximal ICA, with resulting increased velocity. Advantages of carotid Doppler ultrasonography include safety, relatively low cost, portability, and reasonable ability to detect a hemodynamically significant stenosis. Carotid Doppler ultrasonography has a sensitivity of 86% (95% confidence interval [CI] 84–89%) and a specificity of 87% (95% CI 84–90%) compared with the criterion standard of conventional angiography for the diagnosis of greater than 70% stenosis.

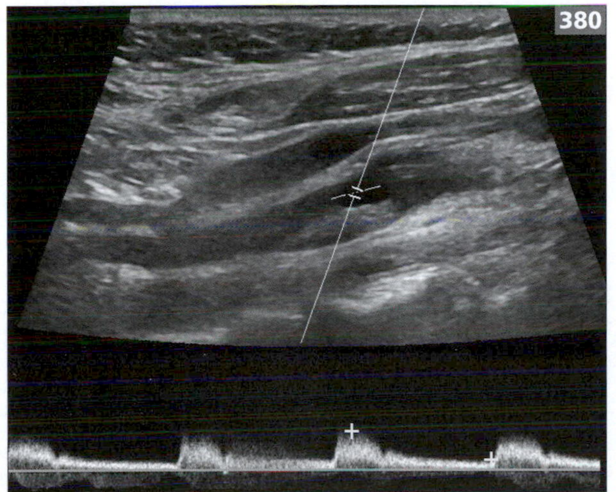

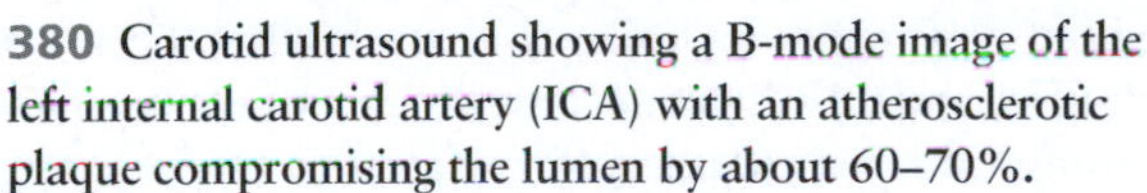

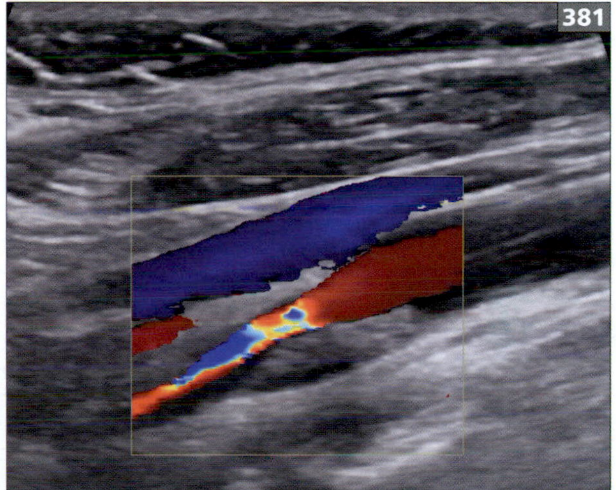

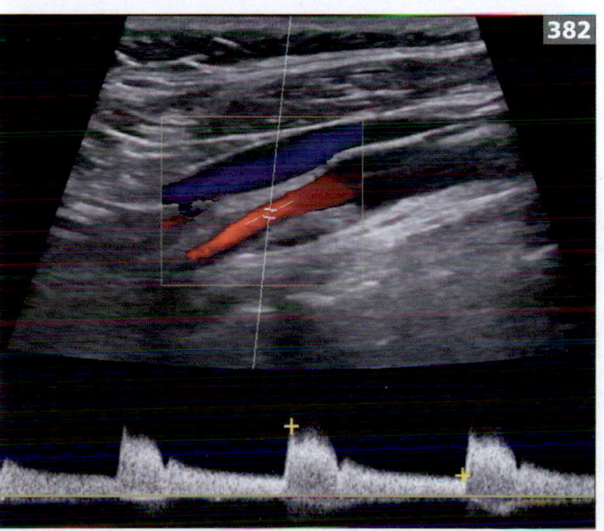

380 Carotid ultrasound showing a B-mode image of the left internal carotid artery (ICA) with an atherosclerotic plaque compromising the lumen by about 60–70%.

381 Colour flow carotid ultrasound of the image in 380, showing arterial flow in the left internal carotid artery (ICA) in red/yellow, and venous flow in the internal jugular vein in blue.

382 Colour flow carotid ultrasound of the image in 380, showing an atherosclerotic plaque compromising the lumen by about 60–70%, arterial flow in the left internal carotid artery (ICA) in red/yellow, and venous flow in the internal jugular vein in blue. Doppler ultrasound measured a peak systolic velocity of 181.8 cm/sec and end diastolic velocity of 53.7 cm/sec.

However, there are limitations. Doppler test results and diagnostic criteria are influenced by several factors, such as the equipment, the specific laboratory, and the technologist performing the test. In addition, factors such as contralateral occlusive disease have been associated with increased carotid volume flow that results in an overestimation of the severity of stenosis. Carotid ultrasonography is insensitive to dissection; it typically demonstrates very poor flow in the artery, giving a 'to and fro' high-resistance signal. Occasionally, the line of the dissection and a double lumen can be imaged. Another limitation of carotid ultrasound is that it evaluates only relatively short segments of the common carotid, carotid bifurcation, and proximal ICA. Thus, stenosis elsewhere along the vascular tree, particularly proximally, is not usually identified.

Therefore, although carotid ultrasound/Doppler imaging is a safe and inexpensive technique, its sensitivity and specificity appear less than that of other modalities (see below). In addition, carotid ultrasound only images a small region of the carotid and vertebral arteries in the neck. Although level A evidence indicates that it remains useful as a screening tool, level B studies indicate that carotid ultrasound should not be used as the sole methodology for the definitive diagnosis of carotid or vertebral artery disease.

Intracranial ultrasound

Transcranial Doppler ultrasonography (TCD) uses energy of 2–4 MHz to insonate cerebral vessels, typically through several bony windows in the skull. This technique can detect intracranial flow velocities, the direction of flow, vessel occlusion, the presence of emboli, and vascular reactivity. The arteries best evaluated are those at the base of the brain (MCA, anterior cerebral artery, carotid siphon, vertebral artery, and basilar artery) and the ophthalmic artery. The primary applications of TCD are to detect and quantify intracranial vessel stenosis, occlusion, collateral flow, embolic events, and cerebral vasospasm (particularly after SAH). TCD is also useful for monitoring patients with sickle cell disease who might benefit from transfusion therapy.

For the diagnosis of intracranial stenosis, compared with the standard criterion of conventional angiography, TCD has a positive predictive value of 36% and a negative predictive value of 86%. The sensitivity and specificity of TCD range from 70% to 90% and from 90% to 95%, respectively. Thus, it is a reasonable, if not perfect, screening tool to help rule out intracranial stenosis.

TABLE 63 **CLASSIFICATION OF ICA STENOSIS BY DOPPLER VELOCITY CRITERIA**

Velocity criteria (cm/sec)	**ICA stenosis** (%)
PSV 110	0–29
PSV 111–130	30–49
PSV >130, EDV 100	50–69
PSV >130, EDV >100	70–99

ICA: internal carotid artery; EDV: end-diastolic velocity; PSV: peak systolic velocity.

CT angiography

Computed tomography angiography (CTA) is an effective means of identifying large vessel stenosis. Given the usual proximity of the CT scanner to the emergency department and round-the-clock availability in many hospitals, CTA has become an important tool in evaluating TIA and stroke patients. CTA source images provide a useful view of vessel anatomy, and multiplanar and 3-dimensional reconstructions are commonly performed, which improve the ease of interpretation. In general, CTA has twice the spatial resolution of magnetic resonance angiography (MRA) but only one-half that of digital subtraction cerebral angiography (DSA). The postprocessing time of CTA images is similar to that of MRA. Because both CTA and MRA produce static images of vascular anatomy, both techniques suffer relative to DSA for the demonstration of flow rates and direction and collateral input into tissues at risk for hypoperfusion.

Drawbacks to using this diagnostic study include exposure to iodinated contrast and ionizing radiation; thus, patients with renal insufficiency or contrast allergies may be excluded from undergoing CTA. Nevertheless, most patients are eligible, and its use is increasing for the reasons mentioned above.

Extracranial CTA

For the evaluation of extracranial carotid artery stenosis, CTA has a sensitivity >80% and specificity >90% for detecting significant lesions compared with DSA[27] (**383, 384**). CTA has similar sensitivity and specificity (close to 100%) compared with DSA for diagnosing severe carotid stenosis, and sensitivity of 89%, specificity of 91%, and accuracy of 90% compared with DSA for diagnosing carotid lesions of >50% stenosis. The differentiation of a very-high-grade stenosis (*string sign*) from a total occlusion is of importance, because a vessel with a high-grade stenosis can be opened with either surgery or angioplasty plus stenting, whereas a total occlusion, unless hyperacute, cannot. CTA has been found to be highly accurate for detecting such a lumen, although not always as good as DSA. However, in some cases, CTA is more accurate than DSA for determining the degree of carotid stenosis, especially the very-high-grade type. CTA is clearly superior to carotid ultrasound for differentiating a carotid occlusion from a very-high-grade stenosis. In terms of identifying plaque morphology, CTA has only 60% sensitivity for detecting significant plaque ulcerations. CTA may also be used if cervicocephalic arterial dissection is suspected, and it is particularly helpful in the posterior circulation in which MRI is less sensitive.

Intracranial CTA

Intracranial CTA is useful for imaging intracranial artery stenoses, aneurysm and arteriovenous malformations. CTA is very reliable for the detection of intracranial occlusions, with sensitivities ranging between 92% and 100%, specificity ranging between 82% and 100%, and a positive predictive value of 91–100%. In acute stroke, the accuracy of CTA for defining the acute intra-arterial thrombus is close to that of DSA. The sensitivities of CTA for intracranial stenoses are slightly lower than those for occlusion, ranging between 78% and 100%, with specificities of 82–100% and a positive predictive value of 93%. CTA therefore has a higher sensitivity and positive predictive value than 3-dimensional time-of-flight (TOF) MRA for both intracranial stenosis and occlusion, including the petrous and cavernous segments of the ICA. CTA appears superior to 3-dimensional TOF MRA, with a higher sensitivity and positive predictive value than MRA for both intracranial stenosis (MRA = 70% and 65%) and occlusion (MRA = 87% and 59%).

CTA is superior to TCD in the detection of stenoses and occlusions. CTA may be as sensitive (>90 to 95%) and specific as DSA for the detection and characterization of intracranial aneurysms. In some cases, a CTA can detect an aneurysm missed by DSA. This ability to detect aneurysms almost as well as or even better than DSA demonstrates the significantly greater spatial resolution of CTA over MRA.

In summary, CTA is a reasonably safe and accurate technique for imaging most extracranial and intracranial vessels for stenoses/occlusions and for the detection of many intracranial aneurysms. In general, the accuracy of CTA is equal to or superior to that of MRA in most circumstances, and in some cases, its overall accuracy approaches or exceeds that of DSA. New CT scanners with even more detectors may further enhance the accuracy of this technique in the future. Because CTA requires the use of substantial amounts of intravenous contrast material, its application may be limited in patients with contrast allergies and renal dysfunction.

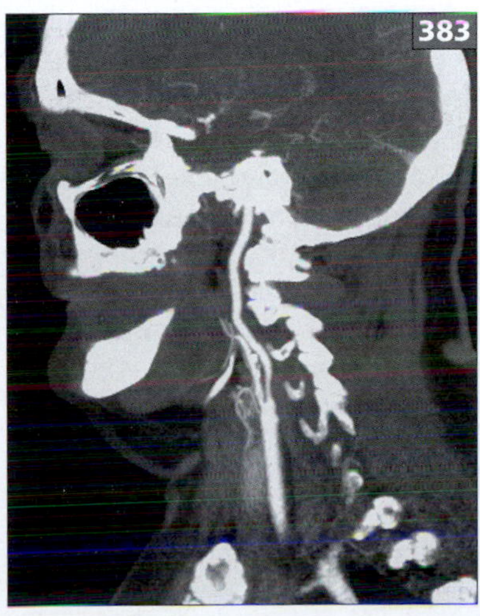

383 CT angiogram of the left common and internal and external carotid arteries, sagittal plane, of the patient in 380, showing 60–70% stenosis of the origin of the left internal carotid artery.

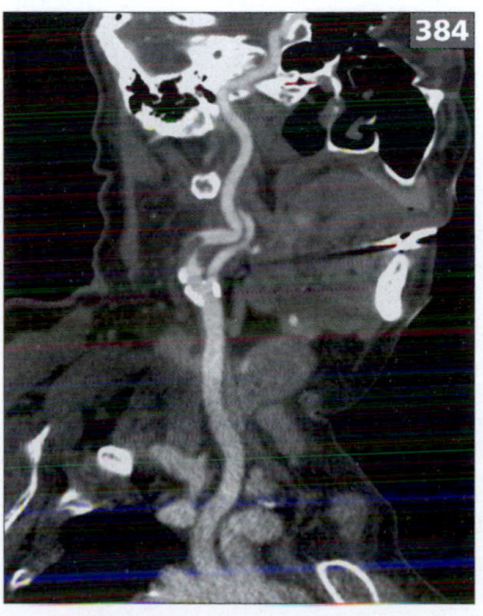

384 CT angiogram showing the aortic arch, left common carotid artery, and left internal and external carotid arteries, with calcification (white) in terminal left common carotid artery, and calcification (white) and thrombus (black) causing very severe stenosis at the origin of the left internal carotid artery.

Magnetic resonance angiography

There are several different MRA techniques that are used for imaging cerebral vessels. They include 2-dimensional TOF, 3-dimensional TOF, multiple overlapping thin-slab acquisition (MOTSA), and contrast enhanced (CE)-MRA.

MRA is also helpful for detecting atherothrombotic lesions in the neck and head, and other, less common causes of ischemic stroke or TIAs, such as arterial dissection, fibromuscular dysplasia, venous thrombosis, and some cases of vasculitis. For hemorrhagic stroke, MRA may be used to detect intracranial aneurysms and arteriovenous malformations.

Extracranial MRA

For the detection of extracranial carotid disease (threshold stenosis typically >70%) nonenhanced MRA shows a mean sensitivity of 93% and a mean specificity of 88% with 2-dimensional or 3-dimensional TOF sequences (**385**)[27].

MRA with gadolinium contrast is rapidly replacing TOF techniques for detecting extracranial carotid stenosis. Studies of CE-MRA compared with DSA (with or without carotid ultrasound) have shown specificities and sensitivities of 86–97% and 62–91%, respectively. The general consensus is that CE-MRA provides more accurate imaging of extracranial vessel morphology and the degree of stenosis than nonenhanced TOF techniques. With a contrast-enhanced protocol, MRA of the neck has a sensitivity of 82% and a specificity of 97% for diagnosis of extracranial carotid stenosis of ≥50%.

Craniocervical arterial dissections of the carotid and vertebral arteries can often be detected with MRA (**386–388**). CE MRA may improve the detection of arterial dissections. Nonenhanced T1-weighted MRI in the axial plane, with fat-saturation techniques, frequently can depict a subacute hematoma within the wall of an artery, which is highly suggestive of a recent dissection. However, an acute intramural hematoma may not be well visualized on fat-saturated T1-weighted MRI until the blood is metabolized to methemoglobin, which may not occur until a few days after ictus. Intramural hemorrhage is almost pathognomonic of dissection and differentiates dissection from vasospasm in patients with subarachnoid hemorrhage. MRA may also show tapering of the lumen at the dissection.

Intracranial MRA

For identifying intracranial stenosis, MRA of the head is generally performed without gadolinium contrast (unlike the neck) (**389**). Intracranial MRA with nonenhanced TOF techniques has a sensitivity that ranges from 60% to 85% for stenoses and from 80% to 90% for occlusions compared with CTA and/or DSA (sensitivity = 100%). The positive predictive value is 59% and the negative predictive value 91%. Thus, although not every intracranial stenosis observed on MRA is real, a negative study result can be reassuring in that no stenosis is present.

MRA is also used for the diagnosis and serial imaging of cerebral aneurysms, particularly the 3-dimensional TOF technique. The ability of the various MRA techniques to demonstrate an aneurysm is a reflection of their spatial resolution. In general, MRA can reliably detect up to 90% of intracranial aneurysms. Specifically, MRA can detect up to 99% of aneurysms >3 mm; this declines to 38% sensitivity for those <3 mm.

Overall, CE-MRA has greater sensitivity and specificity than Doppler ultrasound for detecting most types of extracranial cerebrovascular lesions. It can also noninvasively detect most significant intracranial vaso-occlusive lesions. CE-MRA is useful for detecting intracranial aneurysms and extracranial arterial dissections; however, it cannot be used in patients with pacemakers, some metallic implants, and those with allergies to MR contrast agents, and its use is limited in patients with severe claustrophobia.

Catheter contrast angiography

Intra-arterial, catheter contrast angiography is an invasive technique which is undertaken by inserting a catheter into the femoral artery under local anesthetic, wriggling it until the tip lies in one of the arteries to the brain, then injecting about 5 ml (a teaspoon) of X-ray contrast through it and taking X-ray pictures rapidly as the contrast passes through the blood vessels. With the aid of computerized images, the bones can be subtracted instantaneously leaving the picture of the contrast outlining the artery and nothing else (DSA).

Intra-arterial angiography with selective injection of the carotid or vertebral arteries has traditionally been the gold standard for the delineation of the cranial vasculature but carries a 1% risk of stroke and 0.1% risk of death. DSA remains the gold standard for the detection of many types of cerebrovascular lesions and diseases. For most types of cerebrovascular disease, the resolution, sensitivity, and specificity of DSA equal or exceed those of the noninvasive techniques. This is true for many cases of arterial narrowing, dissection, small arteriovenous malformations (**390, 391**), vasculopathies/vasculitides, and determination of collateral flow patterns. One exception is intracranial aneurysms, in which case CTA is equal to or better than DSA for large aneurysms and may in some cases detect small aneurysms missed by DSA, because of its multiprojectional capabilities.

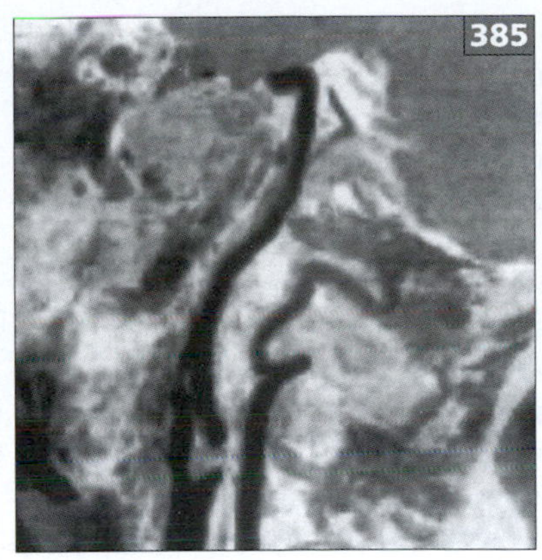

385 MR angiogram, lateral view, showing a flow void, consistent with >70% diameter stenosis, of the origin of the left internal carotid artery.

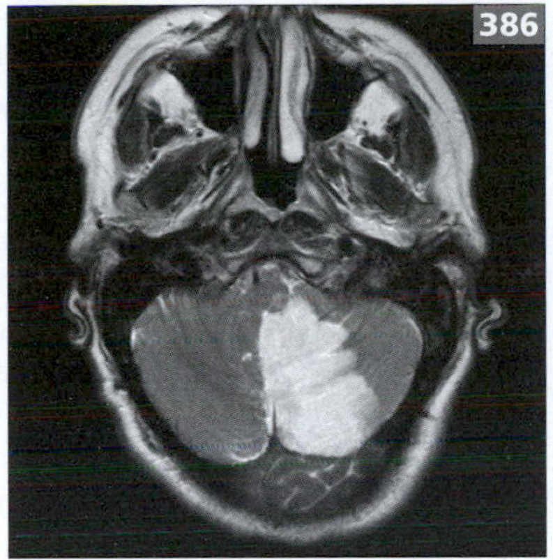

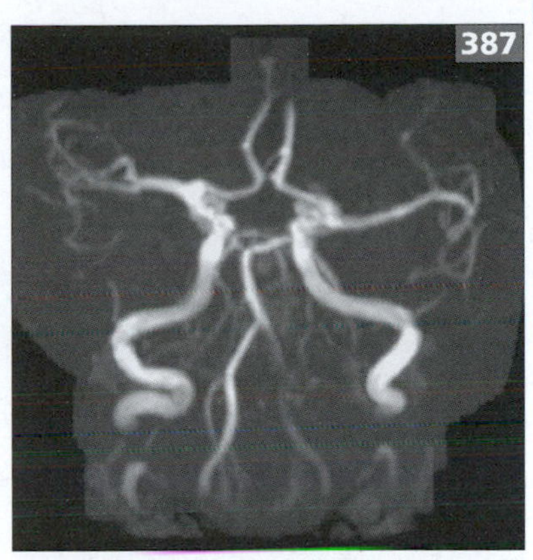

386–388 MRI brain, DWI, axial plane (386) showing an area of restricted diffusion, consistent with infarction, in the left superior cerebellum due to embolic occlusion of the left superior cerebellar artery. MR angiogram, AP view (387), and CT angiogram, lateral view (388) showing a filling defect in the left vertebral artery due to dissection.

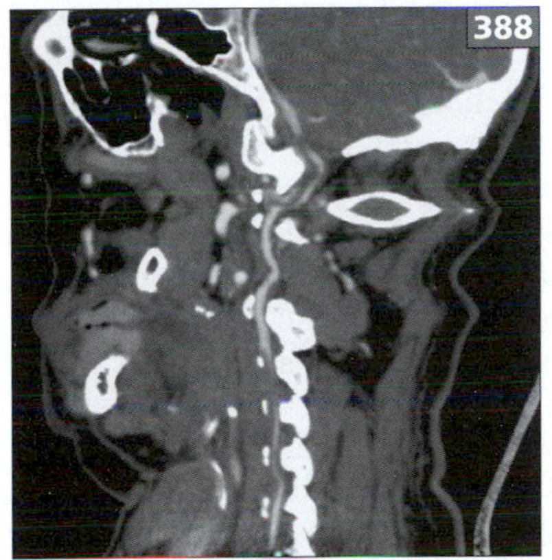

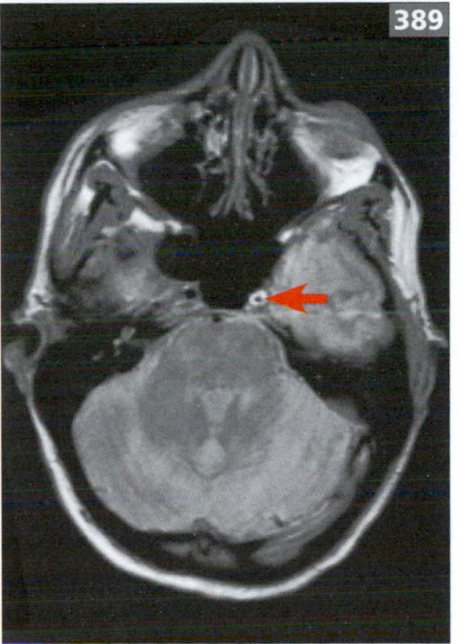

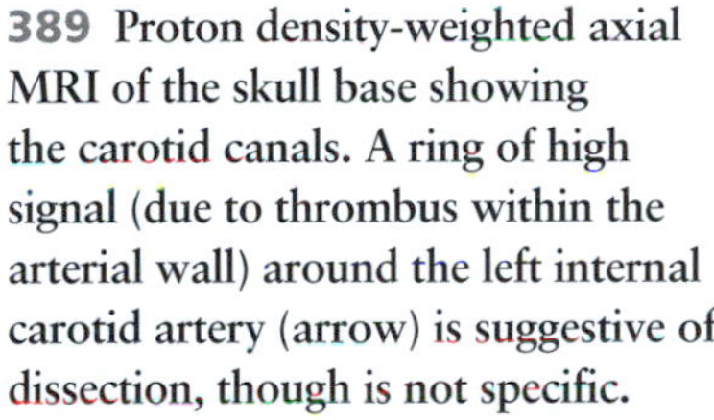

389 Proton density-weighted axial MRI of the skull base showing the carotid canals. A ring of high signal (due to thrombus within the arterial wall) around the left internal carotid artery (arrow) is suggestive of dissection, though is not specific.

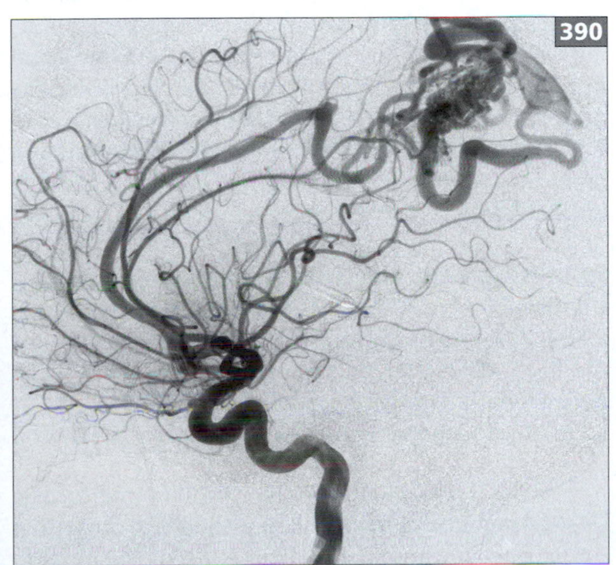

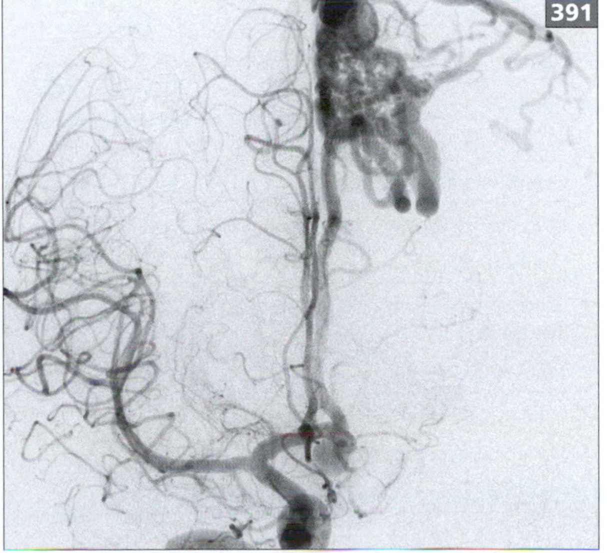

390, 391 Intra-arterial DSA lateral view (390) and AP view (391) showing a parasagittal arteriovenous malformation.

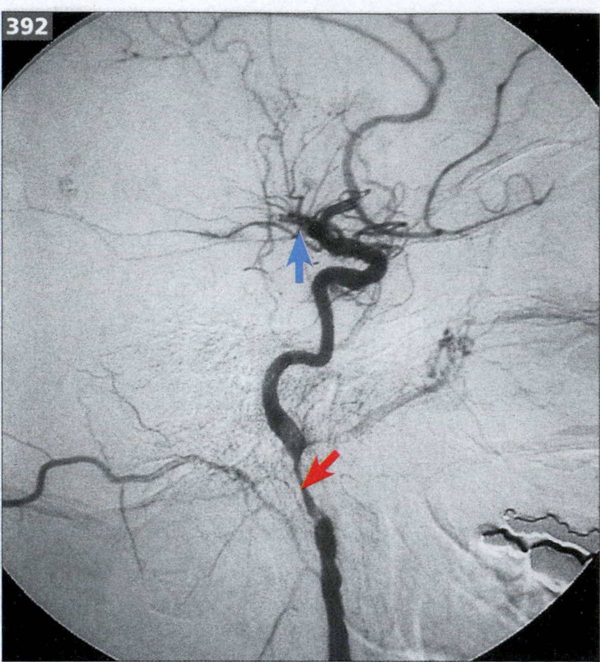

392 **Intra-arterial DSA of an internal carotid dissection (red arrow) following a road accident. Note the occluded middle cerebral artery (blue arrow) due to distal embolization.**

DSA is an invasive test and can cause serious complications such as stroke and death. Most large series have reported permanent deficits or death in <1% of DSA procedures. The largest series of cases to date reported permanent neurologic deficit or death in <0.2%. The use of DSA in patients with a contrast allergy or renal dysfunction is complicated, but DSA can be used with proper medical precautions.

Since the advent of the less invasive MR and CT angiography, the main indications for catheter angiography are now to image intracranial aneurysms (focal little balloon-like outpouchings), vasculitis (focal dilatation and narrowing of the fine branches of the intracranial arteries), arteriovenous malformations (irregular networks of wriggly arteries and veins which fill quickly before the normal cerebral veins and can occur in any part of the head), and dissection.

Angiography of a carotid or vertebral dissection shows a smoothly stenosed artery with a double lumen or intimal flap, or a smooth tapering occlusion (**392**). The 'string sign' is due to hematoma in the wall of the artery compressing the normal lumen to a 'fine thread'. Sometimes the artery is completely occluded but the occlusive stump often has a tapered shape, suggestive of dissection. Other angiographic findings include intraluminal clot, intimal flaps, pseudoaneurysm formation (usually at the base of the skull), and evidence of distal emboli obstructing smaller intracranial arteries.

Angiography of vasculitis may show areas of alternate narrowing and dilatation of intracranial arterial branches ('beading') (**393–395**), or areas of extracranial arterial occlusion (e.g. Takayasu's arteritis). These findings are nonspecific, however (*Table 64*). In primary angiitis of the brain the small intracranial arteries and arterioles are involved, whereas in vasculitis complicating meningitis, tumors, or other causes, the major basal intracranial arteries may be involved. However, the angiogram may be normal even in biopsy-proven vasculitis, particularly if the affected vessels are <500 μm in diameter and too small to be seen, so biopsy is strongly recommended.

TABLE 64 **SOME CAUSES OF SEGMENTAL NARROWING, DILATATION, AND BEADING OF THE CEREBRAL ARTERIES SEEN ON ANGIOGRAPHY**

Cerebral vasculitis
Tumor emboli
Irradiation
Malignant meningitis
Chronic meningeal infections
Drug misuse (cocaine, amphetamines, etc.)
Multiple emboli
Idiopathic reversible cerebral vasoconstriction (puerperal angiopathy)
Arterial dissection
Intravascular lymphoma
Malignant hypertension
Fabry's disease
Pheochromocytoma

Investigating the heart and aortic arch

Imaging

Chest X ray may identify structural abnormalities of the heart such as an enlarged left atrium (**396**) or, in patients with suspected cerebral vasculitis, features of hilar lymphadenopathy (**397**) or pulmonary infiltration (**398**).

Transthoracic echocardiography (TTE) and cardiac (Holter) monitoring for >24 hours, should be considered for patients in whom a proximal source of embolism in the heart or aortic arch is suspected, such as those with a nonlacunar stroke syndrome (e.g. total anterior circulation infarct [TACI], partial anterior circulation infarct

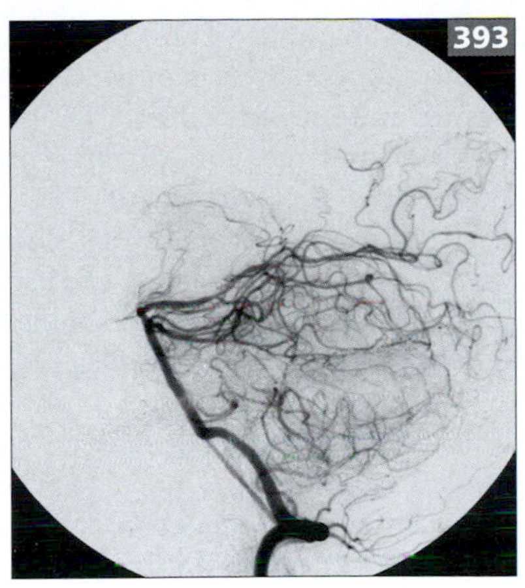
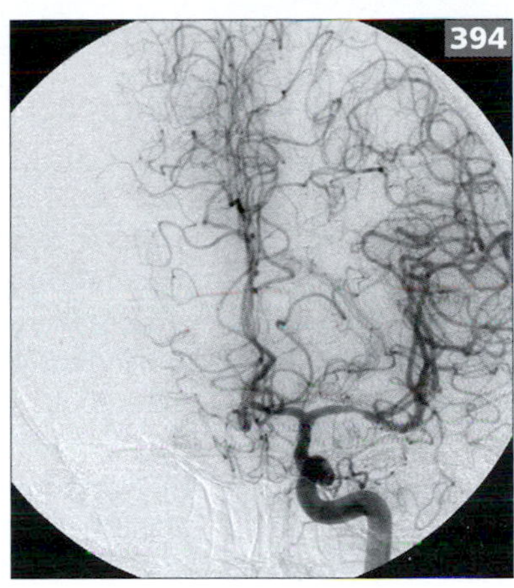
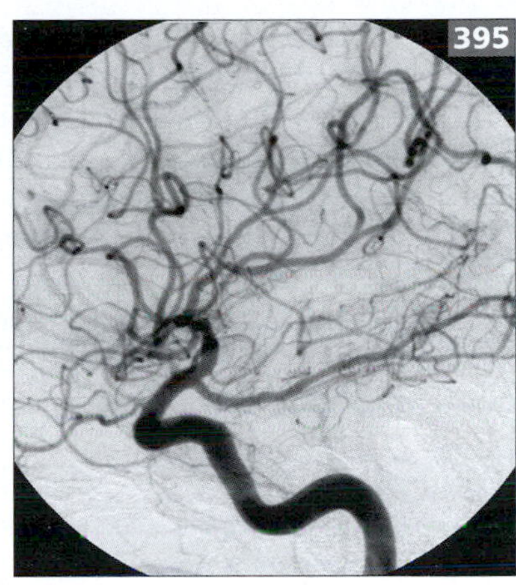

393–395 Intra-arterial DSA right posterior lateral view (393), AP view (394), and left anterior oblique view (395), showing alternate narrowing and dilatation of intracranial arterial branches ('beading') due to intracranial vasculitis.

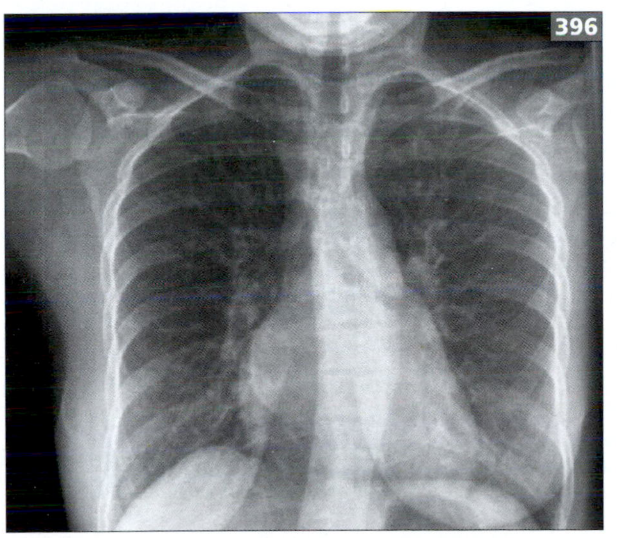
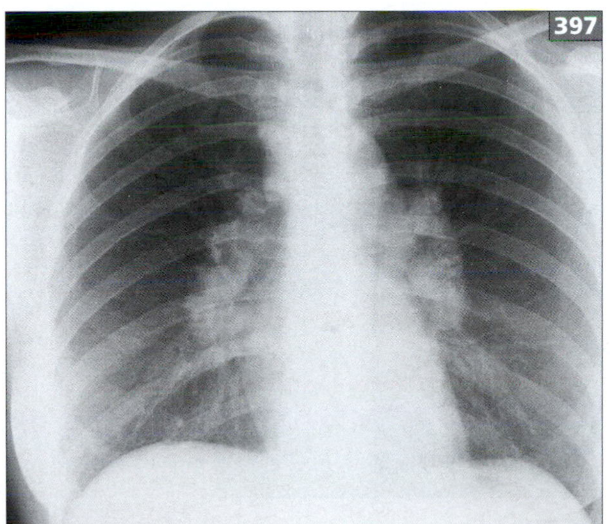

396 Chest X-ray showing straightening of the left heart border due to left atrial enlargement in a patient with rheumatic mitral stenosis and a cardioembolic ischemic stroke.

397 Chest X-ray, postero-anterior view, showing bilateral hilar lymphadenopathy in a patient with sarcoidosis.

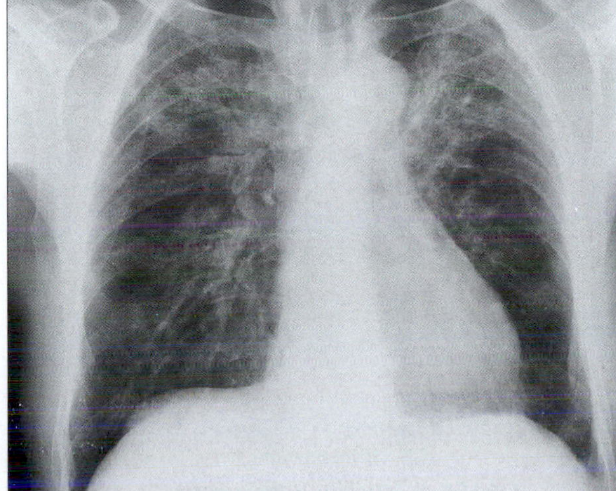

398 Chest X-ray, posterio-anterior view, of a patient with Wegener's granulomatosis, showing a loss of volume in the upper zones of the lungs bilaterally and coarse interstitial infiltrate with confluence and cavitation in the upper zones bilaterally.

[PACI], or posterior circulation infarct [POCI], which are all commonly caused by embolic occlusion of a cerebral artery), an abnormal heart clinically, and abnormal ECG or chest X-ray, and a CT or MRI brain scan showing wedge-shaped cortical/subcortical cerebral infarction (**399, 400**), particularly if there are multiple brain infarcts and in different arterial territories.

For patients with no history or signs of heart disease and a normal ECG, the yield of further cardiac evaluation, by means of TTE, in identifying an abnormality suggestive of a cardioembolic source, is less than 3%. TTE provides good views of the anterior/ventral aspects of the heart, such as the left ventricle (**401, 402**). TTE may also identify a patent foramen ovale (**403, 404**) or valve vegetations due to infective endocarditis (**405**).

Transesophageal echocardiography (TOE) provides better views of the posterior/dorsal aspects of the heart than TTE, and is therefore more sensitive than TTE for detecting atheroma of the aortic arch, abnormalities of the interatrial septum (e.g. atrial septal aneurysm, PFO, atrial septal defect), atrial thrombi and spontaneous echo contrast (**406**), and valvular disease (*Table 65*). The use of contrast increases the detection of right-to-left shunts. TOE is indicated if TTE is negative and there is still a suspected embolic source in the heart, such as in the:

- Venous system (i.e. via a right-to-left shunt, such as a patent foramen ovale).
- Inter-atrial septum (e.g. atrial septal aneurysm).
- Left atrium or left atrial appendage, or
- Aortic arch.

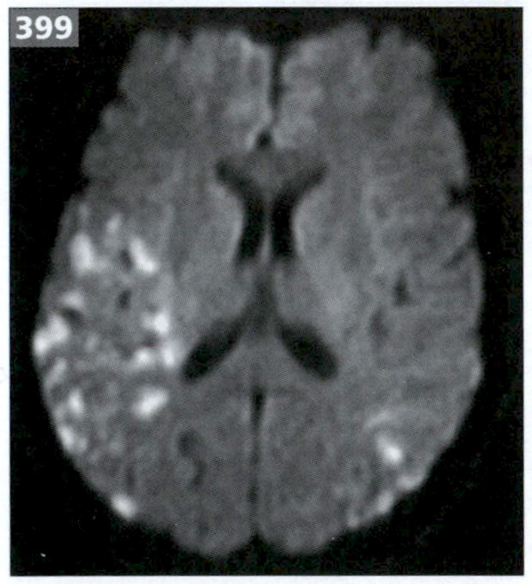

399, 400 Diffusion-weighted MRI brain, axial plane, showing multiple small areas of restricted diffusion in the right and left frontal and parietal lobes due to multifocal infarction in a patient with embolism from the heart due to infective endocarditis.

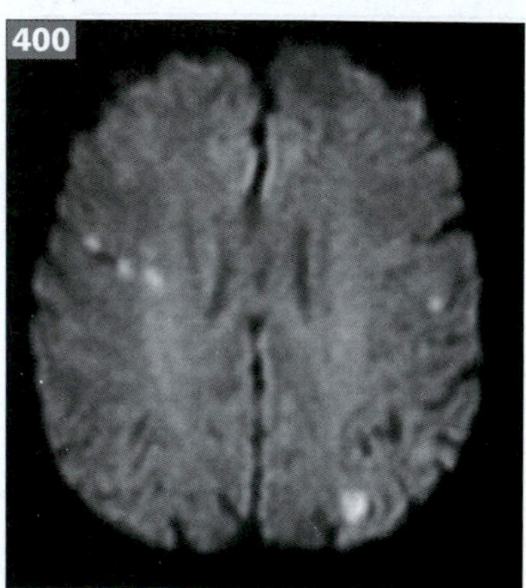

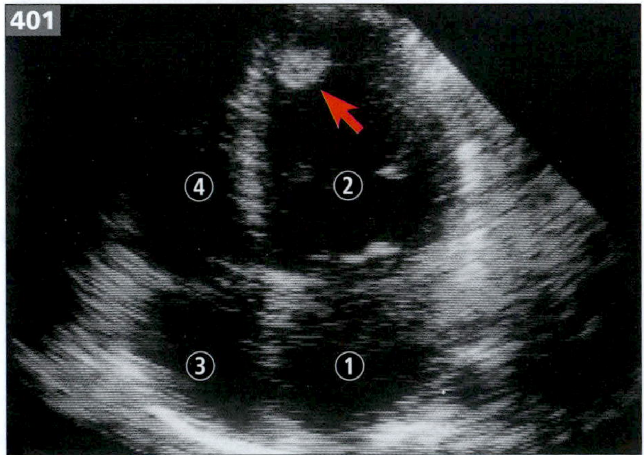

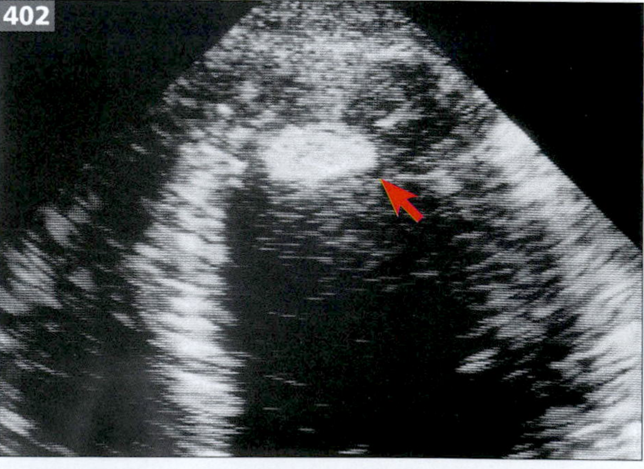

401, 402 Transthoracic 2-dimensional echocardiograph, apical four-chamber view (401), showing thrombus in the apex of the left ventricle (arrow). 1: left atrium, 2: left ventricle, 3: right atrium, 4: right ventricle; (402) higher magnification of the left ventricular apical thrombus. *Reproduced with permission from Hankey GJ, Warlow CP [1994];. Transient Ischemic Attacks of the Brain and Eye. WB Saunders, London.*

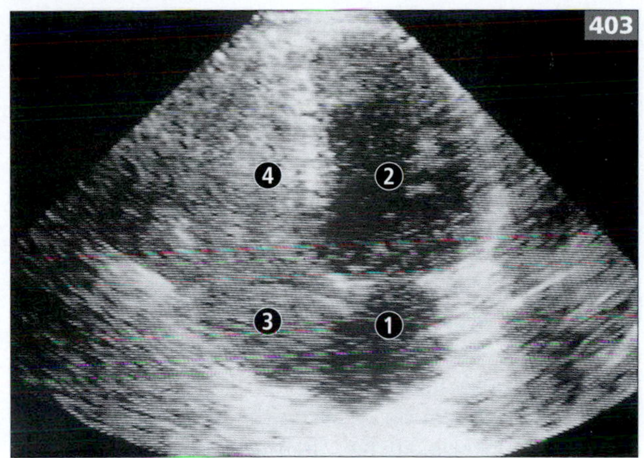

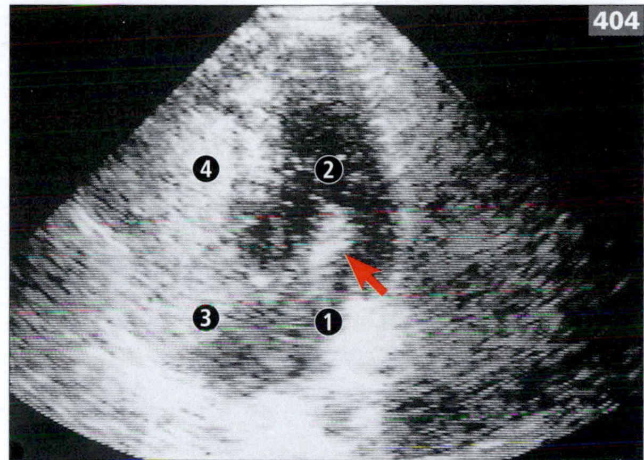

403, 404 Transthoracic 2-dimensional echocardiograph, apical four-chamber view, using contrast (agitated hemaccel) in a patient with a right-to-left shunt due to a patent foramen ovale. 142: Pre-Valsalva maneuver: after intravenous injection of agitated hemaccel, contrast appears in the right atrium and right ventricle without passage across the patent foramen ovale because left atrial pressure is slightly greater than right atrial pressure. Note: contrast does not traverse the pulmonary circulation to appear in the left atrium unless there is a right-to-left shunt such as a pulmonary arteriovenous malformation; 143: Valsalva maneuver: after intravenous injection of agitated hemaccel and during the Valsalva maneuver (which increases right atrial pressure) contrast appears in the right atrium and simultaneously moves into the right ventricle (across the tricuspic valve) and left atrium (through the patent foramen ovale), where it is seen here crossing the mitral valve and entering the left ventricle (arrow). 1: left atrium, 2: left ventricle, 3: right atrium, 4: right ventricle. *Reproduced with permission from Hankey GJ, Warlow CP [1994]; Transient Ischemic Attacks of the Brain and Eye. WB Saunders, London.*

405 Transthoracic 2-dimensional echocardiograph, parasternal long axis view, showing vegetations (arrow) on the anterior leaflet of the mitral valve, which is situated behind the aortic valve. This image is taken during diastole when the mitral valve is open and the aortic valve closed. 1: left ventricle, 2: left atrium. *Reproduced with permission from Hankey GJ, Warlow CP [1994]; Transient Ischemic Attacks of the Brain and Eye. WB Saunders, London.*

406 Biplane transesophageal echocardiograph, longitudinal view, in a patient with atrial fibrillation showing left atrial appendage, an enlarged left atrium, and spontaneous echo contrast. In the absence of regular atrial contractions and the presence of a dilated left atrium, blood flow in the left atrium is slower than normal and is seen on the real-time echocardiography study to be swirling around slowly in the left atrium; slowly flowing or static blood has increased echogenicity and is called spontaneous echo contrast (as opposed to echo contrast that is introduced into the circulation such as agitated hemaccel). 1: left atrium; 2: left ventricle; 3: mitral valve; 4: left atrial appendage. *Reproduced with permission from Hankey GJ, Warlow CP [1994]; Transient Ischemic Attacks of the Brain and Eye. WB Saunders, London.*

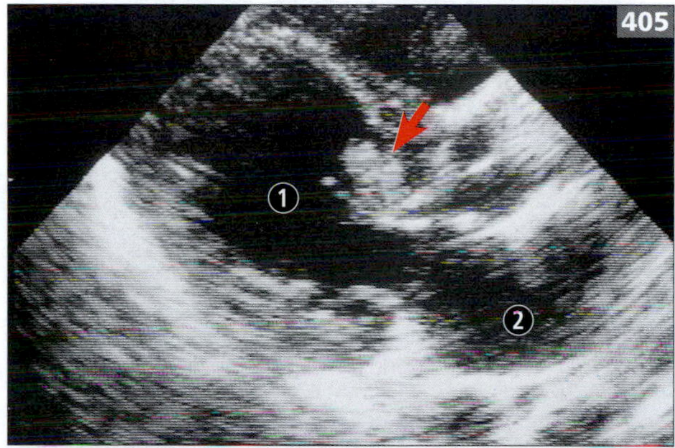

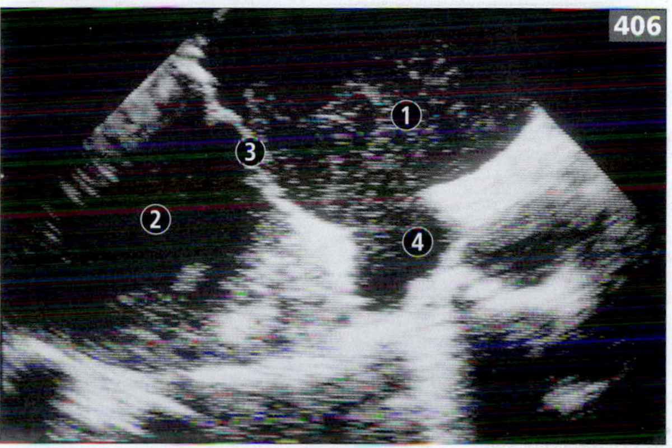

Monitoring of the heart rate and rhythm

A period of continuous and prolonged cardiac monitoring (inpatient telemetry or Holter monitoring) is warranted in patients with an embolic stroke or TIA of uncertain cause, particularly in patients with a history of palpitations or evidence of structural heart diseases by ECG or echocardiogram, even though they present in a sinus rhythm (because patients may have a paroxysmal atrial dysrhythmia). The optimal duration of cardiac monitoring is unknown but the longer the monitoring the greater the yield, albeit with diminishing return.

TABLE 65 **TRANSTHORACIC vs. TRANSESOPHAGEAL ECHOCARDIOGRAPHY FOR DETECTING POTENTIAL CARDIAC SOURCES OF EMBOLISM**

Transthoracic echcocardiography
- Left ventricular thrombus*
- Left ventricular dyskinesis
- Mitral stenosis
- Mitral annulus calcification
- Aortic stenosis

Transesophageal echocardiography
- Left atrial thrombus*
- Left atrial appendage thrombus*
- Spontaneous echo contrast
- Intracardiac tumors
- Atrial septal defect†
- Atrial septal aneurysm
- Patent foramen ovale†
- Mitral and aortic valve vegetations
- Prosthetic heart valve malfunction
- Aortic arch atherothrombosis/dissection
- Mitral leaflet prolapsed

*The detection of an intracardiac thrombus may be a false positive (not all thrombi embolize) and the failure to detect an intracardiac thrombus may be a false negative, either because it is too small to be detected or it has all embolized already.

†A less invasive alternative is to inject air bubbles or other echocontrast material intravenously and, if there is a patent foramen ovale, it can be detected by transcranial Doppler sonography of the mid dle cerebral artery, particularly with a provocative Valsalva maneuver. There is considerable variation in the methods and this influences the diagnostic sensitivity and specificity. It is also uncertain what size of shunt is 'clinically relevant', and some bubbles may pass to the brain through pulmonary rather than cardiac shunts.

Blood tests for thrombophilia

Despite a paucity of evidence supporting a true association between the inherited disorders of coagulation (protein C deficiency, protein S deficiency, antithrombin deficiency, and the factor V Leiden and prothrombin gene mutations) and the occurrence of ischemic stroke, it is common practice for many clinicians to order tests for these thrombophilias as part of the work-up of ischemic stroke, especially in young patients. However, multiple case-control studies have not convincingly shown an association of the inherited thrombophilias with ischemic stroke, even in young patients and patients with PFO. If there is an association between the inherited thrombophilias and arterial stroke, then it is a weak one, likely enhanced by other prothrombotic risk factors. The consequences of ordering these tests and attributing causality to an arterial event can result in significant costs to the health-care system and pose a potential risk to patients, because this may lead to inappropriate use of long-term oral anticoagulants, exposing patients to harm without a clearly defined benefit[28].

Imaging venous infarction, cerebral venous sinuses, and cerebral veins

Plain CT brain scan

Plain CT brain scan will readily show 'venous' infarcts: not corresponding with a known arterial territory (*Table 66*), often with hemorrhagic transformation (**407**); sometimes bilaterally, in the parasagittal area or in the deep regions of the brain, or supra- as well as infratentorial.

CT brain scan also often provides evidence of the underlying sinus thrombosis: the hyperdense sinus sign or the empty delta sign. Hyperdensity of a venous sinus, on a noncontrast CT scan, through filling with fresh thrombus is seen most clearly in the posterior part of the sagittal sinus ('dense triangle sign') or in the straight sinus. In patients with lobar ICH of otherwise unclear origin or with cerebral infarction that crosses typical arterial boundaries, imaging of the cerebral venous system should also be performed.

Post-contrast CT brain scan

The 'empty delta' sign appears only after injection of intravenous contrast material, through which enhancement occurs of the wall but not in the thrombus in the center of the (posterior) part of the sagittal sinus that is perpendicularly imaged on an axial CT slice (**408**). The name of this sign easily sticks in the mind but it is found in only a small number of patients.

TABLE 66 **DIFFERENTIATION OF ARTERIAL FROM VENOUS INFARCTS**

	Arterial	**Venous**
Shape	Wedge or rounded	Usually wedge if cortical, rounded if deep
Number occurring simultaneously	Usually single	May be multiple
Density	Early: slightly hypodense Later: more hypodense	Early obvious hypodensity
Margins	Indistinct early, distinct after several days	Distinct early
Swelling	Develops over days	Marked, appears usually very early
Hemorrhage	Infrequent, peripheral, finger-like	Frequent, central
Additional signs	Hyperdense artery sign	Hyperdense sinus sign,'empty delta' sign (after contrast)

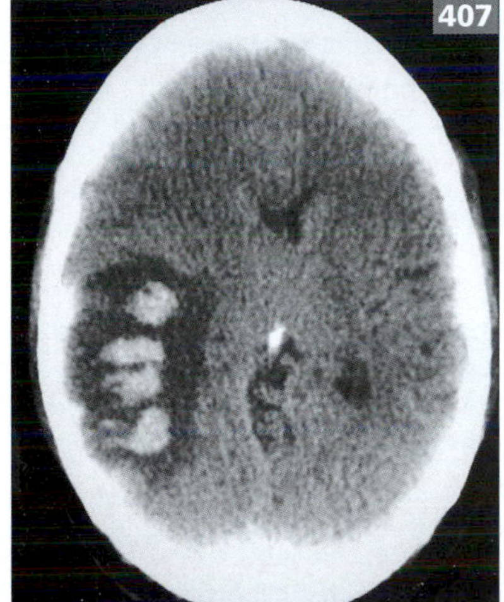

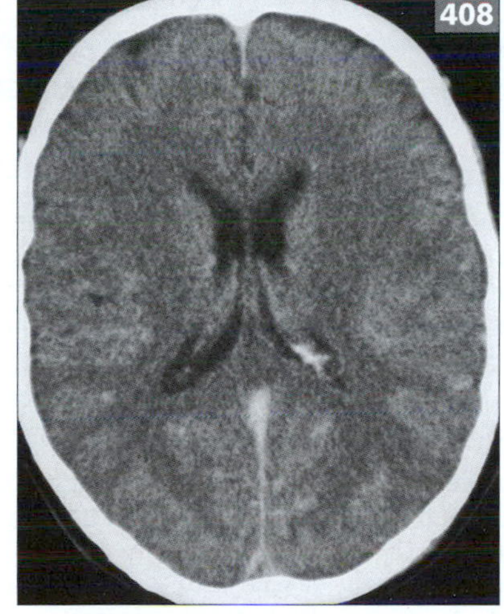

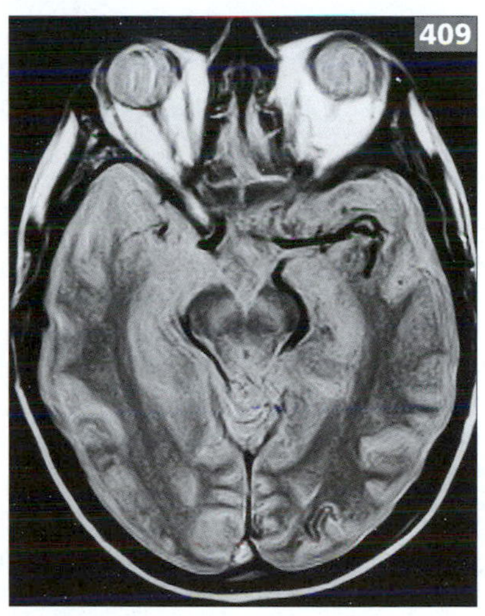

407 CT scan without contrast of a 6-hour-old venous infarct. Note the well defined edges, marked swelling, and central hemorrhage. There was no sinus involvement.

408, 409 CT brain scan (408) showing a triangular filling defect in the venous sinus at the torcula after IV contrast ('empty delta' sign) due to venous sinus thrombosis; 409: MRI brain scan, proton density weighted image, showing hypointense (black) flow voids in the middle and posterior cerebral arteries, and a hyperintense (white) filling defect representing loss of the flow void in the venous sinus at the torcula (due to the thrombus).

MR brain and angiography (venography)

MRI of the brain parenchyma may show early changes of venous congestion on T2-weighted images or with fluid attenuated inversion recovery (FLAIR) techniques, while DWIs show only subtle changes, unlike ischemia from arterial occlusion. MRI imaging of thrombus in the dural sinuses depends very much on the interval from the time the thrombus began to form (409). Three stages can be distinguished in the evolution of thrombus. In the acute stage (days 1–5) it appears strongly hypointense on T2-weighted images and isointense on T1-weighted images (as for arterial thrombi). In the subacute stage (up to day 15) the thrombus signal is strongly hyperintense, initially on T1-weighted images and subsequently also on T2-weighted images. The third stage begins 3–4 weeks after symptom onset: the thrombus signal becomes isointense on T1-weighted images but on T2-weighted images it remains hyperintense, although often nonhomogeneous. Recanalization may occur over months in up to one-third of patients, but persistent abnormalities are common and do not signify recurrent thrombosis.

Catheter contrast angiography

A plain CT or MRI is useful in the initial evaluation of patients with suspected CVT, but a negative plain CT or MRI does not rule out CVT. A venographic study (either CT venography [CTV] or MR venography [MRV]) should be performed in suspected CVT if the plain CT or MRI is negative or to define the extent of CVT if the plain CT or MRI suggests CVT (*Table 67*). Gradient echo T2 susceptibility-weighted images combined with MR can be useful to improve the accuracy of CVT diagnosis.

Catheter cerebral angiography can be useful in patients with inconclusive CTV or MRV in whom a clinical suspicion for CVT remains high. Nonfilling of a sinus, or part of it, on angiogram is in itself insufficient proof of venous thrombosis. Hypoplasia is an alternative explanation, especially in the case of the left lateral sinus or the anterior third of the superior sagittal sinus. To prove occlusion of a sinus, it is necessary to see delayed emptying or dilatation of collateral veins on the angiogram, or to see evidence of thrombus on CT scanning or MRI.

In most centers in the western world, MRA has replaced catheter angiography, especially as MRA in combination with other MR techniques can show the thrombus itself. An early follow-up CTV or MRV is recommended in CVT patients with persistent or evolving symptoms despite medical treatment, or with symptoms suggestive of propagation of thrombus. A follow-up CTV or MRV at 3–6 months after diagnosis is reasonable to assess for recanalization of the occluded cortical vein/sinuses in stable patients. In patients with previous CVT who present with recurrent symptoms suggestive of CVT, repeat CTV or MRV is recommended.

TABLE 67 **COMPARISON OF CT AND MRI IN THE DIAGNOSIS OF CEREBRAL VENOUS THROMBOSIS**

	CT + CTV	MRI + MRV
Advantages	• Good visualization of major venous sinuses • Quick (5–10 min) • Readily available • Fewer motion artifacts • Can be used in patients with a pacemaker, defibrillator, or claustrophobia	• Visualization of the superficial and deep venous systems • Good definition of brain parenchyma • Early detection of ischemic changes • No radiation exposure • Detection of cortical and deep venous thrombosis • Detection of macrobleeding and microbleeding
Disadvantages	• Exposure to ionizing radiation • Risk of contrast reactions • Risk of iodinated contrast nephropathy (e.g. in patients with diabetes, renal failure) • Low resolution for small parenchymal abnormalities • Poor detection of cortical and deep venous thrombosis	• Time consuming • Motion artifacts • Availability • Limited use in patients with cardiac pacemaker or claustrophobia • Confers a low risk of gadolinium-induced nephrogenic systemic fibrosis • Slow flow states, complex flow patterns, and normal anatomic variations in dural sinus flow can affect the interpretation
Sensitivity/specificity	• Small studies comparing multiplanar CT/CTV *vs.* DSA showed 95% sensitivity and 91% specificity • Overall accuracy 90–100%, depending on vein or sinus	• The sensitivity and specificity of DSA MRI/MRV are not known owing to the lack of large MRI/MRV head-to-head studies with DSA • Echoplanar T2 susceptibility-weighted imaging combined with MRV are considered the most sensitive sequences
Practical application	• Acute onset of symptoms • Emergency setting • Multidetector CTV can be used as the initial test when MRI is not readily available	• Acute or subacute onset of symptoms • Emergency or ambulatory setting • Patients with suspected CVT and normal CT/CTV • In patients with suspected deep CVT, because complex basal dural sinuses and their emissary channels are more commonly seen

CT: computed tomography; CTV: CT venography; CVT: cerebral venous thrombosis; DSA: digital subtraction angiography; MRI: magnetic resonance imaging; MRV: magnetic resonance venography.

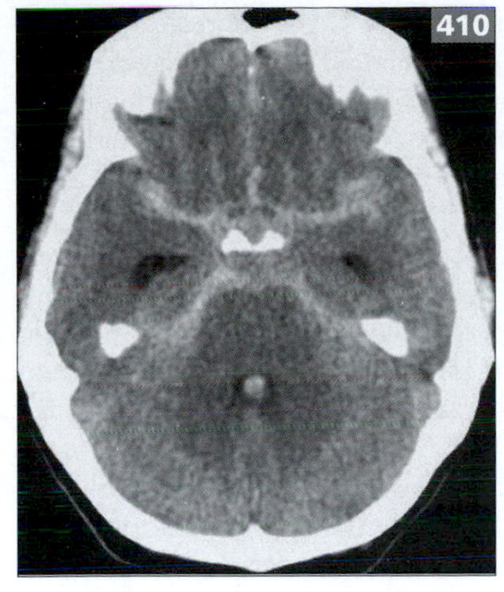

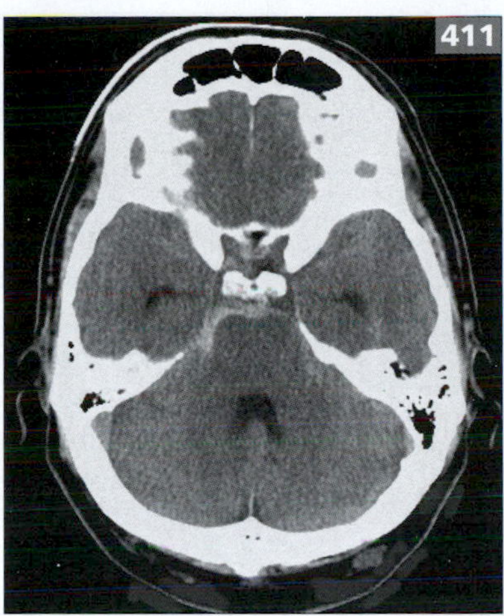

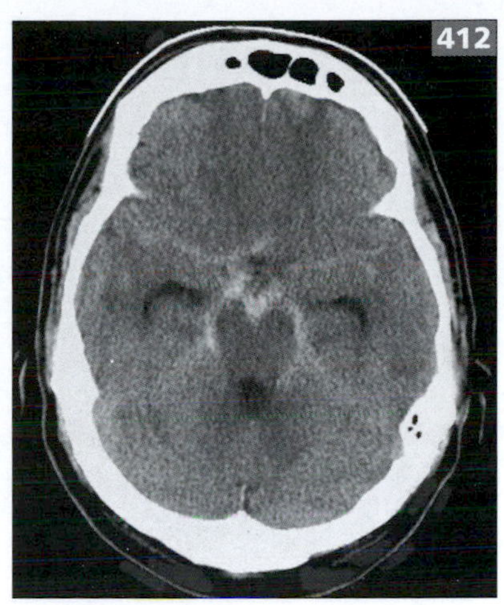

410 Plain cranial CT scan in an unconscious patient following a subarachnoid hemorrhage. Note the high density (blood) in the subarachnoid space (e.g. around the midbrain) and the dilatation of the temporal horns of the lateral ventricles due to secondary communicating hydrocephalus.

411, 412 Plain CT brain scan showing subarachnoid blood in the pre-pontine cistern, interpeduncular and ambient cisterns, around the circle of Willis and interhemispheric (frontal/temporal) fissures. Mild dilatation of the temporal horns of the lateral ventricles is present due to mild hydrocephalus. No aneurysm was identified on two sequential catheter digital subtraction cerebral angiograms.

Imaging subarachnoid hemorrhage

The aims of investigations are to detect subarachnoid blood and to ascertain its source.

Detecting subarachnoid blood

All patients with suspected SAH (including those with a rapid onset, severe headache that is maximal within minutes and lasts more than 1 hour without an alternative explanation) should undergo an immediate plain CT brain scan. The inconvenience and cost of referring the 90% of patients with innocuous sudden, severe headache for a CT brain scan is outweighed by the benefits of diagnosing and treating a ruptured aneurysm before it rebleeds in the other 10% of patients.

On day 1, CT scanning detects SAH in 93–98% of patients, depending on the quantity of subarachnoid blood, the resolution of the scanner, and the skills of the radiologist[19] (**410–412**). In the following days the sensitivity of CT falls dramatically as blood in the subarachnoid space is recirculated and cleared. If the CT brain scan is normal, and SAH is still suspected, lumbar puncture (LP) must be performed. Unless meningitis is also suspected, the LP should be delayed at least 6 hours, and preferably 12 hours, after the onset of symptoms to allow sufficient time for hemoglobin released from erythrocytes in the CSF to degrade into oxyhemoglobin and bilirubin. Bilirubin in the CSF signifies SAH because it is only synthesized *in vivo*, unlike oxyhemoglobin which may result from a traumatic tap or prolonged storage or agitation of blood-stained CSF *in vitro*.

If the CSF looks clear, the pressure should be measured, since a high pressure may signify intracranial venous thrombosis and a low pressure may signify spontaneous intracranial hypotension, both of which can present with sudden, severe headache. Clear CSF should also be sent for culture, because pneumococcal meningitis can present acutely. If the CSF is blood-stained, it should be centrifuged immediately. If the supernatant is yellow (xanthochromia), the diagnosis of SAH is virtually certain because bilirubin causes yellow pigmentation of the supernatant. However, the diagnosis should be established by means of spectrophotometry of the CSF, which confirms or excludes the presence of bilirubin.

If there are delays in centrifuging the CSF, it should be stored in darkness, preferably wrapped in tinfoil, to prevent degradation of any bilirubin by the ultraviolet components of daylight.

If CT brain scan and CSF (including spectrophotometry) are normal within 10 days of symptom onset, the diagnosis of SAH can be excluded and alternative diagnoses considered. However, beyond 10 days, the sensitivity of CT brain scan for SAH is close to zero and the sensitivity of CSF examination declines rapidly; xanthochromia is only detected in 70% of cases after 3 weeks and 40% after 4 weeks.

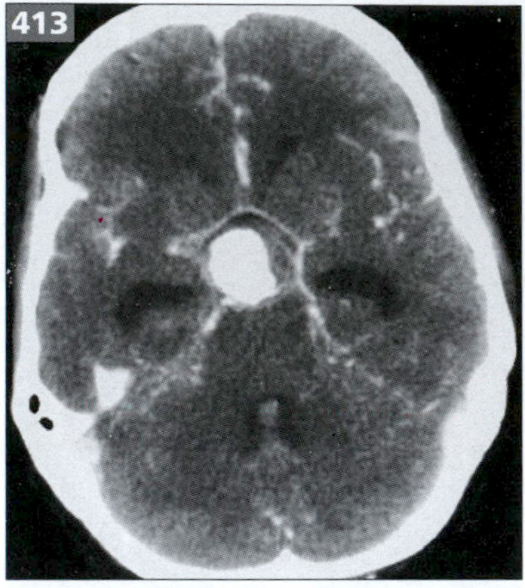

413 CTA showing a large, white, contrast-enhancing central mass measuring 2.5 cm (1 inch) in diameter, which is compressing the upper brainstem anteriorly and the floor of the third ventricle inferiorly, consistent with an aneurysm of the tip of the basilar artery.

Ascertaining the source of subarachnoid blood

The location of the subarachnoid +/– intracerebral +/– intraventricular blood on CT brain scan is a clue to the source of the hemorrhage (e.g. blood in the interhemispheric fissure suggests a ruptured aneurysm on the anterior communicating artery complex, and blood in the Sylvian fissure a ruptured aneurysm of the middle cerebral artery. Multislice CTA with 3-dimensional reconstruction should be performed immediately after the plain CT brain scan, as it identifies aneurysms greater than 3 mm diameter with a sensitivity of about 96% (less for smaller aneurysms) (**413**).

If CTA is normal and aneurysmal SAH is still suspected, four vessel catheter cerebral angiography with views in three dimensions is indicated (**414–416**). If CTA cannot be performed (e.g. contrast allergy), MRA is an option, providing the patient is not restless or requiring mechanical ventilation, as it has similar test characteristics (**417**, **418**).

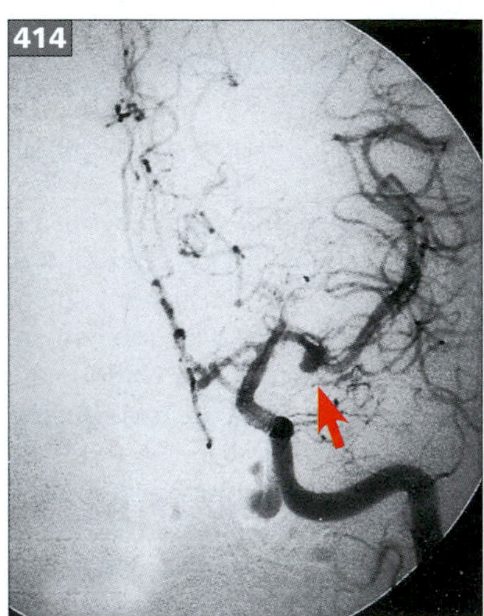

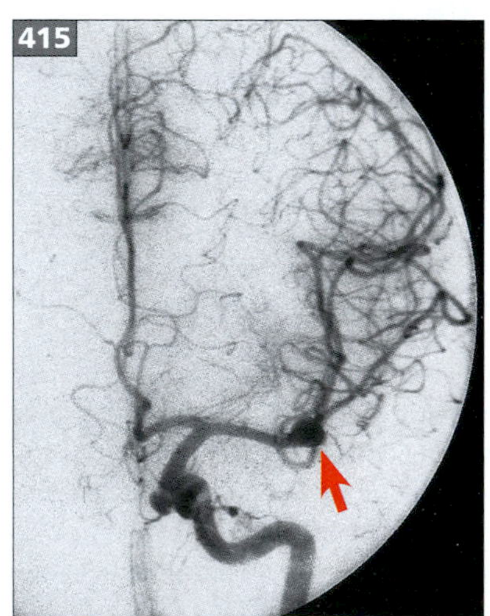

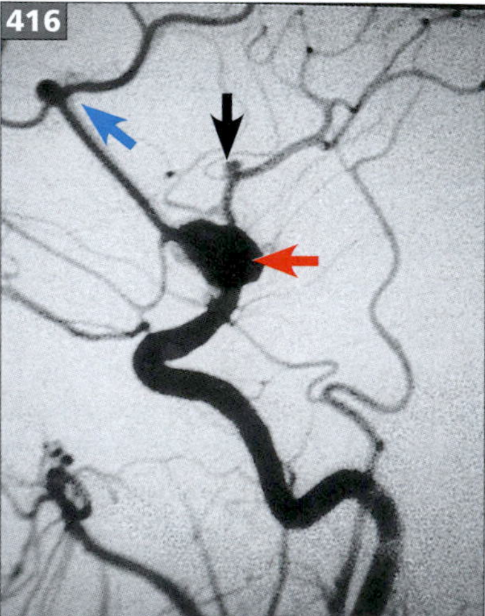

414–416 Intra-arterial angiogram of the left internal carotid artery (414) showing an aneurysm at the trifurcation of the middle cerebral artery (arrow); (415) catheter cerebral angiogram, coronal plane, showing the left middle cerebral artery aneurysm; (416) intra-arterial angiogram of the internal carotid artery showing three aneurysms – a large internal carotid tip (red arrow), a small pericallosal (blue arrow), and a small middle cerebral (black arrow). Multiple aneurysms are not uncommon; usually the largest one is the symptomatic one.

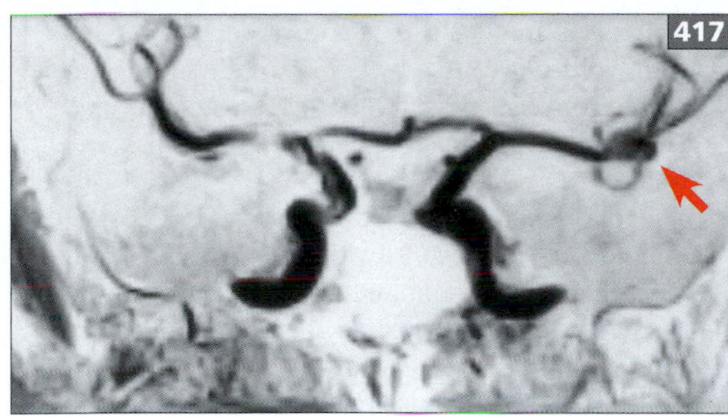

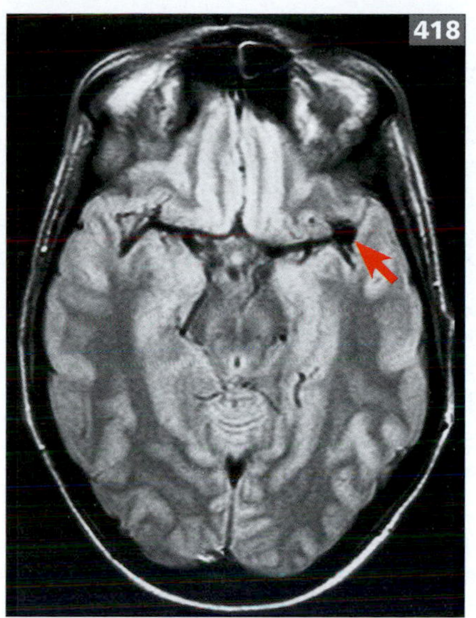

417 MR angiography, coronal plane, showing a left middle cerebral artery aneurysm (arrow).

418 MRI brain scan, proton density image, axial plane, showing hypodense flow voids in the middle cerebral arteries and a left middle cerebral artery aneurysm (arrow).

DIAGNOSIS

The first four stages of clinical assessment listed in *Table 49* and the results of first- and second-line investigations aim to establish a diagnosis of stroke or TIA.

Is the patient having a vascular event of the brain (TIA/stroke) or not?

Community (pre-hospital) diagnosis

Stroke patients (and health professionals) do not always recognize the symptoms of stroke because of the tendency for the focal neurologic symptoms of stroke to be negative rather than positive, and the unreliable relationship between the nature of the clinical symptoms and the nature, site, and severity of the underlying brain and vascular pathology. Therefore, the symptoms and signs of stroke often do not readily lend themselves to autotriage, particularly when compared with symptoms of other conditions such as pain, breathlessness, and bleeding.

TABLE 68 **THE FACE–ARMS–SPEECH TEST (FAST)**

Facial weakness	Can the person smile? Has their mouth or eye drooped?
Arm weakness	Can the person raise both arms?
Speech problems	Can the person speak clearly and understand what you say?

The public and health-care professionals can screen for the diagnosis of a stroke or TIA by means of a simple recognition tool, such as the Face Arm and Speech Test (FAST) (*Table 68*). First responders should be aware however, that the screen is not optimally sensitive or specific, and that hypoglycemia is an important stroke mimic (so blood sugar should be checked at the earliest opportunity).

Primary care or emergency department diagnosis

The Recognition of Stroke in the Emergency Room (ROSIER) score is a more detailed version of the FAST test which can be used to identify patients with likely stroke or TIA in the emergency department (*Table 69*)[29]. However, the sensitivity and specificity of the simpler FAST scale for the immediate diagnosis of acute stroke in the emergency department (sensitivity 81%, specificity 39%) is as good as that of the ROSIER score (sensitivity 83%, specificity 44%)[30].

Ultimately, the diagnosis of a vascular event of the brain is clinical and requires a description by the patient or an eye-witness of symptoms:

- Of sudden onset.
- Of loss of focal neurologic or monocular function (see *Table 50*).
- That are maximal at onset, without spread or intensification.
- That are thought to be due to inadequate blood supply to the relevant part of the brain or eye.

If all of these criteria are met, the likelihood of a vascular disturbance (ischemia or hemorrhage) of brain function is high. The likelihood is even greater if the 'milieu' is appropriate (e.g. an elderly patient with prolonged exposure to several vascular risk factors). About 80% of stroke patients have at least one vascular risk factor, and most are elderly; stroke is uncommon (but not that rare) in young people. All in all, the clinical diagnosis of stroke is accurate about 80–85% of the time, depending on the time since stroke onset and the experience of the examiner.

The clinical diagnosis of stroke is most difficult in the hyperacute phase (e.g. within 6 hours of onset) when symptoms and signs may change rapidly. It is also difficult when the:

- Onset of symptoms is uncertain (e.g. because of coma, dysphasia, confusion, no witness).
- Neuroanatomical localizing value of the symptoms is uncertain (e.g. confusion, amnesia, coma).
- Symptoms are 'positive' in nature, such as hemiballismus caused by lesions of the subthalamic nucleus of Luys in the midbrain, instead of being 'negative' (i.e. with a loss of function, such as weakness).
- The following features are present: anosognosia (inability to recognize any focal neurologic impairment due to nondominant parietal dysfunction), isolated visual field defect (e.g. quadrantanopia or hemianopia); isolated visual–spatial–perceptual dysfunction (e.g. hemispatial neglect or geographical disorientation due nondominant parietal dysfunction); or discriminative sensory loss due to nondominant parietal lobe dysfunction.
- Symptoms are progressing (rather than recovering, as is usually the case after stroke) over hours or even days[31].

TABLE 69 **THE RECOGNITION OF STROKE IN THE EMERGENCY ROOM (ROSIER) SCORE**

Assessment	Date:	Time:	
Symptom onset	Date:	Time:	
Glasgow Coma Scale	Eyes ____	Motor ____	Verbal ____
Blood pressure	____/____ mmHg		
Blood glucose concentration*	________ mmol/l		
Has there been loss of consciousness or syncope?	Yes ____ (–1)	No ____ (0)	
Has there been seizure activity?	Yes ____ (–1)	No ____ (0)	
Is there a *new acute* onset (or on awakening from sleep):			
1. Asymmetric facial weakness?	Yes ____ (–1)	No ____ (0)	
2. Asymmetric arm weakness?	Yes ____ (–1)	No ____ (0)	
3. Asymmetric leg weakness?	Yes ____ (–1)	No ____ (0)	
4. Speech disturbance?	Yes ____ (–1)	No ____ (0)	
5. Visual field defect?	Yes ____ (–1)	No ____ (0)	
Total Score†: ____ (–2 to +5)			
Provisional diagnosis	Stroke ____	Nonstroke (specify) ____	

*If BG <3.5 mmol/l, treat urgently and reassess once normal.
†Stroke is unlikely but not completely excluded if total scores are <0.

TABLE 70 **DIFFERENTIAL DIAGNOSES OF TIA OF THE BRAIN**

Migraine aura (with or without headache)
- Young to middle-aged patients
- Positive symptoms (visual scintillations, tingling)
- Spread of symptoms to adjacent areas over minutes
- Symptoms resolve gradually and usually within 20–60 minutes
- Headache (often unilateral and pulsatile) and nausea usually accompany or follow the neurologic symptoms
- Past or family history of migraine is common
- Vascular risk factors are uncommon
- Recurrences are usually stereotyped and may be reduced with migraine prophylaxis

Partial (focal) epileptic seizures
- Positive symptoms (e.g. limb jerking, tingling)
- Symptoms arise over seconds to 1–2 minutes (not abruptly)
- Symptoms spread/march to adjacent areas over several seconds
- Symptoms usually resolve quickly within a few minutes but can be prolonged for hours
- Antecedent partial seizure symptoms may be present (e.g. epigastric discomfort, nausea)
- Impaired awareness (i.e. complex partial seizure), or secondary generalization with a tonic–clonic convulsion, or loss of consciousness may occur
- Persistent focal neurologic signs may be present after symptoms resolve
- Recurrences are usually stereotyped and respond to antiepileptic drugs

Transient global amnesia
- Abrupt onset of loss of anterograde episodic memory for verbal and nonverbal material
- Usually accompanied by repetitive questioning
- Resolves within 24 hours (and usually a few hours) leaving a dense amnesic gap for the duration of the attack
- No clouding of consciousness, loss of personal identity, or ability to recognize familiar individuals or places, other focal neurologic symptoms, or epileptic features
- Recurrent attacks are exceptional
- The diagnosis is all but impossible if there is no witness available

Labyrinthine disorders *(benign recurrent vertigo, benign paroxysmal positional vertigo, acute labyrinthitis)*
- Vertigo is the only neurologic symptom (with secondary nausea and ataxia): see below

Metabolic disorders *(hypoglycemia, hyperglycemia, hypercalcemia, hyponatremia)*
- Hypoglycemic attacks may recur at regular times and can be excluded with appropriately timed tests of blood glucose

Hyperventilation, anxiety or panic attacks, somatization disorder
- Consider reproducing the symptoms (e.g. forced hyperventilation)

Intracranial structural lesion *(meningioma, tumor, giant aneurysm, arteriovenous malformation, chronic subdural hematoma)*
- Usually cause recurrent stereotyped events; exclude with CT or MRI brain scan

Acute demyelination (multiple sclerosis)
- Usually subacute onset in young adults; exclude with MRI brain scan

Syncope
- A nonfocal neurologic symptom
- Often a precipitating circumstance

Drop attacks
- Usually middle-aged women
- Onset when standing or walking
- Legs give way and patient falls to the ground with otherwise preserved neurologic function and consciousness throughout
- Recovery is immediate unless the patient is injured

Mononeuropathy/radiculopathy
- Lower motor neuron signs

Myasthenia gravis
- Fatiguability

Cataplexy
- Brief muscle weakness precipitated by excitement or emotion (e.g. laughter)

The diagnosis of SAH may be missed because the cardinal symptom – sudden, severe headache – is not present in one-quarter of patients (sensitivity 75%) and, when it is present, the characteristic sudden mode of onset might not be elicited (patients tend to focus on the severity rather than onset of the headache) or the headache may be attributed to a more common cause of headache with an atypically rapid onset (e.g. 'crash' migraine, benign sex or exertional headache, tension headache, cluster headache, meningitis, arterial dissection); among patients who present with sudden headache alone in general practice, SAH is the cause in only one in ten (specificity 10%)[32].

The diagnosis of SAH is also missed because of failure to understand the limitations of CT brain scan, to perform LP at least 6–12 hours after symptom onset, and to interpret correctly the CSF findings.

Differential diagnosis

Transient ischemic attack

The differential diagnosis of transient focal neurologic attacks is shown in *Table 70*.

A common clinical issue is distinguishing isolated vertigo (with secondary nausea, vomiting, and ataxia) due to a TIA from nonvascular causes of isolated vertigo. Vertigo is an illusory sense of movement or orientation, and indicates a disorder of the labyrinth or brainstem, in contrast to other disorders with which it is commonly confused, such as presyncope (a sense of a near faint, typically due to transient hypotension), disequilibrium of the elderly (a nonspecific slight 'unsteadiness', particularly on turning, due to poor balance and strength), and lightheadedness (which is often associated with dysfunctional breathing or anxiety). To distinguish vertigo from nonrotatory dizziness, ask the patient: '*Did you just feel lightheaded or did you see the world spin around as though you had just got off a playground roundabout?*' Eliciting the symptom of vertigo narrows the differential diagnosis to a disorder of the labyrinth or its central connections.

The Hallpike maneuver and the 'head thrust test' (head impulse test) are confirmatory tests that enable a positive diagnosis of vestibular as opposed to brainstem disease[33]. The Hallpike maneuver traditionally begins with the patient sitting on the couch with the legs along the couch; the head is turned to one side (the side of the ear being examined) and then the patient is laid down with the head hanging over the edge of the couch with head still turned to the one side. The doctor can help the patient open the eyes fully for optimally viewing the eye movements and nystagmus, if present. The sideways Hallpike maneuver begins with the patient sitting on the couch with the legs hanging over the couch and the head turned to one side. The patient then lies down sideways to achieve the same final head position as with the traditional Hallpike manouevre. The onset of positional vertigo and torsional nystagmus after a short latent interval of a few sections and which fatigues in 30 seconds is a positive test and diagnostic of benign positional vertigo.

The head thrust test assesses the vestibular ocular reflex. The examiner turns the patient's head with a high acceleration but low amplitude head thrust, to one side. Normally, head movement towards a semicircular canal will cause activation of that canal, and reflex movement of the eyes in the opposite direction – that is, away from the canal. The test is positive when the patient makes a catch-up saccade to refixate the visual target (usually toward the examiner's nose). In a patient with acute vestibular neuritis, head movement towards the defunct semicircular canal will result in failure of activation of the vestibular–ocular reflex and the visual target will be lost from fixation during sudden head movements. In one study of 101 patients with acute vestibular syndrome, the presence of normal horizontal head impulse test, direction-changing nystagmus in eccentric gaze, or skew deviation (vertical ocular misalignment), as identified by a 3-step bedside oculomotor examination (HINTS: Head-Impulse–Nystagmus–Test-of-Skew) was 100% sensitive and 96% specific for stroke[34].

Tip

▸ *Even experienced neurologists with an interest in cerebrovascular disease show considerable interobserver variability in the diagnosis of TIA. This does not imply lack of skill, but rather it is inherent in the clinical assessment of symptoms and signs. Sometimes the available information does not suggest a 'right answer' as to whether the event was a TIA or not – in which case one ends up working on the basis of probability.*

TABLE 71 **DIFFERENTIAL DIAGNOSIS OF STROKE**
(in approximate order of frequency, according to referral patterns)

- Systemic illness, or seizure, causing apparent deterioration of previous stroke
- Epileptic seizure (postictal Todd's paresis) or nonconvulsive seizures
- Structural intracranial lesion:
  - Subdural hematoma
  - Brain tumor or abscess
  - Arteriovenous malformation
- Metabolic/toxic encephalopathy:
  - Hypoglycemia
  - Nonketotic hyperglycemia
  - Hyponatremia
  - Wernicke's encephalopathy
  - Hepatic encephalopathy
  - Alcohol and drug intoxication
  - Septicemia
- Functional/non-neurologic (e.g. hysteria)
- Hemiplegic migraine
- Encephalitis (e.g. herpes simplex virus)/brain abscess
- Head injury
- Spinal cord lesion(s), particularly when presenting with asymmetric limb weakness
- Peripheral nerve lesion(s), Miller Fisher syndrome and other partial forms of Guillain–Barré syndrome
- Myasthenia gravis
- Hypertensive encephalopathy
- Demyelination (multiple sclerosis)
- Creutzfeldt–Jakob disease
- Wilson's disease

Stroke

Sustained focal neurologic symptoms that may mimic stroke can be caused by the conditions listed in *Table 71*.

When patients with a long-standing focal neurologic deficit (e.g. due to a previous stroke) present with an increase in severity of the same focal neurologic deficit, they are often diagnosed with a recurrent stroke in the same vascular territory. However, more often than not, the cause of the deterioration is a systemic illness such as a pneumonia or urinary tract infection, causing temporary decompensation. Diagnosis and treatment of the systemic illness (e.g. infection, hypoglycemia) is usually accompanied by recovery of the focal neurologic dysfunction to the pre-presentation state.

Tip

▶ *The diagnosis of functional (i.e. non-neurologic) motor and sensory symptoms depends on demonstrating positive functional signs as well as the absence of signs of disease. Most of these signs relate to inconsistency, either internal (for example, Hoover's sign reveals discrepancies in leg power) or external (for example, tubular field defect is inconsistent with the laws of optics). However, although inconsistency may be evidence that the signs are functional, it does not indicate whether they are consciously or unconsciously produced, and a positive functional sign does not exclude the possibility that the patient also has disease.*

The final diagnosis of stroke 'mimics' in patients presenting with suspected TIA and stroke in two studies are listed in *Table 72*[29,35].

TABLE 72 **FINAL DIAGNOSIS OF STROKE MIMICS IN TWO STUDIES OF PATIENTS PRESENTING WITH SUSPECTED TIA AND STROKE**

Stroke 'mimic'	Nor *et al.* 2005[29] (n = 59)	Hand *et al.* 2006[35] (n = 109)
Seizure	8 (14%)	23 (21%)
Sepsis	8 (14%)	14 (13%)
Metabolic/toxic encephalopathy	–	12 (11%)
Space-occupying brain lesion	7 (12%)	10 (9%)
Tumor	4 (7%)	–
Subdural hematoma	3 (5%)	–
Syncope/presyncope	13 (22%)	10 (9%)
Acute confusional state	–	7 (6%)
Vestibular dysfunction (labyrinthitis)	3 (5%)	7 (6%)
Acute mononeuropathy	–	6 (5%)
Functional/somatization	7 (12%)	6 (5%)
Dementia	–	4 (4%)
Migraine	–	3 (3%)
Spinal cord lesion	–	3 (3%)
Other	13 (22%)	3 (3%)

Subarachnoid hemorrhage

Differential diagnoses are presented in *Table 73* and include:

- Meningitis or encephalitis.
- Intracerebral hemorrhage (particularly posterior fossa hemorrhage).
- Obstruction of the cerebral ventricles.
- Rapid rise in blood pressure.

Tip

▶ *The top five differential diagnoses of a 'brain attack' (TIA and stroke) are the '5 S's:*

- *Seizures*
- *Syncope*
- *Sepsis*
- *Subdural hematoma*
- *Somatization.*

TABLE 73 **DIFFERENTIAL DIAGNOSIS OF SUDDEN UNEXPECTED HEADACHE**

With neck rigidity

- Subarachnoid hemorrhage
- Acute painful neck conditions
- Meningitis
- Cerebellar or intraventricular hemorrhage
- Pituitary apoplexy
- Recent head injury

Without neck rigidity

- Migraine
- Thunderclap headache
- Pressor responses
- Benign orgasmic cephalalgia
- Benign exertional headache
- Reaction while on monoamine oxidase inhibitors
- Pheochromocytoma
- Expanding intracranial aneurysm
- Carotid or vertebral artery dissection
- Intracranial venous thrombosis
- Occipital neuralgia
- Acute obstructive hydrocephalus

TABLE 74 **CLASSIFICATION OF ETIOLOGIC SUBTYPES OF ACUTE ISCHEMIC STROKE**

Large artery disease

CLINICAL
- Embolic syndrome: cerebral cortical, brainstem or cerebellar symptoms (e.g. TACS, PACS, POCS [*Table 54*])
- Supported by other evidence of large artery disease (*Table 35*); e.g. atherosclerosis: presence of vascular risk factors (hypertension, diabetes, smoking, hypercholesterolemia), family history of symptomatic atherosclerotic events, history of intermittent claudication, previous TIA in same vascular territory, myocardial infarction, carotid bruits, diminished peripheral pulses

BRAIN IMAGING
- Cerebral cortical or cerebellar lesions or brainstem/ subcortical lesions >1.5 cm diameter on CT/MRI brain

VASCULAR IMAGING
- Stenosis >50% of appropriate intracranial or extracranial artery on duplex ultrasound or arteriography (CT, MRI, or digital subtraction)

ECG, HOLTER MONITOR, AND CARDIAC IMAGING
- Potential sources of embolism from the heart (*Table 37*) excluded

Cardiac embolism

CLINICAL
- Embolic syndrome: cerebral cortical, brainstem or cerebellar symptoms (e.g. TACS, PACS, POCS [*Table 54*])
- Supported by other evidence of cardiac embolism: history of stroke or TIA in more than one arterial territory in the brain, or systemic embolism to other arterial territories; heart murmur; potential source of embolism from the heart present (*Table 37*), calcific emboli in the retina or on brain imaging

BRAIN IMAGING
- Cerebral cortical or cerebellar lesions or brainstem/ subcortical lesions >1.5 cm diameter on CT/MRI brain

VASCULAR IMAGING
- Potential sources of thrombosis or embolism in large arteries (e.g. atheroma, dissection, moyamoya disease) should be excluded

ECG, HOLTER MONITOR, AND CARDIAC IMAGING
- At least one cardiac source of embolism should be identified (from high-risk group for 'probable' or medium-risk group for 'possible' cardiac embolism [*Table 37*])

Small artery disease

CLINICAL
- Patient should have one of the traditional clinical lacunar syndromes (*Table 54*) and no evidence of cerebral cortical dysfunction
- Supported by risk factors for, or clinical and laboratory features of, a small artery disease (*Table 36*)

BRAIN IMAGING
- Normal CT/MRI or relevant brainstem or subcortical hemispheric lesion <1.5 cm diameter

VASCULAR IMAGING
- Potential large artery sources of thrombosis or embolism (e.g. atheroma, dissection) excluded

ECG, Holter monitor, and cardiac imaging
- Cardiac sources of embolism excluded

Other determined etiologies

CLINICAL
- Any symptoms compatible with an acute stroke

BRAIN IMAGING
- CT/MRI findings of acute ischemic stroke regardless of the size or location

Vascular imaging
- Potential large artery sources of thrombosis or embolism (e.g. atheroma, dissection) excluded

ECG, HOLTER MONITOR, AND CARDIAC IMAGING
*Cardiac sources of embolism excluded

OTHER INVESTIGATIONS
- Includes patients with non-atherosclerotic vasculopathies, hypercoaguable states, or hematologic disorders (*Table 38*)

Undetermined etiology
- Patients with two or more potential causes of stroke
- No etiology determined despite extensive evaluation
- No etiology determined but cursory evaluation

CT: computed tomography; ECG: electrocardiogram; MRI: magnetic resonance imaging; PACS: partial anterior circulation syndrome; POCS: posterior circulation syndrome; TACS: total anterior circulation syndrome; TIA: transient ischemic attack.

The most distinctive feature of SAH headache is its sudden onset (maximal within seconds) but, even so, only about 25% of patients with sudden headache in general practice prove to have SAH, falling to 10% if sudden headache is the only symptom. This is because headache with a much more common cause, such as migraine and tension headache, can occasionally arise suddenly. None the less, always be careful; missed SAH can be fatal.

Where in the brain and vasculature is the lesion causing the stroke or TIA?

The location of the neurologic lesion is often determined by the neurologic examination and confirmed by brain imaging. The location of the underlying cardiovascular lesion is usually suggested by the neurologic examination and brain imaging, and confirmed by imaging of the heart, aortic arch, and cerebral circulation.

What type of stroke is it and what is the underlying cause?

The pathologic subtype of stroke (ischemic or hemorrhagic) is determined by brain imaging (CT or MRI) and, in the case of suspected SAH with negative brain imaging, by CSF examination (LP).

What is the cause of the stroke or TIA (etiology)?

The cause of the ischemic or hemorrhagic stroke can be determined from the clinical syndrome (*Tables 53, 54*), the patient's risk factor profile (*Tables 45–49*), the location of the brain infarct or hemorrhage on brain imaging, and results of special investigations.

Ischemic stroke

For acute ischemic stroke, a commonly used classification of stroke etiology is the Trial of Org 10172 in Acute Stroke Treatment [TOAST] criteria[36], which aims to identify the most probable pathophysiological mechanism on the basis of clinical findings and results of investigations.

A modification of the TOAST criteria is presented in *Table 74*.

Intracerebral hemorrhage

The biggest clues to the cause of a primary intracerebral hemorrhage are the age of the patient and location of the hematoma. Arteriovenous malformations are the most common cause in the young, degenerative small vessel disease in middle and old age, and amyloid angiopathy in old age (*Table 75*).

TABLE 75 **MOST COMMON CAUSES OF INTRACEREBRAL HEMORRHAGE**
(in approximate rank order, coagulopathies and hemodynamic factors excluded, according to the patient's age and the location of the hematoma)

Location of hematoma	Age <45 years	45–69 years	>70 years
Basal ganglia/thalamus	• AVM or cavernoma • Small vessel disease • Moyamoya syndrome • Amphetamines/cocaine	• Small vessel disease • AVM or cavernoma • Atherosclerotic moyamoya • Tumor • Amyloid angiopathy • Cerebral venous thrombosis† • Infective endocarditis‡	• Small vessel disease • Tumor • AVM or cavernoma • Cerebral vein thrombosis • Infective endocarditis‡
Lobar	• AVM or cavernoma • Saccular aneurysm* • Tumor • Cerebral vein thrombosis† • Amphetamines/cocaine • Infective endocarditis†	• Small vessel disease • AVM or cavernoma • Saccular aneurysm* • Amyloid angiopathy	• Amyloid angiopathy • Small vessel disease • Saccular aneurysm* • AVM or cavernoma
Cerebellum/brainstem	• AVM or cavernoma • Small vessel disease • Tumor	• Small vessel disease • AVM or cavernoma • Tumor	• Small vessel disease • Amyloid angiopathy • Tumor

AVM : arteriovenous malformation; cavernoma: cavernous malformation;
*hematomas in specific locations; †hematoma usually in parasagittal area; ‡with history of valvular heart disease.

On T2-weighted MRI, cavernous malformations are characterized by a combination of a reticulated core of mixed signal intensity with a surrounding rim of decreased signal intensity, corresponding to hemosiderin. Smaller lesions appear as areas of decreased signal intensity (black dots) and are picked up even better by T2-weighted gradient echo MRI.

Subarachnoid hemorrhage

The most common causes of SAH is a ruptured intracranial aneurysm (see *Table 44*).

How severe is the stroke?

The severity of the stroke can be graded according to the:

- Glasgow Coma Scale (GCS).
- National Institutes of Health (NIH) Stroke Scale (*Table 57*).
- Modified Rankin Scale score (mRS) (*Table 58*).

PROGNOSIS

Survival

Case fatality rates

The case fatality rates after a first-ever stroke (all types combined) are about:

- 10% at 7 days.
- 20% at 30 days.
- 30% at 1 year.
- 60% at 5 years.
- 80% at 10 years[37].

Causes of death

Although death within a few hours of stroke onset is not common, when it occurs is usually due to the direct effects of ICH or SAH, and rarely massive brainstem infarction, causing brain herniation.

Death occurring within the first week after stroke is also most commonly due to the direct effects of the brain damage, but the cause is as likely to be cerebral infarction as cerebral hemorrhage; ischemic cerebral edema is maximal about day 2–3 (but can occur up to day 9). Later on, the complications of immobility (e.g. bronchopneumonia, venous thromboembolism) and recurrent vascular events of the brain and heart are the common causes of death.

TABLE 76 **PROBABILITY OF SURVIVAL FREE FROM DEPENDENCY IN ACTIVITIES OF DAILY LIVING 1 YEAR AFTER A STROKE**

Variable†	Parameter coefficient, *b* (SE)	Odds ratio (95% CI)
Constant	15.586 (1.748)	
Age	–0.085 (0.014)	0.92‡ (0.89–0.94)
Living alone	–0.384 (0.259)	0.68 (0.41–1.14)
Independent pre-stroke	–3.174 (0.639)	25.00 (6.67–100)
Normal GCS verbal score (i.e. 5)	–2.177 (0.504)	9.09 (3.33–25)
Able to lift arms	–2.319 (0.513)	10.00 (3.70–25)
Able to walk	–1.154 (0.402)	3.12 (1.45–7.14)

Derived from the Oxfordshire Community Stroke Project using logistic regression, and externally validated on two independent cohorts of stroke patients. Calculating the probability of an outcome is complex (see equation), but easily achieved using a programmable calculator or a nomogram. (Age and Ageing [2010];**39**:360–6.)

Probability of outcome is calculated by: $p = eY/(1 + eY)$, where $Y = a + b1X1 + b2X2 + \ldots + biXi$.

$Y = 15.586 - (0.085 \times \text{age}) + (0.384 \times \text{living alone}) - (3.174 \times \text{independent prestroke}) - (2.177 \times \text{normal GCS verbal}) - (2.319 \times \text{able to lift arms}) - (1.154 \times \text{able to walk})$, where dichotomous variables have numeric values of 1 or 2 as described above.

GCS: Glasgow Coma Scale; †Dichotomous variables were coded 1 = yes, 2 = no; ‡per year of age.

Prognostic factors for survival

The chance of surviving after a stroke depends on the location, size, and pathology of the stroke lesion, and the patient's age and other comorbidities (i.e. handicap) present before the stroke[38–40].

The clinical features at presentation which are indicators of a *poor chance of survival* after stroke include:

- Preadmission comorbidities (dependency, cancer, congestive heart failure, and AF).
- Increased age.
- Reduced level of consciousness.
- Severe/total limb weakness with aphasia or neglect[39].

Another major adverse prognostic factor is hemorrhagic stroke; in the first 30 days after stroke, hemorrhagic stroke (ICH and SAH) carries a much higher risk of death (50%) than ischemic stroke (10%)[38]. For patients with SAH, up to one-half of patients die within 3 weeks after SAH (and one-third of survivors remain dependent, often with cognitive impairment).

Functional ability

Clinical course and recovery after stroke

Among stroke survivors, neurologic function begins to improve within the first few days and continues most rapidly in the first 3 months and more slowly over the next 6–12 months, with some gains still being realized 1–2 years after stroke (not all of which are functional adaptations). The pattern of recovery varies among individuals and doesn't always follow that implied by grouped data. Comorbidities, mood, and motivation are some of several factors that influence an individual's rehabilitation and recovery. Only repeated assessments in individual patients can indicate their pattern of recovery.

Disability rates

The risk of being physically or cognitively disabled and dependent at 1 year after a stroke is about 20–30%. Therefore, at 12 months after first-ever stroke, about one-third of all stroke patients have died, about 20–30% are dependent on another person for everyday activities (e.g. washing, dressing, mobilizing), and 40–50% are independent. For 30-day survivors of first-ever stroke, the 10-year cumulative risk of death or new disability is about 87% (95% CI: 81–92%)[41].

Prognostic factors for survival free of disability

The major clinical factors soon after a stroke which are predictive of being alive and functionally independent at 6 months after a stroke are:

- Younger age at the time of stroke.
- Not living alone (somebody permanently living with the patient before the stroke).
- Independent in activities of daily living before the stroke (Oxford Handicap score ≤2 before stroke).
- Normal verbal GCS score (=5).
- Able to lift both arms to horizontal.
- Able to walk without the help of another person (can use stick/Zimmer frame)[39,40].

These factors seem to be equally predictive whether they are assessed within 48 hours of stroke onset or later, whether the stroke is ischemic or hemorrhagic in type, and whether the patient has had a previous stroke or not (*Table 76*).

Recurrent stroke

Rates of early recurrent stroke

The early risks of recurrent stroke after TIA and minor ischemic stroke are substantially higher than later. Looking forwards from the time of a TIA, the risk of a stroke is as high as 5% within the first 48 hours, 10% within the first week, 12% within the first 30 days, and 18% within the first 3 months[42,43]. Looking back after an ischemic stroke, 23% of patients recall a 'warning' TIA before their stroke, of whom 17% report the TIA occurred on the day of their stroke, 9% on the preceding day, and 43% in the preceding week[44].

Presumably the very high risk of stroke soon after large artery TIA and ischemic stroke is because the symptomatic atherosclerotic plaque in large arteries is still thrombogenic, or inflammed, unstable, and prone to rerupture or recurrent thromboembolism. Understandably, the benefits of carotid endarterectomy for symptomatic carotid stenosis are greatest when endarterectomy (to remove the active atherosclerotic plaque) is undertaken very early.

TABLE 77 **THE ABCD² SCORE, TO IDENTIFY EARLY RISK OF STROKE AFTER TIA**

Variable	**Hazard ratio** (95% CI)	**Score**
Age ≥60 years	1.5 (1.2–2.0)	1 point
Blood pressure at presentation (≥140/90 mmHg)	1.6 (1.2–2.0)	1 point
Clinical features		
• Unilateral weakness	3.2 (2.5–4.1)	2 points
• Speech disturbance without weakness	1.7 (1.2–2.3)	1 point
Duration of symptoms		
• ≥60 minutes	2.1 (1.5–3.0)	2 points
• 10–59 minutes	1.7 (1.1–2.5)	1 point
Diabetes	1.7 (1.3–2.1)	1 point
	Total scores range from 0 (low risk) to 7 (high risk)	

ABCD score	**Patients** (%)	**Strokes** (%)	**7-day risk of stroke** (%, 95 % CI)
≤1	1	0	0
2	15	0	0
3	17	0	0
4	24	5	2 (0–6)
5	26	40	16 (6–27)
6	16	55	35 (19–52)
Total	100	100	10.5 (6–15)

SUMMARY

Score	**Patients**	**Risk of stroke within 2 days** (% [95% CI])	**Risk status**
6–7	21%	8.1%	High risk
4–5	45%	4.1%	Moderate risk
0–3	0–3	1.0%	Low risk

(*Lancet* [2007]; ***369***:283–92.)

Predictors of early recurrent stroke

Some of the factors that are associated with an increased risk of *early* stroke, within the *first weeks*, after a TIA or minor ischemic stroke are shown in *Table 77* and have been used to derived a prognostic index, the ABCD² score, for use in primary care and by emergency department physicians, that has been validated in independent data sets.

The ABCD² score is a seven-point score based on Age ≥60 years, Blood pressure increase (systolic ≥140 mmHg and/or diastolic ≥90 mmHg), Clinical features of unilateral weakness or speech disturbance, Duration of symptoms ≥10 minutes, and Diabetes[45]. It is a simple scoring system that can be used to stratify TIA patients who are at high risk early recurrent stroke. A score of ≥4 is considered high risk (>4% risk of stroke over the next 2 days). As can be seen from *Table 77*, the overall risk of stroke within 7 days of TIA was 10.5% (95% CI: 6–15%), but 95% of these strokes occurred in the 42% of patients who had an ABCD² score of 5 or 6, and all of the strokes occurred in the 66% of patients with an ABCD² score of 4 or more.

As the ABCD² score was not derived from data sets that included other potentially important prognostic factors for early risk of stroke after TIA, such as the presence of severe, ulcerated arterial stenosis in the symptomatic artery, and fresh ischemic brain lesions on MRI DWI brain scanning, another score, the ABCD³–I score has been derived and validated for use in secondary care where the results of special investigations are available (*Table 78*)[46]. The addition of information from brain and carotid imaging to the ABCD² score can improve risk stratification after TIA in secondary care settings.

Rates of recurrent stroke in the long-term

In the long term over 10 years of follow-up after TIA and ischemic stroke, the cumulative risk of first recurrent stroke is at least 43% (95% CI: 34–51%), which is six times greater than the risk of first-ever stroke in the general population of the same age and sex[41]. The annual risk of stroke and other major vascular events after a TIA and ischemic stroke is not linear; it is high early (as high as 5% in the first 2 days, 10% in the first week, 15% in the first month, and 18% at 3 months), declines to a nadir at 3 years, and then progressively increases[47]. The decline in risk between the first few months and 3 years is also seen in patients with symptomatic carotid stenosis treated medically. This decline presumably reflects healing of the symptomatic plaque. The subsequent increasing risk probably reflects continued exposure to causal risk factors, an increase in atherosclerotic plaque burden, and increasing age. Atherosclerosis is therefore an acute on chronic disease, behaving like a volcano with recurrent episodes of activity punctuated by long periods of a symptomatically 'dormant' state.

The main factor increasing the risk of recurrent stroke is failure to treat the underlying cause of the initial stroke. Most recurrent strokes are of the same pathologic type as the initial stroke, and many of the factors associated with an increased risk of recurrent stroke reflect a lack of control of underlying causal risk factors or diseases.

Cerebral venous thrombosis

Early death

Approximately 3–15% of patients die in the acute phase of the disorder[16]. Most early deaths are a consequence of CVT. The main cause of acute death with CVT is transtentorial herniation secondary to a large hemorrhagic lesion, followed by herniation due to multiple lesions or to diffuse brain edema. Status epilepticus, medical complications, and pulmonary embolism are among other causes of early death.

Risk factors for 30-day mortality are depressed consciousness, altered mental status, and thrombosis of the deep venous system, right hemisphere hemorrhage, and posterior fossa lesions.

Late deaths

Deaths after the acute phase are predominantly related to the underlying conditions, in particular malignancies.

Long-term outcome

About 15% of CVT patients die (9%) or become dependent (6%) after CVT. However, approximately one-half of survivors feel depressed or anxious, and minor cognitive or language deficits may preclude them from resuming their previous jobs. Abulia, executive deficits, and amnesia may result from thrombosis of the deep venous system, with bilateral panthalamic infarcts. Memory deficits, behavioral problems, or executive deficits may persist. Aphasia, in general of the fluent type, results from left lateral sinus thrombosis with temporal infarct or hemorrhage. Recovery is usually favorable, but minor troubles in spontaneous speech and naming might persist.

Risk factors for poor long-term prognosis include CNS infection, any malignancy, thrombosis of the deep venous system, intracranial hemorrhage on admission CT/MRI, GCS score <9, mental status disturbance, age >37 years, and male sex. Brain herniation leading to early death is more frequent in young patients, whereas late deaths due to malignancies and less favorable functional outcome are more frequent in elderly patients. A Glasgow Coma Scale score of 14 to 15 on admission, a complete or partial intracranial hypertension syndrome (including isolated headache) as the only manifestation of CVT, and absence of aphasia are variables associated with a favorable outcome.

TABLE 78 **THE ABCD³–I SCORE, TO IDENTIFY EARLY RISK OF STROKE AFTER TIA**

Variable	Score
Age ≥60 years	1
Blood pressure ≥140/90 mmHg	1
Clinical features	
• Speech impairment without weakness	1
• Unilateral weakness	2
Duration	
• 10–59 min	1
• ≥60 min	2
Diabetes	1
Dual TIA (TIA prompting medical attention plus >1 other TIA in the preceding 7 days)	2
Imaging: ipsilateral ≥50% stenosis of internal carotid artery	2
Imaging: acute diffusion-weighted imaging hyperintensity	2
Total range	0–13

Where the stated criteria are not met, a score of 0 is assigned.

(*Lancet Neurology* [2010];**9**:1060–1069.)

Primary intracerebral hemorrhage

About 25% of patients with ICH die during the first day, and 40% within the first month, usually as a consequence of supratentorial hemorrhage large enough to cause transtentorial herniation, or hemorrhage in the posterior fossa causing direct brainstem compression and herniation upwards and downwards.

Survival and functional outcome depends on the following factors:

- Location of the hematoma: worse outcome with posterior fossa, thalamic and putaminal hematoma, and intraventricular extension of blood.
- Volume of the hematoma: >50 ml, or volume of intraventricular hemorrhage >20 ml.
- Level of consciousness on admission (e.g. Glasgow Coma Scale): stupor or coma is a grim prognostic sign except in thalamic hemorrhage.
- Age of the patient: worse prognosis in the elderly.
- Pulse pressure.
- Extravasation of contrast material during CT scanning is another relatively bad prognostic sign, probably reflecting ongoing hemorrhage. A substantial (>33%) increase in ICH volume occurs in about 26% of patients within 1 hour of onset and an additional 12% between 1 and 20 hours.
- Later progression of neurologic signs and development of raised intracranial pressure, the cause of the hematoma. For example, for patients with ICH due to infective endocarditis, the combined case fatality of ICH and the underlying endocarditis is in the order of 25–50%, which is higher than that of ICH alone in the corresponding age group. In contrast, intracerebral hemorrhage from a cavernous malformation is usually limited and rarely fatal. For patients in whom a cavernous malformation has been detected, estimates of the risk of future hemorrhage vary widely, between 0.25% and 6% per annum[18]. Factors possibly predisposing to a relatively high risk of hemorrhage are a previous hemorrhage, deep location of the cavernous malformation (brainstem, cerebellum, basal ganglia, or thalamus), age below 35 on first presentation, and – not surprisingly – the presence of multiple lesions, which mostly occur in familial forms.

Subarachnoid hemorrhage

About one-half of individuals in the general population who experience a SAH die, one-half of the survivors remain severely disabled, and many functionally independent patients have impaired quality of life.

About 15% of patients die outside hospital within hours of the onset and, of those who reach hospital alive, a further 10–12% die within 24 hours of the first bleed. Rebleeding is the cause of death in 50% of patients who die within the first day of admission to hospital. The other common cause of early death is primary dysfunction of the brainstem from massive intraventricular hemorrhage, including distension of the fourth ventricle with blood. In addition to the 25% of patients who die within 24 hours of the onset of SAH, 35% of patients who survive the first day die within the subsequent 3 months, due to poor condition from the initial hemorrhage (e.g. raised intracranial pressure), rebleeding, and delayed cerebral ischemia (in roughly equal proportions).

The three major prognostic factors associated with a poor outcome are reduced level of consciousness, increasing age and increasing amounts of subarachnoid blood on the CT scan.

The risk of rebleeding after rupture of an intracranial aneurysm, without medical, endovascular, or surgical intervention, is about 40% in the first 3 weeks, i.e. 1–2% per day. Rebleeding of a ruptured aneurysm cannot be predicted reliably.

Cerebral ischemia or infarction tends to peak around days 4–12 after SAH. Its cause remains uncertain. It is not confined to the territory of a single cerebral artery or one of its branches, and it occurs only if the source is a ruptured aneurysm. It is strongly related to the total amount of subarachnoid blood. However, any causal relationship between the amount of extravasated blood and the development of delayed cerebral ischemia is not sufficiently explained by the production of putative toxic substances released from clots around the large arteries at the base of the brain. As loss of consciousness at the time of the hemorrhage is an important and independent predictive factor for delayed cerebral ischemia, it is conceivable that global ischemia during this brief period, along with a massive increase in intracranial pressure, may sensitize neurons to marginal perfusion associated with later complications, such as diffuse vasospasm or hypovolemia.

TREATMENT

Table 79 presents the levels of evidence and grades of recommendations for treatment[48].

Tip

▶ *Although the treatment section of this chapter has been structured into phases of stroke care, in practice we should not arbitrarily divide the treatment of stroke into acute and rehabilitation phases but rather adopt an integrated, goal and problem-orientated approach.*

ACUTE STROKE CARE

Acute stroke care takes place between the time of first contact with a potential stroke patient and admission to hospital or outpatient management in the community.

Emergency medical services

The pre-hospital phase, that starts with symptom onset and includes on-scene management by emergency medical services and transport time, should be 3.5 hours or less. Patients who show signs and symptoms of acute stroke must be treated as a time-sensitive emergency and should be transported without delay to the closest institution that provides emergency stroke care (evidence level C)[49]. Immediate contact with emergency medical services (e.g. telephoning 911/000/999 etc.) by patients or other members of the public is strongly recommended because it reduces time to treatment for acute stroke (compared with going to the general practitioner, for example) (evidence level B).

The emergency medical services system must be set up to categorize patients exhibiting signs and symptoms of a hyperacute stroke as a high priority (evidence level C). Direct Transport Protocols must be in place to facilitate the transfer of eligible patients to the closest and most appropriate facility providing acute stroke care (evidence level C). Direct Transport Protocol criteria must be based on: 1) the local emergency department performance which is recommended as being 60 minutes or less; 2) the pre-hospital phase, including symptom duration and anticipated transport time, being 3.5 hours or less; and 3) other acute care needs of the patient (evidence level B)].

Paramedics should use a standardized acute stroke out-of-hospital diagnostic screening tool (evidence level B)]. Paramedics should obtain a history of the stroke event, including time of onset, signs and symptoms, and previous medical and drug history from the patient if able to, or otherwise from an informant (e.g spouse, child, neighbour) if available (evidence level C).

Paramedics must notify the receiving facility of a suspected acute stroke patient so the facility may prepare for patient's arrival (evidence level C). Transfer of care from paramedics to receiving facility personnel must occur without delay (evidence level C).

Patients who are considered ineligible for time-sensitive revascularization (e.g. thrombolytic) therapy should be transported to the closest emergency department which provides access to neuroimaging and stroke expertise for assessment and initiation of secondary prevention management (evidence level C).

Hospital emergency department

The hospital emergency department phase includes the diagnostic evaluation and consideration of treatment options, which should be 60 minutes or less[49]. All patients presenting to an emergency department with suspected stroke or TIA must have an immediate clinical evaluation and investigations to establish the diagnosis, rule out stroke mimics, determine eligibility for thrombolytic therapy, start treatments to minimize the risk of early stroke recurrence and complications, and develop a plan for further management.

Patients presenting with stroke or TIA should not be discharged without diagnostic evaluations, consideration of functional impairments, initiation or modification of secondary prevention therapy, and a plan for ongoing management.

TABLE 79 **SUMMARY OF DEFINITIONS FOR LEVELS OF EVIDENCE**

Grade	Level of evidence
A	Evidence from meta-analyses of randomized controlled trials or randomized controlled trials. Desirable effects clearly outweigh undesirable effects, or *vice versa*
B	Single randomized controlled trial or well-designed observational study with strong evidence; or well-designed cohort or case–control analytic study; or multiple time series or dramatic results of uncontrolled experiment. Desirable effects closely balanced with undesirable effects
C	At least one well-designed, nonexperimental descriptive study (e.g. comparative studies, correlation studies, case studies) or expert committee reports, opinions and/or experience of respected authorities, including consensus from development and/or reviewer groups

(*Chest* [2008];**133**(6 Suppl):123S–31S.)

Initial evaluation

Patients with suspected acute stroke should have a rapid initial evaluation for airway, breathing, and circulation (evidence level B). A neurologic examination should be conducted to determine focal neurologic deficits and assess stroke severity (evidence level B). A standardized stroke scale should be used, such as the NIHSS or Scandinavian Stroke Scale (SSS).

Monitoring in the acute phase should include heart rate and rhythm, blood pressure, temperature, oxygen saturation, hydration, swallowing ability, and presence of seizure activity (evidence level B). Blood chemistry, electrolytes, hematology, and coagulation should be conducted as part of the initial evaluation (evidence level B). Electrocardiogram and chest X-ray should be completed, especially where the patient has a clinical history or evidence of heart disease or pulmonary disease (evidence level B).

Neurovascular imaging

All patients with suspected acute stroke or TIA should undergo brain imaging (MRI or CT) immediately (evidence level A), and vascular imaging of the brain and neck arteries as soon as possible (evidence level B). If MRI is performed, it should include diffusion-weighted sequences to detect recent ischemia and gradient echo and FLAIR sequences to determine the extent of infarct or presence of hemorrhage (evidence level B). If MRI is not possible as the initial imaging, a noncontrast CT scan of the brain should be performed (evidence level B).

Vascular imaging of the carotid and vertebral arteries by duplex ultrasonography, CTA, MRA, or catheter angiography should be performed within 24 hours of a TIA or ischemic stroke unless the patient is clearly not a candidate for revascularization (evidence level B). Ideally, CTA or MRA is performed at the time of the initial CT or MRI.

If not done as part of the original assessment in the emergency department, extracranial vascular imaging should be done as soon as possible to understand better the cause of the stroke event and guide management decisions. Imaging of the intracranial vessels might be warranted in some cases. Duplex ultrasonography, CTA, or MRA of the extracranial and intracranial vessels may be considered. In some circumstances catheter angiography of the extracranial and intracranial vessels should be considered (evidence level B).

Cardiovascular investigations

Following an initial ECG, serial ECGs (i.e. daily) should be done over the first 72 hours post-stroke to detect AF and other acute arrhythmias (evidence level B). Holter monitor during hospitalization may be considered in order to increase detection of AF (evidence level C).

Echocardiography, either 2-dimensional or transesophageal, should be considered for patients with suspected embolic stroke and normal vascular imaging, particularly if there are no contraindications to anticoagulation or cardiac surgery, should they be required (evidence level B).

TABLE 80 **EFFECTIVENESS OF THE FOUR TREATMENTS FOR ACUTE STROKE**

Intervention	Death or dependency		Odds ratio (95% CI)	Absolute risk reduction
	Control	*Intervention*		
Thrombolysis with r-tPA (alteplase)	53.0%	47.1%	0.78 (0.68–0.88)	5.9%
Aspirin	46.2%	45.0%	0.95 (0.91–0.99)	1.2%
Stroke unit	58.7%	54.4%	0.82 (0.73–0.92)	4.3%
Decompressive hemicraniectomy	76.5%	60.2%		16.3%

r-tPA: recombinant tissue plasminogen activator.

Acute ischemic stroke due to arterial thromboembolism

Systematic reviews of randomized controlled trials indicate that there are four effective treatments for acute ischemic stroke: thrombolysis within 4.5 hours, aspirin/acetylsalicylic acid, organized care in a stroke unit, and decompressive hemicraniectomy (*Table 80*)[50,51].

Acute thrombolytic therapy

Rationale

Most (approximately 80%) of strokes are ischemic in nature and caused by acute occlusion of an artery leading to immediated reduction in blood flow within the corresponding cerebrovascular territory. The site and size of the occlusion, and the efficiency of compensatory collateral blood flow, determine the extent of impaired blood flow and resulting focal brain ischemia and neurologic symptoms. Early spontaneous recanalization may occur due to endogenous release of tissue plasminogen activator (tPA), a serine protease of the fibrinolytic system which converts the zymogen plasminogen into the active protease plasmin, leading to cleavage of fibrin and the dissolution of newly formed thrombin 'clot'. However, for many patients, and particularly those with large thrombotic occlusions, this natural physiological function fails to recanalize the artery before the brain tissue it supplies becomes infarcted. The goal of exogenous fibrinolytic therapies is to serve as an adjunct to endogenous fibrinolysis and speed-up the reperfusion process.

Evidence

A recent systematic review of 26 randomized controlled trials of any thrombolytic agent (compared with control) in a total of 7,152 patients with definite ischemic stroke showed that, overall, thrombolytic therapy, mostly administered up to 6 hours after ischemic stroke, increased the risk of symptomatic intracranial hemorrhage at 7–10 days by 5.6% (2.1% control *vs.* 7.7% thrombolysis, odds ratio [OR]: 3.49, 95% CI: 2.81–4.33, absolute risk increase [ARI]: 5.6%) and death at 3–6 months after stroke by 2.6% (13.9% control *vs.* 16.5% thrombolysis, OR: 1.31, 95% CI: 1.14–1.50, ARI: 2.6%), yet significantly reduced death or dependency (modified Rankin scale score 3–6) at 3–6 months after stroke by 4.9% (55.8% control, 50.9% thrombolysis, OR: 0.81, 95% CI: 0.73–0.90, absolute risk reduction [ARR]: 4.9%) (*Table 81*). Treatment within 3 hours of stroke appeared more effective in reducing death or dependency (OR: 0.71, 95% CI: 0.52–0.96) with no statistically significant adverse effect on death (OR: 1.13, 95% CI: 0.86–1.48)[52].

Among the 55% of patients who were enrolled in trials testing intravenous recombinant tissue plasminogen activator (r-tPA; alteplase), random assignment to tPA was associated with a reduction in death or dependency at the end of follow-up from 53.0% (placebo) to 47.1% (tPA); ARR: 5.9%; OR: 0.78, 95% CI: 0.68–0.88 (*Table 81*)[52].

An updated pooled analysis of data from 12 randomized controlled trials of r-tPA (alteplase) given intravenously within 6 hours of stroke onset in 7012 patients reaffirms the time-dependent benefits of r-tPA. In up to 12 trials (7012 patients), r-tPA given within 6 h of stroke significantly increased the odds of being alive and independent (modified Rankin Scale, mRS 0–2) at final follow-up (1611/3483 [46.3%] *vs.* 1434/3404 [42.1%], OR: 1.17, 95% CI: 1.06–1.29, p=0.001), absolute increase of 42 (19–66) per 1000 people treated, and favorable outcome (mRS 0–1) absolute increase of 55 (95% CI: 33–77) per 1000. The benefit of r-tPA was greatest in patients treated within 3 h (mRS 0–2, 365/896 [40.7%] *vs.* 280/883 [31.7%], OR: 1.53, 95% CI: 1.26–1.86, p<0.0001), absolute benefit of 90 (46–135) per 1000 people treated, and mRS 0–1 (283/896 [31.6%] *vs.* 202/883 [22.9%], OR: 1.61, 95% CI: 1.30–1.90, p<0.0001), absolute benefit 87 (46–128) per 1000 treated. Numbers of deaths within 7 days were increased (250/2807 [8.9%] *vs.* 174/2728 [6.4%], OR; 1.44, 95% CI: 1.18–1.76, p=0.0003), but by final follow-up the excess was no longer significant (679/3548 [19.1%] *vs.* 640/3464 [18.5%], OR: 1.06, 95% CI: 0.94–1.20, p=0.33). Symptomatic intracranial hemorrhage (272/3548 [7.7%] *vs.* 63/3463 [1.8%], OR: 3.72, 95% CI: 2.98–4.64, p<0.0001) accounted for most of the early excess deaths. Patients older than 80 years achieved similar benefit to those aged 80 years or younger, particularly when treated early[53,54].

These data strengthen previous evidence to treat patients as early as possible after acute ischemic stroke, although some patients might benefit up to 6 h after stroke. Any extension of the time window should not be reason to delay, however; the correlation between onset to treatment time and benefit is exponential, and the odds of a favorable outcome are greatest (36%) in the first 90-minute window, falling to 18% in the second 90-minutes, and 9% in the third 90-minutes. Time from symptom onset is not the only predictor of outcome in patients undergoing fibrinolysis, however, in the same way that carotid stenosis is not the only predictor of outcome in patients undergoing carotid revascularization. Ongoing research will hopefully help to identify other independent, important clinical,

TABLE 81 **RELATIVE/ABSOLUTE BENEFITS AND HAZARDS WITH ANY THROMBOLYTIC THERAPY AND WITH r-tPA WITHIN 6 HOURS, 3 HOURS, AND 3–6 HOURS**

Outcome	**Thrombolysis within 6 hr** (%)	**Control** (%)	**Odds ratio** (95% CI)	**Absolute risk difference**	**Heterogeneity** (I^2)
Early death (≤10 days)	11.9%	7.7%	1.76 (1.44–2.16)	+4.2%	44%
[r-tPA]	6.7%	5.5%	1.23 (0.9–1.871)	+1.2%	0%
Fatal intracranial hemorrhage	4.5%	0.7%	4.40 (3.21–6.03)	+3.8%	0%
[r-tPA]	3.5%	0.8%	3.70 (2.36–5.79)	+2.7%	0%
Symptomatic intracranial hemorrhage	7.7%	2.1%	3.49 (2.81–4.33)	+5.6%	5%
[r-tPA]	8.3%	2.4%	3.28 (2.48–4.33)	+5.9%	24%
At final follow-up (3–6 months)					
Death	16.5%	13.9%	1.31 (1.14–1.50)	+2.6%	43%
[r-tPA]	13.3%	12.0%	1.14 (0.95–1.38)	+1.3%	40%
Death or dependency	50.9%	55.8%	0.81 (0.73–0.90)	–4.9%	38%
[r-tPA]	47.1%	53.0%	0.78 (0.68–0.88)	–5.9%	62%
Outcome	**Thrombolysis within 3 hr** (%)	**Control** (%)	**Odds ratio** (95% CI)	**Absolute risk difference**	**Heterogeneity** (I^2)
At final follow-up (3–6 months)					
Death	20.9%	19.4%	1.13 (0.86–1.48)	+1.5%	67%
[r-tPA]	17.3%	17.4%	0.97 (0.69–1.36)	–0.1%	38%
Death or dependency	49.7%	59.1%	0.71 (0.52–0.96)	–9.4%	0%
[r-tPA]	49.9%	60.2%	0.64 (0.50–0.83)	–10.3%	0%
Outcome	**Thrombolysis within 3–6 hr** (%)	**Control** (%)	**Odds ratio** (95% CI)	**Absolute risk difference**	**Heterogeneity** (I^2)
At final follow-up (3–6 months)					
Death or dependency	53.7%	56.0%	0.95 (0.82–1.10)	–2.3%	13%
[r-tPA]	45.8%	49.7%	0.85 (0.73–0.99)	–4.1%	34%

r-tPA: recombinant tissue plasminogen activator.

imaging, and biological factors that can distinguish which patients might benefit, not benefit, or be harmed by fibrinolysis, and which reperfusion and adjunctive strategies might improve on the current 40% recanalization rate achieved with alteplase within 24 hours. These may include patients who are of younger age with less severe stroke, absent or less acute ischemic change and leukoaraiosis on CT brain scan immediately before thrombolysis, normal blood glucose and renal function, no recent use of antiplatelet agents, no prior AF, heart failure, cancer, or physical dependency; and shorter time since stroke onset[55,56].

Recommendations

For individuals who have an acute ischemic stroke, the key to treatment is early reperfusion of ischemic, yet salvageable, brain without causing adverse effects, such as hemorrhage and orolingual angioedema. Thrombolysis with intravenous r-tPA, alteplase, should be considered in all patients with a definite disabling ischemic stroke who can be treated within 4.5 hours of onset of focal neurologic symptoms that have been present for at least 30 minutes without significant improvement (evidence level A).

Exclusion criteria

Past history of:

- Any intracranial hemorrhage.
- Disease of the CNS (e.g. neoplasm, aneurysm, past intracranial or spinal surgery).
- Stroke, serious head injury, myocardial infarction, ulcerative gastrointestinal disease in the previous 3 months.
- Gastrointestinal or urinary bleeding within the previous 21 days.
- Major surgery within the previous 14 days.
- Traumatic external heart massage, childbirth, puncture of a noncompressible blood vessel (e.g. subclavian vein or artery) within the previous 10 days.
- Heparin exposure in the preceding 48 hours and partial thromboplastin time not normal.

Current (i.e. pre-treatment) evidence of:

- Intracranial hemorrhage on brain imaging.
- Seizure at onset of focal neurologic symptoms (i.e. could the presentation be a manifestation of a seizure [due to a tumor, for example] and not a stroke?).
- Symptoms suggestive of SAH, even if the CT brain scan is normal.
- Neurologic deficits are mild or improving rapidly.
- Neurologic deficits have been present for longer than 4.5 hours (unless randomizing in clinical trials).
- Systolic blood pressure >185 mmHg or diastolic blood pressure >110 mmHg, or the need to treat aggressively with IV medication to achieve these levels.
- Known hemorrhagic diathesis (e.g. hemorrhagic retinopathy, infective endocarditis, pericarditis, acute pancreatitis, severe liver disease, esophageal varices, neoplasms with increased bleeding risk).
- Oral anticoagulant use or INR >1.7.
- Platelet count $<80 \times 10^9$/l.
- Prolonged partial thromboplastin time.
- Blood glucose <2.8 mmol/l (50 mg/dl) or >22 mmol/l (400 mg/dl).
- Caution should be used in patients with severe stroke (NIHSS score >22), and patients with a past history of stroke *and* concomitant diabetes.

Features on the initial CT brain scan of an otherwise alteplase-eligible ischemic stroke patient that modify the response to treatment remain poorly defined. Some of the trials of alteplase excluded patients with severe hemispheric stroke if the initial CT scan showed early signs of infarction involving more than one-third of the territory of the MCA (i.e. a score of <5 on the Alberta Stroke Program Early CT Score [ASPECTS]). In clinical practice, the decision to treat such a patient with alteplase should be based on the clinical judgment of the treating physician, and the wishes of the patient and family, until such time as additional data from randomized controlled trials are made available (evidence level B).

- Discuss treatment and adverse effects with the patient and family before treatment.
- Delay placement of indwelling bladder catheters and nasogastric tubes (for at least 90 minutes after alteplase infusion completed, if possible) if time to alteplase treatment will be delayed by undertaking these procedures before alteplase.
- Thrombolytic therapy should be administered by, or under the supervision of, clinicians with expertise in stroke medicine, and who have access to a suitable stroke service, with facilities for immediately identifying and managing hemorrhagic complications.
- All eligible patients should receive intravenous alteplase as soon as possible after hospital arrival, with a target door-to-needle time of less than 60 minutes (evidence level C).
- Recommended dose of alteplase is 0.9 mg/kg up to a maximum of 90 mg, the first 10% of the dose (0.09 mg /kg) is given IV as a bolus over 1 minute, the rest (0.81 mg/kg) as an IV infusion over 60 minutes.
- Perform neurologic assessments every 15 minutes during infusion of alteplase, every 30 minutes for the next 6 hours, and every 60 minutes for the next 16 hours. If severe headache, acute hypertension, neurologic deterioration, or nausea and vomiting occur, discontinue the infusion and obtain an emergency CT brain scan.
- Measure blood pressure every 15 minutes for 2 hours, every 30 minutes for 6 hours, and every 60 minutes for 16 hours; repeat measurements more frequently if systolic blood pressure is >180 mmHg or diastolic blood pressure is >105 mmHg, and administer antihypertensive drugs as needed to maintain blood pressure at or below those levels.
- Obtain a follow-up CT brain scan at 24 hours before starting antiplatelet therapy.

There remain situations where there are sparse or no clinical trial data to support the use of thrombolytic therapy: pediatric stroke, adults who present within the first few hours of onset of an acute ischemic stroke but do not meet current criteria for treatment with intravenous alteplase, and intra-arterial thrombolysis. In clinical practice, the decision to use alteplase in these situations should be based on the clinical judgment of the treating physician, and the wishes of the patient and family, until such time as additional data from randomized controlled trials are available (evidence level A).

Management of elevated blood pressure complicating alteplase treatment

If blood pressure is elevated on two readings 10 minutes apart (i.e. systolic BP >185 mmHg, or diastolic BP >110 mmHg), consider treatment with glyceryl trinitrate (GTN) infusion administered via separate IV line, as per local hospital protocol (PVC containers and lines should be avoided). For GTN infusion, 50 mg/100 ml, start at 3 ml/hr, and titrate until BP <180/110 (6 ml/hr = 50 μg/min). After switching off the infusion, the blood pressure-lowering effect abates in minutes. If GTN fails to lower blood pressure adequately, consider IV metoprolol or labetalol, and, failing that, consider IV hydralazine (*Table 82*). If blood pressure is still high, >180/110, consider admission to the intensive care unit for treatment with IV sodium nitroprusside.

Management of intracranial hemorrhage complicating alteplase treatment

Suspect intracranial hemorrhage if:

- Acute neurologic deterioration.
- New headache.
- Nausea or vomiting.
- Acute increase in blood pressure.

If intracranial hemorrhage is suspected:

- Discontinue alteplase administration.
- Organize CT brain.
- Bloods: full blood count (FBC), activated partial thromboplastin time (aPTT), INR, fibrinogen, cross match.
- Call hematology to provisionally request cryoprecipitate and platelets.

If hemorrhage is observed:

- Administer cryoprecipitate 1 unit/10 kg bodyweight.
- If alteplase is still circulating at the time of the bleeding onset and immediate control of bleeding is required, consider antifibrinolytic therapy (e.g. IV aminocaproic acid 0.1 g/kg over 30 minutes or aprotinin 2 million kallikrein inhibitory units over 30 minutes), while awaiting cryoprecipitate.
- Consult Neurosurgery if indicated. The outlook is poor with or without surgery, occasionally salvage evacuation may have a limited role. Discuss with Neurosurgery on a case-by-case basis.
- Recheck FBC, aPTT, INR, fibrinogen after administration of cryoprecipitate and platelets, and target further administration of cryoprecipitate if fibrinogen levels remain <1.0 g/l, in consultation with the hematologist.
- Factor VIIa may have a controversial role. Consider if the patient continues to deteriorate despite the above measures and in discussion with Hematology.

In case of bleeding elsewhere, cease alteplase and investigate and treat as clinically indicated. The principles regarding use of cryoprecipitate, platelets, and antifibrinolytic therapy do not vary after administration of alteplase. In addition, call blood bank to arrange cross-match in case transfusion of fresh frozen plasma is required. Consult Gastroenterology or Urology as clinically indicated.

Management of perioral angioedema complicating alteplase treatment

Perioral angioedema is an uncommon complication of alteplase treatment of acute ischemic stroke, occurring in 1–5% of treated patients. It may occur during, or up to 2 hours after, the infusion and may be hemilingual, contralateral to the side of the stroke. Concurrent angiotensin-converting enzyme (ACE) inhibitor use and involvement by the stroke of the insular cortex in the brain may be risk factors for its development.

The main differential diagnosis is a tongue hematoma. Management is empirical, based on expert opinion. Suggested principles include:

- Early anesthetic consultation; intubation may be required for progressive airway obstruction.
- Tracheostomy must be avoided due to the thrombolytic effects of the alteplase.
- IV hydrocortisone 100 mg.
- IV promethazine 25 mg (must take care to avoid tissue extravasation and intra-arterial administration).
- IV ranitidine 50 mg.
- Adrenaline should be avoided for fear of inducing hypertension.

TABLE 82 **APPROACHES TO ARTERIAL HYPERTENSION IN ACUTE ISCHEMIC STROKE PATIENTS WHO ARE CANDIDATES FOR ACUTE REPERFUSION THERAPY**

Patient otherwise eligible for acute reperfusion therapy, except that BP is >185/110 mmHg

- If heart rate >55 beats per minute:
  - Labetalol 10–20 mg IV over 1–2 minutes; may repeat one time

or

  - Metoprolol 5 mg IV over 3–5 minutes; may repeat in 5 minutes, two times, if necessary

or

- Nicardipine 5 mg/hr IV; titrate up by 2.5 mg/hr every 5–15 minutes, maximum 5 mg/hr; when desired BP reached, adjust to maintain proper BP limits

or

- Hydralazine 5 mg IV over 1 minute; may repeat 5 mg IV bolus in 5 minutes
  - If systolic BP still >180 mmHg, give 10 mg IV bolus every 5 minutes until target systolic BP reached
  - Increase to 20 mg bolus if required
  - Maximum hydralazine dose = 240 mg

or

- Other agents (e.g. enalaprilat) may be considered when appropriate

If BP is not maintained at or below 185/110 m mHg, do not administer r-tPA

Management of BP during and after r-tPA or other acute reperfusion therapy to maintain BP at or below 180/105 mmHg:

- Monitor BP every 15 minutes for 2 hours from the start of r-tPA therapy, then every 30 minutes for 6 hours, and then every hour for 16 hours

- If systolic BP >180–230 mmHg or diastolic BP >105–120 mmHg:
  - Labetalol 10 mg IV followed by continuous IV infusion 2–8 mg/min

or

  - Nicardipine 5 mg/hr IV; titrate up to desired effect by 2.5 mg/hr every 5–15 minutes, maximum 15 mg/hr

or

  - Hydralazine 50–150 μg/min

or

  - Glyceryl trinitrate 1–100 μg/kg/min (or topical glyceryl trinitrate [paste or patch] at a rate of 5–10 mg/24 hr [approximates 200–400 μg/hr])

Note: labetalol and hydralazine may be used together during the maintenance phase.

BP: blood pressure; IV: intravenously; r-tPA, recombinant tissue plasminogen activator.

Implementation

The most recent national sentinel audit of the treatment of patients with stroke admitted to hospital for inpatient care in the UK indicated that in 2008, 1.4% of all inpatients with acute ischemic stroke received intravenous thrombolysis. As this was less than 10% of those deemed eligible (arrived at hospital within 3 hours of stroke onset [now 4.5 hours] and younger than 80 years), it is theoretically possible that at least 10%, if not 15%, of patients hospitalized with acute ischemic stroke could be treated with thrombolysis.

Antiplatelet therapy with aspirin/ acetylsalicylic acid

Evidence

Among 12 randomized controlled trials (RCTs) of antiplatelet therapy in 43,041 participants with acute ischemic stroke, two trials testing aspirin 160–300 mg once daily, started within 48 hours of stroke onset and continuing for 2–4 weeks, contributed 94% of the data[57]. After a maximum follow-up of 6 months, random allocation to early aspirin was associated with a 23% reduction in odds of recurrent ischemic stroke (3.1% [control] *vs.* 2.4% [aspirin]; OR: 0.77, 95% CI: 0.69–0.87), 12% reduction in recurrent stroke of any type (3.9% [control] *vs.* 3.4% [aspirin]; OR: 0.88, 95% CI: 0.79–0.97), 29% reduction in pulmonary embolism (0.48% [control] *vs.* 0.34% [aspirin], OR: 0.71, 95% CI: 0.53–0.97), 8% reduction in death (12.9% [control] *vs.* 12.1% [aspirin], OR: 0.92, 95% CI: 0.87–0.98), and 5% reduction in death or dependency at the end of follow-up (46.2% [control] *vs.* 45.0% [aspirin], OR: 0.95, 95% CI: 0.91–0.99) (see *Table 80*). Subgroup-specific analyses found no significant heterogeneity of the benefits of early aspirin over 2–4 weeks among 28 subgroups examined, which included the elderly, gender, and ischemic stroke subtypes. Against these benefits, random assignment to aspirin was associated with a 22% increase in odds of symptomatic intracranial hemorrhage (0.8% [control] *vs.* 1.0% [aspirin], OR: 1.22, 95% CI: 1.00–1.50) and 69% increase in major extracranial hemorrhage during the treatment period (0.6% [control] *vs.* 1.0% [aspirin], OR: 1.69, 95% CI: 1.35–2.11).

Recommendations

After brain imaging has excluded intracranial hemorrhage, all acute stroke patients not already on an antiplatelet agent should be given at least 160 mg of aspirin immediately as a one-time loading dose (evidence level A). In patients treated with r-tPA, aspirin should be delayed until after the 24-hour post-thrombolysis scan has excluded intracranial hemorrhage (evidence level B). Aspirin (75–150 mg daily) should then be continued indefinitely or until an alternative antithrombotic regime is started (evidence level A). In dysphagic patients, aspirin may be given by enteral tube or by rectal suppository (evidence level A).

In patients already on aspirin prior to ischemic stroke or transient ischemic attack, clopidigrel may be considered as an alternative (evidence level B). If patients have a recent (within the past 24 hours) TIA or minor ischemic stroke, clopidogrel may be added to aspirin for the first 21–90 days (evidence level B) (see page 393). If rapid action is required, then a loading dose of 300 mg or 600 mg of clopidogrel could be considered, followed by a maintenance dose of 75 mg once a day.

Implementation

The national sentinel audit of treatment of hospitalized stroke patients in the UK indicated that, in 2008, 85% of inpatients with acute ischemic stroke were treated early with aspirin.

Anticoagulation therapy

Evidence

A systematic review and meta-analysis of 24 randomized trials comparing early anticoagulant therapy (started within 2 weeks of stroke onset) with control, in 23,748 patients with acute presumed or confirmed ischemic stroke, reported that there was no evidence that anticoagulant therapy reduced the odds of death from all causes (OR: 1.05; 95% CI: 0.98–1.12) or the odds of being dead or dependent at the end of follow-up (OR: 0.99; 95% CI: 0.93–1.04)[58]. Although anticoagulant therapy was associated with fewer recurrent ischemic strokes (OR: 0.76; 95% CI: 0.65–0.88), it was also associated with an increase in symptomatic intracranial hemorrhages (OR: 2.55; 95% CI: 1.95–3.33). Similarly, anticoagulants reduced the frequency of pulmonary emboli (OR: 0.60; 95% CI: 0.44–0.81), but this benefit was offset by an increase in extracranial hemorrhages (OR: 2.99; 95% CI: 2.24–3.99). These data indicated that, in patients with acute ischemic stroke, immediate anticoagulant therapy is not associated with net short- or long-term benefit[51,58]. Treatment with anticoagulants reduced recurrent stroke, deep vein thrombosis, and pulmonary embolism, but increased bleeding risk.

Recommendations

The data do not support the routine use of any of the currently available anticoagulants in acute ischemic stroke to prevent early recurrent stroke.

Ischemic stroke due to cerebral venous thrombosis

Thrombolytic and anticoagulant therapy

Evidence

There is currently no available evidence from RCTs regarding the efficacy or safety of thrombolytic therapy in dural sinus thrombosis. An RCT is justified to test this therapy, especially in patients predicted to have a poor prognosis.

A systematic review and meta-analysis of two small unconfounded RCTs in which anticoagulant therapy was compared with placebo or open control in 79 patients with cerebral sinus thrombosis (confirmed by intra-arterial contrast or MRA) reported that one trial (20 patients) examined the efficacy of IV, adjusted-dose, unfractionated heparin (UFH) and the other trial (59 patients) examined high-dose, body weight-adjusted, subcutaneous, low-molecular weight heparin (LMWH; Nadroparin). Anticoagulant therapy was associated with a pooled relative risk of death of 0.33 (95% CI: 0.08–1.21) and of death or dependency of 0.46 (95% CI: 0.16–1.31). No new symptomatic intracerebral hemorrhages were observed. One major gastrointestinal hemorrhage occurred after anticoagulant treatment. Two control patients (placebo) had a diagnosis of probable pulmonary embolism (one fatal). Based upon the limited evidence available, anticoagulant treatment for cerebral sinus thrombosis appeared to be safe and was associated with a potentially important reduction in the risk of death or dependency which did not reach statistical significance[16].

Recommendations

- Patients with CVT and a suspected bacterial infection should receive appropriate antibiotics and surgical drainage of purulent collections of infectious sources associated with CVT when appropriate (Class I; level of evidence C).
- In patients with CVT and increased intracranial pressure, monitoring for progressive visual loss is recommended, and when this is observed, increased intracranial pressure should be treated urgently (Class I; level of evidence C).
- In patients with CVT and a single seizure with parenchymal lesions, early initiation of antiepileptic drugs for a defined duration is recommended to prevent further seizures (Class I; level of evidence B).

- In patients with CVT and a single seizure without parenchymal lesions, early initiation of antiepileptic drugs for a defined duration is probably recommended to prevent further seizures (Class IIa; level of evidence C).
- In the absence of seizures, the routine use of antiepileptic drugs in patients with CVT is not recommended (Class III; level of evidence C).
- For patients with CVT, initial anticoagulation with adjusted-dose UFH or weight-based LMWH in full anticoagulant doses is reasonable, followed by vitamin K antagonists (VKAs), regardless of the presence of ICH (Class IIa; level of evidence B).
- Admission to a stroke unit is reasonable for treatment and for prevention of clinical complications of patients with CVT (Class IIa; level of evidence C).
- In patients with CVT and increased intracranial pressure, it is reasonable to initiate treatment with acetazolamide. Other therapies (LP, optic nerve decompression, or shunts) can be effective if there is progressive visual loss (Class IIa; level of evidence C).
- Endovascular intervention may be considered if deterioration occurs despite intensive anticoagulation treatment (Class IIb; level of evidence C).
- In patients with neurologic deterioration due to severe mass effect or intracranial hemorrhage causing intractable intracranial hypertension, decompressive hemicraniectomy may be considered (Class IIb; level of evidence C).
- For patients with CVT, steroid medications are not recommended, even in the presence of parenchymal brain lesions on CT/MRI, unless needed for another underlying disease (Class III; level of evidence B).
- In patients with provoked CVT (associated with a transient risk factor), VKAs may be continued for 3–6 months, with a target INR of 2.0–3.0 (Class IIb; level of evidence C).
- In patients with unprovoked CVT, VKAs may be continued for 6–12 months, with a target INR of 2.0–3.0 (Class IIb; level of evidence C).
- For patients with recurrent CVT, venous thromboembolism (VTE) after CVT, or first CVT with severe thrombophilia (i.e. homozygous prothrombin G20210A; homozygous factor V Leiden; deficiencies of protein C, protein S, or antithrombin; combined thrombophilia defects; or APS), indefinite anticoagulation may be considered, with a target INR of 2.0–3.0 (Class IIb; level of evidence C).
- Consultation with a physician with expertise in thrombosis may be considered to assist in the prothrombotic testing and care of patients with CVT (Class IIb; level of evidence C).

Hemorrhagic stroke – primary intracerebral hemorrhage

General care

Recommendations

- Patients with suspected ICH should undergo a CT or MRI immediately to confirm diagnosis, location and extent of hemorrhage (evidence level A).
- Evaluation of patients with acute ICH should include questions about anticoagulant therapy, measurement of platelet count, partial thromboplastin time (PTT), and INR (evidence level A).
- Patients with acute ICH and an established coagulopathy or a history of anticoagulant use should be treated appropriately to reverse the coagulopathy (prothrombin complex concentrate, vitamin K, or fresh-frozen plasma (evidence level B).
- If there is a persisting strong indication for anticoagulation (e.g. mechanical heart valve), the decision about when to restart anticoagulant therapy should be made on a case-by-case basis (evidence level C).
- Patients with acute ICH should be considered for CTA or other imaging modality, such as MRI, to exclude an underlying lesion such as an aneurysm, arteriovenous malformation, or tumor (evidence level B).
- Medically stable patients with an acute ICH should be admitted to a stroke unit (evidence level B), *and* undergo interprofessional stroke team assessment to determine their rehabilitation and other care needs (see subacute care below).
- Beyond the acutely symptomatic period, patients with ICH should be managed similarly to those with ischemic stroke, except for avoidance of antithrombotics.
- ICH should not be considered an indication for statin therapy (A). Continued use in patients previously on a statin for another appropriate indication should be reviewed following ICH because of a potential increased risk of recurrent hemorrhage. Currently, there is insufficient evidence to determine whether the potential increased risk of hemorrhage outweighs the potential benefits for prevention of ischemic cardiovascular disease in ICH survivors with other appropriate indications for statins.

Surgical evacuation of supratentorial intracerebral hemorrhage

Evidence

A systematic review of 10 randomized trials of routine medical treatment plus intracranial surgery compared with routine medical treatment alone in 2059 participants with CT-confirmed primary supratentorial intracerebral hematoma revealed that surgery was associated with statistically significant reduction in the odds of being dead or dependent at final follow-up (OR: 0.71, 95% CI: 0.58–0.88; $2p = 0.001$), with no significant heterogeneity among the study results (evidence level A). Surgery was also associated with significant reduction in the odds of death at final follow-up (OR: 0.74, 95% CI: 0.61–0.90; $2p = 0.003$); however, there was significant heterogeneity for death as outcome. An individual patient data subgroup meta-analysis from 2186 patients enrolled in eight trials indicated that there was improved outcome with surgery if it was undertaken early, within 8 hours of ictus, before the patient deteriorates (p=0.003), or the volume of the hematoma was 20–50 ml (p=0.004), or the Glasgow Coma Score was between 9 and 12 (p = 0.0009), or the patient was aged between 50 and 69 years (p=0.01). In addition, there was some evidence that more superficial hematomas with no intraventricular hemorrhage might also benefit (p=0.09)[59]. The Surgical Trial in Intracerebral Hemorrhage II (STICH II) results confirm that early surgery does not increase the rate of death or disability at 6 months and might have a small but clinically relevant survival advantage for conscious patients with superficial lobar intracerebral hemorrhage of 10–100 ml and no intraventricular hemorrhage, who are admitted within 48 hours of ictus[60].

Cavernous malformations, whether in a cerebral hemisphere or in the brainstem, carry a moderate risk of (re)bleeding, while the functional deficits from such hemorrhages are limited. Surgical treatment or stereotactic radiation is regularly performed but there are no randomized controlled studies.

Recommendations

Most patients with acute supratentorial ICH will not require, or benefit from, neurosurgical evacuation of the hemorrhage. However, *selected* patients with acute supratentorial ICH may be considered for surgical intervention including placement of an extraventricular drain (EVD) for treatment of hydrocephalus, or craniotomy for evacuation of superficial lobar ICH (evidence level B).

Surgical evacuation of infratentorial intracerebral hemorrhage

Evidence

Cerebellar hemorrhage

For decades there has been a strong impression that surgical evacuation saves lives in patients with cerebellar hemorrhages who have clinical evidence of progressive brainstem compression. The need for timely surgical treatment in patients who are in danger of progressive brainstem compression is dictated by the potentially fatal outcome and the often surprisingly mild sequelae after operation. So strong is this notion, that a clinical trial in this category of patients is unlikely to ever be mounted. However, some patients can be managed conservatively, but there is uncertainty about the selection criteria. In general, an impaired level of consciousness seems a sound indication for operative intervention, provided corneal and oculocephalic reflexes have not been lost, in which case the outcome is invariably fatal. Some neurosurgeons advocate surgery with large hemorrhages (>3–4 cm in diameter), even in alert patients, on the basis of experience that delayed deterioration of consciousness may be so rapid that the patient cannot be salvaged at this later stage. Others maintain that such rapid deterioration depends not so much on the absolute size of the hemorrhage as on the degree of effacement of the fourth ventricle, and that operative evacuation is indicated in all patients in whom the fourth ventricle is completely obliterated. Since effacement of the fourth ventricle is associated with hydrocephalus and location of the hemorrhage in the midline (vermis), it is not surprising that these features also predispose to secondary deterioration. If the patient has a depressed level of consciousness and hydrocephalus, without signs of brainstem compression and with a hemorrhage <3 cm, ventriculostomy can be carried out as an initial (and perhaps only) procedure.

As with supratentorial hemorrhage, some patients with cerebellar hemorrhage have been successfully treated by stereotactic aspiration, with or without instillation of fibrinolytic drugs. Any advantage of these techniques over the conventional approach with suboccipital craniotomy remains to be proved. The same applies to ventriculostomy by endoscopic perforation of the third ventricle towards the basal cisterns, rather than by the conventional method of a catheter inserted in the lateral ventricle.

Recommendations

Patients with cerebellar hemorrhage should be referred for urgent neurosurgical consultation and consideration of evacuation of ICH particularly in the setting of altered level of consciousness or new cranial neuropathy (evidence level B).

Pontine hemorrhage

Pontine hemorrhages are frequently fatal; the case fatality is still around 50%. The outcome depends to an important extent on the cause, since hemorrhage in the pons from a cavernous malformation is rarely fatal. The management of patients with 'hypertensive' pontine hemorrhage is usually conservative, but some case reports have documented successful stereotactic aspiration. The natural history may or may not have been influenced by these interventions. There is a narrow margin of uncertainty between patients with poor prognosis because of absent corneal and oculocephalic reflexes and those with small hemorrhages who will do well with conservative management.

Hemostatic drug therapy

Evidence

A systematic review of five phase II, and one phase III, RCTs of hemostatic drug therapies within 4 hours of onset of acute spontaneous (nontraumatic) ICH involving 1398 adults found that 423 participants received placebo and 975 participants received hemostatic drugs (two received epsilon-aminocaproic acid [EACA] and 973 received recombinant activated factor VII [rFVIIa]). Hemostatic drugs did not significantly reduce 90-day case fatality after ICH (risk ratio [relative risk, RR]: 0.85, 95% CI: 0.58–1.25), and rFVIIa did not significantly reduce death or dependence on the modified Rankin Scale (grades 4–6) within 90 days of ICH (RR: 0.91, 95% CI: 0.72–1.15) (evidence level A). There was a trend towards more participants on rFVIIa experiencing thromboembolic serious adverse events (RR: 1.37, 95% CI: 0.74–2.55).

Recommendations

Administration of rFVIIa (NiaStase®) is not recommended for routine use (evidence level A). Although administration of rFVIIa prevents hematoma growth, it increases the risk of arterial thromboembolic phenomena and does not provide a clinical benefit for survival or outcome (evidence level A).

Blood pressure reduction

The blood pressure is usually increased in patients with ICH, through pre-existing hypertension, a response to a sudden increase in intracranial pressure, or both these factors. There are theoretical arguments in favor of decreasing the blood pressure (in the hope of stopping ongoing bleeding from ruptured small arteries), as well as in favor of increasing it further (in the hope of salvaging marginally perfused areas of brain that are compressed around the hemorrhage).

Evidence

The INTERACT 2 trial randomly assigned 2839 patients who had had a spontaneous intracerebral hemorrhage within the previous 6 hours and who had elevated systolic blood pressure to receive intensive treatment to lower their blood pressure (with a target systolic level of <140 mmHg within 1 hour) or guideline-recommended treatment (with a target systolic level of >180 mmHg) with the use of agents of the physician's choosing[61].

Among the 2794 participants for whom the primary outcome could be determined, 719 of 1382 participants (52.0%) receiving intensive treatment, as compared with 785 of 1412 (55.6%) receiving guideline-recommended treatment, had death or major disability – defined as a score of 3–6 on the modified Rankin scale (odds ratio with intensive treatment: 0.87, 95% confidence interval [CI]: 0.75–1.01; p=0.06). The ordinal analysis showed significantly lower modified Rankin scores with intensive treatment (odds ratio for greater disability: 0.87, 95% CI: 0.77–1.00; p=0.04). Mortality was 11.9% in the group receiving intensive treatment and 12.0% in the group receiving guideline-recommended treatment. Nonfatal serious adverse events occurred in 23.3% and 23.6% of the patients in the two groups, respectively[61].

Recommendations

In patients with intracerebral hemorrhage, blood pressure should be lowered to a target systolic level of <140 mmHg as soon as possible.

Hemorrhagic stroke – subarachnoid hemorrhage

General care

Recommendations

- Patients with suspected SAH should have a noncontrast CT scan as soon as possible after hospital arrival to confirm the diagnosis (evidence level B). If the noncontrast CT scan is negative, as reported by a radiologist, the patient should undergo LP for CSF analysis.
- Xanthochromia evaluation may be more sensitive after a delay of 12 hours from symptom onset, but such a delay may not be practical or clinically appropriate (evidence level B). CSF analysis for xanthochromia by spectrophotometry is preferable to visual inspection, but is not routinely available (evidence level B).
- Patients with SAH should undergo high-quality noninvasive CTA to identify the source of the bleed, such as a ruptured aneurysm (evidence level B). If CTA is negative, consider further imaging with catheter angiography (evidence level C).
- Patients with confirmed SAH should have an urgent consultation with a neurosurgeon (evidence level B).

- Patients with SAH should have their blood pressure closely monitored and maintained as normotensive (evidence level B). Treatment for high blood pressure should be initiated while the aneurysm is unsecured to reduce the risk of hypertension-induced rebleeding (evidence level B).
- A high fluid intake of 2.5–3.5 liters per day of isotonic saline is recommended in patients with aneurysmal SAH to compensate for 'cerebral salt wasting' and to prevent hypovolemia which predisposes to cerebral ischemia.
- Although it is reasonable to prevent a decrease in plasma volume, there is no good evidence to support prevention of cerebral ischemia after SAH through increasing plasma volume by infusion of albumin or colloids, or by the administration of fludrocortisone.
- Hyponatremia after SAH usually reflects cerebral salt wasting (sodium depletion) and not secretion of antidiuretic hormone (sodium dilution). Because hyponatremia may lead to hypovolemia, it should not be treated with fluid restriction.
- In patients with a decreased level of consciousness headache may present as restlessness. The 'analgesic staircase' consists of frequent doses of paracetamol, then codeine if necessary, tramadol or, as a last resort, piritramide.
- Antifibrinolytic drugs prevent rebleeding after aneurysmal rupture, but because they increase the risk of cerebral ischemia they have no useful effect on overall outcome.
- For SAH patients with intraparenchymal extension at the time the aneurysm is secured, urgent evacuation of the hematoma should be considered (evidence level C).
- Patients with SAH and CT evidence of hydrocephalus that is clinically symptomatic should undergo urgent placement of an EVD or other CSF diversion technique (evidence level B).
- Patients with aneurysmal SAH should receive venous thromboembolism prophylaxis.

Nimodipine

Evidence

Randomized trials indicate that the calcium antagonist oral nimodipine reduces the risk of secondary ischemia and a poor outcome after aneurysmal SAH by one-third (RR: 0.67, 95% CI: 0.55–0.81).

Recommendation

Patients who present within 96 hours of a SAH and have an adequate blood pressure should immediately be started on oral nimodipine 60 mg every 4 hours by mouth for 14–21 days (evidence level A). Intravenous administration of calcium antagonists cannot be recommended for routine practice on the basis of the present evidence.

Magnesium

Evidence

A meta-analysis of seven randomized trials involving 2047 patients shows that magnesium is not superior to placebo for reduction of poor outcome after aneurysmal subarachnoid hemorrhage (RR: 0.96, 95% CI: 0.86–1.08).

Recommendation

As intravenous magnesium sulfate does not improve clinical outcome after aneurysmal subarachnoid hemorrhage, routine administration of magnesium cannot be recommended.

Endovascular coiling vs. neurosurgical clipping of the ruptured aneurysm

Evidence

A systematic review of three trials involving a total of 2272 aneurysmal subarachnoid hemorrhage patients, who were technically eligible for either endovascular coiling or neurosurgical clipping of the ruptured aneurysm, and most of whom were in good clinical condition and had an aneurysm on the anterior circulation, demonstrated that outcomes were better among those treated by endovascular methods than by microsurgery (evidence level A). After 1 year of follow up, the RR of poor outcome for coiling *vs.* clipping was 0.76 (95% CI: 0.67–0.88). The ARR was 7% (95% CI: 4–11%). In the worst-case scenario analysis for poor outcome overall, the RR for coiling *vs.* clipping was 0.81 (95% CI: 0.70–0.92) and the ARR was 6% (95% CI: 2–10%). For patients with anterior circulation aneurysm the RR of poor outcome was 0.78 (95% CI: 0.68–0.90) and the ARR was 7% (95% CI: 3–10%). For those with a posterior circulation aneurysm the RR was 0.41 (95% CI: 0.19–0.92) and the ARR 27% (95% CI: 6–48%).

Recommendations

Patients with an aneurysmal SAH should have the aneurysm secured urgently by endovascular coiling or microsurgical clipping within 24–48 hours (evidence level B). For patients with poor prognosis for neurologic recovery, an initial course of supportive nonsurgical management may be appropriate (evidence level B).

Decisions regarding modality of treatment should be based on patient-specific characteristics, which include consideration of patient age, clinical grade, morphology of the aneurysm, medical comorbidity, and institutional experience and resources (evidence level B).

SUBACUTE STROKE CARE

Organized multidisciplinary care in a geographically defined stroke unit

Evidence

Among 31 trials which compared organized multidisciplinary care in a stroke unit with an alternative service in a total of 6936 participants, more organized care in a stroke unit was associated with a significant reduction in death or dependency at final (median 1 year) follow-up from 58.7% (general ward) to 54.4% (stroke unit) (ARR: 4.3%, OR: 0.82, 95% CI: 0.73–0.92) (*Table 80*)[62]. Outcomes were independent of patient age, sex, or stroke severity, but appeared to be better in stroke units based in a discrete ward. There was no indication that organized stroke unit care resulted in a longer hospital stay.

TABLE 83 **CAUSES OF DETERIORATION AFTER STROKE**

Neurologic
- Recurrent stroke (ischemic or hemorrhagic)
- Hemorrhagic transformation of an infarct
- Edema around the infarct or hemorrhage*
- Obstructive hydrocephalus
- Epileptic seizures*
- Delayed ischemia* (in SAH)
- Incorrect diagnosis of stroke (*Table 71*):
  - Intracranial tumor*
  - Cerebral abscess*
  - Encephalitis (e.g. herpes simplex)
  - Chronic subdural hematoma*
  - Subdural empyema*

Non-neurologic*
- Infection:
  - Respiratory (e.g. aspiration pneumonia)
  - Urinary
  - Septicemia
- Metabolic/nutritional:
  - Dehydration
  - Electrolyte disturbance (e.g. hyponatremia)
  - Hypoglycemia
  - Wernicke's encephalopathy
- Drugs:
  - Major and minor tranquillizers
  - Baclofen
  - Lithium toxicity
  - Antiepileptic drug toxicity
  - Antiemetics
- Hypoxia:
  - Pneumonia/chest infection
  - Pulmonary embolism
  - Chronic pulmonary disease
  - Pulmonary edema
  - Hypercapnea
  - Chronic pulmonary disease
- Limb or bowel ischemia in patients with a cardiac or aortic arch source of embolism

*Remediable causes of deterioration;
SAH: subarachnoid hemorrhage.

Recommendations

Patients with acute stroke should be admitted to a stroke unit which is a specialized, geographically defined hospital unit staffed by a multidisciplinary interprofessional team and dedicated to the management of stroke patients (evidence level A). The core interprofessional team on the stroke unit should consist of health-care professionals with stroke expertise from medicine, nursing, occupational therapy, physiotherapy, speech-language pathology, social work, and clinical nutrition (dietitian) (evidence level A). Additional disciplines may include pharmacy, (neuro)psychology, and recreation therapy (evidence level B). The interprofessional team should assess patients within 48 hours of admission to hospital and formulate a management plan (evidence level C).

Clinicians should use standardized, valid assessment tools to evaluate the patient's stroke-related impairments and functional status (evidence level B). Roving, mobile stroke teams do not provide the same benefit as stroke teams working in geographically defined stroke units.

Implementation

The national sentinel audit of treatment of hospitalized stroke patients in the UK indicated that in 2008, 68% of patients admitted with an acute stroke spent more than one-half of their admission on a stroke unit.

Anticipating and preventing complications after acute stroke

There are several causes of clinical deterioration after stroke, as listed in *Table 83*.

Elevated blood pressure

Raised blood pressure is common in patients with acute stroke, associated with a poor outcome, and how it should be managed is uncertain. In theory, lowering blood pressure in acute ischemic stroke should reduce further vascular damage, cerebral edema, and hemorrhagic transformation of the fresh brain infarct, and forestall early recurrent stroke. In acute hemorrhagic stroke, lowering blood pressure should reduce hydrostatic expansion of the hematoma, perihematoma edema, and early rebleeding into the brain. Conversely, lowering blood pressure could increase the ischemic penumbra and size of any brain infarction or perihematomal ischemia. In healthy individuals, a fall in systemic blood pressure is accompanied by compensatory dilatation of the cerebral arteries to maintain constant cerebral perfusion. However, patients with acute stroke might have impaired cerebral autoregulation in the region surrounding the stroke; so any reduction in systemic blood pressure might be accompanied by a similar reduction in cerebral blood flow to the ischemic brain.

Within the first 24 hours after stroke, systolic blood pressure spontaneously falls by about 28% (SD 11%) in most patients, particularly when they are moved to a quiet room, they are allowed to rest, their bladder is empty, and any pain and increased intracranial pressure is controlled.

Evidence

A systematic review of interventions to alter blood pressure within 1 week of acute ischemic or hemorrhagic stroke, which included 11 randomized trials and 7000 patients, concluded that pharmacologically lowering blood pressure does not have an overall beneficial effect on functional outcome (RR: 1.04, 95% CI: 0.97–1.12, p=0.30; I^2 = 28%)[62]. Since then, the INTERACT 2 trial has shown that, in patients with intracerebral hemorrhage, intensive lowering of blood pressure to a target systolic level of <140 mmHg within 1 hour did not result in a significant reduction in the rate of the primary outcome of death or severe disability. However, an ordinal analysis of modified Rankin scores indicated improved functional outcomes with intensive lowering of blood pressure[61].

Recommendations

The following recommendations reflect the paucity of evidence in this area and indicate the need for further research.

- Ischemic stroke eligible for thrombolytic therapy: very high blood pressure (>185/110 mmHg) should be treated concurrently in patients receiving thrombolytic therapy for acute ischemic stroke in order to reduce the risk of secondary intracranial hemorrhage (evidence level B).
- Ischemic stroke patients not eligible for thrombolytic therapy: treatment of hypertension in the setting of acute ischemic stroke should not be routinely undertaken (evidence level C). Extreme blood pressure elevation (e.g. systolic >220 or diastolic >120 mmHg) may be treated to reduce the blood pressure by ~15%, and not more than 25%, over the first 24 hours with gradual reduction thereafter (evidence level C). Avoid excessive lowering of blood pressure as this may exacerbate existing ischemia or may induce ischemia, particularly in the setting of intracranial arterial occlusion or extracranial carotid or vertebral artery occlusion (evidence level C).
- Hemorrhagic stroke patients: The INTERACT 2 trial showed that in patients with acute spontaneous intracerebral hemorrhage within the previous 6 hours and an elevated systolic blood pressure, early intensive lowering of blood pressure, with a target systolic level of <140 mmHg within 1 hour, was not associated with an increase in the rates of death or serious adverse events compared with guideline-recommended treatment (a target systolic level of <180 mmHg), and did not result in a significant reduction in the rate of the primary outcome of death or major disability[61]. However, an ordinal analysis of scores on the modified Rankin scale did suggest that intensive treatment improved functional outcomes.
- Pharmacologic agents and routes of administration should be chosen to avoid precipitous falls in blood pressure (evidence level C).

Elevated blood glucose

Evidence

One clinical trial of 933 patients presenting within 24 hours of stroke onset and with admission plasma glucose concentration between 6.0 and 17.0 mmol/l, who were randomly assigned to receive variable-dose insulin GKI to maintain capillary glucose at 4–7 mmol/l (intervention) or saline (control) as a continuous intravenous infusion for 24 hours, was stopped due to slow enrolment. In the GKI group, overall mean plasma glucose and mean systolic blood pressure were significantly lower than in the control group (mean difference in glucose 0.57 mmol/l, p<0.001; mean difference in blood pressure 9.0 mmHg, p<0.0001), but there was no significant reduction in mortality at 90 days (GKI *vs.* control: OR: 1.14, 95% CI: 0.86–1.51, p=0.37) and no significant differences for secondary outcomes. These data indicate hat GKI infusions significantly reduce plasma glucose concentrations and blood pressure but were not associated with significant clinical benefit, although the study was underpowered and alternative results cannot be excluded.

Recommendations

- Patients with suspected acute stroke should have their blood glucose concentration checked immediately (evidence level B).
- Blood glucose measurement should be repeated if the first random glucose value is elevated greater than 10 mmol/l. The repeat measures should include a fasting glucose and an A1c (evidence level B).
- Hypoglycemia should be corrected immediately (evidence level B).
- If the repeat glucose levels and the A1c are elevated (fasting glucose >7 mmol/l; A1c >7%), the use of antihyperglycemic agents should be considered (evidence level C), and in the longer term, education on lifestyle changes and diabetes (evidence level A).

Nutrition

Evidence

Oral nutritional supplementation: a RCT of 4023 stroke patients who could swallow and who were randomly allocated normal hospital diet or normal hospital diet plus oral nutritional supplements until hospital discharge found that supplemented diet was associated with a modest, nonsignificant, absolute reduction in risk of death of 0.7% (95% CI: –1.4–2.7) and an increased risk of death or poor outcome of 0.7% (–2.3–3.8)[63].

Timing of enteral tube feeding: a RCT of 859 dysphagic stroke patients who were randomly allocated, within 7 days of admission, to early enteral tube feeding or no tube feeding for more than 7 days (early versus avoid)[64]. Early tube feeding was associated with an ARR of death of 5.8% (95% CI: –0.8–12.5, p=0.09) and a reduction in death or poor outcome of 1.2% (–4.2–6.6, p = 0.7). Early tube feeding might reduce case fatality, but at the expense of increasing the proportion surviving with poor outcome.

Type of enteral tube feeding: a RCT of 321 dysphagic stroke patients who were randomly allocated, within 7 days of admission, to percutaneous endoscopic gastrostomy (PEG) or nasogastric feeding. PEG feeding was associated with a minor, nonsignificant, absolute increase in risk of death of 1.0% (–10.0–11.9, p = 0.9), and a borderline significant increased risk of death or poor outcome of 7.8% (0.0–15.5, p=0.05)[64]. These data do not support a policy of early initiation of PEG feeding in dysphagic stroke patients.

Recommendations

The nutritional and hydration status of stroke patients should be screened within the first 48 hours of admission using a valid screening tool (evidence level B). Results from the screening process should be used to guide appropriate referral to a dietitian for further assessment and ongoing management of nutritional and hydration status (evidence level C).

Stroke patients with suspected nutritional concerns, hydration deficits, dysphagia, or other comorbidities that may affect nutrition (such as diabetes) should be referred to a dietitian for:

- Recommendations to meet nutrient and fluid needs orally, while supporting alterations in food texture and fluid consistency recommended by a speech-language pathologist or other trained professional (evidence level C).
- Consideration of enteral nutrition support (tube feeding) within 1–7 days of admission for patients who are unable to meet their nutrient and fluid requirements orally. This decision should be made collaboratively with the interprofessional team, the patient, and the caregivers and family (evidence level B).

Cerebral edema

Malignant hemispheric infarction, causing substantial edema of a cerebral hemisphere and compression of the ventricular system and upper brainstem, constitutes between 1% and 10% of all supratentorial ischemic strokes.

Evidence

Mannitol: three small RCTs comparing mannitol (an osmotic agent and a free radical scavenger which might decrease edema and tissue damage in stroke) with placebo or open control in 226 patients with acute ischemic stroke (n = 1 trial) or nontraumatic ICH (n = 2 trials) did not provide enough evidence to support the routine use of mannitol in acute stroke patients. Further trials are needed to confirm or refute whether mannitol is beneficial in acute stroke.

Glycerol: Ten randomized trials comparing intravenous administration of a 10% solution of glycerol (a hyperosmolar agent that is claimed to reduce brain edema) and control in 945 patients with acute ischemic and/or hemorrhagic stroke showed that glycerol was associated with a nonsignificant reduction in the odds of death within the scheduled treatment period (OR: 0.78, 95% CI: 0.58–1.06). Among patients with definite or probable ischemic stroke, glycerol was associated with a significant reduction in the odds of death during the scheduled treatment period (OR: 0.65, 95% CI: 0.44–0.97). However, at the end of the scheduled follow-up period, there was no significant difference in the odds of death (OR: 0.98, 95% CI: 0.73–1.31).

Functional outcome was reported in only two studies but there were nonsignificantly more patients who had a good outcome at the end of scheduled follow up (OR: 0.73, 95% CI: 0.37–1.42). Hemolysis seemed to be the only relevant adverse effect of glycerol treatment. Although this systematic review suggested a favorable effect of glycerol treatment on short-term survival in patients with probable or definite ischemic stroke, the CIs were wide and the magnitude of the treatment effect may be only minimal. Due to the relatively small number of patients, and that the trials were performed in the pre-CT era, the results must be interpreted cautiously.

Decompressive hemicraniectomy: among three RCTs of decompressive hemicraniectomy *vs.* conservative therapy in patients ≤60 years of age or less within 48 hours of onset of symptoms of malignant middle cerebral artery territory infarction, random assignment to decompressive surgery was associated with a reduction in death or dependency from 76.5% (conservative) to 60.2% (surgery), ARR: 16.3%, 95% CI: –0.1–33.1%[65,66].

Recommendations

The lack of reliable evidence of benefit does not support the routine or selective use of osmolar agents, such as mannitol or glycerol, to reduce cerebral edema in patients with acute stroke.

Early decompressive hemicraniectomy (within 48 hours) should be considered in any patients ≤60 years of age or less presenting with malignant hemispheric infarction. Further studies are needed to establish objective neuroimaging criteria for aggressive intervention, and to clarify the role of decompressive surgery in older patients (>60 years of age) and, perhaps, when delayed beyond 48 hours.

Venous thromboembolism prophylaxis

Evidence

Graduated compression stockings: a systematic review identified four RCTs of physical methods to reduce the risk of deep vein thrombosis (DVT) and PE, by means of graduated compression stockings or intermittent pneumatic compression (IPC) applied to the legs, within 7 days of the onset of stroke. Overall, among the two trials of graduated compression stockings that included 2615 patients, and two small studies of IPC that included 177 patients, physical methods were not associated with a significant reduction in DVTs during the treatment period (OR: 0.85, 95% CI: 0.70–1.04) or deaths (OR: 1.12, 95% CI: 0.87–1.45). Use of graduated compression stockings was not associated with any significant reduction in risk of DVT (OR: 0.88, 95% CI: 0.72–1.08) or death (OR: 1.13, 95% CI: 0.87–1.47) at the end of follow-up. IPC was associated with a nonsignificant trend towards a lower risk of DVTs (OR: 0.45, 95% CI: 0.19–1.10) with no evidence of an effect on deaths (OR: 1.04, 95% CI: 0.37–2.89)[67]. These data do not support the routine use of graduated compression stockings to reduce the risk of DVT after acute stroke.

Intermittent pneumatic compression: intermittent pneumatic compression (IPC) is an effective method of reducing the risk of DVT and possibly improving survival in a wide variety of patients who are immobile after stroke[68]. Among 2876 patients with acute stroke (day 0 to day 3 of admission) who were immobile (i.e. could not walk to the toilet without the help of another person) and randomly allocated in the CLOTS 3 trial to IPC or no IPC, a DVT in the proximal veins or any symptomatic DVT in the proximal veins occurred within 30 days of randomization in 122 (8.5%) of 1438 patients allocated IPC and 174 (12.1%) of 1438 patients allocated no IPC; an absolute reduction in risk of 3.6% (95% CI: 1.4–5.8) and adjusted OR = 0.65 (95% CI: 0.51–0.84; p=0·001). Deaths in the treatment period occurred in 156 (11%) patients allocated IPC; 189 (13%) patients allocated no IPC died within the 30 days of treatment period (p=0.057); skin breaks on the legs were reported in 44 (3%) patients allocated IPC and in 20 (1%) patients allocated IPC (p=0.002); falls with injury were reported in 33 (2%) patients in the IPC group and in 24 (2%) patients in the no-IPC group (p=0.221)[68].

Heparin: nine randomized trials comparing heparinoids or LMWH with standard UFH, started within 14 days of stroke onset in 3137 people with acute ischemic stroke, revealed that allocation to LMWH or heparinoid was associated with a significant reduction in the odds of DVT compared with standard UFH (OR: 0.55, 95% CI: 0.44–0.70). However, the number of more major events (PE, death, intracranial or extracranial hemorrhage) was too small to provide a reliable estimate of the benefits and risks of LMWHs or heparinoids compared with standard UFH for these, arguably more important, outcomes. Insufficient information was available to assess effects on recurrent stroke or functional outcome. There is insufficient evidence on the safety and efficacy of anticoagulant DVT prophylaxis after ICH (evidence level C).

Recommendations

- All stroke patients should be assessed for their risk of developing venous thromboembolism (DVT and PE). Patients at high risk include those who are unable to move one or both lower limbs and those who are unable to mobilize independently; a previous history of venous thromboembolism; dehydration; and comorbidities such as malignant disease. Early mobilization and adequate hydration should be encouraged for all acute stroke patients (evidence level C).
- Patients at high risk of venous thromboembolism should be started on venous thromboembolism prophylaxis immediately (evidence level A).
- LMWH should be considered for patients with acute ischemic stroke at high risk of venous thromboembolism; or UFH for patients with renal failure (evidence level B).
- The use of antiembolism stockings for post-stroke venous thromboembolism prophylaxis alone is not recommended (evidence level A), but IPC is recommended for reducing the risk of DVT in immobile stroke patients (evidence level A).
- Antithrombotics and anticoagulants should be avoided for at least 48 hours after onset of ICH (evidence level C).

Urinary incontinence

Recommendations

All stroke patients should be screened for urinary incontinence and retention (with or without overflow), fecal incontinence, and constipation (time and frequency) (evidence level C).

The use of a portable ultrasound is recommended as the preferred noninvasive painless method for assessing post-void residual (evidence level C). Possible contributing factors surrounding continence management should be assessed, including medications, nutrition, diet, mobility, activity, cognition, environment, and communication (evidence level C). This should include assessing the stroke patient for urinary tract infections to determine a possible transient cause of urinary retention (evidence level C). Stroke patients with urinary incontinence should be assessed by trained personnel using a structured functional assessment (evidence level B).

The use of indwelling catheters should be avoided due to the risk of urinary tract infection (evidence level A). If used, indwelling catheters should be assessed daily and removed as soon as possible (evidence level A). Excellent perineal care and infection prevention strategies should be implemented to minimize risk of infections (evidence level C).

A bladder-training program should be implemented in patients who are incontinent of urine (evidence level C), including timed and prompted toileting on a consistent schedule (evidence level B). Appropriate intermittent catheterization schedules should be established based on amount of post-void residual (evidence level B).

A bowel management program should be implemented for stroke patients with persistent constipation or bowel incontinence (evidence level A).

Fever

High body temperature in the first 12–24 hours after stroke onset is associated with poor functional outcome.

Evidence

The Paracetamol (Acetaminophen) In Stroke (PAIS) trial randomly assigned 1400 patients with ischemic stroke or ICH and body temperature between 36°C and 39°C to treatment with paracetamol (6 g daily) or placebo within 12 hours from symptom onset;. 260 (37%) of 697 patients receiving paracetamol and 232 (33%) of 703 receiving placebo improved beyond expectation on the modified Rankin scale at 3 months, according to the sliding dichotomy approach (adjusted OR: 1.20, 95% CI 0.96–1.50). In a post-hoc analysis of patients with baseline body temperature 37–39°C, treatment with paracetamol was associated with improved outcome (OR: 1.43, 95% CI: 1.02–1.97). These results do not support routine use of high-dose paracetamol in patients with acute stroke. However, paracetamol might have a beneficial effect on functional outcome in patients admitted with a body temperature 37–39°C, but this post-hoc finding needs further study.

Recommendations

Temperature should be monitored as part of routine vital sign assessments, every 4 hours for the first 48 hours and then as per ward routine or based on clinical judgment (evidence level C).

For temperature greater than 37.5°C, increase frequency of monitoring, initiate temperature-reducing measures, investigate possible infection such as pneumonia or urinary tract infection (evidence level C), and initiate antipyretic and antimicrobial therapy as required (evidence level B).

Infective endocarditis must be treated with extended courses of high-dose antibiotic treatment, ideally guided by microbiological sensitivity testing. Indications for surgery, which is required in about one-third of patients, include failure to control the infection, threatened or actual embolus of septic material, and development of heart failure. Some patients may be suitable for outpatient intravenous antibiotic treatment after an initial inpatient assessment and treatment period. After discharge from hospital, patients need monitoring for relapse or recurrent infection. Patients remain at risk of further episodes of infective endocarditis and should be counselled to report any potentially relevant symptoms.

Immobilization (moving in bed, sitting up, standing, and walking)

Recommendations

All patients admitted to hospital with acute stroke should be mobilized as early and as frequently as possible (evidence level B), and preferably within 24 hours of stroke symptom onset, unless contraindicated (evidence level C). Some contraindications to early mobilization include, but may not be restricted to, unstable medical conditions, low oxygen saturation, and lower limb fracture or injury.

All patients admitted to hospital with acute stroke should be assessed by rehabilitation professionals as soon as possible after admission (evidence level A), preferably within the first 24–48 hours (evidence level C).

TABLE 84 **SUMMARY OF EFFECTIVE STRATEGIES TO PREVENT RECURRENT ISCHEMIC STROKE**

Intervention	**Stroke rate per year**		**RRR** (95% CI)	**ARR**
	Control	*Intervention*		
Carotid revascularization	6.5%	3.5%	48% (38–60%)	3.0%
Aspirin	5.0%	4.3%	13% (6–19%)	0.7%
Aspirin & extended-release dipyridamole	4.3%	3.6%	18% (8–28%)	0.7%
Clopidogrel (same as aspirin & ER dipyridamole)				
Oral anticoagulation for atrial fibrillation	12.0%	4.0%	61% (37–75%)	7.3%
Blood pressure-lowering by 10 mmHg systolic	5.0%	3.3%	34% (21–44%)	1.7%
LDL cholesterol-lowering by 1 mmol/l	5.0%	4.4%	12% (1–22%)	0.6%
HbA1C-lowering by 0.9%	5.0%	4.7%	7% (6–19%)	0.3%

ARR: absolute risk reduction; Hb: hemoglobin; RRR: relative risk reduction.

Poor oral hygiene

Recommendations

Upon or soon after admission, all stroke patients should have an oral/dental assessment, including screening for signs of dental disease, level of oral care, and appliances (evidence level C). For patients wearing a full or partial denture it should be determined if they have the neuromotor skills to wear and use the appliance(s) safely (evidence level C).

An appropriate oral care protocol should be used for every patient with stroke, including those who use dentures (evidence level C). The oral care protocol should address areas such as frequency of oral care (twice per day or more); types of oral care products (toothpaste, floss, and mouthwash); and management for patients with dysphagia.

If concerns with implementing an oral care protocol are identified, consider consulting a dentist, occupational therapist, speech-language pathologist, and/or a dental hygienist (evidence level C). If concerns are identified with oral health and/or appliances, patients should be referred to a dentist for consultation and management as soon as possible (evidence level C).

Prevention of recurrent stroke and other major vascular events

The strategies which have been proven to be effective in preventing recurrent ischemic stroke include early carotid endarterectomy (CEA), antiplatelet therapy, anticoagulation, and vascular risk factor control (*Table 84*)[51].

Carotid revascularization

Evidence for neurologically symptomatic carotid stenosis

A systematic review of pooled data from the three RCTs of endarterectomy for symptomatic carotid stenosis indicated that for patients with recently symptomatic 70–99% stenosis, CEA was associated with a reduction in risk of any stroke or death at 5 years after randomization from about 33% (no surgery) to about 17% (with surgery); relative risk reduction (RRR): 48% (95% CI: 36–60%); ARR: 15.6% (95% CI: 9.8–20.7%)[69]. The effect was more modest for patients with recently symptomatic 50–69% stenosis, in whom CEA was associated with a ARR of any stroke or death at 5 years after randomization by 7.8% (95% CI: 3.1–12.5%), from about 27% (no surgery) to about 19% (with surgery); RRR: 28% (95% CI: 14–42%).

These data indicate that, for patients with recent carotid territory ischemic events, endarterectomy is an effective addition to best medical therapy. The absolute benefit of CEA is greater in men (than women); older (than younger) patients; those with recent ischemic events of the brain (*vs.* the eye), increasing carotid stenosis, and ulcerated (*vs.* smooth) carotid plaque; and those who have endarterectomy sooner (*vs.* later) after the event.

Carotid stenting is a newer, less invasive revascularization strategy, which patients may prefer despite uncertainties about safety and effectiveness compared with endarterectomy. In a meta-analysis of 13 randomized clinical trials randomizing 7477 participants to carotid artery stenting (CAS) or CEA, CAS was associated with an increased risk of periprocedural outcomes of death, myocardial infarction (MI), or stroke (OR: 1.31; 95% CI: 1.08–1.59), 65% and 67% increases in death or stroke and any stroke, respectively, but with 55% and 85% reductions in the risk of MI and cranial nerve injury, respectively, when compared with CEA[70]. Similarly, CAS was associated with 19%, 38%, 24%, and 48% increases in the intermediate to long-term outcomes of SAPPHIRE-like outcome, periprocedural death or stroke, and ipsilateral stroke thereafter, death or any stroke, and any stroke, respectively compared with CEA. Subgroup analyses suggest that age is the only factor that modified the treatment effect: Patients ≥70 years of age had twice the rate of the composite of stroke or death at 120 days with stenting than endarterectomy, whereas rates were similar in patients <70 years of age. These results suggest that endarterectomy is the preferred revascularization strategy for symptomatic carotid stenosis, particularly in patients ≥70 years of age. They are consistent with those of a recently published trial (CREST), which was not included in the meta-analysis, and suggest that stenting may be as safe as endarterectomy in patients <70 years of age. A trial is needed to test this hypothesis a priori.

Long-term follow-up of patients in the International Carotid STenting and CREST trial is awaited and will add substantially to data from four earlier randomized trials, which showed a higher rate of stroke or death over 2–5 years after angioplasty/stenting compared with endarterectomy in symptomatic carotid stenosis (OR: 1.35, 95% CI: 1.06–1.71).

Recommendations for patients with neurologically symptomatic carotid stenosis

Patients with TIA or nondisabling stroke and ipsilateral 50–99% ICA stenosis (measured by two concordant noninvasive imaging modalities) should be evaluated by an individual with stroke expertise, and selected patients should be offered CEA as soon as possible, optimally within 14 days of the incident event once the patient is clinically stable (evidence level A).

- CEA should be performed by a surgeon with a known perioperative morbidity and mortality of less than 6% (evidence level A). CEA is more appropriate than carotid stenting for patients over age 70 who are otherwise fit for surgery because stenting carries a higher short-term risk of stroke and death (evidence level A).
- Carotid stenting may be considered for patients who are not operative candidates for technical, anatomic, or medical reasons (evidence level A). Interventionalists should have expertise in carotid procedures and an expected risk of periprocedural morbidity and mortality rate of less than 5%.
- CEA is more appropriate than CAS for patients over 70 who are otherwise fit for surgery because stenting carries a higher short-term risk of stroke and death (evidence level A).

Evidence for neurologically asymptomatic and remotely symptomatic carotid stenosis

Three randomized controlled trials of CEA (plus best medical therapy) *vs.* no CEA (plus best medical therapy) involving a total of 5223 patients showed that the overall net excess of operation-related perioperative stroke or death was 2.9%. For the primary outcome of perioperative stroke or death or any subsequent stroke, patients undergoing CEA fared better than those treated with only best medical therapy (RR: 0.69, 95% CI: 0.57–0.83). Similarly, for the outcome of perioperative stroke or death or subsequent ipsilateral stroke, there was benefit for the surgical group (RR: 0.71, 95% CI: 0.55–0.90). For the outcome of any stroke or death, there was a nonsignificant trend towards fewer events in the surgical group (RR: 0.92, 95% CI: 0.83–1.02). Subgroup analyses were performed for the outcome of perioperative stroke or death or subsequent carotid stroke. CEA appeared more beneficial in men than in women and more beneficial in younger patients than in older patients although the data for age effect were inconclusive. There was no statistically significant difference between the treatment effect estimates in patients with different grades of stenosis but the data were insufficient.

Despite about a 3% perioperative stroke or death rate, CEA for asymptomatic carotid stenosis reduces the relative risk of ipsilateral stroke, and any stroke, by approximately 30% over 3 years. However, the ARR is small (approximately 1% per annum over the first few years of follow-up).

Recommendations for patients with neurologically asymptomatic and remotely symptomatic carotid stenosis

Asymptomatic patients should be evaluated by a physician with expertise in stroke management (evidence level A). The advantage of revascularization over current medical therapy alone is not well established (evidence level B); the benefit of surgery may now be lower than anticipated based on randomized trial results and the cited 3% threshold for complication rates may be high because of interim advances in medical therapy[71].

If there is a role for carotid revascularization, the usefulness of carotid stenting as an alternative to CEA in asymptomatic patients at high risk for the surgical procedure is uncertain (evidence level C) and is being evaluated in several ongoing clinical trials (e.g. ACST-2, CREST-2, SPACE-2). Selection of asymptomatic patients for carotid revascularization should be guided by an assessment of comorbid conditions and life expectancy, as well as other individual factors, and should include a thorough discussion of the risks and benefits of the procedure with an understanding of patient preferences (evidence level C). Patients should be less than 75 years old with a life expectancy of more than 5 years, and an acceptable risk of surgical complications (evidence level A).

- CEA may be considered for selected patients with 60–99% carotid stenosis who are asymptomatic or were remotely symptomatic (i.e. >3 months) (evidence level A).
- CEA should be performed by a surgeon with a <3% risk of perioperative morbidity and mortality (evidence level A).
- Carotid stenting may be considered in patients who are not operative candidates for technical, anatomic or medical reasons provided there is a <3% risk of periprocedural morbidity and mortality (evidence level A).
- The use of aspirin in conjunction with CEA is recommended unless contraindicated because aspirin was used in all of the cited trials of CEA as an antiplatelet drug (Class I; evidence level C).

Antiplatelet therapy for the prevention of recurrent ischemic stroke of arterial origin

Evidence

Aspirin/acetylsalicylic acid

Aspirin reduces the risk of recurrent stroke and other major vascular events by at least 13% (95% CI: 6–19%) compared with control, when administered acutely and over the long term (**419, 420**). It is affordable, widely available, and reasonably safe. Although aspirin increases the risk of major bleeding by about 70% (RR: 1.71, 95% CI: 1.41–2 08), the absolute annual increase is modest (0.13%, 95% CI:0.08–0.20%), indicating that one additional major bleeding episode will occur each year for every 769 patients (95% CI: 500–1250) treated with aspirin. The increased risk of bleeding is mainly due to an increase in major gastrointestinal bleeding (RR: 2.07, 95% CI: 1.61–2.66; absolute annual increase 0.12%, 95% CI: 0.07–0.19%) and intracranial bleeding (RR: 1.65; 95% CI:1.06–5.99; absolute annual increase 0.03%, 95% CI: 0.01–0.08%)[72].

Clopidogrel

Clopidogrel is significantly but marginally more effective than aspirin: it reduced the long-term risk of stroke and other major vascular events by 8.7% (95% CI: 0.3–16.5%) compared with aspirin among 19 185 patients at high vascular risk, and by 7.3% (–5.7–18.7%) among a subgroup of 6431 patients with ischemic stroke. Clopidogrel also causes less gastrointestinal bleeding than 325 mg aspirin daily (RR: 0.69, 95% CI: 0.48–1.00; AAR: 0.12%, 95% CI: 0.00–0.28%), but does not reduce the risk of other types of bleeding[73]. However, the cost of clopidogrel is substantially greater than that of aspirin.

Aspirin/acetylsalicylic acid plus extended-release dipyridamole

The combination of aspirin and extended-release (ER) dipyridamole is significantly more effective than aspirin alone in reducing the risk of stroke and other major vascular events (hazard ratio [HR]: 0.82, 95% CI: 0.72–0.92), without excessive bleeding or myocardial infarction in patients with previous TIA or ischemic stroke[74]. However, a direct comparison of 75 mg clopidogrel daily with the combination of 25 mg aspirin and 200 mg ER dipyridamole twice daily in 20 332 patients with ischemic stroke showed no significant difference between either regimen in the prevention of recurrent stroke (9.0% on aspirin plus ER dipyridamole *vs.* 8.8% on clopidogrel; HR: 1.01, 95% CI: 0.92–1.11), myocardial infarction (1.7% *vs.* 1.9%; HR: 0.90, 95% CI: 0.73–1.10), and the composite of stroke, myocardial infarction, and death from vascular causes (13.1% *vs.* 13.1%; HR: 0.99, 95% CI: 0.92–1.07)[75].

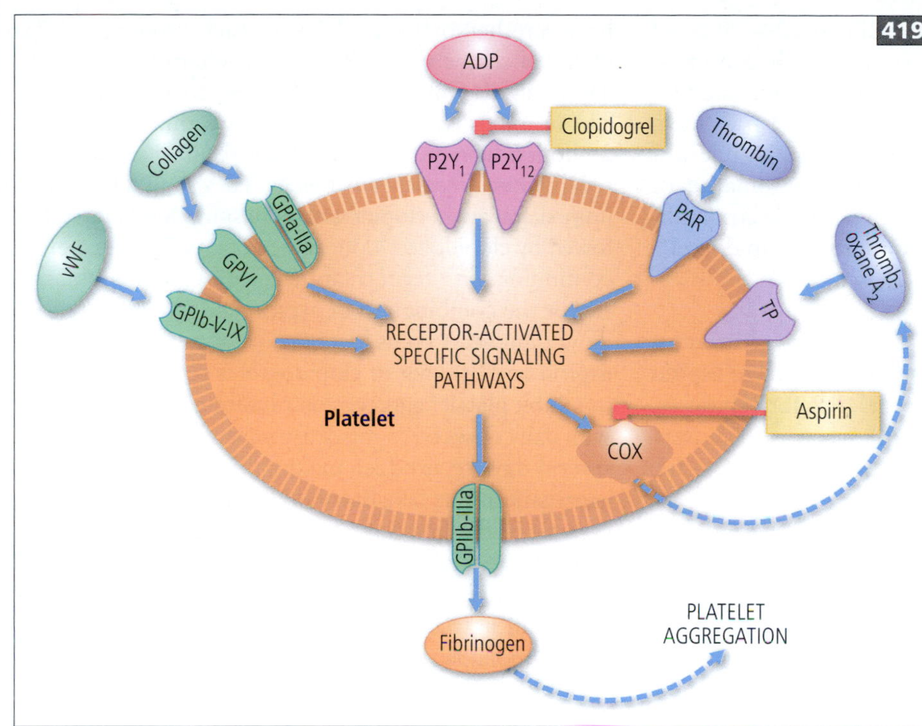

419 Receptors that lead to platelet activation when stimulated, and thereby are potential targets for antiplatelet therapy. ADP: adenosine diphosphate; COX: cyclo-oxygenase; GP: glycoprotein; PAR: protease activated receptor; P2Y1: ADP purinoceptor 1; P2Y12: ADP purinoceptor 12; TP: prostanoid receptor; vWF: von Willebrand factor.

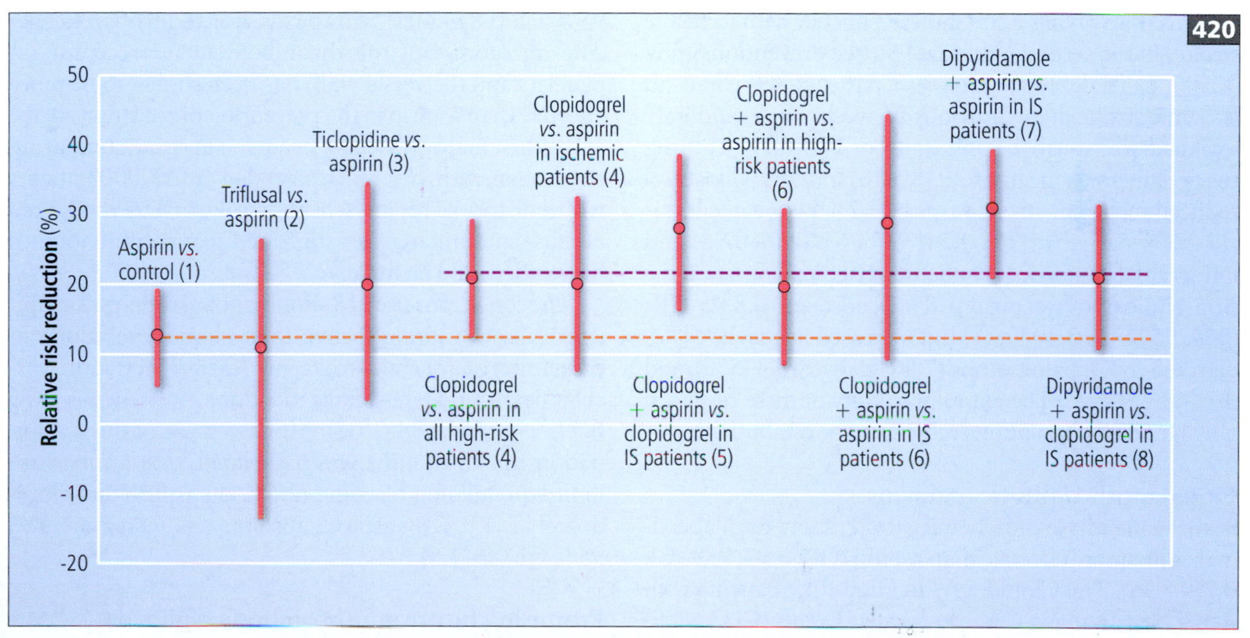

420 Relative effects of antiplatelet regimens *vs.* placebo, aspirin, and clopidogrel in reducing the risk of stroke, myocardial infarction, or vascular death (major vascular events). The y-axis shows the degree of reduction in risk of stroke, myocardial infarction, or vascular death with each antiplatelet regimen. The orange dotted line represents the treatment effect of aspirin (*vs.* placebo).The purple dotted line represents the treatment effect of clopidogrel.The point estimates (circles) and 95% CIs (vertical lines) are shown in comparison with placebo (zero), aspirin (13% relative risk reduction), or clopidogrel (22% relative risk reduction [9% relative risk reduction *vs.* aspirin]), derived from systematic reviews of all trials. 1: Meta-analysis, 10 RCTs, 10,000 patients; 2: Meta-analysis, 4 RCTs; 3: TASS; 4: CAPRIE; 5: MATCH; 6: CHARISMA ; 7: Meta-analysis, 6 RCTs; 8: ProFESS.

Dipyridamole causes headache in 24–70% of patients, which is sufficient to prompt discontinuation in about 10% of patients, usually within the first 3 months. Headache is more likely to occur in women, nonsmokers, and patients with an absence of relevant ischemic lesions on brain imaging. The combination of 25 mg aspirin with 200 mg ER dipyridamole costs substantially more than aspirin but less than clopidogrel.

Triflusal

Triflusal is another antiplatelet drug that is structurally related to aspirin and has similar efficacy to aspirin in the prevention of vascular events (RR for aspirin *vs.* triflusal 1.03, 95% CI: 0.89 –1.20), whereas there were more hemorrhages with aspirin (RR: 1.58, 95% CI: 1.35–1.85).

Cilostazol

Cilostazol reduces platelet aggregation by inhibiting phosphodiesterase 3 and increasing cyclic adenosine-monophosphate (cAMP) concentrations. For longer-term secondary prevention, cilostazol reduced the risk of stroke by about 39% (95% CI: 9–59%) compared with placebo among 1095 Japanese patients with ischemic stroke, and by about 38% (–26–70%) compared with aspirin in a pilot trial involving 720 Chinese patients with ischemic stroke. In the second Cilostazol Stroke Prevention Study (CSPS 2) trial, 2757 Japanese patients who had an ischemic stroke in the previous 26 weeks were randomly assigned to aspirin 81 mg daily or cilostazol 100 mg twice daily for a mean of 29 (SD 16) months. Cilostazol reduced recurrent stroke (aspirin 3.7% per year, cilostazol 2.8% per year; HR: 0.74, 95% CI: 0.56–0.98) and intracranial hemorrhage or hemorrhage leading to admission to hospital (aspirin 1.8%, cilostazol 0.8%; HR: 0.46, 95% CI: 0.30–0.71) but increased headache (7%), diarrhea (6%), palpitations (7%), tachycardia (5%), and dizziness (3%)[75]. The external validity of these results in non-Japanese populations remains to be established.

Other antithrombotic regimens

In the acute phase of ischemic stroke, short-term abciximab is not more effective than aspirin (OR: 0.97, 95% CI: 0.70–1.36). The Clopidogrel in High-Risk Patients with Acute Nondisabling Cerebrovascular Events (CHANCE) trial showed that among 5170 Chinese patients with acute minor ischemic stroke or TIA (onset within the previous 24 hours) at high risk for recurrence, the addition of clopidogrel to aspirin reduced the relative risk of recurrent stroke at 90 days by 32% (8.2% *vs.* 11.7%; hazard ratio: 0.68; 95% CI: 0.57–0.81; absolute risk reduction: 3.5%)[76]. There was no difference between the group that received both clopidogrel and aspirin and the group that received aspirin alone in the incidence of moderate or severe hemorrhage (0.3% in each group; p=0.73) or hemorrhagic stroke (0.3% in each group; p=0.98). These results indicate that Chinese patients with acute TIA or minor ischemic stroke (onset within the previous 24 hours) who are at high risk for recurrence should be regarded as a medical emergency. They should be treated immediately with clopidogrel plus aspirin for 21 days, followed by clopidogrel alone, for a total of 90 days, before continuing long-term treatment with clopidogrel, aspirin, or the combination of aspirin and extended-release dipyridamole. A bolus loading dose of at least 162 mg of aspirin and 300 mg of clopidogrel is required on day 1 to inhibit platelet aggregation rapidly, given that starting with daily doses of 75 mg of aspirin and clopidogrel takes several days to produce maximal inhibition of platelet aggregation. The benefits of dual antiplatelet therapy are greatest in the first days after TIA and ischemic stroke. Clinicians are continuing to enroll non-Chinese patients with acute TIA and minor ischemic stroke into ongoing large clinical trials of the safety and efficacy of dual and triple antiplatelet therapy (e.g. POINT, TARDIS trials).

In the longer term, neither oral anticoagulation (HR: 1.02, 95% CI: 0.77–1.35), dipyridamole (RR: 1.02, 95% CI: 0.88–1.18), triflusal (OR: 0.98, 95% CI: 0.79–1.20), the combination of aspirin and clopidogrel (RR: 0.93, 95% CI: 0.85–1.05), vorapaxar, nor terutroban (a specific antagonist of the thromboxane A2 receptor on platelets and the vessel wall) has been shown to be more effective than aspirin in the prevention of recurrent stroke and other major vascular events. The trial comparing terutroban with 100 mg aspirin daily in 18,000 patients with a history of recent ischemic stroke or TIA was halted because interim analyses suggested that continuation of the study would be futile.

The long-term use (18 months) of aspirin plus clopidogrel is no more effective than clopidogrel alone in prevention of ischemic stroke, myocardial infarction, vascular death, and rehospitalization for acute ischemia (RR: 0.94, 95% CI: 0.84–1.05). Moreover, use of this combination for 18 months was associated with an increase in life-threatening bleeding (2.6% on aspirin and clopidogrel *vs.* 1.3% on aspirin; absolute risk increase 1.3%, 95% CI: 0.6–1.9)[75].

Promising future antithrombotic regimens

In acute TIA and ischemic stroke, the combination of aspirin plus clopidogrel may be more effective than aspirin alone if administered immediately and for only the first few months, when the risk of recurrent stroke is highest, thus not exposing the patient to the long-term risks of bleeding associated with the combination of clopidogrel and aspirin compared with either drug alone[76]. Large Phase 3 trials, such as the POINT (Platelet-Oriented Inhibition in New TIA) trial, are ongoing to establish the relative safety and efficacy of the combination of clopidogrel and aspirin compared with aspirin in patients with acute TIA and mild ischemic stroke. Other antithrombotic agents that have shown efficacy in acute coronary syndromes, such as the newer and more potent thienopyridine, prasugrel, the nonthienopyridine, ticagrelor (a reversible adenosine diphosphate [ADP] receptor antagonist), and the oral factor Xa inhibitors, rivaroxaban and apixaban, may be promising potential treatments for acute TIA and ischemic stroke, but the expected increase in bleeding associated with these drugs may preclude their further development in acute cerebrovascular disease.

Recommendations

All patients with ischemic stroke or TIA should be prescribed antiplatelet therapy immediately for secondary prevention of recurrent stroke unless there is an indication for anticoagulation (evidence level A).

Aspirin, combined aspirin (25 mg) and ER dipyridamole (200 mg), or clopidogrel (75 mg) are all appropriate options and selection should depend on the clinical circumstances (evidence level A). Triflusal is a second-line alternative. The position of cilostazol is not yet established outside of Asia.

For adult patients on aspirin, the usual maintenance dosage is 80–325 mg per day (evidence level A). In children with stroke the usual maintenance dosage of aspirin is 1–5 mg/kg per day for the prevention of recurrent stroke (evidence level B). For 'teens', the maximum dose should be up to 325 mg per day. Clopidigrel may be considered an alternative for pediatric patients with contraindications to aspirin (evidence level C).

Long-term concurrent use of aspirin and clopidogrel is not recommended for secondary stroke prevention unless there is a compelling indication (evidence level B).

The most important priority in the thromboprophylactic management of patients with ischemic stroke and TIA of arterial origin is to ensure that patients are prescribed, taking, and tolerating an effective antiplatelet drug such as aspirin, clopidogrel, or the combination of aspirin and ER dipyridamole. Because aspirin is widely available, affordable, and effective (albeit modestly), it is arguably the first-line treatment of choice. However, if patients are intolerant of or allergic to aspirin, at high risk of a recurrent stroke (more than 15–20% per year), or have experienced a recurrent ischemic event of arterial origin while taking aspirin, then one of the two more effective, although more expensive, regimens is indicated.

The decision to start clopidogrel or the combination of aspirin and ER dipyridamole will be determined by several factors: atherothrombotic vascular disease in other vascular beds (aspirin with ER dipyridamole has not been proven to be effective for the treatment of patients with coronary artery disease, but was not associated with any excess myocardial infarction as an outcome event in stroke patients); a predisposition to adverse effects (e.g. major bleeding in 4.1% of patients on aspirin with ER dipyridamole *vs.* 3.6% on clopidogrel; headache in 6% of patients on aspirin with ER dipyridamole *vs.* 1% on clopidogrel); compliance (aspirin with ER dipyridamole is taken twice daily, whereas clopidogrel is taken once daily); patient preference; and affordability.

Antithrombotic therapy for the prevention of recurrent ischemic stroke of cardiac origin

Evidence

Heparin (in acute cardioembolic stroke)

A meta-analysis of seven randomized controlled trials, involving 4624 patients with acute cardioembolic stroke, showed that, compared with other treatments, anticoagulants were associated with a nonsignificant reduction in recurrent ischemic stroke within 7–14 days (3.0% *vs.* 4.9%, OR: 0.68, 95% CI: 0.44–1.06, p=0.09, number needed to treat = 53), a significant increase in symptomatic intracranial bleeding (2.5% *vs.* 0.7%, OR: 2.89, 95% CI: 1.19–7.01, p=0.02, number needed to harm = 55), and a similar rate of death or disability at final follow-up (73.5% *vs.* 73.8%, OR: 1.01, 95% CI: 0.82–1.24, p=0.9)[77]. These findings indicate that in patients with acute cardioembolic stroke, early anticoagulation is associated with a nonsignificant reduction in recurrence of ischemic stroke, no substantial reduction in death and disability, and increased intracranial bleeding.

Aspirin/acetylsalicyclic acid

Among individuals with prior ischemic stroke or TIA and AF, aspirin reduces the risk of recurrent stroke and other major vascular event by about 17% (HR: 0.83, 95% CI: 0.65–1.05) compared with control. This proportional risk reduction is consistent with the observed effect of antiplatelet therapy for the prevention of first-ever stroke among individuals with AF (HR: 0.78, 95% CI: 0.65–0.94).

Warfarin

Adjusted-dose warfarin (INR 2.0–3.0) reduces the risk of recurrent stroke or systemic embolism by about 61% (95% CI: 37–75%) compared with control in AF patients with recent TIA or ischemic stroke. This proportional risk reduction is consistent with that observed for the prevention of first-ever stroke among individuals with AF, including the elderly. Warfarin also increases the odds of major extracranial hemorrhage (OR: 4.3, 95% CI: 1.5–12.1)[78].

Warfarin (*vs.* aspirin/acetylsalicylic acid)

Adjusted-dose warfarin is significantly more effective than antiplatelet therapy for preventing recurrent stroke (OR: 0.49, 95% CI: 0.33–0.72), consistent with the effect of adjusted-dose warfarin compared with antiplatelet therapy in the prevention of first-ever stroke (RR: 0.61, 95% CI: 0.48–0.78). Although major extracranial bleeding complications occurred more often in patients on anticoagulants (OR: 5.2, 95% CI: 2.1–12.8), the absolute difference was small (1.9%).

Aspirin/acetylsalicylic acid and clopidogrel (*vs.* warfarin)

The combination of aspirin and clopidogrel is not as effective as warfarin, particularly for patients who are taking warfarin without complication.

Aspirin/acetylsalicylic acid and clopidogrel (*vs.* aspirin)

For patients with AF in whom VKA therapy is considered unsuitable, the combination of 75 mg clopidogrel once daily plus aspirin is associated with a modest reduction in stroke, myocardial infarction, non-CNS systemic embolism, or death from vascular causes, after a median of 3.6 years of follow-up, compared with placebo plus aspirin (6.8% *vs.* 7.6% per year; RR: 0.89, 95% CI: 0.81–0.98). However, major bleeding is greater among patients assigned clopidogrel plus aspirin versus those on aspirin alone (2.0% *vs.* 1.3% per year; RR: 1.57, 95% CI:1.29–1.92).

These data suggest that treating 1000 patients with AF for 1 year with clopidogrel plus aspirin prevents eight major vascular events (including two fatal and three disabling strokes) and causes seven major hemorrhages (one fatal) compared with aspirin alone.

Warfarin and aspirin/acetylsalicylic acid combined

Because patients with AF often have coexisting atherosclerotic vascular disease (ischemic heart disease is a common cause of AF), both warfarin and aspirin are thought to be needed to prevent thrombus formation in the left atrium and arteries. Warfarin prevents the formation of fibrin-rich thrombus (so-called 'red clot') associated with AF, whereas antiplatelet treatment prevents the formation of the platelet-rich thrombus (so-called 'white clot') associated with arterial vascular disease. This principle applies particularly to patients with AF who present with unstable vascular disease manifest by an acute coronary syndrome, or who are undergoing vascular injury by means of percutaneous coronary or carotid intervention or stenting, for which aspirin plus clopidogrel is recommended. For such patients with AF, the long-term benefit-to-harm ratio of combination therapy is not known and should be left to the clinician's discretion. However, for patients with AF who have stable vascular disease, there is no reliable evidence to indicate that adding aspirin (or clopidogrel) to warfarin is safe and effective compared with warfarin alone. Indeed, warfarin can be an effective drug for stable coronary and cerebrovascular disease, and the hemorrhage rate seems to be greater with the combination of aspirin and warfarin.

Novel oral anticoagulants

Dabigatran etexilate is a prodrug of the active moiety dabigatran, an oral, reversible, direct thrombin inhibitor that inhibits both clot-bound and circulating thrombin. After oral administration as a fixed-dose, dabigatran etexiltate is rapidly converted by esterases to dabigatran, which has a fast onset of action reaching peak plasma concentrations within 0.5–2 hours, thereby potentially negating the need for initial treatment with a rapidly acting injectable anticoagulant. The anticoagulant effect of dabigatran can be measured by a prolonged thrombin clotting time or aPTT, but the anticoagulation response is sufficiently predictable that routine coagulation monitoring is not required. Dabigatran has a low potential for food and drug interactions, a half-life of 12–14 hours in patients with normal renal function that permits once- or twice-daily administration, and a fast offset of action. About 80% of the drug is excreted unchanged by the kidneys[78].

In a large trial of 18 113 patients with nonvalvular AF, dabigatran etexilate 150 mg bid significantly reduced the rate of the stroke (including hemorrhagic stroke) or systemic embolism compared with warfarin (warfarin: 1.71% per year *vs.* dabigatran 150 mg bid: 1.11% per year; RR: 0.65, 95% CI: 0.52–0.81; $p<0.001$ for superiority), and also death from cardiovascular causes (RR: 0.85, 95% CI: 0.72–0.99) despite a higher discontinuation rate for dabigatran. No significant difference in the same outcomes was found between dabigatran etexilate 110 mg bid and warfarin (stroke or systemic embolism: warfarin 1.71% per year vs. dabigatran 110 mg bid: 1.54% per year; RR: 0.90, 95% CI: 0.74–1.10, $p<0.001$ for noninferiority, $p=0.30$ for superiority)[79].

However, compared with warfarin, the lower dose of dabigatran etexilate, 110 mg bid, significantly reduced the rate of major hemorrhage (warfarin: 3.57% per year *vs.* dabigatran 110 mg bid: 2.87% per year; RR: 0.80, 95% CI: 0.70–0.93; $p=0.003$). No significant difference in major hemorrhage was found between dabigatran etexilate 150 mg bid and warfarin (warfarin 3.57% per year *vs.* dabigatran 150 mg 3.32% per year; RR: 0.93, 95% CI: 0.81–1.07, $p=0.31$ for superiority).

Both doses of dabigatran etexilate were associated with fewer intracranial bleeds than warfarin (warfarin: 0.74% per year *vs*. dabigatran 110 mg bid: 0.23% per year; RR: 0.31, 95% CI: 0.20–0.47], and dabigatran 150mg bid: 0.30% per year; RR: 0.40, 95% CI: 0.27–0.60]). Dabigatran etexilate 150 mg bid significantly increased gastrointestinal bleeding (1.51% per year) compared with warfarin (1.02% per year; RR: 1.50, 95% CI: 1.19–1.89) and dabigatran etexilate 110 mg bid (1.12% per year; RR: 1.36, 95% CI: 1.09–1.70). Coadministration of aspirin and dabigatran increased the risk of major bleeding compared with dabigatran alone (HR: 1.91; $p<0.001$) without any evidence of benefit in reducing stroke and other serious vascular events.

Rates of dyspepsia (including abdominal pain) were elevated with dabigatran (11.8% with 110 mg bid, 11.3% with 150 mg bid) compared with warfarin (5.8%), presumably related to the tartaric acid content of the dabigatran etexilate capsule. The relative effectiveness of dabigatran compared with warfarin was consistent among the subgroup of 3623 patients with prior stroke or TIA and AF and in the whole trial population of AF patients (**421, 422**).

For patients taking dabigatran who bleed, there is no specific antidote. Discontinuation of the drug and supportive measures usually suffice because the anticoagulant effect of dabigatran is short-lived. In emergencies, dabigatran can be dialyzed and, failing that, nonspecific hemostatic agents, such as rFVIIa and prothrombin complex concentrates, can be considered. In case of overdose, the efficacy of early administration of activated charcoal and charcoal filtration are undergoing clinical evaluation.

Rivaroxaban is a direct factor Xa inhibitor with predictable pharmacokinetics, high bioavailability, and rapid onset and offset of action after oral administration (reaching maximum plasma concentrations at 2.5–4.0 hours with a half-life of 5–13 hours) with little variability based on age, sex, or weight[78].

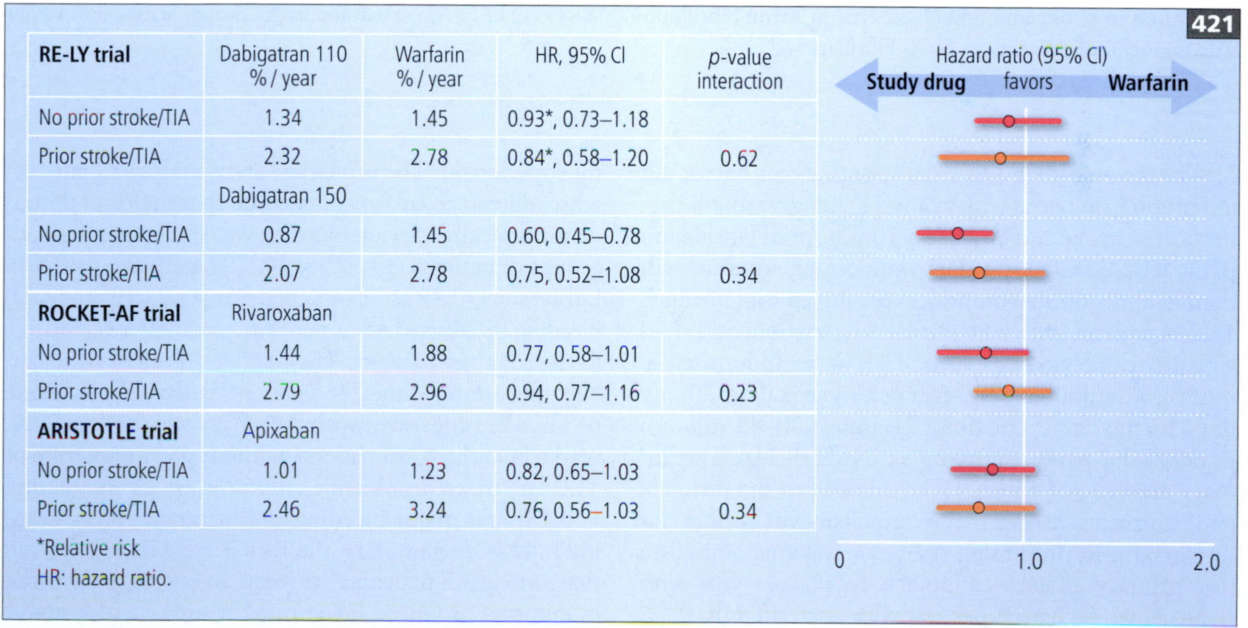

RE-LY trial	Dabigatran 110 % / year	Warfarin % / year	HR, 95% CI	*p*-value interaction
No prior stroke/TIA	1.34	1.45	0.93*, 0.73–1.18	
Prior stroke/TIA	2.32	2.78	0.84*, 0.58–1.20	0.62
	Dabigatran 150			
No prior stroke/TIA	0.87	1.45	0.60, 0.45–0.78	
Prior stroke/TIA	2.07	2.78	0.75, 0.52–1.08	0.34
ROCKET-AF trial	Rivaroxaban			
No prior stroke/TIA	1.44	1.88	0.77, 0.58–1.01	
Prior stroke/TIA	2.79	2.96	0.94, 0.77–1.16	0.23
ARISTOTLE trial	Apixaban			
No prior stroke/TIA	1.01	1.23	0.82, 0.65–1.03	
Prior stroke/TIA	2.46	3.24	0.76, 0.56–1.03	0.34

*Relative risk
HR: hazard ratio.

421 Risk of stroke (ischemic and hemorrhagic) or systemic embolism according to previous stroke or transient ischemic attack (TIA). Summary of the results of the three large Phase 3 warfarin-controlled trials of the new oral anticoagulants for the primary efficacy outcome of stroke or systemic embolism, according to whether or not participants had a history of stroke or transient ischemic attack at the time of randomization[78–81]. RE-LY: Randomised Evaluation of Long-term Anticoagulant Therapy trial[79]; ROCKET-AF: Rivaroxaban Once-daily, oral, direct factor Xa inhibition Compared with vitamin K antagonism for prevention of stroke and Embolism Trial in Atrial Fibrillation[80]; ARISTOTLE: Apixaban for Reduction in Stroke and Other Thromboembolic Events in Atrial Fibrillation[81].

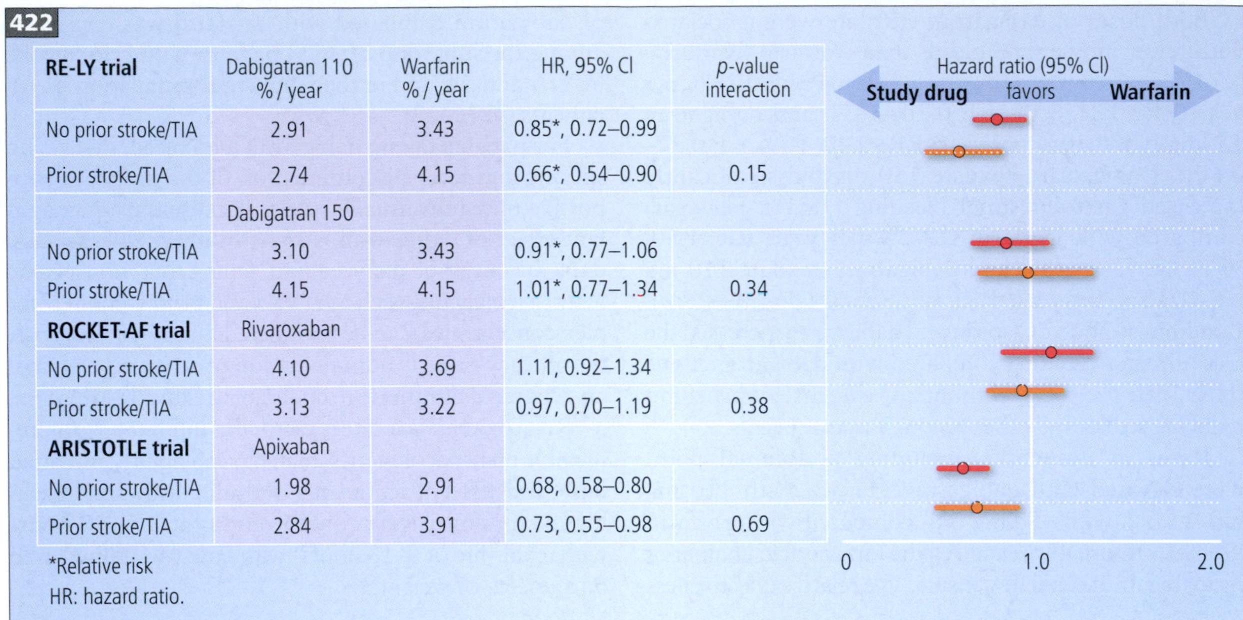

RE-LY trial	Dabigatran 110 % / year	Warfarin % / year	HR, 95% CI	*p*-value interaction
No prior stroke/TIA	2.91	3.43	0.85*, 0.72–0.99	
Prior stroke/TIA	2.74	4.15	0.66*, 0.54–0.90	0.15
	Dabigatran 150			
No prior stroke/TIA	3.10	3.43	0.91*, 0.77–1.06	
Prior stroke/TIA	4.15	4.15	1.01*, 0.77–1.34	0.34
ROCKET-AF trial	Rivaroxaban			
No prior stroke/TIA	4.10	3.69	1.11, 0.92–1.34	
Prior stroke/TIA	3.13	3.22	0.97, 0.70–1.19	0.38
ARISTOTLE trial	Apixaban			
No prior stroke/TIA	1.98	2.91	0.68, 0.58–0.80	
Prior stroke/TIA	2.84	3.91	0.73, 0.55–0.98	0.69

*Relative risk
HR: hazard ratio.

422 **Risk of major bleeding (as defined in each study) according to previous stroke or transient ischemic attack. Summary of the results of the three large Phase 3 warfarin-controlled trials of the new oral anticoagulants for the safety outcome of major bleeding, according to whether or not participants had a history of stroke or transient ischemic attack (TIA) at the time of randomization[78–81]. RE-LY: Randomised Evaluation of Long-term Anticoagulant Therapy trial[79]; ROCKET-AF: Rivaroxaban Once-daily, oral, direct factor Xa inhibition Compared with vitamin K antagonism for prevention of stroke and Embolism Trial in Atrial Fibrillation[80]; ARISTOTLE: Apixaban for Reduction in Stroke and Other Thromboembolic Events in Atrial Fibrillation[81].**

The Rivaroxaban Once-daily, oral, direct Factor Xa inhibition Compared with vitamin K antagonism for prevention of stroke and Embolism Trial in Atrial Fibrillation (ROCKET-AF) study was a multicenter, randomized, double-blind, double-dummy, event-driven trial in which 14,264 patients with nonvalvular AF, of whom 55% had a history of previous stroke or TIA, were randomized to receive, in a double-blind manner, rivaroxaban 20 mg/day (15 mg/day if creatinine clearance 30–49 ml/min) or dose-adjusted warfarin (target INR 2.0–3.0). The primary analysis, of patients who adhered to the protocol and treatment, showed that rivaroxaban was noninferior to warfarin in preventing stroke or systemic embolism (the primary efficacy endpoint); 1.71% per year with rivaroxaban *vs.* 2.16% per year with warfarin (HR: 0.79; 95% CI: 0.66–0.96, $p<0.001$ for noninferiority)[80]. The superiority analysis of patients who adhered to treatment, showed that rivaroxaban was superior to warfarin (1.70 *vs.* 2.15% per year; HR: 0.79, 95% CI: 0.65–0.95, $p = 0.015$). The intention-to-treat analysis of all patients, on and off treatment, showed that rivaroxaban was noninferior to warfarin (2.12 *vs.* 2.42%; HR: 0.88, 95% CI: 0.74–1.03, $p<0.001$ for noninferiority; $p=0.117$ for superiority). The principal safety analysis of patients who adhered to treatment showed that major and nonmajor clinically relevant bleeding was similar among both groups of patients (14.91 *vs.* 14.52% per year, $p=0.57$). Intracranial (0.49 *vs.* 0.74% per year, $p=0.019$) and fatal bleeding (0.24 *vs.* 0.48% per year, $p=0.003$) were lower in rivaroxaban patients. The relative effects of rivaroxaban *vs.* warfarin in the 7468 patients with previous stroke or TIA were consistent with the effects of rivaroxaban *vs.* warfarin in the 6796 patients without previous stroke or TIA for stroke or systemic embolism (p for interaction = 0.23) and major bleeding (p for interaction = 0.36) (**421, 422**). In summary, the ROCKET-AF trial showed that among AF patients, rivaroxaban once daily without monitoring produced lower rates of stroke and systemic embolism while on treatment and similar rates by intention-to-treat compared with warfarin. Overall bleeding was similar; however, rivaroxaban reduced intracranial and fatal bleeding.

Apixaban is also a direct factor Xa inhibitor with predictable pharmacokinetics, high bioavailability, and rapid onset and offset of action after oral administration[78].

The ARISTOTLE (Apixaban for Reduction in Stroke and Other Thromboembolic Events in Atrial Fibrillation) trial compared apixaban with warfarin (target INR 2.0)[81]. Patients with impaired renal function (serum creatinine >221µlmol/l [2.5 mg/dl] or creatinine clearance <25 ml/min) were excluded. Patients who were elderly (80 years or older), had low bodyweight (60 kg or lighter), or a serum creatinine of 133 µmol/l (1.5 mg/dl) or greater received a lower dose of apixaban (2.5 mg twice a day) than did other patients (5 mg twice a day). Apixaban was better than warfarin in reducing the rate of stroke or systemic embolism (p=0.01 for superiority). Apixaban was also associated with significantly less major bleeding (p<0.001), less intracranial hemorrhage (p<0.001), and lower mortality (p=0.047). The occurrence of gastrointestinal hemorrhage and MI was similar in both groups. The relative effects of apixaban *vs.* warfarin in the 3436 patients with previous stroke or TIA were consistent with the effects of apixaban versus warfarin in the 14,765 patients without previous stroke or TIA for stroke or systemic embolism (p for interaction = 0.71) and major bleeding (p for interaction = 0.69) (**421, 422**) [81]. In summary, apixaban reduced the risk of stroke or systemic embolism, major bleeding, intracranial hemorrhage, and mortality compared with warfarin in patients with nonvalvular AF.

Indirect comparisons suggest that the relative effects of each of the new oral anticoagulants compared with warfarin were consistent for stroke and systemic embolism (summary OR: 0.92, 95% CI: 0.83–1.02, I^2 = 22%, p-value for heterogeneity = 0.28), hemorrhagic stroke (OR: 0.43, 95% CI: 0.34–0.55, I^2 = 48%, p for heterogeneity = 0.12) and mortality (OR: 0.90, 95% CI: 0.84–0.96, I^2 = 0%, p for heterogeneity = 0.73) but not for extracranial major bleeding (OR: 0.98, 95% CI: 0.91–1.07, I^2 = 73%, p for heterogeneity = 0.01) and MI (OR: 1.03, 95% CI: 0.89–1.20, I^2 = 73%, p for heterogeneity = 0.01). Heterogeneic effects of apixaban *vs.* warfarin on major and gastrointestinal bleeding seemed more favourable than for dabigatran or rivaroxaban *vs.* warfarin. However, indirect comparisons of the new anticoagulants should be interpreted cautiously because the trials had different designs, participants, and interventions (e.g, time in therapeutic range [TTR] in those assigned warfarin differed between the trials)[78].

The AVERROES (Apixaban Versus Acetylsalicylic Acid [ASA] to Prevent Stroke in Atrial Fibrillation Patients Who Have Failed or Are Unsuitable for Vitamin K Antagonist Treatment) Trial was a double-blind study in which 5599 patients with AF who were at increased risk for stroke and for whom VKA therapy was unsuitable were randomly assigned to receive apixaban (at a dose of 5 mg twice daily) or aspirin (81–324 mg per day), to determine whether apixaban was superior[82]. Before enrolment, 40% of the patients had used a VKA. The mean follow-up period was 1.1 years. The primary outcome was the occurrence of stroke or systemic embolism. The data and safety monitoring board recommended early termination of the study because of a clear benefit in favor of apixaban. There were 51 primary outcome events (1.6% per year) among patients assigned to apixaban and 113 (3.7% per year) among those assigned to aspirin (HR with apixaban, 0.45, 95% CI: 0.32–0.62, p<0.001). The rates of death were 3.5% per year in the apixaban group and 4.4% per year in the aspirin group (HR: 0.79, 95% CI: 0.62–1.02, p=0.07). There were 44 cases of major bleeding (1.4% per year) in the apixaban group and 39 (1.2% per year) in the aspirin group (HR with apixaban, 1.13, 95% CI: 0.74–1.75, p=0.57); there were 11 cases of intracranial bleeding with apixaban and 13 with aspirin. The risk of a first hospitalization for cardiovascular causes was reduced with apixaban as compared with aspirin (12.6% per year *vs.* 15.9% per year, p<0.001). The treatment effects were consistent among important subgroups. In summary, in patients with AF for whom VKA therapy was unsuitable, apixaban reduced the risk of stroke or systemic embolism without significantly increasing the risk of major bleeding or intracranial hemorrhage.

Recommendations

Patients with TIA and AF should begin oral anticoagulation (warfarin, dabigatran, rivaroxaban, or apixaban) immediately after brain imaging has excluded intracranial hemorrhage or large infarct (evidence level B).

For patients treated with dabigatran, a dose of 150 mg twice daily is appropriate for most individuals; 110 mg twice daily is recommended for patients aged 80 or more years and for patients at risk of bleeding (evidence level B). The median duration of treatment in the RE-LY trial was 20 months. The long-term safety and effectiveness of dabigatran are currently under investigation.

For patients presenting with acute ischemic stroke and AF, the immediate use of heparin/heparinoid anticoagulation is not recommended (evidence level A). Most patients with acute ischemic stroke and AF should receive oral anticoagulant therapy (warfarin, dabigatran, rivaroxaban, or apixaban) (evidence level A). The decision to start anticoagulant therapy is optimally made during the acute phase of hospitalization. The optimal timing of oral anticoagulation following acute stroke for patients in AF is unclear; it is common practice to wait 2–14 days and repeat brain imaging (CT or MRI) to rule out asymptomatic intracranial hemorrhage before starting warfarin (evidence level C).

The decision to prescribe oral anticoagulation, and the net clinical benefit of oral anticoagulation, is based on an accurate assessment of the likely absolute annual risk of stroke without oral anticoagulation, and whether the likely benefits of oral anticoagulation (at least a two-thirds reduction in absolute stroke risk) are likely to outweigh the risks of bleeding associated with oral anticoagulation use. The threshold stroke rate for which oral anticoagulation prophylaxis is indicated is more than 2% per year (provided the risk of life-threatening or intracranial bleeding with warfarin is predicted to be <1% per year).

For some patients with acute ischemic stroke and AF, the individual's preferences, level of disability, prognosis, and overall clinical status, including the size of the infarct on neuroimaging, may contraindicate oral anticoagulant therapy (evidence level C). The combination of aspirin and clopidogrel should not be considered as a safer alternative to anticoagulant therapy for patients with AF, and should be reserved for patients in whom anticoagulant therapy is not feasible (e.g. patient refusal or inability to access INR monitoring) or when there are problems maintaining a stable, therapeutic INR (evidence level A).

Enhancing anticoagulation therapy and minimizing bleeding complications

Patients prescribed warfarin, dabigatran, rivaroxaban, or apixaban for AF should be educated about the diagnosis of AF, the risk of stroke with AF, the importance of medication adherence, and compliance with INR monitoring, if required (evidence level B).

For patients with AF who are taking warfarin, careful dosing and consistent INR monitoring are recommended to minimize adverse events; warfarin efficacy is dependent on maintaining therapeutic INR control, and declines significantly when the INR falls below 2.0 (evidence level A). Concomitant antiplatelet therapy with warfarin is not recommended in patients with AF unless there is a specific medical indication such as a coronary stent (evidence level B).

With the exception of patients with mechanical heart valves, the addition of aspirin to warfarin in patients with AF has not been shown to be of benefit in stroke prevention (evidence level B).

Concomitant antiplatelet therapy with dabigatran, rivaroxaban, or apixaban is not recommended in patients with AF (evidence level B).

Patent foramen ovale closure for the prevention of recurrent ischemic stroke of cardiac origin

Strategies to reduce the risk of stroke and systemic embolism in the presence of cryptogenic stroke and PFO include antiplatelet agents, anticoagulation, and percutaneous closure of the PFO with a device. Observational studies indicate that the incidence rate of recurrent stroke is about 0.36 per 100 person years after PFO closure and 2.53 per 100 person years with medical therapy. However, not only may these relative estimates be confounded by imbalances in the underlying risk of recurrent events between the two groups, but periprocedural major complications occur in about 1.1% (95% CI: 0.9–1.3) of cases, most commonly device embolization requiring surgery, and long-term complications occur, most commonly cerebrovascular events (1.3%; 95% CI: 1.1–1.6%) and device thrombosis (1.2%; 95% CI: 1.0–1.4%).

Three randomized controlled trials of PFO closure have reported results in a total of 2303 patients[83–85]. The CLOSURE-I trial randomized 909 patients with PFO and cryptogenic stroke or TIA to device closure of the PFO using the Starflex device combined with medical therapy (aspirin) *vs.* medical therapy alone (aspirin or warfarin or both)[83]. Successful implantation of a device was achieved in 81% of patients assigned to PFO closure. At 2 years there was no significant difference in the rate of stroke, TIA, or death from neurologic causes between the treatment groups (5.5% in the PFO closure group versus 6.8% in the medical therapy group). In most cases the recurrent neurologic events were attributed to causes unrelated to the PFO and it is noteworthy that left atrial thrombus was detected in 1.1% of patients who underwent transesophageal echocardiography at 6 months. Moreover, protocol-defined major vascular complications occurred in 3.2% of the PFO closure group and AF was significantly more frequent in the closure group than in the medical therapy group (5.7% *vs.* 0.7%)[17].

The RESPECT trial (NCT00465270) randomized 980 patients with PFO and cryptogenic stroke to PFO closure with the Amplatzer PFO occluder (St Jude Medical) or to medical therapy alone (with anticoagulation or antiplatelet therapy). A device was successfully implanted in 92.6% of the closure group with effective closure at 6 months in 93.5%. Over a mean 2.6 years follow-up there was no significant difference in the rate of recurrent stroke between the PFO closure arm (nine events) and the medical therapy arm (16 events). The investigators reported different durations of follow-up in the two arms of the trial because some patients in the medical arm withdrew from the study and underwent nonassigned PFO closure. Exploratory survival analyses by treatment received suggested that PFO closure might have reduced the risk of recurrent stroke. The rate of serious adverse events did not differ between the two groups although there was a nonsignificant excess of new AF (3.0% *vs.* 1.5%) and pulmonary embolism (1.2% *vs.* 0.2%) in the PFO closure group[18].

The PC trial (NCT00166257) randomized 414 patients with PFO and ischemic stroke, TIA, or extracranial peripheral thromboembolism to closure of the PFO using the Amplatzer PFO occluder (St Jude Medical) or to standard medical care (antiplatelet therapy or anticoagulation). A device was successfully implanted in 92.1% of the closure group. At a mean follow-up of around 4 years, PFO closure was associated with a nonsignificant 37% reduction in the primary composite endpoint (death, nonfatal stroke, TIA, and peripheral embolism). As with RESPECT, there was a slightly higher rate of new-onset AF in the PFO closure group (2.9% *vs.* 1.0%) but there was no evidence of device-associated thrombus[19].

The individual trials have relatively small sample sizes and short follow-up times, and the low event rates are bounded by wide confidence intervals that encompass clinically relevant treatment effects. Interpretation of the trial results is further complicated by treatment crossovers and incomplete follow-up. Adverse event rates varied across the trials, perhaps because rates of AF and device-related thrombosis differ between closure devices.

In a pooled analysis of the published intention-to-treat data, stroke rates tended to be lower (56 events, 2303 patients, OR: 0.66, 95% CI: 0.37–1.19), and the development of AF higher (40 events, 2254 patients, OR: 3.22, 95% CI: 0.87–11.92), in those patients randomized to PFO closure. Compared with medical therapy, the incidence of clinical AF was increased 10-fold with the STARFlex device in CLOSURE and 2–3-fold with the Amplatzer device in RESPECT and the PC trial.

In the absence of definitive evidence about PFO closure in patients with cryptogenic stroke, it is ethical, indeed imperative, that the three ongoing randomized trials of PFO closure to prevent recurrent stroke in patients with cryptogenic stroke continue to recruit patients [CLOSE (NCT00562289), DEFENSEPFO (NCT01550588), REDUCE (NCT00738894)] and realise their target sample sizes, so that data will be available from the six trials of PFO closure for 4000 patients.

Lowering blood pressure

The greatest potential for reducing the incidence of stroke is by means of blood pressure reduction (see *Table 45*; INTERSTROKE). This is because high blood pressure predisposes to both pathologic subtypes of stroke (hemorrhagic and ischemic) and most subtypes (aneurysmal SAH, hypertensive ICH, large artery atherosclerotic ischemic stroke, small artery ischemic stroke, and cardioembolic ischemic stroke due to AF, and ischemic and hypertensive heart disease).

Evidence

A meta-analysis of 13 RCTs of blood pressure-lowering interventions in patients with a history of stroke indicates that a blood pressure reduction of 10 mmHg systolic and 5 mmHg diastolic is associated with a reduction in the RR of recurrent stroke by 34% (21–44%)[86].

For patients with recent, but nonacute, lacunar stroke, a target systolic blood pressure of less than 130 mmHg is acceptably safe and more effective in preventing recurrent stroke than a target range of 130–149 mmHg[87]. Life-style interventions such as regular physical exercise for 30 minutes daily, alcohol reduction, a low salt diet, and potassium supplementation can realize reductions in blood pressure of 10 mmHg systolic or 5 mmHg diastolic.

Taking one antihypertensive drug at a standard dose, or three drugs at half standard dose, can also reduce the blood pressure by 10 mmHg systolic or 5 mmHg diastolic in patients with a pre-treatment systolic blood pressure of 150 mmHg (and would be associated with a reduction in the RR of recurrent stroke by 34% [21–44%]).

Traditionally, clinicians have relied on measuring the mean blood pressure (the average of several blood pressure readings [as distinct from mean arterial pressure]) to assess the risk of stroke and the benefits of antihypertensive drugs. In a post-hoc analysis of randomized trials in patients with vascular disease, visit-to-visit variability in systolic blood pressure and maximum systolic blood pressure were strong predictors of stroke, independent of mean blood pressure. Information from a systematic review of several randomized trials of antihypertensive treatments indicated that calcium channel blockers and diuretics led to the greatest reduction in visit-to-visit blood-pressure variability and were associated with the greatest reduction in risk of stroke, independent of mean systolic blood pressure. Beta blockers increased the variability of blood pressure in a dose-dependent manner and were the least effective in the prevention of stroke.

These data suggest that blood pressure variability, as well as mean blood pressure, should be measured to assess the risk of stroke and benefits of antihypertensive drugs, and that these drugs should reduce blood pressure variability and mean blood pressure to optimize prevention of stroke.

Recommendations

Blood pressure should be managed in all patients to reach optimal control as follows:

- For patients who have had a stroke or TIA, blood pressure lowering treatment is recommended to achieve a target of 130–139 mmHg systolic and 80–89 mmHg diastolic (evidence level C).
- For patients with recent, but nonacute, lacunar stroke, a target systolic blood pressure of less than 130 mmHg is recommended (evidence level A).
- The specific agents and sequence of agents for the secondary prevention of stroke depend on other patient comorbidities, but generally the combination of an ACE inhibitor (or angiotensin II receptor antagonist) and calcium channel blocker (or diuretic in the elderly) is optimal (evidence level C).
- RCTs have not defined the optimal time to initiate blood pressure lowering therapy after ischemic stroke or TIA. Blood pressure lowering treatment should be initiated or modified before discharge from hospital (evidence level B).
- For patients with stable symptoms of nondisabling stroke or TIA not requiring hospitalization, blood pressure lowering treatment should be initiated or modified to achieve target levels (evidence level B).

Lowering blood cholesterol

Evidence

A meta-analysis of 4 RCTs of statins in patients with a history of stroke or TIA shows that random assignment to a statin is associated with a reduction in LDL concentration by about 1 mmol/l and a reduction in the RR of recurrent stroke by about 12% (95% CI: 1–21%), compared with controls[88].

Recommendations

Patients with ischemic stroke or TIA should be managed with lifestyle modification and dietary guidelines as part of a comprehensive approach to achieve LDL cholesterol of <2 mmol/l (evidence level A). Other parameters may be considered including a 50% reduction in LDL concentration or apolipidprotein B level of <0.80 g/l (evidence level B). Statin agents should be prescribed for most patients who have had an ischemic stroke or TIA to achieve current recommended lipid levels (evidence level A).

Lowering blood glucose

Evidence

Random assignment of individuals with type 2 diabetes mellitus to an intensive blood glucose-lowering regimen that lowers the mean hemoglobin A1c (HbA1c) concentration by 0.9% compared with a standard regimen is associated with a nonstatistically significant trend toward a reduction in stroke by 7% (OR: 0.93, 95% CI: 0.81–1.06).

Recommendations

Glycemic targets must be individualized; however, therapy in most patients with type 1 or type 2 diabetes should be targeted to achieve a glycated hemoglobin (Hb_{A1C}) level ≤7.0% to reduce the risk of microvascular complications (evidence level A) and, in individuals with type 1 diabetes, macrovascular complications (evidence level C).

To achieve an Hb_{A1C} ≤7.0%, patients with type 1 or type 2 diabetes should aim for a fasting plasma glucose or pre-prandial plasma glucose target of 4.0–7.0 mmol/l (evidence level B).

The 2-hour post-prandial plasma glucose target is 5.0–10.0 mmol/l (evidence level B). If Hb_{A1C} targets cannot be achieved with a post-prandial target of 5.0–10.0 mmol/l, further post-prandial blood glucose lowering, to 5.0–8.0 mmol/l, can be considered (evidence level C).

Adults at high risk of a vascular event should be treated with a statin to achieve a LDL cholesterol ≤2.0 mmol/l (evidence level A).

Unless contraindicated, low-dose aspirin therapy (80–325 mg/day) is recommended in all patients with diabetes with evidence of cardiovascular disease, as well as for those individuals with atherosclerotic risk factors that increase their likelihood of cardiovascular events (evidence level A).

B-vitamins

Epidemiologic studies suggest that raised plasma concentrations of total homocysteine might be a risk factor for major vascular events.

Evidence

Among 8164 patients with prior stroke or TIA who were randomized to receive one tablet daily of placebo or B vitamins (2 mg folic acid, 25 mg vitamin B6, and 0.5 mg vitamin B12), and followed-up for a median duration of 3.4 years, 616 (15%) patients assigned to B vitamins experienced a stroke, myocardial infarction, or death from vascular causes compared with 678 (17%) assigned to placebo (RR: 0.91, 95% CI: 0.82–1.00, p=0.05; ARR: 1.56%, 95% CI:–0.01–3.16). There were no unexpected serious adverse reactions and no significant differences in common adverse effects between the treatment groups[89].

Recommendations

Daily administration of folic acid, vitamin B6, and vitamin B12 to patients with recent stroke or TIA is safe but did not seem to be more effective than placebo in reducing the incidence of major vascular events (evidence level A). The results of ongoing trials and an individual patient data meta-analysis will add statistical power and precision to present estimates of the effect of B vitamins in stroke patients.

Life-style behaviors

Persons at risk of stroke and patients who have had a stroke should be assessed for vascular disease risk factors and life-style management issues (smoking, diet, sodium intake, physical activity, body weight, and alcohol intake). They should receive information and counseling about possible strategies to modify their life-style and risk factors (evidence level B)[21].

Recommendations

- **Smoking:** provide unambiguous, nonjudgmental, and personally relevant advice regarding the importance of cessation to all smokers, and offer assistance with the initiation of a smoking cessation attempt, either directly or through referral to appropriate resources (evidence level A).
- A combination of pharmacologic therapy and behavioral therapy should be considered (evidence level A). The three classes of pharmacologic agents that should be considered as first-line therapy for smoking cessation are nicotine replacement therapy, bupropion, and varenicline (evidence level A).
- **Diet:** a healthy, balanced diet high in fresh fruits, vegetables, low-fat dairy products, dietary and soluble fiber, whole grains, and protein from plant sources and low in saturated fat, cholesterol, and sodium (evidence level B).
- **Sodium intake:** the recommended adequate daily sodium intake from all sources for persons 9–50 years is 1500 mg, decreasing to 1300 mg for persons 50–70 years and to 1200 mg for persons over 70 years. A daily upper consumption limit of 2300 mg should not be exceeded by any age group (evidence level B).
- **Alcohol consumption:** limiting consumption to two or fewer standard drinks per day; fewer than 14 drinks per week for men; and fewer than nine drinks per week for women (evidence level C).
- **Physical activity:** participating in moderate exercise (an accumulation of 30–60 minutes) such as walking (ideally brisk walking), jogging, cycling, swimming, or other dynamic exercise 4–7 days each week in addition to routine activities of daily living. High-risk patients (e.g. those with cardiac disease) should engage in medically supervised exercise programs (evidence level A).
- **Body weight:** maintain a body mass index (BMI) of 18.5–24.9 kg/m^2 or a waist circumference of <80 cm (31.5 inch) for women and <94 cm (37 inch) for men (evidence level B).

Rehabilitation

Most patients who experience a stroke or TIA will require some form of physical or cognitive rehabilitation. Rehabilitation begins on day one when brain repair and recovery also begin. Early consultation with rehabilitation professionals not only contributes to reductions in complications from immobility such as joint contracture, falls, aspiration pneumonia, and DVT, but also facilitates brain repair and recovery. There is evidence that an interprofessional approach bringing together clinicians with different skill sets is one of the factors that results in reduced deaths in specialized stroke units[49,90].

Tip

▶ *Rehabilitation is not synonymous with physical therapies such as physiotherapy or occupational therapy – it is a more complex process including multidisciplinary assessment, goal-setting, physical and cognitive therapies, vocational training, social planning, reassessment, and teamwork.*

Stroke rehabilitation unit care

Stroke unit care

All patients with stroke who are admitted to hospital and who require rehabilitation should be treated in a comprehensive or rehabilitation stroke unit by an interprofessional team (evidence level A):

- Post-acute stroke care should be delivered in a setting in which rehabilitation care is formally coordinated and organized (evidence level A).
- All patients should be referred to a specialist rehabilitation team on a geographically defined unit as soon as possible after admission (evidence level A). Pediatric acute and rehabilitation stroke care should be provided on a specialized pediatric unit (evidence level B).
- The interprofessional rehabilitation team should consist of a physician, nurse, physical therapist, occupational therapist, speech-language pathologist, psychologist, recreation therapist, patient, and family and/or caregivers (evidence level A). For children, this should also include educators and child-life workers. This core interprofessional team should consist of appropriate levels of these disciplines, as identified by the Stroke Unit Trialists' Collaboration (evidence level B).

All settings (hospital, clinic, community) where stroke rehabilitation is provided

Post-acute stroke care should be delivered by a variety of treatment disciplines, experienced in providing post-stroke care, to ensure consistency and reduce the risk of complications (evidence level C).

The interprofessional rehabilitation team should assess patients within 24–48 hours of admission and develop a comprehensive individualized rehabilitation plan which reflects the severity of the stroke and the needs and goals of the stroke patient (evidence level C).

- Clinicians should use standardized, valid assessment tools to evaluate the patient's stroke-related impairments and functional status (evidence level B).
- Patients with moderate or severe stroke who have rehabilitation goals and are ready to participate in rehabilitation should be given an opportunity to participate in inpatient stroke rehabilitation (evidence level A).
- Stroke unit teams should conduct at least one formal interprofessional meeting per week to discuss the progress and problems, rehabilitation goals, and discharge arrangements for patients on the unit (evidence level B). Individualized rehabilitation plans should be regularly updated based on patient status reviews (evidence level C).
- Where admission to a stroke rehabilitation unit is not possible, a less optimal solution is inpatient rehabilitation on a mixed rehabilitation unit (i.e. where interprofessional care is provided to patients disabled by a range of disorders including stroke) (evidence level B)[49].

Delivery of inpatient stroke rehabilitation

All patients with stroke should begin rehabilitation therapy within an active and complex stimulating environment (evidence level C) as early as possible once medical stability is reached (evidence level A).

- Patients should receive the intensity and duration of clinically relevant therapy defined in their individualized rehabilitation plan and appropriate to their needs and tolerance levels (evidence level A).
- Stroke patients should receive, through an individualized treatment plan, a minimum of 3 hours of direct task-specific therapy by the interprofessional stroke team for a minimum of 5 days per week (evidence level A). The team should promote the practice of skills gained in therapy into the patient's daily routine in a consistent manner (evidence level A).
- Therapy should include repetitive and intense use of novel tasks that challenge the patient to acquire necessary motor skills to use the involved limb during functional tasks and activities (evidence level A).

The care management plan should include a pre-discharge needs assessment to ensure a smooth transition from rehabilitation back to the community. Elements of discharge planning should include a home visit by a health-care professional, ideally before discharge, to assess home environment and suitability for safe discharge, determine equipment needs and home modifications, and begin caregiver training for how the patient will manage activities of daily living and instrumental activities of daily living in their environment (evidence level C)[49].

Mobility and transfer skills

Therapeutic goal: improve basic mobility and transfer skills

- Task-oriented training (i.e. training that is progressively adapted, salient, and involves active participation) is recommended to improve transfer skills and mobility (evidence levels: early – level C; late – level C).
- Task-oriented training consisting of an extra 11–13 repetitions/day of sit-to-stand practice with eyes open and minimal use of arm support should be included in the patient's therapy program (evidence levels: early – level A; late – level C).
- Spasticity should not limit the use of strength training in the leg (evidence levels: early – level C; late – level C).
- Assess the need for special equipment on an individual basis. Once provided, equipment should be evaluated on a regular basis (evidence levels: early – level C; late – level C).
- Ankle foot orthoses may help some patients with foot drop; they should not be used routinely without proper assessment prior to prescription and follow-up to establish their effectiveness in the individual (evidence levels: early – level A; late – level A).
- Lower extremity orthotic devices may be helpful if ankle or knee stabilization is needed to help the patient walk. Prefabricated bracing can be used initially, and more expensive customized bracing reserved for patients who demonstrate a long-term need (evidence levels: early – level C; late – level C).
- Functional electrical stimulation (FES) should be considered for use in improving muscle force, strength and function (gait) in selected patients. FES must not be assumed to have sustained effects (evidence levels: early – level A; late – level A).
- There is insufficient evidence to recommend for or against neurodevelopmental therapy (NDT) in comparison to other treatment approaches for motor retraining following an acute stroke (evidence levels: early – level B; late – level B).
- Recommend that wheelchair prescriptions be based on careful assessment of the patient and the environment in which the wheelchair will be used (evidence levels: early – level C; late – level C).

Spasticity following stroke

Therapeutic goal: maintain range of motion and reduce spasticity of the leg

- Spasticity and contractures should be treated or prevented by antispastic pattern positioning, range-of-motion (ROM) exercises, stretching and/or splinting (SCORE) (evidence levels: early – level C; late – level C).
- For post-acute stroke patients with focal and symptomatically distressing spasticity, consider use of chemodenervation using botulinum toxin injection to increase ROM (evidence levels: early – level C; late – level A).
- Consider use of tizanidine in patients with generalized spasticity (evidence levels: early – level B; late – level B).
- Recommend against prescription of benzodiazepines during stroke recovery period due to possible deleterious effects on recovery, in addition to deleterious sedation side-effects (evidence levels: early – level C; late – level C)[49].

Lower limb gait following stroke

Therapeutic goal: improve walking ability and speed

- Task-specific training is recommended to improve performance of selected tasks for the lower extremity (evidence levels: early – level B; late – level B).
- Consider treadmill-based gait training (without body support) to enhance walking speed, endurance, and walking distance in persons post stroke. Treadmill training is suggested for 30 minutes, 5 days per week for 2–3 weeks (evidence levels: early – level C; late – level B).
- There is no conclusive evidence that body weight supported treadmill training (BWSTT) is superior to over ground training to enhance walking abilities. BWSTT could be considered when other strategies for walking practice are unsuccessful in those patients with low ambulatory function (evidence levels: early – level B; late – level B).
- Following appropriate medical evaluation, patients should participate regularly in an aerobic exercise program that takes into consideration the patient's comorbidities and functional limitations, to improve gait speed, endurance, stroke risk factor profile, mood, and possibly cognitive abilities (evidence levels: early – level B; late – level B)[49].

Management of the arm and hand

Therapeutic goal: improved arm and hand skill for independence

- Exercise and functional training should be directed towards enhancing motor control for restoring sensorimotor and functional abilities (evidence levels: early – level A; late – level A).
- Engage in repetitive and intense use of novel tasks that challenge the patient to acquire necessary motor skills to use the involved limb during functional tasks and activities (evidence levels: early – level A; late – level A).
- The upper extremity program should include strength training to improve impairment and function after stroke for upper extremity. Spasticity is not a contraindication to strength training (evidence levels: early – level A; late – level A).
- Therapists should provide a graded repetitive arm supplementary program for patients to increase activity on the ward and at home. This program should include strengthening of the arm and hand (small wrist weight, putty, hand gripper), ROM (stretching, active exercises), and gross, fine motor skills (e.g. blocks, Lego®, pegs), repetitive goal and task-oriented activities designed to simulate partial or whole skill required in activities of daily living (e.g. folding, buttoning, pouring, and lifting). The *GRASP* protocol suggests 1 hour per day, 6 days per week (evidence levels: early – level A; late – level C).
- Following appropriate cognitive and physical assessment, mental imagery should be used to enhance sensory–motor recovery in the upper limb (evidence levels: early – level A; late – level B).
- FES can be used for the wrist and forearm to reduce motor impairment and improve functional motor recovery (evidence levels: early – level A; late – level A).
- Intensive constraint-induced movement therapy (CIMT) should not be used for individuals in the first month post stroke until further research is completed (evidence levels: early – level A; late – N/A).
- Consider the use of intensive CIMT for a select group of patients who demonstrate at least 20° of wrist extension and 10° of finger extension, with minimal sensory or cognitive deficits. Intensive training should involve restraint of the unaffected arm for at least 90% of waking hours, and at least 6 hours a day of intense upper extremity training of the affected arm for 2 weeks (evidence level: 3– 6 months – level A; late – level A).
- Consider the use of modified CIMT for a select group of patients who demonstrate at least 20° of wrist extension and 10° of finger extension, with minimal sensory or cognitive deficits. Modified CIMT consists of constraint of the unaffected arm with a padded mitt or arm sling for a minimum of 6 hours a day with 2 hours of therapy for 14 days (evidence levels: early – level A; late – level A).
- Electromyography (EMG) biofeedback systems should not be used on a routine basis. (evidence levels: early – level A; late – level A).
- For patients whose arm and hand are predicted to be less than stage three as measured by the Chedoke–McMaster Stroke Assessment, enhance sensory–motor recovery of the upper limb by using sensory motor stimulation (evidence levels: early – level B; late – level B). This consists of passive- and active-assisted range of movement that also includes placement of the upper limb in a variety of positions within the patient's visual field. (Adapted from HSF-AH 1.2a). (Evidence levels: early – level C; late – level C.)
- Use adaptive devices for safety and function if other methods of performing specific tasks are not available or cannot be learned (evidence levels: early – level C; late – level C).
- Assess the need for special equipment on an individual basis. Once provided, equipment should be re-evaluated on a regular basis (evidence levels: early – level C; late – level C)[49].

Range-of-motion and spasticity

Therapeutic goal: maintain range-of-motion and reduce spasticity in the shoulder, arm, and hand

- Spasticity and contractures should be treated or prevented by antispastic pattern positioning, ROM exercises, stretching and/or splinting (evidence levels: early – level C; late – level C).
- For patients with focal and/or symptomatically distressing spasticity, consider use of chemodenervation using botulinum toxin to increase ROM and decrease pain (evidence levels: early – level C; late – level A).
- Consider use of tizanidine or baclofen for spasticity in patients with generalized, disabling spasticity resulting in poor skin hygiene, poor positioning, increased caregiver burden, or decreased function (evidence levels: early – level C; late – level B).
- Recommend against prescription of benzodiazepines during stroke recovery period due to possible deleterious effects on recovery, in addition to deleterious sedation side-effects (evidence levels: early – level B; late – level B).

Management of shoulder and arm pain

Therapeutic goal: maintain pain-free shoulder and arm

Assessment and prevention of shoulder pain:

- The presence of pain and any exacerbating factors should be identified early and treated appropriately (evidence level C).
- Joint protection strategies include:
    - Positioning and supporting the limb to minimize pain (evidence level B).
    - Protection and support for the limb to minimize pain during functional mobility tasks using slings, pocket, or by therapist and during wheelchair use by using hemi tray or arm troughs) (evidence level C).
    - Teaching patient to respect the pain (evidence level C).
    - Overhead pulleys should not be used (evidence level A).
    - The shoulder should not be passively moved beyond 90° of flexion and abduction unless the scapula is upwardly rotated and the humerus is laterally rotated (evidence level A).
    - Educate staff and caregivers about correct handling of the hemiplegic arm (evidence level A).
- Treat shoulder pain and limitations in ROM through gentle stretching and mobilization techniques focusing especially on external rotation and abduction (evidence level B).
- Reduce hand edema by:
    - Active self ROM exercises in conjunction with elevation (evidence level C) to gain full range of movement of the fingers, thumb, and wrist.
    - Retrograde massage (evidence level C).
    - Gentle grade 1–2 mobilizations for accessory movements of the hand and fingers (evidence level C).
    - Cold water immersion (evidence level B) or contrast baths (evidence level C).
- Consider using FES to increase pain-free ROM of lateral rotation of the shoulder (evidence level A).
- Consider use of acetaminophen or other analgesics for pain relief (evidence level C).
- Consider the use of botulinum toxin injections into subscapularis and pectoralis muscles for individuals with hemiplegic shoulder pain (evidence level C)[49].

Assessment and management of complex regional pain syndrome

(Also known as shoulder–hand syndrome, reflex sympathetic dystrophy, Sudecks atrophy.)

- A bone scan may be used to assist diagnosis of this condition (evidence level C).
- Oral corticosteroids in tapering doses may be used to reduce swelling and pain due to this condition (evidence level B).

Tip

▶ *When a patient is failing to achieve his or her goals (or milestones) then we must seek and identify the reason, and if possible rectify it.*

Outpatient care

Outpatient and community-based stroke rehabilitation

After leaving hospital, stroke survivors must have access to specialized stroke care and rehabilitation services appropriate to their needs (acute and/or inpatient rehabilitation) (evidence level A).

- Early supported discharge should be considered for patients discharged to the community (evidence level A).
- People who have difficulty in activities of daily living, including self-care, productivity and leisure, should receive occupational therapy or interprofessional interventions targeting activities of daily living (evidence level A for adults; evidence level C for pediatrics).
- Patients who are identified as high risk for falls in the community should have a comprehensive set of interventions implemented, such as an individually prescribed exercise program, in order to prevent or reduce the number and severity of falls (evidence level A).
- People with difficulties in mobility should be offered an exercise program specific to those difficulties and monitored throughout the program (evidence level B).
- Patients with aphasia should be taught supportive conversation techniques (evidence level A).
- Patients with dysphagia should be offered swallowing therapy and opportunity for reassessment as required (evidence level A).
- Children affected by stroke should be offered advice on and treatment aimed at achieving play, self-care, leisure, and school-related skills that are developmentally relevant and appropriate in their home, community, and school environments (evidence level B).
- Stroke survivors should be provided with a cardiovascular fitness program to maximize functional outcomes after stroke (and as part of overall vascular risk reduction). Patients should be prescribed modified activities to allow age-appropriate target heart rates to be achieved for 20–30 minutes three times per week (evidence level B)[49].

Advance care planning and palliative care

Advance care planning is a process of helping a patient reflect on and communicate his or her goals, values, and preferences for future health-care, to be used should they become incapable of giving informed consent. Central to this process are conversations between the patient, his or her family, and the health-care providers. For stroke patients, the goal of advance care planning is a shared understanding of the stroke, comorbidities, and prognosis; the benefits and burdens of potential treatments; types and location of care; and the individual's goals and values as they pertain to such care. It is an ongoing process that should be reviewed regularly or as the situation changes. These conversations may lead to a written document, often called a personal or advance directive, which names a substitute decision-maker, proxy, or agent, and outlines the person's desired medical interventions. Advance care planning can also result in rich conversations about meanings and fears around illness and dying, spirituality, and after-death religious practices.

Palliative care is an approach that focuses on comfort and quality of life for those affected by life-limiting illness. It aims to prevent and relieve physical, social, psychologic, or spiritual suffering of stroke patients and their families. Palliative care can complement life-prolonging or disease-modifying therapies post stroke, and need not be reserved for those whose death is imminent.

End-of-life care or terminal care is part of the palliative approach and is the management and treatment of dying patients and their families. The end-of-life period often involves a period of change (e.g. worsening diagnosis) rather than an acute event.

Patients surviving a stroke and their families should be approached by the stroke health-care team to participate in advance care planning (evidence level C).

Advance care planning

- Advance care planning may include identifying a substitute decision-maker (proxy or agent), implementing a personal directive (evidence level C), and discussion of the patient's preferences and the medical appropriateness of therapies such as feeding tubes, hydration, treatment of the current illness, admission to intensive care, ventilation, cardiopulmonary resuscitation, and place of care (evidence level B).
- The goals of therapy should be revisited periodically and when there is a change in health status (evidence level B).
- The interprofessional team should have the appropriate communication skills and knowledge to address the physical, spiritual, psychologic, ethical, and social needs of palliative or dying patients and their families (evidence level C).

Palliative and end-of-life care

The palliative approach should be used with those experiencing significant morbidity after a stroke, or to optimize end-of-life care for dying stroke patients and their families (evidence level B). Communication with patients and their families should provide, on an ongoing basis, information and counseling regarding diagnosis, prognosis, and management, including:

- The appropriateness of life-sustaining measures including mechanical ventilation, enteral/intravenous feeding, and intravenous fluids (evidence level B).
- Oral care (evidence level C).
- Assessment and management of: pain (evidence level B), delirium (evidence level C), respiratory distress (evidence level B), and incontinence, nausea, vomiting, constipation, and skin and wound care (evidence level C).
- Patients and the health-care team should have access to palliative care specialists for consultation on all palliative stroke patients (evidence level C).
- Palliative care specialists should be involved in the care of all patients with difficult-to-control symptoms, complex or conflicted end-of-life decision making, or complex psychosocial family issues (evidence level C).
- The interprofessional team should have the appropriate communication skills and knowledge to address the physical, spiritual, psychologic, and social needs of palliative or dying patients and their families (evidence level C).
- Palliative care pathways should be considered to introduce and monitor standards of care provided to palliative or dying stroke patients (evidence level B)[49].

Outpatient management of TIA and nondisabling stroke

All patients with TIA or nondisabling ischemic stroke who are not on an antiplatelet agent at time of presentation should be started on antiplatelet therapy immediately after brain imaging has excluded intracranial hemorrhage (evidence level A). A loading dose of aspirin should be at least 160 mg. If clopidogrel is used, a loading dose of 300 mg should be given, then maintenance therapy of 75 mg daily (evidence level A).

Patients with TIA or nondisabling ischemic stroke with a 50–99% carotid stenosis on the side implicated by their neurologic symptoms, who are otherwise candidates for carotid revascularization, should have CEA performed as soon as possible, ideally within 2–14 days (evidence level A). Patients with TIA or nondisabling ischemic stroke with AF should begin anticoagulation (heparin, warfarin, or dabigatran) immediately after brain imaging has excluded intracranial hemorrhage or large infarct. For patients on warfarin, the target therapeutic INR is 2.5, with a range of 2.0–3.0 (evidence level A).

All risk factors for cerebrovascular disease must be aggressively managed through pharmacologic and nonpharmacologic means to achieve optimal control (evidence level A). While evidence of the benefit of modifying individual risk factors in the acute phase is lacking, there is evidence of benefit when adopting a comprehensive approach, including antihypertensives and statin medication (evidence level C). Patients with TIA or nondisabling ischemic stroke who smoke should be strongly advised to quit immediately, and be provided with the pharmacologic and nonpharmacologic means to do so (evidence level B).

REFERENCES

1 Rothwell PM, Coull AJ, Silver LE, for the Oxford Vascular Study (2005). Population-based study of event-rate, incidence, case fatality, and mortality for all acute vascular events in all arterial territories (Oxford Vascular Study). *Lancet* **366**:1773–1783.

2 Strong K, Mathers C, Bonita R (2007). Preventing stroke: saving lives around the world. *Lancet Neurol* **6**:182–187.

3 Feigin VL, Lawes CM, Bennett DA, Barker-Collo SL, Parag V (2009). Worldwide stroke incidence and early case fatality reported in 56 population-based studies: a systematic review. *Lancet Neurol* **8**:355–369.

4 Geddes JML, Fear J, Tennant A, *et al.* (1996). Prevalence of self-reported stroke in a population in northern England. *J Epidemiol Commun Health* **50**:140–143.

5 Ferro JM, Massaro AR, Mas JL (2010). Aetiological diagnosis of ischaemic stroke in young adults. *Lancet Neurol* **9**(11):1085–1096.

6 Debette S, Leys D (2009). Cervical-artery dissections: predisposing factors, diagnosis, and outcome. *Lancet Neurol* **8**(7):668–678.

7 Testai FD, Gorelick PB (2010). Inherited metabolic disorders and stroke Part 1. *Arch Neurol* **67**:19–24; Part 2. *Arch Neurol* **67**:148–153.

8 Scott RM, Smith ER (2009). Moyamoya disease and moyamoya syndrome. *N Engl J Med* **360**:1226–1237.

9 Salvarani C, Brown RD Jr, Hunder GG (2012). Adult primary central nervous system vasculitis. *Lancet* **380**(9843):767–777.

10 Pantoni L (2010). Cerebral small vessel disease: from pathogenesis and clinical characteristics to therapeutic challenges. *Lancet Neurol* **9**:689–701.

11 Dichgans M (2007). Genetics of ischaemic stroke. *Lancet Neurol* **6**:149–161.

12 Baird AE (2010). Genetics and genomics of stroke. Novel approaches. *J Am Coll Cardiol* **56**:245–253.

13 Lip GY, Tse HF, Lane DA (2012). Atrial fibrillation. *Lancet* **379**(9816):648–661.

14 Mas JL, Arquizan C, Lamy C, *et al.*; Patent Foramen Ovale and Atrial Septal Aneurysm Study Group (2001). Recurrent cerebrovascular events associated with patent foramen ovale, atrial septal aneurysm, or both. *N Engl J Med* **345**(24):1740–1746.

15 Cohen D, Berger SP, Steup-Beekman GM, Bloemenkamp KW, Bajema IM (2010). Diagnosis and management of the antiphospholipid syndrome. *BMJ* **340**:c2541.

16 Saposnik G, Barinagarrementeria F, Brown RD Jr, *et al.*; American Heart Association Stroke Council and the Council on Epidemiology and Prevention (2011). Diagnosis and management of cerebral venous thrombosis: a statement for healthcare professionals from the American Heart Association/American Stroke Association. *Stroke* **42**(4):1158–1192.

17 Al-Shahi Salman R, Labovitz DL, Stapf C (2009). Spontaneous intracerebral haemorrhage. *BMJ* **339**:b2586.

18 Al-Shahi Salman R, Hall JM, Horne MA, *et al.*; Scottish Audit of Intracranial Vascular Malformations (SAIVMs) collaborators (2012). Untreated clinical course of cerebral cavernous malformations: a prospective, population-based cohort study. *Lancet Neurol* **11**(3):217–224.

19 van Gijn J, Kerr RS, Rinkel GJE (2007). Subarachnoid haemorrhage. *Lancet* **369**: 306–318.

20 Wermer MJ, van der Schaaf IC, Algra A, Rinkel GJ (2007). Risk of rupture of unruptured intracranial aneurysms in relation to patient and aneurysm characteristics: an updated meta-analysis. *Stroke* **38**(4):1404–1410.

21 O'Donnell MJ, Xavier D, Liu L, *et al.*; on behalf of the INTERSTROKE investigators (2010). Risk factors for ischaemic and intracerebral haemorrhagic stroke in 22 countries (the INTERSTROKE study): a case-control study. *Lancet* **376**:112–123.

22 Klijn CJ, Kappelle LJ (2010). Haemodynamic stroke: clinical features, prognosis, and management. *Lancet Neurol* **9**(10):1008–1017.

23 Bamford J, Sandercock P, Dennis M, *et al.* (1991). Classification and natural history of clinically identifiable subtypes of cerebral infarction. *Lancet* **337**:1521–1526.

24 Chalela JA, Kidwell CS, Nentwich LM, *et al.* (2007). Magnetic resonance imaging and computed tomography in emergency assessment of patients with suspected acute stroke: a prospective comparison. *Lancet* **369**(9558):293–298.

25 Doubal FN, Dennis MS, Wardlaw JM (2011). Characteristics of patients with minor ischaemic strokes and negative MRI: a cross-sectional study. *J Neurol Neurosurg Psychiatry* **82**(5):540–542.

26 Wallis A, Saunders T (2010). Imaging transient ischaemic attack with diffusion weighted magnetic resonance imaging. *BMJ* **340**:c2215.

27 Brott TG, Halperin JL, Abbara S, *et al.*; American College of Cardiology Foundation/American Heart Association Task Force on Practice Guidelines; American Stroke Assocation; American Association of Neuroscience Nurses; American Association of Neurological Surgeons; American College of Radiology; American Society of Neuroradiology; Congress of Neurolgocial Surgeons; Society of Atherosclerosis Imaging and Prevention; Society for Cardiovascular Angiography and Interventions; Society of Interventional Radiology; Society of NeuroInterventional Surgery; Society for Vascular Medicine; Society for Vascular Surgery; American Academy of Neurology and Society of Cardiovascular Computed Tomography. ASA/ACCF/AHA/AANN/AANS/ACR/ASNR/CNS/SAIP/SCAI/SIR/SNIS/SVM/SVS guideline on the management of patients with extracranial carotid and vertebral artery disease. *Stroke* **42**(8):e464–540.

28 Morris JG, Singh S, Fisher M (2010). Testing for inherited thrombophilias in arterial stroke: can it cause more harm than good? *Stroke* **41**(12):2985–2990.

29 Nor AM, Davis J, Sen B, *et al.* (2005). The Recognition Of Stroke In the Emergency Room (ROSIER) Scale: development and validation of a stroke recognition instrument. *Lancet Neurol* **4**:727–734.

30 Whiteley WN, Wardlaw JM, Dennis MS, Sandercock PA (2011). Clinical scores for the identification of stroke and transient ischaemic attack in the emergency department: a cross-sectional study. *J Neurol Neurosurg Psychiatry* **82**(9):1006–1010.

31 Edlow JA, Selim MH (2011). Atypical presentations of acute cerebrovascular syndromes. *Lancet Neurol* **10**(6):550–560.

32 Hankey GJ, Nelson MR (2009). Easily missed? Subarachnoid haemorrhage. *BMJ* **339**: b2874.

33 Barraclough K, Bronstein A (2009). Vertigo. *BMJ* **339**:b3493.

34 Kattah JC, Talkad AV, Wang DZ, Hsieh YH, Newman-Toker DE (2009). HINTS to diagnose stroke in the acute vestibular syndrome: three-step bedside oculomotor examination more sensitive than early MRI diffusion-weighted imaging. *Stroke* **40**(11):3504–3510.

35 Hand PJ, Kwan J, Lindley RI, Dennis MS, Wardlaw JM (2006). Distinguishing between stroke and mimic at the bedside: the brain attack study. *Stroke* **37**:769–775.

36 Adams HP Jr, Bendixen BH, Kappelle LJ, *et al.* (1993). Classification of subtypes of acute ischemic stroke. Definitions for use in a multicenter clinical trial. TOAST. Trial of Org 10172 in Acute Stroke Treatment. *Stroke* **24**(1):35–41.

37 Hardie K, Hankey GJ, Jamrozik K, Broadhurst R, Anderson C (2003). Ten-year survival after first-ever stroke in the Perth Community Stroke Study. *Stroke* **34**:1842–1846.

38 van Asch CJ, Luitse MJ, Rinkel GJ, van der Tweel I, Algra A, Klijn CJ (2010). Incidence, case fatality, and functional outcome of intracerebral haemorrhage over time, according to age, sex, and ethnic origin: a systematic review and meta-analysis. *Lancet Neurol* **9**(2):167–176.

39 O'Donnell MJ, Fang J, D'Uva C, *et al.*; for the Investigators of the Registry of the Canadian Stroke Network (2012). The PLAN Score: a bedside prediction rule for death and severe disability following acute ischemic stroke. *Arch Intern Med* **172**(20):1548–1556.

40 Reid JM, Gubitz GJ, Dai D, *et al.* (2010). Predicting functional outcome after stroke by modelling baseline clinical and CT variables. *Age Ageing* **39**(3):360–366.

41 Hardie K, Hankey GJ, Jamrozik K, Broadhurst R, Anderson C (2004). Ten-year risk of first recurrent stroke and disability after first-ever stroke in the Perth Community Stroke Study. *Stroke* **35**:731–735.

42 Giles MF, Rothwell PM (2007). Risk of stroke early after transient ischaemic attack: a systematic review and meta-analysis. *Lancet Neurol* **6**:1063–1072.

43 Chandratheva A, Mehta Z, Geraghty OC, Marquardt L, Rothwell PM; Oxford Vascular Study (2009). Population-based study of risk and predictors of stroke in the first few hours after a TIA. *Neurology* **72**:1941–1947.

44 Rothwell PM, Warlow CP (2005). Timing of TIAs preceding stroke: time window for prevention is very short. *Neurology* **64**(5):817–820.

45 Johnston SC, Rothwell P, Nguyen-Huynh MN, *et al.* (2007). Validation and refinement of scores to predict very early stroke risk after transient ischaemic attack. *Lancet* **369**:283–292.

46 Merwick A, Albers GW, Amarenco P, *et al.* (2010). Addition of brain and carotid imaging to the ABCD² score to identify patients at early risk of stroke after transient ischaemic attack: a multicentre observational study. *Lancet Neurol* **9**(11):1060–1069.

47 van Wijk I, Kappelle LJ, van Gijn J, *et al.*; LiLAC study group (2005). Long-term survival and vascular event risk after transient ischaemic attack or minor ischaemic stroke: a cohort study. *Lancet* **365**(9477):2098–2104.

48 Guyatt GH, Cook DJ, Jaeschke R, *et al.* (2008). Grades of recommendation for antithrombotic agents: American College of Chest Physicians Evidence-Based Clinical Practice Guidelines (8th edition). *Chest* **133**(6 Suppl):123S–131S. (Erratum in *Chest* 2008;**34**:47.)

49 Canadian Stroke Network and Strategy(2010). *Canadian Best Practice Recommendations for Stroke Care.* www.strokebestpractices.ca

50 European Stroke Organisation (ESO) Executive Committee; ESO Writing Committee (2008). Guidelines for management of ischaemic stroke and transient ischaemic attack 2008. *Cerebrovasc Dis* **25**(5):457–507.

51 Hankey GJ (2010). Ischaemic stroke – prevention is better than cure. *J R Coll Physicians Edinb* **40**:56–63.

52 Wardlaw JM, Murray V, Berge E, Del Zoppo GJ (2009). Thrombolysis for acute ischaemic stroke. *Cochrane Database Syst Rev* **4**:CD000213.

53 IST-3 collaborative group, Sandercock P, Wardlaw JM, Lindley RI, *et al.* (2012). The benefits and harms of intravenous thrombolysis with recombinant tissue plasminogen activator within 6 h of acute ischaemic stroke (the third international stroke trial [IST-3]): a randomised controlled trial. *Lancet* **379**(9834):2352–2363. (Erratum in *Lancet* 2012;**380**(9843):730.)

54 Wardlaw JM, Murray V, Berge E, *et al.* (2012). Recombinant tissue plasminogen activator for acute ischaemic stroke: an updated systematic review and meta-analysis. *Lancet* **379**(9834):2364–2372.

55 Saposnik G, Fang J, Kapral MK, *et al.*; Investigators of the Registry of the Canadian Stroke Network (RCSN); Stroke Outcomes Research Canada (SORCan) Working Group (2012). The iScore predicts effectiveness of thrombolytic therapy for acute ischemic stroke. *Stroke 43*(5):1315–1322.

56 Whiteley WN, Slot KB, Fernandes P, Sandercock P, Wardlaw J (2012). Risk factors for intracranial hemorrhage in acute ischemic stroke patients treated with recombinant tissue plasminogen activator: a systematic review and meta-analysis of 55 studies. *Stroke* **43**(11):2904–2909.

57 Sandercock PAG, Counsell C, Gubitz GJ, *et al.* (2008). Antiplatelet therapy for acute ischaemic stroke. *Cochrane Database Syst Rev* **3**:CD000029. doi: 10.1002/14651858.CD000029.pub2.

58 Sandercock PAG, Counsell C, Kamal AK (2008). Anticoagulants for acute ischaemic stroke. *Cochrane Database Syst Rev* **4**:CD000024. DOI: 10.1002/14651858.CD000024.pub3.

59 Gregson BA, Broderick JP, Auer LM, *et al.* (2012). Individual patient data subgroup meta-analysis of surgery for spontaneous supratentorial intracerebral hemorrhage. *Stroke* **43**(6):1496–1504.

60 Mendelow AD, Gregson BA, Rowan EN, Murray GD, Gholkar A, Mitchell PM; for the STICH II Investigators (2013). Early surgery versus initial conservative treatment in patients with spontaneous supratentorial lobar intracerebral haematomas (STICH II): a randomised trial. *Lancet* May 29. DOI:PII: S0140-6736(13)60986-1. 10.1016/S0140-6736(13)60986-1. [Epub ahead of print] PMID: 23726393.

61 Anderson CS, Heeley E, Huang Y, *et al.*; the INTERACT2 Investigators (2013). Rapid blood-pressure lowering in patients with acute intracerebral hemorrhage. *N Engl J Med.* May 29. [Epub ahead of print] PMID: 23713578.

62 Stroke Unit Trialists' Collaboration (2007). Organised inpatient (stroke unit) care for stroke. *Cochrane Database Syst Rev* **4**:CD000197. doi: 10.1002/14651858.CD000197.pub2

63 The FOOD Trial Collaboration (2005). Routine oral nutritional supplementation for stroke patients in hospital (FOOD): a multicentre randomised controlled trial. *Lancet* **365**: 755–763.

64 The FOOD Trial Collaboration (2005). Effect of timing and method of enteral tube feeding for dysphagic stroke patients (FOOD): a multicentre randomised controlled trial. *Lancet* **365**:764–772.

65 Vahedi K, Hofmeijer J, Juettler E, *et al.*; DECIMAL, DESTINY, and HAMLET investigators (2007). Early decompressive surgery in malignant infarction of the middle cerebral artery: a pooled analysis of three randomised controlled trials. *Lancet Neurol* **6**(3):215–222.

66 Hofmeijer J, Kappelle LJ, Algra A, Amelink GJ, van Gijn J, van der Worp HB; HAMLET investigators (2009). Surgical decompression for space-occupying cerebral infarction (the Hemicraniectomy After Middle Cerebral Artery infarction with Life-threatening Edema Trial [HAMLET]): a multicentre, open, randomised trial. *Lancet Neurol* **8**(4):326–333.

67 CLOTS Trials Collaboration (2009). Effectiveness of thigh-length graduated compression stockings to reduce the risk of deep vein thrombosis after stroke (CLOTS trial 1): a multicentre, randomised controlled trial. *Lancet* **373**:1958–1965.

68 CLOTS (Clots in Legs Or sTockings after Stroke) Trials Collaboration (2013). Effectiveness of intermittent pneumatic compression in reduction of risk of deep vein thrombosis in patients who have had a stroke (CLOTS 3): a multicentre randomised controlled trial. *Lancet* May 30. DOI:PII: S0140-6736(13)61050-8. 10.1016/S0140-6736(13)61050-8. [Epub ahead of print] PMID: 23727163.

69 Rothwell PM, Eliasziw M, Gutnikov SA, *et al.* (2003). Pooled analysis of individual patient data from randomised controlled trials of endarterectomy for symptomatic carotid stenosis. *Lancet* **361**:107–116.

70 Bangalore S, Kumar S, Wetterslev J, *et al.* (2011). Carotid artery stenting vs carotid endarterectomy: meta-analysis and diversity-adjusted trial sequential analysis of randomized trials. *Arch Neurol* **68**(2):172–184.

71 Abbott A (2009). Medical (nonsurgical) intervention alone is now best for prevention of stroke associated with asymptomatic severe carotid stenosis. Results of a systematic review and analysis. *Stroke* **40**:e573–583.

72 Algra A, van Gijn J (1999). Cumulative meta-analysis of aspirin efficacy after cerebral ischaemia of arterial origin. *J Neurol Neurosurg Psychiatry* **66**:255.

73 Sudlow CL, Mason G, Maurice JB, Wedderburn CJ, Hankey GJ (2009). Thienopyridine derivatives versus aspirin for preventing stroke and other serious vascular events in high vascular risk patients. *Cochrane Database Syst Rev* **4**:CD001246.

74 Halkes PH, Gray LJ, Bath PM, *et al.* (2008). Dipyridamole plus aspirin versus aspirin alone in secondary prevention after TIA or stroke: a metaanalysis by risk. *J Neurol Neurosurg Psychiatry* **79**:1218–1223.

75 Hankey GJ, Eikelboom (2010). Antithrombotic drugs for patients with ischaemic stroke and transient ischaemic attack to prevent recurrent major vascular events. *Lancet Neurol* **9**:273–284.

76 Wang Y, Wang Y, Zhao X, *et al.* (2013) Clopidogrel with aspirin in acute minor stroke or transient ischemic attack. *N Engl J Med* DOI: 10.1056/NEJMoa1215340.

77 Paciaroni M, Agnelli G, Micheli S, Caso V (2007). Efficacy and safety of anticoagulant treatment in acute cardioembolic stroke: a meta-analysis of randomized controlled trials. *Stroke* **38**:423–430.

78 Alberts MJ, Eikelboom JW, Hankey GJ (2012). Antithrombotic therapy for stroke prevention in non-valvular atrial fibrillation. *Lancet Neurol* **11**(12):1066–1081.

79 Connolly SJ, Ezekowitz MD, Yusuf S, *et al.*; for the RE-LY Steering Committee and Investigators (2009). Dabigatran versus warfarin in patients with atrial fibrillation. *N Engl J Med* **361**:1139–1151.

80 Patel MR, Mahaff ey KW, Garg J, *et al.*; for the ROCKET AF Investigators (2011). Rivaroxaban versus warfarin in nonvalvular atrial fibrillation. *N Engl J Med* **365**:883–891.

81 Granger CB, Alexander JH, McMurray JJV, *et al.*; for the ARISTOTLE Committees and Investigators (2011). Apixaban versus warfarin in patients with atrial fibrillation. *N Engl J Med* **365**:981–992.

82 Connolly SJ, Eikelboom J, Joyner C, *et al.*; for the AVERROES Steering Committee and Investigators (2011). Apixaban in patients with atrial fibrillation. *N Engl J Med* **364**: 806–817.

83 Furlan AJ, Reisman M, Massaro J, *et al.* (2012). Closure or medical therapy for cryptogenic stroke with patent foramen ovale. *New Engl J Med* **366**(11):991–999.

84 Carroll JD, Saver JL, Thaler DE, *et al.* (2013). Closure of patent foramen ovale versus medical therapy after cryptogenic stroke. *New Engl J Med* **368**(12):1092–1100.

85 Meier B, Kalesan B, Mattle HP, *et al.* (2013). Percutaneous closure of patent foramen ovale in cryptogenic embolism. *New Engl J Med* **368**(12):1083–1091.

86 Law MR, Morris JK, Wald NJ (2009). Use of blood pressure lowering drugs in the prevention of cardiovascular disease: meta-analysis of 147 randomised trials in the context of expectations from prospective epidemiological studies. *BMJ* **338**:b1665.

87 The SPS3 Study Group (2013). Blood-pressure targets in patients with recent lacunar stroke: the SPS3 randomised trial. *Lancet* May 28. DOI:PII: S0140-6736(13)60852-1. 10.1016/S0140-6736(13)60852-1. [Epub ahead of print] PMID: 23726159.

88 Amarenco P, Labreuche J (2009). Lipid management in the prevention of stroke: review and updated meta-analysis of statins for stroke prevention. *Lancet Neurol* **8**:453–463.

89 Hankey GJ (2012). Vitamin supplementation and stroke prevention. *Stroke* **43**:2814–2818.

90 Langhorne P, Bernhardt J, Kwakkel G (2011). Stroke rehabilitation. *Lancet* **377**: 1693–1702.

Further reading

Chimowitz MI, Lynn MJ, Derdeyn CP, *et al.*; SAMMPRIS Trial Investigators (2011). Stenting versus aggressive medical therapy for intracranial arterial stenosis. *N Engl J Med* **365**(11):993–1003.

Kipps CM, Hodges JR (2005). Cognitive assessment for clinicians. *J Neurol Neurosurg Psychiatry* **76**(Suppl 1):i22–i30.

Kleinloog R, Regli L, Rinkel GJ, Klijn CJ (2012). Regional differences in incidence and patient characteristics of moyamoya disease: a systematic review. *J Neurol Neurosurg Psychiatry* **83**(5):531–536.

Lozano R, Naghavi M, Foreman K, *et al.* (2012). Global and regional mortality from 235 causes of death for 20 age groups in 1990 and 2010: a systematic analysis for the Global Burden of Disease Study 2010. *Lancet* **380**:2095–2128.

Morgenstern LB, Hemphill JC 3rd, Anderson C, *et al.*; American Heart Association Stroke Council and Council on Cardiovascular Nursing (2010). Guidelines for the management of spontaneous intracerebral hemorrhage: a guideline for healthcare professionals from the American Heart Association/American Stroke Association. *Stroke* **41**(9):2108–2129.

Munot P, Crow YJ, Ganesan V (2011). Paediatric stroke: genetic insights into disease mechanisms and treatment targets. *Lancet Neurol* **10**:264–274.

Murray CJ, Vos T, Lozano R, *et al.* (2012). Disability-adjusted life years (DALYs) for 291 diseases and injuries in 21 regions, 1990–2010: a systematic analysis for the Global Burden of Disease Study 2010. *Lancet* **380**:2197–223. (Erratum in: *Lancet* 2013;**381**:628.)

Rothwell PM, Giles M, Chandrathevea A, *et al.* (2007). Effect of urgent treatment of TIA and minor stroke on early recurrent stroke (EXRESS study): a prospective population-based sequential comparison. *Lancet* **370**:1432–1442.

Sacco RL, Kasner SE, Broderick JP, *et al*; on behalf of the American Heart Association Stroke Council, Council on Cardiovascular Surgery and Anesthesia, Council on Cardiovascular Radiology and Intervention, Council on Cardiovascular and Stroke Nursing, Council on Epidemiology and Prevention, Counc (2013). An updated definition of stroke for the 21st century: A statement for healthcare professionals from the American Heart Association/American Stroke Association. *Stroke*. May 7. [Epub ahead of print] PMID: 23652265.

Sandset EC, Bath PM, Boysen G, *et al.*; SCAST Study Group (2011). The angiotensin-receptor blocker candesartan for treatment of acute stroke (SCAST): a randomised, placebo-controlled, double-blind trial. *Lancet* **377**(9767):741–750.

Saposnik G, Lanthier S, Mamdani M, *et al.*; Canadian Stroke Consortium; Stroke Outcome Research Canada (SORCan) Working Group (2012). Fabry's disease: a prospective multicenter cohort study in young adults with cryptogenic stroke. *Int J Stroke* **7**(3):265–273.

Shi Q, Presutti R, Selchen D, Saposnik G (2012). Delirium in acute stroke: a systematic review and meta-analysis. *Stroke* **43**(3):645–649.

van Beijnum J, van der Worp HB, Buis DR, *et al.* (2011). Treatment of brain arteriovenous malformations: a systematic review and meta-analysis. *JAMA* **306**(18):2011–2019.

INFECTIONS OF THE CENTRAL NERVOUS SYSTEM

Jeremy D. Young, James L. Cook

ACUTE BACTERIAL MENINGITIS

Definition

Bacterial meningitis causes acute inflammation of the leptomeninges, with an onset of signs and symptoms over the course of hours to days. The median duration of symptoms at the time of clinical presentation is only 24 hours, and tends to not be greater than 2 weeks.

Epidemiology

Worldwide, approximately 1.2 million cases of acute bacterial meningitis occur each year, resulting in 135,000 deaths. Overall, there has been a decrease in the incidence of bacterial meningitis in the USA from 1.9 to 1.5 cases per 100,000 between 1998 and 2003, in part due to the advent of the heptavalent pneumococcal conjugate vaccine (PCV7) in 2000 for use in infants. Of note, the USA Food and Drug Administration (FDA) approved a new 13-valent pneumococcal vaccine in February, 2010, to replace PCV7 in the childhood immunization schedule. Among infants in the first month of life, the incidence of bacterial meningitis is approximately 0.25 per 1000 live births.

The history and epidemiology of the patient is a vital component in predicting the pathogen, and therefore in choosing the appropriate empiric antimicrobial therapy (*Table 85*). The most common etiology of community-associated bacterial meningitis in the USA overall remains *Streptococcus pneumoniae*, which is responsible for approximately 50% of all cases and a larger proportion

TABLE 85 **EPIDEMIOLOGIC FACTORS ASSOCIATED WITH SPECIFIC PATHOGENS IN ACUTE BACTERIAL MENINGITIS**

Pathogen	Epidemiologic factors
Streptococcus pneumoniae	Underlying pneumonia, otitis media, sinusitis, mastoiditis, basilar skull fracture, endocarditis, immunoglobulin deficiency (e.g. congenital), multiple myeloma, asplenia, alcoholism, malnutrition, chronic renal or liver disease
Neisseria meningitidis	Children and young adults age 2–18 years, late complement deficiencies, crowded living conditions (college dormitories, military bases)
Listeria monocytogenes	Age ≥60 years or neonates, immunosuppression (e.g. organ transplantation, cytotoxic drugs, corticosteroids) particularly deficiencies in cell-mediated immunity, chronic renal or liver disease, diabetes mellitus, consumption of unpasteurized or raw foods
Streptococcus agalactiae (group B streptococcus)	Neonates
Gram-negative bacilli	Post-neurosurgical, head trauma, enterics associated with invasive strongyloidiasis, *Escherichia coli* in neonatal meningitis
Staphylococcus aureus	Post-neurosurgical, head trauma
Haemophilus influenzae	Pneumonia, sinusitis, otitis media, epiglottitis, alcoholism, diabetes mellitus, asplenia, hypogammaglobulinemia, head trauma with CSF leak

with increasing age. Other common pathogens in adults include *Neisseria meningitidis* (35–40%), *Listeria monocytogenes* (5%), *Haemophilus influenzae*, *Staphylococcus aureus*, and enteric Gram-negative bacilli.

The proportion of *L. monocytogenes* increases with age and in those with defects in cell-mediated immunity, and it causes about 20% of acute bacterial meningitis in those older than 60 years. It is acquired by eating foods contaminated with this ubiquitous organism, including meats (e.g. packaged meats, hot dogs), unpasteurized milk and cheese, and raw vegetables. This makes taking a dietary history an important component in the work-up, as well as eliciting symptoms of concomitant gastroenteritis.

The institution of routine childhood immunization with conjugate *H. influenzae* type b vaccine (Hib) in 1990 has almost eliminated childhood bacterial meningitis caused by this organism, and shifted the epidemiology of infection from childhood to adults. The median age of *H. influenzae* bacterial meningitis in the USA is now 39 years[1]. *H. influenzae* was previously the cause of about 45% of all cases of bacterial meningitis in the USA, but is now isolated only 7% of the time[2].

N. meningitidis of serogroups B, C, and Y accounts for most invasive meningococcal disease in the USA. Patients with terminal complement deficiencies (C5, C6, C7, C8, and C9) have a notably increased risk of invasive infection with meningococcus.

Health-care-associated acute bacterial meningitis primarily occurs after neurosurgical interventions. The pathogens shift in post-neurosurgical infections towards methicillin-resistant *S. aureus* (MRSA), coagulase-negative staphylococci, *Propionibacterium acnes*, and Gram-negative bacilli, including Enterobacteriaeceae and *Pseudomonas aeruginosa*.

Bacterial meningitis complicates up to 1.5% of neurosurgical procedures[3].

Etiology and pathophysiology

Most bacterial pathogens implicated in community-associated meningitis begin with nasopharyngeal colonization of the host. Bacterial pili are involved in adherence of certain organisms to the nasopharyngeal epithelial cells, such as with *N. meningitis* and *H. influenzae*. Several specific virulence factors, along with host factors, can lead to local invasion, bacteremia, meningeal invasion, and subsequent replication of organisms in the subarachoid space. The host immune response causes inflammation, with a neutrophil and cytokine response.

The other mechanisms of central nervous system (CNS) infection include direct inoculation from a contiguous focus following head trauma, neurosurgical procedures, or head and neck space infections, and hematogenous spread during an episode of bacteremia.

Acute inflammation of the leptomeninges with purulent exudates is seen grossly (**423**) and on microscopic examination of tissue specimens (**424**).

423 Base of the brain of a patient who died from acute pyogenic meningitis showing purulent meningeal exudate. *Courtesy of Professor BA Kakulas, Royal Perth Hospital, Western Australia.*

424 Histologic section of the meninges and cerebral cortex of a patient who died of acute pyogenic meningitis, showing neutrophilic infiltration of the subarachnoid space, pia, arachnoid, and Virchow–Robin spaces of the outer part of the brain. Bacteria are numerous, lying free in the subarachnoid space and inside neutrophilic leukocytes (phagocytosis).

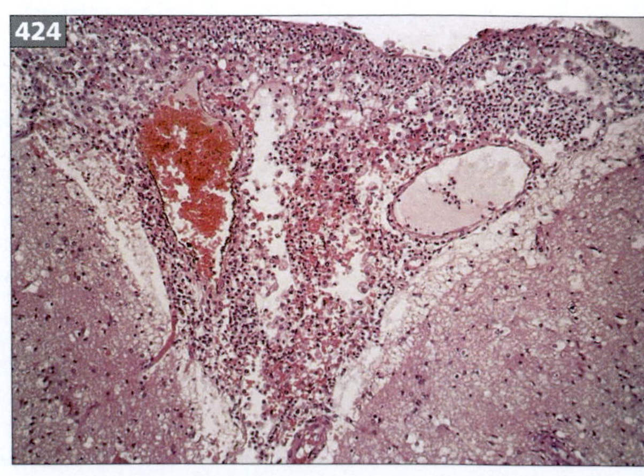

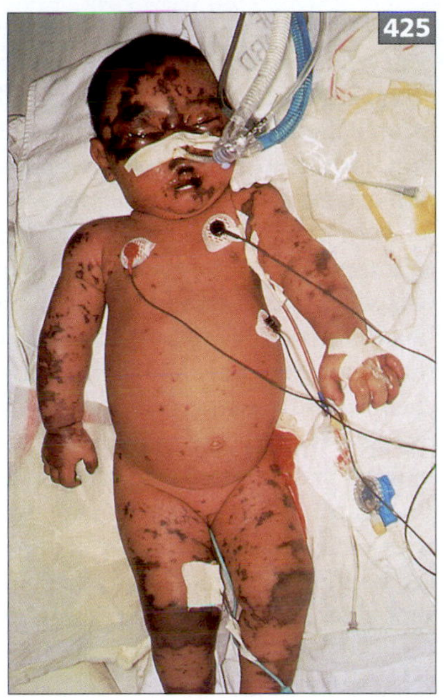

425, 426 **Purpuric skin rash. Rash in an unconscious child (425) and adult (426) with meningococcal meningitis and septicemia.** *Courtesy of Dr AM Chancellor, Tauranga, New Zealand.*

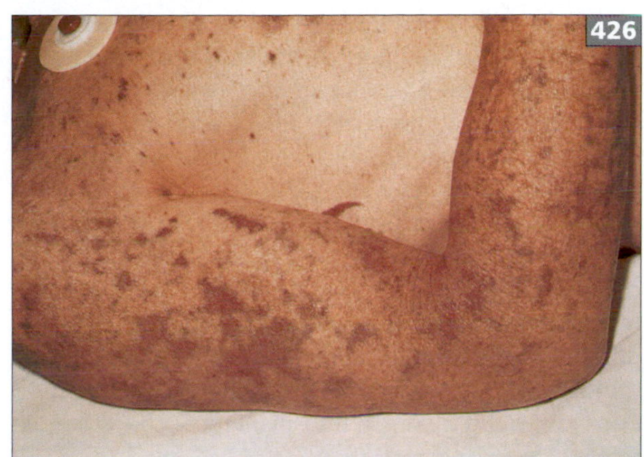

Clinical features

The classic signs and symptoms of acute bacterial meningitis are fever, nuchal rigidity, altered mental status, and headache. Fever is present in 95% of patients at the time of presentation. Hypothermia is an alarming sign. Only 40–50% of patients present with all of the classic signs, but 95% display at least two and almost all have at least one[4].

Confusion, lethargy, or even obtundation are common, making it difficult to distinguish between meningitis and the cerebral dysfunction se en with encephalitis. Other common findings include photophobia, nausea, and vomiting. Seizures, signs of increased intracranial pressure (ICP), such as papilledema, focal deficits, and ataxia may be prominent, particularly if meningitis is complicated by brain abscess. Other signs include cranial nerve palsies and sensorineural deafness, particularly later in the course of disease.

Brudzinski's sign can also be seen, with spontaneous hip flexion during the same chin-to-chest maneuver. Assessing for Kernig's sign involves attempted extension of the knee when the hip is flexed to 90°, revealing reluctance on the part of the patient to extend the knee. These examination findings are insensitive, but are specific.

Listeria spp. have a predilection to cause cerebritis and form brain abscesses. Therefore, delirium, confusion, and focal deficits are common early in the course of disease. Indeed, brain abscess accounts for approximately 10% of CNS listerial infections overall. Another form of CNS listeriosis is rhombencephalitis (encephalitis of the brainstem), which causes cerebellar signs in addition to the classic presentation of bacterial meningoencephalitis.

Meningococcal meningitis can cause petechiae and palpable purpura, or a maculopapular rash (**425, 426**). While the presence of rash is nonspecific, it occurs in 10–60% of patients with invasive *N. meningitidis* infection[4–6].

Differential diagnosis

- Brain abscess.
- Early 'aseptic' meningitis caused by a virus, toxins, or medication.
- Tuberculous meningitis.
- Fungal meningitis.
- Rocky Mountain spotted fever (RMSF).
- Lyme meningitis.
- Neurosyphilis.
- Eosinophilic meningitis.
- Parameningeal (e.g. epidural) abscess.
- Subarachnoid hemorrhage.

Investigations

Physical examination for meningismus can be performed in several ways. Nuchal rigidity can usually be elicited with a simple chin-to-chest maneuver, with the patient displaying resistance to passive flexion of the neck.

Obtaining a detailed travel history is important, since outbreaks of *N. meningitidis* occur worldwide at much higher rates than in the USA, endemic mycoses may be in the differential (e.g. *Coccidiodes immitis* in patients traveling to the southwestern USA), and certain pathogens (e.g. arboviruses, rickettsiae) can be suspected based upon geography and season. It is also important to obtain a detailed history of recent sick contacts, risk of exposure to tuberculosis (TB), recent symptoms of other infections (e.g. pneumonia, sinusitis, otitis media), recent antibiotic use, drug allergies, neurosurgical procedures or head trauma, and the presence of an underlying immunocompromised state (e.g. human immunodeficiency virus [HIV], organ transplantation, corticosteroid therapy).

Lumbar puncture (LP) should be performed in all patients, if feasible, and cerebrospinal fluid (CSF) sent for cell count and differential, protein, glucose, Gram stain and culture. An opening pressure (OP) should be measured and documented. Consideration should be given in certain patients to acid-fast stain and culture, TB polymerase chain reaction (PCR), fungal stains and cultures, cryptococcal antigen, venereal disease research laboratory (VDRL) testing, viral PCR assays for herpesviruses and arboviruses, and cytology.

Brain imaging with computed tomography (CT) should be done prior to LP in patients with a risk of increased ICP or mass lesions, which may be suspected in immunocompromised patients (e.g. HIV infection, hematologic malignancy, cytotoxic chemotherapy), those with focal neurologic deficits, papilledema on physical examination, a seizure in the previous week, or obtundation. However, imaging studies should not delay initiation of empiric antibiotic therapy.

Two sets of blood cultures should be sent, ideally prior to antibiotic therapy, which reveal a pathogen in 50–90% of cases[4,7]. Blood should be drawn and sent for complete blood count (CBC) to assess for leukocytosis, leukopenia, thrombocytopenia, and 'left-shift' in the differential, chemistries to assess renal function and for the presence of acidosis or hyponatremia, and coagulation studies to look for disseminated intravascular coagulation (DIC).

A screening test for terminal complement deficiency with CH_{50} should be performed in all patients presenting with invasive meningococcal infection. HIV testing should be done if the patient's status is unknown.

Diagnosis

LP reveals CSF with >5 white blood cells/µl (usually >1000 cells/µl) with a neutrophil predominance, high protein (100–500 mg/dl [1–5 g/l]) and low glucose (CSF-to-serum glucose ratio <0.4). The sensitivity of Gram stain alone is 60–90% with a specificity of 97–100%[4]. The Gram stain is positive in 10–15% of patients who have a negative culture and can suggest a pathogen within minutes of performing the LP (*Table 86*).

In the case of a 'traumatic,' bloody tap, the true white blood cell (WBC) count in the CSF can be calculated as:

$$\text{true WBC in CSF} = \text{measured WBC in CSF} - \left[\frac{(\text{WBC in blood} = \text{RBC in CSF})}{\text{RBC in blood}}\right]$$

TABLE 86 **SUSPECTED PATHOGENS IN ACUTE BACTERIAL MENINGITIS BY FINDINGS ON GRAM STAIN**

Gram stain	Suspected pathogens
Gram-positive diplococci	*Streptococcus pneumoniae*
Gram-negative diplococci	*Neisseria meningitidis*
Gram-positive bacilli	*Listeria monocytogenes*, *Propionibacterium acnes*
Gram-negative bacilli	*Haemophilus influenzae*, Enterobacteriaceae, *Pseudomonas aeruginosa*, *Acinetobacter baumannii*
Gram-positive cocci in clusters	Staphylococci
Gram-positive cocci in chains	Streptococci, enterococci

However, for a useful approximation, one may also just subtract one WBC for every 750 red blood cells (RBC) in the CSF analysis. PCR tests are available to look for the deoxyribonucleic acid (DNA) of common bacterial pathogens, and appear to have excellent sensitivity and specificity, but false-positives have been reported and there are not enough clinical data to recommend routine PCR testing.

Treatment

Acute bacterial meningitis is a medical emergency. If a CT scan must be performed prior to LP, it should not delay the first dose of appropriate empiric antibiotic therapy, since delayed treatment is associated with a greater risk of morbidity and mortality[8–10]. If LP is deferred temporarily while obtaining an imaging study, blood cultures should be drawn immediately and administration of the first dose of antibiotic and dexamethasone should be given prior to sending the patient for brain imaging.

Tip

▶ *Always be aggressive with antibiotic dosing in acute bacterial meningitis, particularly with cephalosporins. Administer a loading dose of vancomycin and calculate the maintenance dose based upon the patient's weight. The target vancomycin trough is 15–20 μg/ml.*

Important factors in choosing empiric therapy include: appropriate spectrum to cover the most likely pathogens; clinician knowledge of institutional antibiograms and local susceptibility patterns; use of bactericidal therapy; and administration of antibiotics that penetrate the blood–brain barrier. Empiric antibiotic therapy for *community-associated* acute bacterial meningitis in adults should include:

- Ceftriaxone (2 g IV every 12 hours) has good blood–brain barrier penetration and is bactericidal against susceptible pneumococci, meningococci, *H. influenzae*, and group B streptococci (GBS). It does not have activity against *Listeria* spp. Cefotaxime is also an excellent option. Either cefepime or ceftazidime should be the cephalosporin of choice if there is a risk of *Pseudomonas* spp. infection.

Plus:

- Vancomycin (load 25 mg/kg IV once, then at least 15 mg/kg IV every 12 hours, adjusted for renal dysfunction) should be included in the empiric regimen until culture and susceptibility results return due to the rise in β-lactam-resistant *S. pneumoniae*. If there is an indication to continue therapy, a trough should be measured prior to the third or fourth dose, with the goal of 15–20 μg/ml.

Plus:

- Dexamethasone (0.15 mg/kg IV every 6 hours) given before or with the first dose of antibiotic. Adjunctive dexamethasone reduces mortality and the risk of unfavorable outcome, particularly in patients with pneumococcal meningitis. In patients with proven *S. pneumoniae*, dexamethasone should be continued for the first 4 days of antibiotic therapy. Adjunctive corticosteroids are not recommended in neonatal meningitis.

Plus:

For patients who are immunocompromised or >50 years old, include:

- Ampicillin (2 g IV every 4 hours) to provide coverage for *Listeria* spp. If the patient has a severe β-lactam allergy, a reliable and efficacious alternative is trimethoprim–sulfamethoxazole (TMP-SMX, 5 mg/kg of the trimethoprim component IV every 6–8 hours). For proven *Listeria* meningitis, gentamicin (1.7 mg/kg IV every 8 hours) should be added to ampicillin for synergy.

Empiric antibiotic therapy for *post-neurosurgical* acute bacterial meningitis should include:

- Cefepime (2 g IV every 8 hours) OR ceftazidime (2 g IV every 8 hours) OR meropenem (2 g IV every 8 hours).

Plus:

- Vancomycin (load 25 mg/kg IV once, then at least 15 mg/kg IV every 12 hours, adjusted for renal dysfunction) to provide coverage for MRSA. If there is an indication to continue therapy, a trough should be measured prior to the third or fourth dose, with the goal of 15 to 20 μg/ml.

In neonatal meningitis, the most common pathogen is GBS. Empiric therapy generally consists of ampicillin plus gentamicin, which also treats *Listeria* spp; however, enteric Gram-negatives such as *Escherichia coli* are frequently resistant to ampicillin. Many experts include cefotaxime in the initial empiric regimen, particularly if the onset of meningitis occurs after the first week of life. Vancomycin is often added if a hospital-acquired infection (e.g. MRSA) is suspected.

Once a pathogen is identified on Gram stain, antibiotics can be tapered to focus on the likely etiology and further modified using culture and susceptibility data. A total of 14–21 days of therapy should be completed, depending upon the pathogen, and infectious diseases consultation is recommended.

Patients may also require a decrease in the ICP if the OP is >20 cmH_2O. This can require repeated LP, elevating the head of the bed to 30°, hyperventilation to maintain PaCO2 between 27 and 30 mmHg, and/or hyperosmolar agents such as mannitol and glycerin. Supportive care should be provided with antipyretics, aggressive intravenous fluid management, maintaining a patent airway, and antiepileptics if seizures occur.

Prognosis

Risk factors for death include: age >60 years old, hypotension, altered mental status, leukopenia, thrombocytopenia, or seizures within the first 24 hours. Case fatality rates can be as high as 15–25% per episode despite antibiotic therapy, with a similar proportion of survivors experiencing permanent neurologic sequelae, depending upon the pathogen and the timing of antibiotic therapy. Hearing loss is an important late complication, particularly with *S. pneumoniae* meningitis. Other neurologic sequelae include seizures, focal neurologic deficits, and cerebrovascular abnormalities.

BRAIN ABSCESS

Definition and epidemiology

Brain abscess represents a focal area of intracerebral infection. In the early stages, a localized cerebritis is seen; however, within 2–3 weeks, an abscess can organize, which is characterized by a collection of pus surrounded by a vascularized capsule.

Risk factors include head and neck infections, trauma, neurosurgery, immunocompromise, and bacteremia from any source. It is not a reportable infectious disease, so the incidence is difficult to quantify. An estimated 1500–2500 cases are diagnosed each year in the USA[11]. Brain abscess is twice as common in men as women, and there is no difference in racial distribution.

Etiology and pathophysiology

The microbiology of bacterial brain abscesses, while often mixed, is fairly predictable based upon the likely source of infection. Solitary brain abscess, which occurs in 20–60% of cases[12], is generally a complication of head and neck infections, including otitis media, mastoiditis, sinusitis, or dental abscesses.

Aerobic, anaerobic, and microaerophilic streptococci comprising the oropharyngeal microbiota have been isolated most commonly (70% of infections)[13]. These organisms are not only in anatomic proximity to the CNS, but have a predilection for abscess formation. Solitary abscesses are often polymicrobial, involving Gram-negative anaerobes (e.g. *Prevotella*, *Bacteroides* spp.), enteric Gram-negative bacilli (e.g. *E. coli*, *Klebsiella*, *Enterobacter* spp.), and mixed Gram-positives.

When brain abscess follows neurosurgical procedures, the clinician must consider direct inoculation of MRSA and *Pseudomonas aeruginosa*. Post-neurosurgical brain abscesses are more often monomicrobial infections. Compromise of the immune system from HIV infection, transplantation, or malignancy and chemotherapy expand the differential diagnosis to fungi (*Aspergillus* spp., mucormycosis, *Cryptococcus* spp., *Nocardia* spp.), and *Toxoplasma gondii*. Depending upon the epidemiologic setting, other protozoa, helminths, and mycobacteria must be kept in mind.

Despite the fact that *Streptococcus pneumoniae*, *Neisseria meningitidis*, *Haemophilus influenzae*, and *Listeria monocytogenes* are common pathogens seen in bacterial meningitis, they are uncommon causes of brain abscess. However, about 10% of CNS infections with *L. monocytogenes* present with brain abscess.

Multiple abscesses in the watershed vascular areas of the brain are more typically the result of septic emboli from hematogenous spread. Bacteremia from any cause may lead to brain abscess, but the most common underlying factors are endocarditis, lung abscess, empyema, and intra-abdominal infections. Congenital heart disease is a particularly prevalent predisposing factor in children. With hematogenous spread, the most common vascular site involved is the middle cerebral artery (MCA)[14].

Brain abscess is cryptogenic, with no identified source, in about 20–40% of patients[15,16].

Clinical features

Most of the presenting clinical features of brain abscess result from the space-occupying lesion itself, and the specific signs and symptoms are a manifestation of the size and location of the abscess as well as the virulence of the pathogen(s) involved. The most common symptom is headache, occurring in approximately 70% of patients. The classic triad of fever, headache, and focal neurologic deficits occurs in less than 50% of patients at presentation[17]. Papilledema may be seen if there is increased ICP.

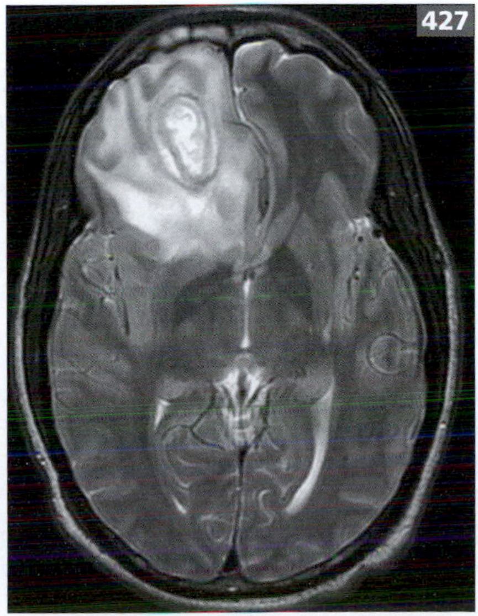

427 **T2-weighted MRI image of the brain, showing bright, vasogenic edema surrounding the pyogenic abscess in the right frontal lobe. The abscess wall is relatively darker than the contents or surrounding edema.** *Courtesy of Dr. Edward Michals, University of Illinois at Chicago.*

Differential diagnosis

- Fungal abscess (e.g. cryptococcoma, *Coccidiodes immitis*, *Aspergillus* spp.).
- Tuberculoma.
- Neurocysticercosis.
- *Paragonimus*.
- *Angiostrongylus* or *Gnathostoma*.
- Toxocariasis.
- Echinococcosis.
- Neurosyphilis with gumma formation.
- Malignancy.

Investigations

Brain imaging is a vital part of the work-up of brain abscess. CT should be performed with contrast, and may reveal early cerebritis or well-circumscribed enhancing lesions with surrounding, ring-enhancing edema and a hypodense center. CT scanning can also help visualize the sinuses, mastoids, and middle ear. Magnetic resonance imaging (MRI) with gadolinium is more sensitive, with improved resolution of small abscesses, and is the best imaging method for brain abscess (**427**). On T1-weighted images, there is enhancement of the abscess capsule and surrounding edema. Diffusion-weighted MRI imaging may help differentiate abscess from malignancy. Multiple brain abscesses from hematogenous spread may be seen at the junction of gray and white matter and localize to any lobe of the brain (frontal, temporal, parietal, occipital) or the cerebellum.

LP is contraindicated if there are focal neurologic signs or evidence of mass effect on imaging. If performed, CSF should be submitted for cell count and differential, protein, glucose, Gram stain, aerobic and anaerobic cultures, mycobacterial smears and cultures, fungal stains and cultures, VDRL, and cytology. Also consider CSF cryptococcal antigen, *Toxoplasma* PCR, and Epstein–Barr virus (EBV) PCR (for CNS lymphoma) in immunocompromised patients, particularly those with HIV/aquired immunodeficiency syndrome (AIDS).

Aspiration of abscess material with stereotactic brain biopsy is often necessary to define the pathogen and for optimal therapy. Abscess material should be sent for Gram stain, aerobic and anaerobic cultures, mycobacterial smears and cultures, fungal stains and cultures, modified acid-fast stain for *Nocardia*, and cytology. Serum anti-*Toxoplasma* immunoglobulin (Ig) G may be helpful in immunocompromised patients to risk-stratify for reactivation CNS infection (see section on toxoplasmosis).

TABLE 87 **APPROPRIATE EMPIRIC ANTIBIOTIC CHOICES BASED UPON RISK FACTORS FOR BRAIN ABSCESS**

Risk factors	Empiric therapy
Head and neck infections such as sinusitis, mastoiditis, otitis media, and dental abscess[a]	Ceftriaxone (2 g IV q12hr) *or* Cefotaxime (2 g IV q4–6hr) *plus* Metronidazole (500 mg IV q6hr)
Penetrating head trauma	Vancomycin[b–d] (25 mg/kg IV load, followed by 15 mg/kg IV q12hr) *plus* Ceftriaxone (2 g IV q12hr)
Post-neurosurgical	Vancomycin[b–d] (25 mg/kg IV load, followed by 15 mg/kg IV q12hr) *plus* Ceftazidime (2 g IV q8hr) *or* Cefepime (2 g IVq8hr)
Infective endocarditis	Vancomycin[b–d] (25 mg/kg IV load, followed by 15 mg/kg IV q12hr) *plus* Ceftriaxone (2 g IV q12hr)
Unknown source	Vancomycin[b–d] (25 mg/kg IV load, followed by 15 mg/kg IV q12hr) *plus* Ceftriaxone (2 g IV q12hr) *plus* Metronidazole (500 mg IV q6hr)

[a] There has been increasing resistance to penicillin G among Gram-negative anaerobes in the oral microbiota (e.g. *Bacteroides fragilis* and *Prevotella*); therefore, it is no longer a good empiric choice.
[b] Change to nafcillin (2 g IV every 4 hours or 12 g over 24 hours continuous infusion) if methicillin-sensitive *Staphylococcus aureus*, due to superior activity.
[c] Adjust for renal dysfunction.
[d] Monitor serum trough concentration, with a goal of 15–20 μg/ml.

Avoid clindamycin, first generation cephalosporins, macrolides and tetracyclines, since they do not achieve adequate concentrations in the CSF.

Diagnosis

A detailed history and physical examination is important to elucidate potential sources of infection and should focus on head and neck space infections, trauma, recent neurosurgery, endocarditis, pneumonia, intra-abdominal infections, and other potential causes of bacteremia.

Brain imaging using CT scan or MRI with contrast findings is consistent with brain abscess. LP will typically show neutrophilic pleocytosis, high protein, and low glucose. Gram stain, aerobic and anaerobic cultures, mycobacterial smears and cultures, and fungal stains and cultures may prove helpful to identify the offending pathogen.

Stereotactic aspiration of abscess material is often enlightening diagnostically and therapeutically beneficial.

Pathology

Histologic findings depend upon whether the infection is acute or chronic. Early, the abscess is poorly demarcated with acute inflammation and edema, reflecting cerebritis. However, liquefaction occurs over the first 2–3 weeks, followed by organization inside a fibrotic capsule.

Gram stains, acid-fast, and modified acid-fast smears, fungal staining, and cultures often reveal a pathogen when abscess material is sent to the microbiology laboratory.

Tips

- *The predictive value for toxoplasmic encephalitis is approximately 85% in a patient with HIV/AIDS and a CD4 count of <100 cells/µl, detection of anti-Toxoplasma IgG antibodies, absence of prophylaxis, and the presence of multiple, ring-enhancing brain lesions on CT or MRI.*
- *It is appropriate, therefore, to presumptively treat a patient presenting with this clinical syndrome for toxoplasmic encephalitis. Brain biopsy should generally be deferred unless the patient does not respond clinically and radiographically to empiric therapy.*

Treatment

Adequate, curative therapy often involves a combination of surgical drainage and antibiotic therapy. Early neurosurgical consultation is encouraged. Stereotactic aspiration or open resection is often necessary for diagnosis and also may be therapeutic. All lesions >2.5 cm (1 in) in diameter should be drained or excised, since there is a higher risk of failure with antibiotic therapy alone. Stereotactic needle aspiration through a burr hole is safer and therefore may be the prudent choice over open surgical excision[18]. If the lesion is <2.5 cm (1 in), medical therapy alone has a greater chance of success[19], and aspiration of the largest lesion can be performed for diagnostic purposes with a focus on antibiotic therapy.

Empiric antibiotic therapy is always necessary, even if a prompt drainage is performed (*Table 87*). Therapy should be directed towards likely pathogens, with a preference given to antimicrobials which cross the blood–brain barrier adequately. Antibiotic therapy should always be tailored based upon stain, culture, and susceptibility testing results.

The duration of therapy recommended is usually 6–8 weeks. However, antibiotics should be continued until there has been adequate clinical improvement and resolution of abscess on CT or MRI. Residual radiographic signs of inflammation may persist for several months, and this is not a reason to continue therapy. Dexamethaxone (10 mg IV every 6 hours) may be considered as adjunctive therapy, if a substantial mass effect is present due to surrounding edema[20].

NEUROSYPHILIS

Definition

Syphilis is a multi-system illness with protean clinical manifestations. Infection of the CNS with the spirochete *Treponema pallidum* leads to neurosyphilis. Like other spirochete syndromes, syphilis is divided into discrete clinical stages with characteristic manifestations; however, neurosyphilis can occur during any phase of illness.

Epidemiology

Syphilis is usually transmitted by sexual interactions, but also can be transmitted by contacts with other active skin or mucous membrane lesions or by transplancental (congenital) infection or transfusion.

There was a decline in reported syphilis cases in the USA during the 1990s. However, the annual incidence of syphilis began increasing in the year 2001 and reached 7.6 cases per 100,000 in men and 1.5 cases per 100,000 in women by 2008[21]. It is more prevalent in the southeastern USA, urban areas, and among men who have sex with men (MSM). The MSM population now accounts for approximately 63% of primary and secondary syphilis in the USA[22]. Neurosyphilis, and especially early neurosyphilis, is most common among those immunosuppressed by infection with HIV. The incidence of late neurosyphilis has declined in the antibiotic era due to the ease of treating early and late latent syphilis with penicillin[23].

Etiology and pathophysiology

Syphilis is caused by the spirochete *T. pallidum* subspecies *pallidum*. The organisms are unicellular, coiled, corkscrew-shaped bacteria.

After direct contact with abraded skin or an intact mucous membrane, spirochetes enter the local lymphatics and bloodstream, disseminating to multiple organ systems. After approximately 3 weeks, a primary chancre develops, which contains many spirochetes. Invasion of the CNS can occur quickly after acquisition of *T. pallidum*, and evidence of neurosyphilis can be found in approximately 25% of patients with untreated early syphilis[24].

Clinical features

Like diseases caused by other spirochetes, infection with *T. pallidum* can be divided into active phases, separated by periods of latency. The clinician should consider whether the patient has early (first year) or late (after 1 year) syphilis. However, neurologic manifestations can occur during any stage of infection and should always be treated with intravenous (IV) penicillin.

Incubating

Mean incubation period, prior to signs and symptoms, is approximately 3 weeks, with a range of 3–90 days.

Primary

The patient develops a painless papule at the site of inoculation, which develops into a chancre with a smooth base and raised, firm borders. A chancre does not develop in every case, and may go unnoticed due to its painless nature. Inguinal lymphadenopathy is often present. The chancre will typically heal spontaneously in 2–8 weeks, followed by a period of clinical latency.

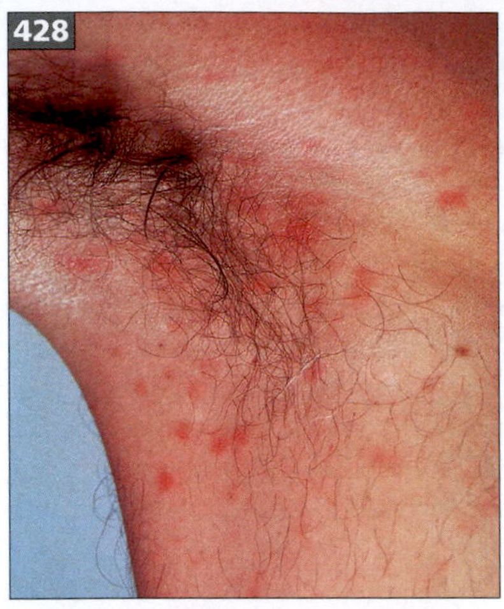

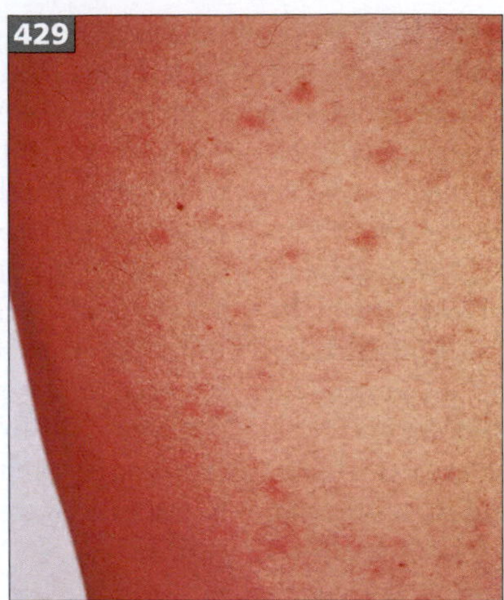

428, 429 Skin rash on the axilla and trunk of a patient in the initial stages of secondary syphilis. The lesions are bilaterally symmetric, pale red/pink, nonpruritic, discrete, round macules, about 5–10 mm (0.2–0.4 in) in diameter, distributed on the trunk and proximal extremities. After 1–2 months, red, papular lesions 3–10 mm (0.1–0.4 in) in diameter also appear on the palms, soles, face, and scalp.

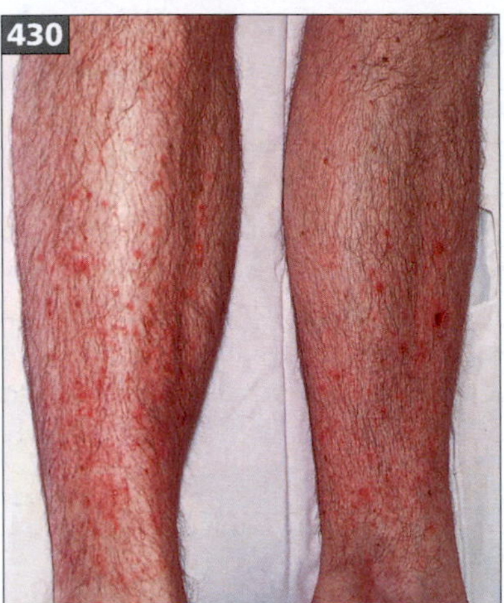

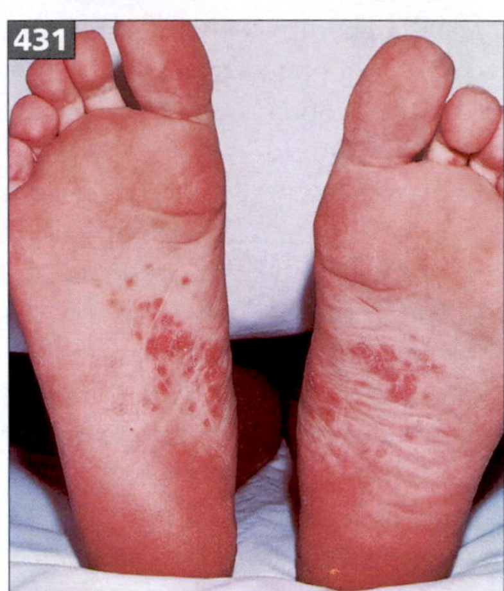

430, 431 Skin rash on the legs and foot soles of a patient in the later stages of secondary syphilis. The lesions are red/copper-colored, papular and papulosquamous, about 3–10 mm (0.1–0.4 in) in diameter and were also present on the palms, face, and scalp.

Secondary

Disseminated infection develops 6–12 weeks after inoculation, although it can occur earlier, with the primary chancre still present[25]. This stage is characterized by a diffuse rash consisting of nonpruritic macules, papules, or pustules, often involving the palms and soles (**428–431**), and mucocutaneous lesions. Patchy alopecia is a frequent finding.

Tip

▶ *The mucocutaneous lesions of primary and secondary syphilis contain many spirochetes and are potentially infectious. Always wear gloves and observe standard precautions when examining a patient who may have mucocutaneous findings of syphilis.*

Because of spirochetemia and dissemination, the CNS becomes involved in up to 40% of patients with secondary syphilis[24,25]. Symptoms of meningitis, such as headache, nuchal rigidity, and photophobia, are common. If an LP is performed, an elevated protein (100–200 mg/dl [1–2 g/l]) and lymphocytic pleocytosis (200–400 cells/µl) are the norm[26]. Oligoclonal bands are frequently present. Other signs and symptoms include cranial neuropathies, visual disturbances, hearing loss, tinnitus, syphilitic paraplegia (Erb's paralysis), and myelitis with lower motor neuron manifestations. Signs of encephalitis are rarely present. Meningeal inflamation can be either diffuse (leptomeningitis) or can present as more focal inflammatory areas called syphilitic gummas. In some cases, early meningovascular disease can result in ischemia, infarction, or seizures.

Latency follows infection in untreated patients, during which time the patient is asymptomatic and can only be diagnosed with serologic testing for syphilis. When possible, based upon known timing of initial infection, the differentiation between early latent (<12 months after infection) and late latent (>12 months after infection) disease can be useful for treatment decisions. When the timing of initial infection is unknown (often the case), the patient is 13–35 years old, and the nontreponemal serology titer is >32, the patient is classified as having latent syphilis of unknown duration.

Tertiary (late)

8–10% of untreated patients will progress to late neurosyphilis, a chronic, slowly progressive inflammatory disease. Late neurosyphilis is divided into parenchymatous and meningovascular, but overlap occurs betweeen these categories. Parenchymal infection may manifest as general paresis and/or tabes dorsalis. Meningovascular syphilis presents as ischemia with focal neurological deficits.

General paresis usually develops 10–25 years after the initial infection, but can occur as early as 2 years. In the pre-penicillin era, this accounted for approximately 10% of all inpatient psychiatric admissions. It may manifest as deficits in memory with progressive dementia, personality change, impaired judgment, depression, mania, or even frank psychosis with delusions and hallucinations.

Tabes dorsalis occurs due to *T. pallidum* infection of the posterior columns of the spinal cord and dorsal root ganglia, usually developing 20 years after initial exposure. Ataxia, focal pain syndromes, or parasthesias are common complaints. The Argyll–Robertson pupil, which occurs commonly, is a small pupil that does not respond to light, but only accommodation and convergence. Physical examination reveals decreased lower extremity reflexes, impaired proprioception, loss of fine touch and vibratory sensation, and sensory ataxia.

Differential diagnosis

- Primary syphilis: genital warts, herpes simplex virus (HSV) infection, chancroid, granuloma inguinale (donavanosis), lymphogranuloma venereum (LGV), community-associated MRSA, tularemia, cutaneous anthrax, sporotrichosis, rat bite fever, Behçet's disease. and others.
- Secondary syphilis: RMSF, viral exanthems, condylomas, psoriasis, drug eruption, pityriasis rosea, lichen planus, vasculitis, and others.
- Neurosyphilis: aseptic meningitis from viruses or medications, progressive multifocal leukoencephalopathy (PML), parameningeal abscess, ischemic stroke, vascular or Alzheimer dementia, transverse myelitis, and others.

Investigations

First, obtain a serum nontreponemal test, such as the rapid plasma reagin (RPR) or VDRL assay and, if positive, a specific treponemal test, such as the fluorescent treponemal antibody (FTA) or microhemagglutination for antibodies to *Treponema pallidum* (MHA-TP) assay. If there is a very high load of spirochetes, such as with secondary syphilis, the prozone effect may be present, creating a false-negative RPR. If this is supected, the lab should dilute the sample and repeat the test.

If there are signs or symptoms of neurosyphilis, ocular manifestations, hearing loss, a patient with HIV infection – particularly with a CD4 T-cell count <350 cells/µl, or high serum RPR titer (>1:32)[27], perform an LP and send CSF for: cell count and differential, protein, glucose, Gram stain, culture, and VDRL[28]. Other studies to consider include HSV PCR, enteroviral PCR, West Nile virus PCR or antibodies, John Cunningham virus (JCV) PCR, cryptococcal antigen, and mycobacterial stains and cultures.

Imaging is often unnecessary; however, CT or MRI can reveal diffuse meningeal enhancement, ischemic stroke in meningovascular syphilis, and many other nonspecific findings. Syphilitic gummas appear as focal nodules. Angiography may show arterial narrowing or occlusion in meningovascular disease.

All patients diagnosed with syphilis should be tested for HIV infection.

Diagnosis

The diagnosis of neurosyphilis is highly dependent upon clinical suspicion. The CSF VDRL is highly specific, but only about 30% sensitive[29]. The CSF FTA is much more sensitive but less specific because of possible cross contamination by blood (and therefore antibody) in the CSF. Due to the insensitivity of CSF VDRL and the high prevalence of asymptomatic neurosyphilis in HIV-infected patients with low CD4 T-cell counts, most experts will treat HIV-infected patients with a positive serum RPR and negative CSF VDRL, but with abnormalities on CSF examination consistent with neurosyphilis (e.g. WBC > 20/µl and increased protein concentration).

If the diagnosis is unclear, CSF can be tested by PCR for *T. pallidum*, but this is not usually necessary and is not widely available. The CSF cell count and protein tend to be more abnormal in early neurosyphilis and late parenchymal infection, but have fewer abnormalities in tabes dorsalis.

CT or MRI of the brain is often performed prior to LP in immunocompromised patients or those with focal deficits. Otherwise, imaging is not usually required to make the diagnosis.

Pathology

T. pallidum cannot be cultured *in vitro*. Therefore, diagnosis depends mainly on serology but can be supported by pathologic findings. A lymphocytic infiltrate is seen on histopathology in all stages of syphilis. Obliterative endarteritis appears as concentric endothelial and fibroblastic proliferative thickening (**432**) – a pathognomonic finding in neurovascular syphilis. Neuronal degeneration in the dorsal columns of the spinal cord is seen in tabes dorsalis (**433**).

Staining with direct immunofluorescent antibody (DFA), immunoperoxidase, or silver may reveal *T. pallidum*, and darkfield microscopy can be used to visualize spirochetes, particularly from primary chancres. Darkfield microscopy should not be performed for oral lesions, since commensal spirochetes are part of the normal oral microbiota and can result in false positives.

Treatment

Treatment of neurosyphilis should be the same at all stages of infection. The genome of *T. pallidum* is extremely conserved and lacks transposable elements, likely explaining its continued susceptibility to penicillin despite decades of use. Penicillin G, 24 million units (MU) intravenously over 24 hours, is usually given as either 4 MU every 4 hours or via continuous infusion, for 10–14 days. Syphilitic otitis should be treated by extending the course to 6 weeks and up to 3 months and, unless contraindicated, corticosteroids should be included for the first week of therapy. In patients with penicillin allergy, desensitization should be performed. While doxycyline may be an option for immunocompetent patients with other forms of syphilis, it is never recommended for CNS infection[30].

As with other spirochete infections, one should be aware of the potential for the Jarisch–Herxheimer reaction. This systemic inflammatory reaction can resemble sepsis with abrupt onset of fevers, chills, myalgias, tachycardia, and vasodilation. This reaction is observed in 70–90% of patients with secondary syphilis because of the high load of treponemes in that phase of infection.

Many experts recommend an LP at 6 months after therapy to check for normalization of CSF parameters, and re-treatment if abnormalities persist.

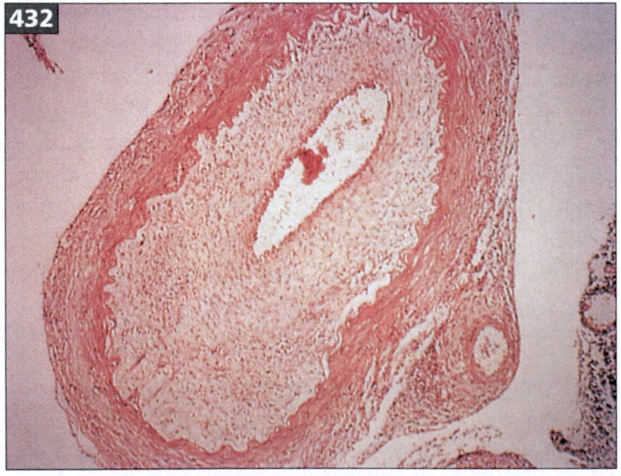

432 Cross- section of a branch of the middle cerebral artery, showing intimal hyperplasia due to meningovascular syphilis.

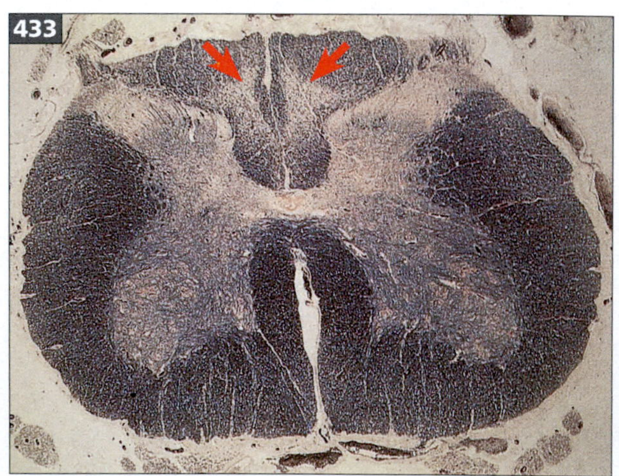

433 Transverse section of the spinal cord in a patient with tabes dorsalis, showing degeneration of the posterior columns (arrows) secondary to *Treponema pallidum* infection and inflammation along the dorsal roots. *Courtesy of Professor BA Kakulas, Royal Perth Hospital, Western Australia.*

LYME DISEASE

Definition

Lyme disease is a tick-borne infectious disease caused by the spirochete *Borrelia burgdorferi* in the USA and other *Borrelia* species in Europe and Asia. After hematogenous dissemination of spirochetes, Lyme disease of the CNS may develop. Neuroborreliosis has myriad potential neurologic manifestations. The disease is named after Lyme, Connecticut, where the disease was first recognized.

Epidemiology

Lyme disease is the most common tick-borne infection in the USA and Europe. The incidence of Lyme disease has steadily increased over the past three decades, likely due to an increase in recognition of the clinical syndrome, climate change, and an increase in the deer population in the northeastern USA[31].

The true incidence of Lyme disease is difficult to quantify due to regional differences in reporting requirements. From 1992 to 2006, almost 250,000 cases were reported in the USA[32], and approximately 20,000 cases are now reported annually[33]. Lyme disease can occur in all ages, but tends to be preferentially distributed in the extremes of age, affecting the very young and some older adults. Just over one-half of cases occur in males, likely due to greater exposure to the outdoors and therefore the tick vector.

Lyme disease tends to occur more commonly in temperate areas of North America, Europe, and Asia[34]. In the USA, the highest incidence is primarily in three geographic foci: the northeast, the northern midwest and occasionally in northern California. These areas harbor the *Ixodes* tick vectors, particularly *I. scapularis*[35].

The tick vectors are most active in early summer, with less activity in late summer. Therefore, Lyme disease has a seasonal distribution, with cases peaking in early summer and beginning to wane in mid to late summer.

Etiology and pathophysiology

B. burgdorferi is a spirochete transmitted by the bite of *Ixodes* species ticks, all of which are part of the *Ixodes vicinus* complex. In the northeastern and northern midwest USA, the blacklegged or deer tick (*I. scapularis*) is the tick vector. *I. pacificus* is the western vector. In endemic areas, 10–50% of nymphal and adult *I. scapularis* ticks harbor *B. burgdorferi*[36]. Spirochetes are motile, corkscrew-shaped, flagellated bacteria.

Tick larvae hatch in the early summer and obtain a blood meal from an infected mouse. The mice are not affected, but remain spirochetemic and infectious. The next spring, larvae develop into persistently infected nymphs. Nymphs and adult ticks seek a blood meal in low-lying shrubs or grass, latching onto an animal when they sense warmth and carbon dioxide. Ticks may obtain a blood meal from many different animals, including humans, mice, deer, other mammals, reptiles, and birds. When a human blood meal occurs, infectious spirochetes exit the salivary gland of the tick and enter the human host.

An important pathophysiologic and historical factor is that a tick must be attached for at least 48 hours in order to transmit *B. burgdorferi*[37]. Therefore, a patient who presents with a tick latched for less time is very unlikely to have Lyme disease. Adult ticks can transmit the spirochete, but the nymph is primarily responsible for human transmission. Due to its small size (<2 mm), the nymph is more likely to remain attached undetected for the full 48 hours, and most patients in fact do not recall a tick bite.

Clinical features

After an incubation period of 3–32 days following the tick bite, several stages of infection, separated by periods of latency, tend to occur in the untreated patient.

Early localized

This typically begins in summertime with the characteristic, localized erythema migrans (EM) rash, possibly accompanied by constitutional symptoms. EM occurs at the site of the tick bite and manifests as an expanding erythematous, warm, indurated lesion with central clearing. EM develops in about 70–80% of patients but may go unnoticed[38].

Early disseminated

Within days to weeks, untreated patients become spirochetemic, and *B. burgdorferi* may disseminate to other areas of the skin, the heart, and the CNS. Multiple secondary EM lesions often occur, accompanied by fever, chills, fatigue, myalgias, and lymphadenopathy.

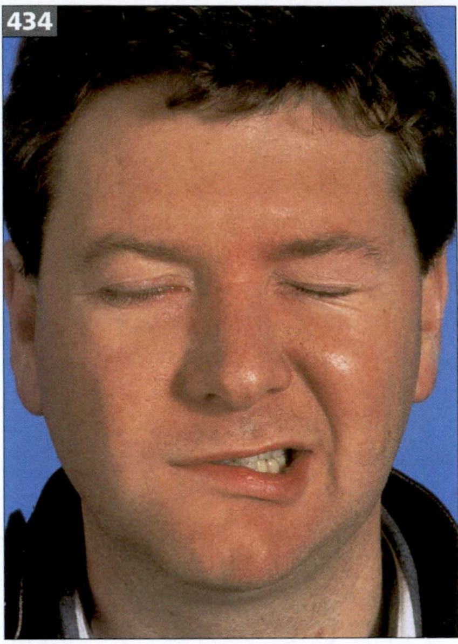

434 Right lower motor neuron facial nerve palsy in a patient with neuroborreliosis (Lyme disease).

Approximately 15% of untreated patients develop neurologic abnormalities, such as lymphocytic meningitis, encephalitis, cranial nerve abnormalities (particularly facial nerve palsies, (**434**), cerebellar ataxia, encephalitis, radiculoneuritis, or myelitis. The classic triad of neuroborreliosis is meningitis, cranial nerve palsies, and motor or sensory radiculoneuropathy[39].

Late persistent

Months to years after primary infection, and usually after a long period of clinical latency, intermittent arthritis may occur, involving one or multiple large joints. The knee is the joint most frequently involved. About 5% of untreated patients develop chronic neurologic manifestations, including spinal radicular pain, localized parasthesias, encephalopathy, and polyneuropathy[40].

Differential diagnosis

- Bell's palsy.
- Ramsay Hunt syndrome.
- Neurosyphilis.
- Cranial nerve palsy from TB, sarcoidosis, or trauma.
- Viral 'aseptic' meningitis (enteroviruses, arboviruses, herpesviruses, HIV).
- Guillain–Barré syndrome.

Investigations

- A detailed physical examination and exposure history.
- Serum Lyme antibodies, including enzyme-linked immunosorbent assay (ELISA) with confirmatory Western blot.
- LP for CSF cell count with differential, protein, glucose, Lyme PCR and antibody testing, cytology, VDRL, PCR for enteroviruses, PCR for herpesviruses (particularly HSV), West Nile virus PCR, or antibody testing and PCR for arboviruses.
- Complete blood count with differential to assess for cytopenias.
- Erythrocyte sedimentation rate (ESR).
- Hepatic transaminases and liver function testing (LFT).
- Serum HIV antibody testing with viral load if acute retroviral syndrome is suspected.
- Serum RPR with FTA if positive.
- Peripheral blood smear if coinfection with anaplasmosis or babesiosis is suspected.

Diagnosis

B. burgdorferi is very difficult to culture but can occasionally be seen on specimens from skin biopsy or CSF with special staining. A culture diagnosis is very insensitive and usually not feasible. The diagnosis of Lyme disease is therefore clinical, relying on the presentation and epidemiology. Most patients do not recall a tick bite, making this is an insensitive historical factor.

A positive antibody against *B. burgdorferi* is highly supportive of the diagnosis. Serology is first tested by ELISA and, if positive, confirmatory Western blot. Serology is relatively insensitive during the first 2 weeks of infection, but by 4 weeks, 70–80% of patients will be seroreactive.

LP tends to show a CSF lymphocytic pleocytosis, usually <100 cells/µl, elevated protein, and normal glucose. CSF IgG, IgM, or IgA directed against *B. burgdorferi* may be present. Lyme antibodies are more often present in the CSF during acute neuroborreliosis than chronic CNS infection.

Pathology

B. burgdorferi is quite fastidious; therefore, culture is insensitive and not widely available. The organism is occasionally grown in Barbour–Stoenner–Kelly (BSK) medium, but a large load of spirochetes is needed, such as from a biopsy of an EM lesion. The organism occasionally grows from blood or CSF, but this is a highly unreliable means of making the diagnosis.

Treatment

- Early localized disease: oral doxycycline (100 mg every 12 hours) for 14–21 days. Doxycycline should not be used in children (less than 8 years old) or pregnant or lactating women. Alternatives are amoxicillin (500 mg every 8 hours) or cefuroxime (500 mg twice daily).
- Neuroborreliosis: isolated cranial nerve palsies can be treated with oral doxycycline (100 mg every 12 hours). However, most CNS Lyme disease should not be treated with oral therapy. The first-line choice for neuroborreliosis is ceftriaxone (2 g IV every 24 hours) for 14–28 days. Alternatives are IV cefotaxime or penicillin G.

When treating any form of Lyme disease, clinicians should be aware of the risk for the Jarisch–Herxheimer reaction. Up to 15% of patients experience a transient worsening of symptoms in the first 24 hours of therapy, which results from the host inflammatory reaction to dying spirochetes.

TUBERCULOSIS (TB)

Definition and epidemiology

TB is an infectious disease of antiquity, with remnants of spinal TB found in early Egyptian remains. The vast majority of TB throughout the world presents as pulmonary disease. Infection of the CNS can manifest as meningitis, spinal arachnoiditis, or tuberculoma.

In 2008, there were approximately 9 million new cases and 1.3 million deaths worldwide from TB, a statistic that has been stable for several years[41,42]. TB is the second leading cause of death worldwide from a single infectious agent, following HIV. A total of 12,904 cases of *Mycobacterium tuberculosis* infection were reported in the USA in 2008, with an incidence of 4.2 cases per 100,000 population, and CNS disease accounted for approximately 1% of all cases[43].

An overall decline has occurred in the incidence of TB in the USA population over the past two decades, but not among foreign-born persons, who account for approximately 50% of new cases nationwide[44]. Among USA-born individuals, TB tends to concentrate in indigent and underserved populations who often cluster in proximity, such as the urban poor, homeless, alcoholics, intravenous drug users, those infected with HIV, and prison inmates. Two-thirds of cases occur in racial and ethnic minorities, including African-Americans, Hispanic-Americans, Asian Pacific Islanders, and Native Americans. In the USA, the incidence is higher in men than women.

TB meningitis develops as part of a continuum following primary infection in children and in adults who are highly immunosuppressed at the time of primary infection (e.g. patients with untreated AIDS). Otherwise, TB meningitis in adults is usually the result of reactivation of latent TB, years after primary infection. Such reactivation TB is more likely in adults with reduced cellular immune defenses as a consequence of aging, alcoholism, immunosuppressive conditions (e.g. HIV infection, organ transplantation), or cytotoxic chemotherapy.

Etiology and pathophysiology

M. tuberculosis is an aerobic, nonspore-forming, nonmotile, acid-fast bacterium. Almost all infections are initially acquired from inhalation of droplet nuclei containing the organism. The bacilli are ingested by alveolar macrophages and may subsequently spread to regional lymph nodes or hematogenously throughout the body. This can result in a subcortical or meningeal focus of *M. tuberculosis* infection that can rupture, releasing organisms into the subarachnoid space. In most cases, the initial infection is controlled by the development of cellular immunity, and clinical disease represents reactivation.

Clinical features

TB meningitis is a nonspecific clinical entity, and a high index of suspicion is required to consider this infection in the differential diagnosis. Initially, the patient presents with the subacute onset of low-grade fevers, weight loss, malaise, headache, and encephalopathy. This frequently progresses to meningismus, worsening headache, nausea, vomiting, lethargy, confusion, and cranial neuropathies.

In late stage disease, the patient may develop stupor, coma, and seizures. Despite antimycobacterial therapy, TB meningitis causes death or severe neurologic deficits in more than 50% of those affected, making early diagnosis key to improving survival[45,46]. An extrameningeal focus of infection is seen in three-quarters of cases, which may be helpful in isolating the pathogen[47].

Spinal arachnoiditis is rare in the USA and manifests as an inflammatory cord compression syndrome with radicular pain, parasthesias, lower motor neuron dysfunction, and bowel or bladder dysfunction. If vasculitis is present, infarction of the spinal cord can result in hemiparesis.

Tuberculomas present with focal neurologic deficits and seizures from the mass effect of the lesion. Meningismus is not a prominent feature with these space-occupying lesions, although it may be present.

Clinical staging is used, to assist with prognosis and to assist with decisions regarding the length and intensity of adjunctive corticosteroid therapy:

- Stage I: Glasgow Coma Scale (GCS) of 15, no focal neurologic deficits, no hydrocephalus on imaging.
- Stage II: GCS 11–14, confusion or focal neurologic deficits.
- Stage III: GCS <10, stupor, dense paraplegia, or hemiplegia.

Differential diagnosis

- Cryptococcosis.
- Neurosyphilis.
- Neurobrucellosis.
- Bacterial brain abscess.
- Parameningeal abscess.
- Viral meningitis or encephalitis (e.g. herpesviruses, West Nile virus, enteroviruses).
- Primary CNS malignancy or meningeal carcinomatosis.

Investigations

LP is a very important test in the work-up of CNS TB. CSF should be sent for cell count and differential, protein, glucose, acid fast stain and culture, VDRL, HSV PCR (and consider PCR for other herpesviruses), cryptococcal antigen, enteroviral PCR, and cytology. Multiple, large-volume samples will increase the sensitivity of acid-fast bacilli (AFB) smear, and many experts recommend daily LP for 3 days to increase the yield of CSF stains. Nucleic acid amplication testing (NAAT), using PCR to look for *M. tuberculosis* DNA, should be sent if there is reasonably high clinical suspicion[48,49]. All positive cultures for *M. tuberculosis* should be tested for antibiotic susceptibility.

Other investigations include:

- Blood cultures using lysis-centrifugation to increase the yield for intracellular pathogens.
- Sputum for AFB smears and mycobacterial cultures. Antibiotic susceptibility testing should be performed on all positive cultures.
- A chest X-ray reveals changes compatible with concomitant pulmonary TB in 50–80% of cases.
- CT or MRI of the brain with contrast. MRI is more sensitive and the preferred modality, particularly if spinal arachnoiditis is suspected.
- Tuberculin skin testing or interferon-γ release assay (IGRA) can be considered (see Diagnosis).
- Chemistries to look for hyponatremia, which may result from the syndrome of inappropriate antidiuretic hormone secretion (SIADH), a relatively common finding in CNS TB. An assessment of renal function is also an important component of the work-up and therapeutic decision-making.
- Hepatic transaminases and LFTs.

Diagnosis

On Ziehl–Neelsen staining, *M. tuberculosis* appears as beaded, AFB. It may be seen occasionally on Gram stain as weakly Gram-positive bacilli, but it is most often colorless. It is a very slow-growing organism with a generation time of 15–20 hours. Culture of *M. tuberculosis* from the CSF is the gold standard for diagnosing CNS TB.

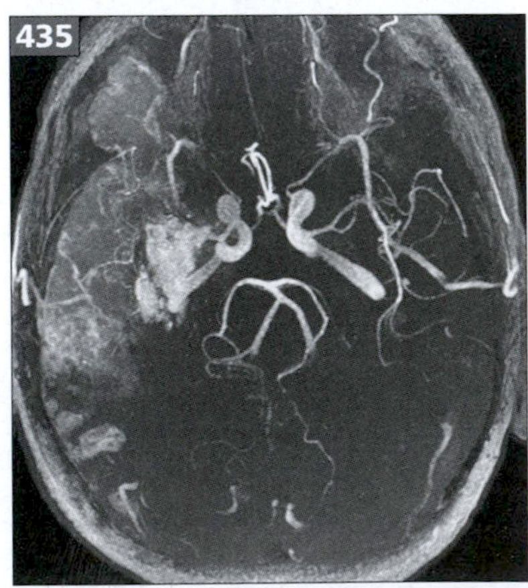

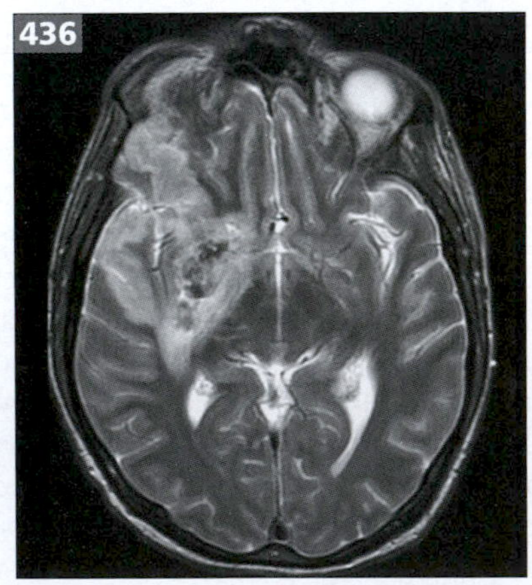

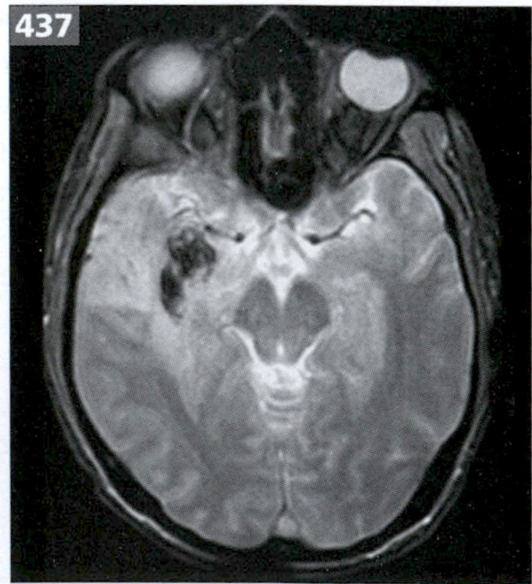

435–437 In this patient, CNS tuberculosis has caused occlusion of the right middle cerebral artery (MCA) with hemorrhagic infarction of the right MCA territory. The MR angiogram (MRA) demonstrates lack of flow enhancement in the right MCA. The T2-weighted (T2W) and T2*W images demonstrate the right MCA territory infarction. The gray matter is clearly increased in signal on the T2W image and the dark area of hemorrhage is better seen on the T2*W image. On the MRA, the area of hemorrhage is bright due to T1 effects. *Courtesy of Dr. Edward Michals, University of Illinois at Chicago.*

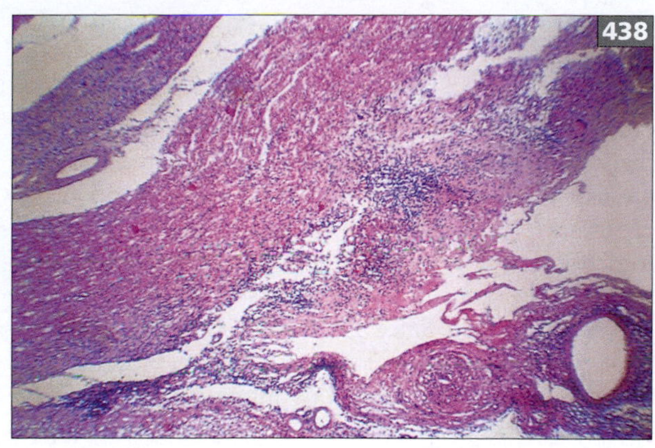

438 **Microscopic examination of the mononuclear inflammatory cell exudate involving the trigeminal nerve root as it traverses the subarachnoid space of a patient with tuberculous meningitis. An artery in the lower part of the field has become inflamed and occluded.**

Tip

▶ *Note that there is a difference between acid-fast (Ziehl–Neelsen) staining, which is used primarily to detect mycobacteria, and modified acid-fast staining, which is used to visualize other pathogens, such as Nocardia and some intestinal protozoa. This is an important distinction when submitting samples to the microbiology laboratory.*

Spinal fluid reveals a lymphocytic pleocytosis (cell count 0–1500/μl), elevated protein (100–500 mg/dl [1–5 g/l]), and low glucose. Early in infection, there may be a predominance of neutrophils, but repeated LP shows a conversion to lymphocyte predominance.

CT or MRI may show a variety of findings, including meningeal inflammation, the rounded, nodular lesions of tuberculomas, basilar arachnoiditis, vasculitis with infarction, and hydrocephalus (**435–437**). Tuberculomas can be single or multiple, appearing as avascular masses with surrounding edema and tend to be more prevalent in HIV-infected patients.

Diagnostic testing for latent TB infection, such as tuberculin skin testing or IGRA (e.g. QuantiFERON®-TB gold) can be supportive of the diagnosis, but the clinician should be cautious in interpreting the results. Sensitivity and specificity data are based upon latent TB infection, not active TB. These tests do not allow for the diagnosis of active TB, merely stratification of the differential diagnosis and assessment of risk.

Pathology

Meningeal involvement tends to be most prominent at the base of the brain where proliferative arachnoiditis may be observed. Vasculitis with thrombosis and infarction is another common pathologic feature (**438**). Tuberculomas appear as well-circumscribed, caseous foci of infection.

Treatment

The mortality of CNS TB is 15–40%. Therefore, initiating therapy early is key. Empiric antimycobacterial therapy should be started in a patient with the appropriate history, epidemiology, and CSF findings while awaiting specific diagnostic testing.

TB of the CNS is treated with the same initial regimen used for pulmonary infection. For the first 2 months, patients should be treated with a four-drug regimen consisting of isoniazid (INH) + rifampin (RIF) + pyrazinamide (PZA) + ethambutol (ETH).

- INH: 10 mg/kg per day initially. Once a clinical response has occurred, the dose can be reduced to 5 mg/kg per day, generally 300 mg per day in adults. INH penetrates well into the CNS, is the cornerstone of therapy, and should always be included in the therapeutic regimen unless a high degree of resistance is present. Pyridoxine (vitamin B6) should be given with INH to help avoid peripheral neuropathy. Follow serum transaminase levels when administering INH.
- RIF: 600 mg daily. Rifamycins are another vital component of antimycobacterial therapy and are essential for short-course therapy (i.e. reduction of therapy from 18 to 6 months).
- PZA: 15–30 mg/kg per day with a maximum dose of 2 g.
- ETH: 15–25 mg/kg per day. The lower dose appears to be efficacious with less ocular toxicity, so 15 mg/kg per day is preferred. Due to the potential for optic neuritis, patients should undergo baseline Snellen visual acuity and red–green color perception testing.

Alternatives include:

- Streptomycin: 15 mg/kg per day intramuscularly with a maximum dose of 1 g. This injectable agent was an important component of therapy prior to the advent of INH, but is used as an alternative agent now due to the route of administration and the potential for adverse effects. If an aminoglycoside antibiotic is needed, amikacin in the same dosage is usually preferred, since it can be given intravenously and serum drug level monitoring is commonly available.

- Fluoroquinolones. Based upon *in vitro* activity, animal model studies, and emerging clinical trial data, fluoroquinolone antibiotics, particularly levofloxacin and moxifloxacin, may be as effective as some first-line agents. However, they should generally be reserved for use in cases of multi-drug-resistant TB.
- Second-line alternatives. These are likely less efficacious and/or more toxic, and include ethionamide, cycloserine, kanamycin, capreomycin, and para-aminosalicylic acid (PAS).

For the continuation phase of therapy, INH and RIF can be given if the isolate is susceptible to both drugs. The total duration of therapy recommended for TB meningitis is 9–12 months. If PZA cannot be used for the initial 2 months of therapy or if RIF cannot be used as part of the multi-drug regimen, treatment should be extended to 18 months. The intensive phase is the same for CNS tuberculoma, but the continuation phase should always be extended to give a total of 18 months of therapy.

Approximately 10% of isolates worldwide are resistant to at least one first-line agent. It should be suspected in patients from TB-endemic areas or in those who have previously been treated. Anti-TB therapy should be modified based upon the results of drug susceptibility testing. If multi-drug-resistant TB is present (i.e. resistance to both INH and RIF), the clinician should consult with an expert in TB therapy for advice about the regimen, and treatment should be extended to 18–24 months.

In addition to antimycobacterial drugs, high-dose corticosteroids should be used as adjunctive therapy, since studies have shown improved survival and fewer serious adverse events with the use of corticosteroids[50]:

- Dexamethasone:
  - 12 mg per day for 3 weeks, *then*
  - 9 mg per day for 1 week, *then*
  - 6 mg per day for 1 week, *then*
  - 3 mg per day for 1 week.
- Prednisone:
  - 60 mg per day for 3 weeks, *then*
  - 40 mg per day for 1 week, *then*
  - 20 mg per day for 1 week, *then*
  - 10 mg per day for 1 week.

In addition, early surgical consultation may be required to manage hydrocephalus and elevated ICP. A ventriculoperitoneal shunt may need to be placed to avoid herniation or other devastating neurologic sequelae.

Treatment of the obtunded patient with TB meningitis

In advanced disease, patients may have markedly suppressed mental status, and it may not be possible to treat them with standard oral regimens. This requires consideration of alternative drug formulations and routes of delivery to initiate therapy, until the patient can be converted to oral therapy. This problem should be approached by seeking consultation from experts in TB therapy and pharmacokinetics. Since TB meningitis in the obtunded patient is a medical emergency, it may be necessary to broaden the coverage to include antibiotics that could be useful for multi-drug-resistant TB, until antibiotic susceptibility testing data are available. Drugs that can be considered in discussion with expert consultants include the following:

- INH: available as an intramuscular preparation and 'INH for injection', that can be given by the IV route. For example, the standard dose can be diluted in 25 ml of normal saline and given by a 5–10 minute IV infusion. This formulation may not be readily available through the hospital pharmacy, requiring special order.
- RIF: available as an IV formulation, which can be given in the standard dose by a 30 minute infusion. Again, special order from the hospital pharmacy supplier will likely be needed.
- PZA: not available in a parenteral formulation. However, excellent absorption can be achieved by nasogastric tube delivery of a slurry of the crushed tablet form in standard doses.
- Fluoroquinolones. Both levofloxacin and moxifloxacin are available in IV formulations. Treatment of the obtunded patient with TB meningitis is one circumstance where it may be desirable to use these medications for initiation of therapy, especially if INH-resistant disease is a possibility. Levofloxacin 750 mg or moxifloxacin 400–800 mg can be considered for this approach.
- Amikacin: Streptomycin is not usually given by the IV route, although this has been done and appears to be well tolerated. Instead, amikacin 15–25 mg/kg/day may be used, if an aminoglycoside antibiotic is needed for treatment of an obtunded patient.

BOTULISM

Definition and epidemiology

Botulism is a life-threatening, neurotoxin-mediated infectious disease that causes a syndrome of paralysis in infants and adults. *Clostridium botulinum* is a ubiquitous organism in the environment, found in soil, marine sediment, and contaminating the surfaces of fruits and vegetables worldwide. Different modes of transmission occur, depending upon the exposure, which all lead to a similar clinical syndrome. Approximately 145 cases of botulism are reported each year in the USA, with relative proportions of 65% infant botulism, 20% wound botulism, and the vast majority of the remaining 15% being food-borne botulism[51].

Cases of inhalational botulism have been reported, but are quite rare. The major concern with inhalational disease is more theoretical, as it might occur if botulinum toxin were used in an act of bioterrorism.

Etiology and pathophysiology

C. botulinum is a Gram-positive, spore-forming, anaerobic bacterium that produces botulinum toxin, the most potent bacterial toxin known to humankind. Botulinum toxins have been designated as types A–G, based upon their subtle antigenic differences, but only types A, B, E, and F cause human disease[52,53].

Botulinum toxin can enter the body in myriad ways, but regardless of its entry point, the ultimate pathophysiology is consistent. Toxin, consisting of light and heavy chains, binds at the cholinergic synapses of neuromuscular junctions, and the light chain enters the neuron via receptor-mediated endocytosis, irreversibly preventing the release of acetylcholine by presynaptic nerve terminals. Botulinum toxin does not cross the blood–brain barrier, only affecting the peripheral cholinergic nervous system[54].

Infant botulism

This begins with the ingestion of clostridial spores, which then produce toxin *in vivo*. Although raw honey has been the most publicized and popularly known source, the majority of cases likely result from the ingestion of contaminated dust or soil. Indeed, despite a massive public education effort to stop infant ingestion of honey, the number of cases has not appreciably decreased. It generally occurs within the first year of life, with the median age of onset being 3–4 months.

Wound botulism

This occurs when soft tissue is colonized by *C. botulinum*, usually the result of skin trauma, and the organism germinates and elaborates toxin. An emerging cause of wound botulism in the USA is injection drug use, specifically from 'skin popping' (i.e. subcutaneous instead of IV injection of drugs)[55]. It is presumed that the drugs themselves, particularly 'black tar' heroin, are contaminated with the organism. Wounds typically do not have the cardinal features of cellullitis, such as erythema, warmth, or purulent drainage and may appear to be healing while neurologic symptoms are progressing. Any of these signs, combined with fever, would suggest wound coinfection with another organism.

Food-borne botulism

This results from the ingestion of pre-formed botulinum toxin in food. Botulinum toxin is resistant to degradation by gastric acid and digestive enzymes, allowing it to be absorbed from the stomach and small intestine into the bloodstream, to target peripheral cholinergic synapses. Exposure can result from eating foods from home canning, particularly of fruits and vegetables, and ingestion of fermented fish[56]. In the USA, the majority of cases occur in Alaska, resulting from consumption of contaminated, fermented fish. Toxins of some strains (e.g. types A and B) denature proteins and may cause food spoilage; however, with other strains, spoilage does not occur and contamination cannot be inferred based upon the appearance, smell, or taste of food. The toxin itself has no smell or taste, further making contamination difficult to detect.

Clinical features

Botulinum toxin affects the peripheral cholinergic nervous system. This classically leads to acute onset cranial neuropathy with symmetric, bilateral, descending weakness. There is no loss of consciousness. Patients are responsive and quite aware of their surroundings. Sensory deficits other than blurry vision (from parasympathetic involvement and papillary dilation) tend not to occur. Unless there is coinfection in wound botulism, patients lack fever or other constitutional signs or symptoms.

Cranial nerve dysfunction can manifest as paralysis in the distribution of cranial nerves III, IV, and VI, dysphagia, dysarthria, or hypoglossal weakness. Weakness is symmetric and descending, spreading from the head and neck to the upper extremities, trunk, and finally the lower extremities. Nausea, vomiting, and diarrhea may also be present from autonomic dysfunction, although they are nonspecific.

Infant botulism commonly presents as feeding difficulties and constipation, followed by drooling, descending weakness and hypotonia, and weak cry. It is important for the clinician to have a high index of suspicion in the infant patient, as the manifestations may be less apparent.

Food-borne botulism classically develops between 12 and 36 hours following toxin ingestion, a classic incubation period for an illness from the ingestion of preformed toxin. A gastrointestinal prodrome frequently occurs, with nausea, vomiting, diarrhea, and abdominal pain.

Wound botulism presents with similar symptoms but lacks the gastrointestinal prodrome and tends to have a longer incubation period of 1–2 weeks.

Differential diagnosis

- Myasthenia gravis.
- Lambert–Eaton myasthenic syndrome (LEMS).
- Tick paralysis.
- Guillain–Barré syndrome.
- Poliomyelitis.
- Brainstem infarction.
- Heavy metal intoxication.
- Shellfish poisoning.

Investigations

- Perform a thorough physical examination for the presence of ticks. In tick paralysis, the *Dermacentor* tick will still be attached at the time of neurologic symptoms.
- Obtain aerobic and anaerobic cultures from wounds. Toxin assays can be performed on serum, stool, and any available implicated food. Confirmation and toxin typing is obtained in approximately 75% of patients[52].

Diagnosis

A careful physical examination and exposure history are vital to make the diagnosis. There are no classic findings on tissue or other pathologic examination in botulism. The diagnosis is supported by isolation of *C. botulinum* in the stool or wound and/or toxin in the stool. However, tests take days to return, and one should not wait for anaerobic cultures or the toxin assay to begin therapy. A presumptive diagnosis and the initiation of therapy as soon as possible are key aspects for improving morbidity and mortality.

For foodborne botulism, a serum toxin assay is diagnostic. Stool and suspected food items can be cultured. In a case of suspected wound botulism, ask about injection drug use, particularly 'skin popping,' and trauma. Growth of *C. botulinum* on anaerobic cultures of the wound is diagnostic.

Pathology

It is usually easy to isolate *C. botulinum* from wounds and the gastrointestinal tract using anaerobic cultures. Gram-positive, rod-shaped bacteria are seen on stain.

Treatment

Ventilatory support, including a low threshold for intubation, is a key aspect of management. The clinician should assess upper airway competency as well as vital capacity. Do not wait for the oxygen saturation to fall or $PaCO_2$ to rise to intubate the patient. Purgatives are occasionally used if there is a suspicion that contaminated food remains in the gastrointestinal tract. Patients with wound botulism should undergo aggressive wound debridement.

Antitoxin trivalent (types A, B and E) equine serum can be obtained through state health departments or the Centers for Disease Control and Prevention (CDC). Retrospective data suggest that administration of antitoxin may decrease mortality[57,58]. However, there have been no controlled clinical trials of antitoxin effectiveness. Skin testing should be performed, and desensitization may be prudent prior to administering antitoxin, since toxin hypersensitivity rates (including anaphylaxis) are 9–20%[59]. One vial of antitoxin is given IV, and one vial is given intramuscularly.

Human botulinum immune globulin, 50 mg/kg IV, is FDA-approved for the treatment of infant botulism in infants less than 1 year of age, and should be given as soon as possible in the clinical course.

Although antimicrobials are of unproven benefit, most experts recommend administering a course of intravenous penicillin G (3 MU IV every 4 hours) or metronidazole (500 mg every 8 hours) to decrease the organism burden in wound botulism. Therapy should be broadened if a coinfection of the wound with another organism is suspected. There is some concern that antibiotics may lead to an increase in elaborated toxin in gastrointestinal tract infection, particularly infant botulism, and this should be considered when deciding about adjunctive antibiotic therapy. Antibiotics cannot be recommended in cases of infant or food-borne botulism.

Return of synaptic function requires the sprouting of a new presynaptic terminal, which requires approximately 6 months.

TETANUS

Definition and epidemiology

Tetanus is a clinical syndrome that has been recognized and described for centuries, characterized by tonic muscular spasms, particularly of the jaw and neck. It is caused by the production of tetanospasmin ('tetanus toxin') produced by the anaerobic bacterium *Clostridium tetani*, a ubiquitous environmental saprophyte.

Tetanus is rare in the developed world due to widespread vaccination and modern medical care of wounds and traumatic injuries; however, it still occurs with relative frequency in areas of the world where tetanus toxoid availability or administration are less common. The incidence has dropped dramatically over the past few decades. The most recent surveillance data place the annual rate of tetanus in the USA at 0.16 cases per million, or approximately 43 cases per year[60]. Incidence rates are similar in other industrialized countries[61,62]. World-wide, tetanus is much more common, with approximately 1,000,000 cases of tetanus occurring each year leading to over 300,000 deaths[63–65].

Neonatal tetanus is extremely rare in the USA, but is a particular problem in the developing world, causing about 180,000 infant deaths in 2002 alone[66].

Approximately 75% of reported tetanus cases in the USA occur after a recognized acute injury, and 15% are associated with injection drug use. Most patients with tetanus have not received the full immunization series. There are reports of patients who have developed tetanus despite pre-existing antibodies, although this appears to be extremely rare, and the vaccine remains quite efficacious[67]. At one time, the majority of USA cases occurred in patients older than 60 years of age, but the proportion of cases in those 25–59 years old has increased over the past decade, likely due to injection drug use.

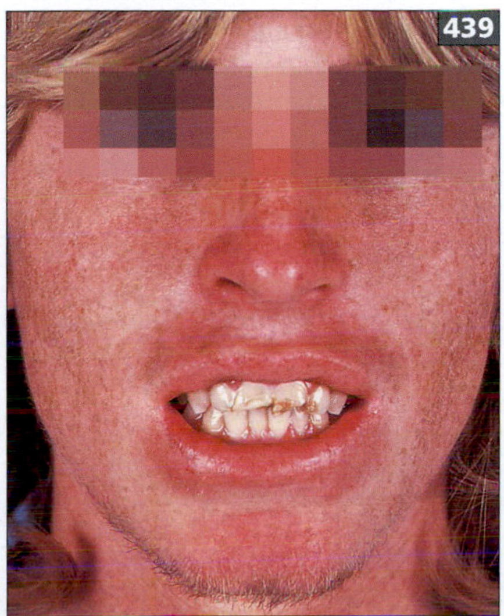

439 Facial photograph of a patient with facial muscle stiffness and grimacing (risus sardonicus) and difficulty opening the jaw (trismus) due to tetanus.

Etiology and pathophysiology

C. tetani is an anaerobic, spore-forming, Gram-positive rod that is commonly present in soil and the gastrointestinal tract of some mammals. Penetrating wounds that are contaminated with dirt or feces are at particular risk for becoming inoculated with tetanus spores. Production of tetanospasmin, a metalloproteinase toxin, leads to the cardinal neuromuscular manifestations of tetanus.

Tetanospasmin ('tetanus toxin') binds at the presynaptic terminals of lower motor neurons, causing peripheral neuromuscular failure (localized tetanus). The toxin is then carried by retrograde axonal transport to neurons in the spinal cord and brainstem, where toxin binds irreversibly. In the CNS, tetanus toxin enters the terminals of inhibitory (e.g. gamma-aminobutyric acid [GABA]-ergic) neurons. Synaptobrevin is degraded by the toxin, inhibiting the docking of vesicles containing neurotransmitters with the synaptic membrane, preventing neurotransmitter release. Tetanospasmin produces muscular rigidity by raising the resting firing rate of motor neurons, and generates spasms by failing to limit reflex responses to afferent stimuli. In the autonomic nervous system, a hypersympathetic state predominates, with a failure to inhibit the adrenal release of catcholamines. Toxin binding is a terminal and irreversible event. Recovery from tetanus appears to depend on the sprouting of a new axon terminal.

A major predisposing factor is tissue injury, particularly with devitalized tissue, which explains some of the at-risk populations, including neonates (umbilical stump infection), obstetric patients (septic abortion), and patients with post-operative tissue necrosis, diabetic foot ulcers, or injection drug use.

Clinical features

The incubation period can be from days to months, with a median of 7 days. Four common clinical patterns occur.

Generalized

This is the most well-known, 'classic' clinical syndrome. It begins as trismus ('lockjaw'), spasm of the masseters, and risus sardonicus ('sardonic smile') which is caused by increased muscular tone of the periorbital and facial muscles (439). This is followed by generalized spasm, a painful tonic contraction of skeletal muscles characterized by opisthotonic posturing (arched back, flexed arms, extended legs, clenched fists), abdominal rigidity ('board-like') and nuchal rigidity. Dysphagia may also be prominent. There is no loss of consciousness, and spasms can be triggered by external sensory stimuli (e.g. startle, cough, touch), making sedation a vital part of management. Autonomic dysfunction also occurs commonly, leading to irritability, restlessness, hypertension, tachycardia, and diaphoresis.

Localized

This is characterized by muscular rigidity at the site of inoculation and can occur at any anatomic location. Lower motor neuron dysfunction predominates, with focal weakness and decreased muscle tone, differentiating this presentation from generalized tetanus. It may resolve spontaneously or be a prodrome to generalized tetanus.

Cephalic

This is a form of localized tetanus specifically involving the muscles innervated by the cranial nerves. This presentation typically results from a head wound. As with other localized disease, facial muscle weakness without spasm is the rule. However, these patients often subsequently develop generalized tetanus.

Neonatal

Neonates may acquire infection of the umbilical stump with *C. tetani*, generally within 14 days of birth. The hypertonic signs and symptoms of generalized tetanus predominate, with trismus, rigidity and spasms of the skeletal muscles, inability to nurse, and occasionally seizures.

Neonatal tetanus results from the failure of aseptic technique and subsequent contamination of the umbilical stump. In certain cultures, substances may be applied to the umbilical stump after birth (e.g. cow dung, mud, straw) exposing the tissue to clostridial organisms. A high index of suspicion is required to make an early diagnosis of neonatal tetanus.

Differential diagnosis

Given its classic, well described clinical manifestations, the differential diagnosis is extremely limited and the diagnosis is usually obvious with a suspicious exposure history. Differentials include:

- Strychnine poisoning.
- Neuroleptic malignant syndrome.
- Dental infection with trismus.
- Mandibular fracture with the appearance of trismus.
- Stiff-person syndrome (very rare, associated with autoantibodies against glutamic acid decarboxylase and other autoimmune disorders, particularly type 1 diabetes mellitus).
- Rabies.

Investigations

A thorough history should be obtained for penetrating trauma, particularly with soil or fecal contamination. Considering the differential diagnosis, a history should also be explored for neuroleptic drugs (e.g. haloperidol, phenothiazines), strychnine ingestion, or the bite of a potentially rabid animal. It is prudent to perform serum and urine toxicology studies for strychnine poisoning in most cases. If stiff-person syndrome is suspected, anti-glutamic acid decarboxylase (GAD) antibodies can be tested, although this is a rare disorder and anti-GAD antibodies are only present in about 60% of patients[68,69].

Diagnosis

Tetanus is a clinical diagnosis, and there is no specific laboratory, histologic, or radiographic test used for definitive diagnosis. There are no pathognomonic findings on histology or other pathologic specimens in tetanus. The organisms are Gram-positive rods that develop terminal spores, often being described as a 'squash racquet' appearance.

While antitetanus antibodies are undetectable in most patients, there have been multiple case reports of tetanus in patients with 'protective' antibody levels. *Clostridium* spp. are notoriously difficult to culture from wounds, even if careful anaerobic cultures are performed. In addition, the presence of *C. tetani* in a wound culture does not confirm that the organism is a toxin-producer.

Treatment

The treatment for tetanus is supportive. Several aspects of the patient should be of immediate concern to the clinician. There are several phases of therapy:

- Airway: before modern critical care, and still in many developing countries without these resources, respiratory failure was a major cause of mortality. Blockade of the neuromuscular junction with adequate sedation is often necessary. Caution must be used, as the introduction of an endotracheal tube may exacerbate spasms, and consideration should be given to early tracheostomy.
- Spasm: IV benzodiazepines are the mainstay of therapy (lorazepam or diazepam). These are GABA agonists that antagonize the effect of tetanus toxin and also provide sedation. Propofol is a reasonable alternative.
- Recurrent tetanus can occur if the patient does not receive human tetanus immune globulin (HTIG) as soon as the diagnosis is suspected.

Phases of therapy

Immediate (first hour)

- Stabilize the patient's airway. Sedation and neuromuscular blockade (pancuronium or vecuronium) are often necessary, with consideration given to early tracheostomy.
- Administer IV benzodiazepine to help alleviate spasm and rigidity and keep the patient sedated.
- Send serum for strychnine and dopamine agonist assays.
- Assess for rhabdomyolysis and resultant renal insufficiency with serum creatinine kinase and chemistries, including blood urea nitrogen and creatinine.
- Determine the portal of entry, incubation period, and immunization history.

Early (first 24 hours)

- Administer HTIG intramuscularly.
- At a different site, administer tetanus toxoid. This can be in the form of either diphtheria–tetanus (Td) or tetanus–diptheria–acellular pertussis (Tdap, 0.5 ml IM). All patients should have active immunization, since infection does not confer immunity. A total of three doses of Td should be administered, and Tdap can be used for the initial dose.
- Metronidazole (500 mg every 6 hours) for 7–10 days is preferred, but penicillin G (2–3 MU every 4 hours) is a reasonable alternative.
- Debride wounds to eradicate spores and necrotic tissue.
- Continue benzodiazipines aggressively to control spasms and for sedation.
- Manage autonomic dysfunction as necessary with magnesium sulfate, beta blockade, atropine, morphine sulfate, or clonidine.

Intermediate

- Treat sympathetic hyperactivity with labetalol (0.25–1.0 mg/min) as needed for blood pressure control. Avoid diuretics, which can worsen autonomic instability.
- Early cardiology consultation for any arrhythmias, which may require temporary pacemaker placement.
- Continue benzodiazepines and neuromuscular blockade as needed. Stop neuromuscular blockade every 24–48 hours to assess the patient's status without these agents.
- Supportive care with ventilation, avoid decubitus ulcers, venous thromboembolic disease, gastrointestinal hemorrhage. Consider early tracheostomy as these patients often require prolonged mechanical ventilation.

Convalescent

- Wean from benzodiazepines and neuromuscular blockage as feasible, and taper slowly to avoid withdrawal.
- Begin physical therapy.
- Complete tetanus toxoid vaccine series. The tetanus vaccine can be given in a series of three intramuscular injections. Children younger than 7 years old should receive combined Tdap vaccine. Older children and adults should receive combined Td vaccine. Routine booster injections are indicated every 10 years. Whereas the full series is ideal, even one or two injections confers substantial protection.

ASEPTIC MENINGITIS

Definition

Aseptic meningitis is a very general term with a broad differential diagnosis. The clinical picture is that of acute meningitis and abnormal CSF parameters indicating meningeal inflammation, but the Gram stain and bacterial cultures are negative with no other obvious infectious etiology, such as fungi. The differential diagnosis includes infectious and noninfectious causes, but viruses are the usual offenders. The most common viral pathogens are discussed individually in this section.

Etiology and pathophysiology

Aseptic meningitis is most commonly associated with several viral pathogens, described below. Most of these begin by colonizing either the respiratory, genital, or gastrointestinal epithelium. If host innate and adaptive immune defenses fail to control epithelial infection, viral replication, invasion, and viremia, breaching of the blood–brain barrier can lead to infection of the CNS.

The inflammatory response detected in the spinal fluid tends to be predominantly lymphocytic, with release of cytokines, such as interleukin (IL)-6, tumor necrosis factor (TNF)-α and interferon (IFN)-γ that amplify the inflammatory response and mediate the symptoms and signs of presentation.

Clinical features

Whereas pathognomonic findings for specific pathogens are discussed below, most patients with aseptic meningitis present with some combination of the classic signs and symptoms of meningitis, including fever, headache, nuchal rigidity, photophobia, nausea, vomiting, and various levels of confusion or delirium.

It is important to differentiate between meningitis and encephalitis (see 'Encephalitis' for details), although this can be difficult based upon history and physical examination alone. In general, patients with meningitis retain normal cerebral function, despite feeling acutely ill or experiencing mild lethargy. In contrast, encephalitis can cause confusion, delirium, behavioral changes, paralysis, and motor or sensory deficits. The difficulty for the clinician is that these two entities often overlap, with pathogens causing both meningitis and cerebritis – so-called meningoencephalitis.

Differential diagnosis

- Enteroviruses.
- Herpesviruses (HSV, cytomegalovirus [CMV], varicella-zoster virus [VZV], EBV, human herpesvirus [HHV]-6, -7, and -8).
- HIV.
- Mumps virus.
- Lymphocytic choriomeningitis virus (LCMV).
- Mollaret's meningitis.
- Arboviruses (e.g. West Nile virus).
- Influenza virus.
- RMSF.
- Neurosyphilis.
- Neuroborreliosis (Lyme disease).
- Partially treated bacterial meningitis.
- Tuberculous meningitis.
- Cryptococcosis.
- Coccidioidomycosis.
- Parameningeal (e.g. epidural) abscess.
- Medication-induced aseptic meningitis (e.g. nonsteroidal anti-inflammatory drugs, IV Ig, TMP–SMX, rofecoxib, OKT3 antibodies).
- Seizures.
- Malignancy.

Investigations

A comprehensive history and physical examination can give clues to the etiology. Inquire about travel, sexual activity, medications, TB exposures, recent tick or mosquito exposures, sick contacts, and animal contact. On physical examination, certain features are suggestive of particular pathogens, including rash (syphilis, HIV, enteroviruses, HSV, VZV, RMSF), parotitis (mumps), and asymmetric flaccid paralysis (West Nile virus).

LP should be performed in all patients, and CSF should be sent for cell count and differential, protein, glucose, Gram stain and bacterial cultures, HSV PCR, enterovirus PCR, viral cultures and VDRL. Depending on the season and epidemiology of the patient, work-up for arboviruses and coccidioidomycosis may also be considered (see appropriate sections). If the patient is known to be immunocompromised, send CSF cryptococcal antigen.

A complete blood count should be performed to look for atypical lymphocytes, leukocytosis, leukopenia, and thrombocytopenia; renal function, hepatic transaminases, RPR with FTA if positive, HIV ELISA with confirmatory Western blot, and HIV viral load if acute retroviral syndrome is suspected. Consider serum cryptococcal antigen, acute and convalescent antibody titers for mumps or LCMV if suspected.

Brain imaging with CT or MRI can be helpful.

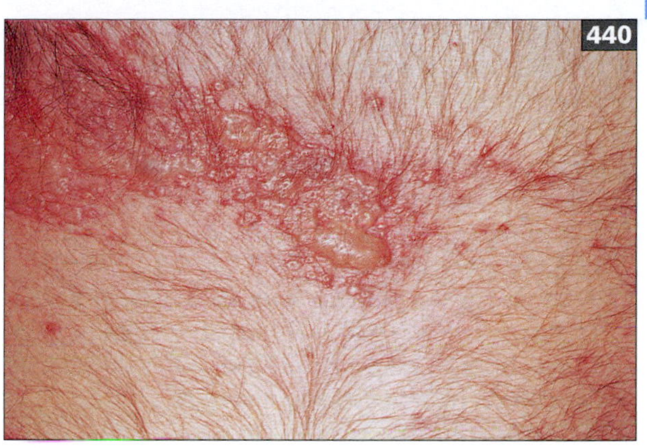

440 Herpes zoster skin rash in a patient with aseptic meningitis.

Enteroviruses

Enteroviruses are the most common cause of aseptic meningitis, accounting for 85–95% of all cases for which a pathogen is identified[70,71]. Approximately 30,000–75,000 cases of enteroviral meningitis occur each year in the USA[72], but this is likely an underestimate since the diagnosis is not always made, and reporting is inconsistent. In the USA and other temperate climates, there is a marked increase in cases in the summer and fall, with a peak in August. The warmer weather likely facilitates fecal–oral transmission of virus. However, enteroviruses still cause 6–10% of cases in the winter and spring, so the season of presentation is helpful but nonspecific[73].

Several different 'nonpolio' enteroviruses can cause infections of the CNS, but various strains of echoviruses, coxsackie B virus, and enterovirus 71 are the most common. Infants and young children are most affected by enteroviral meningitis because of increased exposure to fecally contaminated fomites and lack of immunity.

The presence of a diffuse, maculopapular rash can be a clue to the diagnosis of enteroviral meningitis. Herpangina, with painful vesicles in the oropharynx, has been associated with coxsackievirus A, and pericarditis or pleurisy with coxsackievirus B. Diarrhea, while not pathognomonic, is also relatively common.

Neonates can experience a rapid progression of symptoms, with evolution of a sepsis-like syndrome, DIC, encephalitis, and death. Enteroviral infections tend to be more benign and self-limited in older children and adults.

Diagnosis

CSF pleocytosis (100–1000 cells/μl) with lymphocyte predominance is seen, although there may be a neutrophil response during the first 6–48 hours. Mild elevations of CSF protein with slightly low or normal glucose are common. Enterovirus culture is positive in 4–8 days in the laboratory in 65–75% of cases[71,74]. Culture of enterovirus from the oropharynx or gastrointestinal tract is suggestive, but viral shedding occurs in 7–8% of healthy controls during epidemics of enterovirus. Enterovirus PCR from the CSF is more sensitive (86–100%) and specific (92–100%) than culture, with a faster time to results, and is the diagnostic test of choice[71,75–77].

Treatment

Pleconaril has *in vitro* activity against enteroviruses and may be beneficial for serious infections[78]. However, there are not enough clinical data to recommend its use. Therefore, management of enteroviral meningitis is supportive, with no indication at this time for antiviral agents.

Herpesviruses

Herpesviruses are a group of DNA viruses to which humans are commonly exposed, including HSV types 1 and 2, VZV, CMV, EBV, and HHV-6, -7, and -8.

HSV-1 and -2 account for 0.5–3% of all cases of aseptic meningitis[79]. HSV-2 causes meningitis in an estimated 35% of women and 15% of men with symptomatic primary infections[80]. Herpes meningitis tends to be mild and self-limited, manifesting with headache, nuchal rigidity, photophobia, nausea, and vomiting. Genital lesions are an excellent clue on physical examination, since 85% of patients with primary HSV-2-associated meningitis have lesions present at the time of diagnosis. HSV infection can also cause transverse myelitis and autonomic dysfunction (e.g. urinary retention or constipation), particularly with genital HSV-2 disease. Transverse myelitis manifests as symmetric lower extremity weakness and decreased deep tendon reflexes.

Aseptic meningitis has been associated with primary VZV infection (i.e. chickenpox) and herpes zoster. A vesicular rash, either diffuse or in a dermatomal distribution (**440**), is highly suggestive. EBV and CMV have been reported to cause acute meningitis during a primary mononucleosis syndrome, and pharyngitis, lymphadenopathy, splenomegaly, and the presence of atypical lymphocytes on complete blood count suggest these herpesviruses. CMV may lead to severe meningoencephalitis in immunocompromised hosts; a polyradiculopathy syndrome, with ascending lower extremity weakness, decreased deep tendon reflexes, and bowel or bladder dysfunction, can be seen in patients with HIV/AIDS.

Diagnosis

CSF reveals a lymphocytic pleocytosis, slightly elevated protein, and normal glucose. CSF PCR for HSV, VZV, CMV, and EBV is highly sensitive and specific, and is the diagnostic test of choice for CNS infection with herpesviruses.

Treatment

While trials have not been conducted to allow definitive recommendations, symptomatic, hospitalized patients with HSV meningitis or transverse myelitis should be treated with acyclovir (10 mg/kg IV every 8 hours), and serious VZV infections should be treated similarly. CNS infections with CMV should be treated with ganciclovir (5 mg/kg IV every 12 hours).

Alternatives for patients with ganciclovir-resistant CMV infection may include foscarnet or cidofovir, but infectious diseases consultation is recommended when making the decision to use these antivirals.

Human immunodeficiency virus

Meningitis caused by HIV infection can occur as part of the acute retroviral syndrome with primary infection, or later during the chronic phase of HIV/AIDS. Acute HIV often presents as a mononucleosis-like syndrome with fever, headache, pharyngitis, oral ulcers, cervical lymphadenopathy, myalgias, arthralgias, and a maculopapular rash. Meningoencephalitis occurs in as many as 5–10% of acutely HIV-infected patients, but is often not diagnosed due to the nonspecific nature of the symptoms and the self-limited clinical course[81]. A high index of suspicion should be maintained by the clinician to make the diagnosis.

Diagnosis

CSF shows only a very mild lymphocytic pleocytosis, elevated protein, and normal glucose. HIV ribonucleic acid (RNA) can be detected by PCR in the CSF of most patients with untreated HIV infection, and is therefore not recommended to make the specific diagnosis of HIV meningitis. Patients with acute HIV have often not begun to make antibodies, so a negative HIV ELISA in the blood is not helpful in excluding the diagnosis. Plasma HIV RNA testing should be sent in suspected acute retroviral syndrome. The clinician should be cautious if the HIV viral load is <10,000 copies/ml, since it may represent a false positive because values tend to be high (>100,000 copies/ml) during acute infection. Subsequent seroconversion should be documented.

Treatment

Antiretroviral therapy will not affect the acute course of HIV-associated meningitis. Whether patients ultimately benefit from initiation of antiretrovirals during acute infection is unclear. Although patients appear to have improved markers of disease progression, experts consider antiretrovirals optional at this time.

Mumps virus

Symptomatic meningitis occurs in 10–30% of patients with mumps[82]. The incidence of infection has decreased significantly since the institution of mumps vaccine as part of routine childhood immunizations. Mumps vaccine has reduced the number of cases in the USA from almost 200,000 to less than 500 annually. However, the nonimmunized are at high risk when exposed to mumps virus. The incidence is two to five times higher in males than in females, peaking between the ages of 5 and 9 years old. Mumps meningitis frequently follows parotitis, which is present in about 50% of patients. This virus can lead to severe encephalitis, but this is rare.

Diagnosis

A CSF pleocytosis with lymphocyte predominance is seen in more than 90% of patients, but only about one-half of patients have an elevated protein, and 25% have a low glucose. Serum testing for acute and convalescent antibodies should show a fourfold rise in titer. Viral cultures can be sent, but are only 30–50% sensitive[82].

Treatment

Supportive care. Live-attenuated mumps vaccine (as a component of mumps, measles, rubella [MMR]) is given routinely in childhood, and has been very effective in prevention, although large USA outbreaks involving several thousand cases have occurred in vaccinated individuals in 2006, 2009, and 2010.

Lymphocytic choriomeningitis virus

LCMV is an arenavirus found in the urine and feces of rodents, such as mice, rats, and hamsters. It does not cause disease in rodents, but is chronically excreted into the environment. Humans acquire the virus by direct contact with, or aerosol exposure to, the excreta of infected rodents or contaminated fomites. Mouse bites have also likely transmitted infection.

Due to increased exposure to the enclosed spaces rodents infiltrate for shelter, LCMV is more common during the fall and winter months. There is also an increased risk with exposure to structures infested with rodents, such as urban housing, mobile homes, and barns.

The illness is often biphasic. After a 5–10-day incubation period, LCMV causes fevers and headache, with laboratory studies frequently showing leukopenia and thrombocytopenia. A maculopapular rash may also been seen. A patient then typically improves for 2–4 days, followed by frank meningitis. Several organ systems can be involved, and patients with LCMV occasionally develop myocarditis, arthritis, and orchitis 1–3 weeks after onset.

Diagnosis

The CSF findings are classic for aseptic meningitis, with a lymphocytic pleocytosis, with cell counts >1000/µl commonly seen. Culture from the CSF, blood, throat swabs, or urine is possible, but very difficult. Most diagnoses are made by a fourfold rise in acute and convalescent ELISA antibody titers.

Treatment

Supportive care with no antiviral therapy available.

Mollaret's meningitis

Mollaret's is the name given to a self-limited, recurrent form of lymphocytic meningitis. The DNA of different viruses has been isolated from the CSF of patients, but by far the most common is HSV-2, and occasionally HSV-1[83]. Mollaret's meningitis is considered by most to be a benign form of relapsing HSV meningitis, and symptoms tend to resolve in 2–5 days. Unlike primary HSV-2 meningitis, Mollaret's is not associated with genital herpetic lesions. Rare patients experience severe symptoms with a suggestion of encephalitis, including seizures, delirium, and hallucinations.

Diagnosis

Greater than three episodes of meningismus and fevers, lasting 2–5 days, with spontaneous resolution is highly suggestive of the diagnosis, particularly if HSV PCR is positive with a lymphocytic pleocytosis in the CSF. Large, granular plasma cells on Papanicolaou's stain of the CSF are pathognomonic.

Treatment

No trials have been performed, but no antiviral therapy can be recommended at this time.

Tip

► *Some case reports suggest that acyclovir prophylaxis may be beneficial in decreasing the frequency of Mollaret's meningitis in those with previous episodes. However, there are not enough data to recommend such prophylaxis at this time.*

VIRAL ENCEPHALITIS

Definition, etiology, and pathophysiology

Encephalitis signifies inflammation of the brain parenchyma. Since several processes, infectious and noninfectious, can cause encephalitis, there is a broad differential diagnosis. The most common viral etiologies are discussed in this section.

Various pathogens of the viral encephalitides enter the host through myriad ways, including the respiratory tract, gastrointestinal tract, genital tract, and subcutaneous tissue (e.g. mosquito or tick bite). Subsequent viremia or retrograde neural transport allows virions to gain access to the CNS, inducing an inflammatory response. Inflammation may be prominent in the meninges, perivascular tissue, and neuropil, with neuronal degeneration and phagocytosis, causing the clinical manifestations of encephalitis or meningoencephalitis. On pathologic examination, multi-nucleated giant cells containing viral inclusions and cytopathic changes may be seen.

Post-infectious encephalitis, also called acute disseminated encephalomyelitis (ADEM), is an immune-mediated inflammatory disorder of the CNS. In contrast to viral encephalitis, no pathogens can be identified and, although perivascular inflammation and demyelination occur, the neurons are spared. Measles, mumps, rubella, VZV, St. Louis encephalitis, and influenza have all been linked to ADEM[84].

Clinical features

Patients with encephalitis often have signs and symptoms of both meningitis and parenchymal disease, making it difficult to differentiate clinically between meningitis and encephalitis. However, assessing for the signs and symptoms of encephalitis is a vital component in attempting to distinguish between meningitis and parenchymal infection, which carry distinct differential diagnoses and prognoses.

Unlike solitary meningitis, encephalitis manifests with cerebral dysfunction including delirium, lethargy, confusion, stupor and, at times, frank coma. Seizures are common, and focal neurologic deficits may develop. Certain physical examination findings may suggest a specific pathogen (*Table 88*).

CSF studies typically show an increased WBC count, but less than 250 cells/µl, with a lymphocytic pleocytosis. There may be an early predominance of neutrophils, but there is generally a shift to lymphocytes within hours. CSF also demonstrates a slightly elevated protein, but tends to remain <150 mg/dl (1.5 g/l) and normal glucose. The presence of a significant number of RBCs without a traumatic tap suggests necrotizing infection, such as that caused by HSV-1 encephalitis.

Differential diagnosis

- Herpesviruses (HSV-1 and -2, VZV, CMV, EBV, HHV-6, -7, and -8).
- Flaviviruses (St. Louis encephalitis virus, West Nile virus, dengue fever virus, yellow fever virus, Japanese encephalitis virus, tick-borne encephalitis).
- California encephalitis (e.g. La Crosse encephalitis virus).
- Togaviruses (Eastern equine encephalitis, Western equine encephalitis).
- Mumps.
- Measles.
- LCMV.
- Enteroviruses (e.g. coxsackieviruses and echoviruses).
- HIV.
- Influenza virus.
- PML.
- Rabies virus.
- Lyme disease.
- RMSF.
- Neurosyphilis.
- Brain abscess.
- Tuberculoma.
- Cryptococcal meningoencephalitis.
- Endemic mycoses (e.g. coccidioidomycosis, histoplasmosis, blastomycosis).
- Toxoplasmic encephalitis.
- Guillain–Barré syndrome.
- Metabolic encephalopathy.
- Drug- or toxin-induced encephalopathy.
- CNS vasculitis.
- Neoplasm, primary or metastatic.
- Reye's syndrome.

TABLE 88 **CLINICAL CLUES WHICH MAY SUGGEST A PARTICULAR PATHOGEN IN A PATIENT WITH ENCEPHALITIS**

Physical examination finding	Associated pathogens
Vesicular rash	Herpesviruses – oral or genital lesions are associated with HSV, whereas diffuse vesicles suggest chickenpox, and a dermatomal distribution is associated with zoster
Maculopapular rash	WNV, St. Louis encephalitis virus, syphilis, HIV
Petechial rash	Meningococcus, RMSF
Flaccid paralysis	WNV, St. Louis encephalitis virus
Tremors	WNV, St. Louis encephalitis virus
Parotitis	Mumps virus
Hydrophobia, aerophobia, muscular rigidity, pharyngeal spasms	Encephalitic rabies

HIV: human immunodeficiency virus; HSV: herpes simplex virus; RMSF: Rocky Mountain spotted fever; WNV: West Nile virus.

Investigations

As with aseptic meningitis, a thorough history and physical examination can provide major diagnostic clues in patients presenting with encephalitis. Epidemiologic information, such as travel history, sexual history, insect or animal contact (e.g. tick, mosquito, or bat bites), sick exposures, and vaccination history can lead the astute clinician toward a likely etiology. The season of illness is also important, since the incidence of some forms of viral meningoencephalitis increase as their vectors, such as mosquitoes or ticks, become most active.

All patients should have an LP, with measurement of OP, and have CSF analyzed for cell count and differential, protein, glucose, Gram stain and culture, acid-fast smear and culture, fungal stains and culture, PCR for HSV, PCR for enteroviruses, VDRL, and cytology. In general, viral cultures are insensitive and have largely been replaced by PCR testing. It is very important to test for HSV by PCR since this entity is often fatal if untreated. During the appropriate season, and depending upon geography, consider anti-West Nile virus (WNV) IgM and testing for antibodies against other arboviruses (see below).

If the patient is immunocompromised, consider sending *Toxoplasma* PCR, cryptococcal antigen, and PCR testing for VZV, CMV, EBV, HHV-6 and JC virus. In general, CSF will show a slightly increased WBC count, but tends to remain <250 cells/μl with lymphocyte predominance, slightly increased protein (but still <150 mg/dl [1.5 g/l]) and normal glucose.

In the appropriate season and depending upon travel, consider sending serum ELISA for anti-WNV and St. Louis encephalitis IgM antibodies or other arboviruses. All patients should have a serum HIV ELISA and confirmatory Western blot. Send a serum RPR, with FTA if positive, to work-up for neurosyphilis. Send serum for comprehensive chemistries and transaminases to assess for renal dysfunction, hyponatremia from SIADH, liver dysfunction, and hepatitis.

Consider electroencephalography (EEG), particularly in patients presenting with seizures. Consider performing electromyography (EMG) with nerve conduction studies (NCS) in patients with focal weakness or flaccid paralysis.

Herpesviruses

HSV-1 is the most common cause of sporadic viral encephalitis, and can occur any time of year. Both HSV-1 and -2 cause 10–20% of viral encephalitis cases in the USA, and almost all beyond the neonatal period are caused by HSV-1[85,86]. Neonates are at risk for HSV-2 encephalitis, if the mother has active genital lesions at the time of birth, an entity which can lead to severe neurologic sequelae. Other herpesviruses causing meningoencephalitis include VZV, EBV, CMV, and HHV-6. EBV is a common cause in children, accounting for 10% of cases[87].

HSV-1 can invade the CNS via retrograde transport (trigeminal or olfactory nerves), viremia, or reactivation of latent infection within the CNS. Infection most often leads to necrosis of the temporal lobes. HSV-1 encephalitis manifests as acute onset of fever, headache, aphasia, delirium, focal neurologic signs, and seizures. Behavioral abnormalities associated with HSV-1 encephalitis include mania, Klüver–Bucy syndrome (KBS), and amnesia, all of which are the result of temporal lobe inflammation and necrosis[88]. KBS manifests with varying behavioral changes including diminished anger or fear, dietary changes including overeating, hypersexuality, and visual agnosia.

CSF findings are typical of viral encephalitis, with a lymphocytic pleocytosis, elevated protein, and normal glucose. However, approximately 85% of patients also have increased RBC, indicating cerebral necrosis[89].

Diagnosis

CSF typically shows a lymphocytic pleocytosis and high protein. The presence of RBC may be from a traumatic tap, but are also suggestive of HSV-1 encephalitis. HSV PCR in the CSF is 98% sensitive and 94–100% specific[90].

In HSV encephalitis, MRI classically shows increased signal on T2-weighted images in the temporal and inferior frontal lobes, due to edema, necrosis, and hemorrhage (**441–444**). Temporal lobe lesions are often unilateral but can be bilateral. MRI is the most sensitive modality and the imaging test of choice. EEG abnormalities

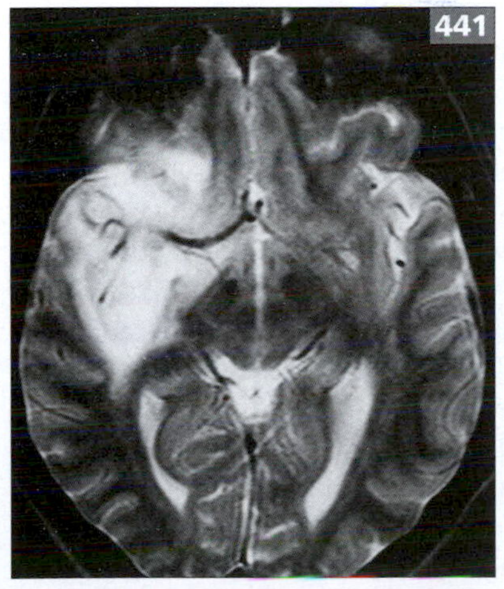

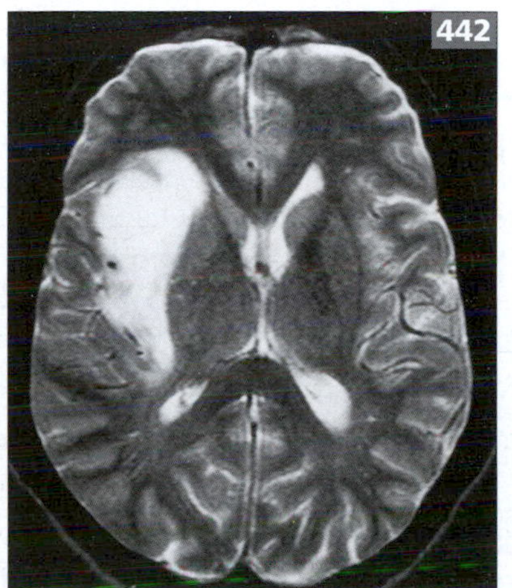

441, 442 MRI brain scan, T2-weighted images in the axial plane of a patient with herpes simplex encephalitis involving the right inferior frontal and antero-medial temporal lobe. The lesion extends to involve the external capsular region and the associated mass effect is seen to compress the frontal horn of the right lateral ventricle.

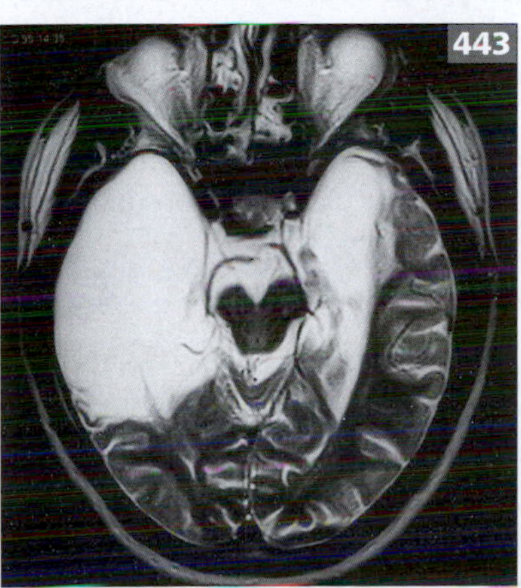

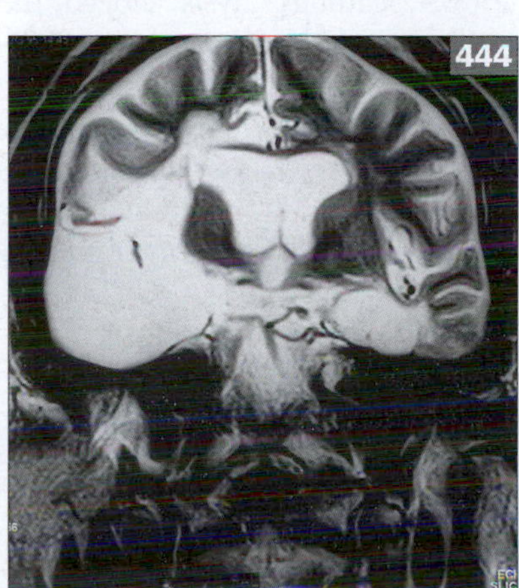

443, 444 MRI brain scan, T2-weighted images in the axial (443) and coronal (444) planes, showing extensive high density due to cystic gliotic change in the anterior three-quarters of the right temporal lobe, the medial left temporal lobe, the inferior and lateral right frontal lobe, the right insular cortex, and the right cingular gyrus of a patient with severe amnesia due to bilateral herpes simplex encephalitis several years previously. The right cerebral peduncle has atrophied.

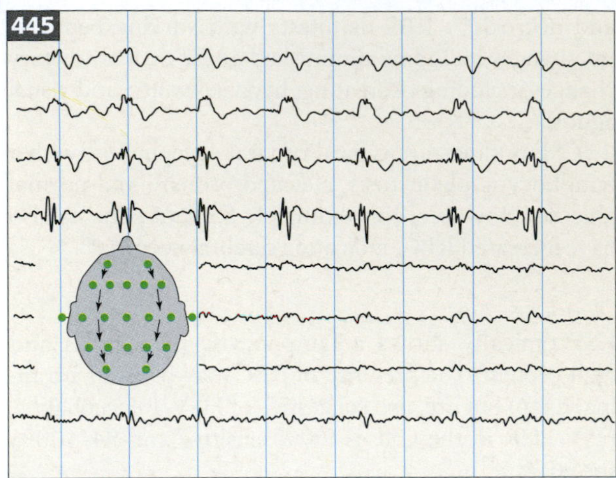

445 Electroencephalogram of a patient with herpes simplex encephalitis, showing complex discharges composed of spiky elements mixed with slower waveforms diffusely over the left hemisphere and recurring at not quite regular intervals. Periodic lateralized epileptiform discharges (PLEDs) usually indicate an acute or rapidly progressive focal brain lesion such as infarction, hemorrhage, glioblastoma, abscess, or encephalitis. Rarely, a severe metabolic disturbance may be present. Occasionally, PLEDs may be bilateral, such as in patients with severe brain injury due to hypoxia, encephalitis, and status epilepticus. PLEDs are usually short lived and disappear within a few weeks, irrespective of etiology and intervention, but a chronic seizure disorder may remain.

occur in more than 80% of patients and may be non-specific during the first few days with slow wave activity, but there is often evolution of characteristic periodic lateralized epileptiform discharges (PLED), consisting of paroxysmal, high voltage sharp waves, sharp and slow waves, spikes or multiple spikes with an amplitude of 50–100 mV (**445**).

Treatment

Clinicians should maintain a high index of suspicion of HSV encephalitis because antiviral therapy is available. In patients with suspected viral encephalitis, empiric therapy should always be initiated with high-dose IV acyclovir. Empirically begin acyclovir (10 mg/kg IV q8 hours) for a suspected diagnosis, and complete a 14–21 day course in patients with confirmed HSV encephalitis.

West Nile virus

WNV is by far the most common arbovirus to cause meningoencephalitis in the USA. It is a relatively recent clinical and epidemiologic phenomenon in the western hemisphere, with the first major outbreak occurring in 1999 in the northeastern portion of the USA, leading to 62 documented cases of encephalitis in New York[91]. Since that time, the virus has spread throughout the nation, causing sporadic infection and annual outbreaks in the summer and early fall.

In 2009, there were 339 cases of meningoencephalitis reported to the CDC, with 30 deaths; however, the incidence varies greatly from year to year[92]. Outbreaks caused more than 2000 WNV cases in 2002 and 2003 in the USA, but this is likely an underestimate since most patients are either asymptomatic or do not seek care. The most current estimates of USA incidence are available from the CDC ArboNET surveillance system at: http://cdc.gov/ncidod/dvbid/westnile/surv&control.htm.

WNV causes cases of encephalitis worldwide, including Africa, the Middle East, Europe, South Asia, and Australia[93]. Risk factors for encephalitis include older age, alcoholism, and diabetes mellitus[94].

Disease follows the bite of *Culex* spp. mosquitoes. Birds are the major amplifying host, particularly North American corvids (e.g. crows and ravens), with humans serving as incidental, dead-end hosts. There have also been reports of infection from organ transplantation[95] and transfusion of blood, platelets, and fresh frozen plasma[96], but universal screening of blood products has essentially eliminated this risk.

Only about 20% of patients with WNV infection have symptoms and fewer than 1% develop meningoencephalitis. After an incubation period of 2–14 days, patients present with fever, fatigue, headache, myalgias, and back pain, a clinical entity known as West Nile fever. A maculopapular rash develops in about 50% of patients with West Nile fever, and in a smaller proportion of those with neuroinvasive disease[97]. In a small number of patients, CNS disease can develop, presenting as meningitis, encephalitis, meningoencephalitis, and/or flaccid paralysis. Indeed, the presence of flaccid paralysis is highly suggestive of WNV infection.

Patients may also present with a variety of other neurologic signs and symptoms, including cranial nerve palsies, tremor, myoclonus, muscular rigidity, postural instability, and ocular manifestations including chorioretinitis and vitritis.

Diagnosis

CSF findings are typical of the viral encephalitides, including a lymphocytic pleocytosis, high protein, and normal glucose, although a neutrophil predominance is not uncommon. Testing for anti-WNV IgM antibodies in the CSF provides a sensitive and specific diagnosis.

Treatment

There is no specific treatment for WNV encephalitis and supportive care is standard. Ribavirin does possess *in vitro* activity against WNV, and other therapies such as interferon and intravenous immune globulin (IVIG) have been attempted; however, none has proven beneficial, and they cannot be recommended.

St. Louis encephalitis

St. Louis encephalitis is a mosquito-borne arbovirus causing disease in North and South America. It is a flavivirus, resembling WNV antigenically, pathophysiologically, and clinically. It is the second most common cause of epidemic viral encephalitis in the USA, following WNV.

Only 1 in 300 infections lead to clinical illness, resulting in a median of 100 reported cases of neuroinvasive disease each year in the USA; during epidemics however, thousands of clinically apparent infections may occur[98]. Elderly persons are at the greatest risk for this encephalitis following an exposure. Additionally, the mortality overall is 8%, but is around 20% in patients over 60 years of age.

The highest incidence is in the summer and early fall months, when mosquitoes are most active. As with WNV, female *Culex* spp. mosquitoes are the primary vectors, transmitting infection to humans through the saliva during a bite. Viremia leads to invasion of the brain or infection of olfactory neurons or peripheral nerves and subsequent retrograde axonal transport with rapid spread from cell to cell throughout the brain and spinal cord.

Most infections are subclinical. However, St. Louis encephalitis can result in a lymphocytic meningitis or rapidly progressive encephalitis with neuronal degeneration, particularly in the hypothalamus, hippocampus, cerebellum, cerebral cortex, basal ganglia, periventricular portions of the brainstem, and the anterior spinal cord.

After an incubation period of 4–21 days (mean of 7 days), patients experience a prodrome of fever, malaise, myalgias, and often a concomitant cough. Dysuria, urgency, and urinary incontinence are also common. CNS infection may lead to delirium, somnolence, tremors, cranial nerve abnormalities, myoclonus, nystagmus, dysarthria, or seizures.

As with WNV infection, some patients also experience a polio-like syndrome of flaccid paralysis. Post-infection clinical presentations include ADEM or Guillain–Barré syndrome[99]. One-third of patients have an increased OP, typically with a lymphocytic pleocytosis, elevated protein, and normal glucose. EEG reveals diffuse, generalized slowing and delta waves, with occasional focal discharges or seizure activity[100]. There are no specific findings on CT or MRI imaging.

Diagnosis

St. Louis encephalitis virus can occasionally be isolated from the blood prior to the development of an antibody response, typically in the first 7 days. However, virus is rarely cultured from the CSF. A positive CSF ELISA for anti-St. Louis encephalitis IgM antibodies in the setting of an appropriate clinical presentation and epidemiology provides a presumptive diagnosis. A definitive diagnosis requires a fourfold change in acute and convalescent serum antibody titers. However, St. Louis encephalitis antibodies do cross-react with other flaviviruses, including WNV, which has a similar clinical presentation and geographic distribution.

Treatment

No specific antiviral therapy is available, and management involves supportive care including fluids and electrolytes and attention to the patient's airway.

California encephalitis viruses

California encephalitis viruses are the most common cause of childhood encephalitis in the USA, with 60–130 cases annually; La Crosse virus is the cause of most cases. More than 90% of CNS disease occurs in children <15 years old, with males affected more than females[101].

La Crosse virus is transmitted in saliva via the bite of the female *Aedes triseriatus* mosquito. The highest incidence is in the upper midwest, although it does occur throughout the eastern USA[102,103].

Human disease occurs mainly in the summer and early fall, particularly in forested areas. Most infections are asymptomatic. However, after an incubation of 3–7 days, patients can experience a wide range of symptoms from a nonspecific febrile illness, to mild aseptic meningitis, to severe meningoencephalitis. The signs and symptoms of CNS disease are typical of the viral encephalitides, including fever, headache, nausea, vomiting, lethargy, confusion, focal neurologic deficits, and seizures. The CSF shows a mild pleocytosis with a slightly increased protein.

Diagnosis

ELISA for IgM in blood and CSF in the appropriate clinical scenario provides a presumptive diagnosis.

Treatment

While La Crosse virus is sensitive *in vitro* to ribavirin[104], and its use has been reported, there is a lack of clinical trials or sufficient experience using this agent to recommend its use in the management of La Crosse encephalitis.

RABIES

Definition and epidemiology

Rabies is a zoonotic infectious disease that has been well described for millennia. It is a neurotropic viral infection that can cause severe encephalitis which is almost uniformly fatal. Rabies virus is distributed world-wide, on all continents except Antarctica. The epidemiology of human rabies is correlated with the prevalence of, and exposure to, animal rabies in a given region. According to the World Health Organization (WHO), rabies causes approximately 55,000 deaths annually, with 30–50% of these occurring in children <15 years of age[105]; however, this is likely an underestimate because most cases occur in locations with limited resources and reporting.

Potential exposures are quite common world-wide, as represented by the observation that an estimated 4 million persons receive post-exposure treatment each year[106]. In the USA, human rabies is relatively rare, with only about three cases reported annually[107]. World-wide, dog bites account for the majority of human exposures. In the developing world, more than 90% of reported cases in humans are transmitted by canines[108]. However, in the USA, domestic animals are immunized against rabies, shifting the main vector from dogs to either unknown sources or bats. Indeed, bats are now thought to be the primary source of human rabies in the USA, with rabid bats documented in all 49 continental states[108,109]. From 1991–2007, only 34 naturally acquired, bat-associated human cases of rabies were reported in the USA, and most submitted bats (approximately 94%) will not be rabid[110]; however, the high mortality of rabies encephalitis necessitates a timely and thorough evaluation for all potential bat bite exposures.

Raccoons, skunks, coyotes, and foxes are the terrestrial mammals most often infected with rabies in the USA[111]. Raccoon rabies has greatly increased in incidence there since the 1970s, but has not caused a significant number of human cases. Rodents, including rats, mice, squirrels, and chipmunks, and lagomorphs (rabbits and hares) have not been known to transmit rabies to humans. Reliable reports of human-to-human transmission have exclusively been the result of organ transplantation from a rabies virus-infected donor[112], particularly in corneal transplants[113].

Etiology and pathophysiology

Rabies virus is a neurotropic pathogen in the family Rhabdoviridae, genus Lyssavirus, with *lyssa* being Greek for 'madness'. It is an enveloped, bullet-shaped virion with a single negative-stranded RNA genome.

Rabies virus is present in high concentrations in the saliva of clinically ill mammals due to viral shedding from nerve endings in the oral mucosa and local replication in the salivary glands[106]. Rabies is typically acquired from an animal bite, but can rarely be transmitted via large mucous membrane exposures or aerosolized virus.

Once rabies virus is deposited in peripheral wounds, it infects local myocytes, replicates, and spreads to the peripheral nerves innervating those muscle spindles. Retrograde passage then occurs from the periphery to the dorsal root ganglia and then to the brain. Rabies virus tends to localize to the spinal cord, brainstem, thalamus, and basal ganglia.

Clinical features

The average incubation period is 1–3 months, but can range from several days to several years[106,114].

Initially, the symptoms of rabies resemble those of other systemic viral infections, with fevers, chills, headache, sore throat, nausea, anorexia, and malaise. Pain or paresthesias at the site of inoculation may be the only early neurologic symptoms. This prodrome typically lasts less than 1 week. Once symptoms develop, rabies is almost universally fatal, leading to death an average of 18 days following symptom onset. The classic acute neurologic features of rabies are generally categorized as either encephalitic rabies ('furious') or paralytic rabies ('dumb').

Encephalitic rabies ('furious')

This is the most well-known clinical presentation, occurring in approximately 80% of patients with classic rabies. Hydrophobia (fear of water), agitation, hyperactivity, autonomic stimulation (e.g. hypersalivation), and progressive delirium are common manifestations. Hydrophobia results from exaggerated, reflexive, painful muscular spasms of the pharynx and upper airways when attempting to swallow liquids. Because of difficulties swallowing saliva, paroxysms may occur without exposure to water. The irritation caused by a simple gust of air may trigger upper airway spasms. Anxiety and anticipation may lead to acute spasms at the mere sight or sound of dripping water. Encephalitic rabies progresses to coma and death.

Paralytic rabies ('dumb')

This form manifests as an ascending paralysis and may evolve to a symmetric quadriparesis, resembling Guillain–Barré syndrome. The spinal cord and brainstem are predominantly affected, with little evidence of cerebral involvement until late in the course. No hydrophobia is seen. Like 'furious' rabies, it eventually progresses to coma and death.

Atypical neurologic presentations of rabies include meningitis, neuropathic pain, sensory or motor deficits, focal brainstem signs, cranial nerve palsies, myoclonus, and seizures. The non-neurologic manifestations are dominated by myocarditis and cardiac arrhythmias, but gastrointestinal symptoms may be prominent early in the course.

Differential diagnosis

The differential diagnosis is somewhat limited in a patient with encephalitis and hydrophobia following a feral animal bite; however, many patients do not give a history of significant zoonotic exposure. The differential varies with specific neurologic manifestations.

- Encephalitic rabies ('furious'): other viral causes of encephalitis (enteroviruses, arboviruses, herpesviruses), tetanus, strychnine poisoning, PML, prion diseases.
- Paralytic rabies ('dumb'): Guillain–Barré syndrome, poliomyelitis, transverse myelitis, botulism, tick paralysis.

Investigations

Since rabies is a clinical diagnosis, the clinician should always take a detailed history and perform a comprehensive physical examination. An LP should be performed, but routine analysis is nonspecific and typically resembles aseptic meningoencephalitis, with a modest lymphocytic pleocytosis, normal glucose, and a slightly elevated protein (<100 mg/dl [1 g/l]).

To establish the diagnosis, one or more of the following rabies-specific investigations should be performed:

- Skin biopsy (test of choice): a full thickness biopsy of skin should be taken from the posterior neck at the hairline, containing a minimum of ten hair follicles and associated cutaneous nerves. Real time PCR (RT-PCR) and DFA staining for viral antigens can be performed.
- Saliva: send for RT-PCR to detect viral RNA.
- Serum and CSF: send both for antibody testing, which is essentially diagnostic if the patient has not been immunized previously. If there is a history of immunization, the clinician can compare serum titers for a rise after a few days. The presence of antibodies in the CSF is highly suggestive of rabies.
- Brain biopsy: rarely performed unless post-mortem. RT-PCR and DFA staining can be performed.

Diagnosis

The early diagnosis of rabies is clinical, and based on history, signs, symptoms, and nonspecific testing modalities (e.g. radiography, LP). However, to have an effect on mortality, the patient should be given post-exposure treatment prior to the entry of virions into peripheral nerves.

Therefore, most diagnoses of rabies are made after exposure, but prior to symptom onset. A history of a bite from a potentially rabid animal or other significant zoonotic exposure should prompt post-exposure treatment.

A definitive diagnosis requires at least one of the above rabies-specific tests from a skin biopsy, saliva, or brain biopsy. Antibody testing may be suggestive, but does not provide a definitive diagnosis. DFA staining of brain tissue on necropsy is the gold standard for a definitive diagnosis. On histology of brain tissue, infection typically appears as encephalitis with Negri bodies, which are eosinophilic neuronal cytoplasmic inclusions. Negri bodies are pathognomonic for rabies, but are not always present in tissue specimens.

Treatment

Once the virus has entered peripheral nerves, administration of Ig and vaccine likely does not prevent central spread, neurologic disease, or mortality. Therapy for symptomatic rabies is entirely supportive, with a focus on comfort care, pain control, and sedation. Timely administration of human rabies immune globulin (HRIG) and rabies vaccine for prophylaxis of infection in the asymptomatic patient can provide passive and active immunity following an exposure, preventing spread of rabies virus to the CNS[108,115]. Following a risky zoonotic exposure, the CDC and WHO both recommend prompt and thorough wound cleansing, followed by post-exposure treatment with HRIG and rabies vaccine. The decision to provide treatment should be made on a case-by-case basis. Infectious diseases consultation and the advice of public health authorities are recommended. Details are beyond the scope of this text.

Prevention

The CDC Advisory Committee on Immunization Practices (ACIP) offers detailed, evidence-based, up-to-date recommendations regarding human rabies prevention[108]. Vaccine (1.0 ml) is given intramuscularly for both pre- and post-exposure prophylaxis. An effective antibody response requires about 7–10 days, and detectable, neutralizing antibodies persist for several years.

Pre-exposure vaccine

Three separate doses are given for pre-exposure prophylaxis (days 0, 7, and 21 or 28). Vaccination is generally limited to high-risk groups, such as veterinarians, laboratory workers who may come into contact with rabies virus, and international travelers who are likely to come into contact with animals in countries where dog rabies is enzootic and rapid access to post-exposure treatment is limited.

Post-exposure prophylaxis

Infection with rabies can be prevented with timely post-exposure treatment. Passive immunization with HRIG provides immediate virus-neutralizing antibodies, lasting a short time (half-life about 21 days)[116]. All healthy persons should develop neutralizing antibodies 2–4 weeks after receiving vaccine. The clinician should weigh the risk-*vs*.-benefit ratio and consult with infectious diseases and public health specialists in deciding whether or not to administer post-exposure treatment. Several aspects of the exposure need to be considered:

- Type of exposure (bite or nonbite).
- Circumstances (provoked or unprovoked bite).
- Species and vaccination status of the animal.
- Epidemiology of animal rabies in the region.
- Whether the animal can be captured and observed or tested for rabies.
- Vaccination status of the patient.
- Reliability of the reporter (e.g. children).

POLIOMYELITIS

Definition and epidemiology

Poliomyelitis is a systemic viral infectious disease, primarily affecting motor neurons of the brain and spinal cord, resulting in flaccid paralysis. Poliovirus infection is a vaccine-preventable disease that has essentially been eradicated in the developed world, but clinicians should still be cognizant of its epidemiology and clinical manifestations.

Through the first half of the 20th century, polio epidemics were common world-wide, including in the USA. Outbreaks occurred most often during the summer months, with a higher incidence in temperate climates and areas with poor sanitation.

Poliovirus is acquired by the oropharyngeal route and can spread rapidly through communities, since most cases are asymptomatic, yet virus can be shed in the feces for weeks following initial infection. Age and gender do not directly influence transmission, but there is a higher incidence in children, with more than 50% of cases occurring in those under 3 years old[117].

There has been a very successful global effort to eradicate disease, beginning with licensure of the Salk trivalent inactivated vaccine (1955) and the Sabin trivalent oral live attenuated vaccine (1961). Mass vaccination programs have had a particularly great impact over the last two decades. In 1988, there were more than 350,000 cases world-wide, which dropped dramatically to approximately 1500 reported cases in 2009[118]. Due to prevention programs and universal vaccination, the western hemisphere, Europe, and most of Asia are free from endemic ('wild-type') poliomyelitis. The last cases of naturally occurring poliomyelitis in the USA occurred in 1978–79[119].

According to the WHO, poliomyelitis is now only endemic in four countries: India, Pakistan, Afghanistan, and Nigeria[117]. However, due to the ease of world-wide travel, there continues to be importation of cases from endemic areas that may lead to outbreaks in countries thought to previously be free of polio.

Etiology and pathophysiology

Poliovirus is a member of the genus Enterovirus, a group of human viral pathogens that also includes coxsackieviruses, echoviruses, and other nonpolio enteroviruses. Poliovirus is further subclassified into three different serotypes (types 1, 2, and 3).

The main route of transmission for poliovirus is fecal–oral, although oral–oral transmission occurs as well, particularly during epidemics. The virus initially undergoes replication in the gut and gastrointestinal lymphatic tissue, followed in 7–14 days by an asymptomatic 'minor' viremia, during which time the virus spreads to the reticuloendothelial system. In approximately 5% of individuals, a second 'major' viremia occurs, causing symptoms that are not easily distinguished from those induced by many other viral infections, such as headache, pharyngitis, fever, nausea, vomiting, abdominal pain, listlessness, malaise, and fatigue. This viral syndrome is known as the 'minor illness' or abortive poliomyelitis.

In a fraction of these patients, involvement of the CNS then occurs, heralded by signs and symptoms of meningitis, including severe headache, fever, nuchal rigidity, and photophobia. In some of these patients, poliovirus then causes selective destruction of motor neurons, characterized by the development of motor weakness. Overall, paralysis occurs in only about 0.1% of all poliovirus infections[120].

The mechanism of spread to the CNS is not well understood. After invading the CNS, viral replication occurs, destroying motor neurons and leading to paralysis of the muscle fibers they innervate. Spread of virus to the neighboring motor neurons may occur laterally, independent of axonal transport or by transneuronal spread. Other neurons may be affected, including autonomic fibers, leading to signs and symptoms of vascular collapse and respiratory insufficiency.

Clinical features

Over 90% of poliovirus infections are asymptomatic. In children, the clinical course is often biphasic, first consisting of 'minor illness' (abortive poliomyelitis) with a typical viral syndrome, which then resolves leaving the patient symptom-free for 2–5 days. This may be followed by the 'major illness', which encompasses the neurologic manifestations of polio. The pre-paralytic 'major illness' manifests classically as aseptic meningitis, with headache, fever, photophobia, nuchal rigidity, nausea, and vomiting. The neurologic manifestations are generally classified into three types.

Spinal paralytic poliomyelitis (>60% of cases)

Classic paralytic polio often begins with severe muscle pain and spasms. This is followed by fasciculations and weakness of the lower limbs (more than upper limbs) and proximal muscles (more than distal muscles). Progression of the patient's weakness peaks in 48 hours, halting after 5–7 days.

The clinician observes flaccid muscle tone, nearly always in an asymmetric distribution. Reflexes are initially brisk, but then become absent as neuronal destruction progresses. The paralytic manifestations may be minor (one muscle or group of muscles) or severe (quadriplegia and respiratory failure). The sensory examination is usually normal, and sensory loss should suggest another diagnosis, such as Guillain–Barré syndrome. The flaccid paralysis of poliomyelitis remains stable for several days or weeks, followed by a slow recovery over months to years.

New sprouting and re-innervation of muscle by surviving motor neurons must occur for recovery. Approximately two-thirds of patients with acute flaccid paralysis do not regain full strength.

Bulbar paralytic poliomyelitis (20% of cases, range of 5–35%)

Poliovirus may also destroy motor neurons of the brainstem, resulting in bulbar paralytic manifestations. Most commonly, the lower cranial nerve nuclei are affected, including those neurons innervating the soft palate and pharynx, resulting in dysphagia, dysphonia, dysarthria, and difficulty handling secretions. Tongue wasting and fasciculations are seen on physical examination (**446**).

Bulbar polio may result in respiratory failure and vasomotor disturbances (hypo- and hypertension, circulatory collapse) requiring aggressive supportive care in an intensive care unit.

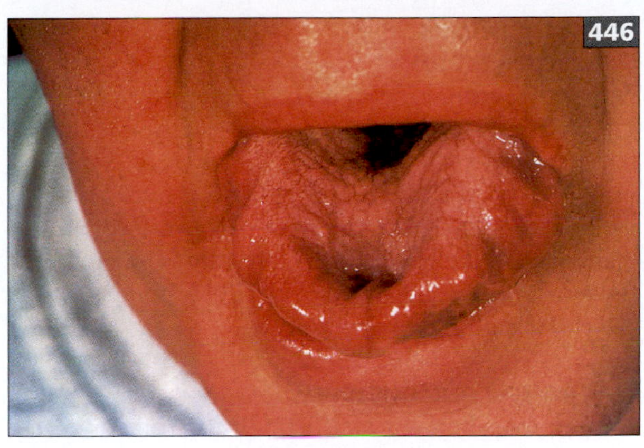

446 Tongue wasting and fasciculation due to necrosis of neurons in the hypoglossal (XIIth cranial) nerve nucleus.

Polioencephalitis

Frank encephalitis from poliovirus is relatively rare, but occasionally occurs in infancy. It is clinically indistinguishable from other forms of viral encephalitis, presenting with signs and symptoms such as agitation, confusion, disturbances of consciousness, stupor, coma, and seizures. A very high index of suspicion is required to make the diagnosis. Polioencephalitis carries a high risk of infant mortality.

Differential diagnosis

- Vaccine-associated paralytic poliomyelitis (VAPP).
- Nonpolio enteroviruses (coxsackie A and B, echovirus, enterovirus 70 and 71).
- WNV.
- Transverse myelitis
- Gullain–Barré syndrome (distinguished by symmetry, a disparate sensory examination, and lack of preceding signs and symptoms of meningitis or CSF pleocytosis).
- HIV encephalitis.
- PML.
- Diphtheria.
- Botulism.
- Lyme disease (*Borrelia burgdorferi*).
- Tick paralysis.
- Neurosyphilis.
- Acute porphyria.
- Ischemia or infarction of the spinal cord.
- Spinal cord compression.
- Myasthenia gravis.
- Disorders of muscle (various myopathies or rhabdomyolysis, distinguished by symmetry and high creatine kinase in serum, normal CSF parameters).

Investigations

Lumbar puncture

Early in the 'major illness' of poliomyelitis, a CSF pleocytosis may be seen (neutrophilic in the first few days, converting to a lymphocytic predominance) with increased protein and normal glucose. It essentially presents as aseptic meningitis. Send fluid for cell count with differential, protein, glucose, PCR for enteroviruses, PCR for herpesviruses and WNV. RT-PCR for poliovirus may be helpful if it is available.

Culture and serology

Culture may be used to isolate virus from the nasopharynx (in the first week) or stool (shed for several weeks). Nonpolio enteroviruses are in the differential diagnosis, and the lab should be notified of this when ordering viral cultures.

It is difficult to make a definitive diagnosis using serum antibody testing, but the lab can compare acute and convalescent sera.

EMG

Early in poliomyelitis, there is a reduced recruitment and interference pattern with voluntary muscle activation. Later, at rest, EMG is electrically silent, with fibrillations developing in 2–4 weeks and persisting indefinitely. Motor unit action potentials are reduced in number but return during recovery, becoming abnormally large in amplitude, with increased duration and a polyphasic pattern due to reinnervation. Motor conduction velocities remain normal.

Other studies

Other studies to consider in acute flaccid paralysis: serum HIV antibodies, serum creatine kinase, Lyme titers if the epidemiology is suggestive, examination of the skin for ticks, ESR and autoimmune serologies for vasculitis, MRI of the brain and spinal cord, nerve or muscle biopsy.

Diagnosis

The diagnosis of poliomyelitis relies on a high clinical suspicion. It is based on the clinical presentation of acute, asymmetric, flaccid paralysis and early CSF findings consistent with aseptic meningitis.

Poliomyelitis is confirmed by isolation of the virus from oropharyngeal swabs or stool cultures. CSF RT-PCR for poliovirus RNA can be used as well, although clinical experience is somewhat limited[121].

Pathology

Poliovirus principally affects motor, and sometimes autonomic, neurons of the brain and spinal cord. Neuronal destruction is followed by inflammatory infiltration with polymorphonuclear leukocytes (PMN), lymphocytes, and macrophages. After inflammation subsides, necrosis predominates on histologic examination. Lesions mainly affect the gray matter of the anterior, intermediate, and posterior horns of the spinal cord and motor nuclei of the pons and medulla.

Treatment

The treatment of poliomyelitis is supportive, including pain control, mechanical ventilation (if necessary), management of secretions, cardiovascular support if autonomic dysfunction occurs, and physical therapy during the recovery phase. There is no role at this time for antiviral therapy. Pleconaril is an oral antiviral with activity against enteroviruses[122] that has shown mixed results for the treatment of enteroviral encephalitis[123]. Pleconaril cannot currently be recommended for treatment of poliomyelitis.

Post-polio syndrome

Post-polio syndrome is the onset of functional deterioration after a prolonged period of stability in a patient with a history of polio, and may occur many years after the initial episode. It generally manifests as progressive muscle pain, weakness, wasting, and fatigue. It occurs in about 25–30% of patients who previously experienced paralysis[124]. Approximately two-thirds of these patients have another potential contributing cause that can be identified (e.g. osteoarthritis, weight gain, atrophy from lack of use); however, one-third of patients have no other explanation. The exact cause remains unknown, but there is no evidence of intrinsic neuromuscular disease.

Post-polio syndrome can present complex management issues, with patients experiencing chronic pain, contractures, depression, fatigue, and sleep disorders. Treatment options include physical therapy for strength conditioning, nutritional education, and antidepressants.

Prevention

Jonas Salk created the highly effective trivalent intramuscular inactivated poliovirus vaccine (IPV) using killed virus in 1952, and routine use began in 1956. IPV is the only vaccine available in the USA for routine childhood immunization, and is preferred in many other countries due to the small but real risk of VAPP with oral poliovirus vaccine (OPV). Because of the risk of VAPP with OPV, IPV is always the preferred formulation in pregnancy and for immunocompromised patients and people over age 50 years. IPV is available alone or in other formulations which include DTaP, hepatitis B, or Hib vaccines.

In the USA, the IPV series is recommended universally in children. It consists of four separate injections at 2 months, 4 months, 6–18 months, and a fourth dose prior to entering school. Neutralizing antibodies are detectable to all three serotypes of poliovirus in >90% of IPV recipients after two doses, 100% after the third dose[125,126], and detectable antibodies persist for at least 5 years[127].

The Sabin trivalent live attenuated OPV became available in 1962. It is taken orally, leading to both serum antibody and local secretory IgA production. OPV is the vaccine currently recommended by the WHO Program on Immunization. It has been reported (rarely) to cause VAPP in both recipients and their contacts[128]. Therefore, it is no longer licensed in the USA, but it remains important in developing countries due to lower cost, ease of administration, induction of mucosal immunity, and secondary immunization of others resulting from transmission of vaccine virus to unimmunized contacts. The efficacy with three doses is nearly 100%[122], and antibodies persist for at least 5 years in the vast majority of patients[129].

OPV is recommended for infants starting at 2 months of age, given in three separate doses, with intervals of 1 month between doses. Where poliomyelitis is endemic, primary immunization with Sabin OPV causes disease in 1:900,000 on the first dose[130]. The risk is higher in those with immunodeficiency and it is contraindicated in these patients.

PROGRESSIVE MULTIFOCAL LEUKOENCEPHALOPATHY (PML)

Definition and epidemiology

PML is an aggressively demyelinating disease of the CNS, preferentially manifesting in immunosuppressed patients. It results from reactivation of remote JCV infection and subsequent destruction of myelin-producing oligodendrocytes.

JCV infection is ubiquitous and usually acquired in childhood, with approximately 70–85% of adults in the USA possessing antibodies to the virus[131,132]. PML was once quite rare, but the HIV pandemic has changed the epidemiology dramatically. PML was seen occasionally in patients with hematologic malignancies[133,134], steroid use[135], or the rare patient of advanced age. It has also been reported in presumably immunocompetent individuals. However, PML is currently considered a disease of the immunocompromised, particularly those with AIDS and patients receiving cytotoxic chemotherapy or other immunosuppressive agents. More than 50% of all deaths from PML occur in HIV-infected individuals, and it is estimated that 1–4% of patients with HIV will develop PML[136].

Since the advent of highly active antiretroviral therapy (HAART) and the ability to improve cellular immune function in patients with AIDS, the incidence of PML has decreased among HIV-infected patients. PML is an AIDS-defining disease, and most patients have a CD4 T-cell count of <200 cells/μl. The incidence of PML has been estimated to be 0.07% among patients with hematologic malignancies[137].

Etiology and pathophysiology

JCV is a small, nonenveloped, polyomavirus (a DNA virus), similar to BK virus. The letters 'JC' refer to the initials of the patient from whom the initial viral isolate was obtained (John Cunningham). It is unclear exactly how JCV is contracted, but acute infection appears to begin in the tonsils and oropharynx, followed shortly by viremia.

The pathophysiology of active CNS infection in PML has not been defined. Infection of mononuclear cells may play a role in transporting JCV into the CNS after reactivation of infection in the kidneys. Alternatively, PML may result from reactivation of infection in the CNS. JCV can be found in the brain tissue of patients without PML, suggesting latent infection[138].

Clinical features

The classic clinical picture of PML is that of subacute onset of focal neurologic deficits without fever or other constitutional manifestations. Common signs and symptoms include hemiparesis, visual field defects, cortical blindness, cognitive impairment, ataxia, aphasia, and cranial nerve dysfunction. Rapid progression occurs following diagnosis, resulting in quadraparesis, severe dementia, seizures, and coma.

Disease is localized to the cerebral white matter, although there can also be involvement of the cerebellum, brainstem, and spinal cord. Many patients experience death within 6 months of the initial diagnosis, although the prognosis has improved with the advent of HAART[134].

Differential diagnosis

- HIV/AIDS-associated dementia.
- Neurosyphilis.
- Toxoplasmosis.
- Herpesvirus encephalitis (HSV, CMV).
- Multiple sclerosis.
- Cerebral infarction.
- CNS lymphoma (EBV-associated) or other malignancies.
- Immunosuppression-induced leukoencephalopathy from tacrolimus, cyclosporine, fluorouracil, or levamisole.

Investigations

- Imaging with CT or MRI of the brain: MRI is more sensitive and the preferred modality.
- LP may be deferred until imaging has been performed to rule out mass effect. However, CSF analysis can be helpful in making the diagnosis, and should include cell count and differential, protein, glucose, JCV PCR, HSV PCR, CMV PCR, EBV PCR, VDRL, *Toxoplasma* PCR, and cytology.
- If it is a diagnostic possibility, serum anti-*Toxplasma* IgG may help stratify this pathogen in the differential diagnosis.
- Serum RPR.
- HIV ELISA and confirmatory Western blot if not already performed.
- Brain biopsy may be necessary.

Due to the high prevalence in the general population, serum antibodies against JCV are *not* helpful in making the diagnosis.

Diagnosis

CT scans reveal hypodense, nonenhancing lesions in the bilateral cerebral white matter. There is no mass effect or surrounding edema. MRI is more sensitive and preferred. On MRI, PML appears as white matter lesions with *decreased* signal intensity on T1-weighted images and *increased* signal on T2-weighted images (**447–449**).

CSF parameters are typically normal in PML, although there may be a mild lymphocytic pleocytosis or high protein. PCR to amplify JCV DNA can be performed on spinal fluid, and the sensitivity is 60–100%, depending upon the study[139]. JCV has been detected by PCR in patients without PML, and is nonspecific in patients without neurologic deficits consistent with the diagnosis. However, if the pre-test probability is high, it is highly specific. Detection of JCV DNA in the CSF of a patient with a compatible clinical syndrome and radiologic imaging is highly supportive of the diagnosis of PML.

Pathology

A definitive diagnosis is made with brain biopsy, and sterotactic biopsy may be required in some circumstances. However, brain biopsy is usually unnecessary. Histologic examination reveals multiple asymmetric foci of demyelination in differing stages of evolution, found in the cortical and subcortical white matter (**450**). JC virus infects oligodendrocytes, resulting in decreased myelin production and demyelination. The enlarged oligodendrocytes show nuclear enlargement and intranuclear hyperchromatic inclusions (**451**) with homogenous staining. Astrocytes may have undergone marked enlargement with irregularly shaped nuclei[133,134]. In general, there are minimal inflammatory changes, but perivascular inflammation has been described, particularly in patients on antiretroviral therapy presenting with immune reconstitution inflammatory syndrome (IRIS).

Treatment

Several medical therapies have been investigated, including cidofovir[140,141], cytarabine[142], interferon[143], and interleukin-2[144], but several trials have been disappointing and there are not enough good clinical data to recommend any of these agents. The best therapy is re-establishment of immune function by treating AIDS patients with antiretroviral therapy, which results in an increase in 1-year survival to approximately 50%[145]. There have been several reports of worsening symptoms caused by IRIS in HIV-positive PML patients treated with antiretroviral therapy.

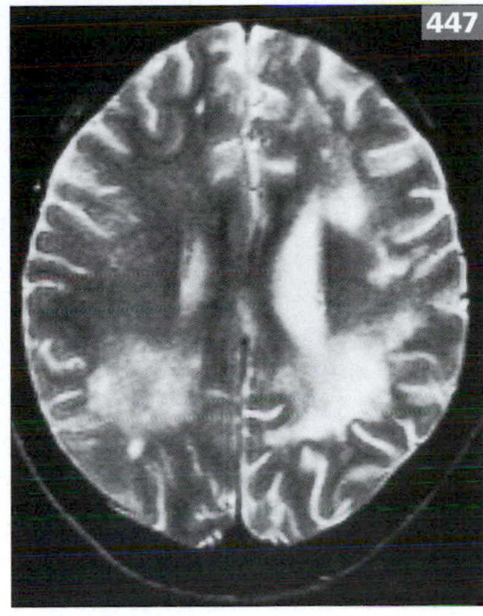

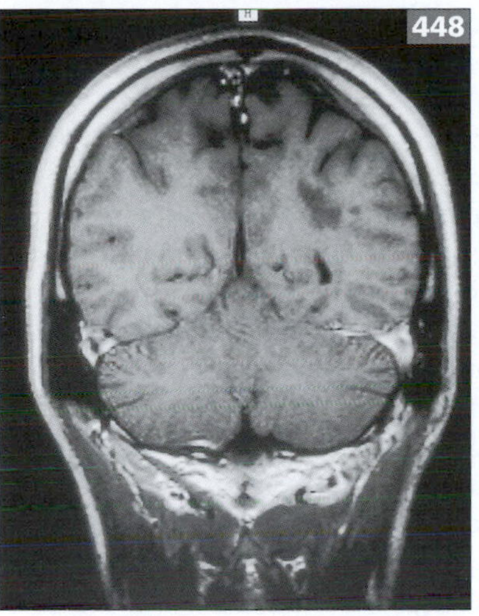

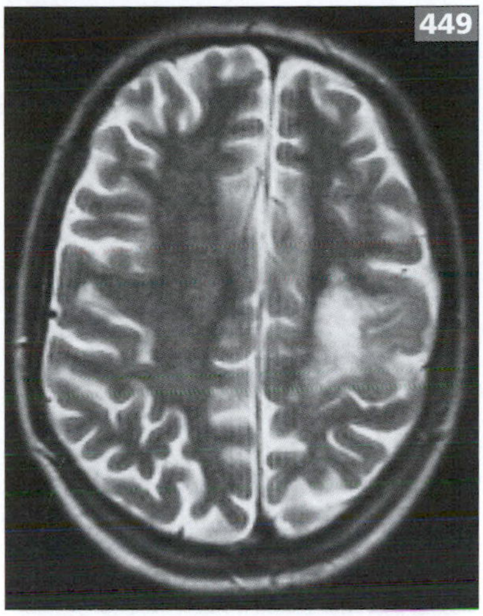

447, 448 T2-weighted axial (447) and T1-weighted coronal (448) MRI with contrast, showing a nonenhancing area on T1-weighted image and high intensity on T2-weighted image in the parietal region typical of PML. *Courtesy of Professor J. Best, Department of Medical Radiology, Royal Infirmary, Edinburgh, UK.*

449 T2-weighted MRI of the brain, showing biopsy-proven progressive multifocal leukoencephalopathy in an HIV-infected patient. Note the T2-weighted high-signal abnormalities involving the parietal subcortical white matter and sparing the cerebral cortex.

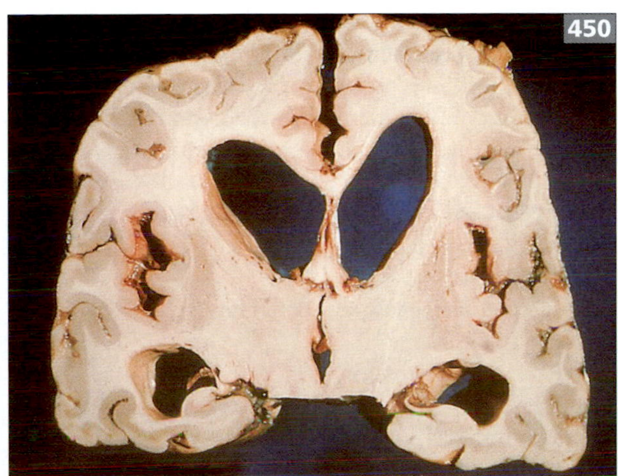

450 Microscopic low power section of cerebral cortex and subcortical white matter, myelin stain, showing multiple foci of demyelination (i.e. lack of staining) in a patient with progressive multifocal leukoencephalopathy.

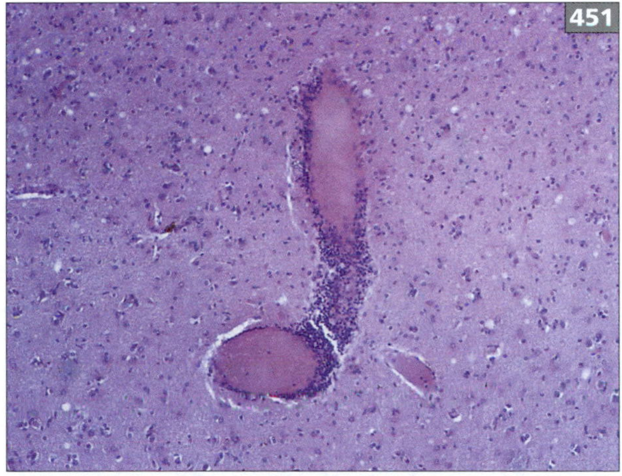

451 Histologic section of cerebral white matter, showing large 'ballooned' oligodendroglial cells with hyperchromatic, enlarged nuclei, and nuclear inclusions which contain many virions.

CRYPTOCOCCOSIS

Definition and epidemiology

Cryptococcal meningoencephalitis represents invasive CNS infection with the encapsulated yeast *Cryptococcus neoformans*. The term 'meningoencephalitis' is often used instead of 'meningitis,' and appropriately so, since the infection almost always involves the brain parenchyma.

C. neoformans is a ubiquitous environmental saprophyte, found in soil and decaying vegetation world-wide. These yeasts thrive in the gastrointestinal tract of some birds, such as pigeons and chickens, and are often found near bird roosts. Organisms do not cause disease in these intermediate hosts, but can become infectious to humans when inhaled.

C. gattii is an occasional human pathogen. It is not associated with bird guano, but occupies a specific environmental niche in some tropical and subtropical regions, particularly associated with Eucalyptus trees in Australia.

Cryptococcal meningoencephalitis is almost always a disease of the immunocompromised host, and is most commonly associated with underlying conditions such as HIV/AIDS, solid organ and stem cell transplantation, malignancy and chemotherapy, sarcoidosis, systemic lupus erythematosus, and the sustained use of moderate-to high-dose glucocorticoids or monoclonal antibodies (e.g. alemtuzumab and infliximab). The most common underlying predisposing condition is HIV/AIDS. Isolated pulmonary disease is seen in healthy individuals, but disseminated or CNS infection is rare in the normal host.

The incidence of infection in patients with HIV/AIDS has decreased significantly in the era of HAART, but remains a common AIDS-associated opportunistic infection. In patients with AIDS, the highest risk of infection begins with CD4 T-cell counts <100 cells/µl. Worldwide, an estimated 1 million cases of cryptococcal meningitis occur annually, resulting in more than 600,000 deaths and making it the fourth most common opportunistic infection in people with AIDS[146].

Etiology and pathophysiology

Cryptococci are unicellular, encapsulated yeasts. Nineteen species have been identified; however, *C. neoformans* (variety *neoformans* or *gattii*) causes the vast majority of human infections. Several virulence factors have been identified, including the polysaccharide capsule, the production of melanin, and rapid growth at human body temperature (37°C [98.6°F]). These traits allow the organism to evade host immunity, deplete complement, cause cytokine dysregulation, protect cryptococci from temperature changes and antifungals, and inhibit phagocytosis[147]. The susceptibility to, and severity of, infection are related to the host immunologic status and the size of the fungal inoculum. Inhalation of infectious propagules initiates infection, followed often by dissemination, including to the CNS. There has been no documented person-to-person transmission.

Clinical features

A defining feature of CNS cryptococcosis is the indolent nature of symptom onset. The typical picture is that of a subacute course of fever, headache, photophobia, nuchal rigidity, nausea, vomiting, malaise, and even frank coma. Patients often complain of progressive symptoms for 1–3 weeks, or occasionally a matter of months. Approximately 25% of patients present with altered mentation, suggesting clinically apparent encephalitis.

A prominent clinical finding is increased ICP, which is often the cause of severe headache and focal neurologic deficits. Cryptococcosis is known to cause vasculitis and ischemic stroke[148], and it should be considered in the differential diagnosis of cerebrovascular disease in the immunocompromised patient.

Patients with disseminated infection can present with signs and symptoms at multiple sites, most commonly the lungs and skin, but any organ system can be involved. Concomitant pulmonary disease is suggested by cough, shortness of breath, crackles on lung examination, and infiltrates on chest X-ray. The classic skin rash presents as umbilicated papules resembling molluscum contagiosum, but with a greater tendency to have central ulceration.

Differential diagnosis

- Toxoplasmosis.
- Nocardiosis.
- Tuberculous meningoencephalitis.
- Neurosyphilis.
- Bacterial brain abscess.
- Endemic mycoses (e.g. CNS histoplasmosis, blastomycosis, coccidioidomycosis).
- CNS lymphoma.
- Metastatic malignancy.
- CNS vasculitis.

Tip

▶ *Several pathogens are known to cause vasculitis, particularly Cryptococcus spp. Always consider cryptococcal vasculitis, as well as neurosyphilis and TB meningitis, in the young adult immunocompromised patient presenting with stroke.*

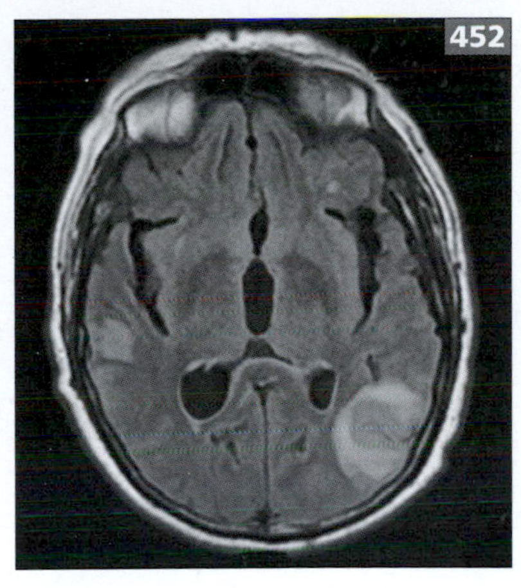

452, 453 **T2 FLAIR images from the same patient with cryptococcoma. (452) Leptomeningeal enhancement with areas of edema, hydrocephalus, and ventriculitis. (453) Cystic mass with surrounding T2 bright signal abnormality in the left cerebral peduncle.** *Courtesy of Dr. Edward Michals, University of Illinois at Chicago.*

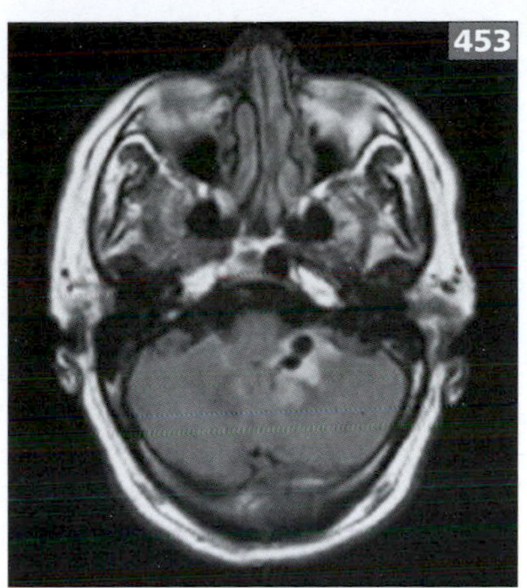

Investigations

LP is the most important test for the diagnosis of CNS cryptococcosis. Standard Gram staining, cultures, glucose, and protein should be sent on the CSF, as well as India ink staining (or other fungal stains) to look for encapsulated yeast. Considering the high organism burden in patients with HIV and low CD4 T-cell counts, fungal stains are often diagnostic, with about 75% sensitivity of India ink on pre-treatment spinal fluid. If cryptococcosis is suspected, a vital component of LP is the assessment of OP. CSF pressures are often quite high, with more than 70% of patients presenting with an OP of >20 cmH_2O. Patients with a pre-treatment opening pressure <25 cmH_2O tend to have increased short-term survival[149].

Another important study is the CSF cryptococcal antigen, both for diagnosis and prognosis. For those patients in whom CSF stains and cultures are negative, cryptococcal antigen testing provides a sensitive and specific adjunct, with a sensitivity of 93–100% and specificity of 93–98%[150]. Higher titers correlate with a greater organism burden and a worse prognosis.

Patients presenting with cryptococcal meningoencephalitis should always be tested for HIV infection, as it is often the presenting, AIDS-defining diagnosis.

In general, neuroimaging should be performed in immunocompromised patients prior to performing an LP. This is particularly true in cryptococcal infection, since patients can have focal lesions and high ICP and hydrocephalus, which may require a shunting procedure.

If LP cannot be performed, a serum cryptococcal antigen is highly suggestive of invasive disease outside the lungs, being more than 90% sensitive and specific[151]. Use in bronchoalveolar lavage fluid or urine is not recommended. While the titer has some prognostic use, with initially high titers suggesting a higher burden of infection and a greater risk of treatment failure, serial antigen titers are not specific and values may vary widely. Therefore, they should not be used to make treatment decisions.

Blood cultures should be sent. Standard automated blood culture methods should be adequate to grow the organism, but lysis-centrifugation can increase the yield of *Cryptococcus* and some other fungal and intracellular pathogens.

Diagnosis

The inflammatory response is blunted in the spinal fluid of patients with AIDS and cryptococcal meningoencephalitis. WBC counts are characteristically low (<50 cells/μl) with a mononuclear predominance. CSF protein levels are slightly elevated with hypoglycorrhachia. Indeed, the CSF glucose can be quite low. However, a normal spinal fluid profile does not rule out infection, since 25–30% of patients with AIDS and CNS cryptococcosis have no CSF abnormalities[152].

CT of the brain can be normal or reveal various abnormalities, including hydrocephalus and focal nodules in the parenchyma. MRI is more sensitive, often revealing inflammatory nodules in the parenchyma and leptomeninges (**452**, **453**).

Pathology

Cryptococci are often easily seen on Gram stain of spinal fluid; however, special stains are more specific for the organism. The polysaccharide capsule can be observed using India ink, methenamine silver, or mucicarmine stains. India ink staining is less often available in laboratories, but mucicarmine stains are almost always available, because they are also used to diagnose adenocarcinomas. More than 80% of patients with AIDS and cryptococcal meningoencephalitis have a positive India ink examination of the CSF[147]. Calcofluor white is a sensitive fluorescent stain that can be used to detect yeast by microscopy. Narrow-based budding yeasts with a polysaccharide capsule, approximately 5–10 µm in size, can be seen on most histopathologic specimens with standard tissue and fungal stains. Inflammation can be highly variable, including relatively little infiltration to frank granulomas. In the lab, *C. neoformans* grows well at 37°C [98.6°F], forming white-to-cream colored, mucoid-appearing colonies.

Treatment

Appropriate antifungal therapy for CNS cryptococcosis includes three phases: induction, consolidation, and maintenance[153].

Induction

Amphotericin B (0.7–1.0 mg/kg/day) or a lipid formulation of amphotericin (3–5 mg/kg/day) intravenously **PLUS** flucytosine (100 mg/kg/day in four divided doses) by mouth for 14 days. Consideration may be given to a longer induction phase if the patient has not improved clinically or CSF cultures remain positive after 14 days of appropriate therapy. If the induction phase does not contain flucytosine, some experts recommend extending the course of amphotericin B to 4–6 weeks total. Alternative regimens have been studied including amphotericin B plus fluconazole, fluconazole plus flucytosine, and fluconazole alone, but these regimens are less fungicidal and therefore less desirable. In patients without known immunocompromise from HIV infection or organ transplantation, 4 weeks of induction therapy is recommended with amphotericin B and flucytosine.

It is ideal to monitor serum flucytosine levels, with the goal of a 2-hour post-dose level of 30–80 µg/ml, measured after 3–5 days of therapy; however, this is often not feasible or timely. Therefore, most clinicians monitor toxicities, such as cytopenias and gastrointestinal tract side-effects, by checking frequent blood counts and monitoring the patient's signs and symptoms.

Consolidation

Fluconazole (400–800 mg/day) by mouth for 8 weeks. The consolidation phase is the same in HIV-infected, solid organ transplant, and presumed nonimmunocompromised patients.

Maintenance

Fluconazole (200 mg/day). Low-dose fluconazole is continued for at least 12 months in HIV-infected patients and until there is reasonable immune reconstitution with antiretroviral therapy as indicated by a CD4 T-cell count >100 cells/µl for at least 3 months. Reinstitution of maintenance fluconazole is considered if the CD4 T-cell count subsequently decreases to <100 cells/µL and /or the serum cryptococcal antigen titer increases. Maintenance therapy is continued in patients without HIV infection, including in patients with solid organ transplantation, for 6–12 months.

A key component of managing cryptococcosis is re-establishing immune function, either with antiretroviral therapy in HIV infection or the decrease of immune suppression as is feasible in organ transplantation. One must remain aware of immune reconstitution syndrome, leading to an exacerbation of symptoms or development of acute meningeal signs or lymphadenopathy.

A particularly important point in the management of CNS cryptococcosis is that of reducing high ICP. Aggressive control of CSF pressure improves clinical outcomes[153]. An initial LP should always be performed, with assessment of OP. The presence of focal neurologic symptoms, new seizures, or other signs and symptoms concerning for space-occupying lesions should prompt imaging of the brain with CT or MRI prior to LP.

During induction therapy, progression of headache, new alterations in sensorium, focal deficits, cranial nerve palsies, or other signs and symptoms of meningoencephalitis should alert the clinician that a therapeutic LP may be required. In general, daily LPs are performed to achieve a target closing pressure of <20 cmH_2O (or half the OP if >40 cmH_2O). An LP should be repeated daily until the OP has been normal and stable for at least 2–3 days. There is no role for mannitol, acetazolamide, or glucocorticoids. A permanent CSF shunt may need to be placed if the patient has progressive symptoms despite appropriate therapy and daily LP. The presence of active infection (i.e. nonsterile CSF) should not delay placement of a shunt if it is clinically indicated.

Of note, the echinocandins (e.g. caspofungin, micafungin, anidulafungin) do not possess reliable activity against *Cryptococcus* spp. and should never be used to treat this infection. *Cryptococcus gattii* is treated with the same antifungal regimens and adjunctive therapy as *C. neoformans*.

Prognosis

Predictors of serious disease and death, at initial presentation include[153,154]:

- Altered sensorium.
- CSF WBC count <20 cells/µl.
- CSF cryptococcal antigen titer >1:1024.

A persistently positive CSF culture at 14 days of appropriate therapy suggests a worse outcome. Therefore, most experts recommend an LP after 2 weeks of antifungal therapy to assess for the need to prolong the induction phase. The mortality approaches 100% without therapy. The 3-month mortality during treatment of the acute phase of cryptococcal meningoencephalitis is approximately 20% despite antifungal therapy, therapeutic LP, and antiretroviral therapy to assist with immune reconstitution.

COCCIDIOIDOMYCOSIS

Definition and epidemiology

Coccidioidomycosis is a common systemic fungal infection. The most frequent site of primary infection is the lungs, and subacute pneumonia is often referred to as 'valley fever'. However, dissemination is not uncommon, and there may be involvement of the CNS with extrapulmonary disease. It is caused by two species of dimorphic fungi, *Coccidioides immitis* and *C. posadasii*.

It is estimated that 150,000 *Coccidioides* spp. infections occur annually, but most of these are subclinical[155]. The organism has a characteristic geographic distribution, living in the soil of semiarid portions of the southwestern USA, Mexico, and South America. Exposure is exceedingly common and, in endemic areas, 10–50% of persons have evidence of exposure by antibody testing[156]. Risk of exposure is highest during dry weather following the rainy season, when soil and dust are most likely to become airborne.

In the USA, fewer than 100 cases of meningitis occur each year. Extrapulmonary disease is the presenting clinical syndrome in only 0.5% of Caucasians, but the risk of dissemination is much higher in other racial groups, including persons of Filipino or African ancestry.

Those with depressed cell-mediated immunity are also at high risk for disseminated infection, such as persons with HIV infection and those treated with high-dose corticosteroids, TNF-α inhibitors[157], or immunosuppressive medications following organ transplantation. Pregnancy, particularly during the third trimester, also predisposes to extrapulmonary coccidioidomycosis[158,159].

Etiology and pathophysiology

Coccidioides spp. are dimorphic fungi, ubiquitous in the topsoil of endemic areas. Fungal spores become airborne with disruption of dry soil from construction, wind storms, earthquakes, and other phenomena which disturb the soil. After humans inhale the arthroconidia, there is transformation in the lung to the characteristic spherules. These spherules enlarge, rupture, and release endospores that can gain access to the bloodstream and disseminate to multiple organs, including the meninges of the brain and spinal cord.

In immunosuppressed persons, coccidioidomycosis can present as reactivation of latent infection, and the risk is correlated with the level of immune compromise. There has been no documentation of person-to-person spread.

Clinical features

There is no clinical distinction between disease caused by *C. immitis* and *C. posadasii*. Classic signs and symptoms of meningitis typically begin within several weeks of exposure, but intervals as long as 2 years have been reported[160]. The most frequent symptom is headache, occurring in 75% of patients. Concomitant blurry vision, nausea, vomiting, and changes in mental status are also common at presentation. Increased ICP can develop, particularly in those with late stage disease and children, leading to hydrocephalus, papilledema, cranial nerve palsies, and other focal neurologic deficits. CNS vasculitis can cause cerebral ischemia and infarction.

While primary infection occurs in the lungs, patients with meningitis may have no symptoms of concomitant pneumonia, and the chest X-ray is often normal. About one-half of all patients with meningitis also have evidence of disseminated infection elsewhere, including the skin, bones, and joints, and these foci can be helpful in making the diagnosis. Erythema nodosum occurs in 5% of patients overall, and a higher proportion of those with disseminated infection[161].

Differential diagnosis

- Cryptococcal meningoencephalitis.
- Meningitis from other endemic mycoses (e.g. histoplasmosis, blastomycosis).
- Tuberculous meningitis.
- Acute bacterial meningitis.
- Eosinophilic meningitis from parasitic infection (e.g. *Angiostrongylus*).
- Brain abscess.
- Neurosyphilis.
- Neurobrucellosis.
- Viral or 'aseptic' meningitis.
- CNS infarction.
- Neoplasm, primary or metastatic.
- Sarcoidosis.

Investigations

- Perform an LP and send CSF for cell count and differential, protein, glucose, Gram stain, culture, acid-fast smear and culture, and fungal stains and culture. Laboratory personnel should be warned of the suspected diagnosis, since plate growth of *Coccidioides* spp. is highly infectious and must be handled with care. High-volume taps may increase the diagnostic yield of fungal culture. Also send CSF for testing of anticoccidioidal antibodies by complement fixation or immunodiffusion. Consider cryptococcal antigen, VDRL, PCR for *Mycobacterium tuberculosis*, and cytology.
- Brain imaging using CT or MRI with contrast. MRI is more sensitive, and is the imaging test of choice.
- Complete blood count with differential.
- Chemistries to assess renal function and look for hyponatremia resulting from SIADH.
- Serum anticoccidioidal antibodies by complement fixation and/or immunodiffusion. The absence of detectable antibodies early in the course of disease does not exclude the diagnosis, since it may take weeks or months to develop a response, particularly in immunocompromised hosts. A positive result may be quite helpful in persons who are not from endemic areas, but most be interpreted with caution in patients who reside in regions with a high seroprevalence.
- Serum for HIV ELISA and confirmatory Western blot, cryptococcal antigen, and RPR with FTA if positive.
- Blood cultures, including fungal isolation and mycobacterial cultures.
- Consider urine *Histoplasma* and *Blastomyces* antigen testing.

Diagnosis

CSF often shows an increased number of WBCs which can be lymphocyte, neutrophil, or eosinophil predominant[162]. There is typically a slight elevation in protein with a profound hypoglycorrhachia. CT or MRI findings are nonspecific, but include meningeal enhancement, hydrocephalus, pseudotumor, and acute infarction (**454**). Hydrocephalus is the most common complication, and is seen in up to 50% of patients with coccidioidal meningitis.

Detecting anticoccidioidal antibodies in the CSF by complement fixation or immunodiffusion allows for a presumptive diagnosis, and is typically how coccidioidal meningitis is identified. Serum positivity for antibodies is suggestive, but not 100% specific, and must be interpreted with caution. Antibody testing of the CSF or serum testing may yield a false negative in early disease, and repeat testing may be needed.

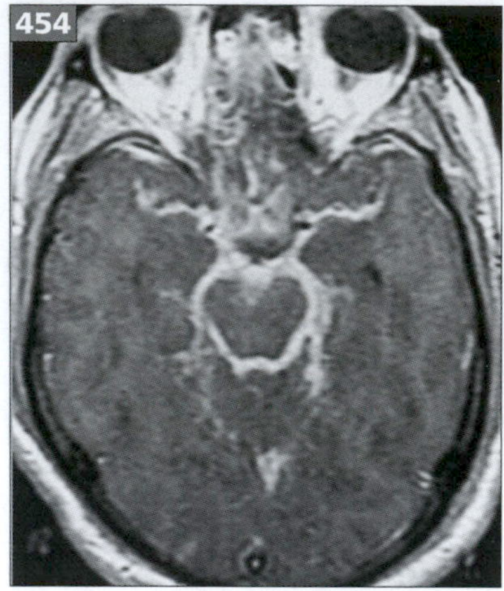

454 Axial T1-weighted image with gadolinium, showing marked basal cistern and meningeal enhancement in coccidioidal meningitis. *Courtesy of Drs. Antonino Catanzaro and John Hesselink. Used with permission from: http://spinwarp.ucsd.edu/NeuroWeb.*

Pathology

Direct examination of tissue specimens shows an acute inflammatory response, often with a mixture of neutrophils, lymphocytes, and eosinophils, along with the spherules characteristic of *Coccidioides* spp. If the infection is chronic, granulomatous inflammation with multinucleated giant cells may be seen. Patients with HIV/AIDS and other forms of immunosuppression may have a poor granulomatous response to infection. *Coccidioides* spp. appears as large, nonbudding spherules, 20–200 µm in diameter, with a refractile double wall encasing multiple endospores. Organisms are occasionally seen on 'wet preparation' with potassium hydroxide or when CSF is stained with calcofluor white or other fungal stains such as Gomori–methenamine silver, periodic acid–Schiff, or hematoxylin and eosin. A definitive diagnosis is made by isolating *Coccidioides* spp. from the CSF. The organisms grow in 5–7 days on most fungal media, but culture is only 15% sensitive.

Treatment

Fluconazole, 400–800 mg IV or orally each day is the drug of choice. Alternative agents include:

- Itraconazole, 200 mg every 8–12 hours appears to be equally efficacious[163]. If itraconazole is used, serum levels should be measured to assure adequate absorption and optimize therapy.

- Voriconazole has excellent *in vitro* activity against *Coccidioides* spp. and case reports suggest clinical efficacy[164,165], but experience with this antifungal is not as extensive as with other azoles. It is far more expensive, and it is not approved by the USA FDA for use in the treatment of coccidioidomycosis.
- Posaconazole may be effective for disseminated, non-meningeal disease, but there is little experience with this agent, and it cannot be recommended without further data.
- Due to the high risk of relapse, indefinite and often lifelong suppressive therapy with one of the above oral azole agents should be given.
- During the first trimester of pregnancy, intrathecal amphotericin B (range of 0.1–1.5 mg per dose, daily to weekly) should be used due to the potential for teratogenic effects of azoles.
- Amphotericin B deoxycholate (0.5–1.5 mg/kg IV every 24–48 hours) or a lipid formulation of amphotericin B (2–5 mg/kg IV every 24 hours) are alternatives in patients who cannot tolerate an azole or occasionally as part of combination therapy in patients with severe disease.
- Echinocandins, such as caspofungin, micafungin, and anidulafungin have unreliable *in vitro* activity against *Coccidioides* spp. and clinical data are lacking. Therefore, drugs from this antifungal class cannot be recommended as a therapeutic option at this time.

If the patient has hydrocephalus, a CSF shunt may be needed to relieve high ICP, and early neurosurgical consultation is recommended. Some experts give adjunctive corticosteroids for vasculitis, but this practice has not been validated in clinical trials.

TOXOPLASMOSIS

Definition and epidemiology

Toxoplasmosis results from infection with the protozoan parasite, *Toxoplasma gondii*. Primary infection is typically asymptomatic, but latency in neural tissue and myocytes persists for life.

Toxoplasmic encephalitis can follow if there is reactivation in the CNS of an immunocompromised patient.

T. gondii is considered a zoonosis; however, most human infections do not occur after direct contact with infected animals. In patients with AIDS-related toxoplasmic encephalitis, there is no epidemiologic association with cat ownership, and it is an unreliable historical factor[166]. Transmission is often remote and unrelated to contact with a felid.

The protozoan is present in the environment world-wide, and the majority of human infections in the USA begin with ingestion of undercooked meat containing tissue cysts, particularly pork and lamb, and water or vegetables contaminated with oocysts. In France, where consumption of raw meat is common, the prevalence of latent infection is relatively high. *T. gondii* is commonly present in many food and game animals, and tissue cysts can survive for several years. Of note, commercial meat is not routinely inspected for the presence of *T. gondii* in the USA and many other regions.

In humans, the prevalence of anti-*Toxoplasma* IgG antibodies increases with age, and is similar in the HIV-positive and HIV-negative populations in the USA, ranging from 10% to 45%[167]. The prevalence is decreasing, with more recent data indicating about 15% of Americans are seropositive[168]. There is no gender predilection. Seroprevalence is lower in the USA than in the developing world, where the proportion of the public with latent infection can be quite high.

Toxoplasmic encephalitis most often occurs in patients with defects in T-cell immunity such as HIV/AIDS, hematologic malignancies, solid organ transplantation, or those taking corticosteroids or cytotoxic medications. The most common predisposing factor is HIV/AIDS, with a CD4 T-cell count below 100 cells/µl.

Encephalitis is the result of reactivation disease in patients with immunosuppression, but solid organ transplant recipients may acquire acute, disseminated toxoplasmosis from the transplanted organ if the donor is positive and the recipient is negative (D+/R−). Although patients with AIDS may have involvement of multiple organs, the most common presentation is encephalitis.

Acute, primary infection in a pregnant woman with subsequent parasitemia and transplacental transmission results in congenital infection. The risk of fetal transmission increases with gestational age.

Etiology and pathophysiology

T. gondii is essentially a parasite of felids, which act as significant reservoirs of infection. Humans and other animals are intermediate hosts. After oral ingestion, the fecal excretion of oocysts is estimated to occur in approximately 1% of the world's cats at any given time[169], contaminating soil and water. Up to 10 million oocysts can be shed in the feces each day[170], and they may remain viable for up to 18 months in moist soil. Oocysts become infectious with sporulation, which occurs in the environment outside of the cat.

Human ingestion of oocysts is followed by invasion of the intestinal epithelium, parasitemia, and dissemination to the brain, spinal cord, skeletal muscle, eyes, and many other organs. Being an intracellular organism, tachyzoites invade target cells and convert into the bradyzoite form. These replicating bradyzoites form tissue cysts, which persist in tissues for the life of the host. In the vast majority of immunocompetent patients, this is without consequence.

T. gondii lies dormant and reactivation is suppressed by the host's immune system. However, with deficiencies in cell-mediated immunity, tissue cysts can rupture with proliferation of organisms and enlarging, necrotic CNS lesions.

Congenital, transplacental, mother-to-child transmission occurs with parasitemia after the mother is acutely infected during gestation. Human-to-human transmission has not been documented definitively, other than from mother to fetus.

Clinical features

Approximately 80–90% of acute infections in immunocompetent hosts are asymptomatic. Symptoms of primary infection often include symmetric, nontender cervical lymphadenopathy that can be mistaken for a mononucleosis syndrome, particularly if constitutional symptoms, pharyngitis, rash, and an atypical lymphocytosis are present. Following acute infection, some patients experience complications such as chorioretinitis, lymphadenitis, myocarditis, or polymyositis.

In the normal host, chronic, latent CNS infection with *Toxoplasma* spp. is asymptomatic, but in immunocompromised individuals, reactivation CNS disease can cause encephalitis with abscesses. Classically, patients present with headache, fever, and varying severity of mental status change. Because of the presence of mass lesions, focal deficits and seizures are common, and if the patient has increased ICP, nausea and vomiting may be prominent.

Other signs and symptoms include hemiparesis, abnormalities of speech, delerium, lethargy, coma, tremor, panhypopituitarism, diabetes insipidus, SIADH, and neuropsychiatric symptoms (e.g. psychosis, dementia, and mood disorders). Diffuse encephalitis without focal lesions has been reported, resulting in generalized cerebral dysfunction without focal signs[171].

Reactivation disease can present in multiple other organ systems, including the eye (chorioretinitis), gastrointestinal tract, musculoskeletal system, heart, bone marrow, and spinal cord. Spinal involvement manifests as motor or sensory disturbances and/or incontinence of bladder or bowel.

Fetal infection can result in calcified CNS lesions, ventricular dilation, and severe neurologic impairment, including neonatal seizures and cerebral palsy.

Differential diagnosis

- Bacterial brain abscess.
- CNS lymphoma.
- Cryptococcoma.
- Histoplasmosis.
- Coccidioidomycosis.
- Aspergillosis.
- Mycobacterial infection (most commonly *M. tuberculosis*).
- Syphilis.
- PML.

Investigations

- Anti-*Toxoplasma* serum IgG.
- Serum RPR or VDRL with FTA test if positive.
- LP with cell count and differential, protein, glucose, *Toxoplasma* PCR, Gram stain and culture, fungal stain and culture, mycobacterial stain and culture, cryptococcal antigen, PCR testing for herpesviruses, PCR for JCV, and cytology.
- Brain imaging, preferably MRI with contrast.
- If HIV diagnosis not established, test for HIV antibodies and if positive, ELISA and Western blot, assess CD4 T-cell count, and HIV viral load.

Diagnosis

A definitive diagnosis is made with pathologic examination of an appropriately stained biopsy specimen. However, open or stereotactic brain biopsy is invasive, and the predictive value for toxoplasmic encephalitis is approximately 80% in a patient with HIV/AIDS and a CD4 count of <100 cells/μL, anti-*Toxoplasma* IgG antibodies, absence of prophylaxis, and the presence of multiple, ring-enhancing brain lesions on CT or MRI[172]. Therefore, it is appropriate to presumptively treat a seropositive patient with AIDS and the appropriate clinical syndrome. Brain biopsy is deferred unless the patient does not respond to empiric therapy.

Specific serum IgG forms during the first 2 weeks of primary infection and usually persists for life. The majority of patients with CNS toxoplasmosis are seropositive; however, serology is not 100% sensitive, and the absence of antibodies does not exclude the diagnosis. Anti-*Toxoplasma* IgG only indicates previous primary infection with latency (i.e. possible reactivation disease). Therefore, the clinician should test for seropositivity in immunocompromised patients in order to stratify toxoplasmosis in the differential diagnosis and make decisions regarding prophylaxis in the asymptomatic patient, not to make a definitive diagnosis.

Toxoplasmic encephalitis classically presents with multiple, ring-enhancing lesions on CT or MRI. On MRI, the focal abscesses appear as high signal abnormalities on T2-weighted images (**455**), with a rim of enhancement surrounding the edema on T1-weighted,

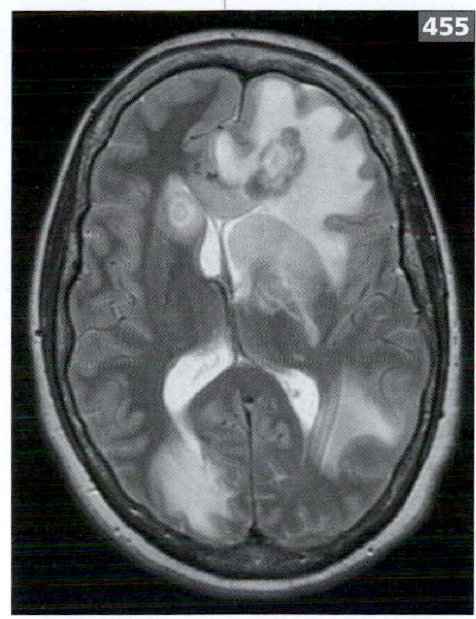

455 **T2-weighted MRI of the brain at the level of the basal ganglia, showing multiple areas of bright, vasogenic edema. Rounded masses of *Toxoplasma gondii* organisms are seen within the right caudate nucleus and adjacent to the left side of the corpus callosum.** *Courtesy of Dr. Edward Michals, University of Illinois at Chicago.*

contrast-enhanced studies. However, due to the broad differential diagnosis, the classic findings are not 100% specific. Lesions may be solitary, and CT scans are normal or only reveal mild cerebral atrophy in the diffuse encephalitic form of CNS toxoplasmosis. The finding of cerebral calcifications in a newborn should raise the suspicion of *T. gondii*, particularly with biventricular dilation.

CSF analysis may show a mild pleocytosis and elevated protein. Organisms are rarely seen on stain. A *Toxoplasma* PCR can be performed; PCR testing has a low sensitivity (50–60%), but high specificity (close to 100%)[173] and can be helpful, if positive, in establishing the diagnosis without a brain biopsy.

Pathology

On biopsy, organisms can be seen on hematoxylin and eosin (H&E) or immunoperoxidase staining, which improves the sensitivity of identifying organisms. Necrosis is the most prominent feature on brain biopsy, and tachyzoites and tissue cysts may be seen adjacent to necrotic areas. Autopsy studies have shown a marked predilection for the basal ganglia. If lymph nodes are biopsied in acute, primary infection, follicular hyperplasia and irregular clusters of tissue macrophages with eosinophilic cytoplasm are seen.

Treatment

Immunocompetent patients with acute lymphadenitis induced by *T. gondii* do not require therapy, since this is a self-limited infection. More severe visceral disease in an immunologically normal host is treated with a regimen listed below for 2–4 weeks, depending upon the patient and extent of organ involvement. In immunocompromised patients with CNS toxoplasmic encephalitis, appropriate treatment regimens have been established.

Pyrimethamine, a folic acid antatgonist, is the most active drug and should always be included in the regimen if possible. A 200 mg loading dose is given followed by 75 mg by mouth each day. Folinic acid (leucovorin, 10–25 mg by mouth daily) is given concurrently, to reduce bone marrow suppression. Folic acid (*not* folinic acid) inhibits the effects of pyrimethamine on tachyzoites and should not be used. Although pyrimethamine is teratogenic in animals, human data are inconclusive, and pregnant women should be treated with the same regimen.

There is no role for monotherapy. The preferred choices for a second antimicrobial are:

- Sulfadiazine (first choice) works synergistically with pyrimethamine. Other sulfonamides may have activity, but are inferior. If the patient has a sulfa allergy, desensitization has been performed successfully[174,175]. Give 6–8 g per day by mouth divided into four doses.
- Clindamycin may be used as a second agent in patients who cannot tolerate sulfadiazine or have a documented sulfa allergy. Clindamycin is efficacious, but sulfadiazine is a superior choice. The clindamycin dose is 600–1200 mg IV or 450 mg orally every 6 hours.

Several other antimicrobials have *in vitro* activity against *Toxoplasma* spp., but clinical data do not allow for definitive recommendations regarding their use as second agents: azithromycin (1200 mg once daily), clarithromycin (500 mg every 12 hours), atovaquone (750 mg by mouth every 6 hours), and dapsone (100 mg by mouth daily). If any of these drugs are used, they should also be given in combination with pyrimethamine. Some data suggest that TMP/SMX (5 mg/kg of trimethoprim component IV every 6–8 hours) alone may be efficacious as compared with standard therapy[176].

The appropriate duration of induction therapy is 6 weeks at high doses, followed by chronic suppressive therapy with pyrimethamine (25–50 mg daily) plus sulfadiazine (2–4 g daily in 2–4 divided doses) and folinic acid. If the CD4 count has risen above 200 cells/μl for 6 months, suppressive therapy ('secondary prophylaxis') can be discontinued[177].

Corticosteroids (dexamethasone, 4 mg IV every 6 hours) may be given if edema causes midline shift or there are clinical signs and symptoms of increased ICP. Anticonvulsants are given if seizures occur.

A detailed neurologic examination should be performed daily to assess for subtle signs of clinical improvement. Serial imaging (every 2 weeks unless otherwise indicated) should be performed. Clinical improvement is seen in 90% of patients after 2–3 weeks of therapy[178,179], but complete resolution on MRI often requires up to 6 months, and radiologic response lags behind clinical response. A lack of improvement, and particularly deterioration, should suggest an alternative diagnosis and lower the threshold for brain biopsy.

Prevention

Patients with HIV/AIDS and CD4 T-cell counts <100 cells/µl who are seropositive for *Toxoplasma* spp. are at risk for developing reactivation CNS toxoplasmosis, unless they are receiving appropriate prophylaxis. Options for prophylactic therapy include:

- TMP/SMX (1 DS tablet thrice weekly or 1 SS tablet daily).
- Dapsone (50 mg daily) + pyrimethamine (50 mg weekly) + folinic acid (25 mg weekly).
- Dapsone (200 mg weekly) + pyrimethamine (75 mg weekly) + folinic acid (25 mg weekly).
- Atovaquone (1500 mg daily).

Immunocompromised patients and pregnant women should be advised to avoid eating undercooked meats or unwashed vegetables and, if they must clean a cat litter box, should use gloves and wash their hands meticulously.

NEUROCYSTICERCOSIS

Definition and epidemiology

Cysticercosis represents tissue infection with the larval cysts of *Taenia solium*, the pork tapeworm. An individual patient will usually harbor multiple cysts in many different anatomic locations. Neurocysticercosis is the term for CNS infection with tissue cysts.

The estimated prevalence of cysticerosis is approximately 50 million people world-wide. However, most infections are asymptomatic, so this is an underestimate. Infection with *T. solium* is endemic in Mexico, Central and South America, and portions of southern Europe, Africa, India, and Asia. Individual risk is correlated with the chances of exposure to the parasite. Therefore, in endemic areas, prevalence increases with age and poor sanitation.

In regions where *T. solium* is highly endemic, 30–50% of patients with new onset seizures have antibodies, compared with 2–10% of the general population[180]. In the USA, where *T. solium* infestation is less common, approximately 2% of patients presenting to emergency departments with seizures have neurocysticercosis[181]. It is more common in areas with a relatively high proportion of immigrants from endemic areas.

Etiology and pathophysiology

Infection is acquired by oral ingestion of food or water contaminated with *T. solium* eggs (fecal–oral transmission from a tapeworm carrier). Humans can function as definitive or intermediate hosts:

- *Definitive host*: a person consuming raw or undercooked pork containing infectious cysticerci can experience intestinal (noninvasive) infection with the adult tapeworm. These definitive hosts are most often asymptomatic. During this 'intestinal phase' of infection, the helminth is attached to the lumen of the small intestine where it can survive for decades. These adult worms produce eggs that are excreted in the feces. These infectious ova may contaminate food or water, which are then ingested by a new (intermediate) host.
- *Intermediate host*: eggs hatch in the small intestine, invade through the intestinal epithelium, and disseminate hematogenously to many tissues, including the brain. The cysticerci that develop can result in neurocysticercosis decades later.

Some humans carry both adult tapeworms and cysticeri, and cysticercosis can develop from autoinfection; that is, a patient can harbor mature organisms that lay infectious ova, and subsequent fecal–oral transmission of the ova in the same patient allows a single person to function as both the definitive and intermediate host.

Neurocysticercosis can involve any region of the CNS. Lesions are subclinical for years or decades. Symptom onset begins when cysticerci can no longer evade the host immune response and begin to die, lose osmoregulatory function, and begin to enlarge. Cysts may leak antigenic material that induces an inflammatory response with subsequent cerebritis, ventriculitis, meningitis, and seizures. Ventricular lesions can cause obstruction and symptomatic hydrocephalus.

Clinical features

Most neurocysticerci never cause symptoms, and lesions are found incidentally on brain imaging. The onset of symptoms peaks 3–5 years after infection, but can be delayed for decades[182,183]. Fever is uncommon in neurocysticercosis. The clinical presentation depends upon the involved anatomic location of the CNS:

- Parenchymal (>60%): focal neurologic deficits from mass lesions, seizures, headache, and psychiatric disorders. Seizures are the most common presenting symptom.
- Intraventricular (10–20%): signs and symptoms of hydrocephalus with nausea, vomiting, headache, and papilledema.
- Subarachnoid: chronic meningitis, arachnoiditis, or vasculitis with infarcts.
- Spinal cord (1%): cord compression with focal deficits or, less often, meningitis.
- Racemose cysticercosis: an aggressive form of basilar neurocysticercosis where cysts proliferate at the base of the brain resulting in rapid mental deterioration, coma, and death.

Differential diagnosis

- Meningoencephalitis caused by other parasites (e.g. *Angiostrongylus cantonensis*, *Gnathostoma*, or *Paragonimus* spp.). Infection with these organisms usually presents as an eosinophilic meningitis and not a focal neurologic lesion.
- Hydatid cysts of *Echinococcus granulosus*, although these are more typically seen in the liver or lung.
- Malignancy, either primary or secondary.
- Tuberculomas.
- Bacterial brain abscesses.
- Toxoplasmosis, although lesions are typically not cystic in appearance.
- Noninfectious seizure disorder.

Investigations

First-line investigations are CT or MRI of the brain. Serologic testing for antibodies should be performed using the enzyme-linked immunoelectrotransfer blot assay (EITB). An LP is usually not necessary. Brain biopsy should be deferred if neurocysticercosis is very likely, but it may be prudent to pursue early if the diagnosis is in question.

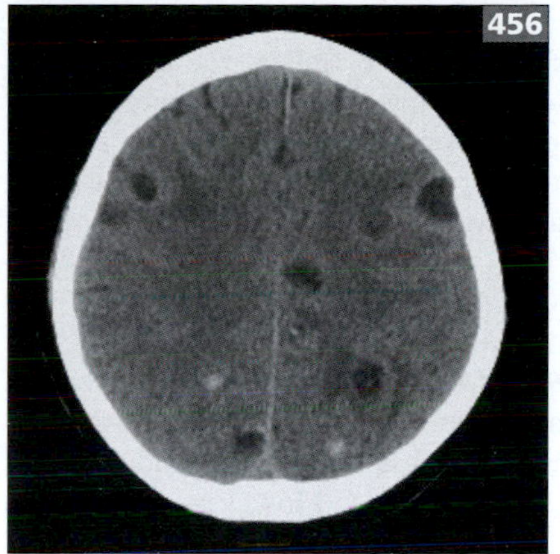

456 CT without contrast in a patient with neurocysticercosis, showing multiple round, cystic-appearing lesions, some with a central punctate density suggestive of the active stage of the disease. Several intraparenchymal calcifications in both cerebral hemispheres are consistent with old cysticercosis lesions. *Courtesy of Dr. Edward Michals, University of Illinois at Chicago.*

Diagnosis

The diagnosis of neurocysticercosis is based on a combination of clinical presentation, radiologic findings, and the appropriate epidemiology. The diagnosis is supported by antibody testing. Intestinal infection is easily diagnosed by finding characteristic eggs and proglottids in the stool. However, stool studies are insensitive and nonspecific for tissue infection (cysticercosis).

The sensitivity of EITB antibody testing is high in patients with multiple cysts (94%) but much lower in those with a solitary cyst (28%)[184], and the sensitivity decreases if cysts are calcified. Therefore, in the scenario where neurocysticercosis is highly suspected based upon presentation, epidemiology, and radiographic findings, seronegativity does not exclude the diagnosis. A positive serology only indicates prior exposure to *T. solium*. Therefore, seropositivity is only supportive and does not allow for a definitive diagnosis. However, with a high pre-test probability, a positive serology is very suggestive. The only way for a definitive diagnosis is brain biopsy, which is usually unnecessary.

CT or MRI of the brain typically shows multiple enhancing and nonenhancing unilocular cysts (**456**)[180]. On imaging, multiple cysticerci are the rule, with an average of 7–10 per patient. Identification of a scolex in a cystic lesion is pathognomonic; they appear as bright structures within the cavity.

The classic CSF profile in neurocysticercosis reveals a lymphocytic or eosinophilic pleocytosis with hypoglycorrhachia and a slightly elevated protein.

Pathology

Brain biopsy is not necessary unless the diagnosis is in question. However, histopathology reveals fluid-filled membranous structures that may contain scolices (anatomic structures of the tapeworm). Occasional granulomatous inflammation is seen around degenerating cysts.

Treatment

Treatment for neurocysticercosis is complex and controversial. Initial case series suggested that medical therapy with antihelminthic agents accelerated the radiographic clearance of CNS lesions[185]. However, subsequent randomized trials indicated that neither praziquantel nor albendazole therapy hastens clinical cure, abatement of seizures, or resolution of parenchymal lesions on CT or MRI[180]. Indeed, there have been reports of exacerbation of inflammatory changes when treating CNS disease with antihelminthic therapy[186,187]. Therefore, the benefit of treating parenchymal lesions remains questionable, with suggestion of potential harm. However, treatment of intraventricular cysts is still recommended by some experts.

Initially, the clinician should focus on seizure control with antiepileptics and treatment of symptomatic hydrocephalus. Most experts recommend 6–12 months of antiepileptic therapy after radiographic resolution, but the optimal duration has not yet been defined by randomized, controlled studies.

If the choice is made to treat a patient with neurocysticercosis using an antihelminthic medication, the preferred agents are:

- Albendazole (15 mg/kg/day in two divided doses) for 7–14 days. Patients with subarachnoid lesions may benefit from a longer duration of therapy of at least 4 weeks.

  or
- Praziquantel (50–100 mg/kg/day in three divided doses) for 2–4 weeks.

Because cyst death may cause increased inflammation and neurologic sequelae, concurrent administration of dexamethasone (0.1 mg/kg/day) for 7–10 days, followed by a rapid taper, should be used. Caution should be used in giving high-dose corticosteroids if the patient could have tuberculomas. Many experts advise screening for latent tuberculosis infection (LTBI) with skin testing or an interferon-γ release assay and at least treating for LTBI if positive. Because corticosteroid therapy may lower levels of praziquantel in the serum and CNS, some experts favor albendazole[188]. In addition, albendazole does not interact with antiepileptic medications, unlike praziquantel.

Individualized therapy, with a combined medical–surgical approach and early consultation with infectious diseases and neurosurgery, is ideal in most patients. Surgery is often necessary to treat hydrocephalus (ventriculostomy or ventriculoperitoneal shunt), spinal lesions, or giant cysticerci with mass effect. Patients should have follow-up radiographic imaging to evaluate improvement and resolution.

EOSINOPHILIC MENINGITIS

Definition and epidemiology

Eosinophilic meningitis is not a specific microbiological diagnosis and can certainly result from noninfectious causes; however, a CSF eosinophilic pleocytosis implies infection with a relatively limited number of pathogens. It is defined as >10 eosinophils/µl, or at least 10% eosinophils in a spun sample of CSF[189].

The zoonotic helminths *Angiostrongylus cantonensis*, the rat lungworm, and *Gnathostoma spinigerum* are the most common infectious agents causing eosinophilic meningitis[190]. *A. cantonensis* is the most likely etiology outside of the USA and Europe. It is endemic in Asia (particularly Thailand and Malaysia), the Pacific basin, Africa, Australia, and the Carribean. *G. spiningerum* is endemic to southeast Asia, China, South and Central America, Africa, and the Middle East[191,192].

Etiology and pathophysiology

The parasitic infections leading to an eosinophilic response are the helminths (i.e. worms), not protozoans. The most common parasites causing eosinophilic meningitis are *A. cantonensis*, *G. spinigerum*, baylisascariasis, *Toxocara canis*, and neurocysticercosis, but many helminthic pathogens can invade the CNS.

A. cantonensis larvae are passed in the stool by rodents. These larvae then penetrate a mollusk, with freshwater shrimps, crabs, snails, and slugs functioning as intermediate hosts. *Angiostrongylus* spp. is quite neurotropic, and when humans ingest these intermediate hosts in undercooked or raw form, the larvae can penetrate the bowel wall, lead to parasitemia and travel to the CNS[193].

The definitive hosts for *G. spinigerum* are dogs and cats, from which eggs are passed in the feces[190]. Larvae are ingested by crustaceans, which are eaten by other animal hosts. When humans ingest the muscle tissue of these hosts, parasitemia can lead to cutaneous, visceral, or CNS infection. Clinical symptoms occur with migration of the parasite within host tissues. *Gnathostoma* spp. are not as neurotropic and can manifest in many tissues.

Clinical features

Neurologic manifestations of eosinophilic meningitis typically develop 2–35 days following ingestion of the parasite and include fever, headache, photophobia, nausea, vomiting, and nuchal rigidity. Headache is often from increased ICP and can frequently be relieved by LP. Migrating painful parasthesias are particularly common in *Angiostrongylus* spp. infection. CNS gnathostomiasis is often more clinically severe than *A. cantonensis* infection, with fulminant meningitis, myelitis, or encephalitis, and a predominance of parasthesias, radicular pain, paresis or paralysis, with or without cranial nerve palsies[194]. Gnathostomiasis is often recognized by its dermatologic manifestations including migratory panniculitis and creeping eruptions.

Differential diagnosis

- Angiostrongyliasis.
- Gnathostomiasis.
- Baylisascariasis.
- Toxocariasis.
- Neurocysticercosis.
- Schistosomiasis.
- Trichinellosis.
- Echinococcosis.
- Paragonimiasis.
- Coccidioidomycosis.
- Malignancy, particularly Hodgkin's lymphoma.
- Aseptic meningitis due to medications.
- Foreign bodies.

Investigations

- LP with CSF for cell count and differential, protein, and glucose.
- Complete blood count to look for peripheral eosinophilia, which may be present.
- Radiologic imaging (CT or MRI) of the brain.
- Serologic testing for some or all of the above causative parasites, if available and depending on the epidemiology.

Diagnosis

The definitive diagnosis of a specific causative agent requires identification of a likely organism in host tissues. However, identification of these agents in the CNS can require brain biopsy, and LP is an insensitive method of visualizing parasites. The diagnosis of *A. cantonensis* and *G. spinigerum* eosinophilic meningitis is typically made with history, epidemiology, physical examination, and the presence of a CSF eosinophilia. Serologic assays have been developed to diagnose *A. cantonensis* and *G. spinigerum*, but the sensitivity and specificity of these assays varies, and they are not widely available in the USA and elsewhere.

Pathology

Wright or Giemsa staining are preferred to differentiate eosinophils from other leukocytes in the CSF[195]. Some pathogens may be seen in tissues with special stains, but this is rarely done. The specific histologic findings in eosinophilic meningitis are dependent upon the etiology.

Treatment

Angiostrongylus spp. infection of the CNS is often self-limited, and the use of antihelminthic agents for angiostrongyliasis or gnathostomiasis is controversial. However, corticosteroid therapy may be beneficial and is frequently used to decrease meningeal inflammation from dying helminths[196]. Albendazole therapy for 14 days may result in a shorter duration of symptoms, particularly headache[197], but there have been reports of exacerbation of CNS inflammation with the use of antihelminthic agents[198]. Therefore, albendazole is not routinely recommended as a component of therapy. Serial LPs are an important part of management, if increased ICP is present.

CREUTZFELDT–JAKOB DISEASE (CJD)

Definition

Creutzfeldt–Jakob disease is a neurodegenerative condition that is the most common subtype of transmissible spongiform encephalopathy (TSE), or prion disease. TSEs are all characterized by the deposition of an abnormal, protease-resistant isoform of a membrane-bound glycoprotein, the prion protein (PrP), in the brain. CJD and other TSEs have long incubation periods, but are rapidly progressive and universally fatal. Prion diseases should be in the differential diagnosis of any patient presenting with a rapidly progressive dementia.

Four known prion diseases affect humans: CJD, Gerstmann–Straüssler–Scheinker syndrome (GSS), fatal familial insomnia (FFI), and kuru. This section will focus on the various forms of CJD. There are several different types of CJD, each characterized by its distinct epidemiology, pathophysiology, clinical presentation, radiologic findings, and/or pathologic patterns: sporadic (sCJD), variant (vCJD), familial (fCJD), and iatrogenic (iCJD).

Epidemiology

CJD is the most common of the human prion diseases. World-wide, the annual incidence is approximately 1 case per million population. The median age of onset for sCJD is about 61 years; however, vCJD has a much younger age of onset, with a mean of 26 years[199,200]. There is no gender predilection. Each type of CJD has a characteristic epidemiology.

Sporadic

sCJD is the presenting type in 85–90% of cases. In epidemiologic analyses, the significant risk factors associated with sCJD appear to be: family history of CJD or psychosis[201], multiple surgical procedures, and more than 10 years of residence on a farm[202]. Unlike vCJD, sCJD is not linked to bovine spongiform encephalopathy (BSE). The overall incidence is just under 1 per million per year, but in people over 50, the risk increases to 3.4 per million per year. In the USA, fewer than 300 cases are reported annually[203].

Variant

vCJD is a phenomenon of the past 15 years, first described in 1996. It has affected considerably younger patients as compared to sCJD, although the age range at onset is wide. It is associated with BSE, linked epidemiologically and pathologically to a large epidemic of this prion disease among beef cattle in the UK.

The vast majority of people who have developed vCJD have either lived in the UK or were thought to have contracted the disease there at some point[204]. As of February, 2010, there have been a worldwide total of 216 cases reported, with 169 from the UK and others distributed in France, Italy, Spain, Japan, Canada, and other regions, with three cases in the USA[205]. However, some estimates have suggested that there may eventually be as many as 3000 cases from exposures during the 1990s. This is likely an overestimate, given that the number of new cases has decreased significantly over the past few years of incubation time.

Familial

fCJD accounts for 5–15% of cases. This form is caused by inherited mutations in the prion protein gene (*PRNP*).

Iatrogenic

iCJD has resulted in very few cases. However, the associations are notable and have led to changes in practice. It has been linked with the administration of cadaveric human pituitary hormones[206], dural graft transplants[207,208], corneal transplants[209], liver transplants[210], and the use of contaminated neurosurgical instruments or stereotactic depth electrodes[211]. Newer surgical techniques, caution in preparation of dural grafts, and using recombinant hormones (rather than those derived from cadaveric pituitary pools) have largely eliminated the risk.

Etiology and pathophysiology

sCJD causes randomly distributed cases, and the exact etiology and pathophysiology are unknown.

There is now excellent evidence linking vCJD to BSE, also known as 'mad cow disease'. Strong data indicate that vCJD is the result of bovine-to-human transmission of BSE[212–214].

fCJD results from inherited point mutations or insertions in the PrP gene (*PRNP*). There is an autosomal dominant pattern of inheritance with variable penetration. *PRNP* is located on the short arm of chromosome 20. The substitution of lysine for glutamine in codon 200 is the most common *PRNP* mutation. Codon 200^{Lys} and 178^{Asp} mutations lead to neuropathologic changes essentially indistinguishable from sCJD. Other forms of CJD are not associated with *PRNP* gene mutations.

iCJD represents human-to-human transmission, either directly from neural tissue or due to contaminated surgical instruments.

Clinical features

Following symptom onset, there is rapidly progressive mental deterioration. Prominent signs include dementia, behavioral abnormalities, difficulty with concentration and judgment, sleep disturbances (insomnia and hypersomnia), and changes in mood such as depression, anxiety, and emotional lability. With disease progression, dementia becomes the dominant sign. Of note, psychiatric symptoms may be more prominent in younger patients. The average time to death from onset of symptoms is 6–9 months.

Myoclonus is very common, and is particularly provoked by startle. It is present in more than 90% of patients with sCJD at some point. sCJD should always be considered in a patient with rapidly progressive dementia and myoclonus. Extrapyramidal signs, such as hypokinesia, and cerebellar manifestations occur in about two-thirds of patients. Corticospinal tract abnormalities also may develop, such as hyper-reflexia, the Babinski sign, and spasticity.

Patients with vCJD tend to present differently than sCJD. They are younger, with the mean age of onset being 26 years[200], and the duration of illness is longer (14 months compared with 4.5 months in sCJD). vCJD presents more frequently with sensory disturbances and psychiatric manifestations, whereas both are rather unusual in sCJD. However, psychiatric symptoms are often later obscured by dementia.

Differential diagnosis

- Metabolic or toxic encephalopathies.
- Alzheimer dementia.
- Multi-infarct dementia.
- Nonconvulsive status epilepticus.
- CNS vasculitis.
- Subacute sclerosing panencephalitis (SSPE).
- CNS malignancy and paraneoplastic syndromes.
- Huntington's disease.
- Psychiatric illness (severe depression and anxiety).
- Viral, fungal, or tuberculous meningoencephalitis.
- Neurosyphilis.

Investigations

- Detailed history, including family and exposure history, and physical examination.
- MRI is preferred over CT scan.
- LP, and send CSF for cell count and differential, bacterial cultures, acid-fast stain and culture, fungal stains and culture, cryptococcal antigen, VDRL, PCR for herpesviruses (HSV, CMV, EBV, VZV), PCR for enteroviruses, PCR for JCV, 14-3-3 protein.
- EEG.
- Brain biopsy should be considered.
- Genetic analysis can be performed for mutations in the *PRNP* gene.
- Tonsil biopsy.

Diagnosis

The gold standard is brain biopsy, which shows the typical pathologic findings (neuronal loss, gliosis, spongiform degeneration) and positive immunostaining for PrP plaques.

To support the diagnosis without biopsy:

- MRI shows abnormally increased T2 (**457**) and FLAIR signal intensity, particularly in the putamen and caudate, but at times in the globus pallidus, thalamus, and cerebral and cerebellar cortex. MRI is superior to CT in sensitivity, and diffusion-weighted imaging may be the most sensitive for detecting abnormalities. Increased T2 signal in the posterior thalamus (the 'pulvinar sign') may be seen in up to 70% of cases of vCJD[215,216].

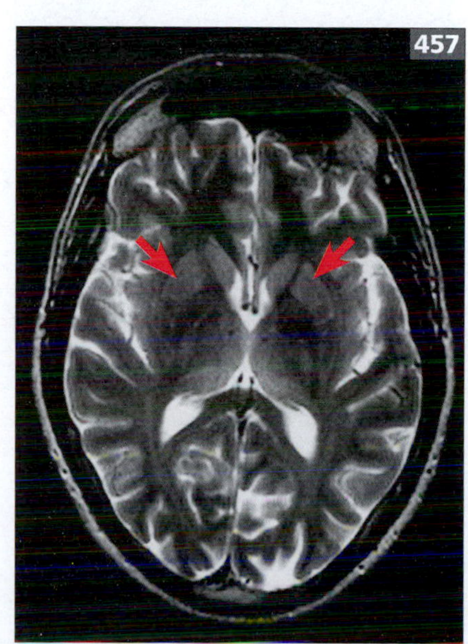

457 T2-weighted MRI from a patient with pathologically proven Creutzfeldt–Jakob disease (CJD). Note increased signal (whiteness) of the basal ganglia (arrows). Normally the basal ganglia become darker due to iron deposition with age. There is also a minor degree of atrophy. These features are suggestive of CJD but are nonspecific.

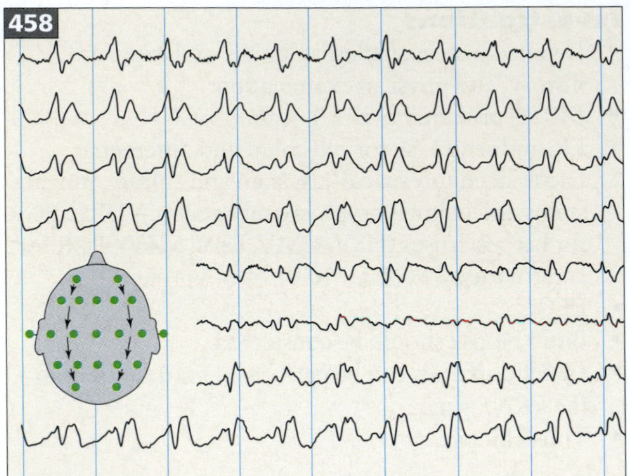

458 Electroencephalograph showing periodic triphasic wave complexes that are rather simple in contour and recurring every 0.7–0.8 seconds, against a slow polymorphous background, in a patient with rapidly progressive dementia and myoclonus due to Creutzfeldt–Jakob disease. Occasionally, the periodic discharges begin unilaterally and may resemble periodic lateralized epileptiform discharges.

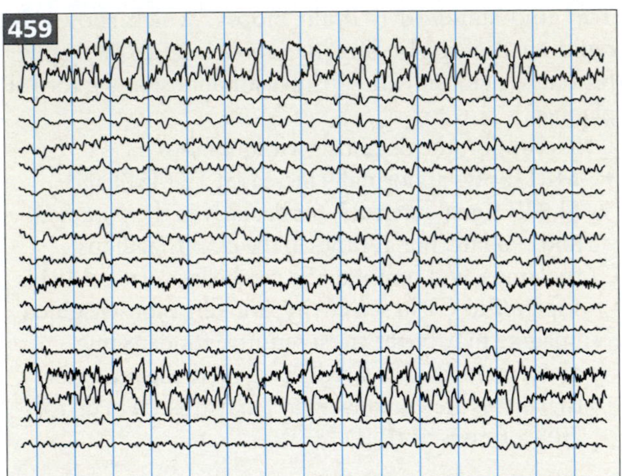

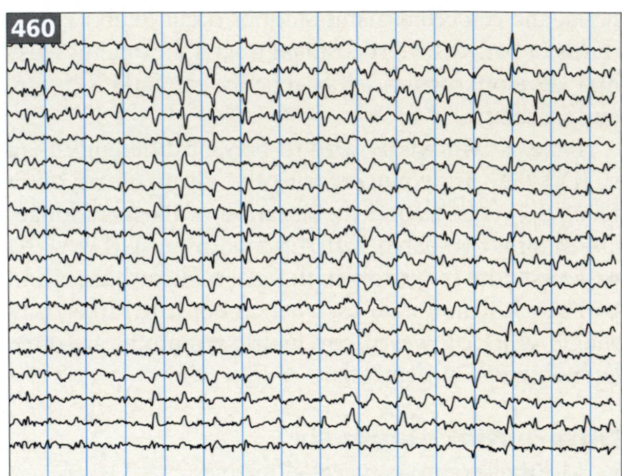

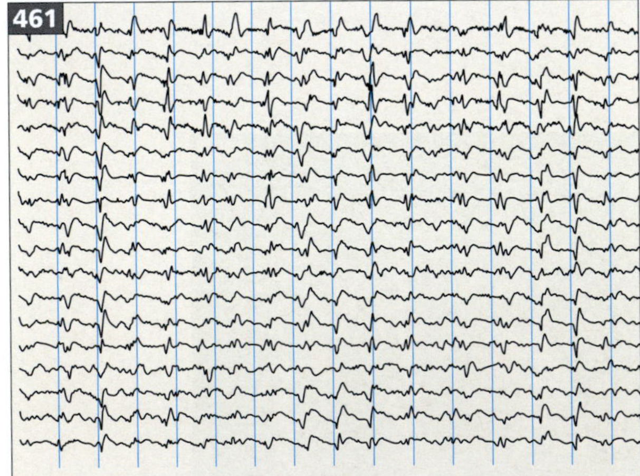

459–461 Serial electroencephalographs, every 3 days, from a patient with Creutzfeldt–Jakob disease showing the progressive evolution of periodic triphasic wave complexes and the background rhythm.

- EEG (**458–461**) can provide supportive evidence of sCJD with the characteristic pattern of periodic synchronous bi- or triphasic sharp wave complexes (PSWC). PSWCs have a high specificity for the diagnosis of sCJD, and do not occur in vCJD, helping to distinguish the two.
- ELISA and Western blot for abnormal CSF protein 14-3-3 may be a sensitive and specific test for sCJD[217], but this remains controversial and not yet established by quality studies. False-positive tests may occur with HSV encephalitis, neoplastic disease, and hypoxic and metabolic encephalopathies. 14-3-3 may also be seen in approximately 50% of cases of vCJD[216].
- Routine tests are typically normal. CSF studies show normal cell counts and a normal glucose, but there is an elevated protein in about 40% of cases.

The WHO has established diagnostic criteria for probable sCJD:

- Progressive dementia.
- At least two of the following: myoclonus, visual or cerebellar disturbance, pyramidal or extrapyramidal dysfunction, akinetic mutism.
- Suggestive EEG and/or positive 14-3-3 protein in CSF.
- Thorough work-up does not suggest an alternative diagnosis.

Pathology

Grossly, there is atrophy of the brain. On histology, CJD classically reveals neuronal loss, reactive glial cell proliferation, and spongiform degeneration (**462–464**), with an absence of inflammation. Spongiform change consists of small, round vacuoles within neurons and the surrounding neuropil. Amyloid plaques may also be present, which are eosinophilic, compact extracellular accumulation of PrP. These plaques are pathognomonic of prion disease but not always present on histologic examination.

PrP can also be detected by immunohistochemical staining. The specific pattern, distribution and type of PrP deposition can be associated with individual types of prion diseases.

Treatment

No effective treatment exists for CJD or other prion diseases, and management is entirely supportive. CJD is uniformly fatal, with most deaths occurring within 1 year of presentation.

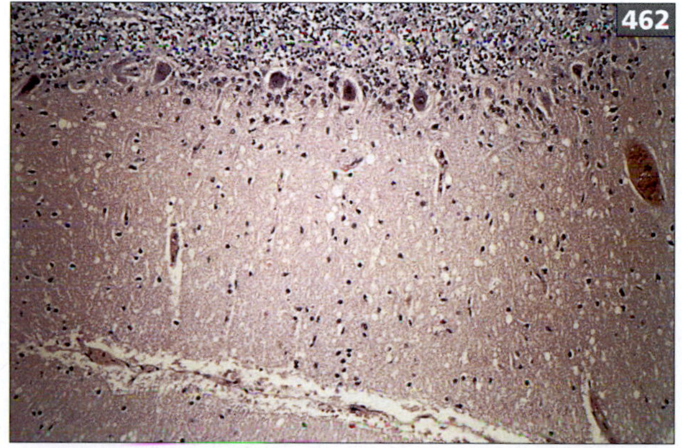

462 Microscopic section of the gray matter of cerebellum of a patient with Creutzfeldt–Jakob disease, showing neuronal loss, reactive astrocytic proliferation and gliosis, and spongiform degeneration (vacuolation of the neurophil).

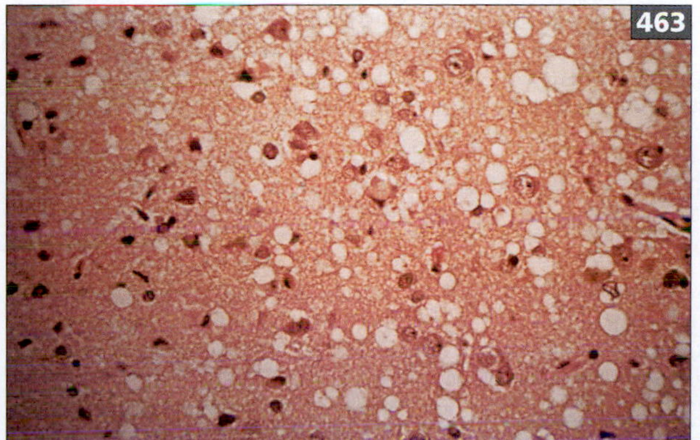

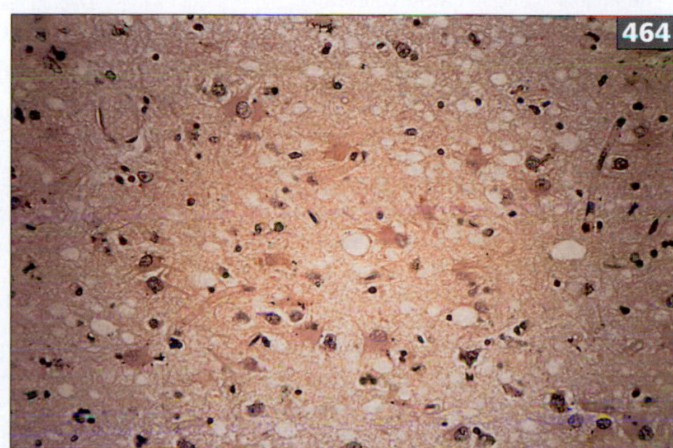

463, 464 Neuronal vacuolation and spongiform change in the brain of a patient with Creutzfeldt–Jakob disease.

REFERENCES

1 Thigpen M, Rosenstein NE, Whitney CG, *et al.* (2005). Bacterial meningitis in the United States 1998–2003. Presented at the 43rd Annual Meeting of the Infectious Diseases Society of America, San Francisco, CA, Abstract #65.

2 Schuchat A, Robinson K, Wenger JD, (1997). Bacterial meningitis in the United States in 1995. *N Engl J Med* 337:970–976.

3 Korinek AM, Baugnon T, Golmard JL, van Effenterre R, Coriat P, Puybasset L (2006). Risk factors for adult nosocomial meningitis after craniotomy: role of antibiotic prophylaxis. *Neurosurgery* **59**:126–133.

4 Van de Beek D, de Gans J, Spanjaard L, Weisfelt M, Reitsma JB, Vermeulen M (2004). Clinical features and prognostic factors in adults with bacterial meningitis. *N Engl J Med* **351**:1849–1859.

5 Durand ML, Calderwood SB, Weber DJ, *et al.* (1993). Acute bacterial meningitis in adults: a review of 493 episodes. *N Engl J Med* **328**:21–28.

6 Heckenberg SG, de Gans J, Brouwer MC, *et al.* (2008). Clinical features, outcome, and meningococcal genotype in 258 adults with meningococcal meningitis: a prospective cohort study. *Medicine* (Baltimore) 87:185–192.

7 Aronin SI, Peduzzi P, Quagliarello VJ (1998). Community-acquired bacterial meningitis: risk stratification for adverse clinical outcome and effect of antibiotic timing. *Ann Intern Med* **129**:862–869.

8 Proulx N, Frechette D, Toye B, Chan J, Kravcik S (2005). Delays in the administration of antibiotics are associated with mortality from adult acute bacterial meningitis. *QJM* **98**:291–298.

9 Auburtin M, Wolff M, Carpentier J, *et al.* (2006). Detrimental role of delayed antibiotic administration and penicillin-nonsusceptible strains in adult intensive care unit patients with pneumococcal meningitis: the PNEUMOREA prospective multicenter study. *Crit Care Med* **34**:2758–2765.

10 Lepur D, Barsic B (2007). Community-acquired bacterial meningitis in adults: antibiotic timing in disease course and outcome. *Infection* **35**:225–231.

11 Mamelak AN, Mampalam TJ, Obana WG, Rosenblum ML (1995). Improved management of multiple brain abscesses: a combined surgical and medical approach. *Neurosurgery* **36**:76–85.

12 Chun CH, Johnson JD, Hofstetter M, Raff MJ (1986). Brain abscess. A study of 45 consecutive cases. *Medicine* (Baltimore) **65**:415–431.

13 Wispelwey B, Dacey RG, Scheld WM (1997). Brain abscess. In: Scheld WM, Whitley RJ, Durack DT (eds). *Infections of the Central Nervous System*, 2nd edn. Lippincott-Raven, Philadelphia, pp. 463–493.

14 Bakshi R, Wright PD, Kindel PR, *et al.* (1999). Cranial magnetic resonance imaging findings in bacterial endocarditis: the neuro-imaging spectrum of septic brain embolization demonstrated in twelve patients. *J Neuroimaging* **9**:78–84.

15 Schliamser SE, Backman K, Norrby SR (1988). Intracranial abscesses in adults: an analysis of 54 consecutive cases. *Scand J Infect Dis* **20**:1–9.

16 Yang SY, Zhao CS (1993). Review of 140 patients with brain abscess. *Surg Neurol* **39**:290–296.

17 Tunkel AR (2005). Brain abscess. In: Mandell GL, Bennett JE, Dolin R (eds). *Principles and Practice of Infectious Diseases*, 6th edn. Elsevier-Churchill-Livingstone, Philadelphia, pp. 1150–1163.

18 Duma CM, Kondziolka D, Lundsford LD (1992). Image-guided sterotactic management of non-AIDS-related cerebral infection. *Neurosurg Clin N Am* **3**:291–302.

19 Rosenblum ML, Hoff JT, Norman D, Edwards MS, Berg BO (1980). Nonoperative treatment of brain abscesses in selected high-risk patients. *J Neurosurg* **52**:217–225.

20 Quartey GR, Johnston JA, Rozdilskyy B (1976). Decadron in the treatment of cerebral abscess: an experimental study. *J Neurosurg* **45**:3.

21 Centers for Disease Control and Prevention (CDC) (2008). Sexually transmitted diseases surveillance, syphilis. Accessed February 22, 2010 from: http://www.cdc.gov/std/stats08/syphilis.htm

22 Heffelfinger JD, Swint EB, Berman SM, Weinstock HS (2007). Trends in primary and secondary syphilis among men who have sex with men in the United States. *Am J Public Health* **97**:1076–1083.

23 Wolters EC (1987). Neurosyphilis: a changing diagnostic problem? *Eur Neurol* **26**: 23–28.

24 Hook EW 3rd, Marra CM (1992). Acquired syphilis in adults. *N Engl J Med* **326**: 1060–1069.

25 Lukehart S, Hook EW, Baker-Zander SH, Collier AC, Critchlow CW, Handsfield HH (1988). Invasion of the central nervous system by *Treponema pallidum*: implications for diagnosis and therapy. *Ann Intern Med* **109**:855–862.

26 Merritt HH, Moore M (1935). Acute neuro-syphilitic meningitis. *Medicine* (Baltimore) **14**:119–183.

27 Marra CM, Maxwell CL, Smith SL, *et al.* (2004). Cerebrospinal fluid abnormalities in patients with syphilis: association with clinical and laboratory features. *J Infect Dis* **189**:369–376.

28 Workowski KA, Berman SM (2006). Sexually transmitted diseases treatment guidelines. *MMWR Recomm Rep* **55**:1–94.

29 Hart G (1986). Syphilis tests in diagnostic and therapeutic decision-making. *Ann Intern Med* **104**:368–376.

30 Silberstein P, Lawrence R, Pryor D, Shnier R (2002). A case of neurosyphilis with florid Jarisch–Herxheimer reaction. *J Clin Neurosci* **9**:689–690.

31 Spielman A (1994). The emergence of Lyme disease and human babesiosis in a changing environment. *Ann NY Acad Sci* **740**:146–156.

32 Bacon RM, Kugeler KJ, Mead PS (2008). Surveillance for Lyme disease – United States, 1992–2006. *MMWR Surveill Summ* **57**:1.

33 Dennis DT, Hayes EB (2002). Epidemiology of Lyme borreliosis. In: Kahl O, Gray JS, Lane RS, Stanek G (eds). *Lyme Borreliosis: Biology, Epidemiology, and Control*. CABI, Oxford, p. 251.

34 Steere AC (2001). Lyme disease. *N Engl J Med* **345**:115–125.

35 Falco RC, McKenna DF, Daniels TJ, *et al.* (1999). Temporal relation between *Ixodes scapularis* abundance and risk of Lyme disease associated with erythema migrans. *Am J Epidemiol* **149**:771–776.

36 Bosler EM, Coleman JL, Benach JL, *et al.* (1983). Natural distribution of the *Ixodes dammini* spirochetes. *Science* **220**:321–322.

37 Falco RC, Fish D, Piesman J (1996). Duration of tick bites in a Lyme disease-endemic area. *Am J Epidemiol* **143**:187–192.

38 Steere AC, Sikand VK (2003). The presenting manifestations of Lyme disease and the outcomes of treatment (Letter). *N Engl J Med* **384**:2472–2474.

39 Pachner AR, Steere AC (1985). The triad of neurologic manifestations of Lyme disease: meningitis, cranial neuritis, and radiculo-neuritis. *Neurology* **35**:47–53.

40 Logigian EL, Kaplan RF, Steere AC (1990). Chronic neurologic manifestations of Lyme disease. *N Engl J Med* **323**:1438–1444.

41 Dye C, Scheele S, Dolin P, Pathania V, Raviglione MC (1999). Consensus statement. Global burden of tuberculosis: estimated incidence, prevalence, and mortality by country. WHO Global Surveillance and Monitoring Project. *JAMA* **282**:677–686.

42 World Health Organization (WHO) (2008). Tuberculosis: estimated incidence, prevalence and mortality. Accessed March 20, 2010 from: http://www.who.int/mediacentre/factsheets/fs104/en/index.html

43 Centers for Disease Control and Prevention (CDC) (2008). Tuberculosis: data and statistics. Atlanta, GA. Accessed March 20, 2010 from: http://www.cdc.gov/tb/statistics/default.htm

44 Centers for Disease Control and Prevention (CDC) (2002). Tuberculosis morbidity among US-born and foreign-born populations – United States, 2000. *MMWR Morb Mortal Wkly Rep* **51**:101–104.

45 Hosoglu S, Geyik MF, Balik I, *et al.* (2002). Predictors of outcome in patients with tuberculous meningitis. *Int J Tuberc Lung Dis* **6**:64–70.

46 Kennedy DH, Fallon RJ (1979). Tuberculous meningitis. *JAMA* **241**:264–268.

47 Pfyffer GE, Kissling P, Jahn EM, Welscher HM, Salfinger M, Weber R (1996). Diagnostic performance of amplified *Mycobacterium tuberculosis* direct test with cerebrospinal fluid, other nonrespiratory, and respiratory specimens. *J Clin Microbiol* **34**: 834–841.

48 Piersimoni C, Scarparo C, Piccoli P, *et al.* (2002). Performance assessment of two commercial amplification assays for direct detection of *Mycobacterium tuberculosis* complex from respiratory and extrapulmonary specimens. *J Clin Microbiol* **40**:4138–4142.

49 World Health Organization (WHO) (2004). *Global Tuberculosis Control: surveillance, planning, financing*. WHO, Geneva.

50 Thwaites GE, Duc Ban N, Huy Dung N, *et al.* (2004). Dexamethasone for the treatment of tuberculous meningitis in adolescents and adults. *N Engl J Med* **351**:1741–1751.

51 Centers for Disease Control and Prevention (CDC) (2010). Botulism. Retrieved 1/21/10 from http://www.cdc.gov/nczved/divisions/dfbmd/diseases/botulism/.

52 Bleck T (2005). *Clostridium botulinum* (botulism). In: Mandell GL, Bennett JE, Dolin R (eds). *Principles and Practice of Infectious Diseases*, 6th edn. Elvesier, Churchill, Livingstone, Philadelphia, Chapter 243, pp. 2822–2828.

53 Oguma K, Yokota K, Hayashi S, *et al.* (1990). Infant botulism due to *Clostridium botulinum* type C toxin. *Lancet* **336**: 1449–1450.

54 Sugiyama H (1980). *Clostridium botulinum* neurotoxin. *Microbiol Rev* **44**:419–448.

55 Passaro DJ, Werner SB, McGee J, Mac Kenzie WR, Vugia DJ (1998). Wound botulism associated with black tar heroin among injecting drug users. *JAMA* **279**:859–863.

56 Sobel J, Tucker N, Sulka A, McLaughlin J, Maslanka S (2004). Foodborne botulism in the United States, 1990–2000. *Emerg Infect Dis* **10**:1606–1611.

57 Tacket CO, Shadera WX, Mann JM, Hargrett N, Blake P (1984). Equine antitoxin use and other factors that produce outcomes in type A food borne botulism. *Am J Med* **76**:794–798.

58 Kongsaengdao S, Samintarapanya K, Rusmeechang S, *et al.* (2006). An outbreak of botulism in Thailand: clinical manifestations and management of severe respiratory failure. *Clin Infect Dis* **43**:1247–1256.

59 Black RE, Gunn RA (1980). Hypersensitivity reactions associated with botulinal antitoxin. *Am J Med* **69**:567–570.

60 Pascual FB, McGinley EL, Zanardi LR, Cortese MM, Murphy TV (2003). Tetanus surveillance – United States, 1998–2000. *MMWR Surveill Summ* **52**:1–8.

61 Rushdy AA, White JM, Ramsay ME, Crowcroft NS (2003). Tetanus in England and Wales, 1984–2000. *Epidemiol Infect* **130**:71–77.

62 Pedalino B, Cotter B, Ciofi degli Atti M, Mandolini D, Parroccini S, Salmaso S (2002). Epidemiology of tetanus in Italy in years 1971–2000. *Euro Surveill* **7**:103–110.

63 Thwaites CL, Rarrar JJ (2003). Preventing and treating tetanus. *BMJ* **326**:117–118.

64 Bhatia R, Prabhakar S, Grover VK (2002). Tetanus. *Neurol India* **50**:398–407.

65 Vandelaer J, Birmingham M, Gasse F, Kurian M, Shaw C, Garnier S (2003). Tetanus in developing countries: an update on the maternal and neonatal tetanus elimination initiative. *Vaccine* **21**:3442–3445.

66 World Health Organization (WHO) Position Paper (2006). Tetanus vaccine. *Wkly Epidemiol Rec* **81**:198–208.

67 Berger SA, Cherubin CE, Nelson S, Levine L (1978). Tetanus despite preexisting antitetanus antibody. *JAMA* **240**:769–770.

68 Solimena M, Folli F, Aparisi R, Pozza G, DeCamilli P (1990). Autoantibodies to GABA-ergic neurons and pancreatic beta cells in stiff-man syndrome. *N Engl J Med* **322**: 1555–1560.

69 Dinkel K, Meinck HM, Jury KM, Karges W, Richter W (1998). Inhibition of gamma-aminobutyric acid synthesis by glutamic acid decarboxylase autoantibodies in stiff-man syndrome. *Ann Neurol* **44**:194–201.

70 Connolly KJ, Hammer SM (1990). The acute aseptic meningitis syndrome. *Infect Dis Clin North Am* **4**:599–622.

71 Rotbart HA (1997). Viral meningitis and the aseptic meningitis syndrome. In: Scheld WM, Whitley RJ, Durack DT (eds). *Infections of the Central Nervous System*, 2nd edn. Lippincott-Raven, Philadelphia, pp. 23–46.

72 Centers for Disease Control and Prevention (CDC) (2000). Entervovirus surveillance – United States, 1997–1999. *JAMA* **284**:2311–2312.

73 Meyer HM Jr, Johnson RT, Crawford IP, Dascomb HE, Rogers NG (1960). Central nervous system syndromes of 'viral' etiology. A study of 713 cases. *Am J Med* **29**:334–347.

74 Chonmaitree T, Baldwin CD, Lucia HL (1989). Role of the virology laboratory in diagnosis and management of patients with central nervous system disease. *Clin Microbiol Rev* **2**:1–14.

75 Romero JR (2002). Diagnosis and management of enteroviral infections of the central nervous system. *Curr Infect Dis Rep* **4**:309–316.

76 Rotbart HA (1990). Diagnosis of enteroviral meningitis with the polymerase chain reaction. *J Pediatr* **117**:85–89.

77 Sawyer MH, Holland D, Aintablian N (1994). Diagnosis of enteroviral central nervous system infection by polymerase chain reaction during a large community outbreak. *Pediatr Infect Dis J* **13**:177–182.

78 Rotbart HA, Webster AD (2001). Treatment of potentially life-threatening enterovirus infections with pleconaril. *Clin Infect Dis* **32**:228–235.

79 Corey L, Spear PG (1986). Infections with herpes simplex viruses (2). *N Engl J Med* **314**:749–757.

80 Corey L, Adams HG, Brown ZA, Holmes KK (1983). Genital herpes simplex virus infection: clinical manifestations, course, and complications. *Ann Intern Med* **98**:958–972.

81 Berger JR, Simpson DM (1997). Neurological complications of AIDS. In: Scheld WM, Whitley RJ, Durack DT (eds). *Infections of the Central Nervous System*, 2nd edn. Lippincott-Raven, Philadelphia, pp. 255–271.

82 Gnann JW Jr (1997). Meningitis and encephalitis caused by mumps virus. In: Scheld WM, Whitley RJ, Durack DT (eds). *Infections of the Central Nervous System*, 2nd edn. Lippincott-Raven, Philadelphia, pp. 169–180.

83 Kojima Y, Hashiguchi H, Hashimoto T, Tsuji S, Shoji H, Kazuyama Y (2002). Recurrent herpes simplex virus type 2 meningitis: a case report of Mollaret's meningitis. *Jpn J Infect Dis* **55**:85–88.

84 Sejvar JJ, Bode AV, Curiel M, Marfin AA (2004). Post-infectious encephalomyelitis associated with St. Louis encephalitis virus infection. *Neurology* **63**:1719–1721.

85 Levitz RE (1998). Herpes simplex encephalitis: a review. *Heart Lung* **27**:209–212.

86 Whitley RJ (1990). Viral encephalitis. *N Engl J Med* **323**:242–250.

87 Doja A, Bitnun A, Jones EL, *et al.* (2006). Pediatric Epstein–Barr virus-associated encephalitis: 10-year review. *J Child Neurol* **21**:385–391.

88 Hart RP, Kwentus JA, Frazier RB, Hormel TL (1986). Natural history of Kluver–Bucy syndrome after treated herpes encephalitis. *South Med J* **79**:1376–1378.

89 Nahmias AJ, Whitley RT, Visintine AN, Takei Y, Alford CA Jr (1982). Herpes simplex virus encephalitis: laboratory evaluations and their diagnostic significance. *J Infect Dis* **145**:829–836.

90 DeBiasi RL, Kleinschmidt-DeMasters BK, Weinberg A, Tyler KL (2002). Use of PCR for the diagnosis of herpesvirus infections of the central nervous system. *J Clin Virol* **25** (Suppl 1):S5–S11.

91 Nash D, Mostashari F, Fine A, *et al.*; 1999 West Nile Outbreak Response Working Group (2001). The outbreak of West Nile virus infection in the New York City area in 1999. *N Engl J Med* **344**:1807–1814.

92 Centers for Disease Control and Prevention (CDC) (2009). 2009 West Nile virus activity in the United States. Accessed March 17, 2010 from: http://www.cdc.gov/ncidod/dvbid/westnile/surv&controlCaseCount09_detailed.htm

93 Gubler DJ (2007). The continuing spread of West Nile virus in the western hemisphere. *Clin Infect Dis* **45**:1039–1046.

94 Bode AV, Sejvar JJ, Pape WJ, Campbell GL, Marfin AA (2006). West Nile virus disease: a descriptive study of 228 patients hospitalized in a 4-county region of Colorado in 2003. *Clin Infect Dis* **42**:1234–1240.

95 Iwamoto M, Jernigan DB, Guasch A, *et al.*; West Nile Virus in Transplant Recipients Investigation Team (2003). Transmission of West Nile virus from an organ donor to four transplant recipients. *N Engl J Med* **348**:2196–2203.
96 Pealer LN, Marfin AA, Petersen LR, *et al.*; West Nile Virus Transmission Investigation Team (2003). Transmission of West Nile virus through blood transfusion in the United States in 2002. *N Engl J Med* **349**:1236–1245.
97 Watson JT, Pertel PE, Jones RC, *et al.* (2004). Clinical characteristics and functional outcomes of West Nile fever. *Ann Intern Med* **141**:360–365.
98 Centers for Disease Control and Prevention (CDC) (2010). Saint Louis encephalitis: epidemiology and geographic distribution. Accessed March 17, 2010 from: http://www.cdc.gov/sle/technical/epi.html
99 Sanders M, Blumberg A, Haymaker W (1953). Polyradiculopathy in man produced by St. Louis encephalitis virus (SLE). *South Med J* **46**:606–608.
100 Brinker KR, Paulson G, Monath TP, Wise G, Fass RJ (1979). St. Louis encephalitis in Ohio, September 1975. Clinical and EEG studies in 16 cases. *Arch Intern Med* **139**:561–566.
101 McJunkin JE, de los Reyes EC, Irazuzta JE, *et al.* (2001). La Crosse encephalitis in children. *N Engl J Med* **344**: 801–807.
102 McJunkin JE, Khan RR, Tsai TF (1998). California-La Crosse encephalitis. *Infect Dis Clin North Am* **12**:83–93.
103 Jones TF, Erwin PC, Craig AS, *et al.* (2000). Serological survey and active surveillance for La Crosse virus infections among children in Tennessee. *Clin Infect Dis* **31**: 1284–1287.
104 McJunkin JE, Khan R, de los Reyes EC, *et al.* (1997). Treatment of severe La Crosse encephalitis with intravenous ribavirin following diagnosis by brain biopsy. *Pediatrics* **99**: 261–267.
105 World Health Organization (2009). Human and animal rabies. Retrieved December 9, 2009 from: http://www.who.int/rabies/en/
106 Bleck TP, Rupprecht CE (2005). Rhabdoviruses. In: Mandell GL, Bennett JE, Dolin R (eds). In: *Principles and Practice of Infectious Diseases*, 6th edn. Churchill Livingstone, Phildelphia, pp. 2047–2056.
107 Centers for Disease Control (2009). Rabies epidemiology in the United States. Retrieved December 10, 2009 from: http://www.cdc.gov/rabies/epidemiology.html
108 Manning SE, Rupprecht CE, Fishbein D, *et al.* (2008). Human rabies prevention – United States, 2008: recommendations of the Advisory Committee on Immunization Practices. *MMWR Recommend Rep* **57**:1–39.
109 Blanton JD, Hanlon CA, Rupprecht CE (2007). Rabies surveillance in the United States during 2006. *J Am Vet Med Assoc* **231**:540–556.
110 Mondul AM, Krebs JW, Childs JE (2003). Trends in national surveillance for rabies among bats in the United States (1993–2000). *J Am Vet Med Assoc* **222**:633–639.
111 Krebs JW, Mandel EJ, Swerdlow DL, Rupprecht CE (2005). Rabies surveillance in the United States during 2004. *J Am Vet Med Assoc* **227**:1912–1925.
112 Srinivasan A, Burton EC, Kuehnert MJ, *et al.* (2005). Transmission of rabies virus from an organ donor to four transplant recipients. *N Engl J Med* **352**:1103–1111.
113 Centers for Disease Control and Prevention (CDC) (2004). Update: investigation of rabies infections in organ donor and transplant recipients – Alabama, Arkasas, Oklahoma, and Texas, 2004. **53**:586–589.
114 Rupprecht CE, Hanlon CA, Hemachudha T (2002). Rabies re-examined. *Lancet Infect Dis* **2**:327–343.
115 World Health Organization (WHO) (2005). WHO expert committee on rabies. *World Health Organ Tech Rep Ser* **931**:1–121.
116 Cabasso VJ, Loofbourow JC, Roby RE, Anuskiewicz W (1971). Rabies immune globulin of human origin: preparation and dosage determination in non-exposed volunteer subjects. *Bull World Health Organ* **45**:303–315.
117 World Health Organization (WHO) (2009). Poliomyelitis, the disease and the virus. Retreived December 4, 2009 from: http://www.polioeradication.org/disease.asp
118 World Health Organization (WHO) (2009). Wild poliovirus weekly update. Retreived December 4, 2009 from: http://www.polioeradication.org/casecount.asp.
119 Kim-Farley RJ, Bart KJ, Schonberger LB, *et al.* (1984). Poliomyelitis in the USA: virtual elimination of disease caused by wild virus. *Lancet* **2**:1315–1317.
120 Modlin JF (2005). Poliovirus. In: Mandell GL, Bennett JE, Dolin R (eds). *Principles and Practice of Infectious Diseases*, 6th edn. Elsevier, Philadelphia, pp. 2141–2148.
121 Casas I, Klapper PE, Cleator GM, Echevarria JE, Tenorio A, Echevarria JM (1995). Two different PCR assays to detect enteroviral RNA in CSF samples from patients with acute aseptic meningitis. *J Med Virol* **47**:378–385.
122 Pevear DC, Tull TM, Seipel ME, Groarke JM (1999). Activity of pleconoril against enteroviruses. *Antimicrob Agents Chemother* **43**:2109–2115.
123 Desmond RA, Accortt NA, Talley L, Villano SA, Soong SJ, Whitley RJ (2006). Enteroviral meningitis: natural history and outcome of pleconaril therapy. *Antimicrob Agents Chemother* **50**:2409–2414.
124 Ramlow J, Alexander M, LaPorte R, Kaufmann C, Kuller L (1992). Epidemiology of the post-polio syndrome. *Am J Epidemiol* **136**:769–786.
125 McBean AM, Thoms ML, Albrecht P, Cuthie JC, Bernier R (1988). Serologic response to oral polio vaccine and enhanced-potency inactivated polio vaccines. *Am J Epidemiol* **128**:615–628.
126 Simoes EA, John TJ (1986). The antibody response of seronegative infants to inactivated poliovirus vaccine of enhanced potency. *J Biol Stand* **14**:127–131.
127 Swarz TA, Handsher R, Stoeckel P, *et al.* (1989). Immunologic memory induced at birth by immunization with inactivated polio vaccine in a reduced schedule. *Eur J Epidemiol* **5**:143–145.
128 Henderson DA, Witte JJ, Morris L, Lanmuir AD (1964). Paralytic disease associated with oral polio vaccines. *JAMA* **190**:41–48.
129 Krugman RD, Hardy GE, Sellers C, *et al.* (1977). Antibody persistence after primary immunization with trivalent oral poliovirus vaccine. *Pediatrics* **60**:80–82.
130 Alexander LN, Seward JH, Santibanez TA, *et al.* (2004). Vaccine policy changes and epidemiology of poliomyelitis in the United States. *JAMA* **292**:1696–1701.
131 Padgett BL, Walker DL (1973). Prevalence of antibodies in human sera against JC virus, an isolate from a case of progressive multifocal leukoencephalopathy. *J Infect Dis* **127**:467–470.
132 Weber T, Trebst C, Frye S, *et al.* (1997). Analysis of the systemic and intrathecal humoral immune response in progressive multifocal leukoencephalopathy. *J Infect Dis* **176**: 250–254.
133 Aåström K-E, Mancall EL, Richardson EP Jr (1958). Progressive multifocal leukoencephalopathy: a hitherto unrecognized complication of chronic lymphatic leukemia and Hodgkin's disease. *Brain* **81**:93–110.
134 Richardson EP Jr (1961). Progressive multifocal leukoencephalopathy. *N Engl J Med* **265**:815–823.
135 Newton P, Aldridge RD, Lessells AM, Best PV (1986). Progressive multifocal leukoencephalopathy complicating systemic lupus erythematosus. *Arthritis Rheum* **29**:337–343.
136 Holman RC, Janssen RS, Buehler JW, Zelasky MT, Hooper WC (1991). Epidemiology of progressive multifocal leukoencephalopathy in the United States: analysis of national mortality and AIDS surveillance data. *Neurology* **41**:1733–1736.
137 Power C, Gladden JG, Halliday W, *et al.* (2000). AIDS- and non-AIDS-related PML association with distinct p53 polymorphism. *Neurology* **54**:743–746.
138 White FA III, Ishaq M, Stoner GL, Frisque RL (1992). JC virus DNA is present in many human brain samples from patients without progressive multifocal leukoencephalopathy. *J Virol* **66**:5726–5734.

139 Demeter LM (2005). JC, BK, and other polyomaviruses; progressive multifocal leukoencephalopathy. In: Mandell GL, Bennett JE, Dolin R (eds). *Principles and Practice of Infectious Diseases*, 6th edn. Elsevier-Churchill-Livingstone, Philadelphia, pp. 1856–1863.

140 DeLuca A, Giancola ML, Ammassari A, *et al*. (2000). Cidofovir added to HAART improves virological and clinical outcome in AIDS-associated progressive multifocal leukoencephalopathy. *AIDS* **14**:F117–F121.

141 DeLuca A, Giancola ML, Ammassari A, *et al*. (2001). Potent antiretroviral therapy with or without cidofovir for AIDS-associated progressive multifocal leukoencephalopathy: extended follow-up of an observational study. *J Neurovirol* **7**:364–368.

142 Hall CD, Dafni U, Simpson D, *et al*. (1998). Failure of cytarabine in progressive multifocal leukoencephalopathy associated with human immunodeficiency virus infection. *N Engl J Med* **338**:1345–1351.

143 Steiger MJ, Tarnesby G, Gabe S, McLaughlin J, Schapira AH (1993). Successful outcome of progressive multifocal leukoencephalopathy with cytarabine and interferon. *Ann Neurol* **33**:407–411.

144 Przepiorka D, Jaecle KA, Birdwell RR, *et al*. (1997). Successful treatment of progressive multifocal leukoencephalopathy with low-dose interleukin-2. *Bone Marrow Transplant* **20**:983–987.

145 Engsig FN, Hansen AB, Omland LH, *et al*. (2009). Incidence, clinical presentation, and outcome of progressive multifocal leukoencephalopathy in HIV-infected patients during the highly active antiretroviral therapy era: a nationwide cohort study. *J Infect Dis* **199**:77–83.

146 Park BJ, Wannemuehler KA, Marston BJ, Govender N, Pappas PG, Chiller TM (2009). Estimation of the current global burden of cryptococcal meningitis among persons living with HIV/AIDS. *AIDS* **23**(4):525–530.

147 Perfect JR (2005). *Cryptococcus neoformans*. In: Mandell GL, Bennett JE, Dolin R (eds). *Principles and Practice of Infectious Diseases*, 6th edn. Elsevier-Churchill-Livingstone, Philadelphia, Chapter 261, pp. 2997–3012.

148 Kouame-Assouan AE, Cowppli-Bony P, Aka-Anghui DE, *et al*. (2007). Two cases of cryptococcal meningitis revealed by an ischemic stroke. *Bull Soc Pathol Exot* **100**(1):15–16.

149 Grayhill JR, Sobel J, Saag M, *et al*. (2000). Diagnosis and management of increased intracranial pressure in patients with AIDS and cryptococcal meningitis. The NIAID Mycoses Study Group and AIDS Cooperative Treatment Groups. *Clin Infect Dis* **30**(1):47–54.

150 Tanner DC, Weinstein MP, Fedorciw B, Joho KL, Thorpe JJ, Reller L (1994). Comparison of commercial kits for detection of cryptococcal antigen. *J Clin Microbiol* **32**(7):1680–1684.

151 Kauffman CA, Bergman AG, Severance PJ, McClatchey KD (1981). Detection of cryptococcal antigen. Comparison of two latex agglutination tests. *Am J Clin Pathol* **75**:106–109.

152 Garlipp CR, Rossi CL, Bottini PV (1997). Cerebrospinal fluid profiles in acquired immunodeficiency syndrome with and without neurocryptococcosis. *Rev Inst Med Trop Sao Paulo* **39**(6):323–325.

153 Perfect JR, Dismukes WE, Dromer F, *et al*. (2010). Clinical practice guidelines for the management of cryptococcal disease: 2010 update by the Infectious Diseases Society of America. *Clin Infect Dis* **50**:291–322.

154 Dromer F, Mathoulin-Pelissier S, Launay O, Lortholary O; French Cryptococcosis Study Group (2007). Determinants of disease presentation and outcome during cryptococcosis: the CryptoA/D study. *PLos Med* **4**(2):e21.

155 Galgiani JN, Ampel NM, Blair JE, *et al*. (2005). Coccidioidomycosis. *Clin Infect Dis* **41**:1217–1223.

156 Centers for Disease Control and Prevention (CDC) (2010). Coccidioidomycosis. Accessed April 1, 2010 from: http://www.cdc.gov/nczved/divisions/dfbmd/diseases/coccidioidomycosis/

157 Bergstrom L, Yocum DE, Ampel NM, *et al*. (2004). Increased risk of coccidioidomycosis in patients treated with tumor necrosis factor alpha antagonists. *Arthritis Rheum* **50**:1959–1966.

158 Peterson CM, Schuppert K, Kelly PC, Pappagianis D (1993). Coccidioidomycosis and pregnancy. *Obstet Gynecol Surv* **48**:149–156.

159 Wack EE, Ampel NM, Galgiani JN, Bronnimann DA (1988). Cocciodioidomycosis during pregnancy. An analysis of ten cases among 47,120 pregnancies. *Chest* **94**:376–379.

160 Vincent T, Galgiani JN, Huppert M, Salkin D (1993). The natural history of coccidioidal meningitis: VA-Armed Forces Cooperative Studies, 1955–1958. *Clin Infect Dis* **16**:247–254.

161 Body BA (1996). Cutaneous manifestations of systemic mycoses. *Dermatol Clin* **14**:125–135.

162 Ismail Y, Arsura EL (1993). Eosinohilic meningitis associated with coccidioidomycosis. *West J Med* **158**:300–301.

163 Tucker RM, Denning DW, Dupont B, Stevens DA (1990). Itraconazole therapy for chronic coccidioidal meningitis. *Ann Intern Med* **112**:108–112.

164 Prabhu RM, Bonnell M, Currier BL, Orenstein R (2004). Successful treatment of disseminated nonmeningeal coccidioidomycosis with voriconazole. *Clin Infect Dis* **39**:e74–77.

165 Proia LA, Tenorio AR (2004). Successful use of voriconazole for treatment of *Coccidioides* meningitis. *Antimicrob Agents Chemother* **48**:23–41.

166 Wallace MR, Rossetti RJ, Olson PE (1993). Cats and toxoplasmosis risk in HIV-infected adults. *JAMA* **269**(1):76–77.

167 Luft BJ, Remington JS (1992). Toxoplasmic encephalitis in AIDS (AIDS commentary). *Clin Infect Dis* **15**:211–122.

168 Falusi O, French AL, Seaberg EC, *et al*. (2002). Prevalence and predictors of *Toxoplasma* seropositivity in women with and at risk for human immunodeficiency virus infection. *Clin Infect Dis* **35**(11):1414–1417.

169 Dubey J (1994). Toxoplasmosis. *J Am Vet Med Assoc* **205**:1593–1598.

170 Dubey JP, Lindsay DS, Speer CA (1998). Structures of *Toxoplasma gondii* tachyzoites, bradyzoites, and sporozoites and biology and development of tissue cysts. *Clin Microbiol Rev* **11**:267–299.

171 Gray F, Gherardi R, Wingate E, *et al*. (1989). Diffuse 'encephalitic' cerebral toxoplasmosis in AIDS. Report of four cases. *J Neurol* **236**(5):273–277.

172 Liesenfeld O, Wong SY, Remington JS (1999). Toxoplasmosis in the setting of AIDS. In: Bartlett JG, Merigan TC, Bolognesi D (eds). *Textbook of AIDS Medicine*. Williams & Wilkins, Baltimore, pp. 225–259.

173 Cinque P, Scarpellini P, Vago L, Linde A, Lazzarin A (1997). Diagnosis of central nervous system complications in HIV-infected patients: cerebrospinal fluid analysis by the polymerase chain reaction. *AIDS* **11**(1):1–17.

174 Leoung GS, Stanford JF, Giordano MF, *et al*.; American Foundation for AIDS Research (AmFAR) Community-Based Clinical Trials Network (2001). Trimethoprim-sulfamethoxazole (TMP-SMZ) dose escalation versus direct challenge for *Pneumocystis carinii* pneumonia prophylaxis in human immunodeficiency virus-infected patients with a previous adverse reaction to TMP-SMZ. *J Infect Dis* **184**(8):992–997.

175 Soffritti S, Ricci G, Prete A, Rondelli R, Menna G, Pession A (2003). Successful desensitization to trimethoprim–sulfamethoxazole after allogeneic haematopoietic stem cell transplantation: preliminary observations. *Med Pediatr Oncol* **40**(4):271–272.

176 Torre D, Casari S, Speranza F, *et al*. (1998). Randomized trial of trimethoprim–sulfamethoxazole versus pyrimethamine-sulfadiazine for therapy of toxoplasmic encephalitis in patients with AIDS. Italian Collaborative Study Group. *Antimicrob Agents Chemother* **42**:1346–1349.

177 Kaplan JE, Benson C, Holmes KH, Brooks JT, Pau A, Masur H (2009). Guidelines for prevention and treatment of opportunistic infections in HIV-infected adults and adolescents: recommendations from CDC, the National Institutes of Health, and the HIV Medicine Association of the Infectious Diseases Society of America. *MMWR Recomm Rep* **58**:1–207.

178 Porter SB, Sande M (1992). Toxoplasmosis of the central nervous system in the acquired immunodeficiency syndrome. *N Engl J Med* **327**:1643–1648.

179 Levy RM, Rosenbloom S, Perrett LV (1986). Neuroradiologic findings in AIDS: a review of 200 cases. *Am J Neuroradiol* **147**:977–983.

180 Carpio A (2002). Neurocysticercosis: an update. *Lancet Infect Dis* **2**:751–762.

181 Ong S, Talan DA, Moran GJ, *et al.*; EMERGEncy ID NET Study Group (2002). Neurocysticercosis in radiographically imaged seizure patients in US emergency departments. *Emerg Infect Dis* **8**(6):608–613.

182 Del la Garza Y, Graviss EA, Daver NG, *et al.* (2005). Epidemiology of neurocysticercosis in Houston, Texas. *Am J Trop Med Hyg* **73**(4):766–770.

183 Dixon HBF, Lipscomb FM (1961). *Cysticercosis: An Analysis and Follow-up of 450 Cases*. Her Majesty's Stationary Service, London.

184 Wilson M, Bryan RT, Fried JA, *et al.* (1991). Clinical evaluation of the cysticercosis enzyme-linked immunoelectrotransfer blot in patients with neurocysticercosis. *J Infect Dis* **164**(5):1007–1009.

185 Del Brutto OH, Sotelo J (1988). Neurocysticercosis: an update. *Rev Infect Dis* **10**:1075–1087.

186 Evans C, Garcia HH, Gilman RH, Friedland JS (1997). Controversies in the management of cysticercosis. *Emerg Infect Dis* **3**:403–405.

187 Bang OY, Heo JH, Choi SA, Kim DI (1997). Large cerebral infarction during praziquantel therapy in neurocysticercosis. *Stroke* **28**:211–213.

188 Takayangui OM, Jardim E (1992). Therapy for neurocysticercosis: comparison between albendazole and praziquantel. *Arch Neurol* **49**:290–294.

189 Lo Re V, Gluckman SJ (2003). Eosinophilic meningitis. *Am J Med* **114**(3):217–223.

190 Ramirez-Avila L, Slome S, Schuster FL, *et al.* (2009). Eosinophilic meningitis due to *Angiostrongylus* and *Gnathostoma* species. *Clin Infect Dis* **48**:322–327.

191 Slom TJ, Cortese MM, Gerber SI, *et al.* (2002). An outbreak of eosinophilic meningitis caused by *Angiostrongylus cantonensis* in travelers returning from the Caribbean. *N Engl J Med* **346**:668–675.

192 Kuberski T, Wallace GD (1979). Clinical manifestations of eosinophilic meningitis due to *Angiotrongylus cantonensis*. *Neurology* **29**:1566–1570.

193 Jindrak K 91975). *Angiostrongylus cantonensis* (eosinophilic meningitis, Alicata's disease). In: Hornabrook RW (ed). *Topics on Tropical Neurology*. FA Davis, Philadelphia, pp. 133–164.

194 Rusnak JM, Lucey DR (1993). Clinical gnathostomiasis: case report and review of the English-language literature. *Clin Infect Dis* **16**:33–50.

195 Kuberski T (1979). Eosinophils in cerebrospinal fluid. *Ann Intern Med* **91**:70–75.

196 Chotmongkol V, Sawanyawisuth K, Thavaronpitak Y (2000). Corticosteroid treatment of eosinophilic meningitis. *Clin Infect Dis* **31**:660–662.

197 Jitpimolmard S, Sawanyawisuth K, Morakote N, *et al.* (2007). Albendazole therapy for eosinophilic meningitis caused by *Angiostrongylus cantonensis*. *Parasitol Res* **100**:1293–1296.

198 Hidelaratchi MD, Riffsy MT, Wijesekera JC (2005). A case of eosinophilic meningitis following monitor lizard meat consumption, exacerbated by antihelminthics. *Ceylon Med J* **50**:84.

199 Brown P, Cathala F, Raubertas RF, Gajdusek DC, Castaigne P (1987). The epidemiology of Creutzfeldt–Jakob disease: conclusion of a 15-year investigation in France and review of the world literature. *Neurology* **37**:895–904.

200 Spencer MD, Knight RSG, Will RG (2002). First hundred cases of variant Creutzfeldt–Jakob disease: retrospective case note review of early psychiatric and neurological features. *BMJ* **324**:1479–1482.

201 Wientjens DP, Davanipour Z, Hofman A, *et al.* (1996). Risk factors for Creutzfeldt–Jakob disease: a reanalysis of case-control studies. *Neurology* **46**:1287–1291.

202 Collins S, Law MG, Fletcher A, Boyd A, Kaldor J, Masters CL (1999). Surgical treatment and risk of sporadic Creutzfeldt–Jakob disease: a case-control study. *Lancet* **353**:693–697.

203 Centers for Disease Control (CDC) (2010). Creutzfeldt–Jakob disease. Accessed on January 8, 2010 from http://www.cdc.gov/ncidod/dvrd/cjd/

204 World Health Organization (WHO) (2010). Variant Creutzfeldt–Jakob disease. Accessed on January 8, 2010 from http://www.who.int/mediacentre/factsheets/fs180/en/

205 The National Creutzfeldt–Jakob Disease Surveillance Unit (NCJDSU) (2010). Variant CDJ cases worldwide. Accessed on February 25, 2010 from http://www.cjd.ed.ac.uk/

206 Lewis AM, Yu M, DeArmond SJ, *et al.* (2006). Human growth hormone-related iatrogenic Creutfeldt–Jakob disease with abnormal imaging. *Arch Neurol* **63**:288–290.

207 Centers for Disease Control and Prevention (CDC) (1997). Creutzfeldt–Jakob disease associated with cadaveric dura mater grafts – Japan January 1979–May 1996. *MMWR Morb Mortal Wkly Rep* **46**:1066–1069.

208 Centers for Disease Control and Prevention (CDC) (2003). Update: Creutzfeldt–Jakob disease associated with cadaveric dura mater grafts – Japan 1979–2003. *MMWR Morb Mortal Wkly Rep* **52**:1179–1181.

209 Allan B, Tuft S (1997). Transmission of Creutzfeldt–Jakob disease in corneal grafts. *BMJ* **315**:1553–1554.

210 Creange A, Gray F, Cesaro P, *et al.* (1995). Transmission of Creutzfeldt–Jakob disease after liver transplantation. *Ann Neurol* **38**:269–272.

211 Bernoulli C, Siegfreid J, Baumgartner G, *et al.* (1977). Danger of accidental person-to-person transmission of Creutzfeldt–Jakob disease by surgery. *Lancet* **1**:478–479.

212 Collinge J, Sidle KCL, Meads J, *et al.* (1996). Molecular analysis of prion strain variation and the aetiology of 'new variant' CJD. *Nature* **383**:685–690.

213 Bruce ME, Will RG, Ironside JW, *et al.* (1997). Transmissions to mice indicate that 'new vaiant' CJD is caused by BSE agent. *Nature* **389**:498–501.

214 Scott MR, Will R, Ironside J, *et al.* (1999). Compelling transgenetic evidence for transmission of bovine spongiform encephalopathy to humans. *Proc Natl Acad Sci USA* **96**:15137–15142.

215 Collie DA, Sellar RJ, Zeidler M, *et al.* (2001). MRI of Creutzfeldt–Jakob disease: imaging features and recommended MRI protocol. *Clin Radiol* **56**:726–739.

216 Will RG, Zeidler M, Stewart GE, *et al.* (2000). Diagnosis of new variant Creutzfeldt–Jakob disease. *Ann Neurol* **47**:575–582.

217 Zerr I, Bodemer M, Gefeller O, *et al.* (1998). Detection of 14-3-3 protein in the cerebrospinal fluid supports the diagnosis of Creutzfeldt–Jakob disease. *Ann Neurol* **43**:32–40.

INFLAMMATORY DISORDERS OF THE NERVOUS SYSTEM

Neil Scolding

ACUTE DISSEMINATED ENCEPHALOMYELITIS (POST-INFECTIOUS ENCEPHALOMYELITIS)

Definition and epidemiology

Acute disseminated encephalomyelitis (ADEM) is an acute inflammatory demyelinating disease of the brain and spinal cord characterized by widespread perivascular inflammation and demyelination and caused by an autoimmune attack on the brain, most commonly as a reaction to a viral infection which activates autoreactive T cells that recognize myelin-specific proteins. The disease is one of immunoregulatory failure rather than immunosuppression.

- Incidence: uncommon; most frequent after nonspecific upper respiratory tract infections of undetermined etiology.
- Age: any age, but commoner in childhood.
- Gender: either sex.

Etiology and pathophysiology

- Post-infectious:
  - Exanthematous:
    - Measles: complicates 1:1000 cases of measles; in countries where vaccination is not routine.
    - Varicella-zoster: <1:10,000 (more commonly causes acute ataxia).
  - Nonexanthematous:
    - Influenza A upper respiratory tract infection.
    - Mumps.
    - Epstein–Barr virus.
    - Rubella: <1:20,000 (more commonly causes a toxic encephalopathy).
  - Bacterial infection: *Mycoplasma pneumoniae*.
- Post-immunization:
  - Vaccination (vaccinia, rabies).
  - Tetanus antitoxin.
- No recognizable preceding illness sometimes.

ADEM is thought to be an autoimmune disease, partly because of the inability to isolate an infectious agent from the central nervous system (CNS), and because of experimental models of autoimmune diffuse white matter encephalomyelitis that can be induced in animals, or accidentally in humans, by injection of myelin antigens with adjuvant. A very small inoculum of activated T cell clones that recognize small fragments of myelin basic protein and proteolipid protein can induce CNS inflammation and destruction of normal brain white matter by the immune system. The disease can range from acute hemorrhagic leukoencephalitis (Weston Hurst disease) with massive fibrin deposition and a substantial neutrophilic hemorrhagic lesion, to a demyelinating disorder with a lymphocytic infiltrate, which is histologically similar to multiple sclerosis (MS).

It is believed that a viral infection activates circulating autoreactive T cells that recognize myelin-specific proteins, and these T cells migrate into the CNS and recruit neutrophils in a bystander fashion, triggering massive multifocal tissue destruction. The mechanism of T cell activation is unknown.

Clinical features

- Preceding upper respiratory tract or gastrointestinal tract infection is common.
- Latent interval between the acute viral illness and the neurological onset is from a few days to 2–3 weeks.
- Acute/subacute onset.
- Fever, headache, malaise.
- Impaired conscious level.
- Meningismus.
- Seizures.

Progressive focal neurologic signs include:

- Hemiparesis or paraparesis.
- Sensory defects, depending on the location of lesions in the brain and spinal cord.
- Ataxia.
- Optic neuritis (often bilateral; unilateral is uncommon).
- Other cranial nerve palsies.
- Raised intracranial pressure (ICP):
  - Headache.
  - Vomiting.
  - Papilledema.
  - Obtundation.

Tips

▶ *Although the differential is wide, the triad of HEADACHE, IMPAIRED AWARENESS, AND FEVER should always make you think of ADEM.*

▶ *Urgent cerebral imaging, and if safe, a lumbar puncture, are almost always mandatory.*

▶ *High-dose intravenous CORTICOSTEROIDS, followed if there is no rapid response by PLASMA EXCHANGE, are recommended.*

▶ *It is commonly necessary to 'cover' empirically for other possible treatable disorders (e.g. high-dose acyclovir for herpes simplex) until they are formally excluded.*

Special forms: acute hemorrhagic leukoencephalitis

Acute hemorrhagic leukoencephalitis is a more aggressive form of ADEM.

- Epidemiology: affects children and adults and both sexes equally.
- Clinical features:
  - Latent period after the initial illness ranges from 1–20 days but, unlike ADEM, tends to last just a few days or may even be unnoticeable.
  - Fever (temperature up to 42°C [108°F]) and malaise.
  - Mild neck rigidity.
  - Progressive focal neurologic signs and raised ICP.
- Investigations:
  - Peripheral blood neutrophil pleocytosis and a high erythrocyte sedimentation rate (ESR).
  - Computed tomography (CT)/magnetic resonance imaging (MRI) scan: abnormal; brain swelling, similar to ADEM, but with much more extensive lesions, and a hemorrhagic component.
  - Cerebrospinal fluid (CSF):
    - High pressure (>300 mmH_2O).
    - Cells: neutrophil pleocytosis (may be >1000 cells × 10^6/l); hundreds of red cells.
    - Protein: raised.
    - Glucose levels: normal.
- Diagnosis: only confirmed with certainty at autopsy in most cases. Pathology shows:
  - Swollen hemorrhagic brain with herniation.
  - Widespread necrotizing hemorrhagic lesions in the white matter and brainstem.
  - Perivascular neutrophilic infiltrate with varying numbers of lymphocytes.
  - Blood vessels impregnated with fibrin (fibrinoid necrosis).
  - Widespread demyelination, usually in regular patches, and around areas of hemorrhage.
  - Gray matter is also frequently involved.
- Prognosis: rapid clinical course (more rapid than ADEM), progressing to delirium and coma; often fatal.

Differential diagnosis

- Viral encephalitis: direct infection of the CNS (e.g. by arbovirus, herpes simplex virus [HSV], cytomegalovirus [CMV]) rather than activation of autoreactive T cells by the primary infection. The presence of a persistent neutrophilic instead of lymphocytic CSF pleocytosis in ADEM is against a direct viral infection of the CNS.
- Leptospirosis meningoencephalitis: a biphasic illness, with a prodrome of chills and conjunctival suffusion and the presence of leptospires in the blood and CSF. In the second phase, many develop neurologic complications with a neutrophilic pleocytosis in CSF.
- Lyme disease.
- Brain abscess.
- Brain tumor.
- MS: may have partially similar underlying pathophysiology and clinical presentation, but has a chronic relapsing and remitting, or progressive course.
- Meningitis: viral, bacterial, tuberculous, cryptococcal.
- Stroke: massive carotid territory infarction with temporal lobe swelling compressing the posterior cerebral artery against the brainstem and causing additional posterior infarction.
- Transverse myelitis.

Investigations

CT brain scan

Scans show diffuse low attenuation throughout the gray and white matter of one or both hemispheres with mass effect (midline shift, subfalcine herniation, uncal herniation, effacement of basilar cisterns, entrapment of lateral ventricles) *but may be normal.*

MRI brain scan

MRI is much more sensitive than CT. Areas of increased signal on T2-weighted images in the white matter are present which may be quite extensive and enhance with contrast (**465**). The lesions occur mostly in the cerebrum, but are also found in the brainstem and cerebellum and spinal cord. When they predominate in the latter, they may mimic spinal cord or brainstem tumor. The lesions may not resolve completely, and result in diffuse atrophy. No new lesions should appear on MRI after 6 months from the start of the disease.

CSF

CSF is normal in about one-third of patients. Two-thirds show a mild mononuclear cell pleocytosis and protein elevation. Viral and bacterial culture, polymerase chain reaction (PCR) for viral deoxyribonucleic acid (DNA), and immunoglobulin (Ig) G (which may be elevated) are indicated. Oligoclonal band testing is usually negative.

Blood

- Full blood count and ESR.
- Blood biochemistry.
- Blood viral serology: acute and convalescent sera may establish the specific infecting agent but usually are not of help in differentiating acute encephalitis caused by direct infection from encephalitis caused by immune-mediated perivenular demyelination.

Other investigations

- Chest X-ray.
- Throat and rectal swabs.
- Urinalysis.
- Electroencephalogram (EEG): abnormal; nonspecific diffuse slow wave activity.

Diagnosis

There are no consistent abnormalities in the blood or urine. A definitive diagnosis requires pathologic examination; most treated cases are presumed, rather than certain. Macroscopic pathology shows the brain is congested and swollen (**466**).

Microscopic pathology shows perivascular inflammation (macrophages, plasma cells, and T lymphocytes) and demyelination of the white matter tracts of the cerebral hemispheres, brainstem, spinal cord, and optic nerves. There is significant axon destruction.

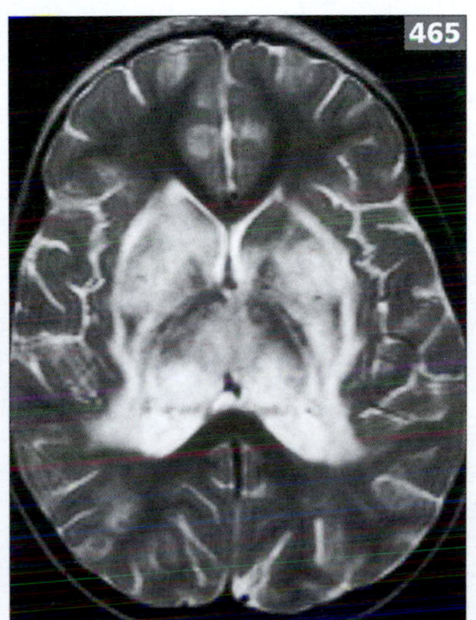

465 T2-weighted MRI from a young patient who became confused and neurologically unwell about 2 weeks after a dose of chickenpox. Note the extensive white matter and basal ganglia increased signal which also extended into the brainstem.

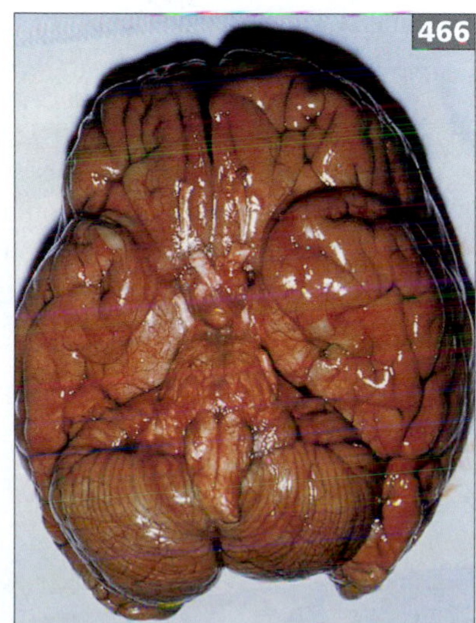

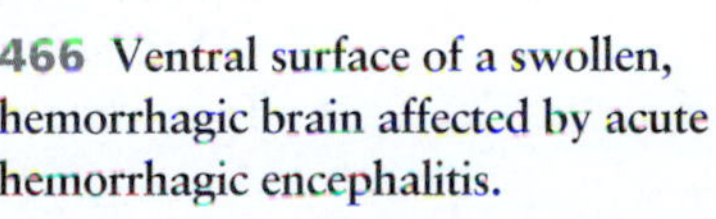

466 Ventral surface of a swollen, hemorrhagic brain affected by acute hemorrhagic encephalitis.

Treatment

Supportive care aims to lower temperature with antipyretic agents, maintain an adequate fluid intake, treat epileptic seizures if they develop, and reduce ICP if raised. Despite the absence of conclusive trial evidence, most authorities recommend intravenous methyl prednisolone, proceeding to plasma exchange in the absence of a therapeutic response[1].

Some patients make remarkable recoveries, even after prolonged periods of profound coma, so very aggressive supportive therapy should almost always be pursued.

Prognosis

Major sequelae include:

- Measles: frequent (case fatality rate 20%).
- Rubella: rare (case fatality rate 20%).
- Vaccinia: 10% (case fatality rate 10%).
- Varicella: very rare (case fatality rate 5%).

Prevention

The cessation of immunization with vaccinia virus and the introduction of vaccines for measles, mumps, and rubella viruses have proved highly effective.

MULTIPLE SCLEROSIS (MS)

Definition and epidemiology

MS is a chronic autoimmune inflammatory demyelinating disease of the CNS in which the lesions are disseminated in time and space (different sites in the CNS are affected at different points in time).

Prevalence is higher in temperate climates further from the equator (e.g. Hobart, Tasmania, Australia, 76:100,000); lower in tropical and subtropical climates close to the equator (e.g. tropical Queensland, Australia, 12:100,000).

- Onset is rare (though increasingly recognized) before puberty and beyond 60 years of age. *Age of onset is <20 years: 20% of cases; 20–50 years: 50–60% of cases; >50 years: 20–30% of cases.
- There is a female propensity (F>M: >3:1).
- MS is most common in patients with northern European ancestry; MS is uncommon in Australian aboriginals, Maori, Chinese, Japanese, and black Africans.

Etiology and pathophysiology

Etiology is unknown, but likely to be a misdirected autoimmune disease (because of the predilection for women, the human leukocyte antigen [HLA] association, the relapsing and remitting course, and the finding of immunologically active cells in the brain, spinal cord, and CSF). This, and other evidence, suggests that MS is an autoimmune disease resulting from an immune attack on the myelin sheaths and axons in the CNS by autoreactive T lymphocytes and autoantibodies. Environmental factors, such as a virus infection (e.g. herpes virus-6), may trigger immune-mediated demyelination in genetically predisposed individuals. Vitamin D is increasingly implicated[2]. The most consistent finding of HLA associations with MS is with DR15 and DQ6. Other loci have shown a possible protective effect, such as HLA-C554 and HLA-DRB1.

Epidemiologic evidence[3] points to environmental factors at a young age:

- Prevalence of MS increases with increasing latitude.
- Risk of MS for an individual corresponds to the risk of their area of residence before the age of about 15 years.

Genetic factors[4] are also likely to be relevant:

- A family history of MS is present in about 10% of people with MS.
- The concordance rate for MS in monozygotic twins is 35% *vs.* 5% in dizygotic twins and nontwin siblings.

One suggestion is that exposure to an unidentified nonself antigen 'mimics' constitutive peptides of myelin and evokes an antigen-specific, T cell-mediated immune response. Lymphocytes, macrophages, and humoral factors enter the CNS and the blood–brain barrier breaks down. B-lymphocytes produce oligoclonal IgG in the CSF. Sensitized T cells produce cytokines which may also damage oligodendrocytes and myelin. Nerve conduction is blocked in demyelinated axons and can be restored by remyelination. In contrast, axonal and neuronal loss lead to a permanent loss of neurologic function, as the CNS axonal regenerative capacity is severely limited.

Clinical features

MS usually has a subacute onset of neurologic symptoms over several hours to days. Infrequently the symptoms evolve quickly over minutes or slowly over weeks or months. The onset is monosymptomatic in about 75% of cases. The remainder have initial symptoms of multiple lesions within the CNS. The symptoms usually reflect dysfunction of the optic nerves, brainstem, or spinal cord.

Vision

Reduced visual acuity, which varies from a slight dulling of color vision to complete monocular blindness, together with pain around the eye that is exacerbated by eye movement or touching the eye, are symptoms of optic neuritis. The signs include a central or paracentral scotoma in most patients, particularly using a red target (most of the optic nerve fibers transmit information from the macular), and a swollen optic disc (papillitis) in the acute phase if there is demyelination of the anterior part of the optic nerve (**467**). Optic disc pallor due to optic atrophy ensues later (**468**).

Internuclear ophthalmoplegia results in double vision, due to lesion of the medial longitudinal fasciculus (MLF), which connects the nuclei of cranial nerves III and VI (**469**). It is elicited by asking the patient to look to one side and noticing a slower rate of adduction, or a failure of adduction, of the adducting eye (ipsilateral to the lesion) and horizontal jerk nystagmus of the fully abducting eye. Subtle forms can be detected if the examiner watches the patient from the side, in the direction of attempted lateral gaze (i.e. not 'front-on'), and following the visual axes during rapid voluntary eye movements (saccades) from one side to the other and back; and then watching from the other side. The lesion may be unilateral (which can be due to cerebrovascular disease or demyelination) or bilateral (which is more commonly due to demyelination). With rostral MLF lesions, near the IIIrd nerve nucleus, vergence (ability to converge the eyes) may be impaired, whereas with caudal MLF lesions, near the VIth nerve nucleus, vergence is preserved.

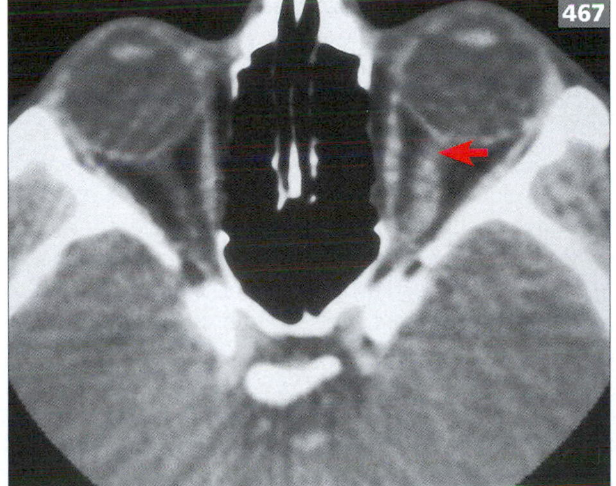

467 Optic neuritis. MRI orbits, axial plane, of the optic nerve, showing swelling of the optic nerve (arrow) in a patient with optic neuritis due to multiple sclerosis.

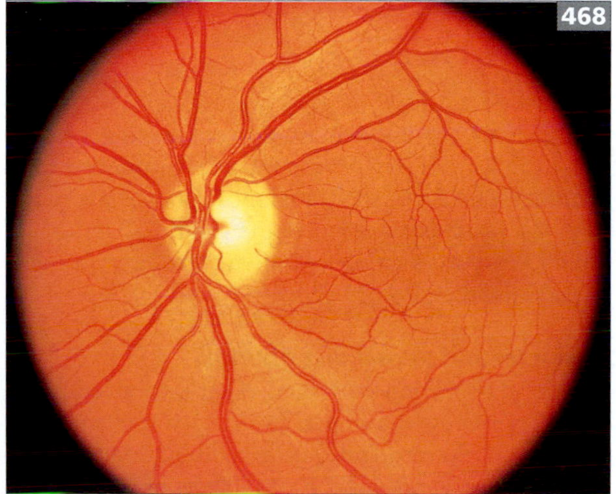

468 Optic atrophy.

469 Bilateral internuclear ophthalmoplegia.

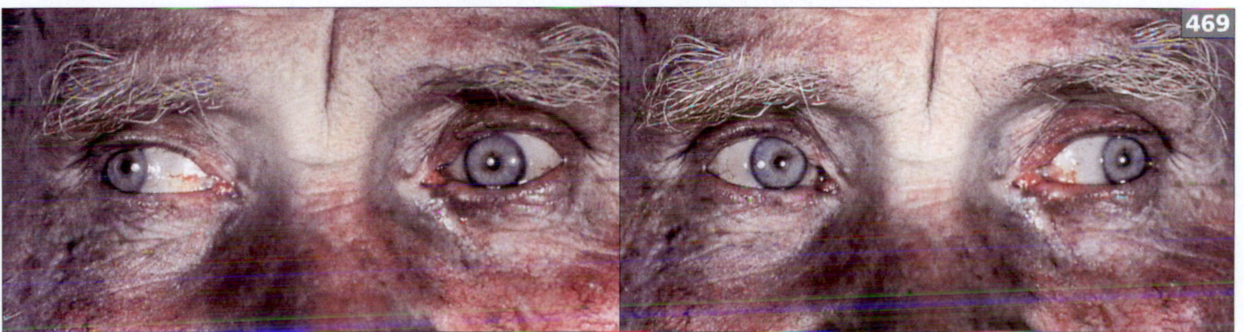

Weakness

Weakness occurs in one or more limbs or the face due to corticospinal tract demyelination. It may be described as heaviness, tiredness, or stiffness, dragging of one leg, or a tendency to fall. Altered sensation of the face, trunk, or one or more limbs includes:

- Trigeminal neuralgia (tic douloureux) (brainstem).
- Lhermitte's symptom: electric shock-like sensation down the back on flexing the neck (cervical spinal cord).
- Numbness starting in the feet and spreading up to the waist (cervical or thoracic cord).
- Reduced temperature sensation, noticed in a warm bath/shower or when swimming (spinothalamic tract).
- Feeling of a tight band wrapped around the trunk or limbs, or swelling of limbs (posterior columns).
- Clumsy or functionally useless hand despite normal power and coordination (posterior columns and dorsal root entry zone).

An unsteady gait, weakness and spasticity, proprioceptive loss (sensory ataxia) results from spinocerebellar dysfunction or vestibular dysfunction, with reduced or double vision, and other comorbidities such as pain and arthritis.

Vertigo

Vertigo is the sensation of rotation or spinning, causing nausea and ataxia (involving intra-axial vestibular nerve, vestibular nucleus in the lateral medulla, and pathways from the vestibular nucleus to the vestibular cortex). It occurs rarely in isolation and often together with other brainstem symptoms.

Sphincter and sexual disturbances

Bladder dysfunction may be divided into a failure to empty (caused at least in part by detrusor sphincter dyssynergia), failure to store, or a combination of both. Frequency, urgency, and precipitancy of micturition (85%), urge incontinence (63%), hesitancy and interrupted stream (45%), and retention of urine may be early symptoms of spinal cord demyelination and are very common in later stages. Bowel dysfunction occurs in more than one-half of patients. Impotence is also common.

Mental changes and seizures

After several years, many patients experience emotional instability, anxiety, depression, euphoria, and impaired cognitive function (short-term memory, attention, and speed of processing). Epileptic seizures may occur but are uncommon.

Fatigue and pain

Many patients with long-standing MS complain of often very severe and debilitating fatigue.

Pain occurs in up to two-thirds of patients. In most it is chronic, but in about 10% it is acute and paroxysmal. Examples include trigeminal neuralgia; brief (1 minute) dysesthetic burning pain in one or more extremities that is provoked by movement, tactile stimulation, or hyperventilation; and painful tonic seizures. The latter can occur with or immediately after the dysesthetic burning pain, or independently. They are brief, frequent, and often intensely painful episodes in which the limbs on one side may adopt a tetanic posture. They may be precipitated by movement or sensory stimulation and usually remit completely after 4–6 weeks. The three main types of chronic pain are dysesthetic extremity pain, chronic back pain, and painful leg spasms.

Precipitating and exacerbating factors in MS include:

- Trauma (including surgery), infections, vaccinations, emotional stress, and fatigue have been suggested to precipitate MS relapses, though this is controversial.
- Pregnancy can reduce the rate of relapses, while the early post-partum period can mildly increase the risk of exacerbations of MS, while the long-term outcome is not affected.
- Physical exercise or other causes of an increase in body temperature (e.g. hot weather, hot baths), may briefly exacerbate neurologic symptoms (Uhthoff's symptom). A reversible conduction block in partially demyelinated nerve fibers secondary to an increase in body temperature is believed to play a role.
- Immunization may, albeit uncommonly, precipitate relapses of MS, so the potential benefits and risks of immunization need to be carefully considered.

Tips

▶ *While a daunting variety of symptoms and signs are possible in MS, a number of clinical patterns are common and diagnostically helpful.*

▶ *In relapse onset MS (around 80–90% of cases), optic neuritis (usually unilateral), a partial spinal cord syndrome, or brainstem events are common.*

▶ *In primary progressive disease, insidiously deteriorating spastic paraparesis, ataxia, or more rarely, cognitive decline are more typical.*

▶ *In consequence, the differential diagnosis is quite different .*

Tip

▶ *For both relapse onset and primary progressive MS it is always important to maintain diagnostic vigilance not just at presentation, but throughout the course of the disease:*

- *A number of mimics may take several years to exclude with certainty.*
- *Having definite MS offers no protection against other neurologic diseases, rather the opposite in some instances (falls are common and may cause subdurals; required drug treatments for pain [e.g. carbamazepine] may cause ataxia, and so on).*

Differential diagnosis[5]

Differentials depend on the clinical presentation.

Multi-focal neurologic syndrome

- Inherited ataxias.
- Vitamin B12 deficiency.
- Mitochondrial disease.
- Vasculitis:
  - Infection: *Borrelia burgdorferi* (Lyme disease), meningovascular syphilis.
  - Isolated granulomatous angiitis of the CNS.
  - Polyarteritis nodosa.
  - Systemic lupus erythematosus (SLE) (facial rash, arthritis, pericarditis, pleuritis).
  - Behçet's disease.
- Granulomatous inflammation:
  - Sarcoidosis.
  - Infection:
    - Bacteria (brucellosis, chlamydia, tularemia), and mycobacteria (tuberculosis, atypical mycobacteria).
    - Fungi (histoplasmosis, coccidioidomycosis, cryptococcosis).
    - Spirochetes (treponemal infections such as syphilis).
    - Parasites (toxoplasmosis, leishmaniasis).
  - Occupational and environmental exposure to organic or inorganic agents (e.g. methotrexate, talc, metals).
  - Neoplasia: lymphoma (e.g. intravascular lymphoma).
  - Autoimmune disorders (Wegener's granulomatosis, Churg–Strauss syndrome).
- Infection:
  - Acute post-infectious encephalomyelitis.
  - Subacute leukoencephalitis caused by human herpesvirus-6.
  - Progressive multifocal leukoencephalopathy (PML; JC papovavirus).
- Leukodystrophy.
- Brain, foramen magnum, or spinal arteriovenous malformation or tumor(s) (primary or metastatic).
- Cervical spondylitic myeloradiculopathy.
- Tethered spinal cord.
- Multiple emboli to the CNS.
- Multiple pathologies.

Optic neuropathy

- Leber's hereditary optic neuropathy: a maternally inherited disease, usually leading to severe bilateral visual loss, and associated with several mitochondrial DNA point mutations; the major ones at nucleotide positions 11778, 3460, and 14484.
- Other hereditary optic neuropathies.
- Ischemic optic neuropathy.
- Neurosyphilis.
- Devic's disease.

Acute noncompressive spinal cord syndrome

- Vascular:
  - Anterior spinal artery infarction: paraparesis with loss of pain and temperature sensation, develops over minutes to hours, and usually persists if infarction occurs.
  - Intramedullary hemorrhage.
- Inflammation of the spinal cord:
  - Devic's disease.
  - MS: usually a partial cord syndrome (e.g. unilateral loss of pain and temperature, deafferentation of one limb, or an asymmetric incomplete paraparesis) develops over hours to days with partial or complete recovery over several weeks.
  - Transverse myelitis: complete loss of sensory and motor function below the level of the lesion, resulting in a flaccid, areflexic paraplegia; develops over hours to days, commonly after an infection (e.g. upper respiratory tract).
  - Acute necrotizing myelitis: tuberculosis, lymphoma, carcinoma.
  - Connective tissue disease: SLE.
  - Sarcoidosis.
- Infection of the spinal cord:
  - Herpes zoster.
  - HSV types I and II.
  - Human immunodeficiency virus (HIV).
  - Tuberculosis (TB).
  - Syphilis.

Chronic noncompressive spinal cord syndrome

- Inherited: hereditary spastic paraparesis: usually a family history of autosomal dominant inheritance.
- Vascular: dural arteriovenous malformation: the most common type of spinal angioma. Usually affects the thoracolumbar segments and tends to present in middle-aged men as a chronic progressive myelopathy with symptoms that may fluctuate or be aggravated by exercise. A combination of upper and lower motor neuron signs may be present.
- Inflammation of the spinal cord:
  - MS.
  - Sarcoidosis.
- Infection of the spinal cord:
  - Herpetic necrotizing myelitis.
  - CMV.
  - Varicella-zoster granulomatous myelitis.
  - Human T lymphocyte virus-1 (HTLV-1) associated myelopathy ('tropical spastic paraparesis') in adults from endemic regions or with other risk factors (e.g. Afro-Caribbeans). A progressive spastic paraplegia develops over a number of years. However, sphincter disturbance is the rule and considerable neuropathic lower limb pain is common.
  - TB.
  - Syphilis.
  - Toxoplasmosis.
  - Schistosomiasis.
- Intramedullary tumor of the spinal cord:
  - Astrocytoma.
  - Ependymoma.
  - Lymphoma.
  - Lipoma.
  - Hemangioma.
  - Metastases.
- Metabolic:
  - Vitamin B12 deficiency: presents over weeks or months as a subacute spinal cord syndrome with intense paresthesia and a combination of pyramidal and dorsal column signs.
  - Adrenomyeloneuropathy: an X-linked inherited disorder that affects males and some heterozygous females with a progressive myelopathy. A peripheral neuropathy and adrenal insufficiency may be present.
- Toxic/iatrogenic:
  - Radiation myelopathy: steadily progressive spastic paraplegia, months to years after radiotherapy. Pathologically there is necrosis of the irradiated cord segments with obliterative changes in blood vessels in the same region.
  - Lathyrism: endemic in parts of India and presents as a subacute or chronic spastic paraparesis in people who regularly ingest chickling pea vetch (*Lathyrus sativus*) over several months. It is thought to be caused by a toxin in the chickling pea.
- Degenerative:
  - Syringomyelia.
  - Motor neuron disease: purely motor; usually a combination of lower and upper motor neuron signs.

Investigations

History

- Establish the onset and nature of the neurologic symptoms, any associated or exacerbating factors, and the clinical course.
- Enquire about previous neurologic symptoms such as blurred vision, blindness, double vision, weakness, altered feeling (numbness, tingling), and disturbances of bladder function.

Physical examination

- Assess the presenting neurologic impairments and functional disabilities (e.g. spastic paraparesis).
- Search for other 'silent' neurologic signs of previous subclinical demyelination (e.g. optic atrophy, internuclear ophthalmoplegia).

MRI of the brain

MRI is the imaging investigation of choice. T2-weighted images show:

- Areas of increased signal (brightness) in the white matter which can be anywhere in the brain but are typically seen in the immediate periventricular white matter and corpus callosum (**470–475**).
- The areas of brightness can be of varying size, may show some swelling, and may be multiple or only a few.
- A small proportion of patients with definite MS will have a normal MRI.
- It is important to differentiate other causes of bright spots which are nonpathologic from MS plaques, for example enlarged perivascular spaces which are usually small. Normal young persons are allowed to have up to three white spots (if small); older individuals have more.

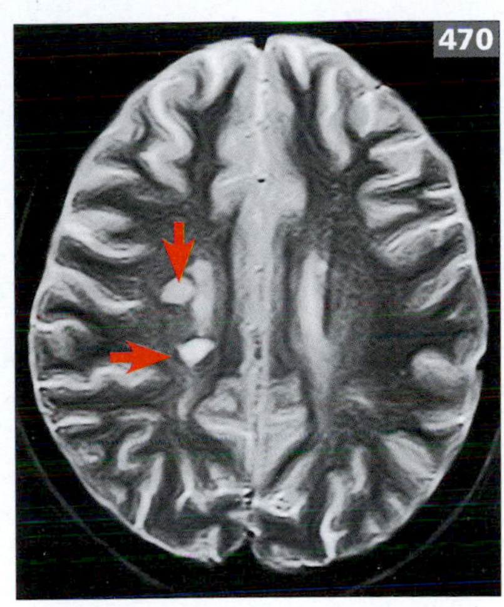

470, 471 MRI of brain in the sagittal plane, proton density image (470), and axial plane T2-weighted image (471), showing multifocal areas of high signal intensity adjacent to the corpus callosum (470) and lateral ventricles (471) due to demyelination (arrows).

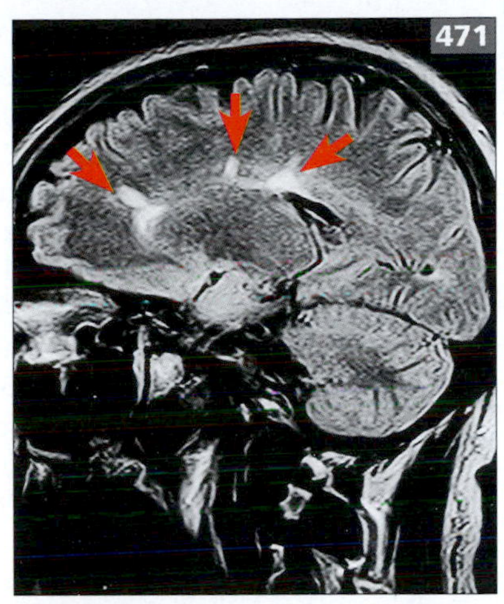

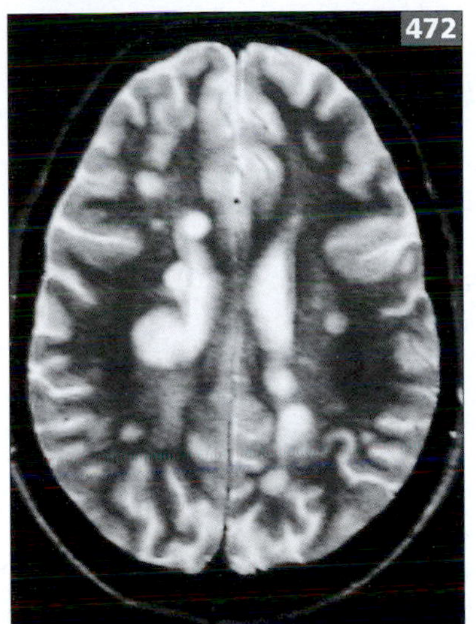

472 T2-weighted MRI showing multiple areas of increased signal in the periventricular white matter. The involvement of the corpus callosum (lesions right at the top of the lateral ventricles) is said to be characteristic of MS.

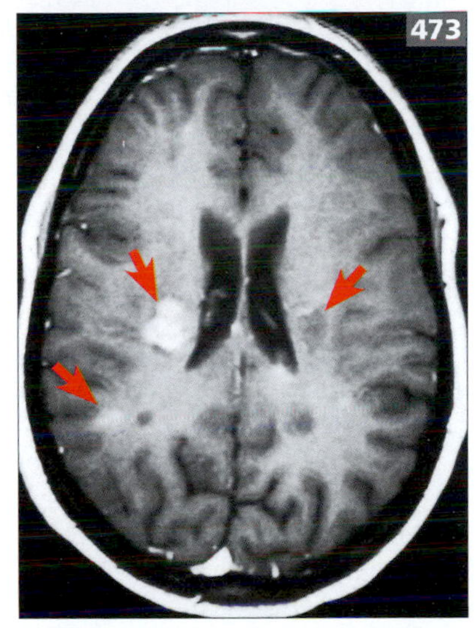

473 T1-weighted MRI following contrast (same patient as 472) shows that some of the lesions enhance (arrows) and some do not, indicating that they are of different ages and confirming the most likely diagnosis to be MS.

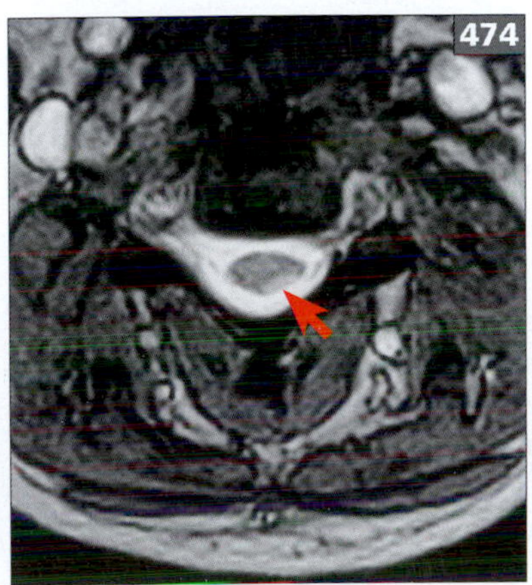

474, 475 MRI cervical spine, T2-weighted image, in the axial plane (474) and sagittal plane (475), showing a focal area of high signal intensity in the high left cervical spinal cord posteriorly (arrows) due to demyelination, in a patient who presented with symptoms and signs of left dorsal column dysfunction (ascending tight feeling in left leg like a stocking around it).

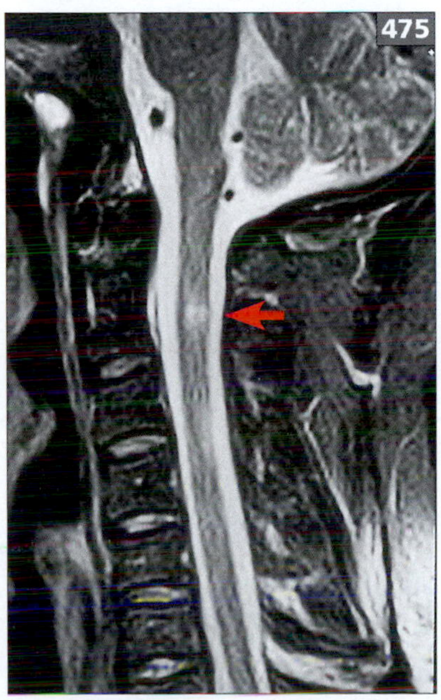

T1-weighted images show:

- Low signal areas (dark spots), but the T1-weighted image is not so sensitive and demonstrates fewer lesions than T2-weighted.
- To differentiate MS from other causes of white matter bright spots it is sometimes necessary to give intravenous contrast; MS will show patchy contrast enhancement suggesting active inflammation of some, but not all, abnormal areas, indirectly reflecting its typical multi-phasic course. Other diseases such as ADEM are monophasic so all the abnormal areas should either enhance or not.

Differential diagnosis

The appearance of MS on MRI, while typical, is nonspecific. A similar picture can occur in other conditions (see below). Differential diagnosis of brain MRI mimicking MS includes:

- Subcortical arteriosclerotic encephalopathy (Binswanger's disease).
- Multiple metastases.
- Vasculitis.
- Sarcoidosis.
- Leukodystrophies.
- Encephalitis:
  - Viral: HIV, PML, subacute sclerosing panencephalitis (measles), ADEM.
  - Bacterial: TB.
  - Spirochetal: syphilis, neuroborreliosis (Lyme disease).
- Alzheimer's disease.
- Radiation therapy.
- Chemotherapy.
- Cyclosporine use.
- Hyperperfusion syndrome.
- Subacute combined degeneration of the spinal cord (vitamin B12 deficiency).

CSF

- Cell count: increased (5–50 lymphocytes/mm^3) in two-thirds of patients during an acute attack; normal (<3–4 cells/mm^3) in two-thirds of patients in remission.
- Protein: mildly elevated, up to 1.0 g/l (100 mg/dl), in about one-third of patients.
- IgG/albumin ratio: raised (>25%), in two-thirds of clinically definite MS.
- IgG index (compares IgG/albumin ratio in the CSF and blood): abnormal in about 90% of patients with clinically definite MS.
- Oligoclonal IgG bands (**476**): present in about 90% of patients with clinically definite MS; not specific; found in other immune-mediated CNS diseases.
- Viral serology and culture.
- Venereal disease research laboratory (VDRL), *Treponema pallidum* hemagglutination assay (TPHA).

Electrophysiologic studies and EEG

At least 90% of patients with clinically definite MS have a persistent abnormality detected by visual, auditory, or somatosensory evoked potentials:

- Visual evoked potentials: delayed conduction in about 90% of clinically definite MS.
- Brainstem auditory evoked potentials: abnormal in one-half of clinically definite MS.
- Somatosensory evoked potentials: abnormal in 70% with clinically definite MS.
- EEG: if considering a diagnosis of encephalitis, but generally not commonly needed in pursuing a diagnosis of MS.

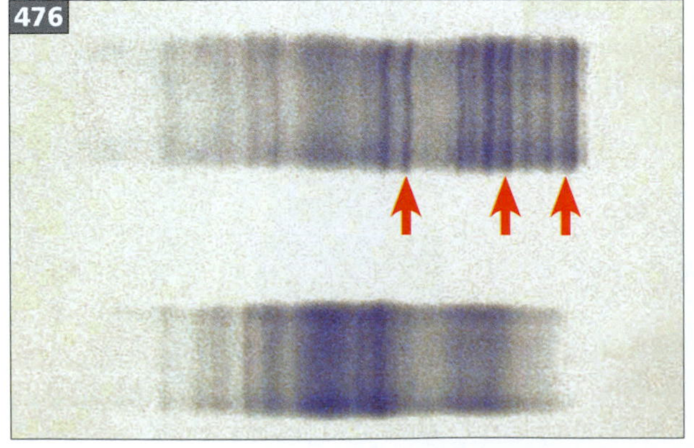

476 Isoelectric focusing in an agarose gel at stable pH (range 5.0–9.5) demonstrating the presence of oligoclonal bands (arrows) in the CSF (above) and not the serum (below). The oligoclonal bands are different clones of IgG that have migrated electrophoretically in the stationary pH gradient until a steady state is reached, when all the components are concentrated or focused as sharp bands at their respective isoelectric points. The bands are visualized by immunofixation. To be positive, two or more oligoclonal bands must be detected in the CSF that are not present in the serum of the patient.

Diagnosis

Diagnosis is from clinical and MRI evidence of at least two CNS lesions that are consistent with demyelination occurring at different sites in the CNS and at different times. The diagnosis can be classified according to the degree of certainty as clinically 'definite', 'probable', or 'possible'.

Tip

▶ *MS should only be considered if all of the symptoms and signs cannot be explained by a single neurologic lesion and the history, examination, and special investigations fail to identify other conditions that can cause multiple CNS lesions.*

Diagnostic criteria for MS

Clinically definite MS:

- Two attacks and clinical evidence of two separate lesions; OR
- Two attacks; clinical evidence of one lesion and paraclinical evidence of another, separate lesion.
  - Paraclinical evidence of a lesion: the demonstration by means of various tests and procedures of the existence of a lesion of the CNS which has not produced signs of neurologic dysfunction but which may or may not have caused symptoms in the past. Such tests and procedures include the hot bath test, evoked response studies, tissue imaging procedures (including MRI), and reliable, expert neurologic assessment.

The two attacks must involve different parts of the CNS, must be separated by a period of at least 1 month, and must each last a minimum of 24 hours.

Laboratory-supported definite MS:

- Two attacks; either clinical or paraclinical evidence of one lesion; and CSF oligoclonal bands or increased IgG (serum levels of either must be normal).
- One attack; clinical evidence of two separate lesions; and CSF oligoclonal bands or increased IgG.
- One attack; clinical evidence of one lesion and paraclinical evidence of another, separate lesion; and CSF oligoclonal bands or increased IgG.

Clinically probable MS:

- Two attacks and clinical evidence of one lesion (the two attacks must involve separate parts of the CNS [historic information cannot be considered as a substitute for the clinical evidence]); *or*
- One attack and clinical evidence of two separate lesions; *or*
- One attack; clinical evidence of one lesion and paraclinical evidence of another, separate lesion.

Laboratory-supported probable MS:

- Two attacks and CSF oligoclonal bands or increased IgG.

Diagnostic criteria for MS[6] incorporate MRI into the overall diagnostic scheme, and add guidelines for the diagnosis of primary progressive disease. Some problems with these criteria are discussed by Poser and Brinar[7]. There is a tendency to use MRI scanning to disclose new lesions, and make a diagnosis of MS after a single clinical event when later new MRI lesions are seen. The utility and accuracy of this remain open to question.

Pathology

Multiple plaques of demyelination are seen in the white matter of the CNS.

- Acute lesion:
  - Demyelination of nerve fibers in the white matter of the CNS.
  - Loss of oligodendrocytes.
  - Perivenular infiltration of T and B lymphocytes, macrophages (filled with myelin debris), and plasma cells.
  - Axonal degeneration.
- Chronic lesion:
  - Some axonal loss and remyelination.
  - Glial cell proliferation resulting in discrete gray colored areas of gliosis (or sclerosis) that are called plaques.

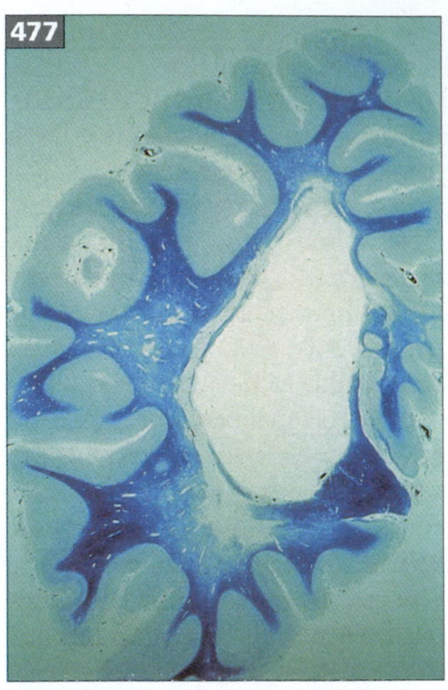

477 Section of one cerebral hemisphere (parietal lobe), showing a lack of staining due to periventricular demyelination in the white matter. *Courtesy of Professor BA Kakulas, Royal Perth Hospital, Western Australia.*

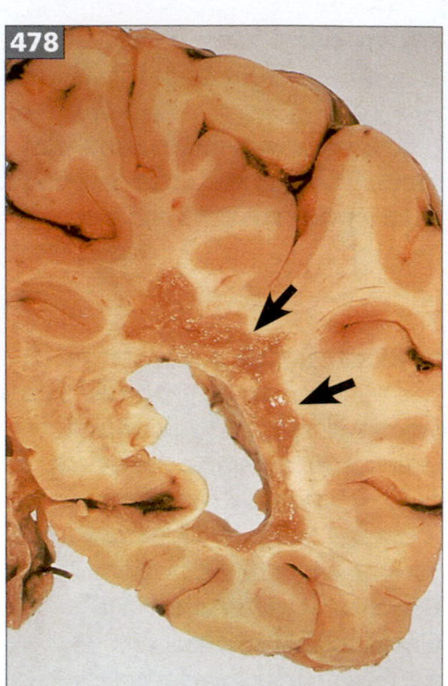

478, 479 Autopsy specimens of brain, coronal sections, showing periventricular demyelination.

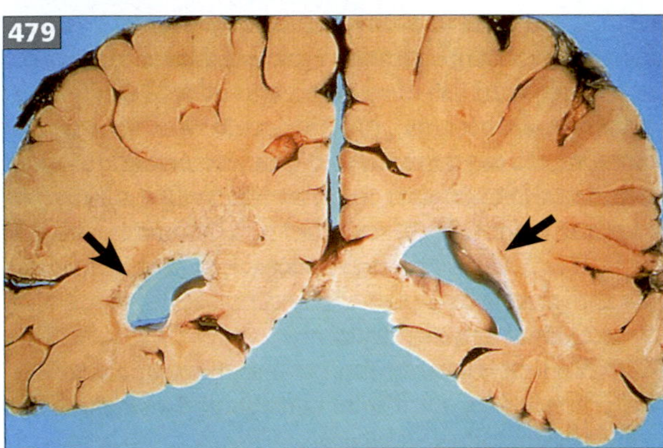

480 Optic neuritis. Transverse section of the optic nerve at autopsy, showing demyelination of the optic nerve in a patient with optic neuritis due to multiple sclerosis.

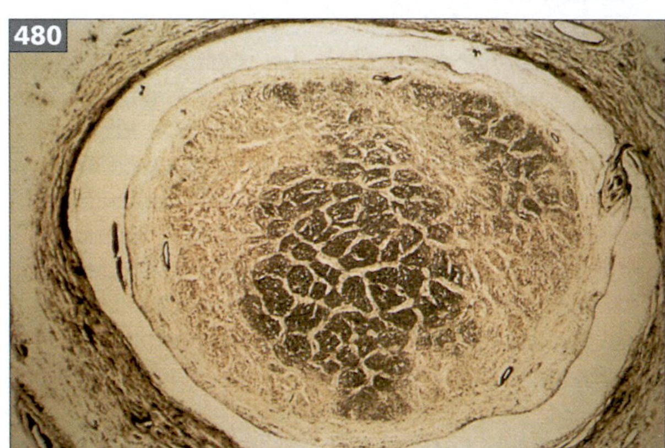

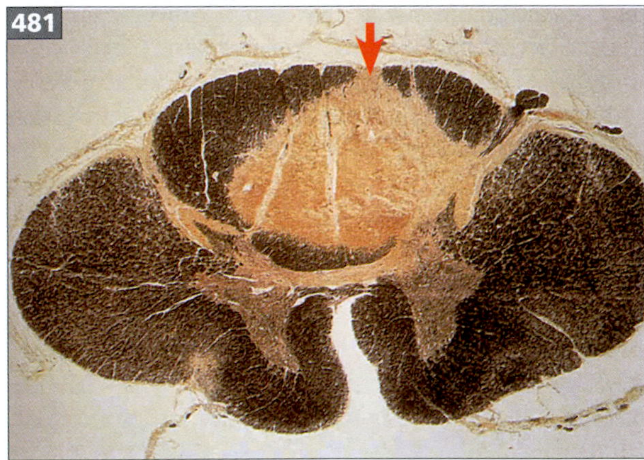

481 Transverse section of the thoracic spinal cord, showing a large plaque of demyelination in the dorsal columns (arrow) in a multiple sclerosis patient who had a high-stepping gait due to sensory ataxia in the lower limbs. *Courtesy of Professor BA Kakulas, Royal Perth Hospital, Western Australia.*

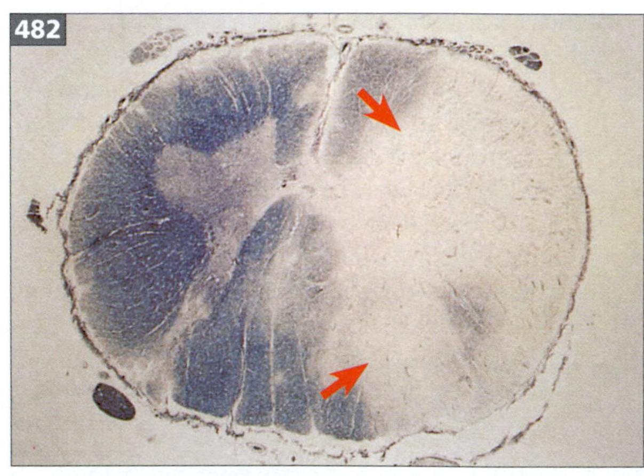

482 Transverse section of the spinal cord, showing a large plaque of demyelination in almost one-half of the spinal cord in a multiple sclerosis patient with a Brown–Sequard syndrome. *Courtesy of Professor BA Kakulas, Royal Perth Hospital, Western Australia.*

Sites of demyelination can be any part of the CNS, particularly:
- Periventricular white matter of the cerebral hemispheres (**477–479**).
- Optic nerves (**480**).
- Cerebellum.
- Brainstem.
- Spinal cord (particularly subpial regions of the spinal cord) (**481, 482**).

It is now clear that gray matter as well as white matter is involved, and that tissue between lesions is also affected. The peripheral nervous system is not affected.

Treatment

Relapsing–remitting MS

Acute treatment is used to accelerate recovery from the acute attack. For mild relapse of relapsing–remitting MS no specific treatment is required, as most resolve spontaneously. For moderate to severe relapse of relapsing–remitting MS, methylprednisolone is given[8], 1000 mg in 100 ml 5% dextrose, infused intravenously over 30–60 minutes, daily for 3 days, or 500 mg daily for 5 days. This therapy accelerates the rate of recovery (i.e. reduces the duration of relapse) but has no effect on long-term outcome. Potential adverse effects include mood alterations, psychosis, acne, fluid retention, hyperglycemia, and osteonecrosis. Equivalent doses of methyl prednisolone given orally appear equally efficacious.

Long-term treatment is given to prevent relapses[9] in relapsing–remitting MS with at least two relapses in the previous 2 years. Several drug treatments to reduce the relapse rate are now available (see below) but they are all expensive, most have to be given by injection, their long-term efficacy is not yet known, and so far none appears to have any useful effect on progression of disability.

Interferon beta-1b [IFN-β-1b], 8 million international units (MIU) subcutaneously every second day, and interferon beta-1a, 6 MIU once a week, intramuscularly; or Rebif 6–12 MIU three times a week subcutaneously, all reduce the frequency of relapses by about one-third. Adverse effects include systemic 'flu-like' symptoms, injection site reactions, liver enzyme elevations, anemia, mild leukopenia, thrombocytopenia, and possibly depressive symptoms. Active, severe depression, pregnancy, and breastfeeding are contraindications to its use. Neutralizing antibodies to IFN-beta are detectable in about 38% of patients by the third year of treatment and have been claimed to attenuate the treatment effect. The mechanism of action of IFN-beta in MS remains unknown. None of these products significantly delays or slows the progression of disability.

Glatiramer acetate, 20 mg per day by daily subcutaneous injection, may reduce relapse rate by about 30%. It, too, has no useful effect on progressive disability. Adverse effects include a transient injection site reaction, sometimes with focal lipoatrophy, and a transient self-limiting systemic reaction characterized by flushing or chest tightness with palpitations, anxiety, or dyspnea. It is a mixture of random polymers of alanine, glutamine, lysine, and tyrosine. It approximates the antigenic structure of myelin basic protein (MBP) sufficiently to be cross-reactive with monoclonal antibodies and T cells generated to MBP, a putative target antigen in MS. Glatiramer acetate is an alternative to IFN-beta therapy in relapsing–remitting MS.

Azathioprine also appears to reduce the relapse rate by approximately one-third[10].

Oral agents[11] (cladribine, fingolimod, teriflunomide, laqinimod, and fumarate) are all at various stages of development for relapsing–remitting MS (cladribine is licensed in Australia; fingolimod in the USA and EU). Their tablet form is a practical advantage, and their potency in preventing relapses may be slightly greater than IFN-beta and glatiramer, but their side-effects are more serious (cladribine has recently been rejected by the European Medicines Agency partly because of the perceived risk of malignancy).

Tips

▶ *The term 'disease modifying treatment' (DMT) is less specific than it might be: it is the frequency, and possibly the severity of relapses that is 'modified', rather than the rate of accumulation of disability in progressive disease.*

▶ *Immunotherapy for MS is a fast evolving field; at present it may be speculated that treatments will come to fall into three categories:*

▶ *First-line DMTs: beta-interferons, glatiramer, and possibly some of the less potent oral agents; these appear extremely safe, but are limited in efficacy, with a 20–30% reduction in relapse rate.*

▶ *Second-line DMTs: oral agents such as fingolimod and perhaps fumarate. These are more potent (50–60% reduction in relapse rate) but may have more side-effects than first-line agents. Many also have the advantage of oral administration, but some of the more recently explored monoclonals may fall in the same efficacy range.*

▶ *Third-line agents: currently, natalizumab and probably soon alemtuzumab. These are more potent still (80% or more reduction in relapse rate vs. placebo) but can have more serious – even occasionally fatal – side-effects.*

Monoclonal antibodies are now available for the prevention of relapses and are used in individuals with particularly aggressive relapsing MS, and (particularly) in those who continue to suffer relapses while treated with glatiramer or IFN-beta. Natalizumab is a humanized monoclonal antibody directed against one of the key adhesion molecules involved in the transmigration of activated lymphocytes across the blood–brain barrier, which traffic it effectively blocks. Treatment results in a substantial (approximately 70%) reduction in relapse rate, and an effect on disease progression is also claimed. There are however risks – around 1 in 1000 patients develops progressive multi-focal leukoencephalopathy[12].

Alemtuzumab is likely to be the next monoclonal antibody to become available in MS; it is directed against the pan-leukocyte marker CD52, decreases relapse rates by around 80–90%, may also limit progression, and can induce often serious autoimmune diseases[13,14].

Primary or secondary progressive MS

Recent accelerated deterioration is treated with intravenous or oral high-dose methyl prednisolone infusion (500 mg over 5 days). (There is very limited evidence that methyl prednisolone pulse can help in this situation.) The chemotherapeutic agent mitoxantrone may have a limited role in the management of patients with recent onset, severe, and rapidly progressive disease. It does carry a significant risk of cardiac toxicity and malignancy (leukemia).

There are no treatments that reliably reverse, halt, or even slow the sustained deteroration and accumulation of disability in primary or secondary progressive MS. Trials are underway exploring neuroprotective agents and/or stem cells with this aim[15].

Symptomatic relief

Rehabilitation by a multidisciplinary team plays a crucial role in management of MS[16].

Spasticity

- Attend to any factors which may exacerbate spasticity, such as noxious stimuli due to urinary tract infection, infected pressure sores or ulcers, tight clothing, or an uncomfortable orthotic.
- Educate patients to understand and manage their spasticity.
- Correct posture: avoid positions which favor the pattern of spasticity.
- Physiotherapy: aims to inhibit spasticity by facilitating a normal pattern of movement, improving postural tone and re-learning selected movements. Muscle stretching is also important.
- Pharmacology:
  - Oral agents:
    - Tizanidine, an L2 alpha adrenergic antagonist.
    - Baclofen, 5 mg bd, increasing slowly to 10–25 mg three times daily if tolerated and required: the most effective oral agent.
    - Diazepam 5–10 mg three times daily.
    - Dantrolene.
    - Gabapentin.
  - Intramuscular injections of botulinum toxin A for focal spasticity (i.e. hip adductors). Effective when combined with regular physiotherapy.
  - Intrathecal baclofen: test with an initial bolus injection for functional benefit and analgesia; abdominal wall subcutaneous reservoir and pump, connected by a catheter to the subarachnoid space between L3/4 with the catheter tip located around T12 or higher.
  - Rarely, nerve blocks are used: preferably on predominantly motor nerves, such as obturator nerves. Pre-test with a reversible local anesthetic such as bupivacaine before resorting to dilute phenol or alcohol.
- Surgery.

Bladder dysfunction[17]

- Detrusor hyper-reflexia:
  - Clean intermittent self-catheterization (CISC) is the most effective.
  - Anticholinergic agents (reduce urgency but may increase residual volume):
    - Oxybutynin hydrochloride 5 mg tablets, 25–5.0 mg every 6–8 hours.
    - Propantheline bromide 15 mg, four times daily.
    - Amitriptyline 25–100 mg daily.
  - Intravesical botulinum toxin is an increasingly promising technique.
  - Intravesical capsaicin, which has a toxic effect on the C-fiber afferents in the bladder wall that drive the abnormal spinal detrusor reflex, reduces detrusor muscle hyperactivity and may help patients with severe detrusor hyper-reflexia whose bladder has very limited storage capacity. The effect lasts 1–5 months, and may respond to repeat infusions.
  - Indwelling suprapubic catheter if the combination of medication and CISC is not effective or practical.
- Nocturia. Desmopressin spray (DDAVP) reduces the volume of urine produced.

Bowel dysfunction
- Diet.
- Lactulose.
- Suppositories.
- Loperamide for urgency.

Sexual dysfunction[18]
- Erectile dysfunction:
  - Psychotherapy and psychosexual counseling.
  - Sildenafil: a phosphodiesterase type-5 (PDE-5) inhibitor which increases cyclic guanosine monophosphate (GMP) levels in the penis and enhances the smooth muscle relaxant effects of the nitric oxide (NO)/cyclic GMP pathway, increasing penile blood flow. There are three doses (25 mg, 50 mg, 100 mg). The usual starting dose is 50 mg; the 25 mg dose is used in younger men, men with renal or hepatic impairment, and those men on CYP3A4 inhibitors (erythromycin, cimetidine, and retroviral drugs). The tablet should be taken at least 1 hour before anticipated sexual activity and will remain effective for up to 4 hours. A large meal and alcohol intake may delay the absorption. It is effective in 70–80% of men with erectile problems. Adverse effects are mild and include headache, facial flushing, indigestion, and rhinitis. It is contraindicated in men who take nitrate medication (including glyceryl trinitrate and amyl nitrate) or any form of NO donors, because of potential hypotensive effects.
  - Surgically implanted prostheses.
- Lack of vaginal lubrication and loss of sensation: lubricating gels.

Bulbar dysfunction
- Speech (dysarthria predominantly): speech pathologist assessment and guidance: advice on breathing and articulation patterns, and augmentative communication aids.
- Swallowing dysfunction (oral and pharyngeal phases):
  - Speech pathologist (± videofluoroscopy) assessment and guidance: education, dietary modification, positioning strategies (e.g. 'chin tuck' and 'head turn'), thermal stimulation (i.e. using ice to stimulate the faucal arches, which delays triggering of the swallow reflex).
  - Assisted feeding, via percutaneous gastrostomy, may be required in severe cases where swallowing is no longer safe and the patient and carer agree.

Visual dysfunction
- Monocular blindness or scotoma, diplopia and oscillopsia: this is difficult to manage, but referral to low vision clinics can be helpful.
- Botulinum toxin injections of oculomotor muscles may reduce persistent oscillopsia.
- Acquired pendular nystagmus may respond to converging prisms and isoniazid (and possibly gabapentin).

Cognitive dysfunction and depression

Adequate assessment and clarification of the deficits allows informed discussion with the patient and carer, constructive planning to minimize or overcome these deficits and, in some cases, cognitive rehabilitation. There is emerging evidence for acetylcholinesterase inhibitors such as donepezil. The treatment of depression is similar to that of a patient who does not have MS, and includes psychologic counseling and serotonin reuptake inhibitors such as tricyclic antidepressants. However, particular attention needs to be paid to adverse effects, as they may exaggerate existing problems such as sexual dysfunction.

Tremor and ataxia
- Physiotherapy: improve the patient's posture and seating and supply adequate support.
- Oral medication – drugs are usually of extremely limited value, but the following can help in some cases:
  - Clonazepam 0.5–2.0 mg two or three times daily.
  - Ondansetron, a 5-hydroxytryptophan-3 (5-HT3) antagonist, 8 mg IV.
  - Carbamazepine.
  - Gabapentin.
  - Isoniazid and pyridoxine.
  - Propranolol.
  - Buspirone.
- Surgery. Deep brain stimulation appears promising for tremor, but not ataxia, in MS.

Fatigue
- Psychologic counseling.
- Amantadine 100 mg in the morning and afternoon can help in some cases.
- 4-Aminopyridine (fampridine), and 3-4-diaminopyridine, a potassium channel blocking agent, may have a role.

Impaired mobility
4-Aminopyridine (fampridine), and 3-4-diaminopyridine, may help marginally in responsive patients[19].

Pain
- Trigeminal neuralgia:
  - Gabapentin, 300 mg bd or tds, increasing as needed.
  - Carbamazepine 200–400 mg three times daily.
  - Baclofen 10–20 mg three times daily.
  - Sodium valproate.
- Dysesthetic burning pain in the extremities:
  - Paroxysmal: avoid precipitating maneuvers such as movement, tactile stimulation, and hyperventilation, if possible; consider bromocriptine 2–5 mg bd.
  - Chronic: tricyclic antidepressants, e.g. amitriptyline, or alternatively gabapentin, may help.
- Painful tonic seizures: phenytoin can be extremely effective. Muscle relaxants, e.g. baclofen, may help.
- Chronic back pain: physiotherapy incorporating heat pads and transcutaneous electric nerve stimulation.
- Painful leg spasms: baclofen.

Clinical course

Symptoms of a relapse usually persist for several weeks and then gradually but incompletely resolve over 1 or 2 months or more. Vision frequently improves in 1 or 2 weeks and often returns to near normal. Occasionally, symptoms are short lived and paroxysmal (e.g. recurrent short episodes of ataxia). The course is relapsing and remitting in about 80% of patients. Relapse may occur at any time. The average relapse rate is about 0.5 attacks per year but is very variable. In most patients, the course becomes progressive with increasing disability, and it is increasingly clear that this progression is unrelated to the frequency or severity of relapses: the mechanisms appear far more complex than simple accumulation of relapse-related disability[20].

A chronic progressive course occurs from onset in the other 20%, particularly if onset occurs after 40 years of age with spastic paraparesis due to spinal cord dysfunction, and usually ataxia. This is primary progressive MS[21]. These patients also tend to have a worse prognosis.

Prognosis

Life expectancy from onset of symptoms is very variable, but on average is only little shortened. Mean survival is 30 years; 10% die within 15 years and a small percentage die within several months or years. In one study, the 25-year survival rate was 74%, compared with 86% for the general population. Most deaths are related to advanced chronic disability (pneumonia, sepsis, thromboembolism) and not acute attacks. After 25 years, one-third of MS patients are still working and two-thirds are still ambulating. Adverse and favorable factors for long-term survival free of disability are show in *Table 89*.

TABLE 89 **ADVERSE AND FAVORABLE FACTORS FOR LONG-TERM SURVIVAL FREE OF DISABILITY IN MULTIPLE SCLEROSIS**

	Adverse	Favorable
Age of onset	Late	Early
Sex	Male	Female
Dysfunction at onset	Cerebellar (ataxia)	Sensory (paresthesia)
Relapse interval	Short	Long
Clinical course	Progressive	Relapsing–remitting
Relapse rate	High	Low
Imaging	Spinal cord neuronal loss on MRI; reduced N-acetyl aspartate on MRS	Fewer lesions on baseline MRI
CSF	–	Oligoclonal band negative

MRI: magnetic resonance imaging; MRS: magnetic resonance spectroscopy.

DEVIC'S DISEASE

This was previously considered a variant of MS, though the extent to which it is fundamentally or mechanistically similar remains poorly understood. The term – or the synonym neuromyelitis optica (NMO) – originally applied to the clinical combination of optic neuritis (usually sequential and bilateral) occurring with transverse myelitis (again simultaneous or with a usually short interval between), both of subacute onset and behaving in many ways initially rather like comparable relapse events in MS. (In fact, however, the clinical picture of transverse myelitis, in contrast with partial cord lesions, is rather uncommon in MS.) However, in NMO patients, recovery is often poor, other types of clinical event do not occur, and spinal fluid analysis does not show the presence of oligoclonal bands. MRI scans show changes outside the spinal cord and optic nerves.

Over the last decade, such cases were found to harbour serum antibodies against the aquaporin-4 water channel, expressed on astrocytes, and the disorder has increasingly come to be both diagnosed and defined according to this antibody. Other clinical features – perhaps particularly brainstem phenomena such as hiccoughs – have come to be associated, and cerebral MRI changes identified[22]. A response to plasma exchange is commonly reported and this is now widely accepted as a useful therapeutic maneuver in this situation. Longer-term treatment with corticosteroids and immunosuppressants such as azathioprine or methotrexate are also often recommended.

NEUROSARCOIDOSIS[23]

Definition and epidemiology

Neurosarcoidosis is a chronic, multisystem, granulomatous, inflammatory disease of unknown etiology in which any part of the nervous system (and indeed any organ of the body) may be affected.

- Prevalence:
  - Systemic sarcoidosis: 1–50:100,000 population.
  - Neurosarcoidosis: 5:100,000.
- Incidence: systemic sarcoidosis: 10.9:100,000 for whites; 35.5:100,000 for blacks.
- Age: any age (3 months to old age), but commonly 20–55 years of age.
- Gender: M=F.

Etiology and pathophysiology

These are uncertain. The involvement of various microorganisms has been suggested, but never proven. An exaggerated helper-inducer T lymphocyte cellular immune response to a variety of antigens or self-antigens is seen. Since the activated helper-inducer T lymphocytes release mediators that attract and activate mononuclear phagocytes, it is likely that the process of granuloma formation is secondary to the exaggerated helper-inducer T cell process.

Clinical features

Systemic manifestations

Systemic manifestations are present in over 90% of patients with neurosarcoidosis. Symptoms include exertional dyspnea and dry cough due to interstitial lung disease. Signs include skin rash (i.e. erythema nodosum), uveitis, lymphadenopathy, and arthritis.

Neurologic manifestations

These are the presenting manifestation in about 2% (0.3–2.5%) of cases of sarcoidosis, concurrent with systemic involvement in about 5% of patients, and may precede systemic involvement by up to 18 months.

- Meningitis:
  - Aseptic meningitis.
  - Chronic granulomatous basal meningitis.
- Epilepsy: secondary to meningitis; mass lesion; cerebral infarction.
- Raised ICP:
  - Intraparenchymal mass lesion.
  - Hydrocephalus.
- Uni- or multifocal neurologic deficits:
  - Stroke syndrome.
  - Multifocal changes in CNS white matter.
  - Vasculopathy: ophthalmoscopy may reveal periphlebitis, as yellowish-white focal or diffuse sheathing of retinal veins. Hard exudates, sometimes termed 'taches de bougie' because of their resemblance to candle-wax drippings, often accompany the periphlebitis and can leave white choreoretinal scars.

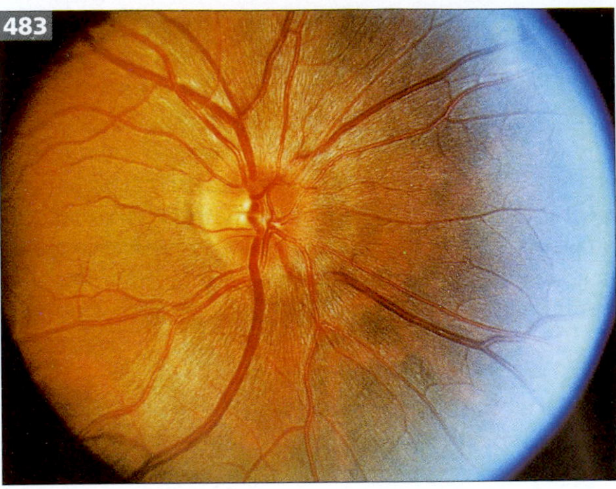

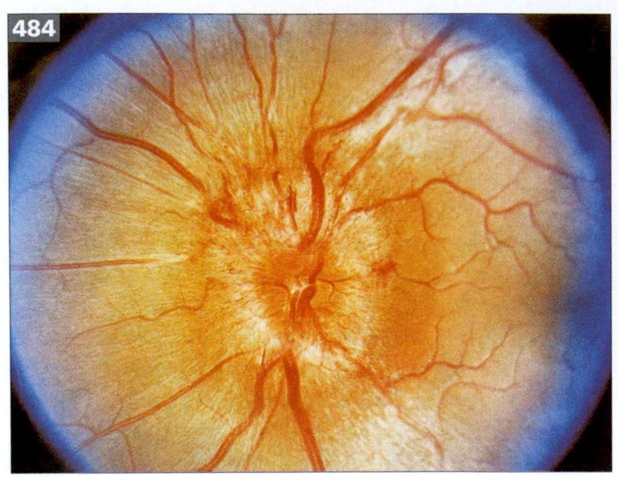

483, 484 Ocular fundi of a patient with anterior optic neuropathy due to sarcoidosis. He presented with subacute onset of an island of blurred vision in the inferior visual field of the left eye and mild ocular pain bilaterally. Examination showed normal visual acuity bilaterally, an enlarged blind spot, and an arcuate scotoma inferonasally on the left, and asymmetric optic disc swelling, being greater in the left eye (484). Note the nerve fiber layer hemorrhages in the left fundus.

- Single or multiple cranial neuropathies:
  - Anterior optic neuropathy (**483, 484**).
  - Facial palsy: with enlarged parotid glands (uveoparotid fever).
- Neuroendocrine (hypothalamic and pituitary dysfunction): diabetes insipidus (polyuria, polydipsia, disordered thirst).
- Subacute or chronic myelopathy.
- Peripheral neuropathy:
  - Guillain–Barré syndrome.
  - Polyradiculopathy.
  - Symmetric polyneuropathy (pure sensory, pure motor, sensorimotor).
  - Mononeuritis multiplex.
- Myopathy.

Investigations

Blood

No peripheral blood findings are diagnostic of the disease:

- Full blood count: anemia, increased number of monocytes.
- Serum urea and electrolytes, glucose, liver function tests, uric acid: may be abnormal.
- Serum calcium: elevated.
- Serum Igs: hypergammaglobulinemia.
- Serum angiotensin-converting enzyme (ACE): elevated in about two-thirds of patients but it is neither sensitive (56–86%) nor specific. The false-positive rate in a normal population is about 2–4%. The level of serum ACE can correlate with the severity of the lung disease and the presence or absence of extrathoracic disease, but also with ACE-inhibitor therapy.

Imaging

- Chest X-ray: may show bilateral hilar adenopathy (**485**) but occasionally a similar pattern is seen in lymphoma, TB, brucellosis, and bronchogenic carcinoma. High-resolution CT thorax is the most sensitive test.
- Gallium scan: more sensitive than chest X-ray and the appearance of diffuse uptake in the lungs (or parotid, salivary, and lacrimal glands), even in the absence of clinical involvement, is relatively specific but not diagnostic. A positive result can guide diagnostic biopsy.

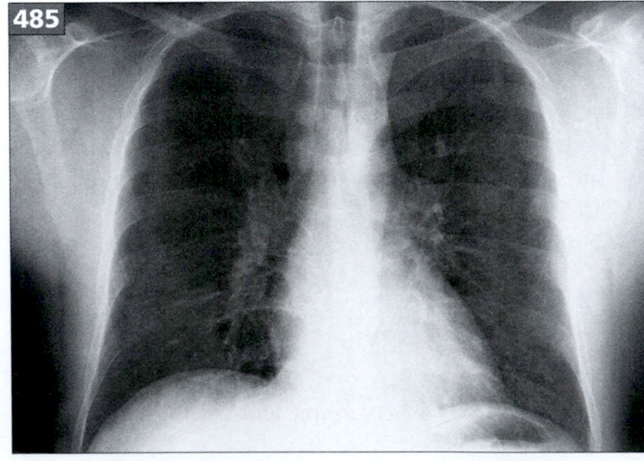

485 Chest X-ray showing bilateral hilar adenopathy due to sarcoidosis.

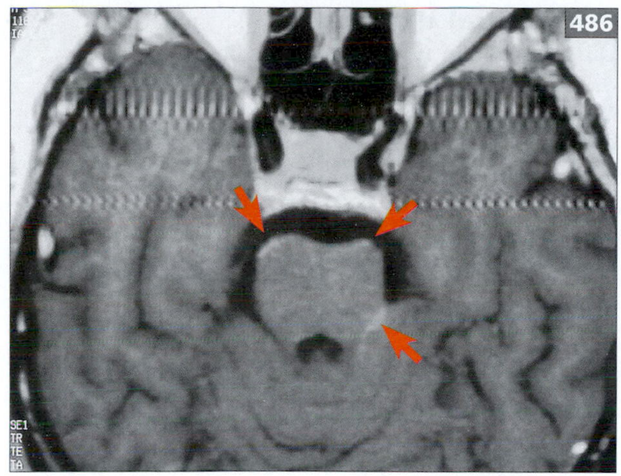

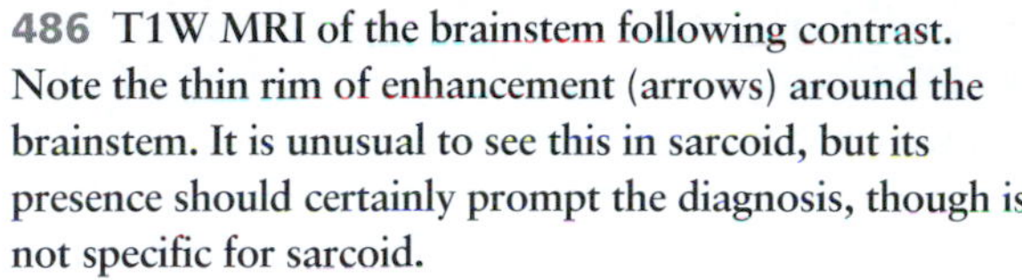

486 T1W MRI of the brainstem following contrast. Note the thin rim of enhancement (arrows) around the brainstem. It is unusual to see this in sarcoid, but its presence should certainly prompt the diagnosis, though is not specific for sarcoid.

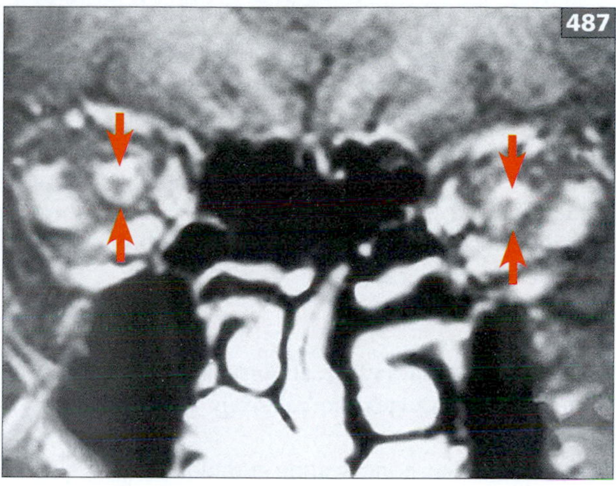

487 MRI of the orbits, coronal plane, after gadolinium injection, showing brightness, due to contrast enhancement, of the dural sheath of the optic nerves (arrows) bilaterally in the patient in 483, 484, with bilateral optic neuropathy due to sarcoidosis.

- CT brain scan without and with contrast: hydrocephalus, leptomeningeal thickening and enhancement, intra-axial mass lesions, extra-axial mass lesions.
- Whole body positron emission tomography (PET) CT can also disclose asymptomatic deep lymphadenopathy (allowing diagnostic biopsy).
- MRI brain/spinal cord scan: several patterns may be visible on cranial MRI (**486**) (CT is much less sensitive):
  - Chronic basal leptomeningitis with thickened enhancing meninges involving the hypothalamus, pituitary stalk, optic nerve (**487**), and chiasm.
  - Communicating hydrocephalus.
  - Involvement of the lenticulostriate arteries by spreading up the Virchow–Robin spaces causing thrombosis and granulomatous angiitis.
  - Parenchymal nodules (granulomas) which may be iso- or hyperdense, may calcify and appear as a mass lesion, and may or may not enhance. These may cause obstruction to the ventricles. They occur particularly around the skull base, pituitary, pons, hypothalamus, and periventricular region.
  - Diffuse high signal areas in the white matter on T2-weighted images indistinguishable from MS may also occur.
  - Extra-axial sarcoid may mimic a meningioma by causing a dural enhancing mass with hyperostosis.
  - Spinal sarcoid may mimic leptomeningeal metastases.
- Cerebral angiography: changes suggestive of cerebral angiitis may sometimes occur.

Tip

▶ *Meningeal thickening and/or enhancement occurs rarely, if ever, in conventional MS, but typically in:*
- *Neurosarcoidosis.*
- *Wegener's disease.*
- *Lymphoma.*

More occasionally it occurs in:
- *CNS rheumatoid disease.*
- *As a core feature of idiopathic hypertrophic cranial pachymeningitis.*

It can offer a very useful biopsy target.

CSF

- Mild pleocytosis (mostly lymphocytes).
- Mild increased protein.
- Increased T4:T8 lymphocyte ratio.
- Low CSF glucose in 20–39% of cases.
- Elevated CSF ACE, oligoclonal banding, and increased IgG index in nearly one-third of patients may occur.

Electromyography (EMG)

- Compound muscle action potentials and sensory nerve action potentials: normal or mild to moderately decreased.
- Motor and sensory nerve conduction velocities: mild to moderately decreased.
- EMG features of chronic partial denervation may be present.

Kveim test

A suspension of sarcoid tissue is injected intradermally and produces a sarcoid granuloma in about 75% of patients with subacute active sarcoidosis, and in about two-thirds of those with chronic sarcoidosis of >2 years duration. False-positives occur in <5% of cases. Kveim tissue is increasingly difficult to access, and with concerns of transmissible disease (e.g. prions) this test is now extremely rarely performed.

Tissue

- Bronchoalveolar lavage: abnormally increased T4:T8 lymphocyte ratio: relatively specific but not diagnostic.
- Bone marrow: noncaseating granuloma.
- Biopsy of muscle (even in the absence of myopathic symptoms), lymph node, conjunctiva, skin, lung, liver, or brain may reveal the diagnosis.
- Nerve biopsy:
  - An axonopathy sparing unmyelinated fibers.
  - Marked loss of myelinated fibers.
  - Demyelination is not prominent nor is it in the usual central predominant pattern seen in vasculitic neuropathies.
  - Epineural and perineural granuloma with or without periangiitis and panangiitis.
- Brain biopsy: in many cases involving intracranial mass lesions which are difficult to access safely with stereotactic brain biopsy, biopsy can be deferred until a trial of steroids is given if sarcoidosis can be inferred clinically.

Other tests

- Skin: skin-test unreactivity (anergy).
- Urine: 24-hour urinary calcium level: typically elevated, but not diagnostic of sarcoidosis.

Tips

▶ *Inflammatory CNS disease from systemic disorders, such as sarcoid, vasculitis, and Behçet's, can be very difficult to distinguish from MS, and from each other.*

▶ *Exhaustive examination and directed history, and to look for systemic manifestions, are vital.*

▶ *In the absence of clinical features, investigation to disclose non-neurologic disease can be highly informative, including CT (chest, abdomen, and pelvis), MRI, and whole body PET-CT.*

▶ *Biopsy of any identified non-neurologic involved tissue should normally follow; CNS biopsy should be seriously considered if no proof is otherwise available and if MS appears unlikely.*

Differential diagnosis

Differentials depend on the clinical presentation.

Meningoencephalitis

- Granulomatous inflammation:
  - Infection by bacteria (brucellosis, chlamydia, tularemia), mycobacteria (TB, atypical mycobacteria), fungi (histoplasmosis, coccidioidomycosis, cryptococcosis), spirochetes (treponemal infections such as syphilis), and parasites (toxoplasmosis, leishmaniasis).
  - Occupational and environmental exposure to organic or inorganic agents (e.g. methotrexate, talc, metals).
  - Neoplasia (lymphoma).
  - Autoimmune disorders (Wegener's granulomatosis, Churg–Strauss syndrome).
  - Histiocytosis X.
- Viral encephalitis: HIV infection.
- Carcinomatous meningitis.
- Granulomatous angiitis of the CNS. The meningeal inflammatory reaction is consistently localized to blood vessel walls and typically produces extensive disruption of the vascular wall.
- Meningiomatosis.
- Limbic encephalitis associated with occult neoplasm.

Multifocal white matter disease

Multiple sclerosis

Mass lesions

- Primary brain tumor: glioma (including optic nerve glioma), meningioma, germ cell tumor, leukemia, primary CNS lymphoma.
- Metastatic brain tumor.
- Granulomatous inflammation: syphilitic gumma, tuberculoma, cryptococcoma, toxoplasmosis, histiocytosis X.
- Spinal cord glioma, ependymoma, myelitis.

Noncaseating granulomas

Nonspecific: found in infections and malignancy.

Increased level of serum ACE

- Youth.
- Hyperthyroidism.
- Diabetes.
- HIV infection.
- Leprosy.
- Tuberculosis.
- Coccidioidomycosis.

- Histoplasmosis.
- Amyloidosis.
- Multiple myeloma.
- Hodgkin's disease.
- Lymphoma (including intravascular lymphoma).
- Malignant histiocytosis.
- Primary biliary cirrhosis.
- Whipple's disease.
- Gaucher's disease.
- Silicosis.
- Asbestosis.

Diagnosis[24]

A positive biopsy finding of noncaseating granulomas in the context of characteristic clinical features, blood test (elevations of serum gamma globulin, ESR, or serum ACE), chest X-ray evidence of enlarged hilar and mediastinal lymph nodes, gallium scan, defects in cell-mediated immunity, and MRI and CSF findings, having excluded other causes of granulomatous inflammation.

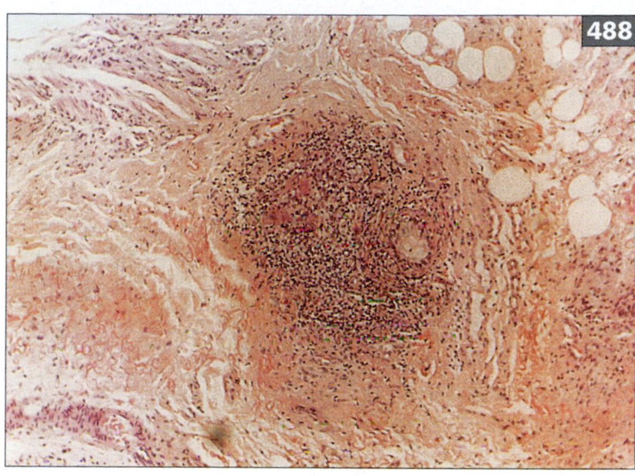

488 Biopsy showing a sarcoid granuloma characterized by an aggregate of tightly clustered mononuclear epithelioid histiocytes and multinucleated giant cells.

Pathology

Sarcoidosis often affects multiple organ systems, including the lungs (about 87%), lymph nodes (28%), skin (18%), eyes (conjunctivae, iris; 15%), and the CNS (5–16%).

- Intracranial CNS:
  - Meningeal: diffuse granulomatous meningitis or meningoencephalitis, or circumscribed granulomas, causing thickening of the arachnoid, anywhere over the surface of the brain or spinal cord but particularly around the optic chiasm, hypothalamus, basal cisterns, and subependymal region of the third ventricle.
  - Parameningeal.
  - Parenchymal lesions: anywhere but particularly in the periventricular regions and in the Virchow–Robin spaces where they form granulomatous masses up to several centimeters in diameter. Cerebral infarction may also occur due to sarcoid angiitis.
  - The hypothalamus and pituitary are characteristically (though inexplicably) vulnerable.
  - Ependymal linings of ventricles and choroid plexus (may cause hydrocephalus).
  - Cranial nerves (any nerve, but mostly facial nerve, involved by granulomatous infiltration or compression by mass lesions).
- Spinal cord: granulomatous meningitis, vasculitis, or circumscribed granulomas within the leptomeninges or parenchyma of the spinal cord.
- Peripheral nervous system (6–18%):
  - Polyradiculopathy.
  - Symmetric polyneuropathy (pure sensory, pure motor, sensorimotor).
  - Mononeuritis multiplex.
- Muscle.
- Liver.
- Kidneys.
- Testes.

Microscopic findings in the nervous system

- Noncaseating epithelioid granulomata (488):
  - An aggregate of tightly clustered mononuclear epithelioid histiocytes (phagocytes) with eosinophilic cytoplasm and oval nuclei surrounded by a rim of T helper-inducer lymphocytes and, to a far lesser extent, B lymphocytes.
  - Giant cells of the Langhans or foreign-body variety may be present in the granulomata. Tend to form in the perivascular spaces and walls of small penetrating arteries and veins of the meninges and parenchyma.

- Lymphocytic infiltrate, often perivascular and associated with neuronal loss, reactive gliosis, loss of myelin, and residual scars.
- Basal leptomeningitis.
- More diffuse leptomeningeal and ependymal disease.
- Intra-axial granulomatous masses.
- A granulomatous necrotizing angiitis that predominantly affects veins (causing a phlebitis or venulitis) and small arteries of the meninges and brain can occur, but is very uncommon.

Treatment

Treatment is inferred from experience with pulmonary sarcoidosis; there are no controlled studies to date.

- Prednisone 60 mg (1 mg/kg) oral, daily for 4–6 weeks, followed by a slow taper over 3–6 months or longer.
- If steroids fail, or cannot be tapered eventually, other immunosuppressive agents, such as cyclophosphamide, azathioprine, and cyclosporine (4–6 mg/kg/day, which inhibits interleukin-2 secretion by T cells) allow reduction of steroids to 30–50% of the original dose.
- The monoclonal antibody infliximab, directed against tumor necrosis factor (TNF)-alpha, may be effective in refractory neurosarcoidosis, as may other TNF blockers.
- Surgery may be indicated for hydrocephalus, expanding mass lesions, or mass lesions causing increased ICP.

Prognosis

Most patients respond to treatment and can have medication withdrawn over months but about one-third will relapse, often in the same location as the initial disease. Neurosarcoidosis limited to peripheral nerves and cranial nerves may improve spontaneously. Intracranial neurosarcoidosis, such as mass lesions or hydrocephalus, has a more malignant course and a higher rate of relapse. Patients with relapsing disease and more ominous clinical features (e.g. intracranial neurosarcoid such as mass lesions or hydrocephalus) should probably remain on low-dose steroids as a maintenance dose between exacerbations.

CAVERNOUS SINUS SYNDROME[25]

Definition and epidemiology

Involvement of two or more of the IIIrd, IVth, Vth (V1, V2), or VIth cranial nerves or oculosympathetic fibers on the same side.

- Incidence: rare.
- Age: any age; mean age: 40 years.
- Gender: M=F.

Etiology and pathophysiology

The cavernous sinus (really a venous plexus) lies within a dural envelope that funnels upper cranial nerves to the orbit. Consequently, small lesions, adjacent to or within the cavernous sinus, can produce dramatic localizing signs. Etiologies include:

- Tumor: 30–70% of all cases, with malignant tumors causing two-thirds:
  - Nasopharyngeal cancer: 22–46% of tumors.
  - Metastases: 16–33%.
  - Lymphoma: 0–18%.
  - Pituitary adenoma: 9–22%.
- Benign tumors; one-third.
  - Meningioma: 4–9% of tumors.
  - Chordoma: 2–11%.
  - Neuroma: 0–8%.
- Aneurysm or fistula: 5–35% of all cases:
  - Cavernous carotid artery aneurysm.
  - Carotid–cavernous fistulas.
- Trauma: 5–25% of all cases.
- Surgery: 10% of all cases.
- Inflammation (idiopathic cavernous sinusitis)[26]: 0–23% of all cases.

The Tolosa–Hunt syndrome eponym, with its promise of making a specific diagnosis on clinical grounds, has not proved reliable. One of the five patients who helped establish the Tolosa–Hunt syndrome later was shown to have a meningioma. A generic description, such as idiopathic cavernous sinusitis, seems preferable. Overlap with orbital inflammatory pseudotumor and idiopathic multiple cranial neuropathy syndromes suggest a similar underlying mechanism.

- Infection: 0–5% of all cases. Spread of fungus or bacteria, usually from the sphenoid sinus:
  - Mucormycosis.
  - Meningitis.
  - Bacterial sphenoid sinusitis.
  - Septic cavernous sinusitis.
- Diabetes: 1% of all cases.

Clinical features

Cranial nerve palsy

- Oculomotor (IIIrd) nerve: almost all patients; pupil is involved in three-quarters of cases and generally parallels the severity of the ophthalmoplegia.
- Abducens (VIth) nerve: 95% of patients.
- Trochlear (IVth) nerve: 30% of patients; may be difficult to confirm in the presence of a partial IIIrd nerve palsy.
- Trigeminal (Vth) nerve: 40% of patients.
- Optic nerve or chiasmal dysfunction: 40% of patients.
- Horner's syndrome: 5–10% of patients. Difficult to diagnose in the presence of IIIrd nerve palsy without pharmacologic pupillary testing. The history is important:
  - Age of onset.
  - Presence or absence of pain.
  - Speed of progression.
  - Past infections and tumors.

Tumor

- Average age: 47 years.
- Nasopharyngeal cancer: preferentially involves the VIth nerve and mandibular division of the Vth nerve.
- Metastases: often present with rapid complete ophthalmoplegia.
- Lymphoma: other signs may be present, such as abdominal mass.
- Pituitary adenoma: lateral extension tends to involve the IIIrd nerve and ophthalmic division of the Vth nerve. Apoplectic onset usually, and involves the oculomotor nerves with a relative frequency ratio of about 4 (IIIrd nerve), 2 (VIth nerve), and 1 (IVth nerve).
- Benign tumors: a single cranial nerve is involved for long periods.

Aneurysm

- Average age: 52 years.
- Typically progressive, painful involvement of multiple cranial nerves.
- Multiple cranial nerves are affected in two-thirds, VIth nerve only in one-quarter, and IIIrd nerve only in 10%.
- Despite IIIrd nerve involvement, the pupil on the involved side is often the same size or smaller than the normal pupil, perhaps because the parasympathetic fibers are less vulnerable within the cavernous sinus.
- Painful onset in almost all patients.
- Sudden onset in about 10% of cases.

Trauma

- Average age: 30 years.
- Usually severe head trauma with basal skull fractures.

Inflammation

(Idiopathic cavernous sinusitis)

- Average age: 35 years.
- Painful, nonspecific inflammation of the superior orbital fissure.

Infection

- Underlying diabetes is common.
- Rapid, complete ophthalmoplegia.
- Life-threatening.

Differential diagnosis

Differentials depend on the presenting clinical features.

Unilateral ophthalmoplegia

- Orbital inflammatory pseudotumor syndrome.
- Idiopathic multiple cranial neuropathy syndrome.
- Wernicke's encephalopathy.
- Myasthenia gravis.

Rapid onset, severe ophthalmoplegia

- Trauma.
- Pituitary apoplexy.
- Carotid aneurysm.
- Mucormycosis.
- Metastatic tumor.

Bilateral cavernous sinus syndrome

(<10% of all cases)

- Nasopharyngeal carcinoma.
- Lymphoma.
- Leukemia.
- Craniopharyngioma.
- Pituitary apoplexy.
- Mucormycosis.

Investigations

Contrast-enhanced MRI brain scan (**489**) is the key investigation: it clearly demonstrates any tumor mass or aneurysm large enough to cause a cavernous sinus syndrome, and usually shows carotid–cavernous fistulas, clues to bacterial or fungal nasal sinusitis, and adjacent basilar meningeal enhancement. Idiopathic cavernous sinusitis is often not apparent on noncontrast imaging but, after contrast injection, the affected cavernous sinus usually appears mildly or moderately enhanced. Abnormal signal tissue, which may have mass effect in the cavernous sinus (similar to muscle on T1-weighted imaging and to fat on T2-weighted imaging), may extend into the orbital apex. The differential diagnosis includes sarcoid, meningioma, lymphoma, metastatic or local spread of tumor, infections like actinomycosis.

Other investigations include MR angiography or catheter contrast carotid angiography, and CSF, including cytology, if meningitis, lymphoma, or leukemia is suspected. The Tensilon test can be performed if myasthenia gravis is suspected.

Diagnosis

Idiopathic cavernous sinusitis is a diagnosis of exclusion, made only after the passage of considerable time (at least 6 months) after the onset of acute painful ophthalmoplegia, to confirm complete or almost complete remission and eliminate the possibility of a subacute infection or a subtle tumor in the cavernous sinus. MRI enhancement of a mildly enlarged cavernous sinus supports, but does not establish, the diagnosis; it may also be caused by infection, lymphoma, meningioma, or dural arteriovenous malformation.

Treatment

Specific medical (antimicrobial, anti-inflammatory) or surgical treatments are used, depending on the cause. Idiopathic cavernous sinusitis may respond to corticosteroid therapy but patients need to be carefully observed for a facilitated fungal infection.

Prognosis

- Tumor: malignant tumors show rapid deterioration; benign tumors have a prolonged course.
- Aneurysm: typically progressive, prolonged course. One-quarter have some recovery of eye movements; residual damage often consists of elevator paresis and mild ptosis due to permanent damage to the superior division of the IIIrd nerve.
- Inflammation (idiopathic cavernous sinusitis): has a remitting course, usually self-limiting.
- Infection: life-threatening and usually fatal, despite intensive antibiotic treatment.

Close clinical follow-up is essential and the MRI should be repeated if a sustained remission is not forthcoming.

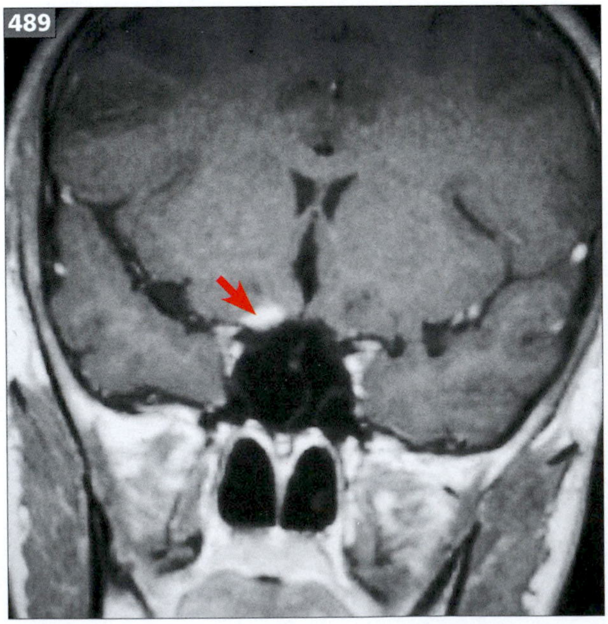

489

489 T1-weighted coronal MRI with contrast of a 20-year-old male with a painful right ophthalmoplegia, visual loss, sensory disturbance in the V1 distribution. This section was taken just posterior to the orbital apex. Note the enhancement (whiteness, arrow) around the right optic nerve which extended from the orbital apex.

REFERENCES

1. Chhibber V, Weinstein R (2012). Evidence-based review of therapeutic plasma exchange in neurological disorders. *Sem Dialysis* **25**:132–139.
2. Weinstock-Guttman B, Mehta BK, Ramanathan M *et al.* (2012). Vitamin D and multiple sclerosis. *Neurologist* **18**:179–183.
3. Handel AE, Giovannoni G, Ebers GC, Ramagopalan SV (2010). Environmental factors and their timing in adult-onset multiple sclerosis. *Nat Rev Neurol* **6**:156–166.
4. Oksenberg JR, Baranzini SE, Sawcer S, Hauser SL (2008). The genetics of multiple sclerosis: SNPs to pathways to pathogenesis. *Nat Rev Genet* **9**:516–526.
5. Scolding N (2001). The differential diagnosis of multiple sclerosis. *J Neurol Neurosurg Psychiatry* **71**(Suppl 2): ii9–15.
6. McDonald WI, Compston A, Edan G, *et al.* (2001). Recommended diagnostic criteria for multiple sclerosis: guidelines from the International Panel on the diagnosis of multiple sclerosis. *Ann Neurol* **50**(1):121–127.
7. Poser S, Brinar VV (2001). Problems with diagnostic criteria for multiple sclerosis *Lancet* **358**(9295):1746–1747.
8. Myhr KM, Mellgren SI (2009). Corticosteroids in the treatment of multiple sclerosis. *Acta Neurol Scand Suppl*:73–80.
9. Duddy M, Haghikia A, Cocco E *et al.* (2011) Managing MS in a changing treatment landscape. *J Neurol* **258**:728–739.
10. Casetta I, Iuliano G, Filippini G (2007). Azathioprine for multiple sclerosis. *Cochrane Dat Syst Rev* CD003982.
11. Gold R (2011). Oral therapies for multiple sclerosis: a review of agents in Phase III development or recently approved. *CNS Drugs* **25**:37–52.
12. Bloomgren G, Richman S, Hotermans C, *et al.* (2012). Risk of natalizumab-associated progressive multifocal leukoencephalopathy. *N Engl J Med* **366**:1870–1880.
13. Cohen JA, Coles AJ, Arnold DL, *et al.* (2012). Alemtuzumab versus interferon beta 1a as first-line treatment for patients with relapsing-remitting multiple sclerosis: a randomised controlled phase 3 trial. *Lancet* **380**:1819–1828.
14. Coles AJ, Twyman CL, Arnold DL, *et al.* (2012). Alemtuzumab for patients with relapsing multiple sclerosis after disease-modifying therapy: a randomised controlled phase 3 trial. *Lancet* **380**:1829–1839.
15. Wilkins A, Scolding N (2008). Protecting axons in multiple sclerosis. *Mult Scler* **14**:1013–1025.
16. Thompson AJ, Toosy AT, Ciccarelli O (2010). Pharmacological management of symptoms in multiple sclerosis: current approaches and future directions. *Lancet Neurol* **9**:1182–1199.
17. Fowler CJ, Panicker JN, Drake M, *et al.* (2009). A UK consensus on the management of the bladder in multiple sclerosis. *Postgrad Med J* **85**:552–559.
18. Kessler TM, Fowler CJ, Panicker JN (2009). Sexual dysfunction in multiple sclerosis. *Expert Rev Neurother* **9**:341–350.
19. Hauser SL, Johnston SC (2010). 4-aminopyridine: new life for an old drug. *Ann Neurol* **68**:A8–A9.
20. Scalfari A, Neuhaus A, Degenhardt A, *et al.* (2010). The natural history of multiple sclerosis: a geographically based study 10: relapses and long-term disability. *Brain* **133**:1914–1929.
21. Montalban X, Sastre-Garriga J, Filippi M, *et al.* (2009). Primary progressive multiple sclerosis diagnostic criteria: a reappraisal. *Mult Scler* **15**:1459–1465.
22. Wingerchuk DM, Lennon VA, Lucchinetti CF, *et al.* (2007). The spectrum of neuromyelitis optica. *Lancet Neurol* **6**:805–815.
23. Joseph FG, Scolding NJ (2007). Sarcoidosis of the nervous system. *Pract Neurol* **7**:234–244.
24. Zajicek JP, Scolding NJ, Foster O, *et al.* (1999). Central nervous system sarcoidosis – diagnosis and management. *Quart J Med* **92**:103–117.
25. Keane JR (1996). Cavernous sinus syndrome. Analysis of 151 cases. *Arch Neurol* **53**: 967–971.
26. Lutt JR, Lim LL, Phal PM, Rosenbaum JT (2008). Orbital inflammatory disease. *Semin Arthritis Rheum* **37**(4):207–222.

Further reading

Acute disseminated encephalomyelitis

Young NP, Weinshenker BG, Lucchinetti CF (2008). Acute disseminated encephalomyelitis: current understanding and controversies. *Semin Neurol* **28**(1):84–94.

Wilkins A (ed) (2013). *Progressive Multiple Sclerosis*. Springer Verlag, London.

Multiple sclerosis (MS)

General

Compston A, Coles A (2008). Multiple sclerosis. *Lancet* **372**(9648):1502–1517.

Pathogenesis and etiology

Confavreux C, Suissa S, Saddier P, *et al.* (2001). Vaccinations and the risk of relapse in multiple sclerosis. *N Engl J Med* **344**:319–326.

Dhib-Jalbut S (2007). Pathogenesis of myelin/oligodendrocyte damage in multiple sclerosis. *Neurology* **68**(22 Suppl 3):S13–S21.

Dutta R, Trapp BD (2007). Pathogenesis of axonal and neuronal damage in multiple sclerosis. *Neurology* **68**(22 Suppl 3):S22–S31.

Clinical entities

Chan JW (2000). Optic neuritis in multiple sclerosis: an update. *Neurologist* **6**:205–213.

Diagnosis, prognosis

Degenhardt A, Ramagopalan SV, Scalfari A, Ebers GC (2009). Clinical prognostic factors in multiple sclerosis: a natural history review. *Nat Rev Neurol* **5**:672–682.

Drug treatment

Ebers GC, Traboulsee A, Li D, *et al.* (2010). Analysis of clinical outcomes according to original treatment groups 16 years after the pivotal IFNB-1b trial. *J Neurol Neurosurg Psychiatry* **81**:907–912.

Gilmore CP, Cottrell DA, Scolding NJ, Wingerchuk DM, Weinshenker BG, Boggild M (2010). A window of opportunity for no treatment in early multiple sclerosis? *Mult Scler* **16**:756–759.

Polman CH, O'Connor PW, Havrdova E, *et al.* (2006). A randomized, placebo-controlled trial of natalizumab for relapsing multiple sclerosis. *N Engl J Med* **354**:899–910.

Rice C, Scolding N (2007). Strategies for achieving and monitoring myelin repair. *J Neurol* **254**:275–283.

Rice GP, Incorvaia B, Munari L, *et al.* (2001). Interferon in relapsing-remitting multiple sclerosis. *Cochrane Dat Syst Rev* CD002002.

Rehabilitation

Khan F, Turner-Stokes L, Ng L, Kilpatrick T (2007). Multidisciplinary rehabilitation for adults with multiple sclerosis. *Cochrane Dat Syst Rev* CD006036.

Neuromyelitis optica

Watanabe S, Nakashima I, Misu T, *et al.* (2007). Therapeutic efficacy of plasma exchange in NMO-IgG-positive patients with neuromyelitis optica. *Mult Scler* **13**:128–132.

Neurosarcoidosis

Newman LS, Rose CS, Maier LA (1997). Sarcoidosis. *N Engl J Med* **336**:1224–1234.

Nikhar NK, Shah JR, Tselis AC, Lewis RA (2000). Primary neurosarcoidosis: a diagnostic and therapeutic challenge. *Neurologist* **6**:126–133.

TUMORS OF THE NERVOUS SYSTEM

Julie E. Hammack, Robert P. Dinapoli

NEOPLASIA

Definition and epidemiology

Neoplasms of the nervous system may be categorized into those that derive from cells of the brain, spinal cord, and peripheral nerve (primary tumors) and those that have metastasized to the central nervous system (CNS) from non-neural tissues (metastatic tumors). Metastatic tumors of the nervous system are more common than malignant brain and spinal cord tumors. By definition, all metastatic tumors to the central and peripheral nervous systems are malignant.

Brain tumors account for 2% of all cancers but produce disproportionate morbidity and mortality when compared with other malignancies.

Tip

▶ *Metastatic tumors are the most common CNS tumors and the risk of brain metastases varies depending on the primary malignancy. The most common tumors to metastasize to the brain are lung, breast, melanoma, renal cell, and colorectal carcinoma.*

Incidence

- Primary brain tumors (malignant and non-malignant):16.5/100,000 person-years (according to the Central Brain Tumor Registry of the United States: 2009 CBTRUS data for data collected for the years 2000–2004):
  - 9.2/100,000 person years for nonmalignant tumors in adults.
  - 7.3/100,000 person years for malignant tumors in adults.
  - In adults, the rate is slightly higher in females than in males (17.2/100,000 person years *vs.* 15.8/100,000 person years respectively).
  - In childhood, the overall incidence of primary malignant and nonmalignant tumors is 4.5/100,000 person years.
  - The rate is slightly higher in males than in females (4.7/100,000 person years and 4.3/100,000 person years respectively).
- Metastatic tumors: 10–25% of systemic malignancies metastasize to the nervous system, making metastatic tumors the most common CNS malignancy:
  - Estimated incidence is 4.1–11.1/100,000 person years.
  - Incidence is likely underestimated, because of inadequate capture, in patients dying of metastatic malignancy.

Systemic malignancies may metastasize to the brain and cord parenchyma, leptomeninges, dura, and epidural space. Breast, lung, melanoma, renal and gastrointestinal (GI) cancers are the most common solid tumors giving rise to CNS metastases. The incidence of nervous system metastases appears to be increasing, likely due to improved ascertainment from more sensitive neuroimaging and also to longer survival, as a result of improved systemic therapies which do not penetrate the blood–brain barrier, of patients with systemic malignancy .

Risk factors for developing nervous system tumors

For metastatic tumors, risk depends on the risk factors for developing primary malignancy (i.e. smoking in lung cancer, family history in breast and colon cancer).

Primary nervous system tumors

- Genetic factors/heritable brain tumors (account for a minority of cases overall):
  - Neurofibromatosis (NF) 1: neurofibroma, glioma (particularly optic nerve glioma).
  - Neurofibromatosis 2: schwannoma, meningioma, ependymoma.
  - Von Hippel–Lindau syndrome: hemangioblastoma, endolymphatic sac adenoma.
  - Nevoid basal cell carcinoma syndrome: medulloblastoma.
  - Tuberous sclerosis: subependymal giant cell astrocytoma (SEGA).
  - Li–Fraumeni syndrome: glioma, medulloblastoma.
  - Turcot syndrome: glioma, medulloblastoma.
  - Multiple endocrine neoplasia: pituitary adenoma.
- Environmental factors:
  - Ionizing radiation: meningioma, glioma, malignant peripheral nerve sheath tumors.
  - No other environmental factors have been conclusively linked to an increased risk of brain tumors in humans (i.e. mobile phone use, chemical exposure, viral exposure).
- Age:
  - In adults, supratentorial tumors predominate (metastases, meningioma, glioma, pituitary adenoma).
  - In children, infratentorial tumors (pilocytic astrocytoma, medulloblastoma, ependymoma) are more common than supratentorial tumors (astrocytoma, primitive neuroectodermal tumor [PNET]).
  - Primary spinal cord and peripheral nerve tumors are rare in adults and children, accounting for less than 5% of primary nervous system tumor (except for patients with neurofibromatosis).

Pathology

Metastatic tumors

Most are epithelial-derived malignancies, e.g. carcinoma (**490**):

- Lung carcinoma.
- Breast carcinoma.
- Melanoma.
- Renal cell carcinoma.
- Colorectal carcinoma.
- Hematopoietic tumors: these tumors usually metastasize to the dura and leptomeninges:
  - Systemic lymphoma (usually non-Hodgkin's lymphoma [NHL]).
  - Leukemia.

Primary nervous system tumors

Neuroepithelial-derived tumors

- Tumors of glial tissue:
  - Astrocytoma (including glioblastoma multiforme [GBM]) (**491**)
    - Low grade astrocytoma.
    - Anaplastic astrocytoma.
    - GBM.
    - Subependymal giant cell astrocytoma.
    - Pilocytic astrocytoma (**492**).
  - Oligodendroglioma.
  - Oligoastrocytoma.
  - Ependymoma/subependymoma.
  - Pleomorphic xanthoastrocytoma (PXA).
  - Choroid plexus papilloma and carcinoma.
- Neuronal and mixed neuronal–glial tumors:
  - Gangliocytoma.
  - Ganglioglioma.
  - Dysembryoplastic neuroepithelial tumor.
  - Paraganglioma.
  - Esthesioneuroblastoma.
- Embryonal tumors:
  - Medulloblastoma.
  - Supratentorial PNET.

Meningothelial-derived tumors

- Meningioma.
- Atypical meningioma.
- Anaplastic meningioma.

Mesenchymal, nonmeningothelial tumors

- Hemangiopericytoma.
- Hemangioblastoma.
- Sarcoma.
- Choroid plexus papilloma/carcinoma.
- Epidermoid tumor.

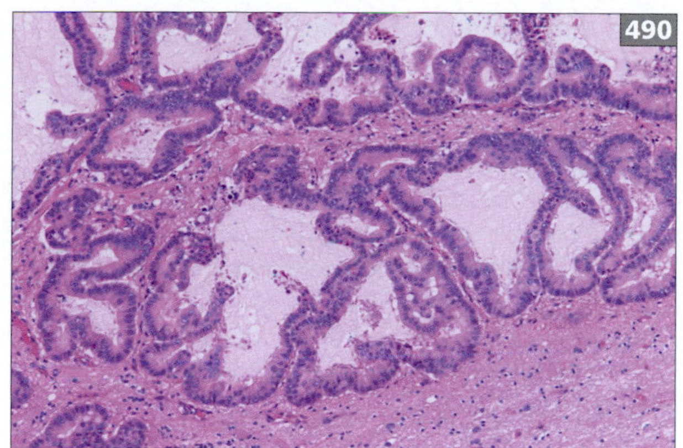

490 Metastasis to brain: adenocarcinoma.

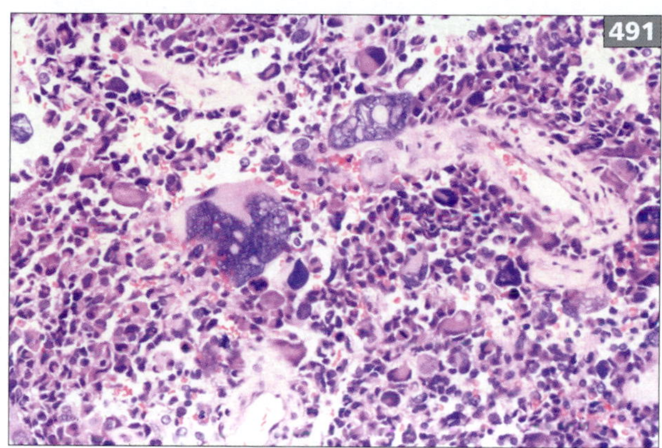

491 Glioblastoma multiforme: demonstrating marked glial atypia.

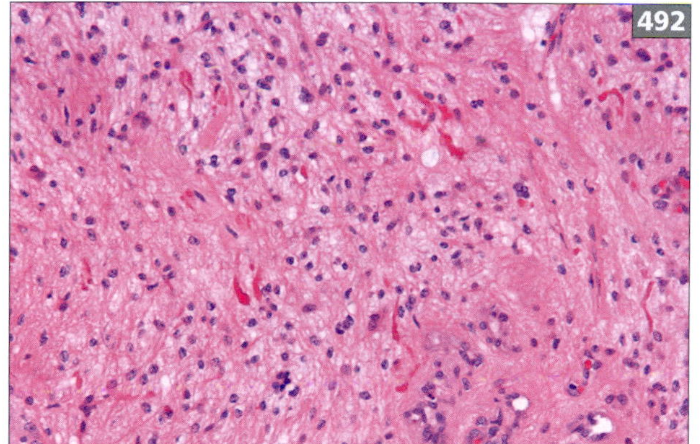

492 Pilocytic astrocytoma: demonstrating hypercellularity and Rosenthal fibers.

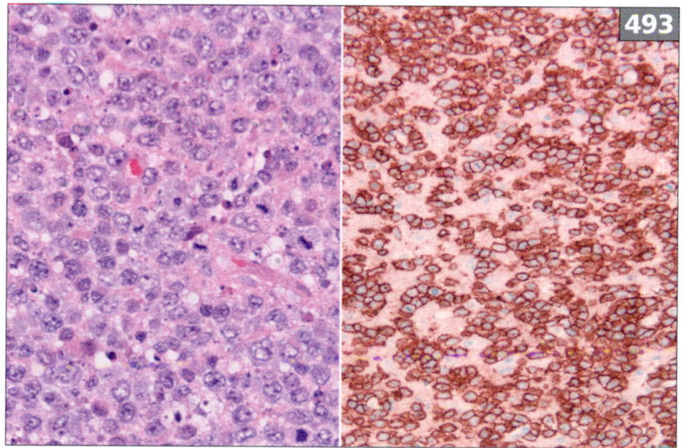

493 Primary CNS lymphoma: polyclonal B cells and positive CD20 staining.

Tumors of peripheral nerve
- Schwannoma.
- Neurofibroma.
- Perineurioma.
- Malignant peripheral nerve sheath tumors (MPNST).

Lymphomas and hematopoietic tumors
- Primary CNS lymphoma (PCNSL) (493).
- Plasmacytoma.

Germ cell tumors
- Germinoma.
- Embryonal carcinoma.
- Yolk sac tumor.
- Choriocarcinoma.
- Teratoma.
- Mixed germ cell tumors.

Tumors of the sellar region
- Pituitary adenoma/carcinoma.

Pineal parenchymal tumors
- Pineocytoma.
- Pineoblastoma.

Tumors of embryonal remnants
- Craniopharyngioma.
- Rathke's cleft cyst.
- Chordoma.
- Colloid cyst.

Clinical features (primary and metastatic tumors)

The clinical features depend on the location and growth rate of the tumor. Symptoms and signs may be divided into three main categories: elevated intracranial pressure (ICP), focal neurologic deficit, and seizures (focal and/or secondarily generalized). Symptoms that are focal, progressive, and subacute or chronic suggest neoplasm as the etiology. Occasionally, nervous system tumors may present acutely as with seizure or tumor hemorrhage.

Tip

▶ *Regardless of whether the tumor is primary or metastatic to the brain, the symptoms and signs of neoplasm are those of elevated ICP, focal (usually progressive) neurologic deficit, and seizure.*

Elevated ICP

The symptoms may be related directly to the tumor mass and the surrounding edema or obstruction of cerebrospinal fluid (CSF) pathways and resulting hydrocephalus. Hydrocephalus is particularly common in tumors involving the posterior fossa or structures adjacent to the 3rd ventricle. Tumors involving the leptomeninges may obstruct the arachnoid granulations and produce communicating hydrocephalus. Signs or symptoms of raised ICP are present in 45% of metastatic brain tumors and 50% of malignant primary brain tumors at the time of presentation.

Symptoms of elevated ICP include:

- Headache:
  - Typically worse when reclining and worse on awakening.
  - Worse with Valsalva maneuver.
- Vomiting:
  - Usually associated with headache.
  - Related to compression/irritation of the area postrema in the medulla.
- Altered level of consciousness.
- Visual obscurations: transient visual loss with Valsalva maneuver; resulting from optic nerve compression.
- Diplopia: usually a false localizing sign from bilateral stretching of the abducens nerves.

Signs of elevated ICP include:

- Papilledema.
- Reduced level of consciousness.
- Meningismus: usually mild and related to cerebellar tonsillar herniation; frequently present in tumors with leptomeningeal involvement.

Signs and symptoms of focal neurologic dysfunction

These signs reflect the tumor location:

- Supratentorial:
  - Hemiparesis.
  - Aphasia.
  - Cognitive impairment/personality change.
  - Visual loss (monocular, bitemporal hemianopia, homonymous hemianopia).
  - Sensory loss (primary sensory loss [thalamic], or cortical sensory loss [parietal lobe]).
- Infratentorial:
  - Ataxia
  - Dysarthria
  - Cranial neuropathies (CN III–XII).
- Spinal tumors:
  - Spine and radicular pain.
  - Paraparesis/paraplegia.
  - Sensory loss with sensory level.
  - Bowel, bladder, and/or sexual dysfunction.

Associated features of nervous system tumors

- Signs and symptoms of systemic metastatic neoplasms:
  - Anorexia, weight loss, adenopathy, hemoptysis, finger clubbing, skin lesions (melanoma).
  - In patients with suspected metastatic brain tumors, a complete history and physical examination are the most useful diagnostic studies.
- Scalp mass in meningioma with hyperostosis.
- Signs of a neurocutaneous syndrome associated with primary nervous system tumors:
  - Café au lait spots (NF-1, less common in NF-2).
  - Cutaneous neurofibromas (NF-1).
  - Adenoma sebaceum, Shagreen patches and periungual fibromas (tuberous sclerosis).
  - Retinal hemangioblastomas (von Hippel–Lindau disease).

Differential diagnosis for nervous system neoplasms

- Subdural hematoma.
- Aqueductal stenosis.
- Arachnoid cyst.
- CNS demyelinating disease.
- Cerebral infarct/hemorrhage.
- CNS hamartoma.
- Cortical migration abnormality.
- Brain abscess.
- Metabolic encephalopathy.

Investigations

Computed tomography (CT) head with and without contrast

- Largely superseded by magnetic resonance imaging (MRI).
- CT is still used in emergency situations to diagnose hemorrhage, acute hydrocephalus, and mass effect.
- CT is superior to MRI in determining the presence of tumor calcification.
- Unless hemorrhage or dense calcification is present, brain tumors typically appear as areas of low density (hypodense) on noncontrast CT of the brain:
  - Very cellular tumors (i.e. primary CNS lymphoma and medulloblastoma) often appear as areas of slight hyperdensity.
  - Malignant tumors often have areas of central necrosis (low density).
- Following IV contrast injection, vascular tumors (i.e. metastases, high-grade gliomas, and meningiomas) enhance.

MRI of the brain/spine

- More sensitive than CT of the brain and much more useful than CT in imaging the posterior fossa and spinal cord.
- Gadolinium enhancement increases the sensitivity of MRI.
- Current technology of MR spectroscopy and perfusion images is not sufficient to replace the need for brain biopsy (tissue diagnosis) in patients without a prior pathologic diagnosis.

Skull X-ray

- Skull X-rays are almost never utilized for the diagnosis of CNS tumors. Historically, skull X-rays were used to demonstrate intracranial calcifications and demonstrate midline shift with lateral deviation of the calcified pineal gland. They may be useful as an adjunct in osteolytic tumors involving the skull (i.e. myeloma, epidermoid tumors) or tumors with associated hyperostosis (i.e. meningioma).

Lumbar puncture

CSF examination must be approached with great caution in patients with intracranial or spinal masses due to the risk of brain or spinal cord herniation. If significant mass effect is absent, the CSF basal cisterns appear open, and a leptomeningeal neoplasm (i.e. leptomeningeal carcinoma, lymphoma, leukemia, medulloblastoma, ependymoma) is suspected, then CSF examination is appropriate and diagnostically useful.

Other investigations

These are guided by the clinical situation. If a metastatic tumor is suspected but not previously confirmed, the following studies may be useful in selected patients:

- CT chest, abdomen, and pelvis with contrast.
- Mammogram.
- Positron emission tomography (PET) scan (utilized primarily to define the presence of systemic neoplasms).
- Metastatic bone survey.
- Blood work: only a few CNS tumors may be definitively diagnosed with blood work (obviating the need for a pathologic diagnosis). These include the following:
  - Germ cell tumor – pineal region mass with elevated serum beta- human chorionic gonadotropin [β-HCG] or alpha fetoprotein.
  - Pituitary prolactinoma – markedly elevated serum prolactin with a sellar mass.

Biopsy/resection and other surgical interventions

The goals of surgery are threefold: 1) to establish a pathologic diagnosis; 2) to treat the patient's symptoms by debulking the tumor, alleviating focal symptoms or symptoms of elevated ICP; or 3) in rare, specific instances to render a surgical cure.

A stereotactic or open biopsy may be required to make a diagnosis in patients with solitary or multiple brain lesions, if there is no evidence or prior history of a metastatic systemic neoplasm and no other clues to suggest a non-neoplastic process which could mimic a brain neoplasm (i.e. demyelination, brain abscess).

Indications include:

- Patients with deep-seated gliomas and PCNSL in whom an aggressive resection is high risk.
- Patients with glioma (low-grade or malignant), medulloblastoma, and PNET have improved survival if a more complete resection takes place at the time of diagnosis, even though these patients are not cured by surgery.
- Patients with large, symptomatic primary or metastatic tumors may benefit from surgical debulking to palliate symptoms, prevent herniation, and allow reduction of corticosteroid dosages.
- Patients with systemic carcinoma who have limited systemic disease have longer survival if a solitary brain metastasis is resected. In this subset of patients, median survival is prolonged and functional status is maintained longer than in those patients not undergoing resection.

- Patients with surgically curable neoplasms (meningioma, pilocytic astrocytoma, dysembryoplastic neuroepithelial tumor [DNET], ganglioglioma, myxopapillary ependymoma, pituitary adenoma, epidermoid, hemangioblastoma) are best treated with gross total resection if it is feasible.
- Ventriculoperitoneal shunting or 3rd ventriculostomy may be required to alleviate symptoms of raised ICP in patients with communicating or obstructive hydrocephalus.

Surgery is not necessary if:

- The patient has a very poor prognosis (i.e. elderly, poor performance status) in whom tumor therapies (radiation and chemotherapy) would be unlikely to offer significant clinical benefit and a non-neoplastic condition has been reasonably excluded.
- CT or MRI reveals multiple centrally necrotic, ring-enhancing lesions in a patient with a known, pathologically confirmed systemic malignancy which has a proclivity to metastasize to the brain (i.e. breast or lung carcinoma).
- A patient with a sellar mass and a markedly elevated serum prolactin (diagnostic of prolactinoma).
- A patient with a pineal region mass, elevated serum or CSF β-HCG and/or alpha fetoprotein (diagnostic of germ cell tumor).
- Patients with small, incidentally discovered meningiomas, particularly if calcified.

Biopsy/resection may be delayed if the lesion is suggestive of a low-grade glioma, the patient is asymptomatic, and imaging was performed for some other reason (i.e. head trauma). In this instance the patient should be followed with serial neuroimaging. Biopsy/resection is indicated if, after serial neuroimaging, the lesion is noted to be enlarging and/or the patient develops symptoms clearly referable to the lesion (i.e. seizures, headache, and focal neurologic deficit).

Surgical morbidity of tumor biopsy or resection is largely related to tumor location and skill of the neurosurgeon. In noneloquent brain (nondominant anterior frontal cortex), the risk of neurologic morbidity is usually <3–5%; in eloquent areas of brain (dominant frontal lobe, thalamus, and brainstem) the risk of neurologic morbidity with resection or biopsy is much higher. However, even in neurologically eloquent areas of the brain, the mortality risk from stereotactic biopsy is usually $<1\%$.

Treatment

For a summary of treatment see *Table 90*.

Tip

▶ *Corticosteroids may be life-saving and improve function in patients with brain tumors. They reduce peritumoral edema and ICP but also often have annoying or life-threatening adverse effects. The latter include gastrointestinal hemorrhage, hyperglycemia, mania, insomnia, and avascular necrosis, among others.*

Medical therapy

Elevated ICP is usually due to a combination of tumor mass and peritumoral edema. Sudden increase in ICP may occur in patients with tumor-associated hemorrhage. Patients with acute and/or severe increases in ICP may develop transtentorial or tonsillar herniation requiring urgent medical and possibly surgical therapy.

- Corticosteroids: dexamethasone 12 mg oral or IV load followed by 4 mg tid or qid. The clinical effect may take 24–48 hours to fully develop. If PCNSL is suspected, corticosteroids should be avoided unless absolutely necessary for the patient's well-being. Even single doses of corticosteroid can render a subsequent biopsy nondiagnostic due to the apoptotic effect of corticosteroids in lymphoma. Corticosteroids should be monitored for acute adverse effects, including mania, insomnia, hyperglycemia, and gastrointestinal hemorrhage.
- IV mannitol 1 g/kg as a 20% solution over 20 minutes with or without IV furosemide 40 mg. This is usually used only as a temporizing measure until a more definitive treatment is available (i.e. placement of an external ventricular drain, ventriculoperitoneal shunting, or surgical resection of a mass lesion).
- Antiemetics and analgesic therapy are appropriate in symptomatic patients. Use caution with potent opioids due to the sedating effects which can complicate monitoring of the patient's mental status.
- Anticonvulsant therapy is required if seizures have occurred.
  - For status epilepticus, IV lorazepam and loading with fosphenytoin is preferred.
  - If IV treatment is not required, oral administration of a nonenzyme inducing anticonvulsant (non-EIAC) (levetiracetam, valproic acid, lamotrigine) is preferred. Non-EIAC drugs do not interfere with corticosteroids or chemotherapy agents the patient may require.

- There is no proven benefit of anticonvulsants when used prophylactically to prevent a first seizure in patients with brain tumors. Patients should receive anticonvulsants pre-operatively to prevent post-operative seizure activity. Anticonvulsants can be tapered quickly 1 week post-operatively in patients who remain seizure free.
- Chemotherapy: if indicated, the type of chemotherapy will be dictated by the specific tumor type (see below).

For surgical therapy, see prior section: Biopsy/resection and other surgical interventions.

Radiation therapy

(See also specific tumor types)

- High-grade glioma (WHO grade III and IV):
  - Involved field external beam radiation therapy (EBRT) is standard (encompassing the T2 signal abnormality plus a 2 cm margin).
  - 50–60 Gy (5000–6000 cGy) in ~30 fractions administered over 6 weeks.
- Low-grade glioma (WHO grade II astrocytoma, oligodendroglioma, oligoastrocytoma, and ependymoma):
  - EBRT is often delayed if a gross total resection has taken place.
  - Usually lower doses of EBRT are used in low-grade glioma (50.4 Gy in 28 fractions).

TABLE 90 **TREATMENT OF TUMORS**

Tumor	Surgery	Adjuvant therapy	Prognosis
Glioblastoma	Maximal resection if tumor is accessible	Radiation therapy and temozolomide	14 months median survival
Low-grade glioma (astrocytoma, mixed glioma and oligodendroglioma)	Maximal resection if tumor is accessible	Radiation therapy if there is post-operative residual or at recurrence	Variable: 5–12 years median survival
Pilocytic astrocytoma	Maximal resection if tumor is accessible	Radiation therapy considered post-operatively if residual tumor is present	95% 10-year survival; potentially curable if a gross total resection has taken place
Primary CNS lymphoma	Biopsy only	IV methotrexate; whole brain radiation therapy at recurrence	30–60 months median survival
Brain metastases	Surgical resection if solitary or primary tumor is unknown	Whole brain radiation therapy	4–7 months median survival
Medulloblastoma/PNET	Maximal resection if feasible	Radiation and platin-based chemotherapy	>50% 5-year survival
Meningioma	Maximal resection if feasible	Stereotactic radiation for recurrence	20% recurrence risk at 5 years even with gross total resection
Vestibular schwannoma	Gross total resection if feasible	Stereotactic radiation for unresectable or recurrent tumors	Very low recurrence if a gross total resection has taken place
Craniopharyngioma	Gross total resection if feasible	Localized radiation for residual or recurrent tumor	Very low recurrence rate if a gross total resection has taken place
Pituitary adenoma	Unnecessary for prolactinoma; for other types, gross total resection if feasible	Radiation therapy for recurrent/ residual tumor; prolactinomas are treated only with cabergoline	Excellent long-term prognosis

Radiation usually is not indicated for WHO grade I tumors which are best treated with surgical resection. These include:

- Pilocytic astrocytoma
- PXA.
- DNET.
- Ganglioglioma.
- Meningioma.

Some primary brain tumor types may benefit from neuraxis radiation because of their tendency to produce leptomeningeal spread. These include the following tumor types:

- Medulloblastoma.
- PNET.
- Germ cell tumors.
- High-grade ependymoma (WHO grade III).

Metastatic carcinoma to the brain is treated with whole brain radiation therapy (WBRT) 20–30 Gy in 10–15 fractions to treat both visible and microscopic tumor deposits. The role of radiation therapy is palliative. Patients with brain metastases survive only 3–7 months on average, usually dying from progression of their systemic disease and not from CNS disease.

Stereotactic radiosurgery (gamma knife, Cyberknife) and particulate radiation therapy (proton beam and boron neutron capture therapy [BNCT]) have the advantage of treating well-circumscribed lesions that are not amenable to surgical resection. The advantage of these treatments is to deliver a therapeutic dose of radiation and reduce radiation exposure to surrounding normal brain. Because of logistical and cost issues, particulate radiation therapy is utilized much less frequently than radiosurgery. Stereotactic radiosurgery has role in the treatment of the following tumor types:

- Meningioma.
- Chordoma.
- Parenchymal brain metastases from carcinoma:
  - In conjunction with WBRT.
  - In patients with limited systemic malignancy and good performance status.
  - Data indicate that the concurrent use of gamma knife radiosurgery improves CNS control in patients with three or fewer brain metastases (but at significantly greater cost).

Adverse effects

Adverse effects depend on the total dose of radiation administered, the extent of the treated area, and the time elapsed from treatment. There is greater risk of acute and chronic adverse effects with WBRT and larger total dose and fraction size. Acute effects include:

- Fatigue: very common, sometimes delayed until after radiation therapy has finished (somnolence syndrome), but self-limited.
- Signs of elevated ICP (headache, vomiting) and focal neurologic deficits may develop or worsen due to edema from acute tumor necrosis – usually best managed with corticosteroids.
- Reduced taste and dry mouth, from effects on salivary glands and glossal papillae.
- Reduced hearing – usually from serous otitis media from swelling of the Eustachian tube. It is best treated with decongestants and steam inhalation.

Subacute (early delayed) effects, weeks or months after radiation include:

- Somnolence syndrome: the most common. Patients show profound fatigue and hypersomnia usually commencing 2–4 weeks after the completion of brain radiation and lasting 4–6 weeks with spontaneous resolution.
- Radiographic ‘pseudoprogression’. There is evidence of increased edema and contrast enhancement within a few months of the completion of brain radiation. It resolves spontaneously in 4–6 weeks but may require corticosteroid treatment if symptomatic. Pseudoprogression is often mistaken for true tumor progression which may lead to inappropriate treatment changes and needless worry for the patient.
- Lhermitte’s phenomenon in patients receiving spinal radiation. This probably results from focal demyelination in the posterior columns. It is self-limited and resolves spontaneously in a few weeks. Sometimes Lhermitte’s phenomenon develops during radiation therapy.

Chronic (late) effects, years after radiation therapy include:

- Neuropsychologic – cognitive impairment:
  - Particularly common in patients receiving WBRT although also seen with EBRT.
  - Pathologically demyelination, gliosis, microcalcification are seen.
  - Particularly common in patients receiving IV or IT methotrexate after radiation therapy.
  - Classic presentation is that of a slowly progressive subcortical dementia with gait apraxia and urinary incontinence.

- Focal necrosis with enhancement and edema (radiation necrosis):
  - A form of 'pseudoprogression'.
  - Radiographically mimics progression.
  - MR spectroscopy and PET are not reliable in differentiating radiation necrosis from tumor progression.
  - Empiric therapy with steroids and repeat imaging in 4–6 weeks may be helpful.
  - Biopsy may be required to differentiate definitively from tumor progression.
- Neuroendocrine:
  - Growth retardation in children.
  - Hypothyroidism.
  - Hypogonadism and infertility.
- Cataracts.
- Deafness (both conductive and neurogenic).
- Radiation therapy-induced tumors (usually 10 or more years after radiation therapy to the brain or spine):
  - Meningiomas are the most common.
  - MPNST.
  - Malignant gliomas.
- Accelerated cerebrovascular atherosclerosis of intra- or extracranial vessels included in the radiation field.

Prognosis

Prognosis is dependent on the type of tumor. For most high-grade gliomas (WHO grade III and grade IV) and brain metastases treatment is noncurative and often only palliative.

See section on individual tumor types for a more complete description of therapy and prognosis.

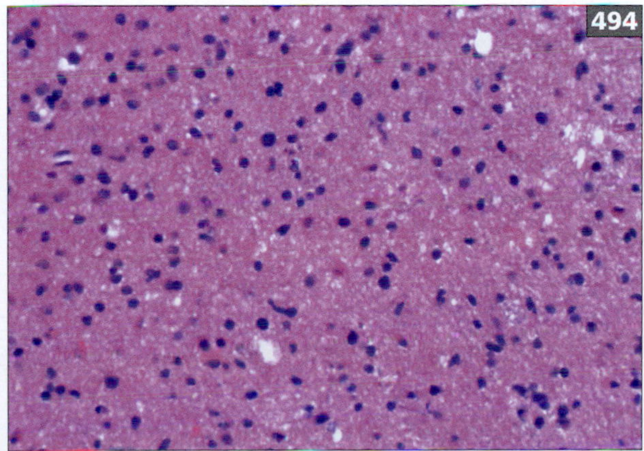

494 Diffuse astrocytoma (grade II–IV).

GLIOMAS

Definition

Gliomas are neuroepithelial-derived lesions of the brain and spinal cord. They arise from astrocytic (astrocytoma), oligodendroglial (oligodendroglioma), mixed (oligoastrocytoma), and ependymal (ependymoma) cell lines. Gliomas also include the rare choroid plexus tumors. Within each category, the tumors are graded by the degree of cellular differentiation (WHO grade I–IV). Rare subtypes are given a designation of WHO grade I (see below).

Classification by cell of origin

Astrocytoma

Astrocytomas are derived from astrocytes. They are the most common intracranial glioma (75% of all gliomas). Subtypes include:

- Diffuse astrocytomas (grade II–IV) (**494**):
  - Low-grade astrocytoma (grade II).
  - Anaplastic astrocytoma (grade III).
  - GBM (grade IV): accounts for 50% of all gliomas.
- Pilocytic astrocytoma (grade I).
- PXA (grade I).
- Subependymal giant cell astrocytomas (grade I).

Oligodendroglioma

These are derived from oligodendroglial cells, and account for 5–15% of intracranial gliomas. Subtypes include:

- Low-grade oligodendroglioma (grade II).
- Anaplastic oligodendroglioma (grade III).
- Oligoastrocytoma (grade II–IV).

Ependymoma

These are derived from ependymal cells. They are more common in children than in adults (6% of adult intracranial gliomas and 9% of childhood intracranial gliomas). Subtypes include:

- Myxopapillary ependymoma (WHO grade I): spinal only (typically develops in the filum terminale).
- Subependymoma (WHO grade I).
- Ependymoma (WHO grade II, III).

Choroid plexus tumors

These include choroid plexus papilloma and choroid plexus carcinoma.

Epidemiology

Glioma is the most common symptomatic primary brain tumor in adults (meningiomas are the most common tumor overall in adults).

- Incidence: 6 per 100,000 adult persons per year for all gliomas. Gender-specific incidence is shown in *Table 91*.
- Age:
  - May occur at any age.
  - Glioblastoma, the most common glioma, has peak incidence in the middle-aged and elderly, with a mean age at diagnosis of 55 years.
  - Anaplastic astrocytoma: mean age 46 years at diagnosis.
  - Oligodendrogliomas: mean age 45 years at diagnosis.
  - Ependymomas:
    - Intracranial ependymomas are more common in children: mean age of 4 years at diagnosis.
    - Spinal ependymomas are more common in adults: mean age of 40 years at diagnosis.

Pathogenesis

The formation and progression of gliomas is typically associated with inactivation of tumor suppressor genes, nullification of apoptotic genes, and dysregulation of DNA repair genes[1].

For low-grade astrocytomas, the inactivation of the tumor suppressor *P53* gene is responsible. This gene codes for a protein that plays an important role in cell cycle regulation and apoptosis and is located on chromosome 17p. Loss of a gene on chromosome 22q is also involved in most low-grade gliomas, although the specific gene has yet to be identified.

The molecular genetics of glioblastoma multiforme (GBM) vary depending on whether the GBM arose *de novo* (primary GBM) or evolved from a low-grade glioma (secondary GBM). Most GBMs are primary and usually occur in older patients.

TABLE 91 **INCIDENCE OF GLIOMAS (PER 100,000 ADULTS PER YEAR)**

	Males	Females
Glioblastoma	3.94	2.38
Anaplastic astrocytoma	0.53	0.37
Oligodendroglioma	0.54	0.45
Ependymoma	0.29	0.24

The transition of low-grade astrocytoma to anaplastic astrocytoma (World Health Organization [WHO] grade III) is associated with loss of chromosome 13q (which includes the retinoblastoma gene locus) and inactivation of genes on chromosomes 9p and 19q. The transition to GBM from anaplastic astrocytoma is associated with inactivation of the tumor suppressor gene *PTEN* on chromosome 10 and amplification of the epidermal growth factor receptor (*EGFR*) gene resulting in overexpression of *EGFR*. *EGFR* amplification or overexpression is found in most primary (*de novo*) GBMs.

In oligodendrogliomas and mixed gliomas (oligoastrocytomas) oncogene overexpression is only rarely observed. Deletions in chromosomes 1p and 19q are the most common abnormalities found in these tumors (40–80%). The precise role that these deletions play in tumorigenesis is unknown. Allelic loss of 1p/19q is a strong predictor of chemosensitivity to alkylating agents and overall portends a better prognosis in tumors that possess these deletions.

Growth factor and growth factor receptor overexpression are common in malignant gliomas and may accelerate tumorigenesis and tumor progression. Most of these are found predominantly in diffuse, high-grade, astrocytic tumors and include the following:

- *EGFR*.
- Platelet-derived growth factor (PDGF).
- Vascular endothelial growth factor (VEGF).
- Insulin-like growth factor (IGF-1).
- Basic fibroblast growth factor (bFGF,FGF-2).
- Transforming growth factor (TGF)-alpha.

Methylguanine-deoxyribonucleic acid (DNA) methyltransferase (MGMT) is an important enzyme in high-grade gliomas necessary for DNA repair following treatment with alkylating agents. Patients whose tumors possess a silenced *MGMT* gene (from promoter methylation) have a better response to alkylating agent chemotherapy and improved survival compared with those with activation of the *MGMT* gene.

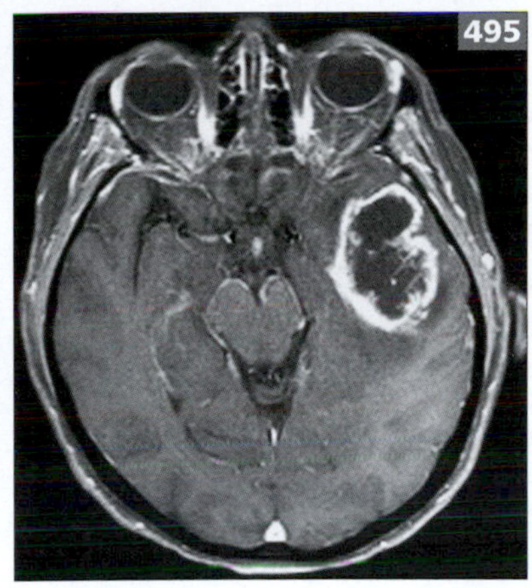

495 Irregularly enhancing supratentorial mass on CT/MRI, indicative of glioblastoma multiforme/anaplastic astrocytoma.

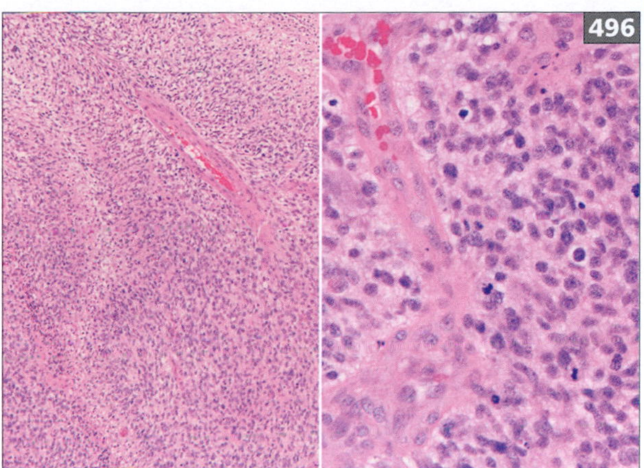

496 Pseudopalisading (arrangement of tumor cells around blood vessels) in glioblastoma multiforme.

GLIOBLASTOMA MULTIFORME (GBM) AND ANAPLASTIC ASTROCYTOMA (AA)

Clinical features

The vast majority are supratentorial in location. Because of the diffuse, infiltrative nature, most occupy more than one lobe of the brain. GBM and AA frequently cross the corpus callosum; 5–10% are multifocal. Tumors are highly vascular, often with evidence of gross or microscopic hemorrhage. They are typically associated with significant vasogenic edema and mass effect. GBM and AA are usually subacute in presentation, with a temporal profile spanning a few weeks or months. The presentation may be acute with seizures (GBM 25%, AA 56%) or tumor hemorrhage. Other features include:

- Headache: 53–57%.
- Focal neurologic deficits, cognitive impairment: 25–50%.

Investigations

CT or MRI demonstrates an irregular enhancing supratentorial mass (**495**).

- Central necrosis is present in GBM but not in AA.
- 90% solitary (10% may be multicentric) (see image).
- May cross the corpus callosum.
- Diffuse brain infiltration (gliomatosis cerebri) is more common with AA and low-grade astrocytoma.
- Leptomeningeal spread (meningeal gliomatosis) occurs in <5% and extraneural metastases are exceedingly rare.
- MR spectroscopy and PET usually do not add diagnostic information.

Diagnosis

The only definitive way to make a diagnosis is by surgical biopsy/resection. Surgery excludes alternative diagnoses (inflammatory disease, metastatic tumor) and allows grading of the tumor.

Pathology

- Infiltrative pleomorphic, mitotically very active cells (**496**).
- Necrosis is always present in GBM but not AA. GBM often shows pseudopalisading (arrangement of tumor nuclei around areas of necrosis) (**496**).
- Endothelial proliferation in GBM is typical.

Treatment

Surgery

The initial treatment for malignant glioma is surgical resection. Biopsy alone should be reserved for patients with glioma in very eloquent brain or those deemed too medically frail to tolerate a more extensive resection. Aggressive surgical resection offers several advantages over biopsy:

- Improved survival, particularly in younger patients with better performance status.
- More accurate diagnosis due to a larger, more representative sample.
- Debulking of the tumor often produces symptomatic improvement and allows more rapid tapering of corticosteroids (with reduced corticosteroid adverse effects).
- Smaller tumor volumes may improve the response to post-operative adjuvant therapies.

Radiation therapy

External beam radiation is the single most effective treatment for GBM and AA. Radiation is delivered to involved fields (T2 signal abnormality with a 2 cm margin). There is no survival benefit from WBRT and significantly more toxicity. The usual course of radiation is 60 Gy in 30 fractions over 6 weeks. There is no proven benefit of stereotactic radiation in the treatment of high-grade glioma.

Chemotherapy

Chemotherapy generally has been disappointing in the treatment of gliomas. The current standard drug for high-grade glioma is oral temozolomide, an alkylating agent[2]. Temozolomide is given in low doses daily during radiation and then in a 5 day/month regimen. A phase III study has demonstrated that the addition of temozolomide prolongs median survival to a modest degree (2.4 months) when compared to radiation therapy alone in GBM[3].

Other drugs with activity against high-grade glioma include bevacizumab (a VEGF receptor antagonist), the alkylating agents (carmustine, lomustine, and procarbazine) and etoposide among others[4].

Prognosis

The most important prognostic factors are patient age, tumor grade, and performance status. Extent of resection also is a lesser determinant of prognosis.

- With surgery alone, median survival for GBM is 12–14 weeks.
- Radiation therapy prolongs median survival to 8–12 months in GBM.
- The addition of temozolomide extends median survival to 14.4 months.
- The median survival for AA (grade III astrocytoma) is 2–3 years with surgery, radiation therapy, and chemotherapy (temozolomide).

ANAPLASTIC OLIGODENDROGLIOMA (AO) AND OLIGOASTROCYTOMA (AOA)

Definition

Anaplastic glioma, completely or partially composed of oligodendroglial-derived cells, deserves a separate discussion from AA and GBM, due to the more favorable natural history and improved response to treatment of these tumors.

AO and AOA are predominantly tumors of adulthood with a peak incidence between the 4th and the 6th decade of life. A high percentage of AO and AOA possess allelic loss of chromosome 1p and/or 19q; 75% of oligodendroglial tumors possess deletion of either 1p or 19q and 60% of oligodendroglial tumors are codeleted for both chromosomes.

The presence of 1p and/or 19q deletion predicts a better response to alkylating agent chemotherapy and a better overall prognosis.

Clinical features

As with AA and GBM, the usual presenting symptoms are seizure, headache, and focal neurologic deficit. Most AO and AOA are supratentorial.

Investigations

On imaging, AO/AOA is indistinguishable from AA. CT typically shows a mass with low attenuation affecting the white and gray matter. Calcification is frequently evident on CT. MRI of the brain reveals increased T2 signal with mass effect. Contrast enhancement may or may not be present.

Diagnosis

As with all glioma, biopsy or surgical resection is required to make a diagnosis of AO and AOA. Once the diagnosis is made, tissue is typically sent for fluorescence *in situ* hybridization (FISH) studies to evaluate the presence of 1p and 19q deletions.

Treatment

An attempt at aggressive resection (preferably gross total resection) is considered the best initial therapy of these tumors.

Post-operative external beam radiation is considered standard in the treatment of AO and AOA, 60 Gy to the area of T2 signal with an additional margin of 2 cm.

Chemotherapy (usually temozolomide) in conjunction with radiation therapy is routinely administered, particularly in patients whose tumors have deletion of 1p and/or 19q. The role of upfront temozolomide before radiation has yet to be determined with a randomized trial.

Procarbazine, CCNU, and vincristine (PCV) is another chemotherapy regimen shown to be effective against AO and AOA. PCV usually is a more toxic regimen and has been supplanted by temozolomide.

Prognosis

Median survival for AO is 5 years with surgery and radiation, and is 3–5 years for AOA with surgery and radiation.

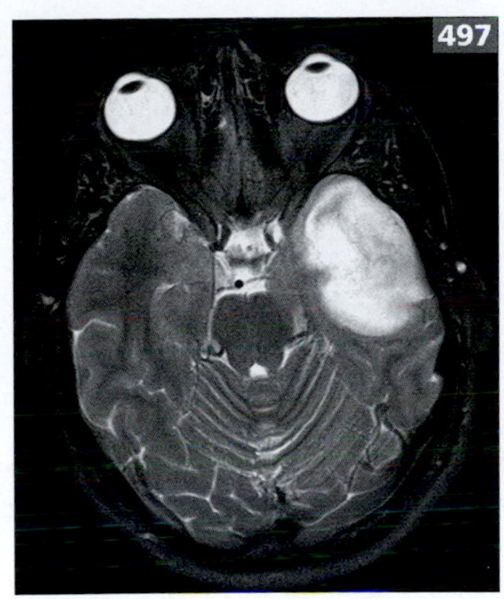

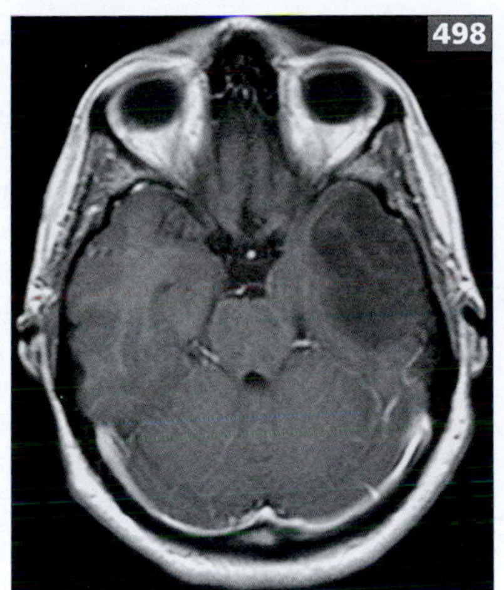

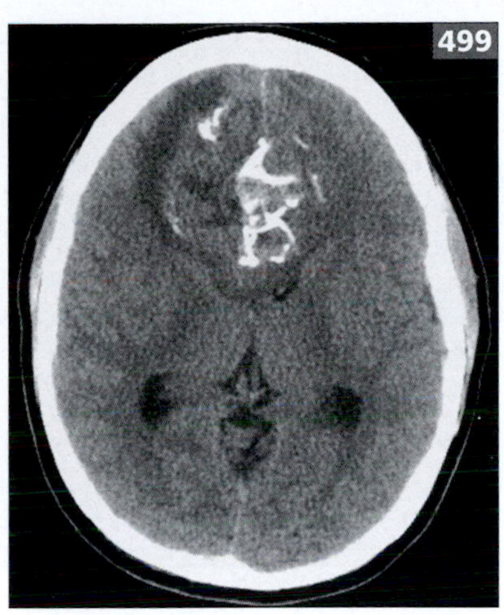

497 Area of intra-axial increased T2 signal on MRI with associated mass effect, indicative of low-grade glioma.

498 Area of low signal on contrasted T1 signal on MRI, indicative of low-grade glioma.

499 Calcification may be present in low-grade oligodendrogliomas.

LOW-GRADE GLIOMA (LGG): ASTROCYTOMA, OA, AND OLIGODENDROGLIOMA (WHO GRADE II)

Definition and epidemiology

LGG describes a spectrum of tumors characterized pathologically by diffuse proliferation of astrocytes, oligodendroglial cells, or mixed astrocytic/oligodendroglial cell types. LGG are far less common than high-grade gliomas in adults, accounting for only 20% of CNS glial tumors. The vast majority of LGG are supratentorial in adults and infratentorial (brainstem and cerebellum) in children.

LGG have a younger median age of onset (35 years) than AA or GBM. Optic nerve glioma is a form of LGG that is more common in children. Pilocytic astrocytoma, ganglioglioma, and PXA are categorized apart from LGG because of their particularly benign behavior and are given a WHO grade I designation.

Clinical features

In some patients, the tumor is asymptomatic and discovered when a CT or MRI of the brain is performed for unrelated reasons (e.g. head trauma). Seizures are more common as a presenting symptom of LGG than AA or GBM (85% *vs.* 56% and 25%). Seizures are particularly common in low-grade oligodendrogliomas. Features include:

- Headache (50%).
- Focal neurologic deficit (40%).

Investigations

LGG usually appears as an area of intra-axial low attenuation on CT and increased T2 signal on MRI with associated mass effect (**497**, **498**). Calcification may be present in some, particularly in low-grade oligodendrogliomas (**499**). Contrast enhancement may be present, but is usually absent in LGG. Cystic change is often present and may be confused radiographically with necrosis.

Diagnosis

As with high-grade glioma, biopsy or surgical resection is required to make a diagnosis of LGG.

Gross total resection obtains more tissue for accurate diagnosis.

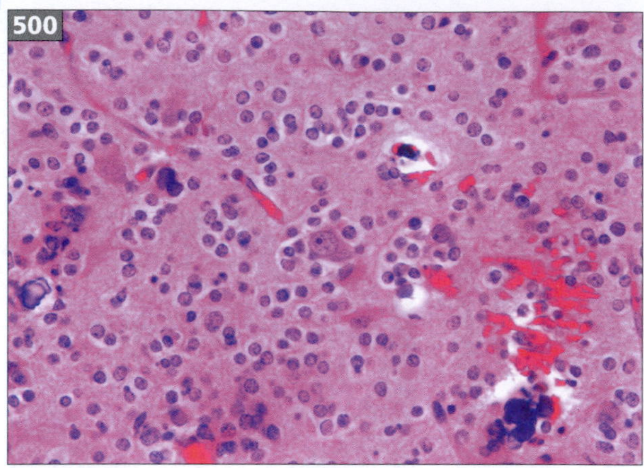

500 Low-grade oligodendroglioma: demonstrating 'fried egg' appearance of nuclei with surrounding halo.

Pathology

LGG lacks frank necrosis although some may contain cystic change. Often the gross appearance may very closely mimic adjacent normal brain tissue. Hemorrhage is rare in LGG. Calcification is more common in low-grade oligodendrogliomas and OA than in low-grade astrocytomas.

LGGs are typically infiltrative and may have a microscopic appearance of hypercellular glial tissue. LGG is distinguished from gliosis by cellular atypia. Low-grade astrocytoma is usually made up of atypical-appearing fibrillary, gemistocytic, or protoplasmic astrocytes.

Low-grade oligodendroglioma contains atypical oligodendroglial cells which have a small, round appearance, often with a halo of surrounding cytoplasm ('fried egg' appearance), as an artifact of fixation (500). Mixed LGG contains a mixture of astrocytic and oligodendroglial cells.

A high proportion (60–80%) of low-grade oligodendrogliomas and low-grade OA have deletions in the short arm of chromosome 1 (1p) and the long arm of chromosome 19 (19q), a feature that predicts a better response to therapy and an overall better prognosis.

Treatment

Aggressive resection is an important first step in therapy for LGG, if it is deemed to be feasible and of acceptable risk. Gross total resection appears to improve survival in patients with LGG. However, in some patients, only a biopsy is possible (i.e. brainstem and thalamic LGG).

In patients whose LGG is asymptomatic at the time of presentation, close observation with surveillance MRI to detect progression is a reasonable alternative to immediate surgery.

Radiation therapy for LGG should be considered in patients who have a biopsy or subtotal resection. Upfront radiation therapy for LGG has been shown to extend the time to radiographic progression (progression-free survival) but does not prolong overall survival when compared to patients receiving radiation only at the time of tumor progression. The radiation port is limited to the area of abnormal T2 signal with a small margin (2 cm) inclusive of the surrounding normal appearing tissue. Slightly lower doses of radiation are typically used in the treatment of LGG as compared to high-grade glioma – 50–55 Gy are typically used for LGG.

The role of chemotherapy in the treatment of LGG is poorly defined and the use of chemotherapy is not considered standard at present in the treatment of LGG.

Prognosis

Even with treatment, most LGG will recur and usually evolve into high-grade glioma at some point in their clinical course. Median survival for low-grade astrocytoma is 8 years and is 10 years for low-grade OA. Median survival for low-grade oligodendroglioma is 12 years.

EPENDYMOMAS

Definition and epidemiology

A glial tumor derived from ependymal cells, usually arising from the ventricular surface or spinal cord. Ependymomas are relatively uncommon, accounting for approximately 1.9% of all primary CNS tumors (6% of gliomas) in adults, 5.9% of all primary CNS tumors (9% of gliomas) in children, and 25% of primary spinal tumors.

Intracranial ependymomas are more common in children (usually infratentorial), while spinal cord ependymomas are more common in adults. Males and females are equally affected.

There is an increased incidence of spinal cord ependymoma in patients with neurofibromatosis type 2 (NF-2).

Clinical features

The clinical presentation depends upon the location of the tumor. Posterior fossa tumors typically present with cerebellar ataxia and signs and symptoms of elevated ICP (headache, vomiting, altered consciousness). Elevated ICP is due to direct mass effect of the tumor or obstructive hydrocephalus.

Spinal cord tumors present with spine and limb pain, upper motor neuron distribution weakness in the limbs, sensory loss, and bowel/bladder/sexual dysfunction.

Myxopapillary ependymomas typically present with a cauda equina syndrome of lower motor neuron weakness in the legs, saddle anesthesia, and bowel/bladder/sexual dysfunction. All grades of ependymoma may be associated with leptomeningeal spread of tumor resulting in radiculopathies, cranial neuropathies, and communicating hydrocephalus.

Differential diagnosis

- Other tumors of the posterior fossa: metastases, hemangioblastoma, choroid plexus papilloma/carcinoma, meningioma, vestibular schwannomas.
- Other tumors of the spinal cord/cauda equina: astrocytoma, hemangioblastoma, schwannoma, metastases, meningioma, paraganglioma.
- Inflammatory disorders: neurosarcoidosis, demyelinating disease (cord and brain lesions), abscess.
- Other leptomeningeal disorders: leptomeningeal carcinoma/lymphoma/leukemia, leptomeningeal gliomatosis, neurosarcoidosis.

Investigations

MRI of the brain and total spine with contrast is the most useful diagnostic study. Patients with intracranial ependymomas should have complete spinal imaging due to the frequent presence of asymptomatic 'drop' metastases. Ependymomas are typically well-demarcated and hyperintense on T2 and fluid attenuated inversion recovery (FLAIR) imaging. Most tumors enhance with gadolinium. Leptomeningeal enhancement may be present if there has been seeding of tumor in the CSF.

CSF examination may be performed unless the patient has a significant intracranial mass lesion. CSF cytology is usually negative in ependymoma, even with leptomeningeal spread. The primary value of CSF examination is to rule out other disorders including leptomeningeal carcinoma, infection, and neurosarcoidosis.

Diagnosis

Ependymomas are usually slow-growing indolent tumors arising from the ventricular system or spinal cord. On gross pathology, calcification and hemorrhage are common. In the spinal cord, most ependymomas are associated with a syrinx.

Pathology

The WHO has designated three pathologic divisions based on histologic appearance:

- WHO grade I:
  - Myxopapillary ependymoma, a benign tumor occurring in the filum terminale. Although benign, myxopapillary ependymoma may seed the CSF.
  - Subependymoma, a very benign relative of ependymoma, usually located in the 4th ventricle or spinal cord, which is often asymptomatic. Subependymomas do not spread to the leptomeninges.
- WHO grade II: cellular, papillary, and clear cell variants. These tumors typically arise from the ventricular surface (4th ventricle is most common) or spinal cord parenchyma.
- WHO grade III: anaplastic ependymoma, a more malignant behaving tumor with a tendency for leptomeningeal spread and even extra-CNS metastases.

Treatment

Although there are no randomized trials evaluating the extent of resection in ependymoma, an attempt at gross total resection (if feasible) is preferred both for intracranial and intraspinal tumors.

For WHO grade I and II tumors, radiation is usually withheld if a gross total resection has taken place and there is no evidence of leptomeningeal spread. In these patients, surveillance with serial MRIs is recommended and radiation administered at the time of recurrence. Patients with incompletely resected WHO grade II tumors and all patients with WHO grade III tumors are radiated after surgery[5]. The radiation fields are limited to the tumor bed and a small margin of adjacent normal brain or spinal cord. Patients with leptomeningeal tumor typically receive radiation to radiographically involved regions. Complete craniospinal radiation is usually avoided secondary to toxicity. Stereotactic radiation is frequently employed for post-operative residual tumor or for small recurrent tumors, although the role for this form of radiation has never been formally defined.

There is no established role for the use of chemotherapy in adults with WHO grade I and II ependymomas. In pediatric patients with WHO grade III ependymomas, chemotherapy may have a role in delaying post-operative radiation therapy. Chemotherapy (cisplatin, VP-16, temozolomide, and bevacizumab among other agents) is often used at the time of recurrence in anaplastic ependymoma after radiation therapy. Individual results are variable and there are no available randomized trial data showing efficacy.

Prognosis

Prognosis depends primarily on tumor grade, extent of resection, and patient performance status[6].

For patients with WHO grade I and II tumors who have undergone gross total resection with good post-operative performance status, median survival is usually many years and even decades. Patients with WHO grade III ependymomas have a much higher rate of recurrence, and usually have median survivals of <5 years.

MENINGIOMA

Definition and epidemiology

A tumor of mesenchymal origin derived from the arachnoid cap cells of the meninges; 90% are benign (WHO grade I).

According to the Central Brain Tumor Registry of the United States (CBTRUS) 2009, meningioma accounts for 32.1% of reported primary CNS tumors, with an incidence of 5.5/100,000. The incidence of meningioma is undoubtedly underestimated as many meningiomas are small, asymptomatic, and are unreported. Age at diagnosis is 40–70 years. Females are at greater risk than males (2–3:1).

Tip

▶ *Meningiomas are one of the most common primary tumors of adulthood. They are most common in middle-aged women and are typically benign. Most meningiomas are sporadic; a minority are associated with NF-2 and exposure to ionizing radiation. If the meningioma is small (2 cm or less), calcified, and asymptomatic, it can usually be observed*[7].

Etiology

Meningiomas express receptors for progesterone, estrogen, and androgens as well as peptide growth factors (IGF, PDGF, VEGF, and EGF)[8]. Patients with NF-2 are at increased risk of developing meningioma. Specific chromosomal mutations have not been linked to sporadic meningiomas, although mutations in the *NF-2* gene on chromosome 22q or the *DAL-1* gene on chromosome 18p are identified in approximately 50% of sporadic meningiomas.

Ionizing radiation to the head increases the risk of developing meningioma, usually with a delay of at least 10 years. Higher doses of radiation increase the risk and shorten the latency of developing meningioma. There is no convincing evidence that head trauma or cell phone use cause meningioma.

Clinical features

Many meningiomas are discovered when small and asymptomatic when a CT or MRI is performed for an unrelated reason (e.g. trauma, migraine, stroke). For symptomatic meningioma, the symptoms will depend on the location and size of the lesion. Most symptoms are of slow and insidious onset; because of slow growth, symptomatic meningiomas are often very large at the time of diagnosis.

- Tuberculum sella/olfactory groove:
  - Anosmia, monocular visual loss, headache (ipsilateral optic atrophy with contralateral papilledema: Foster Kennedy syndrome).
  - If large, abulia, inattentiveness, impaired executive function, and gait apraxia from bilateral frontal lobe involvement.
- Cavernous sinus meningioma:
  - Diplopia (VIth nerve palsy is most common).
  - Trigeminal neuralgia.
  - Occasional hypopituitarism.
  - Exophthalmos if there is invasion of the orbit.
  - Complex partial seizures if extension to the mesial temporal lobe).
- Falcine meningioma:
  - Lower extremity spastic paresis or paraparesis.
  - Focal motor or sensory seizures.
  - Headache from tumor mass or occlusion of the superior sagittal sinus.
- Petrous ridge:
  - Ipsilateral hearing loss.
  - Facial nerve palsy.
  - Trigeminal neuropathy.
  - Cerebellar ataxia.
  - Contralateral hemiparesis if the basis pontis is affected.
- Foramen magnum:
  - Upper cervical/occipital pain and stiffness.
  - Spastic quadriparesis.
  - Ascending sensory loss.
  - Bowel/bladder/sexual dysfunction.
  - Dysarthria/dysphagia.
- Thoracic spine:
  - Spastic paraparesis.
  - Ascending sensory loss.
  - Bowel/bladder/sexual dysfunction.
  - Spine pain with thoracic radicular pain.

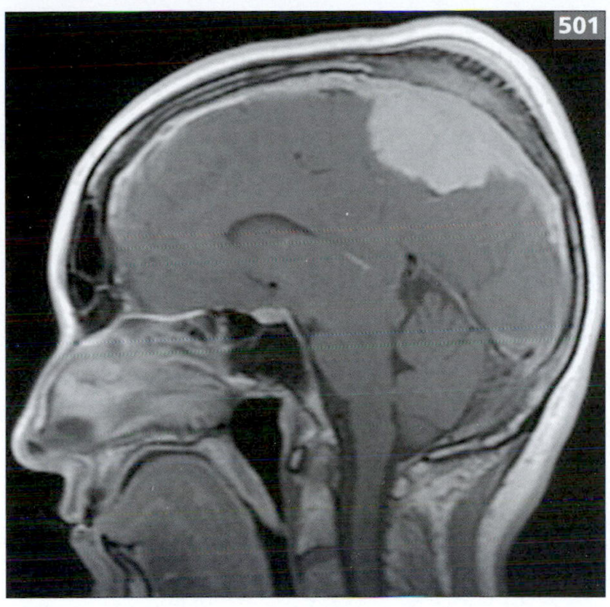

501 CT hyperostosis of the adjacent skull in meningioma.

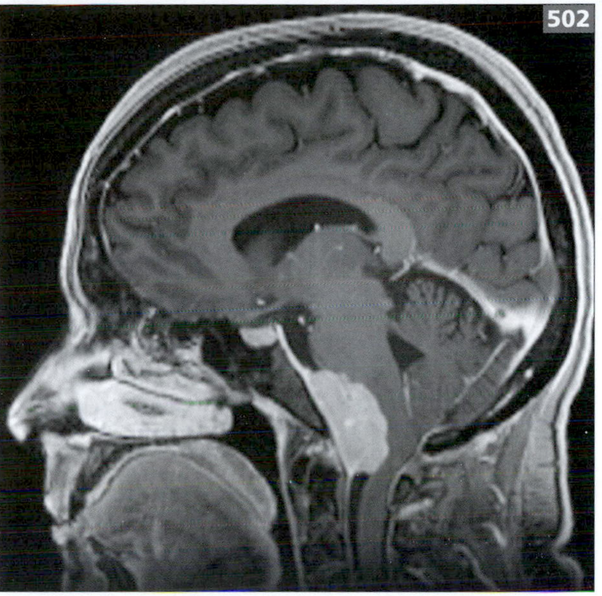

502 MRI of meningioma, showing enhancement and dural tail with gadolinium contrast.

Differential diagnosis

Differential diagnosis depends on the tumor location.

- Parasellar meningioma:
  - Chordoma.
  - Pituitary adenoma.
  - Lymphoma.
  - Retro-orbital pseudotumor.
  - Hemangioma.
  - Trigeminal schwannoma.
  - Metastasis.
  - Cavernous carotid aneurysm.
  - Granulomatous disease:
    - Sarcoidosis.
    - Wegener's granulomatosis.
- Sphenoid ridge:
  - Fibrous dysplasia.
  - Skull or dural metastasis.
  - Optic nerve glioma.
  - Skull sarcoma.
- Petrous ridge (cerebellopontine angle):
  - Vestibular/trigeminal schwannoma.
  - Epidermoid tumor.
  - Metastasis.
  - Hemangioblastoma.
- Cerebral convexity:
  - Dural metastasis from carcinoma.
  - Lymphoma.
  - Solitary fibrous tumor.

Investigations

CT brain

Meningiomas almost always arise from dura (rarely intraventricular). A 'dural tail' of enhancement extending from the tumor margin is typical. Other features on CT include:

- They are extra-axial and displace, but usually do not invade, brain tissue.
- Meningiomas are usually well-circumscribed and lobular.
- The lesions often exhibit calcification (sometimes dense calcification).
- Significant hyperostosis of the adjacent skull is common (**501**).
- Obstruction or narrowing of an adjacent venous sinus may be seen.
- Vasogenic edema of the adjacent brain is variably present and is more common in atypical and anaplastic meningiomas.

MRI brain

MRI is generally superior to CT in imaging meningiomas although CT is better at demonstrating calcification. Meningiomas are frequently (but not always) iso-intense with gray matter on both T1- and T2-weighted imaging. Meningiomas enhance homogeneously with gadolinium contrast and demonstrate dural attachment with the 'dural tail' (**502**). MRI offers the advantage of MR angiography and venography to document the presence of vascular compromise by tumor.

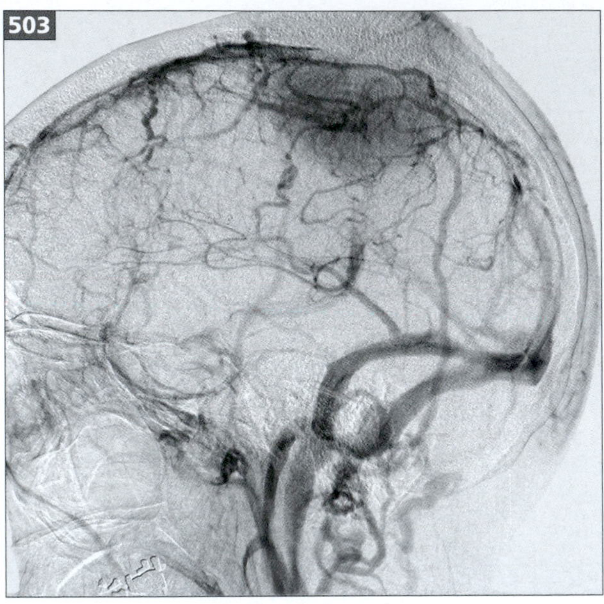

503 Cerebral angiography/venography of meningioma, demonstrating obstruction of the superior sagittal sinus.

Cerebral angiography

Angiography is not essential for diagnosis but may be useful pre-operatively to delineate tumor blood supply or determine if venous sinuses are patent (**503**). Most meningiomas receive their blood supply from branches of the external carotid artery. Occasionally, patients with large meningiomas benefit from pre-operative tumor embolization to reduce tumor vascularity and improve tumor resectability.

Diagnosis

Although the imaging characteristics are highly suggestive of meningioma, surgery is required to make a histologic diagnosis.

Pathology

Meningiomas arise from the arachnoid cap cells and almost always have a dural attachment. A small percentage arise from arachnoidal cells in the choroid plexus and have an intraventricular location. Macroscopically meningiomas are firm, gray, and sharply circumscribed; usually they are clearly demarcated from brain or spinal cord parenchyma. 5–10% have hyperostosis and may invade the adjacent bone (**504**).

Common sites of origin include:

- Skull base:
  - Tuberculum sella/olfactory groove.
  - Sphenoid wing or ridge: may grow into the orbit/optic nerve; cavernous sinus.
  - Petrous ridge: often grows into cerebellopontine angle.
  - Foramen magnum.
- Cerebral convexity.
- Falx cerebri.
- Tentorium cerebelli.
- Spine (usually thoracic and located anterior to the cord).

Microscopically, meningiomas usually comprise uniform sheets of meningothelial cells, often with a whorling pattern. Psammoma bodies may be present (**505**). Most (90%) are benign (WHO grade I) with only mild atypia and rare mitoses; 8% are atypical (WHO grade II) and 2% are malignant/anaplastic (WHO grade III) with marked atypia and many mitoses.

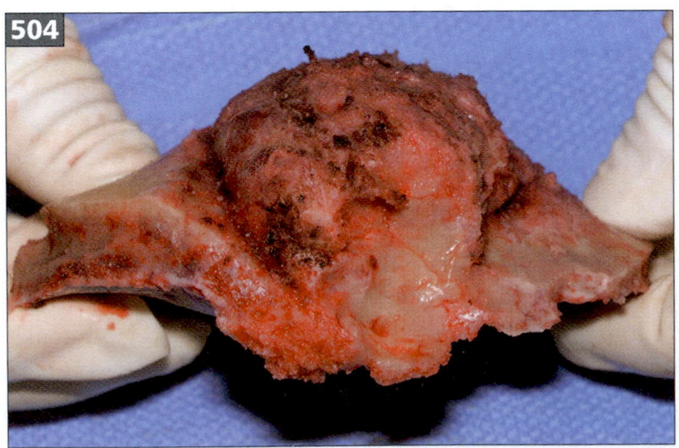

504 Hyperostosis in meningioma.

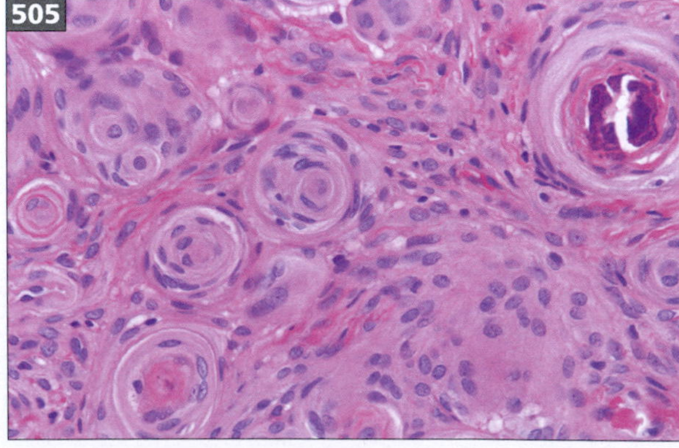

505 Hematoxylin and eosin (H&E) stain, demonstrating Psammoma bodies.

Treatment

Most small asymptomatic meningiomas can be observed with serial imaging (MRI of CT) at 3–6 month intervals. Densely calcified meningiomas are particularly prone to exhibit little or no growth. Women should be advised against the use of female hormones (particularly progestins) given the concern that tumors may grow with exposure to these hormones. Surgery, radiation therapy, and chemotherapy are all used in the treatment of meningiomas.

- Surgery:
  - Gross total resection is the optimal therapy of meningioma if the tumor is symptomatic or radiographically enlarging and if gross total resection is deemed feasible[9].
  - Aggressive resection may not be possible if the tumor is intimately associated with critical neural or vascular structures (i.e. cranial nerves, brainstem, cerebral arteries or veins). In that instance a partial resection may be warranted, with radiation therapy to follow for treatment of the residual tumor.
- Radiation therapy:
  - EBRT or stereotactic radiosurgery can be either the primary treatment of unresectable meningiomas (i.e. those of the cavernous sinus) or as an adjunct to surgery, particularly if an incomplete resection has taken place[10].
  - Radiation therapy may be indicated even after gross total resection of atypical or anaplastic meningiomas, as it reduces risk of recurrence or prolongs the time to tumor recurrence.
- Chemotherapy agents:
  - Chemotherapy is generally ineffective in the treatment of meningioma.
  - Mifepristone (RU-486) a progesterone antagonist, failed to show benefit when subjected to a randomized controlled trial.
  - Hydroxyurea, an alkylating agent, suppresses meningioma cell growth *in vitro* but does not appear to confer significant benefit in patients.
  - Somatostatin receptors are present on most meningioma cells and somatostatin inhibits meningioma growth *in vitro*. Modest anecdotal data of meningioma stability after administration of somatostatin are published in the literature

Alpha-interferon inhibits meningioma growth *in vitro* but has failed to demonstrate clinical benefit in patients with meningioma.

Prognosis

Most meningiomas are benign and exhibit a very slow rate of growth. Small, asymptomatic meningiomas may be observed. The risk of recurrence after gross total resection of a WHO grade I meningioma is approximately 20% at 10 years. The recurrence rate is significantly higher in atypical (WHO grade II) and anaplastic (WHO grade III) meningioma, in which 40% and 60% recur at 10 years even after gross total resection.

Few patients die from WHO grade I and II meningiomas. Most meningioma-related deaths are seen in patients with WHO grade III lesions and in those patients with lower-grade lesions which are large and deemed unresectable.

Age is an important independent prognostic factor for survival.

CRANIOPHARYNGIOMA

Definition and epidemiology

A rare tumor of the sellar region which is usually partially cystic and derives from embryonic remnants of Rathke's cleft. Craniopharyngiomas arise in the region of the sella turcica, suprasellar cistern, or third ventricle. These tumors are presumed to be congenital but gradually enlarge with time, producing symptoms by compression of the optic chiasm and/or pituitary stalk.

Craniopharyngioma represents less than 1% of all new brain tumors diagnosed each year, but 3.6% of brain tumors diagnosed in children aged 0–14 years. Craniopharyngiomas are the third most common primary brain tumor of childhood, behind gliomas and medulloblastomas. They are most common in children in the first decade of life. A second peak occurs between the ages of 55 and 65 years. Males and females are equally affected.

Clinical features

Craniopharyngiomas usually present with one of several syndromes:

- Hypothalamic–pituitary axis dysfunction[11]:
  - Growth failure in children.
  - Amenorrhea.
  - Sexual dysfunction (most common symptom in adults).
  - Adiposity or weight loss.
  - Diabetes insipidus.
  - Galactorrhea from compression of the pituitary stalk and increased prolactin secretion.
  - Impaired temperature regulation or drowsiness from hypothalamic dysfunction.
- Optic nerve or chiasm compression (40–70%):
  - Bitemporal hemianopia; usually inferior quadrants are affected first because of compression of the superior aspect of the chiasm first.
- Symptoms of elevated ICP (tumor mass effect or obstructive hydrocephalus):
  - Headache.
  - Vomiting.
  - Drowsiness.
  - Abulia and personality change (from hydrocephalus or extension of tumor into the frontal lobes).

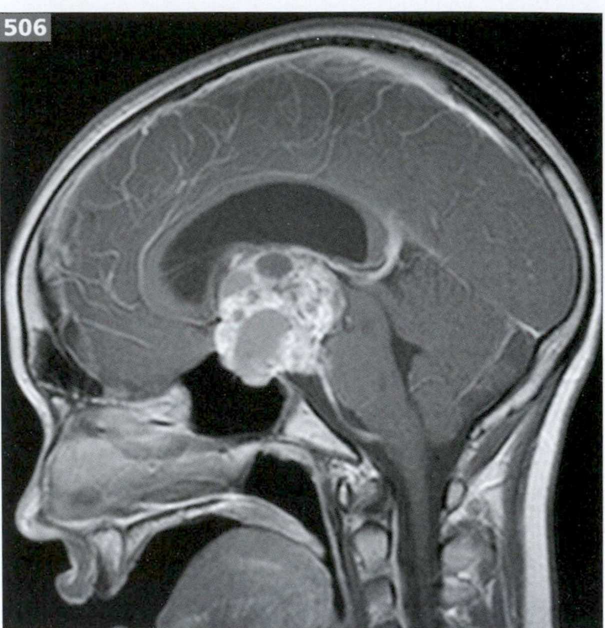

506 Craniopharyngioma: a partially cystic, enhancing mass in the suprasellar cistern on MRI.

Investigations

MRI of the head with contrast is the imaging modality of choice although CT head and even plain X-rays of the skull may be useful to ascertain the presence of calcification (80–90%). T1 noncontrast MRI images occasionally demonstrate increased signal in the tumor cyst secondary to the cholesterol (lipid) content. A partially cystic, enhancing mass is noted, usually in the suprasellar cistern, sometimes extending into the 3rd ventricle (**506**). Compression of the optic chiasm and pituitary stalk is common.

Differential diagnosis

- Rathke's cleft cyst.
- Optic chiasm tumor:
  - Glioma (particularly pilocytic astrocytoma).
  - Germ cell tumor.
- Pituitary adenoma.
- Colloid cyst.
- Parasellar chordoma.
- Langerhan's cell histiocytosis.
- Sarcoidosis.
- Carotid aneurysm.

Diagnosis

Most tumors occur in the suprasellar region, less frequently in the 3rd ventricle or within the sella. The tumor may be infiltrative into the 3rd ventricle (hypothalamus), optic chiasm, or infundibulum.

Pathology

Most craniopharyngiomas consist of a solitary or multiple cysts with well circumscribed solid component. The cyst fluid is typically discolored in appearance and contains cholesterol crystals, hence the description, 'crank case oil'.

Histologically, there are two subtypes of craniopharyngioma:

- Adamantinomatous type: more common in children; typically associated with calcification.
- Papillary type: more commonly seen in adults, and less likely to calcify.

Malignant transformation is very rare. When it occurs it is typically a squamous cell malignancy.

Treatment

Surgery, radiation therapy, and a combination of the two treatments are the options for treating craniopharyngioma. Surgical resection is the best treatment for tumor control if it can be accomplished[12]. Surgical risk includes injury to the hypothalamus, pituitary stalk and gland, and optic chiasm. Radiation therapy is typically used only if residual tumor is present or with recurrence.

An attempt at gross total resection carries greater surgical risk but offers the best chance for long-term tumor control. Radiation therapy is reserved for patients with incomplete resection or those who develop recurrence after surgical resection. Radiation therapy includes conformal EBRT and stereotactic radiosurgery.

Cyst aspiration, with or without instillation of radioactive isotopes, may alleviate symptoms of inoperable cystic tumors. There are no randomized, controlled trial data to establish the efficacy of this treatment.

Prognosis

The most important prognostic factor in patients with craniopharyngioma is the extent of surgical resection accomplished at the initial surgery. There is no evidence that pathologic subtype (adamantinomatous *vs.* papillary) is important in determining prognosis.

Recurrence-free survival is 87% at 5 years after gross total resection of craniopharyngioma and 50% for patients undergoing partial resection.

PITUITARY TUMORS

Definition and epidemiology

Pituitary tumors, primarily benign adenomas, account for 10–15% of primary brain tumors. They are the third most common tumor after meningiomas and gliomas. Etiology is unknown.

Pituitary adenomas have an annual incidence of 0.5–8.2/100,000 persons. Prevalence is higher, however, because autopsy studies suggest 20–25% of the population have silent or unrecognized adenomas. Pituitary tumors occur mostly in adults, with a mean age of 60 years, and more often in males than females.

Clinical features

Depending on tumor type and growth characteristics, patients may present with a variety of endocrinologic and neurologic symptoms and signs.

Hypersecretion of one or more hormones

Hyperprolactinemia

- Women:
  - Infertility.
  - Amenorrhea.
  - Galactorrhea.
  - Reduced libido.
  - Delayed menarche.
- Men:
  - Reduced libido.
  - Impotence.
  - Galactorrhea – unusual.
  - Apathy.
  - Weight gain.

Growth hormone excess

- Gigantism in children.
- Acromegaly in adults.

Adrenocorticotropic hormone (ACTH) excess

- Rare.
- Cushing's disease.

Hyposecretion of pituitary hormones

- Women:
  - Hypogonadism.
  - Amenorrhea.
  - Reduced libido.
  - Dyspareunia.
- Men:
  - Reduced libido and impotence.
  - Reduced facial/body hair.
  - Gonadal atrophy.

- Hypoprolactinemia:
  - Failure to start/maintain lactation.
  - Hypothyroidism with low thyroid stimulating hormone (TSH).
  - Growth hormone deficiency.
  - Poorly defined in adults.
  - Hypoadrenalism.
  - Fatigue.
  - Postural hypotension.

Local pressure

- On optic nerve/chiasm:
  - Visual field defects in one or both eyes (classic bitemporal hemianopia, beginning in the superior quadrants).
  - Scotomas.
  - Blindness.
- On cavernous sinus: cranial nerve palsies III, IV, V, VI.
- On temporal lobes: complex partial seizures.
- On third ventricle: obstructive hydrocephalus.
- Others:
  - Headaches.
  - Asymptomatic: image abnormality only.

Differential diagnosis

- Craniopharyngioma, optic glioma, supraclinoid carotid artery aneurysm.
- Arachnoid cysts.
- Meningioma, metastasis, dermoid, teratoma.
- Cavernous carotid aneurysm, cavernous sinus thrombosis.
- Chordoma, basilar artery aneurysm.
- Sphenoid sinus mucocele, carcinoma, granuloma.
- Empty sella syndrome.

Investigations

- Pituitary hormones determination.
- CT and MRI brain scan:
  - CT best for calcified lesion, i.e. craniopharyngioma.
  - MRI is the most sensitive modality for detecting microadenomas (<10 mm in diameter).
  - Microadenomas appear as low signal with gadolinium; hypointense on MRI.
  - Macroadenomas (>10 mm) arise out of pituitary fossa, and may distort the chiasm and anterior cerebral arteries as well as extend into the cavernous sinus (507).
  - Carotid angiography may be indicated to exclude an aneurysm.

Diagnosis

Diagnosis is from a typical history and neurologic abnormalities, confirmed by CT or MRI and blood tests.

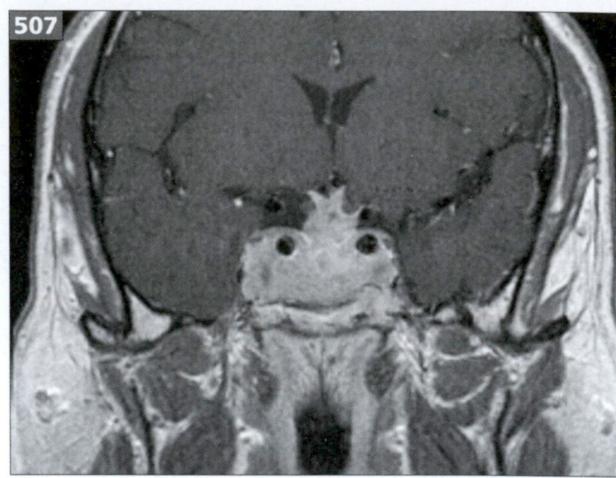

507 Pituitary macroadenoma.

Pathology

- Classified by size, hormonal production, clinical presentation, histologic features, immunohistochemical profile, and ultrastructural features[13].
- Adenomas are usually benign and slow-growing.
- Three-quarters secrete inappropriate amounts of pituitary hormones, one-quarter are ‘nonfunctioning’.
- The most common functioning tumor is prolactin-secreting, followed by adenomas that secrete growth hormone, ACTH, and rarely gonadotropin and TSH.
- Nonsecreting adenomas, 20–25% of all tumors, are usually chromophobe adenomas.

Treatment

- If panhypopituitarism, glucocorticoids should be replaced before thyroid hormone.
- Prolactinomas are treated with dopamine agonists (bromocriptine or cabergoline) which shrink tumors and reduce prolactin secretion.
- Surgical resection is indicated for nonprolactinoma hypersecreting tumors; post-operative endocrine and neurologic evaluation is required.
- Growth hormone secreting tumors can be treated with the somatostatin analog octreotide.
- Radiation therapy may reduce tumor recurrence but has known delayed side-effects (radionecrosis, vaso-occlusive disease, secondary tumors).

Prognosis

Prognosis is excellent with treatment. Metastases are rare. MRI is useful for post-operative surveillance and early detection of recurrences.

VESTIBULAR SCHWANNOMA (ACOUSTIC NEUROMA)

Definition and epidemiology

A Schwann cell-derived benign tumor that most commonly affects the vestibular component of the VIIIth cranial nerve. Vestibular schwannomas account for approximately 8% of all intracranial primary brain tumors and 80% of tumors of the cerebellopontine angle[14].

Neurofibromatosis type 2 (NF-2) is associated with bilateral vestibular schwannomas. Patients with NF-2 and vestibular schwannomas have a median age of diagnosis of 32 years. In patients with sporadic vestibular schwannoma, the median age of onset is 50 years. Incidence is 1/100,000 per year; males and females are equally affected.

Etiology

Most cases are sporadic and have no known underlying cause. In patients with NF-2, an autosomal-dominant syndrome caused by mutations on chromosome 22q (see p. 234), there is a 90% incidence of bilateral vestibular schwannomas. These patients may also have spinal schwannomas and intracranial and spinal meningiomas, ependymomas, and astrocytomas.

There is no definitive evidence that cell phone use increases the risk of developing vestibular schwannomas although this remains a subject of controversy.

Clinical features

Unilateral hearing loss (95%) with or without tinnitus (60%) is the most common initial symptom of vestibular schwannoma. Vertigo is a rare symptom, due to the fact that the tumor is very slow growing and allows compensation of the vestibular system. Unsteadiness of gait without vertigo is a much more common symptom than vertigo.

Trigeminal neuropathy with or without trigeminal distribution pain may be present in larger tumors that extend into the cerebellopontine angle. Facial weakness is present in only 6% of patients. Only very large tumors produce corticospinal distribution weakness (from pontine compression), cerebellar deficits, or symptoms of obstructive hydrocephalus.

Differential diagnosis

- Other tumors/masses of the cerebellopontine angle:
  - Meningioma.
  - Trigeminal schwannoma.
  - Cholesteatoma.
  - Epidermoid cyst.
  - Glomus tumor.
  - Chordoma.
  - Choroid plexus papilloma.

Investigations and diagnosis

Contrast MRI of the brain, particularly with FIESTA (fast imaging employing steady state acquisition sequences), is the definitive study for imaging vestibular schwannomas (508).

In patients who cannot undergo MRI, CT of the brain is a viable alternative. Vestibular schwannomas typically arise from and enlarge the internal acoustic meatus. Larger lesions may fill the cerebellopontine angle.

The vast majority (95%) of patients will have evidence of sensorineural hearing loss on audiometry.

Pathology

Vestibular schwannoma arises from the perineural elements of the vestibular nerve. Only very rarely do they derive from the auditory component of the VIIIth nerve. Grossly this tumor typically grows out of the internal acoustic meatus, enlarging the bony canal.

The tumor may extend into the cerebellopontine angle compressing the VIIth and VIIIth nerves, and ultimately the pons and cerebellum. Very large lesions may compress the 4th ventricle and produce obstructive hydrocephalus.

Pathologically, vestibular schwannoma consists of zones of alternately dense and sparse areas of cellularity (Ansoni A and B areas respectively). Malignant degeneration is exceedingly rare.

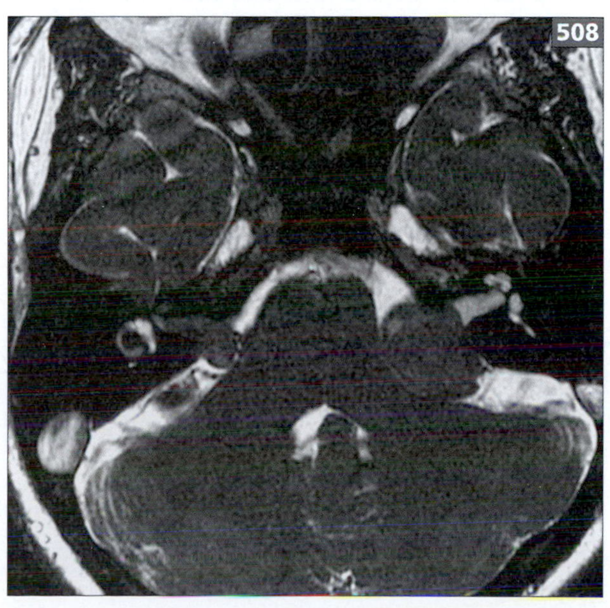

508 MRI (FIESTA view) of a left vestibular schwannoma.

Treatment

The natural history of vestibular schwannoma is to enlarge very slowly and become increasingly symptomatic. Forty percent of tumors may show no evidence of growth or even shrink on serial imaging. Small asymptomatic vestibular schwannomas may be observed with serial MRI, but vestibular schwannomas which are large, symptomatic, and/or are radiographically shown to grow should be treated.

Surgery is the primary modality for treatment of vestibular schwannoma and is usually curative if a gross total resection has taken place. Several operative approaches are possible and depend upon the size of the tumor and whether or not hearing preservation is a realistic goal. In the modern era of neurosurgery, preservation of facial nerve function is usually possible particularly for small tumors. Intra-operative electrophysiologic monitoring of facial and auditory nerve function is routine.

Surgical mortality is low (1–2%) in modern series. Other risks include CSF leak, facial nerve palsy, hearing loss, and brainstem injury (in larger tumors).

Stereotactic radiation and proton beam therapy is a reasonable alternative to conventional surgery in patients with smaller tumors[15]. The risk of increased hearing loss and facial nerve injury is lower than that associated with surgical resection. The overall tumor control rate at 10 years is 97% with radiation therapy.

Prognosis

The prognosis of vestibular schwannoma is usually excellent. Yearly surveillance MRIs are indicated for patients with small, incidentally discovered lesions, those who have undergone surgical resection, and those who have received radiation therapy.

PRIMARY CENTRAL NERVOUS SYSTEM LYMPHOMA

Definition and epidemiology

Primary central nervous system lymphoma (PCNSL) is non-Hodgkin lymphoma (NHL) arising *de novo* from the brain, spinal cord, or leptomeninges, and comprises 1–2% of cases of all NHL and 3% of all intracranial tumors.

PCNSL represents an aquired immunodeficiency syndrome (AIDS)-related malignancy but AIDS-related PCNSL is decreasing in frequency since highly active antiretroviral therapy (HAART) is available.

The incidence of non-human immunodeficiency virus (HIV)- related PCNSL is continuing to increase in immunocompetent and older patients, for unknown reasons[16]. The median age for PCNSL is 57 years (non-AIDS); males are affected more frequently than females (1.5:1).

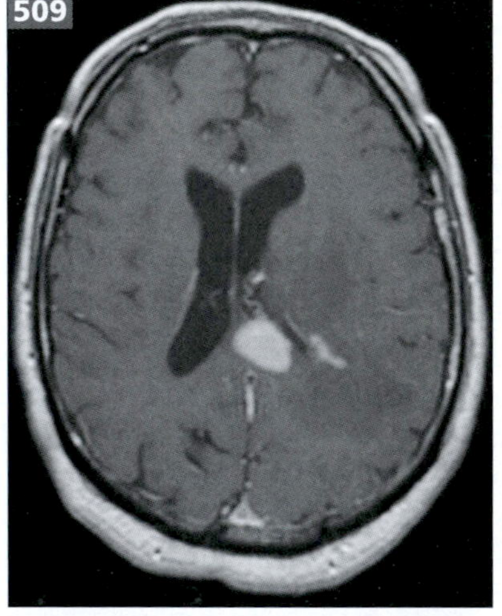

509 'Snowball' lesion on CT of a primary CNS lymphoma.

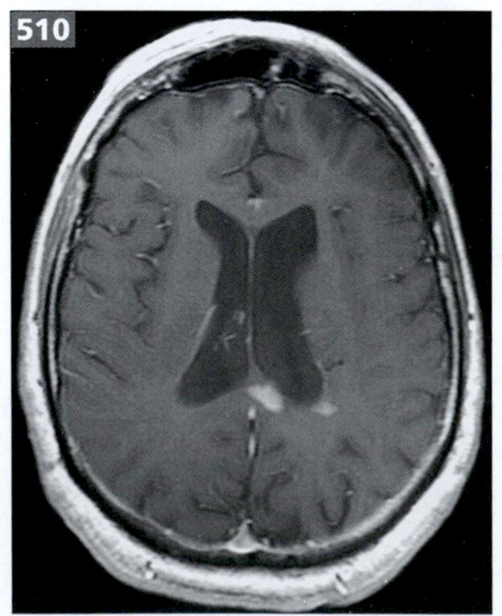

510 Primary CNS lymphoma, demonstrating improvement with corticosteroids.

Etiology and pathophysiology

Predisposing factors include:

- Immunosuppression, inherited or acquired.
- Congenital immunodeficiencies.
- Combined immunodeficiency syndrome.
- Immunodeficiency associated with systemic lupus erythematosus, rheumatoid arthritis, and organ transplant recipients.
- Long-term corticosteroid treatment.
- Immunosuppression related to HIV infection.
- HIV or other viruses (Epstein–Barr virus [EBV]), growth factors, aberrant oncogene or tumor-suppressor gene expression, and factors that promote genetic instability or DNA damage or alter host or viral genome repair may all promote cell hyperproliferation and clonal expansion.
- Hyperactivation of B cells is believed to contribute to lymphoma development associated with HIV infection.

Clinical features

- Subacute onset and progression with one or more intracranial masses.
- Specific symptoms and signs dependent on location, size, and number of lesions.
- Prompt and usually brief dramatic clinical and imaging response to corticosteroid therapy.
- Personality, behavioral, cognitive change occurs in 24%.
- Cerebellar signs in 21%.
- Headache in 15%.
- Motor dysfunction in 11%.
- Seizures in 13%.
- Visual problems: 'floaters' (usually from vitreous involvement) occur in 8%.
- Leptomeningeal involvement is often silent, but can present with multiple cranial and peripheral nerve root deficits.

Investigations

CT shows a homogeneously enhancing mass or masses in the corpus callosum or central gray matter, sometimes referred to as a 'snowball lesion' (**509**).

MRI is usually preferred to CT because of its greater resolution and its ability to show the meninges and posterior fossa. There is usually an isointense or hyperintense mass or masses on T1, T1–T2, and T2 scans with contrast enhancement. Both CT and MRI may show improvement with corticosteroid therapy (**509, 510**).

CSF is usually abnormal with elevated protein, lymphocytic pleocytosis, and malignant lymphocytes on cytologic examination.

Diagnosis

Diagnosis is preferably by CT-guided stereotactic biopsy, with no role for surgical resection. Immunohistochemical markers should be done to demonstrate the malignant infiltrate.

Tip

▶ *The diagnosis of PCNSL should be considered in elderly and immunocompromised patients with homogeneously enhancing masses in a periventricular distribution. These tumors are often steroid-sensitive and pretreatment with corticosteroids may render a subsequent biopsy nondiagnostic.*

Pathology

- Deep-seated bulky tumor without corresponding mass effect, often with contact with CSF surface along the ventricles.
- Poorly defined with infiltration into brain tissue.
- Immunocompromised patients (organ transplant recipients and AIDS patients) usually have multiple lesions with hemorrhage, neovascularity, and necrosis.
- Supratentorial in 75%, infratentorial in 20%, diffuse leptomeningeal in 5%.
- Involvement of posterior segment of eye (retina and vitreous) is present in 25%.
- Most common histologic subtype is diffuse large B-cell lymphoma in 80% of cases.
- Lower-grade B-cell and T-cell forms are rare compared to systemic lymphoma.
- Highly cellular, numerous mitotic figures; large centroblasts or immunoblasts expressing B-cell markers CD19, CD20, and CD79a; cells in a background matrix of reticulum and microglia (see **493**).
- Tumor cells in immunocompromised patients are always B-cell, polyclonal, high-grade, associated with necrosis and hemorrhage, and usually EBV driven.
- Lymphocytes express either kappa or lambda light chain immunoglobulin.
- Usual pattern, regardless of cell type, is a perivascular infiltration with malignant cells around blood vessels in concentric layers.

Treatment

Management depends on the immunologic status of the patient. Although treatable, results of multiple trials show that the results are very different than similar patients with large B-cell lymphomas at other extranodal sites[17].

In immunocompetent patients, chemotherapy with high-dose methotrexate, followed by whole brain radiation at relapse, is the usual current approach with response rates of 90% and median survivals of 30–60 months.

Immunosuppressed patients (transplant recipients or patients with AIDS), do very poorly and present major problems in management. Reversal of immunosuppression with HAART (in patients with HIV infection) or discontinuance of immunosuppressive medication is usually the best initial approach.

Prognosis

Although treatable, PCNSL is almost always a fatal disease. Approximately 10–15% do not respond to any treatment and responding patients almost always recur. With the aging population and the incidence of PCNSL increasing for unknown reason, effective treatment remains a future goal.

GERM CELL TUMORS OF THE CNS

Definition and epidemiology

Primary intracranial germ cell tumors arise in midline CNS locations, primarily in pineal and suprasellar regions, and are generally indistinguishable histologically from systemic sites[18]. They are rare in Western countries; 1% of adult and 3% of pediatric brain tumor diagnoses, and are much more frequent in Japan, especially in children (16% of pediatric brain tumors). Germ cell tumors are more common in males than in females

Clinical features

- Hypothalamic dysfunction – diabetes insipidus, sleep disturbance, precocious puberty.
- Midbrain compression – Parinaud's syndrome (supranuclear paresis of upward gaze, dilated pupils that accommodate but do not react to light), hydrocephalus secondary to obstruction of the posterior 3rd ventricle and aqueduct.
- Gait and limb ataxia.
- Spastic quadriparesis.

Investigations

Brain and spine MRI with gadolinium show an enhancing mass in pineal region, anterior 3rd ventricle, or optic chiasm, often with obstructive hydrocephalus (**511**). Tumor markers alpha fetoprotein (AFP) and a subunit of β-HCG are found in serum and in CSF. Pituitary function studies should be performed in patients with anterior 3rd ventricular involvement, and visual field testing.

Diagnosis

Following initial diagnostic evaluations, the presence of hydrocephalus is determined and a decision for surgical-biopsy or resection is appropriate. An endoscopic biopsy of the tumor can be accomplished at the time of the 3rd ventriculostomy.

Serum and/or CSF tumor markers are pivotal. If either β-HCG or alpha fetoprotein is positive, this confirms nongerminoma (NGGCT) and tissue may not be required for diagnosis. If negative, tissue is definitely required for diagnosis. This may include stereotactic biopsy, open craniotomy with biopsy, or endoscopic biopsy.

Pathology

Tumors arise from totipotential germ cells, capable of producing several different cell types; tumors can be composed of more than one tumor cell type. Tumors are classified by cell of origin into two basic types: undifferentiated germinoma (GCT) and nongerminoma (NGGCT).

Pineal and suprasellar location is most common. Multifocal germinoma or multiple lesions may be seen: pineal, hypophyseal, cavernous sinus, optic chiasm, third ventricle wall. Disseminated germinoma or metastatic disease can be present.

Generally there is rapid growth; clinical features depend on age at presentation and location of tumor. Tumors spread by direct infiltration or along CSF pathways, seeding cranial and peripheral nerve roots.

GCT are the most primitive, but are most readily curable by radiation therapy. NGGCT are composed of several histopathologic variants, are relatively more radioresistant, with generally a worse prognosis (malignant teratoma, embryonal carcinoma, yolk sac tumor, choriocarcinoma, or mixed tumors).

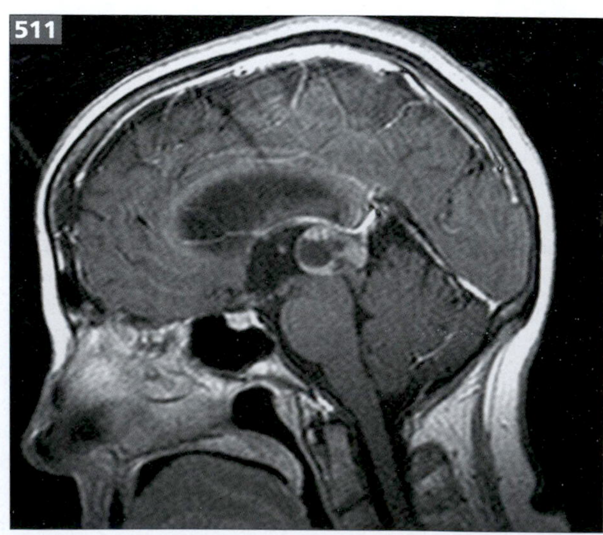

511 MRI with gadolinium shows an enhancing mass in the pineal region.

Treatment

If hydrocephalus is present, endoscopically guided third ventriculostomy, external ventricular drain, or ventriculoperitoneal shunt is appropriate.

Post-operatively, with tissue diagnosis confirmed, patients should have tumor staging with brain and spine MRI with gadolinium, and tumor markers. Accurate histologic diagnosis guides the extent of adjuvant therapy:

- For GCT, radiation therapy with possible dose reduction with chemotherapy.
- For NGGCT surgery, chemotherapy, and radiation therapy are appropriate.

Prognosis

Intracranial germinoma may be cured using craniospinal radiation with a local boost to the primary site. The main question currently is whether standard dosage and volumes known to cure can be reduced or eliminated by substituting chemotherapy.

Unfortunately, the outcome for intracranial NGGCT remains poor with radiation therapy alone. Chemotherapy has been added or used alone in an effort to improve survival. The optimal chemotherapy, radiation dose and volume, and the role and timing of surgery remain to be determined in a large cooperative group setting.

VON HIPPEL–LINDAU DISEASE

Definition and epidemiology

Von Hippel–Lindau disease (VHL) is an inherited, autosomal-dominant disorder associated with specific tumors in multiple organs including the retina, brain, spinal cord, pancreas, adrenal gland, kidney, epididymis, and endolymphatic sac.

Eugen von Hippel, a German ophthalmologist, originally described the retinal lesions. Later, Arvid Lindau, a Swedish pathologist, described the relationship between retinal and cerebellar hemangioblastomas and tumors of other viscera, and noted that the disorder was inherited. Harvey Cushing first named the disorder Lindau's disease and it was only later that von Hippel's earlier contribution was recognized with the renaming of the disease von Hippel–Lindau disease.

- Prevalence 1/36,000 newborns are born with the genetic abnormality.
- Gender: M=F.
- Age of onset of initial symptoms: 26 years:
  - Retinal lesions are usually the first sign of the disease.
  - Cerebellar and spinal hemangioblastomas and renal cell carcinoma are usually detected 5–10 years later.
  - It is unusual that signs of the disease are detected before puberty.

Tip

▶ *The VHL gene is located on the short arm of chromosome 3 and is a tumor-suppressor gene regulating the activity of HIF-1, VEGF, and PDGF. Patients with VHL develop hemangioblastomas, renal cell carcinomas, pheochromocytomas, pancreatic and endolymphatic sac cystadenomas.*

Etiology and pathophysiology

VHL has an autosomal-dominant inheritance – 20% of cases result from a spontaneous *de novo* mutation. The *VHL* gene is located on the short arm of chromosome 3 (3p25). The gene product, pVHL, functions as a tumor suppressor protein, which regulates the activity of hypoxia-inducible factor-1 (HIF-1) which in turn regulates the activity of VEGF, PDGF, and TGF[19].

Families with VHL disease have been divided into types I and II based on the likelihood of developing pheochromocytoma. Kindreds with type I disease typically do not develop pheochromocytoma, although they do develop the other tumors associated with VHL; kindreds with type II disease are at high risk of developing pheochromocytoma. Type IIA and type IIB families are at high and low risk of developing renal cell carcinoma, respectively.

VHL has a high penetrance (i.e. a high proportion of people possessing the gene will develop the disease; penetrance is in excess of 90% by age 60. There is variable expression, with the severity and expression of the disease varying even within the same kindred.

Patients with VHL inherit the germline mutation which inactivates one copy of the *VHL* gene in all cells. For *VHL*-associated tumors to develop, there must be loss of the second normal allele (the so-called '2 hit hypothesis').

Clinical features

Symptoms usually do not appear before late adolescence[20].

- Visual loss:
  - Due to enlargement of retinal hemangioblastoma.
  - Exudative retinopathy/macular edema.
  - Retinal detachment.
  - Vitreous hemorrhage.
  - Retinal lesions are often in the periphery of the retina but large draining veins may be seen at the disc.
- Cerebellar signs: gait and limb ataxia, dysarthria, nystagmus, vertigo.
- Signs and symptoms of elevated ICP:
  - From cystic mass in the cerebellum.
  - Obstructive hydrocephalus may be present from obstruction of the 4th ventricle.

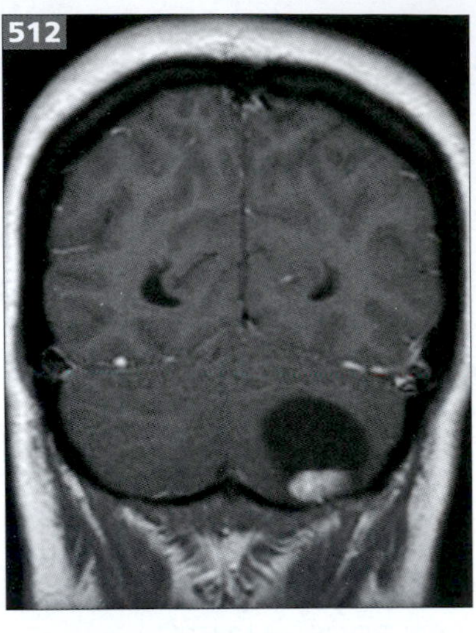

512 MRI showing cystic mass in the cerebellum with enhancing mural nodule.

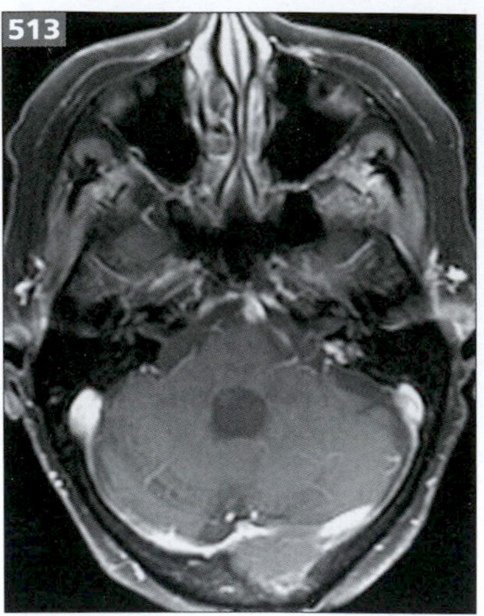

513 Endolymphatic sac adenoma in the petrous temporal bone on MRI.

- Spine pain and progressive myelopathy (spinal hemangioblastoma).
- Polycythemia due to secretion of erythropoietin by cerebellar hemangioblastomas and/or renal cell carcinomas.
- Symptoms of pheochromocytoma (from sudden release of catecholamines); these tumors are most commonly present in younger patients:
  - Sudden elevation of blood pressure.
  - Sweating.
  - Tachycardia.
  - Anxiety.
- Hearing loss with or without vertigo – endolymphatic sac cystadenoma.

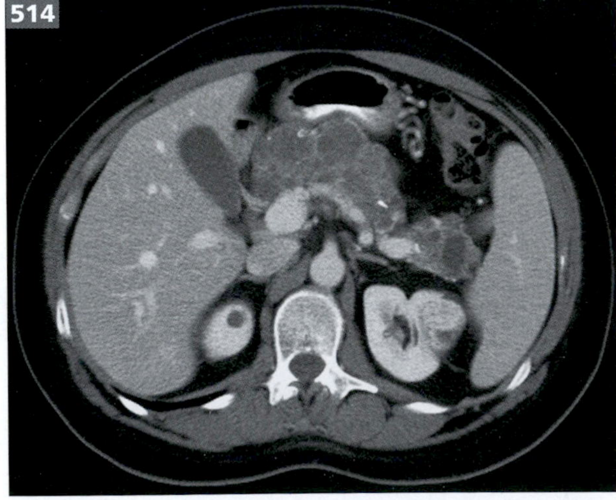

514 CT abdomen, demonstrating renal cell carcinoma and pheochromocytoma in a patient with von Hippel–Lindau syndrome.

Differential diagnosis

- Cerebellar tumors: pilocytic astrocytomas and metastases may have a very similar radiographic appearance to hemangioblastomas.
- Spinal/brainstem tumors: ependymoma and astrocytoma.

Investigations

- Complete blood count to determine the presence of polycythemia (present in 20% of patients).
- Ophthalmologic examination for retinal hemangioblastomas.
- MRI of the brain and total spine with contrast:
  - Classic appearance: cystic mass with enhancing mural nodule (**512**).
  - Tumor hemorrhage is rare.
  - Hydrocephalus may be present in larger cerebellar lesions.
  - Petrous temporal bone lesion(s): endolymphatic sac cystadenoma is present in 25% of patients (**513**).
- Audiogram (endolymphatic sac cystadenoma may produce hearing loss)[21].
- Screening tests for pheochromocytoma; serum fractionated metanephrines or 24-hour urine catecholamines.
- CT abdomen and pelvis: screening for renal cell carcinoma and pheochromocytoma (**514**).
- Genetic testing (performed on peripheral blood leukocytes, virtually 100% sensitive and specific):
  - DNA analysis identifies a mutation on chromosome 3p25, inherited in most but in 20% of patients the mutation arises *de novo*.
  - Deletions, nonsense, frameshift, and missense mutations may be responsible.

- Potentially affected family members of patients with a known VHL mutation should undergo genetic testing for the disease to determine if they require regular surveillance testing for hemangioblastomas, renal cell carcinoma, and pheochromocytoma.
- Skilled counseling based on full knowledge of the disease, its natural history, and the impact of the diagnosis on the individual and other family members is essential.
- Somatic mosaicism (a mutation occurring in tissues during embryonic development, after fertilization) rarely occurs in VHL; in these patients the mutation may not be detectable in the peripheral blood leukocytes.

Screening

Patients known to possess the *VHL* mutation or those with known VHL disease require regular (at least yearly) screening for disabling and potentially malignant tumors. Affected persons under the age of 11 rarely develop renal cell carcinoma, brain or spinal cord hemangioblastomas, or pheochromocytoma. Yearly retinal examinations are appropriate in this age group, however.

Surveillance is largely focused on early detection and monitoring of retinal and CNS hemangioblastomas, renal cell carcinoma, and pheochromocytoma:

- Annual physical, ophthalmologic, and neurologic examinations.
- Annual plasma catecholamines.
- Annual CT of the abdomen with contrast.
- Annual MRI of the head and total spine.
- Annual audiogram.

Pathology

Capillary hemangioblastoma are well-circumscribed, benign neoplasms derived from endothelial cells:

- Retinal hemangioblastoma:
  - Present in up to 70% of patients.
  - Often multifocal and bilateral.
  - Untreated lesions may cause retinal hemorrhage or detachment.
  - Best treated with laser photocoagulation or cryotherapy.
- Cerebellum and spinal cord:
  - 60–84% of patients develop these tumors at some point in their illness.
  - Distribution of hemangioblastomas:
    - 51% in spinal cord.
    - May be associated with tumor syrinx.
    - 38% in cerebellum.
    - 10% in brainstem.
    - 2% supratentorial.
  - Frequently cystic with a small mural nodule.
  - Usually multiple.
  - Rarely these tumors develop spontaneous hemorrhage.
  - 20% secrete erythropoietin and may produce polycythemia.

Additional lesions

- Renal cell carcinoma
  - As many as two-thirds of patients will develop these tumors during their lifetime.
  - Mean age of discovery is 44 years.
  - Usually multicentric and bilateral.
  - Tumors <3 cm have a low potential for metastasis.
- Pheochromocytoma:
  - 18% of VHL patients.
  - Kindreds with type II VHL develop pheochromocytoma.
  - Kindreds with type I VHL do not develop pheochromocytoma.
- Endolymphatic sac cystadenoma of the ear:
  - Located in the temporal bone.
  - 5% of patients with VHL.
  - May be bilateral.
  - Often present with vertigo and hearing loss.
- Pancreatic tumors:
  - 77% of patients.
  - Usually benign cystadenomas.
  - No increased risk of pancreatic adenocarcinoma.
  - Neuroendocrine tumors occur rarely and can secrete vasoactive intestinal peptide and insulin.
- Papillary cystadenomas of the epididymis (men) and broad ligament (women):
  - 25% of patients with VHL.
  - Benign and usually asymptomatic.

Treatment

Small peripheral retinal hemangioblastomas are best treated with laser photocoagulation and larger tumors are treated with cryotherapy. These treatments are effective in over 70% of cases, usually with a single treatment.

Cerebellar and spinal hemangioblastomas should be removed if they are symptomatic or noted to be rapidly enlarging. In cystic hemangioblastomas, the mural nodule of tumor must be resected in order to prevent reaccumulation of the cystic mass.

Renal cell carcinomas are rare in patients with VHL under the age of 20 years. Tumors <3 cm have a low metastatic potential. Because of the multiple and often bilateral nature of the tumors, a nephron-sparing approach is usually taken[22]. The goal is to preserve as much renal parenchyma as possible. Small lesions (<3 cm) are usually closely observed; these tumors are treated with radiofrequency ablation and cryotherapy if they enlarge.

Pheochromocytomas are typically treated with adrenalectomy. Pancreatic cysts and cystadenomas are usually observed. Neuroendocrine tumors (i.e. insulinomas) of the pancreas usually require partial pancreatectomy.

Endolymphatic sac cystadenomas are treated surgically if they are symptomatic. Stereotactic radiosurgery may be an option for inoperable or recurrent tumors.

Prognosis

Median survival for patients with VHL is 49 years. The most common cause of death is renal cell carcinoma followed by complications of CNS hemangioblastoma[23]. Most patients retain vision and renal function if they receive appropriate tumor surveillance and medical care.

METASTASES TO THE CNS

Definition and epidemiology

Dissemination of malignant cells from their primary site to the CNS. Incidence is 4.1–11.1/100,000 person years. Metastatic tumor is the most common cause of multiple intracranial masses and the most common cause of a solitary cerebellar mass in adults within the developed world.

The incidence of CNS metastases appears to be increasing due to improved detection and better control of extracerebral cancer with improved systemic therapies; 10–25% of systemic malignancies metastasize to the CNS, and 85% of patients presenting with CNS metastases already have an established diagnosis of systemic malignancy.

Any age and either sex may be affected, depending on the source of the primary malignancy.

Etiology and pathophysiology

Most metastases to the CNS (dural, leptomeningeal, and parenchymal) derive from hematogenous spread of systemic malignancy.

Clinical features

Metastases to the skull and dura

- Skull convexity metastases may be asymptomatic or present with localized head pain and occasional a palpable scalp mass.
- Dural metastases may predispose to subdural hematoma with symptoms of elevated ICP and focal neurologic deficit due to compression or irritation of the underlying brain tissue.
- Skull base metastases often compress/infiltrate exiting cranial nerves and may produce cranial neuropathies (cavernous sinus syndrome, jugular foramen syndrome, 'numb chin' syndrome [mandibular metastases], orbital syndrome, occipital condyle syndrome, and so on).

Metastases to the leptomeninges

Multilevel neurologic dysfunction is the classic presentation.

- Headache (often from communicating hydrocephalus).
- Multiple cranial neuropathies.
- Spinal radiculopathies (particularly cauda equina syndrome).
- Spine pain.
- Myelopathy.

Metastases to the brain parenchyma

- Focal or multifocal progressive neurologic dysfunction (i.e. hemiparesis, aphasia, visual field cut, ataxia).
- Some patients, particularly the elderly, may present with a more diffuse encephalopathy that may mistakenly be attributed to a nonspecific delirium or degenerative dementing illness.
- Symptoms of elevated ICP (positional headache, vomiting, reduced level of consciousness).
- Tumor hemorrhage may produce a stroke-like presentation.
- Seizures are the presenting symptom in 15–20% of patients with brain metastases and 40% of patients with brain metastases will have a seizure at some point in their clinical course.

Differential diagnosis

- Primary brain tumor: GBM; only 10% of GBM are multifocal.
- Brain abscess:
  - Typically ring-enhancing and often multiple.
  - Brain abscess usually shows restricted diffusion on diffusion-weighted MRI images.
- Cerebral infarct:
  - Subacute infarcts may enhance on contrasted CT or MRI.
  - Primary hemorrhages or hemorrhagic infarcts may be difficult to distinguish from hemorrhagic tumor.
- Vasculitis.
- CNS sarcoidosis or other granulomatous inflammatory disease.

Investigations

Contrast MRI of the brain is the most sensitive study to demonstrate skull, dural, leptomeningeal, and parenchymal metastases (**515–517**). On MRI, parenchymal metastases are hyperintense on T2-weighted images with ring enhancement and central necrosis apparent on T1 contrasted images. Leptomeningeal metastases reveal pial enhancement most often in dependent areas of the brain and spine (cerebellum, brainstem, and cauda equina). Communicating hydrocephalus may be present from obstruction of the arachnoid granulations.

CT of the brain is often used in the emergency department setting to detect initially the presence of tumor and hemorrhage in patients presenting with acute neurologic illness. On CT, metastases are typically hypodense to normal brain on noncontrast imaging, with disproportionate hypodense vasogenic edema surrounding them. Mass effect is almost always present, and 70% are multiple. Meningeal metastases may be very difficult to detect on CT. Communicating hydrocephalus is often present due to obstruction of the arachnoid granulation.

CSF examination is primarily indicated for the detection of leptomeningeal metastases. CT or MRI of the brain should be performed initially to exclude focal masses which could predispose the patient to uncal or tonsillar herniation if lumbar puncture were performed. In meningeal metastases:

- Opening pressure is normal or elevated.
- Protein is usually elevated.
- Glucose is normal or low.
- Nucleated cells are usually increased:
  - Lymphocytic pleocytosis is most common.
  - Malignant cells are often designated as 'other' on the differential cell count.

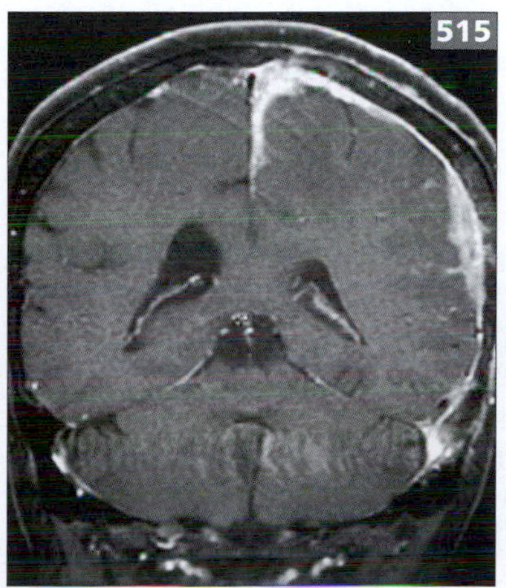

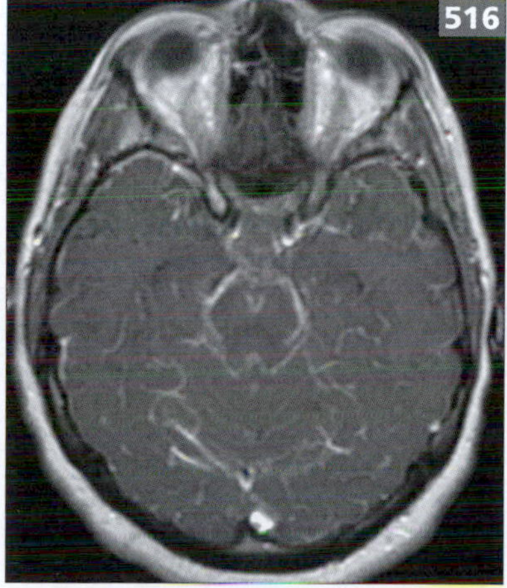

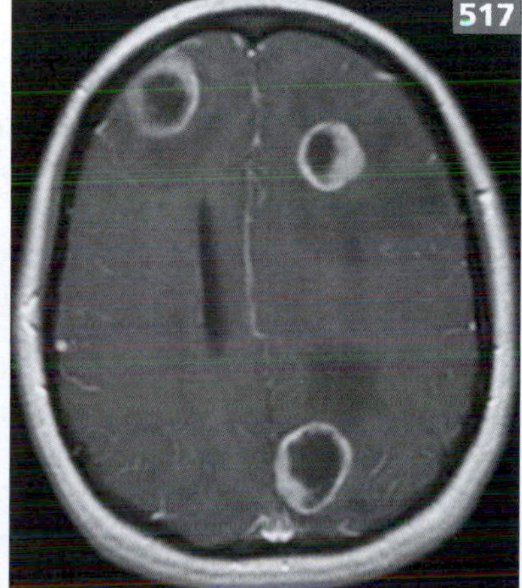

515–517 Contrast MRI of the brain is the most sensitive study to demonstrate dural, leptomeningeal, and parenchymal metastases.

- Tumor markers in the CSF:
  - Carcinoembryonic antigen (CEA) is often elevated in adenocarcinoma.
  - Beta-glucuronidase is frequently elevated in patients with leptomeningeal metastases from epithelial-derived tumors.
  - $Beta_2$-microglobulin is useful in hematopoietic malignancies involving the leptomeninges.
  - Alpha fetoprotein and β-HCG may be noted in metastatic germ cell tumors with leptomeningeal involvement.

Diagnosis

Patients with a known active systemic malignancy presenting with evidence of dural, leptomeningeal, or parenchymal metastases usually do not require biopsy of the intracranial lesion for diagnosis. Surgery (biopsy or resection) is appropriate for the small percentage (15%) of patients whose initial presentation of systemic malignancy is CNS metastases, although a search for systemic malignancy should be performed before resorting to a brain biopsy.

Pathology

- Skull and dura metastases; the most common primary malignancies are:
  - Breast and prostate carcinoma.
  - Myeloma and lymphoma.
- Meningeal metastases; the most common primary malignancies are:
  - Adenocarcinoma of the lung, breast, and gastrointestinal tract.
  - Melanoma.
  - Leukemia and lymphoma.
- Parenchymal brain metastases; the most common primary malignancies are:
  - Carcinomas of the lung, breast, kidney, and gastrointestinal tract.
  - Melanoma.
  - Uncommon malignancies include tumors of the prostate, pancreas, hepatobiliary system, and esophagus (almost never metastasize to the brain parenchyma).
  - 70% of parenchymal metastases are multiple (30% solitary).

Radiographically, metastases are usually well circumscribed, located at the gray–white junction, centrally necrotic, and surrounded by a disproportionately large area of vasogenic edema. Metastases from melanoma, choriocarcinoma, thyroid, and kidney are particularly prone to hemorrhage.

Treatment

Supportive care is appropriate for all patients. This includes:

- Measures to reduce symptoms of elevated ICP and focal neurologic deficits – dexamethasone 12 mg IV or PO initially followed by 4 mg tid–qid.
- Control of seizures if they occur; no role for prophylactic anticonvulsants.
- Prevention of complications of debilitating neurologic illness:
  - Deep venous thrombosis.
  - Aspiration pneumonia.
  - Decubitus ulcers.

Solitary brain metastasis

If the lesion is surgically accessible and the systemic malignancy is limited and/or under good control, surgical resection of the brain lesion prolongs the time to neurologic progression and maintains neurologic function longer[24]. WBRT (2000–3000 cGy in 10–15 fractions) is standard with or without resection of a solitary metastasis. Stereotactic radiation therapy to the solitary lesion may be used in conjunction with WBRT, if the metastasis is surgically inaccessible.

Multiple brain metastasis

Surgery may be indicated to relieve life-threatening mass effect (e.g. cerebellar metastasis with obstruction of the 4th ventricle). WBRT (2000–3000 cGy in 10–15 fractions) is the standard therapy.

Recurrent brain metastases

If the patient's systemic tumor is under control, additional therapy for the brain metastases may be reasonable:

- Stereotactic radiation.
- Re-operation.
- Repeat WBRT may be considered for short-term palliation, but greatly increases the risk of radiation-induced brain necrosis.
- Chemotherapy is ineffective in treating most brain metastases because of a failure of most drugs to cross the blood–brain barrier.

Leptomeningeal metastases

- Radiation to the clinically symptomatic areas.
- Corticosteroids (dexamethasone) are helpful symptomatically.
- There is no established role or documented efficacy for the use of intra-CSF chemotherapy.
- High-dose IV methotrexate can be very useful in the treatment of leptomeningeal lymphoma and leukemia.

Dural metastases

Radiation therapy is usually administered to the whole brain for palliation in these patients.

Prognosis

Most patients with CNS metastases die from complications of their systemic tumor and not from complications of their CNS disease.

Brain metastases

The most important prognostic factors are patient age, functional status, and activity of systemic tumor[25]:

- Patients <65 years, with limited systemic disease and capable of self-care have a median survival of 7.1 months after WBRT.
- Patients >65 years with active systemic malignancy and/or a poor functional status have survival of only 2–4 months after WBRT.
- In patients with a solitary metastasis and limited systemic tumor who undergo surgical resection of their lesion followed by WBRT, survival is improved to a median of 10 months.

Leptomeningeal metastases

Radiation therapy rarely stabilizes neurologic symptoms for more than a few months. Median survival is 4–6 months after radiation therapy.

PARANEOPLASTIC NEUROLOGIC DISEASE

Definition and epidemiology

Paraneoplastic syndromes are a rare, heterogeneous group of neurologic diseases in patients with systemic malignancy in which remote effects of the malignancy produce neurologic signs and symptoms[26]. Less than 1% of patients with cancer will develop paraneoplastic syndromes.

By definition, these effects cannot be ascribed to direct effects of the tumor on the nervous system, injury to vital systemic organs, metabolic or nutritional disorders, infection, coagulation disorders, or the adverse effects of antineoplastic therapies. Some of these neurologic syndromes may occur in the absence of malignancy. Paraneoplastic neurologic disorders may appear before, and therefore presage, the diagnosis of the underlying systemic malignancy. They occur in adults, rarely in children. Males and females are equally affected (depending on the underlying malignancy).

Tip

▶ *Paraneoplastic syndromes are exceedingly rare, and other diagnoses including toxic/metabolic disorders, vascular disease, and metastatic disease must always be considered first. Only a minority of well-characterized paraneoplastic disorders have been associated with typical circulating antibodies.*

Etiology

Any level of the nervous system may be affected. Specific paraneoplastic syndromes typically target specific areas of the nervous system. The pathogenesis of most of these disorders is incompletely understood, although immunologic factors are suspected or known to be involved in the etiology of most, due to the detection of serum antibodies directed against neural antigens in some but not all patients (*Table 92*). The immunologic response in these cases is believed to be directed against tumor antigens which share antigenic similarity with neural proteins.

Associated malignancies

- Paraneoplastic cerebellar degeneration (PCD): ovarian, uterine, breast, small-cell lung, Hodgkin's lymphoma.
- Paraneoplastic encephalomyelitis (PEM): small-cell lung, breast, testicular, Hodgkin's disease, immature teratoma.
- Opsoclonus–myoclonus: breast, small-cell lung, ovarian, neuroblastoma (children only).
- Lambert–Eaton myasthenic syndrome (LEMS): small-cell lung cancer, other small-cell tumors (prostate), lymphoma.
- Paraneoplastic sensory neuropathy (PSN): small-cell lung, breast, Hodgkin's disease.
- Stiff-person syndrome: small-cell lung, breast, Hodgkin's disease.
- Polymyositis/dermatomyositis: ovary, lung, gastrointestinal system, breast, lymphoma. The association of malignancy with dermatomyositis is stronger than with polymyositis.

TABLE 92 **PARANEOPLASTIC SYNDROMES: MOST FREQUENT ASSOCIATED TUMORS AND ANTIBODIES**

Cerebellar degeneration	Breast, ovarian, Hodgkin's disease, SCLC	PCA-1 (anti-Yo), ANNA-1 (anti-Hu), Anti-Tr, ANNA-2 (anti-Ri), CRMP-5 antibody
Paraneoplastic encephalomyelitis	SCLC, non-SCLC, testicular cancer, Hodgkin's disease	ANNA-1 (anti-Hu), PCA-1 (Anti-Yo), ANNA-2 (Anti-Ri), CRMP-5 antibody, Anti-Ma1, Anti-Ma2, anti-NMDA
Opsoclonus–myoclonus	SCLC, breast, neuroblastoma (children)	ANNA-2 (Anti-Ri), ANNA-1 (Anti-Hu), PCA-1 (anti-Yo), CRMP-5 antibody
Paraneoplastic sensory neuronopathy	SCLC	ANNA-1 (Anti-Hu)
Lambert–Eaton myasthenic syndrome	SCLC	Anti-P/Q VGCC, ANNA-1 (Anti-Hu)
Polymyositis/dermatomyositis	Ovarian, gastric, lung, pancreatic, bladder, lymphoma	Anti-Jo-1

SCLC: small-cell lung cancer.

Clinical features/diagnosis/therapy

These vary by syndrome. In approximately two-thirds of patients the symptoms of the paraneoplastic disorder precede the diagnosis of the malignancy. Onset is usually subacute and progressive.

Paraneoplastic cerebellar degeneration

PCD is a pancerebellar syndrome with gait and limb ataxia, dysarthria, vertigo, and nystagmus. It may be part of a more widespread encephalomyelitis with other symptoms of cortical, brainstem, and spinal cord dysfunction. Most patients will have serum or CSF antibodies: anti-YO (PCA-1), anti-Tr, or anti-Hu (ANNA-1) are the most common.

MRI brain with contrast may be normal or show cerebellar atrophy over time (**518**). One-half of patients have elevated protein and CSF pleocytosis.

- Differential diagnosis: cerebellar metastases, nutritional deficiency (vitamin B12, vitamin E deficiency), drug toxicity (5-FU, ARA-C, anticonvulsants), cerebellar infarct, cerebellar abscess, demyelinating disease, inherited cerebellar degeneration.
- Pathology: diffuse loss of Purkinje cells with minimal involvement of the molecular and granular layers. Typically little or no inflammatory change is noted in the brain.

Paraneoplastic encephalomyelitis

Paraneoplastic encephalomyelitis (PEM) comprises limbic encephalitis: confusion, impaired short-term memory, seizures, hallucinations, and behavioral changes. Cerebellar ataxia, dysarthria, pyramidal weakness, and sensory ataxia may be seen in patients with more widespread encephalomyelitis. Associated antibodies (serum or CSF) are: anti-Hu (ANNA-1), CRMP-5 antibody, anti-Ma2, anti-NMDA antibody, and voltage-gated potassium channel antibody.

MRI brain with contrast may be normal or show T2 signal abnormalities in the limbic cortex (with or without enhancement) (**519**). Two-thirds of patients will have elevated protein and CSF lymphocytic pleocytosis. Electroencephalography often demonstrates epileptiform discharges, usually localizing to the temporal lobes.

- Differential diagnosis: multiple cerebral metastases, nonconvulsive status epilepticus, metabolic encephalopathy, nutritional deficiency, drug toxicity (opioids, chemotherapy agents), meningoencephalitis (particularly herpes simplex encephalitis), disseminated intravascular coagulation, venous sinus thrombosis.
- Pathology: characterized by involvement of multiple levels of the CNS:
  - Limbic system.
  - Cerebellum.
  - Brainstem.
  - Spinal cord.
  - Dorsal root ganglia.
  - Autonomic nervous system.
  - Pathologic examination usually shows inflammatory perivascular and interstitial infiltrates of T and B lymphocytes with loss of neurons and gliosis.

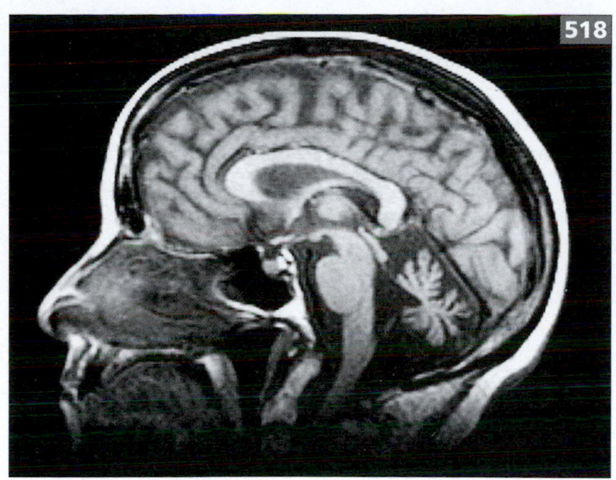

518 MRI of cerebellar degeneration with diffuse cerebellar atrophy.

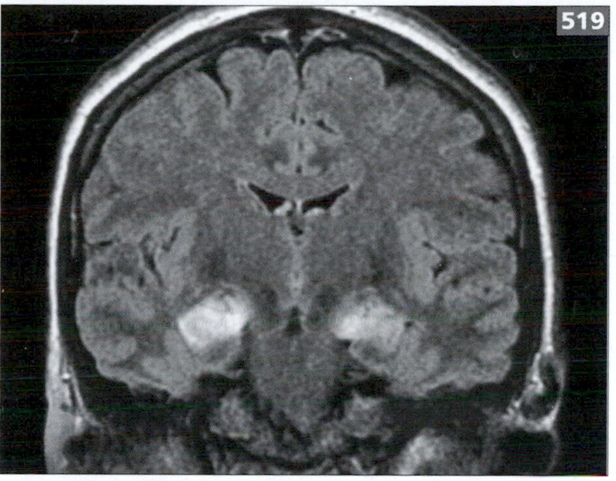

519 MRI brain FLAIR image demonstrating increased T2 signal in the mesial temporal lobe in a patient with limbic encephalitis.

Paraneoplastic sensory neuronopathy

Paraneoplastic sensory neuronopathy (PSN) comprises paresthesia with loss of vibration and joint position sense, followed by loss of pain and temperature sensation. Neuropathic pain and Lhermitte's phenomenon may be present. Profound sensory ataxia is usually present, and most patients are nonambulatory at the time of diagnosis. PSN may be a component of a more widespread paraneoplastic encephalomyelitis. Associated antibodies are anti-Hu (ANNA-1).

Electromyography (EMG)/nerve conduction studies (NCSs) show markedly reduced or absent sensory nerve action potentials (SNAPs) and preserved compound muscle action potentials (CMAPs). There is usually a normal needle examination although signs of motor involvement may be present.

- Differential diagnosis: vitamin B6 toxicity, nutritional deficiency (vitamin B12, copper), leptomeningeal carcinomatosis, epidural cord compression, and chemotherapy toxicity (cisplatin, paclitaxel, vincristine).
- Pathology:
  - Inflammatory infiltrates in the dorsal root ganglia with associated neuronal loss.
  - Degeneration of the dorsal columns and axonal loss in peripheral nerves

Opsoclonus–myoclonus syndrome

Opsoclonus is a disorder of ocular motility characterized by involuntary, rapid, irregular conjugate eye movements in both the vertical and horizontal plane. The patient experiences oscillopsia, and myoclonic movements of the trunk and limbs. Cerebellar and other brainstem signs may be seen.

Associated tumors include neuroblastoma in children, and breast and small-cell lung cancer in adults. Associated antibodies are anti-Ri and occasionally anti-Hu.

MRI of the brain with contrast may be normal or show areas of abnormal T2 signal in the brainstem. One-half of patients have elevated CSF protein and CSF pleocytosis.

- Differential diagnosis: brainstem or leptomeningeal metastases, hypernatremia, drug toxicity (lithium, tricyclic antidepressants, thallium, haloperidol), hydrocephalus, viral brainstem encephalitis.
- Pathology: Purkinje cell loss and perivascular inflammatory infiltrates in the cerebellum have been demonstrated.

Lambert–Eaton myasthenic syndrome

Patients with Lambert–Eaton myasthenic syndrome (LEMS) show symptoms of cholinergic autonomic dysfunction, such as dry mouth, dry eyes, orthostatic hypotension, erectile dysfunction, and constipation. Approximately 40% of patients with LEMS do not have malignancy. There is proximal muscle weakness (which improves with exertion), and reduced and usually absent deep tendon reflexes that may increase after exercise. Associated antibodies (serum) are anti-VGCC antibody and ocassionally anti-Hu.

EMG/NCS show reduced CMAPs, significant increment in amplitude with rapid (50 Hz) repetitive stimulation, and motor unit action potential (MUP) variability on needle examination.

- Differential diagnosis: myopathy (inflammatory, metabolic, congenital), inflammatory polyradiculoneuropathy, critical care neuromyopathy, and leptomeningeal carcinomatosis.
- Pathology: antibodies directed against the voltage-gated calcium channels at the presynaptic motor nerve terminal. This results in reduced acetylcholine release and impaired neuromuscular transmission.

Polymyositis/dermatomyositis

Polymyositis/dermatomyositis comprises subacute proximal greater than distal muscle weakness with muscle tenderness. Ocular and facial muscles are preserved. Dysphagia and dysarthria may occur. Patients with dermatomyositis usually have a violaceous heliotrope rash of the face and a maculopapular rash over the extensor surface of the hands and fingers (Gottran's sign). The rash may be trivial. Polyarthralgia and arthritis may be associated.

Polymyositis/dermatomyositis may be associated with other autoimmune syndromes (particularly the nonparaneoplastic forms). The association of malignancy with dermatomyositis is stronger than with polymyositis. No specific paraneoplastic antibody is associated with polymyositis/dermatomyositis. Anti-Jo antibody is seen in one-fifth of patients with polymyositis, but usually not dermatomyositis.

EMG/NCSs show small CMAPs with normal SNAPs, reduced motor unit size, and rapid recruitment. Patients have elevated creatine kinase levels. Muscle biopsy is diagnostic.

- Differential diagnosis: inflammatory myopathy unassociated with malignancy, corticosteroid-induced myopathy, hypothyroidism, critical care neuromyopathy.
- Pathology: muscle fiber necrosis and atrophy with perifascicular inflammatory infiltrates.
- Dermatomyositis is likely due to a humoral attack on muscle capillaries and arterioles, with associated microinfarction of muscle fibers:
  - Polymyositis is manifested by endomysial infiltrates with muscle fiber necrosis and fiber size variation. Perivascular infiltrates are rare.
  - Dermatomyositis is manifested by perivascular and perimysial inflammation, with muscle fiber necrosis produced by ischemia. Ischemia produces perifascicular atrophy.

Diagnostic approach for a suspected paraneoplastic syndrome

- Rule out other neoplastic, toxic/metabolic, vascular, and inflammatory/infectious etiologies.
- Paraneoplastic antibody testing: directed by syndrome.
- In patients without known malignancy (depending on the neurologic syndrome and probable associated malignancy):
  - CT chest, abdomen, and pelvis.
  - Mammography.
  - Testicular ultrasound.
  - Body PET scan[27].
- The malignancy may be very small and undetectable at the time of presentation of the neurologic syndrome.

Treatment

Treating the underlying malignancy if it can be identified is often the most effective therapy of the paraneoplastic syndrome.

- PCD, PEM, PSN: no specific therapy is known to be effective. Immunosuppression with steroids or intravenous immune globulin (IVIG) is often tried. Even with treatment of the malignancy, most patients are left with significant neurologic disability.
- Opsoclonus–myoclonus: no specific therapy is known to be effective. A significant percentage of patients experience remission of their neurologic symptoms with treatment of the underlying malignancy.
- LEMS: plasma exchange, IVIG, and corticosteroids may improve neurologic symptoms at least in the short term. 3,4-Diaminopyridine, a potassium channel blocker which prolongs the duration of the action potential and improves calcium influx into the nerve terminal, can be helpful.
- Polymyositis/dermatomyositis: treatment of the underlying malignancy and immunosuppressive therapy with corticosteroids, azathioprine, cyclophosphamide, methotrexate, and other potent immunosuppressive agents is usually effective in controlling the disease.

Prognosis

In most patients with paraneoplastic disease the prognosis for neurologic recovery is poor even with treatment of the malignancy and immunosuppressive therapy. Interestingly, many patients with paraneoplastic disease appear to have longer than expected survivals compared with other patients with the same malignancy. This is believed possibly to relate to an improved immunologic response against the malignancy.

REFERENCES

1 Wen PY, Kesari S (2008). Malignant gliomas in adults. *N Engl J Med* **359**:492–507.
2 Chang SM, Parney IF, Huang W, *et al.* (2005). Patterns of care for adults with newly diagnosed malignant glioma. *JAMA* **293**:557–564.
3 Stupp R, Hegi ME, Mason WP, *et al.* (2009). Effects of radiotherapy with concomitant and adjuvant temozolomide versus radiotherapy alone on survival in glioblastoma in a randomized phase II study: 5 year analysis of the EORTC-NCIC trial. *Lancet Oncol* **10**:459–4566.
4 Butowski NA. Sneed PK. Chang SM (2006). Diagnosis and treatment of recurrent high-grade astrocytoma. *J Clin Oncol* **24**(8):1273–1280.
5 Mansur DB, Perry A, Rajaram V, *et al.* (2005). Postoperative radiation therapy for grade II and III intracranial ependymoma. *Int J Radiat Oncol Biol Phys* **61**(2):387–391.
6 Reni M, Brandes AA, Vavassori V, *et al.* (2004). A multicenter study of the prognosis and treatment of adult brain ependymal tumors. *Cancer* **100**(6):1221–1229.
7 Nakamura M, Roser F, Michel J, *et al.* (2003). The natural history of incidental meningiomas. *Neurosurgery* **53**(1):62–70.
8 Whittle IR, Smith C, Navoo P, Collie D (2004). Meningiomas. *Lancet* **363**(9420):1535–1543.
9 Stafford SL, Perry A, Suman VJ, *et al.* (1998). Primarily resected meningiomas: outcome and prognostic factors in 581 Mayo Clinic patients, 1978 through 1988. *Mayo Clin Proc* **73**(10):936–942.
10 Mendenhall WM, Morris CG, Amdur RJ, *et al.* (2003). Radiotherapy alone or after subtotal resection for benign skull base meningiomas. *Cancer* **98**(7):1473–1482.
11 Karavitaki N, Wass JA (2008). Craniopharyngioma. *Endocrinol Metab Clin North Am* **37**(1):173–193.
12 Komotar RJ, Roguski M, Bruce JN (2009). Surgical management of craniopharyngiomas. *Neurosurg Rev* **32**(2):125–132.
13 Saeger W, Ludecke DK, Buchfelder M, *et al.* (2007). Pathohistological classification of pituitary tumors: 10 years of experience with the German Pituitary Tumor Registry. *Eur J Endocrinol* **156**(2):203–216.
14 Propp JM, McCarthy BJ, Davis FG, *et al.* (2006). Descriptive epidemiology of vestibular schwannomas. *Neuro-oncol* **8**(1):1–11.
15 Chan AW, Black P, Ojemann RG, *et al.* (2005). Stereotactic radiotherapy for vestibular schwannomas: favorable outcome with minimal toxicity. *Neurosurgery* **57**(1):60–70.
16 DeAngelis LM (1999). Primary central nervous system lymphoma. *J Neurol Neurosurg Psychiatry* **66**:699–701.
17 O'Brien PC, Seymour JF (2009). Progress in primary CNS lymphoma. *Lancet* **374**(9700):1477–1478.
18 Goodwin TL, Sainani K, Fisher PG (2009). Incidence patterns of central nervous system germ cell tumors: a SEER Study. *J Pediatr Hematol Oncol* **31**(8):541–544.
19 Barry RE, Krek W (2004). The von Hippel-Lindau tumour suppressor: a multi-faceted inhibitor of tumourigenesis. *Trends Mol Med* **10**:466–472.
20 Lonser RR, Glenn GM, Walther M, *et al.* (2003). von Hippel-Lindau disease. *Lancet* **361**:2059–2067.
21 Lonser RR, Kim HJ, Butman JA, *et al.* (2004). Tumors of the endolymphatic sac in von Hippel-Lindau disease. *N Engl J Med* **350**:2481–2486.
22 Steinbach F, Novick AC, Zincke H, *et al.* (1995). Treatment of renal cell carcinoma in von Hippel-Lindau disease: a multicenter study. *J Urol* **153**:1812.
23 Wanebo JE, Lonser RR, Glenn GM, *et al.* (2003). The natural history of hemangioblastomas of the central nervous system in patients with von Hippel-Lindau disease. *J Neurosurg* **98**:82–94.
24 Patchell RA, Tibbs PA, Walsh JW, *et al.* (1990). A randomized trial of surgery in the treatment of single metastases to the brain. *N Engl J Med* **322**(8):494–500.
25 Gaspar LE, Scott C, Rotman M, *et al.* (1997). Recursive partitioning analysis (RPA) of prognostic factors in three Radiation Therapy Oncology Group (RTOG) brain metastases trials. *Int J Radiat Oncol Biol Phys* **37**:745–751.
26 Toothaker TB, Rubin M (2009). Paraneoplastic neurological syndromes: a review. *Neurologist* **15**(1):21–33.
27 Patel RR, Subramaniam RM, Mandrekar JN, *et al.* (2008). Occult malignancy in patients with suspected paraneoplastic neurologic syndromes: value of positron emission tomography in diagnosis. *Mayo Clin Proc* **83**(8):917–922.

Further reading

Bruce JN, Fetell MR, Balmaceda CM, Stein BM (1997). Tumors of the pineal region. In: Black PM, Loeffler JS (eds). *Cancer of the Nervous System*. Blackwell Science, pp. 576–592.

Darnell RB, Posner JB (2006). Paraneoplastic syndromes affecting the nervous system. *Sem Oncol* **33**(3):270–298.

Jane Jr. J, Dumont AS, Vance ML, Laws Jr. ER (2005). Pituitary adenomas and sellar lesions: multidisciplinary management. In: D. Schiff, BP O'Neill (eds). *Principles of Neuro-oncology*. McGraw-Hill.

Levy A, Lightman SL (1994). Diagnosis and management of pituitary tumours. *BMJ* **308**:1087–1091.

Morris PG, Abrey LE (2009). Therapeutic challenges in primary CNS lymphoma. *Lancet Neurol* **8**(6):581–592.

O'Neill BP, Illig JJ (1989). Primary central nervous system lymphoma. *Mayo Clin Proc* **64**:1005–1020.

Posner JB (1995). *Neurologic Complications of Cancer*. FA Davis, Philadelphia.

Shuanshoti S, Rushing EJ, Mena H, *et al.* (2005). Supratentorial extraventricular ependymal neoplasms. *Cancer* **103**: 2598–2605.

Takakura K (1985). Intracranial germ cell tumors. *Clin Neurosurg* **32**:429–444.

DEGENERATIVE DISEASES OF THE NERVOUS SYSTEM

James A. Mastrianni,
Brandon R. Barton, Kathleen M. Shannon,
Sid Gilman, Vikram Shakkottai, Peter Todd

DEMENTIA

ALZHEIMER'S DISEASE (AD)

Definition and epidemiology

Alzheimer's disease is a clinico-pathologic entity comprising clinical evidence of dementia (sufficient to interfere with social and work function) and histopathologic evidence of neurofibrillary tangles and senile plaques in the brain. AD is the most common cause of dementia, accounting for almost one-half of cases.

- Incidence: age-dependent. Rises from 2.8 per 1000 person years for 65–69 year olds to 56.1 per 1000 person years in the older than 90-year-old group.
- Prevalence: approximately 5% of those over the age of 70 have AD and 25–45% of those over 85 years of age have AD. It is predominantly a disease of old age but not an invariable accompaniment of aging. AD seldom presents before 40 years of age, except in Down's syndrome or some inherited forms of AD.
- Gender: the prevalence of Alzheimer's disease is slightly higher in females, partly related to their greater longevity, although hormonal influence appears to contribute to some extent.

Etiology

Most cases are probably polygenic (resulting from the action of several different genes), and the penetrance of disease is influenced by age and environmental factors. The concordance rate is higher (1.2–2.7) in monozygotic and dizygotic twin pairs, suggesting the contribution of genetic factors, but monozygotic twins are not fully concordant, implicating the involvement of nongenetic and environmental factors. Genetic factors appear to lead to quantitatively worse disease but not to a qualitatively different pattern of brain involvement. Amyloid-β (Aβ) deposition seems to be the neuropathologic factor most strongly influenced by genetic factors.

Sporadic (most cases of AD)

A negative family history occurs in 50–75% of cases. There are associations with advanced maternal age, head trauma, depression, cardiovascular disease risk factors, and carriage of apolipoprotein E (ApoE) ε4 allele.

A positive family history in one or more first-degree relatives occurs in 25–50% of cases. This likely results from the influence of multiple risk-associated genes. Major gene effect is the *APOE* gene on chromosome 19q which encodes ApoE[1]. Although this gene occurs as one of three variants including ε2, ε3, and ε4, the ε4 variant substantially increases the risk of AD. This is, therefore, a risk factor or 'susceptibility' gene (see below) rather than a causative gene. In individuals that carry a homozygous *APOE* ε4 allele, the onset of AD is roughly 10–20 years earlier compared to those who carry an ε2 or ε3 allele, and it is 5–10 years earlier in individuals who are heterozygous with ε4 allele. Other recently identified potential genetic risk modifiers include:

- *SORL1* on chromosome 11q 23 encodes a protein involved with amyloid precursor protein (APP) trafficking.
- *CALHM1* on chromosome 10q24 encodes a protein that controls cytosolic calcium concentrations and Aβ levels.
- *GAB2* on chromosome 11q14 encodes a scaffolding protein implicated in growth and differentiation.

A number of additional genes that have been associated with a modification of risk for AD can be found on the AlzGene database (www.alzforum.org/res/com/gen/alzgene/default.asp).

Familial variants of AD (rare)

Only ~1% of all cases of AD are linked to an autosomal dominant inheritance of mutations in one of the three known causative genes of presenile (under 60–65 years of age) AD:

- *APP* gene on the long arm of chromosome 21, encodes *APP*, responsible for <1% of all early-onset AD cases.
- *PSEN-1* gene on chromosome 14q (50% of early-onset cases) encodes presenilin-1 (PS-1): >50 mutations in the gene for PS-1 have been identified in patients with early-onset AD.
- *PSEN-2* gene on chromosome 1 encodes presenilin-2 (PS-2), which accounts for 15–20% of early-onset AD.

Mutations in all these genes result in a shift in the metabolism of APP to produce a 42–43 amino acid form of Aβ.

Down's syndrome

An extra copy of chromosome 21 in Down's syndrome results in an extra copy of the *APP* gene which resides there. This results in Aβ deposition and brain changes associated with AD by around age 40 in most Down's syndrome patients.

Risk factors for AD

Definite

- Aging (accumulation of Aβ in the brain increases with age).
- Family history of dementia (having a first-degree relative with AD increases the risk ~3.5 times, perhaps because vulnerability genes are shared by family members).
- Down's syndrome.
- ApoE gene allele status. ApoE may be involved in neuronal repair:

ApoE is produced predominantly in astrocytes and is carried by low-density lipoprotein (LDL) receptor into neurons, where it binds to neurofibrillary tangles. The three alleles of *APOE* (ε2, ε3, and ε4) vary in their affinity for Aβ. Allele ε4 increases the rate of deposition of fibrillary Aβ, resulting in an increase in amyloid deposits. In the general population, 75–85% have the ε3 allele, 10–15% have ε4, and 5–10% have ε2. In AD, ε4 is over-represented (40%) and ε2 is under-represented (4%). Up to 30-40% of the risk for late-onset AD is attributable to alleles at the ApoE locus.

The ε4 allele is associated with a threefold (heterozygotes) to eightfold (homozygotes) increased risk of sporadic and familial late-onset AD. However, even among homozygotes for ε4, only about 50% develop dementia by age 90 years. The ε2 allele appears to be protective.

Although ε4 is an important risk factor for AD, it is neither essential for the development of the disease, nor specific for the disease. Thus, testing for the *APOE* genotype as a diagnostic marker is not advised.

Possible

- Ethnic group: AD appears to be more common in African Americans, although the basis for this is currently under investigation.
- Head injury: neuronal injury may trigger the deposition of Aβ; however, this appears to be enhanced and related to the presence of an ε4 allele.
- Lower educational attainment and socioeconomic status, which may relate to a reduced 'brain reserve'.
- High blood pressure and other vascular risk factors.
- High plasma homocysteine.

Possible protective factors

Several epidemiologic studies have supported the use of anti-inflammatory drugs, estrogen replacement therapy, and cholesterol lowering drugs (i.e. statins), as protective factors. However, thus far, prospective studies looking at the benefit of anti-inflammatory drugs and statins in AD have not supported that hypothesis. In fact, estrogen replacement in older women appears to promote a higher risk for developing AD. Additional prospective studies are in progress to sort out these relationships.

Pathophysiology

The amyloid hypothesis[2]

APP is a large transmembrane protein from which Aβ is derived. The Aβ motif is a fragment of 40–42 amino acids extending from the exterior to half-way through the plasma membrane. There are at least three different forms of Aβ, depending on the site of ribonucleic acid (RNA) splicing. Mutations found within the APP gene are associated with an increased production of Aβ 1–42, leading to the generation of β-amyloid deposits. The amyloid hypothesis is that mutations present in APP and presenilin genes are associated with increased cellular production of Aβ, which is toxic to neurons. As indicated above, the *APOE* ε4 allele also promotes an increase in the rate of Aβ plaque deposition; however, it does not increase the production of Aβ. Recent evidence suggests that soluble oligomers of Aβ constitute the neurotoxic factor, rather than the Aβ plaques deposited in the extracellular space.

Clinical features

Insidious onset of short-term memory decline is the primary feature of AD. A deficit in episodic memory is observed, with early loss of memory for everyday events. Previously stored long-term memories from the past are preserved early on, in addition to a relative preservation of immediate memory (e.g. digit span). Impaired learning (encoding) of new verbal and visual information is evident on neuropsychologic assessment. This impairment in antegrade episodic memory is thought to correlate with the deposition of tangles in the transentorhinal region, which result in deafferentation of the hippocampal complex.

In addition to memory deficits, visuospatial abilities and language deficits commonly coexist in AD. There may, however, be focal cortical neurologic signs including aphasia, agraphia, dyscalculia, apraxia (ideomotor and dressing), agnosia for objects or faces, and neglect or sensory inattention. These may mark the onset of disease, but generally appear after presentation of memory impairment.

Psychiatric features may include paranoia and other personality or behavioral changes. In particular, patients have a delusion that people may be stealing from them, as a result of their misplacing items. If hallucinations are present, they are typically persecutory or of deceased family members.

On physical examination, primitive reflexes and other frontal release signs may be observed at any stage, but are more evident in later stages of disease. Generally, the remainder of the neurologic examination is benign in early presentations of AD. However, as the disease progresses muscular rigidity (paratonia) may be evident, in addition to reduced gait speed and stride.

In terminal stages of disease, myoclonic jerks and seizures may occur in some patients. Urinary and bowel incontinence will also be evident in later stages of disease. In the end stage of disease, the patient is often in an akinetic and mute state.

Tip

▶ *In the early stages of AD, the neurophysical examination is typically normal. A physical finding, such as unilateral motor or sensory abnormalities or parkinsonian features, suggests another process.*

Differential diagnosis

Dementia

- AD: 50–55%.
- Vascular dementia (VaD) or mixed dementia (AD plus VaD): 15–20%.
- Frontotemporal dementia (FTD), including Pick's complex (~50% of presenile, and approximately 30% of all dementia).
- Dementia with Lewy bodies: 15–25%.
- Parkinson's disease: 5–10%.
- Brain injury: alcohol or head trauma: 5%.
- Other causes: 5%:
  - Normal pressure hydrocephalus (NPH).
  - Tumor.
  - Subdural hematoma, especially bilateral.
  - Toxic/metabolic: chronic drug intoxication (e.g. alcohol, sedatives, barbiturates, bismuth).
  - Chronic hepatic encephalopathy.
  - Endocrine: hypothyroidism, Cushing's syndrome.
  - Autoimmune: systemic lupus erythematosus (SLE), other vasculitides, paraneoplastic syndromes.
  - Nutritional: vitamin B12 deficiency, Wernicke–Korsakoff syndrome.
  - Syphilis, human immunodeficiency virus (HIV).
  - Huntington's disease (HD).
  - Creutzfeldt–Jakob disease (CJD): ataxia, myoclonus, and rapidly progressive dementia.
  - Multiple causes (i.e. combinations of the above) 10–15%.

Familial dementia

- HD.
- Familial prion disease.
- Hereditary cerebral hemorrhages with amyloidosis, Dutch type.
- Chromosome 17- and chromosome 3-linked forms of FTD.
- Cerebral autosomal dominant arteriopathy with subcortical infarcts and leukoencephalopathy (CADASIL).

Pseudo-dementia

Depression is the most common cause of pseudodementia but it should be noted that depression may also accompany the earlier stages of AD. As a general rule, patients with cognitive impairment caused by AD typically underestimate the severity of their cognitive deficit and make an effort during cognitive testing, whereas those with anxiety or depression exaggerate the severity of their symptoms and tend to provide poor effort during cognitive testing.

Anticholinergics may cause dementia-like symptoms; however, it should be cautioned that these may affect patients with AD more significantly than normals in addition to unmasking an underlying AD in the very early stage.

Mild cognitive impairment (MCI)

MCI is a relatively new diagnostic classification that represents a precursor to dementia. Patients who have significant cognitive impairment on formal testing, yet do not show impairment in activities of normal daily function, meet the general diagnostic criteria for MCI[3]. MCI portends an increased risk for developing Alzheimer's disease within several years after the diagnosis:

- Approximately 15% of patients with MCI will convert to AD within 1 year. By 5 years, approximately 80% will convert.
- A distinction of MCI types, including amnestic MCI (principal cognitive deficits are in memory) and/or multidomain MCI (cognitive deficits affecting several domains, not primarily memory), may distinguish risk for AD, and/or VaD, respectively. Studies suggest even further segregation of MCI types for those who will eventually develop FTDs or Parkinson's dementia may be possible.

Investigations

Cognitive evaluation

The Mini Mental State Examination (MMSE) is a 30-point questionnaire that provides a crude assessment of general cognitive function. A score of 24 or less is generally considered abnormal, but this test should only be used as a screening assessment and not a diagnostic test[4]. It is limited by the relatively small proportion devoted to testing memory (3 points) and, as such, it may lack the sensitivity to detect cognitive impairment at the very early stages of AD. Patients may score high on the MMSE, but perform poorly on a detailed neuropsychologic assessment. In addition, because the MMSE is heavily language-based, patients with aphasia due to a non-AD process may perform much worse on the MMSE than their actual potential.

Thus, the MMSE should, at least, be combined with complimentary investigations such as the Functional Assessment Staging Test (FAST), to assess the impact of cognitive impairment on the patient's activities of daily living (ADL). For those subjects that score high on MMSE, but for whom there is a suspicion for cognitive impairment related to early AD, a more extensive neuropsychologic battery should be administered. This limitation of the MMSE is especially important in making a diagnosis of MCI. Despite high MMSE scores, patients with MCI may still demonstrate memory impairment that is greater than 1.5 standard deviations below the age- and education-adjusted norms, one of the general criteria for making a diagnosis of MCI.

While sensitivity for early disease may be low, the MMSE may be useful for staging progression of AD. Typically, patients decline about 2–3 points per year on the MMSE and disease stage is roughly correlated using the following guidlines: mild = 21–24, moderate = 10–20 and severe = <10.

The Montreal Cognitive Assessment (MoCA) is another screening tool that is gaining popularity. It may be more sensitive than MMSE to identify MCI patients, possibly due to the task of word recall that includes five rather than three words. It may not, however, be as useful for staging, compared with the MMSE.

In addition to face-to-face memory assessment with the patient, it is important that the spouse, family, or friends be interviewed, preferably independent of the patient interview. Patients with AD are often unaware of cognitive difficulties that are recognized by their colleagues at work. As such, forgetting appointments, forgetting names of colleagues, or not recognizing them, may be reported by individuals who know the patient at work and at home. A change in the role of the patient is also an important clue: if the patient normally deals with family finances, yet one of the family members has found the need to take over those finances, this represents a loss in functioning. Other examples that are commonly reported include problems with cooking, in particular forgetting pots on the stove to the point that the pots burn, keeping the house clean and organized, and confidence and accuracy while driving. Often patients will report a restriction in their driving radius, providing a clue that they are unsure of themselves with regard to driving.

Other tests

Psychologic, medical, psychiatric, and social factors that may contribute to the patient's intellectual decline should also be evaluated. These factors may contribute greatly to the patient's cognitive status. In particular, other medical conditions need to be ruled out in order to make a diagnosis of AD. A formal diagnosis of AD requires the demonstration of a decline in functional capacity as a result of the cognitive problems, and no other medical condition to explain the symptoms. Thus, the following investigations should be performed on all patients with cognitive impairment and a concern of AD:

- Complete blood count plus platelets.
- Basic medical panel.
- Thyroid function test, (at least thyroid stimulating hormone [TSH], and with abnormalities T3, T4, and T3 uptake).
- Rapid plasma reagin (RPR) and/or fluorescent treponemal antibody (FTA) in patients residing in areas designated as endemic or high-risk for syphilis.
- Serum vitamin B12.
- Antinuclear antibodies (ANA), primarily in younger patients (<65 years) with onset of cognitive impairment.
- HIV serology, for those with appropriate risk factors for HIV.
- Brain magnetic resonance imaging (MRI) scan, although head computed tomography (CT) may be substituted. The main findings of brain imaging include diffuse cortical atrophy that is most prominent in temporal and/or parietal lobes, in addition to enlarged ventricles, sulci, and fissures, due to the overall atrophy of the brain. Although the presence of atrophy in the temporal and parietal lobes is a helpful diagnostic clue, it is often very subtle or not present in early AD. A coronal MRI may allow easier assessment of focal hippocampal atrophy.

The principal purpose of brain imaging is to exclude either a mass (tumor or subdural hemorrhage), NPH, or severe cerebrovascular disease or vasculitis that might be the cause of the patient's cognitive impairment.

A positron emission tomographic (PET) scan demonstrates reduced metabolic activity (reduction in radiolabeled glucose utilization) over the temporal and parietal lobes, as a characteristic feature of AD. The single photon emission tomography (SPECT) scan, which has lower resolution, may sometimes substitute for the PET. It is notable that the US health insurer Medicare covers the cost of a PET scan when discriminating between AD and FTD. Recent developments in tracers have produced agents that can be used to assess amyloid plaque pathology in living patients. However, because amyloid deposition may predate symptoms of AD by up to 10 years, the availability of this test raises concerns about the population to which it should be administered.

- Electroencephalography (EEG): this may be normal in early AD, or may show generalized slow-wave activity that may be more prominent over the temporal parietal regions.
- Cerebrospinal fluid (CSF):
  - Tau levels: total tau level is increased; however, phosphorylated tau is also elevated. This feature helps distinguish AD from FTD, which may also be associated with an increase in total tau, but only nonphosphorylated tau. It should be cautioned that other neurodegenerative diseases can increase CSF tau, as it is an intraneuronal protein released following neuronal death.
  - Aβ42: this is reduced, presumably because the Aβ42 is no longer remaining in solution but is being sequestered into amyloid plaques in the brain, thereby reducing the total levels detectable in the CSF. The ratio of Aβ42 to total tau is used with some commercial assays, as a diagnostic marker of AD.

Although this ratio defines an increased risk for AD, the additional test of phosphorylated tau helps to discriminate AD from other forms of dementia, especially FTD and dementia with Lewy bodies (DLB). CSF Aβ42 reduction may also be present during MCI, and predicts the development of AD.

Genetic testing

In the individual with cognitive impairment, genetic testing can be used to determine whether the disease is genetically transmissible. In the individual without cognitive impairment, the overall very low prevalence of genetic defects that cause AD, especially older onset (greater than age 65), militates against indiscriminate screening for *APP*, *PS-1*, and *PS-2* mutations in clinical practice.

Early-onset familial (autosomal dominant) AD

Transmissibility of disease is often clear based on a strong family history of individuals presenting with early-onset dementia. Detection of a genetic mutation of *APP*, *PS-1*, or *PS-2* in the proband may sensitize the family for concern about other carriers who are currently asymptomatic. While the presence of an autosomal dominant mutation in one of these genes predicts the development of disease with almost 100% probability, the age at onset determination is much less certain, falling within 2.5 standard deviations from the mean age of onset of the family with *APP* mutations.

Late-onset AD with a positive family history

A routine search for known mutations in individual families is limited. Large scale studies looking for genetic risk factors for AD continue to be performed and have revealed some new markers (*Table 93*).

Sporadic AD

The ε4 allele of the *ApoE* gene is more common in patients with sporadic late-onset AD (roughly 40%) than in elderly controls (10–15%). Among people over the age of 60 who have dementia, the pretest probability (prevalence) of AD is about 66%. If the patient has an ε3/ε4 genotype, the probability increases to about 81%. If the patient has an ε2/ε3, the probability of AD is reduced by one-half, i.e. there is double the possibility that there may be another cause for dementia other than AD. Detecting an ε4 allele in a demented patient may therefore increase the likelihood of a diagnosis of AD; however, as noted earlier, the *ApoE* testing should not be relied upon as a diagnostic test for AD in and of itself. *ApoE* genotyping is not useful as a predictive test for AD in an asymptomatic individual; the population at highest risk of developing AD (*ApoE* ε4/ε4 genotype) is only 2% of the normal population and even for this small group, the period of risk extends over five decades (50s to 90s) and some may not develop AD at all.

Diagnosis

The diagnosis of AD is largely one of exclusion of other causes of progressive dementia. Recently, diagnostic criteria for AD have been updated[5]. For clinical use, 'Probable', 'Possible', and 'Definite' AD are defined.

A diagnosis of 'probable AD'can be made if dementia is manifest by the following criteria:

- At least two of the following cognitive domains are affected:
  - Acquisition and recall of new information.
  - Reasoning, judgment, handling complex tasks.
  - Visuospatial abilities.
  - Language function.
  - Personality, behavior, or comportment.

  In addition to documenting:
- An insiduous onset.
- A clear-cut worsening of cognition by report or observation, and
- Initial and most prominent cognitive deficits in either learning and recall or language, visuospatial, and executive dysfunction.

TABLE 93 **GENETIC CLASSIFICATION OF ALZHEIMER'S DISEASE**

Type	Chromosome	Gene	Age at onset	% of cases
Early-onset familial AD	21q21	*APP*	45–66	<0.1% (<1% of early-onset cases)
Early-onset familial AD	14q24.3	*PS-1*	40s mean (28–62)	1–2% (50% of early-onset familial AD)
Early-onset familial AD	lq31–q42	*PS-2*	50s mean (42–68+)	<0.1% (15–20% of early-onset cases)
Late-onset	12	α_2-*macro*	>70	30%
Late-onset familial AD and sporadic; ApoE ε4 allele associated	19q13	*ApoE*	>60	40%
Late-onset familial; and sporadic; not ApoE allele associated	?	?	>75	10–40%
Other				

APP: amyloid precursor protein; α_2-macro: alpha$_2$-macroglobulin mutation; ApoE: apolipoprotein E; PS-1: presenilin-1; PS-2: presenilin-2

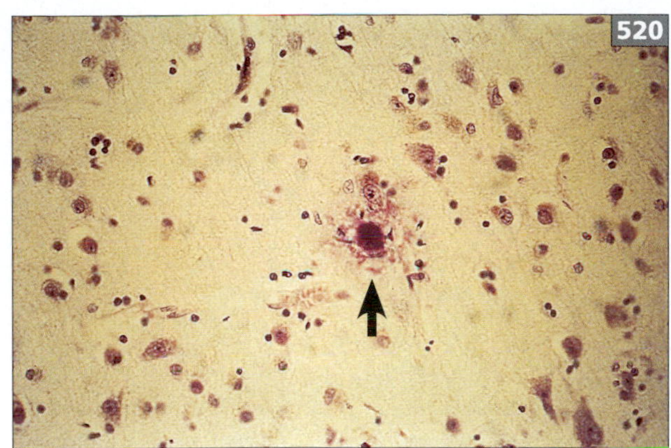

520 Microscopic section of cerebral cortex, cresyl violet stain, showing neuronal loss and an extracellular senile or 'neuritic' plaque containing a homogeneous central core of amyloid (arrow).

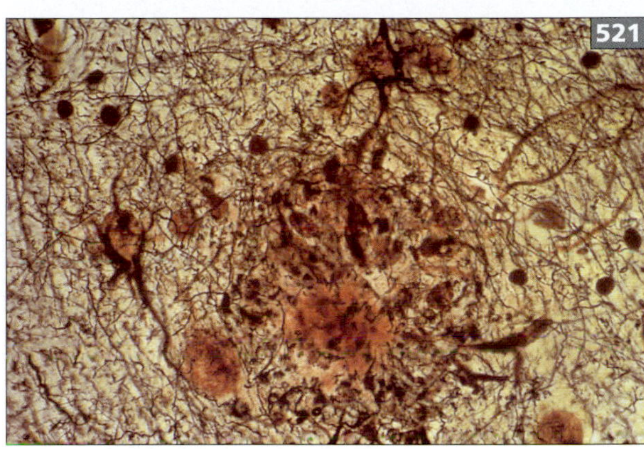

521 Microscopic section of cerebral cortex, silver stain, showing an extracellular senile or 'neuritic' plaque as a deposit of amorphous material with a central core of amyloid surrounded by numerous short fibrils (resembling a bird's nest) that represent products of degenerated nerve terminals, mainly dendritic, containing lysosomes, abnormal mitochondria, and often twisted tubules.

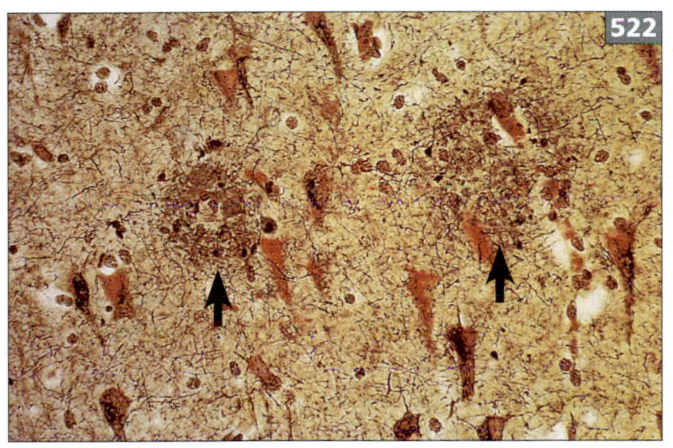

522 Microscopic section of cerebral cortex, Cajal stain, showing two senile or 'neuritic' plaques (arrows).

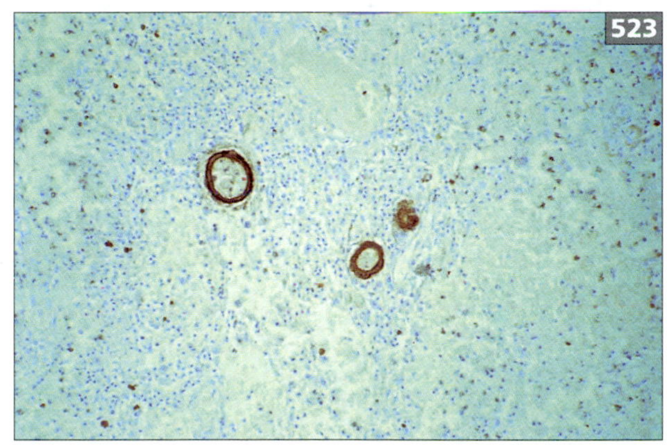

523 Amyloid in the walls of small blood vessels near senile plaques (amyloid or congophilic angiopathy).

In addition, there must be no evidence of an alternate medical cause for the symptoms. In most centers that specialize in AD, the accuracy of diagnosis approaches 90%. The addition of neuroimaging and PET scanning may improve the diagnostic accuracy. Newer diagnostic tests, such as measurement of tau and Aβ42 in the CSF, and PET scans that use radioactive tracers to label amyloid plaques (currently experimental) may provide further confidence in the diagnosis[6].

'Definite AD' is determined only by histology. This diagnosis relies on quantitative and qualitative features that define the presence, location, and number of Aβ plaques and neurofibrillary tangles (NFTs), the pathognomonic histopathologic features of AD.

Pathology

Macroscopically brain atrophy is present: narrowed cerebral convolutions and widened cerebral sulci, enlarged third and lateral ventricles (hydrocephalus ex vacuo). Microscopic pathology shows senile (neuritic) plaques and NFTs.

Plaques (520–523) are large extracellular lesions in which the principal component of the core of the plaque is the insoluble 42–43 amino acid peptide Aβ protein, which is a breakdown product of APP. Plaques result from the accumulation of several proteins and an inflammatory reaction around deposits of Aβ. Amyloid burden and the number of plaques do not correlate directly with the severity of clinical disease.

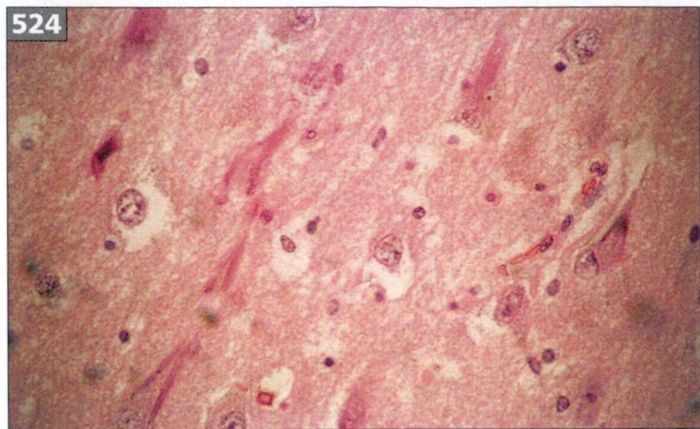

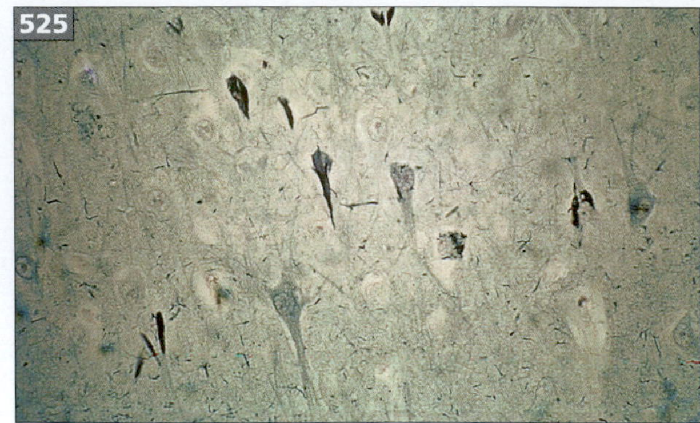

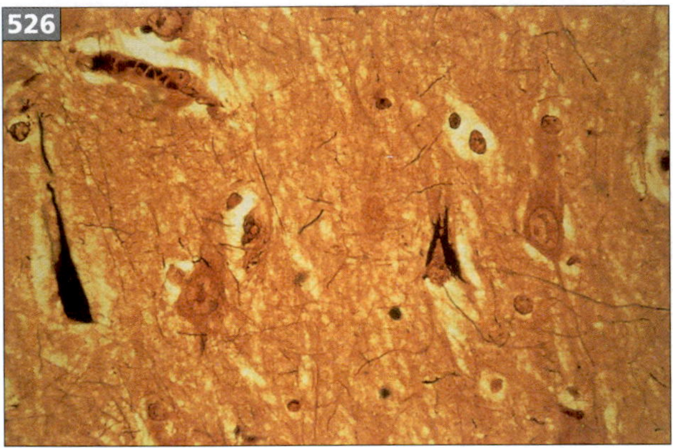

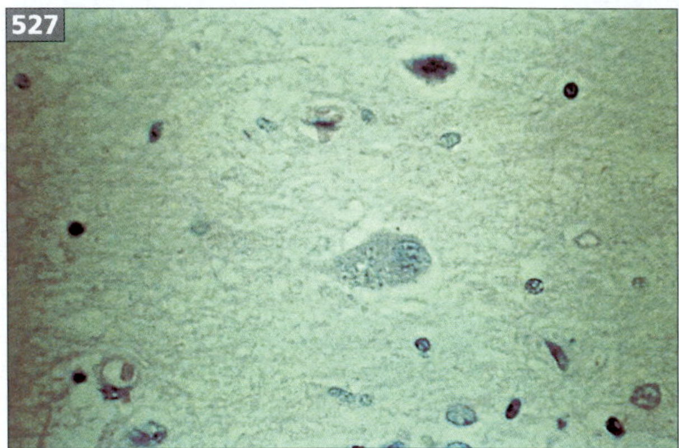

524–526 **Microscopic sections of brain, showing neurofibrillary tangles as thick, fiber-like strands of silver-staining material, often in the form of loops, coils, or tangled masses in the nerve cell cytoplasm.**

527 **Microscopic section of brain, showing granulovacuolar degeneration of neurons in the pyramidal layer of the hippocampus.**

NFTs (**524–527**) are intracellular lesions principally composed of aggregations of an abnormal form of a cytoskeletal-associated microtubular protein, tau, which is hyperphosphorylated. The aggregated neurofibrils are visualized as paired helical filaments on electron microscopy. They are present, together with plaques, in the projection neurons of the limbic and association areas of the cerebral cortex, particularly the parietal cortex and hippocampus, especially the CA1 zone and the entorhinal cortex, subiculum, and transitional cortex of the hippocampus.

The number of tangles increases with the duration and severity of disease. Tangles are not specific for AD, as they are also found in other conditions such as dementia pugilistica, subacute sclerosing panencephalitis (SSPE), tuberous sclerosis, and FTD, among others.

Dystrophic neurites are found, together with loss of neocortical neurons (>40%). Loss is widespread (hippocampus, entorhinal cortex, association areas of neocortex, and nucleus basalis of Meynert [the substantia innominata] and locus ceruleus) and predominantly a loss of cholinergic, noradrenergic, and dopaminergic neurons. There is loss of neuronal synapses, assessed using antibodies to synaptic proteins such as synaptophysin. The degree of synaptic loss best correlates with the severity of dementia.

Chemical pathology

A cholinergic deficit is found secondary to degeneration of subcortical neurons (e.g. in the basal nucleus of Meynert) which project to the cortex and hippocampus. Alterations in some neurotrophic factors, especially brain-derived nerve growth factor (BDNF) and nerve growth factor (NGF), important protective chemicals for the survival of cholinergic cells, are thought to contribute to this degeneration.

Diminution of monoaminergic neurons and noradrenergic, gamma aminobutyric acid (GABA)ergic, and serotonergic functions occurs in affected neocortex, along with decreased neuropeptide transmitters, including substance P, somatostatin, and cholecystokinin.

Treatment

At present, treatment is primarily symptomatic and not curative; however, several treatments geared towards disease modification are currently under development in phase II or phase III clinical trials. Targeting Aβ has been the principal focus of investigational therapies, particularly using monoclonal antibodies against this peptide[7]. Thus far, efficacy has not been demonstrated in mild to moderate AD, although administration at earlier time points, such as during MCI or even a 'prodromal' stage of AD, as predicted by amyloid-detecting PET scans, is being considered as a more effective strategy.

For dementia, compensatory strategies can be taught to patients in the early stages of AD, including note-taking, posting a calendar, and carrying a date book.

Acetylcholinesterase inhibitors

Acetylcholinesterase inhibitors (donepezil, rivastigmine, and galantamine) are used as symptomatic treatment of cognitive and behavioral manifestations in mild to moderate dementia of Alzheimer's type. Donepezil has been approved for all stages of Alzheimer's dementia and rivastigmine has also been approved for Parkinson-related dementia[8,9]. These drugs inhibit acetylcholinesterase and act to decrease acetylcholine breakdown in the synapse. These drugs do not affect the underlying pathophysiologic disease process. Efficacy is generally similar among all of these agents, which amounts to approximately 6–12 months' delay in the course of the disease after 30 weeks' treatment in about two-thirds of the patients with mild to moderate AD.

Donepezil was approved in the USA and UK in 1997. It is easily administered in a once-a-day dose, and has a favorable adverse effect profile and simplified compliance, prescribing, and monitoring. The drug is started at a dose of 5 mg once daily, generally administered at night to avoid some the potential side-effects, for the first 4–6 weeks. The dose can then be increased to 10 mg once daily if the lower dose is well tolerated. Nausea and diarrhea may occur in up to 15% and vomiting in less than 10%. These effects are generally transient, occurring on initiation or up-titration of the drug and tend to recede. If they do not subside, a rest from the medication or a reduction in dose for 1–2 weeks may be necessary and then the dose can be increased again, often without recurrence of side-effects. Other symptoms may include headache, fatigue (8%), insomnia, dizziness (8%), muscle cramps (8%), agitation, hallucinations, unpleasant dreams, and urinary urgency. The drug can also be administered in the morning and may be appropriate in patients with insomnia or vivid dreams. The drug should be used with caution in patients with supraventricular conduction abnormalities, peptic ulcers, and obstructive airway disease. Recently, a 25 mg dose formulation has been made available for late-stage AD. The benefits are minimal and the degree of gastrointestinal side-effects may overshadow the benefits.

Rivastigmine is a pseudo-irreversible acetyl-butyryl-cholinesterase inhibitor selective for the central nervous system (CNS) and has regional selectivity within the brain for the cortex and hippocampus[10]. Dosage is initially 1.5 mg orally twice daily for a minimum of 2 weeks, at which point the dose can be increased by 1.5 mg twice daily every 4 weeks if well tolerated. The patient should be maintained on the highest dose tolerated, up to a maximum of 6 mg twice daily. Adverse effects include nausea (47%), vomiting (31%), diarrhea (19%), headaches (17%), dizziness (21%), and abdominal pain (13%) with 6–12 mg per day. These are usually transient and minimized by gradual titration and administration with food. To offset some of the gastrointestinal side-effects, this drug is now available in patch form. The patch is applied daily. A 4.6 mg dose patch is used to initiate therapy, and after 4–6 weeks, a 9.5 mg patch is applied daily

Galantamine reversibly and competitively inhibits acetylcholinesterase and enhances the response of nicotinic receptors to acetylcholine[11]. Galantamine is available in 4 mg and 8 mg, with a liquid preparation (4 mg/ml), which is useful for titration. The dose can be titrated from 4 mg twice daily to 8 mg twice daily over 4 weeks according to tolerance and benefit, but patients with hepatic impairment should be started with 4 mg daily. Galantamine is contraindicated in patients with severe renal impairment, but no dose adjustment is required for mild to moderate renal impairment (creatinine clearance rate greater than 9 ml/min). It is well tolerated. With 8 mg daily, most adverse effects occur in the first 4 weeks: nausea (6%), vomiting (4%), diarrhea (5%), anorexia (6%), and agitation (15%). A long-acting form of galantamine is now also available that can be given once a day.

If cholinesterase inhibitors are used, they should be given within the first 5 years of the disease, while the patient is still functioning and independent. The main goal of these medications is to delay some end-points associated with AD, including the need for outside caregiver or placement in a nursing home or other facility.

Possible neuroprotective agents

- Memantine: *N*-methyl- D-aspartate (NMDA) receptor antagonist that prevents excess glutamate from binding to NMDA receptors[12].
- Selegiline (10 mg per day): a monoamine oxidase B inhibitor that also facilitates catecholaminergic activity.
- Vitamin E: an antioxidant that traps oxygen free radicals. While vitamin E was shown to be protective

against AD in a large prospective study, more recent evidence using meta-analysis data showed that high doses of vitamin E may cause unexplained death in the elderly. As such, rather than the initial 2000 IU a day that was shown effective for AD, most clinicians suggest a lower dose in the order of 400–600 IU per day, although it is not clear that this dose is of any benefit. Vitamin E may interact with warfarin and lead to bleeding problems. Vitamin C in combination with vitamin E has also been shown to provide some protection, although studies are limited in scope.

Symptomatic treatment

Depression can coexist with AD, and should be treated appropriately (i.e. supportive counseling and, if necessary, antidepressant drug therapy). Selective serotonin reuptake inhibitors (SSRIs) are the preferred choice because of their relatively short half-lives and minimal anticholinergic, adrenergic, and histaminic adverse effects; tricyclic antidepressants may aggravate AD based on their anticholinergic effect.

Behavioral manifestations are often very difficult to treat, and for many behaviors initiation of one of the cholinesterase inhibitors may demonstrate an improvement. Acute behaviors on top of chronic behaviors may relate to an underlying medical condition and, as such, physical symptoms or iatrogenic factors should be sought out and corrected. Infection of either the bladder or lungs often causes a marked change in behavior in patients with AD. Overmedication, or the lack of administration of prescribed medications, may also produce new behavioral symptoms.

Pharmacologic treatment of behavioral symptoms should be reserved for drug responsive symptoms that are causing at least moderate distress to the patient primarily. While hallucinations may be concerning for caregivers, if they are not causing the patient distress, pharmacologic treatment should be witheld. Overall, the best practice is to limit the number of medications or maintain the lowest doses possible, in order to minimize the potential side-effects.

Newer antipsychotic agents such as risperidone, olanzapine, and quetiapine, have very few anticholinergic or extrapyramidal side-effects, and appear to be at least as effective as conventional neuroleptics for those symptoms that might be treatable by neuroleptics. However, these drugs now carry a black box warning in that they have been associated with a higher risk of sudden death and/or stroke in elderly patients with dementia. First-line therapy is education of the caregivers in how to deal with difficult behaviors expressed by the patient. Often, with education by a social worker or nurse experienced in AD, caregivers and family members can learn how to diffuse situations that precipitate aggressive or agitated behaviors.

Tip

▶ *The best management of the behavioral manifestations of AD involves behavior management and training of the caregiver. A negative reaction to the patient's behavior escalates problematic behaviors. A calming, supportive, and reassuring voice that is nonconfrontational works best.*

Prevention

Multiple epidemiologic studies have linked various drug therapies or behaviors with a reduced risk of AD; however, not all have been proven. An example is estrogen replacement therapy, which by epidemiologic assessment appeared to show that this was protective, and reduced the risk and delayed the onset of AD in post-menopausal women. However, randomized trial of estrogen replacement did not bear those findings out and, in some studies, estrogen replacement was associated with an increased risk of AD[13]. Similar studies linking cholesterol-lowering agents, such as simvastatin, with a reduced risk of AD in later life was borne out by prospective studies[14]. A larger study is currently ongoing to test this theory.

There is also insufficient evidence to support the use of antioxidants, anti-inflammatory agents, monoamine oxidase B inhibitors, folic acid, or antihypertensive drugs.

An emerging field is developing to promote healthy life-style and reduce the risk of AD. This field is related to diet, physical exercise and 'brain exercise'. Laboratory rodents that are genetically engineered to develop AD had a significant delay in the onset of disease when their cage was enriched with apparatus to increase their activities, in addition to physical activity. The pathology of disease was clearly delayed by these modifications. Clinical studies have also suggested daily exercise in the form of a brisk walk for 30 minutes or other aerobic exercise might enhance cognitive abilities and reduce the risk for AD.

Omega-3 fatty acids in the diet are heart-healthy and appear also to be beneficial for brain health, and are currently promoted as a way to reduce the risk for developing cognitive impairment in AD. It is still not clear whether challenging the brain with puzzles such as crossword puzzles, Sudoku, word jumbles, word searches, or a variety of other brain exercises that are promoted commercially, are beneficial. However, these can be recommended without concern.

Prognosis

Upon initial presentation and diagnosis of AD, cognitive deficits may be relatively circumscribed and related primarily to memory along with some other minor features in other cognitive domains. However, as the disease progresses, the impairment becomes more generalized to involve all cognitive domains. The average survival after diagnosis ranges from 5 to 20 years.

FRONTOTEMPORAL DEMENTIA (FTD)

Definition

The frontotemporal dementias are a group of neurodegenerative disorders characterized pathologically by anterior frontal and/or temporal lobe degeneration, and clinically by progressive decline in behavior and/or language that begins at a relatively young age. Microscopically, in general, there is neuron loss, astrocytic gliosis, and sometimes intraneuronal inclusions of tau, ubiquitin, and/or TAR-DNA binding protein (TDP-43).

The classification of FTD is still evolving. It has been complicated by the recognition that several diseases once thought to be distinct entities (e.g. Pick's disease and primary progressive aphasia [PPA]) and a single disease that is now split into three subtypes (i.e. PPA) all belong to this family of diseases. A further complication is that several pathologic subtypes (inclusions of tau, ubiquitin, and TDP-43) contribute to the FTDs. Currently, FTD is classified into three major clinical syndromes, including:

- Behavioral variant of FTD (bvFTD).
- Semantic dementia (semantic variant [SV] of PPA) (SD).
- Progressive nonfluent aphasia (PNFA) (nonfluent variant of PPA).

The presence of common pathologies associated with the FTDs has led to the classification of the frontotemporal complex of diseases, also labeled frontotemporal lobar degeneration (FTLD) subtypes:

- Ubiquitin and TDP-43 inclusions, linked to FTLD with motor neuron disease (FTLD-MND or frontotemporal lobar degeneration with amyotrophic lateral sclerosis [FTLD-ALS]).
- Tau pathology linked to:
  - Corticobasal degeneration (CBD).
  - Progressive supranuclear palsy (PSP)[15].

Epidemiology

FTDs are estimated to account for up to 10–20% of all cases of dementias, and they may be the most common dementia that affects patients under the age of 60[16].

- Prevalence is unknown.
- Onset is typically between the ages of 50 and 65; however, the disorder has been observed in patients as young as 21 and as old as 80 years.
- Females and males are equally affected.

The rate of progression is variable with some progressing to dementia over a course of more than 10–15 years, while others may proceed within a few years. In those with concomitant motor neuron disease, the time to death tends to be short, secondary to the more common sequelae of swallowing difficulty and aspiration pneumonia.

Etiology and pathophysiology

Approximately 40–60% of cases are familial. Of these, up to 25% will have a history suggesting an autosomal dominant inheritance pattern; however, 20–40% show instead a polygenic familial inheritance pattern.

At least four genes are associated with FTDs[17–21]:

- *MAPτ* gene on chromosome 17q21–22, encoding the tau protein.
- TAR-DNA binding protein gene (*TDP-43*), on chromosome 1p36.2.
- Progranulin (*GRN*), on chromosome 17q21.32.
- *C9orf72* gene, on the short arm of chromosome 9 that encodes an unknown protein.

Less than 50% of FTD cases are considered tauopathies (FTLD-TAU), based on the presence of NFTs.

FTLD-U are FTDs that demonstrate cytoplasmic or nuclear inclusions that are immunoreactive to ubiquitin. A major constituent of ubiquitin inclusions is *TDP-43*.

Mutations within *GRN* have been associated with the ubiquitin- and *TDP-43*-positive cases that show inheritance.

A hexanucleotide repeat expansion (GGGGCC) greater than the normal length of 30 (up to hundreds) of the *C9orf72* gene is linked to familial FTD and ALS .

Clinical features

- Gradual onset, frequently beginning in the mid 50s to 60s.
- Marked by a range of behavioral, personality, and cognitive changes, and sometimes motor signs.
- Behavioral changes (especially with bvFTD):
  - Changes in personality, flattened affect, loss of empathy.
  - Less involved in routine daily activities, and tend to withdraw emotionally from others.
  - Increasingly inappropriate social behavior, e.g. swearing, overeating or drinking, impulsivity, shoplifting, hypersexual behavior, and poor personal hygiene.
  - Little insight into evolving behavior changes with little or no concern for the effect.
  - Some may perform stereotyped obsessive compulsive disorder (OCD)-like behaviors such as hand clapping, walking to the same place every day, and so on.
- Language changes:
  - Problems with expression of language or severe naming difficulty (e.g. PNFA).
  - Problems with word meaning (e.g. SD or svPPA).

- Cognitive and emotional symptoms: affect the patient's ability to perform complex thinking and reasoning as demonstrated by impairment in 'executive functions'– the ability to plan, organize, and execute activities:
  - Distractibility and impersistence: losing train of thought.
  - Mental rigidity and inflexibility.
  - Planning and problem solving impairments.
  - Poor financial judgment, impulsive spending.
  - Abulia: reduced initiative.
  - Frequent mood changes.
- Motor signs:
  - Parkinsonism: shuffling gait, rigidity, bradykinesia, pseudocontractures of limbs; more common in families with exon 10 *MAPT* mutations, causing selective overproduction of 4-repeat tau isoforms.
  - Dystonia unrelated to medications.
  - Upper or lower motor neuron dysfunction.
  - Myoclonus.
  - Postural or action tremor.
  - Dysphagia/dysarthria.
  - Eyelid opening and closing apraxia.

Behavioral variant FTD (bvFTD)

Progressive deterioration in the ability to control or adjust behavior to different social situations that result in inappropriate social behavior.

- Hyperoral.
- Stereotyped and/or repetitive behavior.
- Poor personal hygiene.
- Hyperactivity: pacing, wandering, outbursts of frustration, aggression.
- Hypersexuality.
- Impulsivity.
- Apathy.
- Lack of insight.
- Emotional blunting.
- Frequent mood changes.

Semantic dementia (SD)

Also known as temporal variant of FTD (tvFTD) or svPPA, SD patients often complain of word-finding difficulties. Most commonly, patients present with difficulty generating or recalling familiar words.

- Lose ability to recognize the meaning of words or recognize words within similar categories.
- Fluency is spared – patients may present with circumlocution early in the disease.
- Word finding pauses become common with difficulty naming in later stages of SD.
- Some may have problems recognizing familiar objects and faces; this can help to confirm the diagnosis. This presentation is associated with disease that starts in the right temporal lobe, in contrast to the more common left-sided involvement, that affects language first.

Progressive nonfluent aphasia (PFNA)

Also known as nonfluent variant of PPA.

- Hesitant, effortful speech.
- Patient's ability to comprehend is preserved longer than the ability to produce speech.
- Eventual decline in reading and writing.
- May also have difficulty swallowing or apraxia of speech.

Corticobasal degeneration (CBD)

- May present with cognitive changes (not seen in all patients).
- Frontal lobe features are evident[22].
- Alien limb syndrome: the patient does not recognize the actions of their limb and cannot control its movement.
- Apraxia.
- Acalculia.
- Visuospatial impairment.
- Motor symptoms: akinesia/bradykinesia, rigidity, tremor, limb dystonia, all of which are more prominent unilaterally.
- Language symptoms: hesitant and halting speech in some patients.

FTD-motor neuron disease (FTD-MND or FTD-ALS)

- Patients can experience similar behavior and language symptoms associated with the other FTD syndromes.
- Motor symptoms: arising from the motor neuron and are similar to those seen in ALS. Not all symptoms are seen in every patient, but may include:
  - Muscle weakness which can include the arms, legs, face, tongue, or neck.
  - Clumsiness, tripping or falling due to weak or stiff legs.
  - Shortness of breath.
  - Muscle atrophy, fasciculations, muscle cramps.
  - Dysphagia.
  - Dysarthria.
  - Spasticity.
  - Hyper-reflexia.
  - Pseudobulbar affect: uncontrollable outbursts of laughing or crying.

Pick's disease

Older terminology, linked to a disease with prominent behavioral features most comparable to current designation of bvFTD. They may or may not experience language abnormalities. Distinguished by the pathology that shows 'Pick bodies' (see Pathology section).

Progessive supranuclear palsy (PSP)[15]

- Patients have difficulty coordinating eye movements: this is the most distinguishing and earliest symptom, manifested as difficulty with voluntary vertical gaze, especially downward gaze.
- Impaired balance and stability.
- Slowness and stiffness of movement.
- Posture generally upright, if not hyperextended, in contrast to flexed posture of Parkinson's disease (PD).
- Dysphagia.
- Dysarthria.
- Alterations of mood and behavior.
- Later in the course of the disease, patients may develop behavioral symptoms such as those seen in bvFTD, but usually milder.

Differential diagnosis

- AD.
- DLB.
- Alcoholic dementia.
- HD.
- CJD.
- Gerstmann–Straussler–Scheinker (GSS) disease.
- Depression.
- Mania.
- Schizophrenia.
- OCD.

Investigations

- Laboratory evaluation: includes testing to rule out other metabolic and infectious causes of dementia – TSH, vitamin B12, HIV, RPR, complete blood count, complete medical panel, as usual for dementia work-up.
- Paraneoplastic panel may be warranted in some individuals, to rule out an autoimmune process related to an occult malignancy.
- Neuropsychologic evaluation: to document frontal and temporal lobe dysfunction.
- Frontal assessment battery: six tasks that assess frontal lobe performance, and may be helpful as a screening tool, although its benefit in distinguishing early AD from early FTD has been challenged.
- MRI of the brain: bilateral or asymmetric atrophy of the cortex and white matter of the frontal and/or temporal lobes (bvFTD), or temporal lobes in isolation (SD), perisylvian atrophy (PNFA), and paracentral gyrus (FTD-MND), may be observed, in addition to enlarged ventricles secondary to cortical and subcortical atrophy. These signs are not always evident on initial scan and vary considerably among the different FTD subtypes (**528, 529**). Coronal section through the hippocampus may best visualize temporal atrophy, while sagittal or axial images demonstrate frontal atrophy.
- Dynamic/functional neuroimaging: PET imaging may show decreased metabolic activity (uptake of fluoro-deoxyglucose) in affected areas of frontal and temporal regions, in contrast to the temporoparietal hypometabolism seen in AD (**530**).
- EEG: normal or nonspecific slowing.
- Electromyography (EMG): FTD-MND may show findings similar to those seen in ALS.

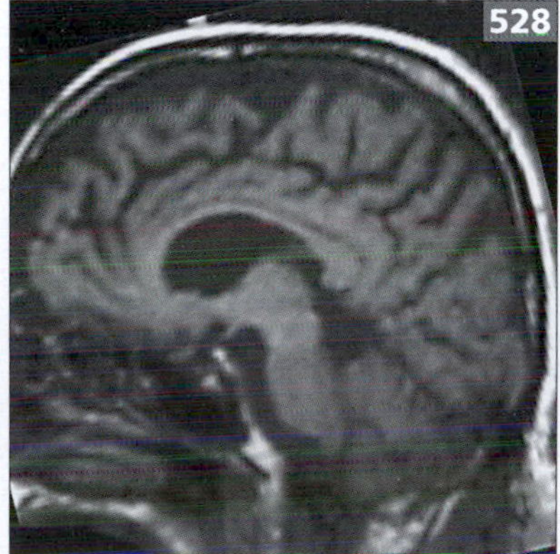

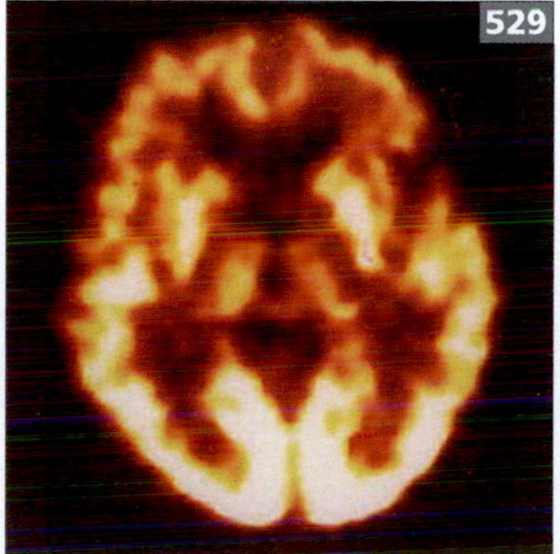

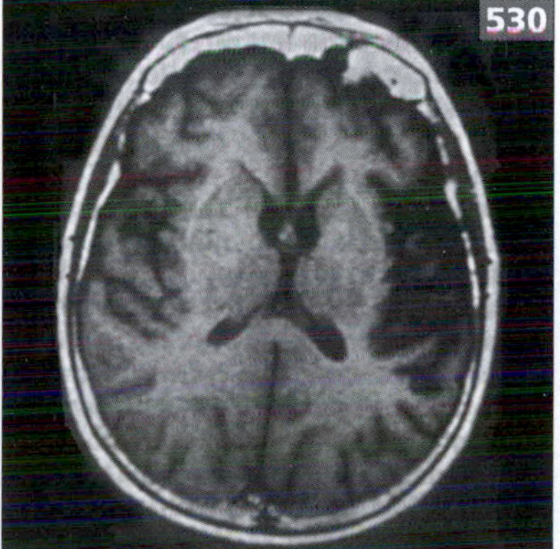

528–530 Brain imaging in FTD. (528) MRI of FTD, showing prominent atrophy of frontal lobe. While a useful diagnostic marker, this finding may be subtle or absent in the early presentation of disease; (529) positron emission tomography (PET) of FTD case displays frontotemporal hypometabolism following radiolabeled fluoro-deoxyglucose injection; (530) a case of primary progressive aphasia, demonstrating focal left perisylvian and temporal lobe atrophy.

Tip

▶ *The neuropsychologic assessment should be focused on distinguishing frontal lobe features (language, executive function, attentional tasks) relative to visuospatial abilities, a parietal function.*

Diagnosis

Diagnosis is made on medical history, detailed neurologic examination, and neuropsychologic pattern of deficits consistent with one of the above syndromes. Neuropathologic diagnosis is determined through autopsy.

Pathology

Underlying pathology varies with the particular subtype of FTD/FTLD. A consistent feature is lack of typical AD pathology. Macroscopic changes include atrophy, with decreased brain weight and frontotemporal atrophy that is most severe in the mesial and temporal area (**531**).

In the subtype FTD-MND (or FTD-ALS), atrophy of the motor strip has been noted on gross examination. Atrophy less frequently affects the hippocampus and parietal lobes. There is a thinned cortical ribbon of affected gyri, with some evidence of left perisylvian atrophy in those with PFNA. Enlarged ventricles and thickened overlying pia–arachnoid are present.

Microscopic pathology is dependent upon the particular subtype, but the following pathologies may be seen[15]:

- Varying degrees of neuronal loss and astrocytosis in the frontal and temporal lobes – most marked in the first three cortical layers with characteristic superficial spongy change in the second layer of the cortex.
- Neuronal loss in the basal ganglia and substantia nigra.
- Loss of medullated fibers in the affected subcortical white matter.
- Astrocytic gliosis of the cortex and subcortical white matter tracts.
- NFTs composed of tau protein found in both neuronal and glial cells (**532**).
- Pick cells: swollen (ballooned or chromatolytic-appearing) neurons found randomly scattered throughout the cortex (**533**).
- Pick bodies: argyrophilic intracytoplasmic inclusions found most frequently in the mesial temporal lobes. They are both tau and ubiquitin positive (**534**, **535**).
- Intranuclear inclusions containing ubiquitin and TDP-43 in FTLD-U diseases, such as FTD-MND, although these are also seen in other forms of FTD.
- Senile plaques are not present.

Treatment

No specific treatment is available to slow or reverse the progression of FTD. Caregiver education regarding the nature of the disease is key to management. Family members should be counseled on how to manage behavioral improprieties, impulsivity, and so on. Support groups for family members should be offered as a mechanism to learn behavioral management techniques.

Early speech therapy and assistive devices may be useful in patients with predominant language difficulties.

Symptomatic treatment:

- Cholinesterase inhibitors, such as donepezil, galantamine, or rivastigmine, have not shown benefit for FTD.
- The role of memantine in FTD is currently under study.
- Behavioral abnormalities, including apathy, depression, and social withdrawal may benefit from SSRIs.
- Parkinsonian features including bradykinesia/akinesia, rigidity, tremor, and limb dystonia may benefit from:
  - L-dopa – start with carbidopa/levodopa 25/100 mg three times a day and titrate upward very slowly. Benefit may not be significant and hallucinations and worsening behavior should be monitored.
  - Other dopaminergics, such as ropinorole, pergolide, or pramipexole, may also be tried, at low doses.

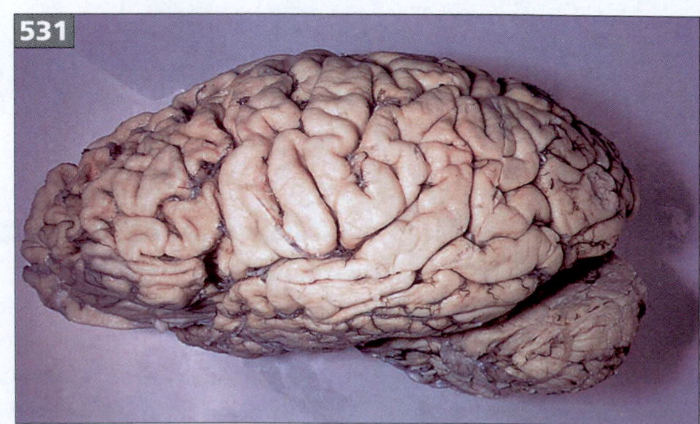

531 Gross brain atrophy in frontal and temporal lobes seen in FTD.

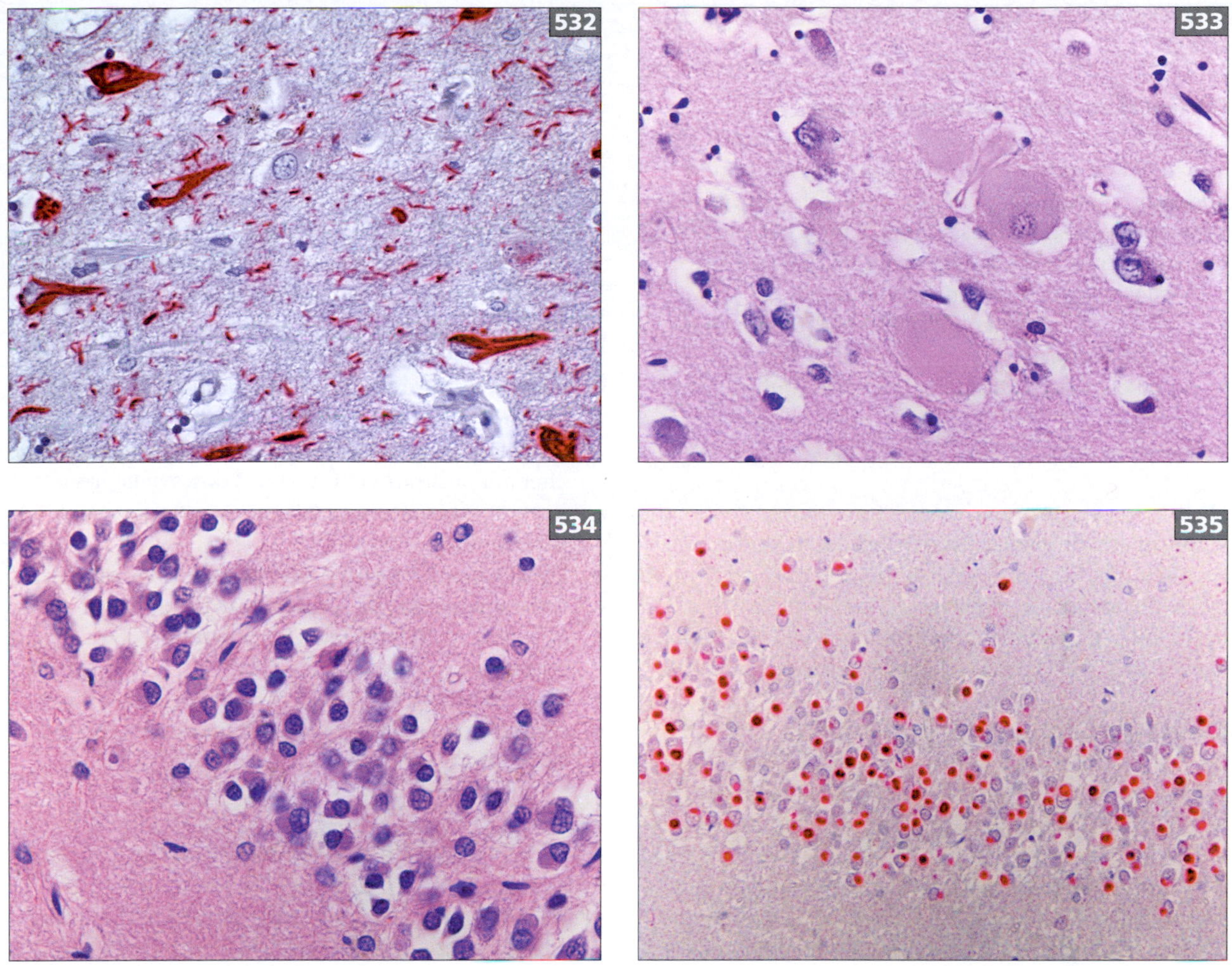

532–535 Histopathologies associated with FTDs. (532) Immunohistochemical staining of the hippocampal pyramidal cell layer for tau shows flame-shaped intracytoplasmic inclusions referred to as neurofibrillary tangles; (533) H&E stained section of temporal neocortex showing cortical neurons with expanded, abnormally pale, pink cytoplasm that corresponds to abnormal aggregation of neurofilament and causes the morphologic appearance of ballooned neurons that are also referred to in the case of Pick's disease; (534) H&E stained section of the dentate granular neurons in the hippocampal formation showing discrete, rounded pink inclusions in the cytoplasm of several cells (Pick bodies); (535) Immunohistochemical staining of the same area for tau highlights the presence of abundant rounded cytoplasmic inclusions (Pick bodies). *Courtesy of Peter Pytel, University of Chicago.*

Prognosis

FTD is progressive, with extreme variability to end stage. Many patients eventually display akinetic mutism in the final stages. Loss of language function to the point of muteness is uncharacteristic of AD and a distinguishing feature of FTD. Patients with FTD-MND may progress faster than other forms of FTD, because of the effects on motor and swallowing function. Patients with isolated PPA may show isolated language impairment, without global development of dementia in as many as 50% of affected individuals. Long-term prognosis is poor.

DEMENTIA WITH LEWY BODIES (DLB)

Definition and epidemiology

Dementia with Lewy bodies was first reported in 1961, as a separate entity from AD. Since recognition, it has undergone several modifications and refinements in the clinical diagnostic criteria, guided by a consortium of investigators. It is chiefly characterized clinically by:

- Visual hallucinations and/or delusions.
- Parkinsonism (axial rigidity and bradykinesia more so than tremor).
- Significant fluctuations in the level of confusion and alertness.
- Progressive dementia.

DLB is not uncommon, and is now recognized as the second most common cause of neurodegenerative dementia after AD, accounting for approximately 20% of all cases of dementia. In addition, Lewy bodies are found in up to 40% of AD cases. Onset is in the elderly, between ages 60 and 90. Males and females are equally affected.

Etiology and pathophysiology

DLB is complex and poorly understood. The features of disease are multifactorial. Motor symptoms likely result from the loss of dopamine-containing neurons within the substantia nigra, the key feature associated with Parkinson's disease. Cognitive dysfunction may be related to the loss of cholinergic neurons within the nucleus basalis of Meynert, as is typically present in AD. The presence of Lewy bodies in cortical layers V and VI likely impairs informational processing from neocortex to subcortical structures. Hallucinations may relate to early impairment in the parietal and occipital association cortices, which may also account for the predominance of visuospatial dysfunction in these patients compared with AD. The extreme fluctuations in alertness have not been explained.

Clinical features

The clinical presentation includes any combination of the following:

- Cognitive decline: cognitive impairment is present, affecting memory, language, visuospatial ability, praxis, and reasoning skills (e.g. early prominent attention deficits, disproportionate difficulties with problem solving, and visual–spatial–perceptual function). Cognitive impairment is persistent and progressive, but characterized by pronounced fluctuation, varying between lucid intervals and episodic confusion. Memory may be relatively spared in early stages compared to AD.
- Hallucinations: usually persistent, well-formed, visual hallucinations, may be accompanied by secondary paranoid delusions. Auditory hallucinations may occur.
- Fluctuating alertness: typically delirium-like, with recurrent falls and/or transient clouding or loss of consciousness. Episodes may last from a few minutes to several days.
- Extrapyramidal syndrome: mild akinetic–rigid parkinsonism occurs in some patients at presentation, but more commonly occurs later or after treatment with neuroleptic drugs. Overall, rest tremor is uncommon and axial features (postural instability, gait difficulty, facial immobility) are most common. Unusually, severe parkinsonism or sedation occurs after administration of standard doses of neuroleptic agents (patients are 'exquisitely' sensitive to neuroleptic agents).
- Dysautonomia: urinary incontinence (may precede, but more commonly soon follows the onset of cognitive decline), orthostatic hypotension, constipation.
- Sleep disorders: excessive daytime sleepiness, rapid eye movement (REM) sleep behavioral disorder may be present.

Tip

▶ *In contrast to the hallucinations of AD, hallucinations of DLB are described as 'benign', often consisting of children or animals. Patients often recognize that these are hallucinations, rather than believing they are real.*

Differential diagnosis

Cognitive decline

- AD: behavioral/psychiatric symptoms and urinary incontinence do not tend to occur early on in AD. Also, it tends not to show marked fluctuations in alertness. NFTs and senile neuritic plaques are common. More prominent signs of aphasia, apraxia, visuospatial abnormalities. May be frequently associated with mild parkinsonsism (6–92%).
- Parkinson's disease with or without dementia: Lewy bodies are predominantly subcortical in location (substantia nigra, locus ceruleus, substantia innominata, and dorsal motor nucleus of the vagus nerve), in contrast to DLB, where immunocytochemically similar Lewy bodies are more widespread and found in the neocortex as well as brainstem neurons.
- VaD: evidence of strokes on clinical examination and/or brain imaging.
- PSP: vertical gaze palsy present.

- NPH: gait dysfunction, urinary incontinence, then dementia.
- CJD: rapidly progressive cognitive decline and myoclonus.
- Fluctuating cognitive function: delirium due to drug toxicity (particularly anticholinergics or catecholaminergics) or intercurrent illness.

Repeated falls, syncope, and transient loss of consciousness

- Transient ischemic attacks.
- Cardiogenic:
  - Orthostatic hypotension.
  - Paroxysmal arrhythmia.
- Seizures.

Delusions and hallucinations

- Complex partial seizures.
- Delusional disorder (late paraphrenia).

Investigations

- Neuropsychologic testing: global cognitive dysfunction with marked impairment of tests sensitive to frontal lobe dysfunction.
- CT/MRI brain scan: normal or generalized cortical atrophy.
- Dopamine transporter imaging: may be able to distinguish DLB from AD, but not DLB from Parkinson's disease or multiple system atrophy (MSA).
- Other ancillary testing (PET, SPECT, EEG, MRI): see below.

Diagnosis

Definite diagnosis is pathologic/post mortem. According to continued revisions of the DLB consortium diagnostic criteria[23], allowing classification into possible and probable DLB.

Progressive cognitive decline of sufficient magnitude to interfere with normal social or occupational function is the central required feature. Prominent or persistent memory impairment may not necessarily occur in the early stages but is usually evident with progression. Deficits on tests of attention, executive function, and visuospatial ability may be especially prominent.

In addition, two of the following core features are essential for a diagnosis of probable DLB, and one is essential for possible DLB:

- Fluctuating cognition with pronounced variations in attention and alertness.
- May include daytime drowsiness/lethargy, daytime sleep >2 hours, staring into space for long periods, episodes of disorganized speech.
- Recurrent visual hallucinations that are typically well formed and detailed.
- Spontaneous motor features of parkinsonism (e.g. not secondary to drugs).

Features suggestive of the diagnosis (which, if one or more present in addition to one or more core features, can be made) include:

- Severe neuroleptic sensitivity (occurs in only ~50%).
- REM sleep behavioral disorder.
- SPECT/PET imaging demonstrating low dopamine transporter uptake in basal ganglia.

Features supportive of the diagnosis (not specific but commonly present) include:

- Unexplained, transient loss of consciousness.
- Repeated falls and syncope.
- Systematized delusions.
- Hallucinations in other modalities.

Ancillary test findings demonstrate:

- EEG: prominent slow-wave activity with temporal lobe sharp waves.
- Metaiodobenzylguanidine (MIBG) myocardial scintigraphy: low uptake.
- SPECT/PET perfusion scans: generalized low uptake, more prominent in posterior parietal and occipital regions.
- CT/MRI: relatively preserved medial temporal lobe structures.

A diagnosis of DLB is less likely in the presence of:

- Cerebrovascular disease, evident as focal neurologic signs or on brain imaging.
- Evidence of any physical illness or other brain disorder sufficient to account for the clinical picture.
- Parkinsonism occurring only in the setting of severe dementia.

Temporal sequence

Dementia occurs before or simultaneous with parkinsonism (if the latter is present). The co-occurrence of cognitive and motor features is defined by a '1-year rule', by which DLB is proposed to be distinguished from PD dementia (PDD); the phenotype of PDD is similar to DLB, but typically occurs after several years of well-established PD. However, it is generally recognized that the 1-year rule is arbitrary and difficult to apply in the clinical setting.

PDD and DLB may be seen as different points on a spectrum of Lewy body-related disease. The complex overlap between AD, DLB, and PD is illustrated in Figure 536.

Tip

▶ *PD, MSA, and DLB are all related to deposition of alpha-synuclein in the brain and are therefore sometimes called 'synucleinopathies'. The symptoms of these disorders have significant overlap, and they are often hard to differentiate from one another clinically*[32].

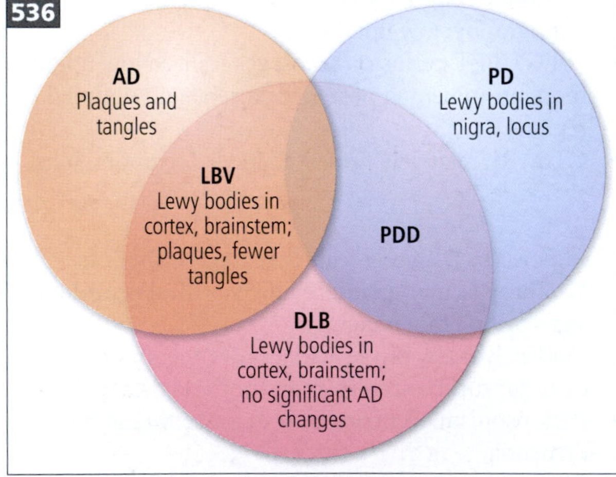

536 Relationship of DLB to Alzheimer's disease and Parkinson's disease. AD: Alzheimer's disease; DLB: Dementia with Lewy bodies; LBV: Lewy body variant of AD; PD: Parkinson's disease; PDD: Parkinson's disease with dementia. *Adapted from Weisman 2007, with permission.*

Pathology

DLB is defined pathologically by the presence of cortical Lewy bodies.

Essential for the pathologic diagnosis of DLB

Lewy bodies in the neocortex (temporal > frontal = parietal), limbic cortex (cingulate, entorhinal, amygdala), subcortical nuclei, and brainstem (as opposed to more prominent nigrostriatal and brainstem Lewy bodies associated with Parkinson's disease). Lewy bodies are intracytoplasmic, spherical, eosinophilic neuronal inclusions composed of abnormally ubiquinated neurofilament proteins (537–542). They are immunoreactive to ubiquitin (hence are more readily visualized with antiubiquitin immunocytochemical detection), and are surrogate markers of neuronal loss. Alpha-synuclein immunocytochemistry is potentially the most sensitive and specific technique for detecting and quantifying Lewy bodies and Lewy neurites.

Associated but not essential for the diagnosis of DLB

- Lewy-related neurites: found by means of ubiquitin staining in the hippocampus (CA2/3 region), amygdala, nucleus basalis of Meynert, dorsal vagal nucleus, and other brainstem nuclei. They are a neurofilament abnormality in which the proteins are present as a diffuse aggregate that does not contain crystallin.
- Plaques (all morphologic types). Senile neuritic plaques, often in similar numbers to those found in AD, and Aβ deposition are common.
- Neocortical NFTs are few or absent.
- Regional neuronal loss occurs, particularly in brainstem (substantia nigra and locus ceruleus) and nucleus basalis of Meynert. There is no evidence of significant neuronal loss in the hippocampus and medial temporal and frontal cortices.
- Microvacuolation (spongiform change) and synapse loss.
- Neurochemical abnormalities and neurotransmitter deficits.

The finding that as many as 60% of AD cases may meet criteria for DLB using the original DLB criteria has led to continued refinement in pathologic diagnosis. The most recent consensus criteria suggests assigning likelihoods of dementia attributed to AD pathology (using NIA-Reagan criteria) in addition to semiquantitative grading of Lewy body pathology. The relative predominance of each pathology may then be correlated to assess the overall likelihood that the pathologic findings are associated with a DLB clinical syndrome.

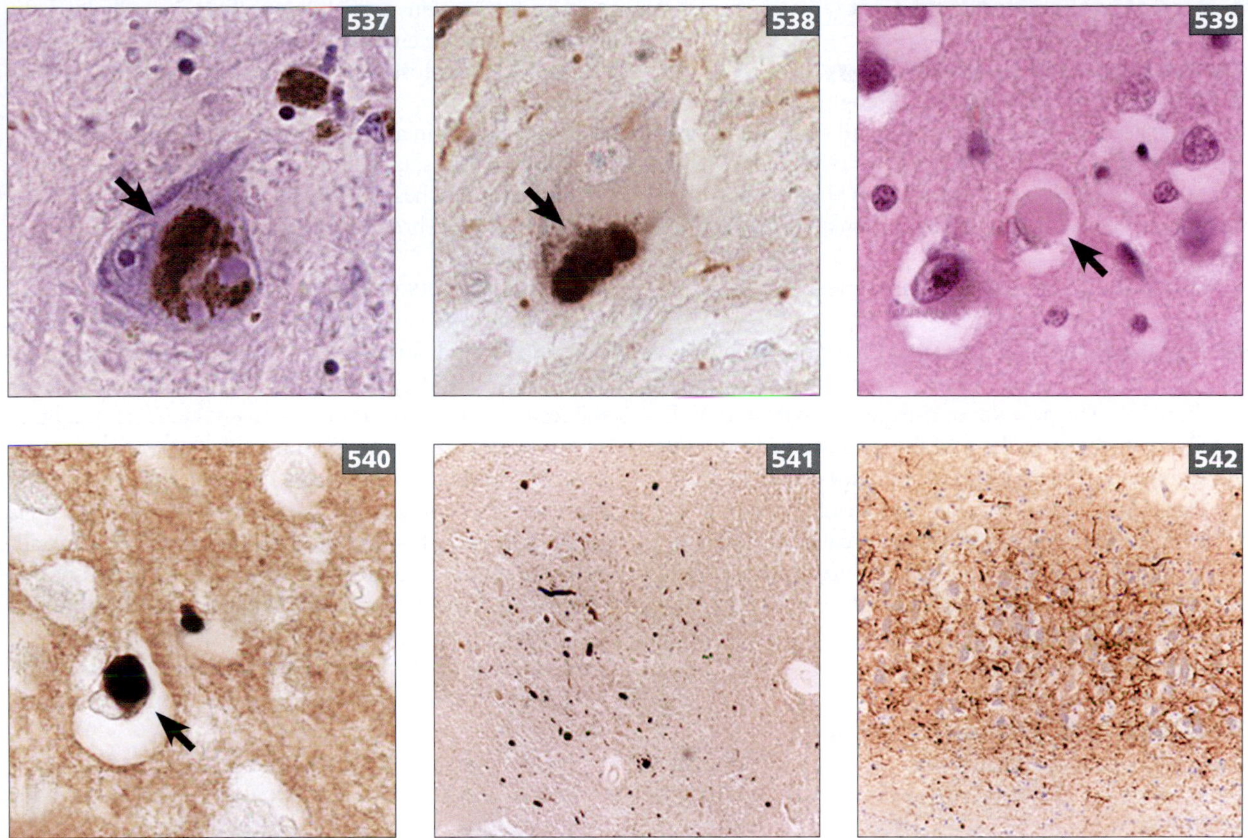

537–542 (537, 538) Multiple Lewy bodies in the same neuron of the substantia nigra (arrows); (539, 540) cortical Lewy bodies in the anterior cingulate cortex (arrows); (541) Lewy bodies and Lewy neurites in the dorsal motor nucleus of the vagus nerve; (542) numerous Lewy neurites in the CA 2–3 field of the hippocampus. (537, 539) haematoxylin–eosin staining; (538, 540, 541, 542) anti-alpha-synuclein immunostaining. *Reproduced from Kovari 2009, with permission.*

Treatment

Treatment is difficult, due to the combination of parkinsonism and neuropsychiatric features: improvement of one symptom is often achieved at the expense of the other. Levodopa may be cautiously and slowly introduced if motor features interfere with function, since it may worsen neuropsychiatric features.

Cholinesterase inhibitors may be effective and relatively safe for neuropsychiatric and cognitive symptoms. All drugs in this class may be effective but there is more evidence to support rivastigmine[24]. Drugs with anticholinergic properties should be avoided.

Antipsychotic drugs, often used as the first choice for psychiatric symptoms and behavioral disturbances in dementia, should also be avoided. DLB patients may develop a sensitivity reaction to these, resulting in exacerbation of motor and mental disability. If antipsychotic therapy is required, atypical agents (quetiapine, clozapine) with fewer extrapyramidal side-effects are preferred.

For REM sleep behavior disorder, clonazepam, melatonin, and cautious use of quetiapine are recommended. There are no systematic studies for treatment of depression in DLB, but SSRIs or seretonin–norepinephrine reuptake inhibitors (SNRIs) are probably preferred.

Prognosis

Progressive deterioration occurs over 5–8 years, with progressive parkinsonism, cognitive decline, and psychiatric symptoms.

VASCULAR DEMENTIA

Definition and epidemiology

VaD is an acquired syndrome of cognitive impairment characterized by the abrupt onset and stepwise progression of deficits of memory and at least two other cognitive functions sufficient to interfere with the person's usual social activities, and caused by vascular diseases of the brain.

- Incidence: 2.5 per 1000 nondemented individuals per year.
- Prevalence: in the Western world, the prevalence is ~1.5%, but slightly higher in Japan, at slightly more than 2%. The prevalence rises steeply with age. VaD accounts for up to 40% of dementia cases, and is the second most common cause of dementia after AD. Please note, however, that estimates of the prevalence of VaD may be unreliable because of different diagnostic and pathologic criteria used in different studies, and the co-occurrence of AD in many[25].
- Onset is in the elderly.
- Males are affected more than females.

Etiology and pathophysiology

The site of brain tissue loss is a more important determinant of cognitive function than the volume of tissue lost.

Single strategically placed infarcts or hemorrhages

A single infarct or hemorrhage, if located in a strategically important brain region, such as the circuits involving the dorsolateral frontal convexity–caudate nucleus–globus pallidus–thalamus, can produce a vascular-related dementia. Examples include:

- Dominant angular gyrus syndrome, from a lesion in the angular gyrus located within the inferior parietal lobule. This is classically characterized as 'Gerstmann's syndrome', which includes acalculia, agraphia, right–left confusion, and finger agnosia. An acute onset of this syndrome resulting from embolic occlusion of the angular branch of the inferior division of the middle cerebral artery may be accompanied by fluent aphasia, when Wernicke's area within the superior temporal gyrus is involved.
- Thalamus, particularly the dominant dorsomedial thalamus, resulting from occlusion of the paramedian thalamic (thalamoperforate) branches of the posterior cerebral artery, causing memory loss, slowness, apathy, ocular palsies, and drowsiness.
- Caudate nucleus and globus pallidus, usually by thrombotic or embolic occlusion of the penetrating lateral lenticulostriate branches of the middle cerebral artery.
- Basal forebrain and dorsolateral pre-frontal cortex.
- Hippocampus, usually by embolic occlusion of the cortical branches of the posterior cerebral artery, or diffuse cerebral ischemia.

Multiple infarcts or hemorrhages

Cortical/subcortical infarcts or hemorrhages may cause a 'cortical' type dementia with signs of amnesia, aphasia, apraxia, and agnosia. The infarcts are commonly the result of thromboembolism from the heart or a large artery (aortic arch, carotid, and vertebrobasilar) to the anterior, middle, or posterior cerebral arteries or their branches, but can also be caused by large vessel disease causing hypoperfusion and infarcts in the borderzones between major arterial territories, and small vessel disease such as microatheroma/lipohyalinosis and vasculitis. Multiple cortical hemorrhages are most commonly due to amyloid angiopathy but can also be seen with vasculitis, bleeding diatheses, metastases, hemorrhagic infarction, and trauma.

Small deep (lacunar) infarcts may cause a subcortical dementia characterized by psychomotor slowing, poor concentration, indecision, and mental apathy. Other features, besides cognitive impairment, include hemiparesis, small stepping gait (marche à petits pas), dysarthria, and dysphagia. Typical patients are elderly, ex- or current smokers, with hypertension and/or diabetes. Rarely, they are part of the syndrome of CADASIL, a hereditary disease linked to the *NOTCH3* gene on chromosome 19.

Diffuse white matter infarction

Also described as subcortical arteriosclerotic leukoencephalopathy, or Binswanger's disease. Occurs as diffuse or multifocal, often periventricular, areas of demyelination, axonal loss, and reactive gliosis in the white matter, probably due to anoxia as a result of arteriosclerotic changes (hyalinization, fibrosis, and thickening) in the long penetrating end arteries and arterioles of the periventricular white matter. White matter lesions are found in about 80% of patients with VaD, but also in about 15% of patients with early-onset AD, and as much as 75% of patients with late-onset AD. They are associated with hypertension and, in some studies, with heart disease and diabetes. They are thought to cause dementia by disconnecting the pathways between the cortical and subcortical areas[26]. Diffuse laminar necrosis (global cerebral ischemia) can also occur.

Vascular pathophysiology includes:

- Hypoxic–ischemic lesions:
  - Large artery atherosclerosis.
  - Small vessel hyaline wall thickening (arteriosclerosis), microatheroma, and lipohyalinosis.
  - Embolism from the heart.
  - Nonatheromatous angiopathies.
- Granular degeneration of the media of small arteries (CADASIL).
- Cerebral vasculitis.
- Neoplastic angioendotheliomatosis (malignant lymphoma of blood vessels).
- Mural dissections.
- Dural arteriovenous malformation.
- Hematologic disease (thrombophilia).
- Hemorrhagic lesions:
  - Subdural hematoma.
  - Subarachnoid hemorrhage: anterior communicating artery aneurysm.
  - Intracerebral hemorrhage: amyloid angiopathy; hypertensive small vessel disease.

Risk factors for vascular dementia

- Increasing age.
- Past history of stroke (symptomatic stroke increases the risk of dementia more than ninefold) or myocardial infarction (one-third of patients).

Other putatitive risk factors include:

- Hypertension (60% of patients).
- Smoking (35%).
- Diabetes (20% of patients).
- Hyperlipidemia (20%).
- Alcohol abuse.
- Family history (CADASIL).
- Cortical infarcts.
- Brain white matter lesions.
- Left hemisphere stroke.
- Early urinary incontinence.
- Falls.
- Abnormal electrocardiogram (ECG) (80% of patients compared with 30% of people with AD).

Clinical assessment

Slowly progressive intellectual impairment, with recurrent stroke-like events.

History

- Presenting symptoms: more commonly, sudden onset and stepwise course of cognitive decline with a history of transient ischemic attacks, strokes, or both. Epileptic seizures occur in 10% of patients. Incontinence of urine and stool is not uncommon.
- Past history of vascular risk factors: hypertension, diabetes, heart disease, smoking.
- Family history: CADASIL.

Neurologic examination

- Focal neurologic deficits such as pyramidal tract signs (hemiparesis, extensor plantar response, pseudobulbar palsy), extrapyramidal signs, hemisensory loss, hemianopsia, and dysarthria.
- Gait abnormality: start and turn hesitation, shuffling, reduced arm swing.
- Grasp reflexes.
- Hypertension and hypertensive retinopathy.
- A source of thromboembolism such as atrial fibrillation, valvular heart disease, heart failure, carotid artery disease.

Neuropsychologic examination

- Concentration and executive function: poor learning strategies, impaired word-list generation, emotional blunting and lability, poor insight and judgment.
- Memory: impaired learning of verbal and visual information, reduced recall following a delay, but better recognition memory (i.e. ability to pick correct items from a list).
- Verbal output: dysarthria, reduced grammatical complexity of spontaneous speech.
- Depression: present in 25% of patients; depressive symptoms in 60%.
- Anxiety: common.
- Delusions: may be present in up to one-half of patients.
- Personality alterations: apathetic, listless, lifeless, quiet, and labile.

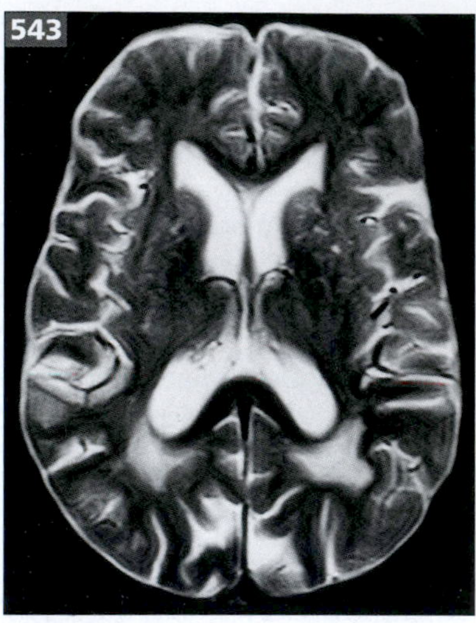

543 T2-weighted MRI in a 78-year-old woman with possible vascular dementia. Note the cerebral atrophy and the diffuse hyperintense areas adjacent to the frontal and posterior horns of the lateral ventricles, representing subcortical ischemic leukoencephalopathy.

544 T2-weighted MRI at the level of the lateral ventricles in a 75-year-old woman with cognitive impairment due to multi-infarct dementia. Note the atrophy and multiple hyperintense areas in the periventricular white matter.

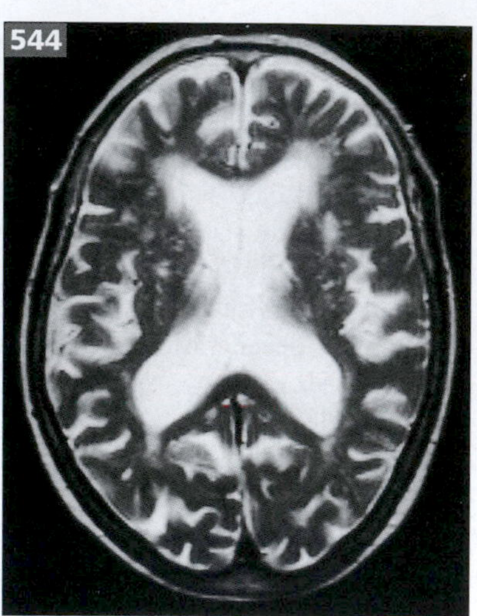

Differential diagnosis

- VaD and AD (mixed dementia).
- Clinical course may be slowly progressive and it may be difficult to interpret the relevance of brain lesions, consistent with infarction, seen on neuroimaging (e.g. white matter lesions).
- All conditions listed in 'Differential diagnosis' of AD pertain here.

Investigations

CT or MR imaging of the brain

Excludes other causes of dementia (e.g. frontal tumor, hydrocephalus) and almost always identifies one or more vascular lesions. These studies are important, as the diagnosis of VaD requires a significant burden of cerebrovascular disease to account for the cognitive disturbance present in the patient. CT brain scan reveals more or less symmetric periventricular and subcortical hypodensity in the cerebral white matter, with or without ventricular dilatation and focal hypodensities thought to be due to 'small vessel' ischemia and infarction.

MRI demonstrates high signal areas of infarction on T2-weighted, or fluid attenuated inversion recovery (FLAIR) imaging (**543, 544**). These radiological appearances (leukoaraiosis [leuko = white, ariosis = rarefaction]) are rather nonspecific and can be found in apparently normal elderly people. However, they are more commonly associated with gradual overall cognitive decline, unsteadiness of gait, and recurrent ischemic, particularly lacunar, or occasionally hemorrhagic, strokes. These changes are more frequent in patients with hypertension, other vascular risk factors, atherosclerosis, and cerebral atrophy. Additional features may include multiple infarcts in the basal ganglia and pons, or cortical infarcts.

Tip

▶ *A key to the diagnosis of VaD is the temporal correlation of strokes and/or brain imaging findings consistent with vascular insults and the dementia. In addition, the degree of white matter disease should be 'sufficient to account for the dementia'. This is sometimes difficult. Pairing the neuropsychologic test results (especially the prominence of retrieval deficits) with the imaging findings is often necessary.*

Blood tests

As described in the section on AD. With suspicion of VaD add:

- Lipid panel.
- Antinuclear antibodies.
- Serum protein electrophoresis.
- Coagulation studies (younger patients).
- Antiphospholipid antibodies.
- Proteins C and S.
- Antithrombin III.
- Factor V Leiden mutation.

Other tests

- ECG.
- Echocardiography: if prosthetic heart valves, rheumatic valvular heart disease, or suspected left atrial myxoma.
- Doppler ultrasonography of the carotid arteries.
- SPECT: asymmetric patchy areas of reduced cerebral blood flow.

Diagnosis

The clinical and laboratory assessments are used to establish the diagnosis of VaD, the cause of the cerebrovascular disease, and other factors that may be contributing to the cognitive compromise.

The diagnosis of VaD is based on a decline in cognitive function that has a clear temporal correlation with a history of strokes. However, the association between dementia and cerebrovascular disease may not be causal; it may be merely contributory or even coincidental. Various diagnostic criteria exist to aid the diagnosis but many have not been validated[27].

The Hachinski ischemia scale may have diagnostic value (*Table 94*). This includes a set of criteria that may distinguish between possible atherosclerotic causes of dementia and AD. A score of 7 or higher in this scale is said to be diagnostic of VaD but this scale has poor inter-rater reliability.

NINDS-AIREN criteria for vascular dementia

Definite VaD is diagnosed with:

- Clinical criteria for probable VaD.
- Autopsy demonstration of appropriate ischemic brain injury and no other cause of the dementia.

Probable VaD is diagnosed with:

- Evidence of dementia, as described for AD.
- Focal neurologic signs consistent with stroke.
- Neuroimaging evidence of extensive vascular lesions that are sufficient to account for the cognitive impairment.
- Relationship between the dementia and the cerebrovascular disease established by abrupt deterioration, a fluctuating course, or stepwise progression of the cognitive deficit.

Possible VaD is diagnosed with:

- Dementia with focal neurologic signs but without neuroimaging confirmation of definite cerebrovascular disease.
- Dementia with focal neurologic signs but without a clear temporal relationship between dementia and stroke.
- Dementia with focal neurologic signs but with a subtle onset and variable course of cognitive deficits.

Treatment

Treat any underlying causes and risk factors that may be remediable[28]:

- Cerebral vasculitis: corticosteroids or immunosuppressives.
- Hyperviscosity syndrome.
- Neoplastic angioendotheliomatosis: chemotherapy.
- Control vascular risk factors such as hypertension, smoking, hypercholesterolemia, and diabetes.
- Long-term antiplatelet therapy such as low-dose aspirin.
- Physiotherapy for motor dysfunction and spasticity or gait instability.
- Speech therapy for dysarthria, aphasia, dysphagia.

Prognosis

- Characteristically, a progressive stepwise course of cognitive decline but in up to one-half of patients it can follow a slow progressive course.
- 50% survival: 6.7 years (cf. 8.1 years for AD).
- Cause of death: heart disease or recurrent stroke.

TABLE 94 **HACHINSKI ISCHEMIA SCALE**

Item	Score value
Abrupt onset*	2
Stepwise course*	1
Fluctuating course	2
Preservation of personality	1
Nocturnal confusion	1
Depression	1
Somatic complaints*	1
Emotional incontinence*	1
History of hypertension*	1
Evidence of associated atherosclerosis	1
History of stroke*	2
Focal neurologic symptoms*	2
Focal neurologic signs*	2

*Discriminating items after validation at post mortem examination.

PRION DISEASES

Definition and epidemiology

A family of fatal neurodegenerative diseases characterized by the CNS accumulation of a misfolded isoform of a membrane-bound glycoprotein, the prion protein (PrP), which acquires the property of transmissibility. Also known as transmissible spongiform encephalopathies (TSEs).

- Incidence: ~1–1.5 cases per million per year (sporadic), 1 per 10 million per year (familial).
- Age: median age of onset: 67 years; rare cases younger than 30 (especially variant CJD), and older than 80 years.
- Gender: M=F.

Etiology and pathophysiology

- Sporadic:
  - Vast majority of cases.
  - Occur spontaneously. Possibly somatic mutation of the PrP gene (*PRNP*), but this is theoretical.
  - No exogenous source of prions identified. Randomly distributed incidence (85–90% of cases).
- Inherited: mutation of the *PRNP* gene located on the short arm of chromosome 20. Familial CJD (10–15% of all cases), GSS (1–2% of cases). Autosomal dominant pattern of inheritance; point mutations or insertions in *PRNP*. The codon 200Lys and 178Asp mutations are associated with neuropathologic changes essentially indistinguishable from sporadic CJD.
- Acquired: iatrogenic transmission of CJD (<0.1% of cases):
  - Human cadaveric pituitary-derived growth hormone (hGH): >150 cases worldwide. Incidence essentially nil since recombinant GH instituted in the 1980s.
  - Dura mater grafts: >100 cases worldwide, derived from a single commercial source.
  - Inadequately sterilized neurosurgical instruments and depth electrodes: 6 cases.
  - Human gonadotrophin: 5 cases.
  - Corneal transplant: 3 cases.
  - Depth electrodes: 2 cases.

Prion disease is transmissible to experimental animals following inoculation or dietary exposure. The long incubation period led to an initial concept that a slow virus was the etiology of these diseases, but it is now clear that they are not due to a conventional infectious agent.

Prion hypothesis

- The transmissible agent is a proteinaceous infectious particle, i.e. prion[29].
- A prion consists principally or entirely of a partially protease-resistant, misfolded isoform of a normal host-encoded cellular glycoprotein, the prion protein (PrP).
- The non-pathogenic, or cellular form of PrP, designated PrP^C, is a normal constituent of the surface of the neuronal cell.
- In disease, PrP^C is converted into a disease-related isoform[30], PrP^{Sc}.
- PrP^{Sc} conformational change can occur spontaneously, be promoted by the presence of a mutation of PRNP, or be induced by exposure to prions.
- The conformational change in protein structure from PrP^C to pathogenic PrP^{Sc} is a critical pathologic event, resulting in either toxicity due to accumulation of PrP^{Sc} or loss of function of PrP^C, more likely the former.
- Clinical heterogeneity in prion disease (see below) appears to reflect differences in PrP^{Sc} structural isoforms and these may be modified by the host genotype, especially with regard to a common polymorphism at codon 129 (e.g. for sporadic CJD, two major protease-resistant subtypes exist – Type 1 and Type 2 – that carry different clinical features and are more commonly associated with 129MM and 129VV, respectively).

Genetic susceptibility to acquired iatrogenic and sporadic CJD

The general population has a common silent protein polymorphism at codon 129 of the *PRNP* gene, where either a methionine (Met) or valine (Val) may be encoded. About 40% of the white population are homozygous for the more frequent Met alleles, 50% are heterozygotes, and 10% are homozygous for the Val allele. Homozygosity at codon 129 appears to confer susceptibility to iatrogenic and sporadic disease:

- More than 80% of patients with sporadic CJD are homozygous for either allele[31].
- All primary cases of variant CJD (see below) are 129Met homozygotes.
- Most patients with iatrogenic CJD (treatment with cadaveric pituitary-derived hGH) are homozygous, mainly for Val.
- Heterozygosity for the *PRNP* gene appears to be protective.

Risk factors

- Family history and/or the presence of a mutation in the *PRNP* gene. Inheritence is autosomal dominant (50% risk of acquiring defective gene if one of the parents carries a mutation).
- Exposure to bovine-derived prions.
- Exposure to known iatrogenic sources of prions.

Clinical features

Variable (particularly with familial cases, and even within the same pedigree). Features can include:

- Insidious onset.
- Early behavioral abnormalities (initial symptom in about 10% of cases):
  - Personality change, withdrawal, apathy, depression, sleep disturbance.
  - Agitation, fear, and paranoia may prompt a psychiatric referral.
- Rapidly progressive and profound dementia: forgetful, confused, visual distortions and hallucinations may occur.
- Myoclonus, usually stimulus-sensitive (>80% of patients with CJD).
- Motor abnormalities:
  - Cerebellar ataxia.
  - Extrapyramidal signs: tremor, rigidity, bradykinesia, dystonic posturing; choreoathetosis.
  - Pyramidal signs: weakness, spasticity, hyper-reflexia, and Babinski signs.
- Generalized seizures may occur.

Clinical variants (the spectrum)

CJD

- Heidenhain variant: early pathologic involvement of the occipital cortex leading to cortical blindness.
- Brownell–Oppenheimer (ataxic) variant: early and prominent ataxia (cerebellar ataxia is also prominent in iatrogenic CJD due to pituitary-derived hormones).

Variant CJD (vCJD)

- Linked causally to bovine spongiform encephalopathy (BSE), vCJD results from consumption of bovine tissues contaminated with BSE prions[32].
- Young age of onset – teens and younger adults (however, a 75-year-old patient was reported).
- Early behavioral/psychiatric disturbance (anxiety, depression, apathy), cerebellar ataxia, and dysesthesias of the lower extremities.
- Absence of typical EEG changes of CJD, although the EEG is abnormal.
- High signal changes in the pulvinar of the thalamus on diffusion-weighted (DWI) and proton-weighted MRI imaging of the brain.
- Clinical course is more protracted, with average duration of 13 months compared with a mean of 6 months in other types.
- Specific neuropathologic profile includes 'florid plaques', identified as a central region of dense core PrP plaques resembling those seen in kuru, but surrounded by a zone of spongiform change.
- Homozygosity for Met at codon 129 of the *PRNP* gene.
- Associated with a specific pattern of protease-resistant PrP^{Sc} on Western blot analysis. The biochemical signature is distinct from other types of CJD and matches that of animals experimentally infected with BSE, supporting the link between vCJD and BSE.

TABLE 95 **INVESTIGATION FINDINGS IN CREUTZFELDT–JAKOB DISEASE**

Disease	'Typical EEG'	14-3-3 +ve CSF*	High signal on MRI brain	Other
Sporadic CJD	+ (65%)	+ (50–90%)	+ (>90%) (basal ganglia and/or cortical ribbon)	
Familial CJD	±	±	±	*PRNP* gene analysis
Iatrogenic CJD				
• CNS route	±	?	?	
• Peripheral route	–	± (50%)	±	
New variant	– (100%)	± (50%)	+ (>70%) (posterior thalamus)	Tonsil biopsy

Percentage of cases with a positive investigation, where known, is in parentheses.
*Total CSF tau protein has similar, if not slightly better, results.

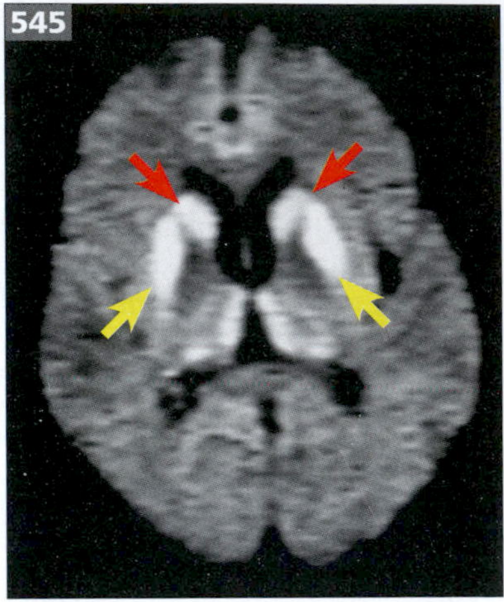

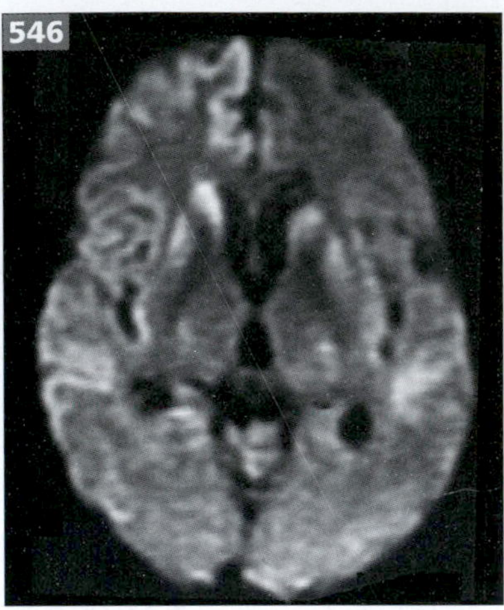

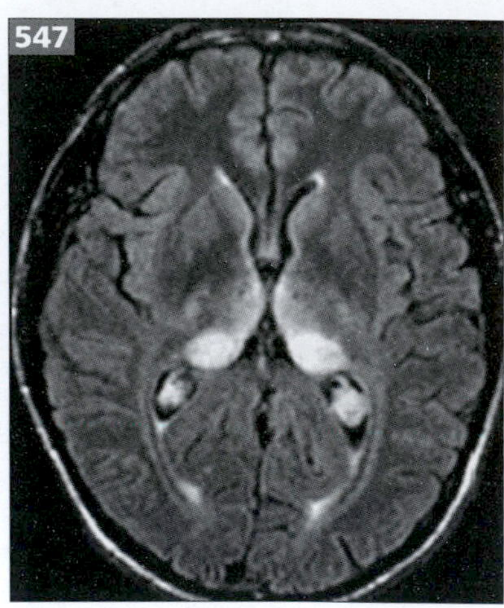

545, 546 Diffusion-weighted MRIs from two patients with sCJD, revealing the two major patterns of restricted diffusion. Hyperintensities of the caudate (red arrows) and putamen (yellow arrows) may be observed in isolation (545), or in combination with cortical hyperintensities (546).

547 Proton-weighted imaging of the brain demonstrates pulvinar hyperintensity in a patient with vCJD.

Fatal insomnia (genetic and sporadic)

In fatal insomnia, the symptoms above may occur, although sleep disturbance is often the presenting feature. The classic phenotype includes initial onset of insomnia (may be mild), that is resistant to sleep medications and progressive in nature, which is followed by autonomic disturbances (blood pressure and heart rate fluctuations, lacrimation, and so on), ataxia, and dementia. Familial FI (FFI) and sporadic FI (sFI) have remarkably similar phenotypes, although the autonomic features may be less common in sFI[33].

The genetic mutation linked to FFI is an aspartate (D) change to asparagine (N) at codon 178, but only when allelic with Met coding at 129. If coding is 129Val on the D178N mutation, the presentation is more typical of familial CJD (fCJD).

GSS

Ataxia is the presenting symptom in most cases, occurring as gait ataxia, dysarthria, ocular dysmetria, or appendicular ataxia. These symptoms are followed by pyramidal and/or extrapyramidal features, and dementia in the later stages.

Variability is great; some patients present with isolated cognitive decline, without prominent ataxia (telencephalic presentation), whereas others may present with behavioral changes that suggest a presentation of FTD.

Variably protease sensitive prionopathy (VPSPr)

A recently identified subtype that is distinguished primarily by the relatively lower protease resistance of the prion protein. Clinical features are similar to CJD, although aphasia and behavioral features seem more common.

Differential diagnosis

- AD with myoclonus, but the course is usually more prolonged.
- Spinocerebellar ataxias.
- Whipple's disease.
- Paraneoplastic syndrome.
- Nonconvulsive status epilepticus.
- Metabolic/toxic encephalopathy (e.g. drugs).
- Bilateral subdural hematomas.
- CNS vasculitis.
- SSPE.
- Infiltrating corpus callosum glioma.
- HD.
- Psychiatric illness (anxiety, depression).

Investigations

(See *Table 95*.)

Brain CT or MRI

- Scans are normal (45%) or show cerebral atrophy (30%) at presentation.
- DWI MRI commonly reveals high-signal changes in the basal ganglia or cortical ribbon in cases of CJD (**545, 546**), while proton density images in vCJD show hyperintensity of thalamus (especially pulvinar) (**547**), although FI and GSS are not well studied with regard to these scans.
- Fluoro-deoxyglucose PET in FI shows reduction in thalamic metabolic activity[34].

EEG

- Early: non-specific disorganization and generalized slow wave activity.
- Later (within 12 weeks of onset of symptoms):
  - Slow background rhythm.
  - Periodic sharp wave complexes (PSWCs) (**548**):
    - Bisynchronous, and most commonly anterior and central (but may be lateralized and localized: occipital preponderance in Heidenhain's variant).
    - Duration: 100–600 ms; repetitive, occurring every 0.5–2.0 seconds.
    - Amplitude up to 300 mV; may be monophasic, biphasic, triphasic, or multiphasic.
    - May be associated with myoclonic jerks; may be activated by startle.
    - Present in >65% of cases, particularly sporadic CJD, rarely in iatrogenic CJD, and generally not present in fCJD, vCJD, GSS, FFI, or sFI.
  - Evolution from intermittent to persistent PSWCs may be detected by serial EEGs (**549–550**)
    - Nonspecific; also occur in several encephalopathies, epilepsy, and post-ictal states, or during barbiturate overdose and deep anesthesia.

CSF

CSF has normal or slightly elevated protein. Immunoassay for the 14-3-3 brain protein is used, which is a nonspecific marker of CNS neuronal injury or death. A positive test is highly sensitive (90%) although specificity has varied widely from study to study, ranging from 30 to 90%, perhaps dependent on the pre-test likelihood that the patient has CJD[35]. This test has also been reported to be elevated in CNS herpes, acute strokes, multiple sclerosis, and other inflammatory conditions.

Neuron-specific enolase (NSE) concentrations may be increased early (>35 ng/ml; sensitivity 80%, specificity 92%) and when myoclonus and periodic sharp complexes appear, and return to normal in the late stage. Raised NSE in CSF is also reported in brain trauma, tumor, and acute stroke including subarachnoid hemorrhage. The enzyme is localized in neurons and neuroendocrine cells and is synthesized completely in the CNS.

Tau (nonphosphorylated) levels in the CSF may be elevated to extremely high levels (>1250 pg/ml)[36].

Tip

▶ *CSF 14-3-3 and/or tau are most likely to be elevated in prion disease that runs a rapidly progressive course.*

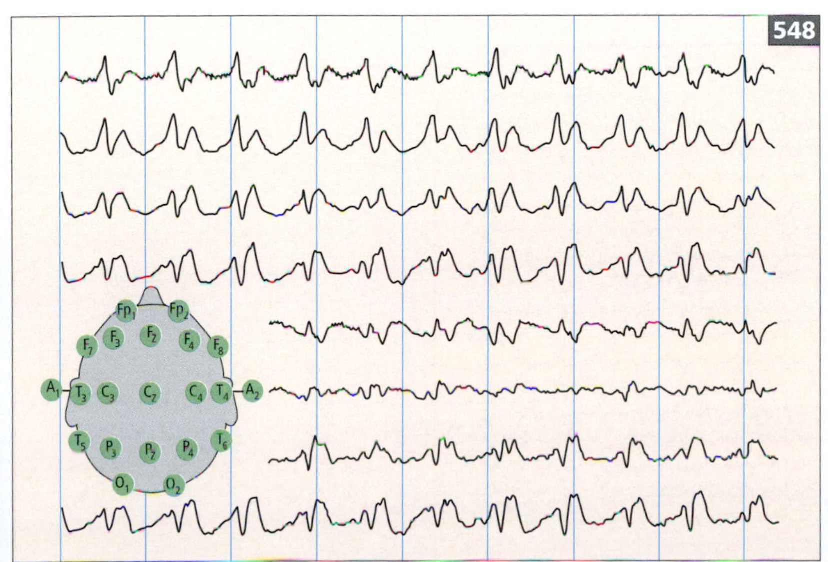

548 Electroencephalograph showing periodic triphasic wave complexes that are rather simple in contour and recurring every 0.7–0.8 seconds, against a slow polymorphous background, in a patient with rapidly progressive dementia and myoclonus due to CJD. Occasionally, the periodic discharges begin unilaterally and may resemble periodic lateralized epileptiform discharges.

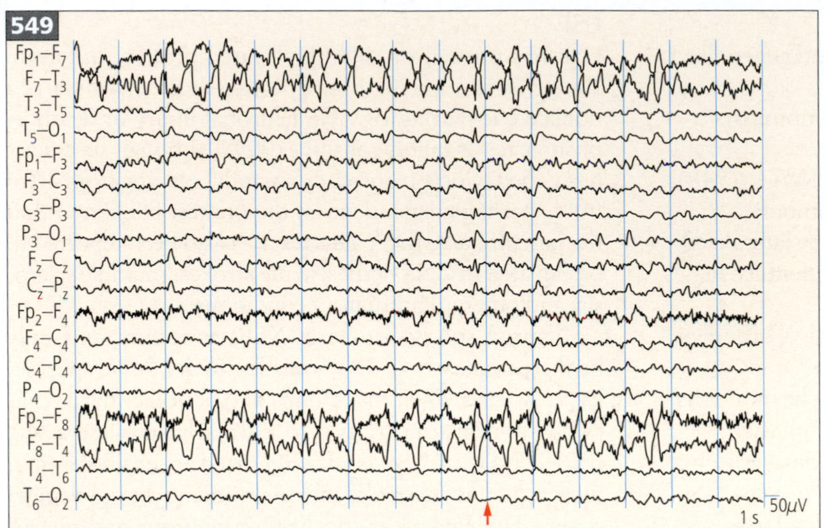

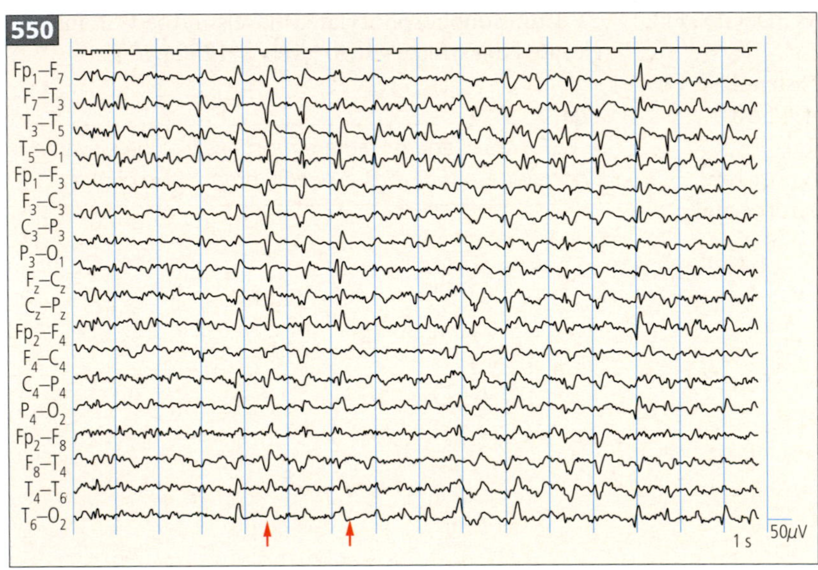

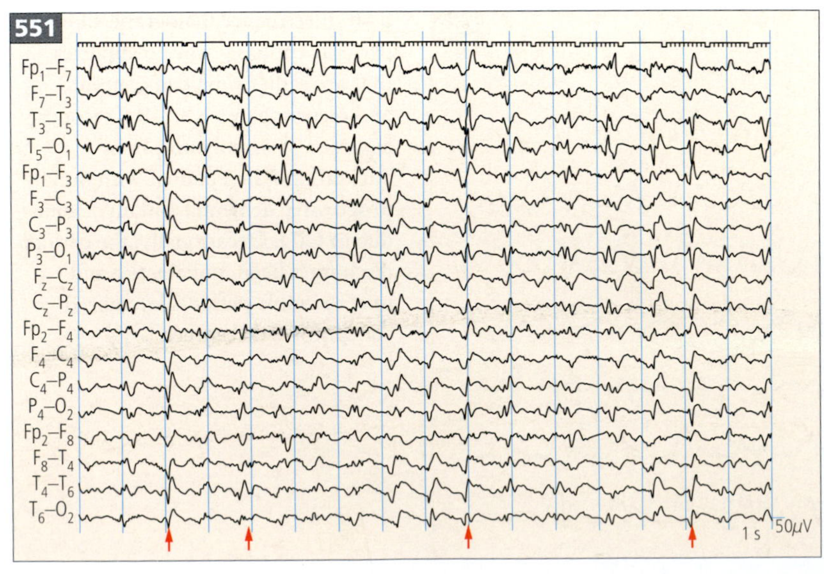

549–551 Serial electroencephalographs, every 3 days, from a patient with CJD, showing the progressive evolution of periodic triphasic wave complexes (arrows) and the background rhythm.

Molecular genetic analysis

The prion protein gene (*PRNP*) blood test is a genetic test for mutations that cause familial prion disease, using DNA analysis from blood or brain. The *PRNP* gene is sequenced for the presence of pathogenic mutations, and the polymorphic risk factor found at codon 129. It is important to perform, even if no family history is apparent, as mutations are occasionally detected in apparently sporadic cases as a result of incomplete penetrance, non-paternity, adoption, or because the gene-carrying parent died from another cause at a young age, prior to the onset of prion disease.

Several mutations occurring throughout the entire length of the *PRNP* gene have been identified. Point mutations that result in single amino acid substitutions are most common. Of these, the two most frequently detected include an asparagine substitution for aspartate at codon 178 (D178N) and a lysine (K) substitution for glutamate (E) at codon 200 (E200K). In addition, four nonsense mutations that result in expression of a truncated PrP, and insertions of one to nine multiples of an eight or nine amino acid repeat segment, known as the octarepeat region, result in expression of a longer PrP.

Tonsil biopsy

Western blot analysis of tonsil material obtained by biopsy of tonsil or lingual tonsillar remnants under local anesthetic can provide the antemortem detection of protease-resistant PrP in the lymphoreticular system of patients with vCJD, but not with other forms of prion disease.

Brain biopsy

Biopsy is mainly indicated to diagnose a suspected treatable cause of the clinical state, such as CNS vasculitis or SSPE. It is rarely indicated to diagnose prion disease because:

- It may miss the diagnosis because the prion immunostaining may be patchy.
- The elaborate preparation and decontamination of the operating suite is often prohibitive.

Diagnosis

Sporadic CJD

Definite:

- Neuropathologically confirmed, and/or
- Immunohistochemically confirmed proteinase-resistant PrP in tissue sections or Western blot.

Probable:

- Progressive dementia.
- Typical periodic EEG, positive MRI, or positive CSF study, and:
- At least two of the following clinical features:
  - Myoclonus.
  - Visual or cerebellar disturbance.
  - Pyramidal/extrapyramidal dysfunction.
  - Akinetic mutism.

Possible:

- Progressive dementia.
- Two of the clinical features listed above.
- Either a negative diagnostic test (EEG, MRI, or CSF) or they are unavailable.
- Duration <2 years.

Iatrogenic CJD

- Progressive cerebellar syndrome in a pituitary hormone recipient.
- Sporadic CJD with a recognized exposure risk (e.g. dura mater transplant).

Familial CJD

- Definite or probable CJD plus definite or probable CJD in a first-degree relative.
- Neuropsychiatric disorder plus disease-specific PRNP mutation.

vCJD

- 1a: Progressive neuropsychiatric disorder.
- 1b: Duration of illness >6 months.
- 1c: Routine investigations do not suggest an alternative diagnosis.
- 1d: No history of potential iatrogenic exposure.
- 2a: Early psychiatric symptoms (especially apathy and depression).
- 2b: Persistent painful sensory symptoms.
- 2c: Ataxia.
- 2d: Myoclonus or chorea or dystonia.
- 2e: Dementia.
- 3a: EEG does not show the (typical) PSWCs of CJD (or no EEG performed).
- 3b: Posterior thalamic (pulvinar) high signal on DWI or proton density MRI brain scan.

Definite vCJD: 1a and neuropathologic confirmation of vCJD.

Probable: 1 and four-fifths of 2, and 3a and 3b.

Possible: 1 and four-fifths of 2.

552 Western blots of the four major prion subtypes. The banding pattern represents the major fractions of the protease-resistant pathogenic prion protein (in essence, the prion). These differences support the notion that the phenotype of each disease is determined by the respective conformational subtype of the prion. Left to right; CJD, FI, vCJD, GSS.

Pathology

The demonstration of protease-resistant PrP in brain is the neuropathologic diagnostic marker of prion disease. Specific banding patterns of the protease-resistant PrP^{Sc} (by Western blot analysis) correspond to the major prion disease subtypes of CJD, GSS, FI, and vCJD (**552**). Proteinase-resistant PrP^{Sc} can also be assessed by immunohistochemistry on brain sections, using antibodies against PrP. Molecular genetic analyses of the *PRNP* gene can be used to confirm a mutation.

Macroscopically, the brain is atrophic. Microscopically, CJD consists of a triad of:

- Neuronal loss.
- Reactive astrocytic proliferation and gliosis.
- Spongiform degeneration (spongiform change): vacuolation of the neuropil, particularly in deeper laminae of the gray matter of the frontal and temporal lobes, but also the gray matter of the striatum, thalamus, tegmentum of the upper brainstem, and cerebellar cortex (**553, 554**).

Ultrastructurally, spongiform degeneration appears as intraneuronal, complex, clear vacuoles whose membranous septa look curled in profile.

Kuru plaques may also be present: eosinophilic, round, compact extracellular depositions of PrP; these are pathognomonic of a prion disease but are found in only a few sporadic cases.

GSS shows mild spongiform degeneration, prominent extracellular amyloid deposits composed of PrP, most prominent within the cerebellum, but also common in frontal and temporal cortex.

FI shows neuronal loss and gliosis typically present within thalamic nuclei, especially anterior and dorsomedial nuclei, in addition to inferior olivary nucleus. There is minimal spongiform degeneration and no amyloid plaque deposits are present.

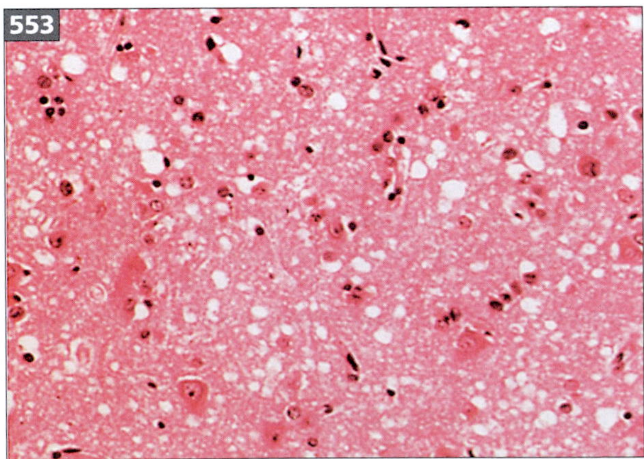

553 Neuronal vacuolation, also known as spongiform degeneration, is the key histopathologic feature of CJD.

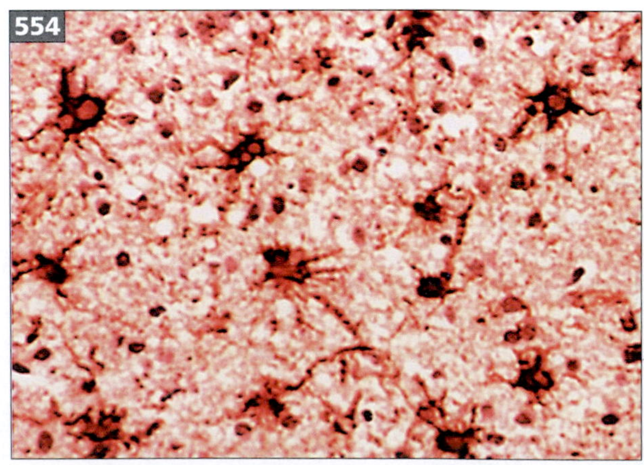

554 Glial fibrillary acidic protein antibody demonstrates the proliferation and hypertrophy of glial cells that commonly occur in prion disease.

Treatment

At present, no effective curative therapy is available, treatment is symptomatic. Patients should be nursed similarly to others with infectious disease, using disposable supplies when possible. Antiepileptic drugs may be required for seizures, intermittent or indwelling bladder catheters for urinary incontinence, and appropriate posturing and regular turning to prevent bedsores.

Prognosis

90% of CJD patients display a rapidly progressive decline to akinetic mutism and death over 2–12 months; about 10% have a protracted clinical course (these usually begin with ataxia rather than dementia). GSS has a significantly more protracted course, lasting over several years, resulting in severe disability from ataxia, whereas FI has a similar, if not slightly more prolonged course, to CJD.

Prevention

hGH is now manufactured using recombinant DNA technology, thereby eliminating the need for human sources. Dura mater source has been identified. The safety of the blood supply, especially within countries where vCJD has been reported, has been under scrutiny. In fact, there have been at least four cases of vCJD transmission attributed to blood product transfusion.

Genetic counseling coupled with prenatal genetic screening is possible, but the apparent incomplete penetrance of some of the inherited prion diseases increases the uncertainty of predicting the future for an asymptomatic individual. Problems common to all predictive testing programs are also likely to arise.

NORMAL PRESSURE HYDROCEPHALUS

Definition and epidemiology

Normal pressure hydrocephalus (NPH) is a clinical syndrome characterized by abnormal gait, urinary incontinence, and dementia. A frequently missed, or late diagnosed condition, NPH is a potentially reversible cause of dementia. First described by Hakim in 1965, NPH was described as hydrocephalus without evidence of papilledema and with normal CSF opening pressure on lumbar puncture.

- Incidence: 5.5 per 100,000.
- Prevalence: ~5% of all dementia cases. Up to 14% in the elderly population living within a care facility.
- Age: predominately seen in the elderly population and incidence as well as prevalence tend to increase with age.
- Gender: M=F.

Etiology and pathophysiology

NPH tends to be idiopathic in up to 50% of patients. Secondary causes may include head injury, subarachnoid hemorrhage, meningitis, CNS tumor, and previously compensated congenital hydrocephalus.

Symptoms of NPH are due to distortion of the corona radiata caused by distention of the lateral ventricles, with ensuing white matter edema and impaired blood flow. Abnormal gait and incontinence are due to distortion of the periventricular white matter which includes sacral motor fibers that innervate the legs and bladder. Abnormal gait may also be due to compression of brainstem structures related to gait. Dementia is due to distortion of the periventricular limbic system.

Hakim theorized that NPH may start with a transient increase in intracranial pressure causing ventricular enlargement. As the ventricles enlarge, the pressure returns to normal. Other theories include the possibility of extraventricular obstructive hydrocephalus where the primary event is decreased resorption of CSF at the level of the arachnoid villi. This then leads to a transient high pressure hydrocephalus with ventricular enlargement. With ventricular enlargement, the CSF pressure returns to normal.

Clinical features

- Progressive disorder.
- Gait disorder: typically the earliest symptom, apraxia of gait characterized as a wide-based, bradykinetic, magnetic, and/or shuffling gait. Patients may experience difficulty or arrest in initiation of ambulation as well as multiple falls.
- Urinary incontinence: 95% have been found to have detrusor overactivity leading to urinary frequency, urgency, or frank incontinence.
- Apathy may be present.
- Dementia: usually of the subcortical type and includes:
  - Memory impairment – primarily retrieval, rather than encoding deficits (patients do better than AD patients on recognition memory tasks).
  - Bradyphrenia – slowness of thought processing.
  - Decreased attention.

Differential diagnosis

- AD: up to 75% may have AD pathology noted at time of shunt surgery.
- Carcinomatous meningitis.
- Chronic alcoholism.
- Multi-infarct dementia.
- Confusional state and acute memory disorders.
- Cortical basal degeneration.
- Dementia with motor neuron disease.
- DLB.
- FTD.
- Marchiafava–Bignami disease.
- Mutiple system atrophy.
- Paraneoplastic encephalomyelitis.
- PD.
- Parkinson-plus syndromes.
- Uremic encephalopathy.
- Wilson's disease.

Investigations

- Laboratory evaluation: includes testing to rule out other metabolic and infectious causes of dementia – complete blood count, liver function tests, HIV, basic metabolic panel, as described in AD work-up.
- Imaging studies: CT or MRI scan of the brain shows ventricular enlargement out of proportion to sulcal atrophy and may show periventricular hyperintensity due to transependymal flow of CSF. There may also be a prominent flow void in the cerebral aqueduct and third ventricle – 'jet sign' – thinning and elevation of the corpus callosum on sagittal images, and narrow CSF space at the high convexities as compared to the Sylvian fissure size. In order to rule out the possibility that the imaging findings may be secondary to hydrocephalus ex vacuo, at least one of the following must be present:
  - Temporal horn enlargement.
  - Periventricular signal changes.
  - Periventricular edema.
  - Aqueductal/fourth ventricle flow void.
- CSF outflow studies: used to evaluate the pressure response to outflow following the infusion of a sterile solution. So far, this type of study has shown inconsistent results from measurement of outflow CSF pressure.
- Lumbar puncture: normal opening pressure; however, some may have transiently elevated CSF pressures; if so, other causes for hydrocephalus must be excluded before diagnosing NPH. Symptom improvement (especially gait) with large volume (~40–50 ml) drainage is supportive of a diagnosis of NPH.

Treatment

Levodopa has been used to rule out the possibility that the clinical picture is due to PD, as NPH may produce extrapyramidal features. Symptoms related to NPH do not respond to dopamine agonists.

CSF shunting is currently the mainstay of treatment. Neuropsychiatric testing is performed before and after (3 hours later) a large volume lumbar puncture. Those with a clear improvement in mental status and/or gait are associated with a favorable response to shunt surgery.

Tip

▶ *Placement of a shunt should be performed before dementia progresses to a significant level, as its cognitive benefit declines with disease progression.*

Prognosis

Overall prognosis is poor as the clinical course is progressive. Between 21 and 90% of NPH patients may show marked improvement after shunt surgery. Complications from shunt surgery are numerous, including: shunt malfunction, intracranial hemorrhage from placement of the ventricular catheter, infection, intracranial hypotensive headaches, subdural hematomas, due to rapid lowering of CSF causing reduction in ventricular size resulting in tension on the bridging veins. For this reason, patients considered for shunt placement must be chosen carefully.

PARKINSON'S DISEASE AND PARKINSONIAN DISORDERS

INTRODUCTION

The term parkinsonism refers to a motor syndrome with any combination of the following cardinal features:

- Bradykinesia/hypokinesia: slowness with decrement and degradation of repetitive movements ('fatigue').
- Rigidity.
- Tremor: usually at rest.
- Loss of postural reflexes.

In addition to the above cardinal features, the following motor signs are frequently associated:

- Gait abnormalities: freezing, festinating, short/shuffling steps.
- Flexed posture of limbs, neck, and trunk.
- Masked facial features, decreased blinking.
- Micrographia.

While the most common cause of parkinsonism encountered by the clinician is Parkinson's disease, a large number of other disorders may cause parkinsonism, often associated with other neurologic or systemic signs and symptoms. Causes of parkinsonism may be grouped into the following four categories:

- Primary (idiopathic) parkinsonism: Parkinson's disease.
- Multisystem degenerations ('parkinsonism plus' or atypical parkinsonism).
- Heredodegenerative parkinsonism.
- Secondary (symptomatic, acquired) parkinsonism.

Figure 555 outlines a basic categorization algorithm for the most common causes of parkinsonism. Neurodegenerative parkinsonian disorders may also be subdivided by the predominant types of proteins found on pathologic examinations of brain tissue, with the most common disorders related to either deposition of tau ('tauopathies') or alpha-synuclein ('synucleinopathies') protein (*Table 96*, next page).

Tip

▶ *Parkinsonian signs are not specific to Parkinson's disease; a patient presenting with parkinsonism should be carefully evaluated. Secondary or atypical causes of parkinsonism are usually differentiated from Parkinson's disease by the history and examination.*

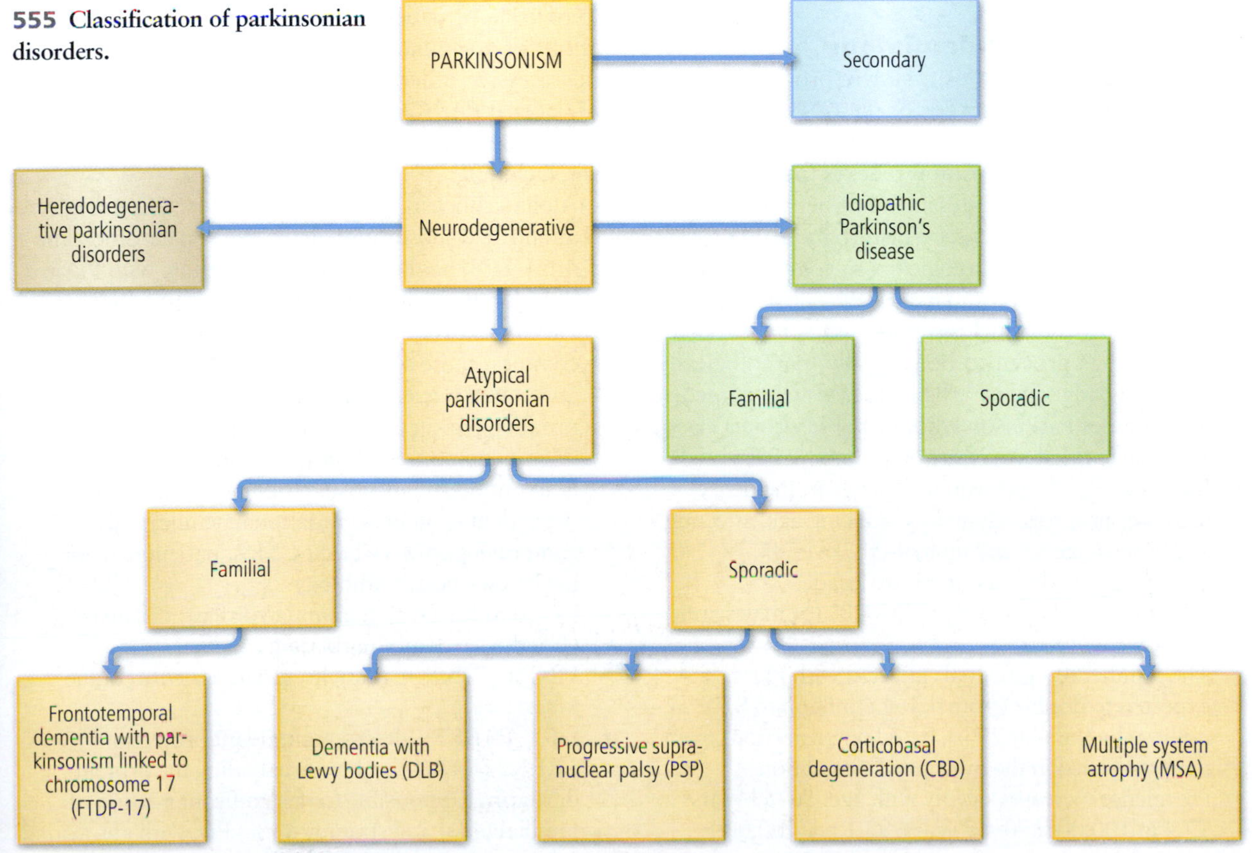

555 Classification of parkinsonian disorders.

TABLE 96 **CLASSIFICATION OF NEURODEGENERATIVE PARKINSONIAN DISORDERS BY PREDOMINANT PROTEIN**

Synucleinopathies	Tauopathies
Parkinson's disease	Corticobasal degeneration
Multiple system atrophy	Progressive supranuclear palsy
Dementia with Lewy bodies/diffuse Lewy body disease	Frontotemporal dementia and parkinsonism linked to chromosome 17
	Pantothenate kinase-associated neurodegeneration
	Postencephalitic parkinsonism
	Dementia pugilistica
	Parkinsonism–dementia complex of Guam

PRIMARY (IDIOPATHIC) PARKINSONISM: PARKINSON'S DISEASE

Definition and epidemiology

Parkinson's disease (PD) is a slowly progressive, age-related, degenerative disorder of the CNS, with motor features characterized clinically by tremor, bradykinesia, rigidity, and disturbed postural reflexes (parkinsonism), as well as non-motor features including neuropsychiatric, sleep, autonomic, and sensory disturbances. PD is classically characterized pathologically by loss of dopaminergic cells in the pars compacta of the substantia nigra with typical neuronal inclusions known as Lewy bodies, although it has proven to be clinically, pathologically, and etiologically diverse[1]. The disease was named in honor of James Parkinson who, in 1817, wrote a classic monograph entitled 'An Essay on a Shaking Palsy'.

- Incidence: 16–19 per 100,000 per year. Incidence increases progressively with advancing age, affecting 1–2% over age 65 and up to 4–5% over 85. Incidence may decrease in ninth decade.
- Lifetime risk of developing PD is 2% for males and 1.3% for women.
- The number of individuals affected with PD is expected to double (from 4.1–4.6 million to 8.7–9.3 million) by the year 2030, based on projections from data published in the most populous nations.
- Prevalence increases steeply with age: 50–59 years: 17.4 in 100,000; 70–79 years: 93.1 per 100,000.
- Median age of onset 60 years; however, onset <45 years of age in about 10% of patients.
- Gender: M>F with a 3:2 ratio; male predominance most reported in elderly, western epidemiologic studies.

Etiology and pathophysiology

PD is a mostly sporadic disease which is likely multifactorial and heterogeneous in etiology. PD is likely due to a complex interaction among genetic, environmental, and other individual factors. Alternatively, PD may not be one condition with a single cause for all patients, but a common clinical manifestation of different types of insults to the substantia nigra (e.g. hereditary, toxic, infectious). The cause of dopaminergic cell death in PD is not clearly understood and probably heterogeneous and multifactorial, related to a probable self-propagating series of reactions involving dopamine, alpha-synuclein, and redox-active metals, including:

- Oxidative stress, reactive species production.
- Mitochondrial dysfunction (recent genetic studies indicate that this may play a major role).
- Excitotoxicity.
- A rise in intracellular free calcium.
- Protein aggregation.
- Inflammation.

Heredity/genetic susceptibility[2]

Up to 10% of patients with PD have a positive family history of a similar disease. Both autosomal dominant and recessive inheritance are known. Many genes for PD (labeled *PARK1–14*) have been characterized among families in which PD is clearly inherited as a Mendelian trait, including:

- Alpha-synuclein gene mutations (*PARK1*): a single amino acid substitution in the gene on chromosome 4q21–q23, has been shown to segregate with PD in a large kindred with autosomal dominant inheritance.
- Parkin gene mutations (*PARK2*): second most common cause of genetic parkinsonism with autosomal recessive inheritance. The parkin gene product, parkin protein, is a ubiquitin protein ligase (E3), a component of the ubiquitin system, which is an important adenosine triphosphate (ATP)-dependent protein degradation machine, and a component of Lewy bodies. Most patients do not have Lewy body pathology.
- Ubiquitin carboxy-terminal hydrolase and ligase (*PARK5*): a de-ubiquitinating enzyme.
- PINK1 (*PARK6*): mitochondrial serine/threonine kinase.
- DJ-1 (*PARK7*): altered antioxidant protection.
- LRRK2 (*PARK8*): a kinase encoding the protein dardarin. Responsible for a significant portion of familial (4%) and sporadic (1%) PD, with autosomal

dominant inheritance, making it as common as MSA and PSP. More benign course with lower incidence of dementia.

- Prevalence of PD in first-degree relatives is 1.3–2.1%, which is about double what is expected.
- The lifetime risk of PD in first-degree relatives of sporadic cases is as high as 17%.
- For the vast majority of patients (98% or more) who have no family history, there may be no genetic contribution or several genes may be responsible.

Environmental toxins

N-methyl-4-phenyl-1,2,3,6,-tetrahydropyridine (MPTP), a synthetic opiate derivative, causes a form of parkinsonism that strongly resembles PD both clinically and in response to levodopa, altering mitochondrial function.

While few individual cases of parkinsonism induced by other toxins (e.g. pesticides, herbicides, solvents, mercury) have been documented, growing evidence suggests a causal association between pesticide exposure and parkinsonism.

Possible risk factors include postmenopausal women not on hormone replacement, rural living (with chronic exposure to well water, chemicals, herbicide/pesticide products), head injury, middle-age obesity, lack of exercise, and infections:

- Epidemics of Von Economo's encephalitis (encephalitis lethargica) swept Europe in the early 1920s with some patients developing progressive parkinsonism, not identical to PD. Post-encephalitic parkinsonism is now very rare.
- Influenza and whooping cough infection have been associated with an increased risk of PD in two ecologic studies but have not been confirmed.
- 'Dual Hit Theory': a neurotrophic (perhaps viral) pathogen enters the brain via both nasal routes (with anterograde progression into the temporal lobe) and gastric routes, secondary to swallowing nasal secretions in saliva and retrograde transport to the medulla through the enteric plexus and preganglionic vagal nerve fibers.
- Prion hypothesis: alpha synuclein misfolding triggers protein aggregation in interconnected neuronal groups.

Individual risk factors

- Older age is the highest risk factor for PD.
- Male sex.
- Personality traits and behaviors: low novelty seeking (may represent early disease features); may relate to risk factors of never smoking, low quantities of daily caffeine.

Classic pathophysiologic model of basal ganglia

The dopamine pathway in the basal ganglia participates in a complex circuit of both excitatory and inhibitory pathways that are part of a loop connecting the cortex to the thalamus via the basal ganglia and back to the frontal cortex, and serves to modulate the motor system (556). The pathophysiologic hallmark of parkinsonism is hyperactivity in the subthalamic nucleus (STN) and internal globus pallidus (GPi).

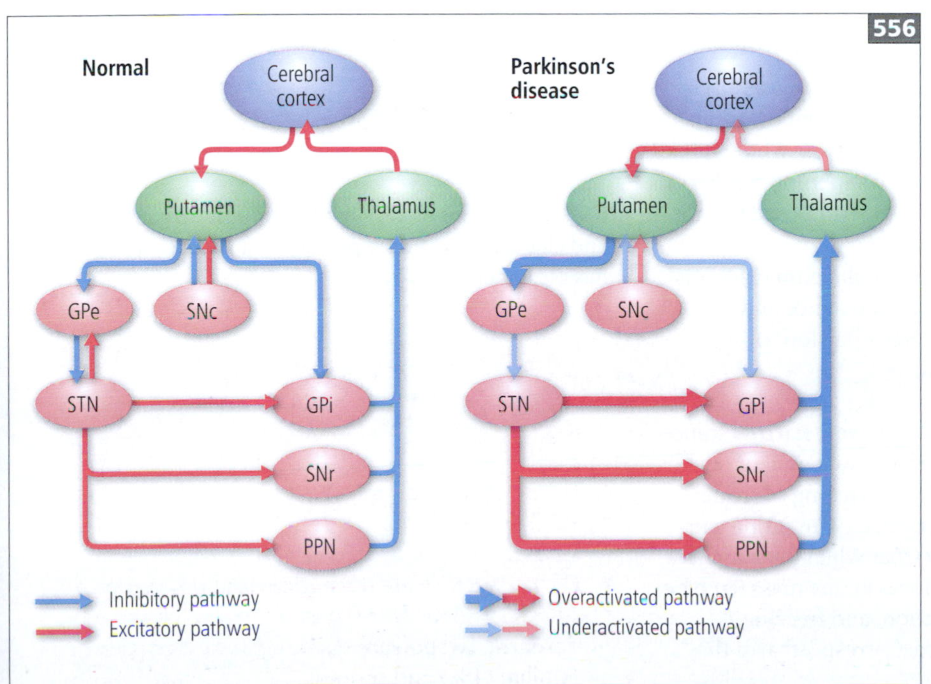

556 Classical schematic representation of basal ganglia circuitry, illustrating the direct and indirect pathways connecting the striatum and globus pallidus, and the modulatory effects of dopaminergic neurons on each of these systems. In PD, the loss of input from the SNc leads to a net increased inhibitory output to the thalamus. GPe: external globus pallidus; Gpi: internal globus pallidus; PPN: pedunculopontine nucleus; SNc: substantia nigra pars compacta; SNr: substantia nigra pars reticularis; STN: subthalamic nucleus.

Despite lack of correlation with animal models of the disease, the classic basal ganglia model proposes that loss of dopaminergic neurons in the substantia nigra pars compacta (SNc) results in dopamine deficiency in the nigrostriatal pathway, which subsequently reduces the normal inhibition of the nigrostriatal pathway on GABA–enkephalin neurons in the putamen. This increases the activity in the GABA/enkephalinergic putaminal neurons that project to, and inhibit, the globus pallidus externus (GPe). The GPe, which sends GABAergic inhibitory projections to the STN and the GPi, is now inhibited and so the inhibitory tone of GPi on the STN and GPi is reduced. The STN, which exerts a powerful excitatory drive on to the GPi and substantia nigra reticulata (SNr), now increases its activity well above normal to excite the GPi/SNr. The GPi and SNr are the major output nuclei of the basal ganglia, and finally project, via inhibitory GABAergic pathways, to the ventrolateral thalamus (VL) on their route to the pre-motor cortices. The increased inhibitory GABAergic outflow from neurons in the GPi/SNr leads to increased inhibition of thalamocortical projection neurons and decreased activation of the precentral motor fields, resulting in bradykinesia. Excessive tonic discharges are not the only physiologic abnormality of the basal ganglia in PD; phasic oscillations in neuronal firing appear to be responsible for tremor.

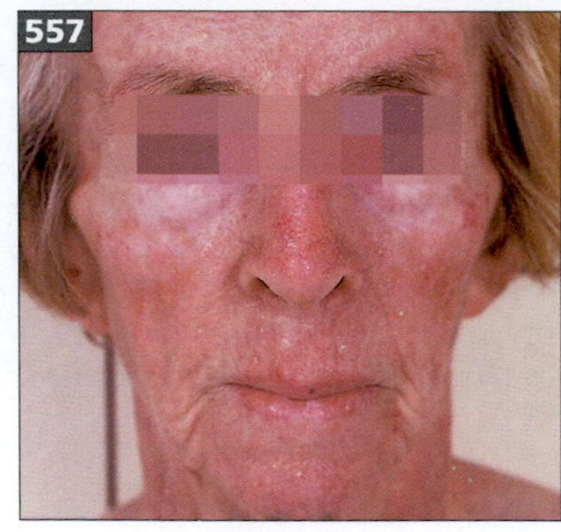

557 **Typical masked facial features of Parkinson's disease.**

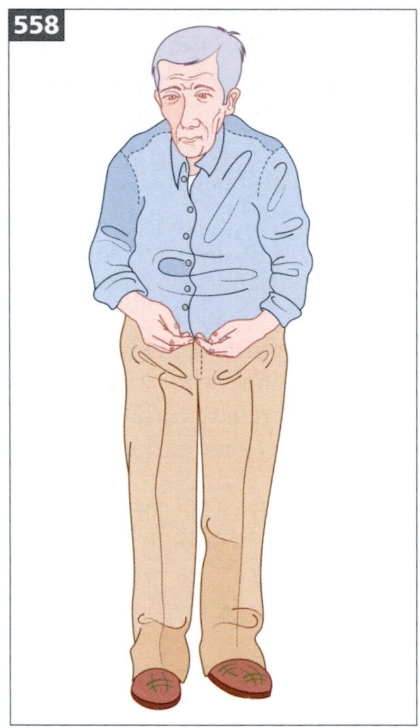

558 **Illustration of the slightly anxious, frozen face and characteristic flexed posture of a Parkinson's disease patient.**

Clinical features[3]

Motor features

Insidious onset of:

- Tremor*: at rest, 4–6 Hz, rhythmic, involves hand ('pill-rolling') ± leg, voice, jaw.
- Bradykinesia: diminished rate and range of movements (e.g. impassive face [hypomimia]; 557), reduced finger tapping and arm swing).
- Rigidity: increased resistance ('lead-pipe' rigidity), to passive movement of the wrist and elbow joints during passive movement through their whole range of movement; with or without a superimposed jerky 'cogwheel' character due to a superimposed tremor that rhythmically interrupts tone.
- Postural instability: impaired equilibrium reactions/righting reflexes: slow to correct balance and tendency to fall backwards (retropulsion) or accelerate forwards (festination).
- Gait disturbance:
  - Stooped posture with arms flexed, narrow stance base (558), reduced or absent swinging of one arm initially, followed by shortening of stride length (shuffling steps), difficulty initiating gait, stiffening of the trunk so that when the patient turns the whole body moves in one mass (en bloc), stooped posture, festination, and freezing.
  - The gait has a narrow base, irrespective of the severity of the disease.

- Asymmetry*: onset is usually unilateral, eventually becoming bilateral after a few years.
- A good response* to levodopa therapy (70–100%).
- Several features of PD may be considered secondary to the core main features: infrequent blinking, facial immobility, soft voice, saccadic ocular pursuit, hypometric ocular saccades, drooling, micrographia, flexed body posture at the trunk, neck, elbows, and knees; joint and muscle pain (e.g. frozen shoulder, and possibly bursitis) are likely a result of muscle rigidity and bradykinesia.
- Treatment-induced dyskinesias*: writhing, swinging movements of the limbs and trunks typically occur in patients with advanced disease and prominent motor fluctuations and are caused by excess levodopa, but may also occur with dopamine agonists. Dystonic dyskinesia (sustained twisting movements) may be painful and necessitate reduction of levodopa dosage.
- The deep tendon reflexes remain preserved and the plantar responses are flexor.

(*Best predictors of PD.)

Non-motor features[4]

Almost all patients experience a combination of the many possible non-motor symptoms (see *Table 97*):

- May occur early, even before motor features[5], and contribute to reduced quality of life, in many cases outweighing disability from motor symptoms.
- More highly prevalent and disabling as disease course advances.
- Result from multifocal pathologic lesions in extra-nigral pathways (e.g. brain, spine, ganglion, visceral organs) and nondopaminergic neurotransmitter systems.
- Pain and sensory phenomena are common. Deep cramping sensations in the limbs may be a primary symptom or related to levodopa medication. Superficial burning dysesthesia also may occur.
- Anxiety and depression (40%).
- Cognitive impairment: common, even in early PD (up to one-third), mainly subcortical features: bradyphrenia, decreased attention, executive dysfunction, memory deficits, visuospatial dysfunction, apathy, decreased verbal fluency.
- Dementia:
  - Occurs in 22–48% of cases, accounting for 3–4% of dementia in general population. Increased relative risk of dementia 1.7–5.9 with PD. 10% of PD population may develop dementia per year.
  - Must be distinguished from depression, physical slowness, and adverse effects of drug treatment.
- Psychosis and hallucinations: often secondary to antiparkinsonian medications.
- Autonomic dysfunction: due to central and peripheral involvement of autonomic regulatory neurons:
  - Orthostatic hypotension and/or supine hypertension.
  - Urinary dysfunction: urinary urgency, frequency, nocturia, delayed emptying, difficulty initiating, recurrent infections. Usually related to detrusor or sphincter muscle hyperactivity, less frequently to hypoactive detrusor; paradoxical co-contraction of urinary sphincter.
  - Erectile dysfunction.
  - Thermoregulatory dysfunction: excessive sweating; may be related to 'on' state (with peak-dose dyskinesias) or 'off' state.

Tip

▶ *Non-motor symptoms of PD are present in nearly all patients, and should not be neglected in evaluation and treatment of the disorder. Often these symptoms contribute more disability to the patient than the motor symptoms, particularly as the disease progresses.*

TABLE 97 **SPECTRUM OF NON-MOTOR SYMPTOMS IN PARKINSON'S DISEASE**

Neuropsychiatric	Depression, apathy, anxiety, anhedonia; dementia; impulse control disorders; psychosis: hallucinations, delusions
Autonomic	Bladder dysfunction; orthostatic hypotension, supine hypertension; hyperhydrosis; dysphagia/sialorrhea; constipation, nausea, vomiting, delayed gastric emptying; sexual dysfunction
Sleep	Insomnia, poor sleep efficiency, excessive daytime sleepiness, sleep fragmentation; primary sleep disorders (restless leg syndrome, periodic limb movement disorder, obstructive sleep apnea); REM behavioral disorder; vivid dreams
Sensory	Pain, paresthesias; olfactory dysfunction, ageusia; visual symptoms: diplopia, blurring
Other	Fatigue; weight loss/gain; seborrhea; respiratory complaints; sialorrhea

REM: rapid eye movement.

Differential diagnosis

Tremor

- Benign essential tremor: upper limb tremor which is worse with posture and action (on attempted writing, the tremor is exacerbated and the script becomes enlarged and irregular, whereas in PD, the tremor usually abates and the writing becomes smaller as the script progresses across the page [micrographia]), positive family history, tremor response to alcohol, later developing head/voice tremor.
- Dystonic tremor: associated with dystonic hand posturing, decreased arm swing, or sometimes cogwheel rigidity at the wrist. May resemble parkinsonian tremor, but typically more irregular with a 'null point'.
- Cerebellar tremor.

Parkinsonism

- Multisystem degenerations ('parkinsonism plus' or atypical parkinsonism) (see later section).
- Heredodegenerative parkinsonism (see later section).
- Secondary parkinsonism (see later section).
- Progressive pallidal atrophy.
- Parkinsonism–dementia–ALS complex of Guam (PDACG), or Lytico–Bodig.
- X-linked dystonia–parkinsonism.
- Rapid-onset dystonia–parkinsonism.
- Pallidopyramidal disease.

Neuropsychiatric features

As either an alternative primary or concurrent diagnosis to PD:

- AD.
- Vascular dementia (VaD).
- Dementia with Lewy bodies (DLB).
- Brain injury: alcohol, head trauma.
- Other causes:
  - NPH.
  - Intracranial mass lesion: frontal or temporal lobe tumor, chronic subdural hematoma.
  - Metabolic/toxic: chronic drug intoxication (e.g. alcohol, barbiturates, sedatives), chronic hepatic encephalopathy.
  - Endocrine: hypothyroidism, Cushing's syndrome.
  - Autoimmune: SLE.
  - Nutritional: vitamin B12 deficiency; Wernicke–Korsakoff syndrome.
  - Infection: syphilis (general paresis of the insane), HIV.
  - FTD.
  - HD.
  - PSP.
  - Prion disease.
- Pseudo-dementia: related to depression.
- Age-related cognitive impairment in 'normal' (not diagnosed with a specific neurologic disease) aged persons.
- Multiple causes (i.e. combinations of the above).

Investigations

Indicated if parkinsonism is atypical for idiopathic PD (see below).

- Serum copper and ceruloplasmin, 24-hour urine copper, slit lamp examination; in younger patients, to exclude Wilson's disease.
- CT brain scan: to exclude hydrocephalus, cerebral infarction, or hemorrhage, and a structural lesion such as an arteriovenous malformation (AVM) or tumor (usually convexity meningioma causing contralateral hemiparkinsonism). Usually shows nonspecific generalized atrophy of the brain.
- MRI brain scan:
  - May show generalized atrophy.
  - Prominent iron deposition (dark signal on T2-weighted imaging) in the substantia nigra may be noted.
  - Some narrowing of part of the substantia nigra has been demonstrated in some cases but both this and the previous feature are very nonspecific and hard to spot.
  - A combination of putamenal hypointensity and brainstem atrophy is a consistent finding in Parkinson-plus syndromes and excludes PD.
- Functional imaging:
  - Positron emission tomography (PET): limited availability/cost precludes use as screening or diagnostic tool.
    - 18F-dopa-PET is a form of metabolic imaging which may indirectly provide a quantitative assessment of presynaptic nigrostriatal dopaminergic function, with early PD patients showing reduced metabolism in the dorsal striatum, though this finding is not entirely specific to PD.
    - 18F-fluoro-deoxyglucose-PET may provide an assessment of regional metabolic rates of glucose, which in addition to 18-F-dopa-PET may help distinguish PD from other atypical parkinsonian disorders.
  - Dopamine transporter imaging (FP-CIT-SPECT DaTSCAN)
    - Sensitive method to detect presynaptic dopamine neuronal dysfunction, assisting in differentiation between PD and other conditions, such as dystonia, essential tremor or secondary etiologies.

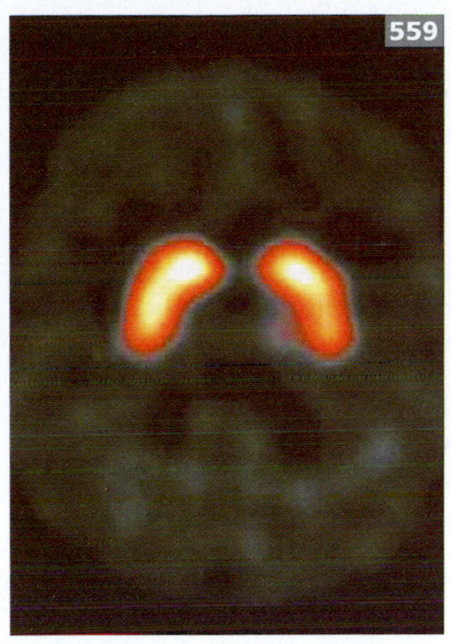

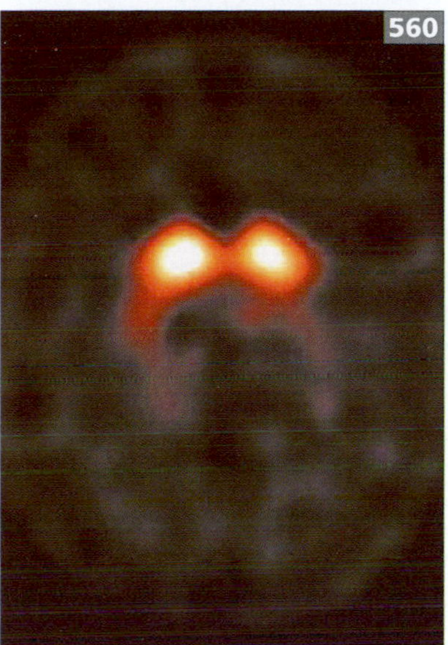

559, 560 FP-CIT-SPECT (DaTSCAN) differentiation of parkinsonian and tremor disorders. A normal test (559) shows the comma-shaped caudate and putamen; this pattern is seen in healthy individuals or patients with other causes of tremor or parkinsonism not involving degeneration of the presynaptic dopaminergic neurons. (560) This abnormal image shows a reduction in the left more than in the right putamen. The scan asymmetry typically corresponds to the asymmetry of parkinsonism in an affected patient. *Courtesy of Donald D. Grosset, Southern General Hospital, Glasgow.*

  - Does not distinguish between PD and other forms of atypical degenerative parkinsonism.
  - More widely available as a clinical diagnostic test, although the cost of the test prohibits widespread use, particularly since clinical examination and history remain the gold standard for the diagnosis of PD.
  - Best applied in cases where diagnosis is unclear, examination is equivocal, or if results would change treatment and prognosis (**559, 560**)
- Transcranial ultrasound of the substantia nigra: shows midbrain hyperechogenicity in 90% of PD patients, but is not specific, also seen in depression and normal individuals.
- Acute drug challenges: apomorphine test, levodopa challenge; no longer considered reliable as a sensitive means of diagnosing PD.
- Bloodwork to exclude secondary causes, as indicated: complete blood count, peripheral blood smear, thyroid function tests, VDRL/RPR/TPHA, vitamin B12, antinuclear antibodies, HIV, serology.

Diagnosis

A clinical diagnosis can be made with confidence when:

- There are two of the four cardinal clinical features of parkinsonism, including bradykinesia and one of the following: tremor (present in 80%), rigidity, and disturbed postural reflexes. However, early impairment of postural reflexes may be a sign of an atypical cause of parkinsonism.
- There is no detectable alternative cause for the parkinsonism.
- The patient responds to levodopa.
- The course is slowly progressive.

However, the clinical diagnosis may be incorrect in up to 25% of patients, particularly early on in the clinical course. Clues to an alternative diagnosis are the presence of additional nonparkinsonian features and a partial or absent response to levodopa and dopamine agonists.

Tip

▶ *The diagnosis of PD is a clinical one, based on the presence of typical symptoms and the absence of atypical features. However, since PD is a heterogeneous disorder, and the spectrum of findings in any single patient can vary significantly, often the diagnosis may be unclear in the beginning. Progression of atypical features over time and response to antiparkinsonian medications usually improve the certainty of diagnosis.*

Early clinical features raising doubts about the diagnosis of idiopathic PD

- Atypical levodopa-induced dyskinesias (e.g. torticollis, antecollis, sustained dystonic spasm of facial musculature).
- Onset before the age of 40 years.
- Strictly unilateral disease.
- Symmetric disease.
- Early, more prominent:
  - Dysphagia.
  - Severe autonomic failure (orthostatic hypotension, incontinence, erectile dysfunction).
  - Speech abnormalities: dysarthria, palilalia, laryngeal stridor.
  - Postural instability and falls.
  - Cognitive signs: dementia, hallucinations, psychosis, pseudobulbar affect, apraxia.
  - Dystonia: disproportionate antecollis.

- Absence of:
  - Rest tremor.
  - Levodopa-induced dyskinesias after several years or despite high levodopa dose.
- Clinical signs outside the spectrum of PD:
  - Oculomotor (e.g. restricted eye movements due to supranuclear gaze palsy).
  - Cerebellar features (nystagmus, dysarthria, wide-based gait, ataxia).
  - Pyramidal tract signs (hyper-reflexia, weakness, Babinski sign).
  - Nondrug-induced myoclonus.
  - Inspiratory stridor.
- Peripheral neuropathy.
- Poor or limited response to adequate doses of levodopa.
- Family history of a movement disorder.
- Rapid or stepwise progression.

Pathology

- Loss (>50%) of melanin-containing, pigmented, dopaminergic neurons in the substantia nigra; preferentially affects the ventrolateral substantia nigra pars compacta which projects to the posterior putamen, with less involvement of the medial tegmental pigmented neurons that project to the caudate nucleus (**561–564**).

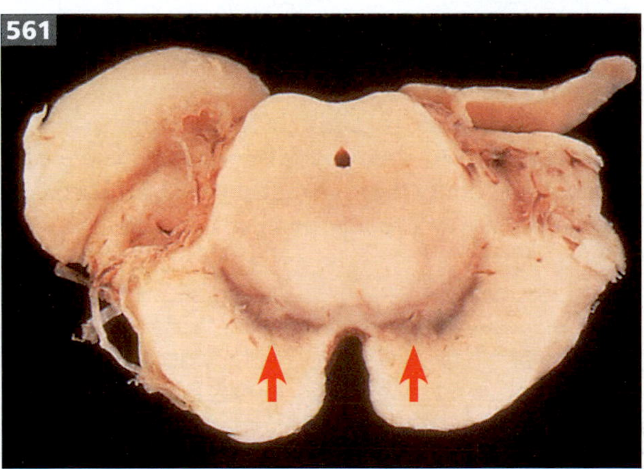

561 Axial section through the midbrain of a normal patient showing normal pigmentation of the substantia nigra.

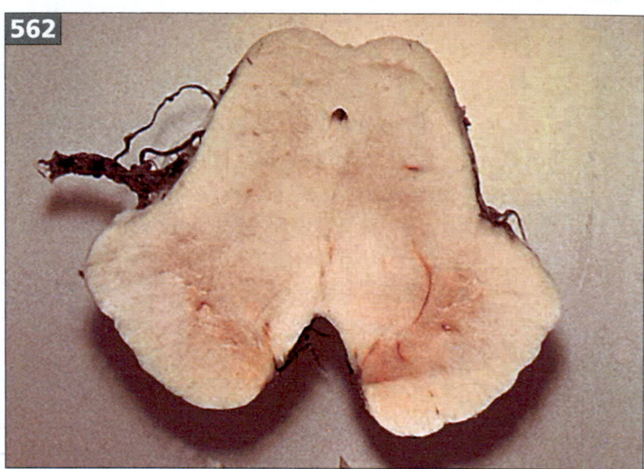

562 Axial section through the midbrain of a patient with Parkinson's disease, showing lack of pigmentation in the substantia nigra due to loss of melanin-containing pigmented dopaminergic neurons.

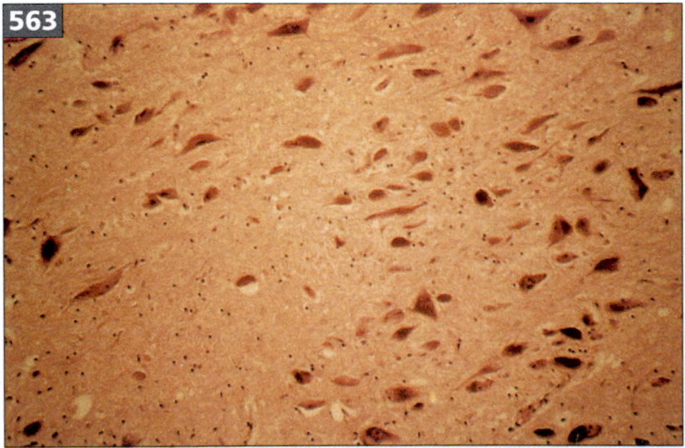

563 Section of the substantia nigra of a normal patient at low magnification power showing normal melanin-containing, pigmented, dopaminergic neurons.

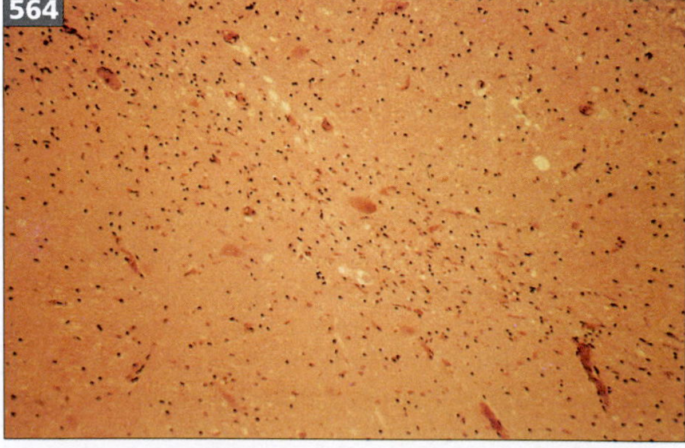

564 Section of the substantia nigra of a patient with Parkinson's disease, showing a reduced number of normal melanin-containing, pigmented, dopaminergic neurons.

565

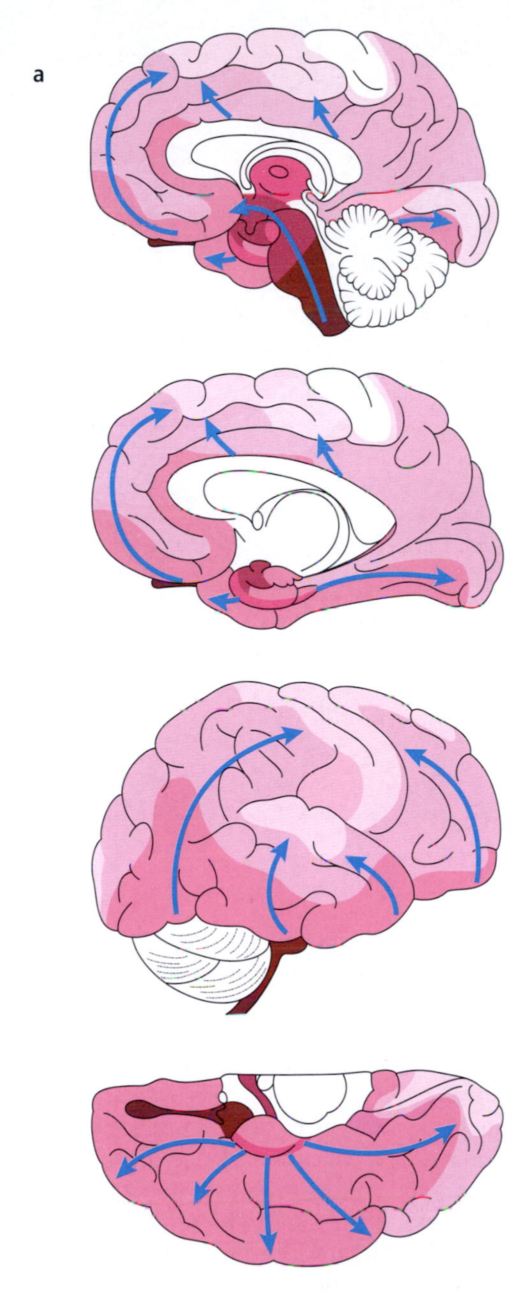

565 Progression of PD-related intraneuronal pathology. (a) The pathologic process targets specific subcortical and cortical induction sites. Lesions initially occur in the dorsal IX/X motor nucleus and frequently in the anterior olfactory nucleus. Thereafter, less susceptible brain structures gradually become involved (arrows). The brainstem pathology takes an upward course with cortical involvement following. (b) Simplified diagram showing the topographic expansion of the lesions (from left to right: dm to fc) and, simultaneously, the growing severity of the overall pathology (from top to bottom: stages 1–6). With the addition of further predilection sites, the pathology in the previously involved regions increases. co: ceruleus–subceruleus complex; dm: dorsal motor nucleus of the glossopharyngeal and vagal nerves; fc: first order sensory association areas, pre-motor areas, as well as primary sensory and motor fields; hc: high order sensory association areas and pre-frontal fields; mc: anteromedial temporal mesocortex; sn: substantia nigra. *Adapted from Braak 2003, with permission.*

b

Sites (columns); PD stages (rows)

dm	co	sn	mc	hc	fc
1					
2					
3					
4					
5					
6					

- Braak hypothesis of early PD pathology progression (**565**)[6]:
  - Stages 1 and 2 (medulla/pontine tegmentum): pathologic process of PD initially affects dorsal motor nucleus of the vagal and glossopharyngeal nerves, anterior olfactory nucleus, and locus ceruleus.
  - Stages 3 and 4 (lower and upper brainstem): thereafter, the disease process ascends in the brainstem, affecting the substantia nigra and mesocortex (transentorhinal region and CA2-plexus).
  - Stages 5–6 (neocortical areas): more severe brain involvement, with neocortical involvement of prefrontal and high order sensory association areas.

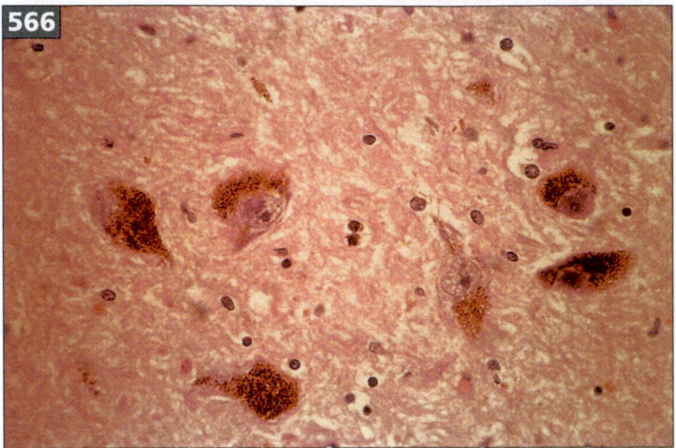

566 Microscopic sections of the substantia nigra at high magnification power showing normal melanin-containing, pigmented, dopaminergic neurons in a normal patient.

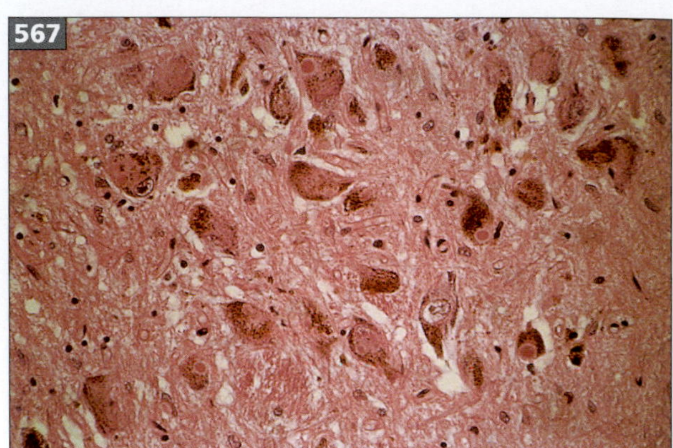

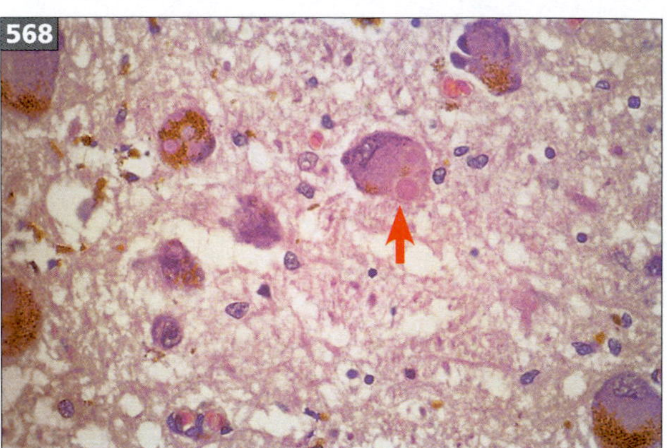

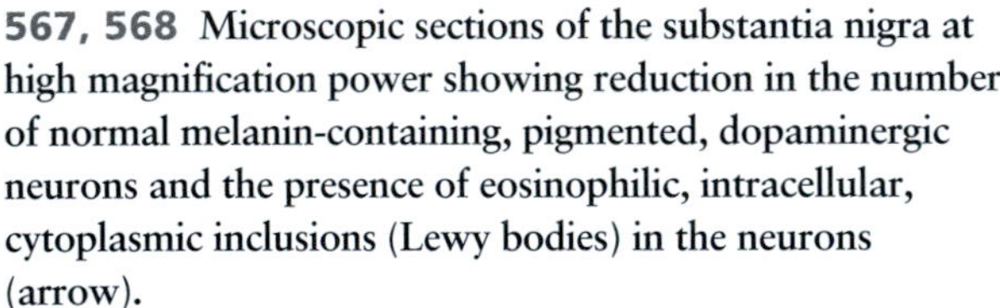

567, 568 Microscopic sections of the substantia nigra at high magnification power showing reduction in the number of normal melanin-containing, pigmented, dopaminergic neurons and the presence of eosinophilic, intracellular, cytoplasmic inclusions (Lewy bodies) in the neurons (arrow).

While the Braak hypothesis has had a profound effect on current models of PD, it is criticized for its lack of explaining other synuclein-related diseases (e.g. DBLD), lack of predictive validity, limitation to CNS structures, the observation of 'silent' stage 4–6 pathology in some subjects at autopsy, and the absence of this pattern in at least 15% of PD patients.

- Presence of eosinophilic intracellular cytoplasmic inclusions, known as Lewy bodies (which contain phosphorylated neurofilaments, ubiquitin, phospholipids, and many other cytoskeletal components) in the brainstem and other parts of the brain (**566–568**). Of note, not all genetically determined Parkinson syndromes include Lewy bodies.
- Dopamine deficiency (>80%) in the nigrostriatal pathway and relative hyperactivity of striatal (putamen and caudate nucleus) cholinergic activity. Clinical features do not emerge until 40–50% of nigral neurons and 60–80% striatal dopamine are lost.

Treatment[7]

The great majority of patients are adequately managed in the outpatient setting. Patients should be encouraged to keep as physically active as possible, with most evidence suggesting that exercise and physical activity may have at least short-term benefit in reducing the severity of many PD symptoms.

Non-motor symptoms of PD are often overlooked. Be aware of and treat concurrent symptoms such as pain (e.g. with tricyclic antidepressants), anxiety (e.g. with benzodiazepines), depression (with antidepressants or electroconvulsive therapy [ECT]), sleep disturbances, cognitive or sensory features.

The decision when to start symptomatic treatment is an individual decision for each patient based on personal needs and disability from PD symptoms. There is no conclusive evidence to suggest that early medical treatment of PD affects the progression of the disease, although some experts advocate that early treatment may reduce potentially harmful compensatory mechanisms related to untreated disease. Treatment-related adverse effects such as motor fluctuations and dyskinesias may be caused partly by the duration and total dose of drug treatment, particularly with levodopa. Compelling indications for starting symptomatic treatment are when employment is in jeopardy or when falling becomes a risk.

Commence medical therapy (dopamine replacement) at the lowest required dose and proceed with dose increases slowly in order to minimize risk of adverse effects such as nausea, dizziness, or confusion, particularly in the elderly (*Table 98*, next page). An hour-by-hour diary of the presence and severity of parkinsonian symptoms and dyskinesias can be helpful in guiding medication schedules for more advanced patients.

Medical therapies

Levodopa[8]

Levodopa is a naturally occurring amino acid, most of which is metabolized by catechol-O-methyltransferase (COMT) to form an inactive metabolite, and some of which is decarboxylated by an aromatic amino acid decarboxylase to form dopamine (**569**). It is still the gold standard drug for PD, after 30 years of use, for improving the cardinal features of the illness. Currently many formulations exist on the market (*Table 99*, next page).

Levodopa is usually combined with a peripheral decarboxylase inhibitor (carbidopa [Sinemet] or benserazide [Madopar]) that does not cross the blood–brain barrier. This combination minimizes production of dopamine in the systemic (peripheral) circulation and helps prevent adverse effects such as nausea and vomiting.

Early in the disease, low-dose levodopa (i.e. 100 mg, in combination with 25 mg of decarboxylase inhibitor, taken three to four times daily) controls most patient's symptoms very well (the 'honeymoon period' of a few years):

- If not effective but tolerated, the dose can be increased slowly to an effective dose (that improves function), which is commonly about 500–600 mg per day, and which does not cause adverse effects such as confusion, nausea, or dyskinesias.
- Failure to evoke substantial benefit should lead to a re-evaluation of the diagnosis.
- In the early stages of PD, the response to levodopa is sustained, despite the relatively short half-life of levodopa (about 90 minutes). Patients are often able to miss doses without any deterioration in clinical response.
- It may take as long as 30 days to achieve maximal benefit at a given dose, an adequate duration therapeutic trial is important.

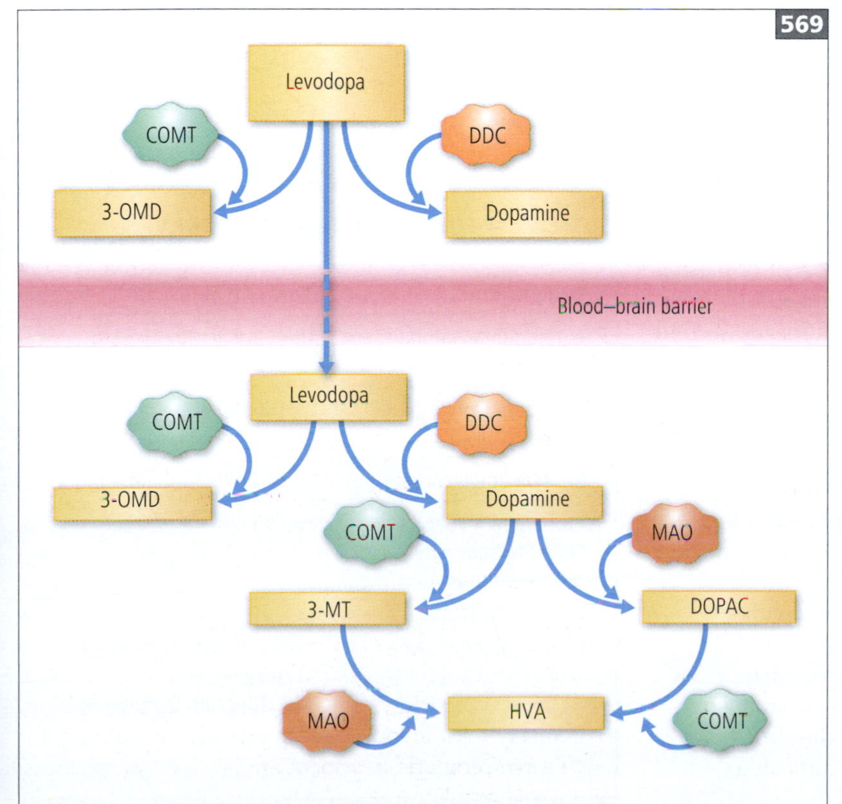

569 Metabolism of levodopa. Dopamine itself is unsuitable as a treatment for PD, as it cannot cross the blood–brain barrier, but its immediate precursor, levodopa, is metabolized to dopamine by the enzymes catechol-O-methyltransferase (COMT) and dopa decarboxylase (DDC). Orally-administered levodopa is converted into dopamine in the GI tract, leaving less available for transport into the CNS, while its generation within the peripheral circulation has adverse effects. 3-MT: 3-methoxytyramine; 3-OMD: 3-O-methyldopa; DOPAC: 3, 4-dihydroxyphenylacetic acid; HVA: homovanillic acid; MAO: monoamine oxidase.

TABLE 98 **COMMONLY USED DOPAMINERGIC DRUGS IN PARKINSON'S DISEASE, AND DOSE RANGES**

Drug	Initial dose	Effective daily dose
Amantadine	100 mg daily	200–400 mg daily
Carbidopa/levodopa	12.5/50 mg bid–tid	36.5/150–500/2000 mg daily
Controlled release carbidopa/levodopa	25/100 mg bid	50/200–500/2000 mg daily
Pramipexole	0.125 mg tid	1.5–4.5 mg daily
Ropinirole	0.25 mg tid	8–24 mg daily
Controlled release ropinirole	2 mg daily	8–24 mg daily
Rotigotine	2 mg daily	6–8 mg daily
Apomorphine subcutaneous	2–6 mg (individual titration)	2–6 mg for sudden 'off'
Entacapone	200 mg tid (give with carbidopa/levodopa)	Up to 1600 mg daily
Selegiline	5 mg daily	5 mg bid
Rasagiline	0.5 mg daily	1.0 mg daily

As the disease progresses, with continued loss of dopaminergic neurons in the substantia nigra, the duration of benefit following a single dose of levodopa diminishes, eventually mirroring the drug's plasma concentration curve. This phenomenon is known as 'end of dose failure' or 'wearing off' and is characterized by increasing bradykinesia and tremor in the hour or two before the next dose of levodopa is due. These predictable motor fluctuations are best managed by aiming for relatively constant levels of levodopa by reducing the time interval between each dose and prescribing more frequent, and sometimes smaller, doses of levodopa.

Subsequently, the patient may develop unpredictable motor fluctuations that are independent of plasma levodopa concentration and are attributed to post-synaptic changes in the dopamine receptors and second messengers:

- Recurrent swings between dyskinetic adverse effects of levodopa ('on') and severe bradykinesia ('off') may occur, as may sudden episodes of 'freezing'.
- Individual levodopa doses may fail to provide any benefit at all, known as 'no-on' phenomenon. The addition of a dopamine agonist or an enzyme inhibitor (see below) may be helpful.
- Controlled release levodopa for patients with motor fluctuations may cause a reduction in end of dose dystonia, and may be particularly helpful for overnight or early morning dystonia or breakthrough symptoms. However, this drug may have less bioavailability and may be difficult to titrate in more advanced patients.
- Increasing the dose of levodopa runs the risk of causing adverse effects which include nausea, postural hypotension, neuropsychiatric problems (mental confusion and hallucinations), and involuntary movements of the mouth, tongue, and limbs (peak dose dyskinesia).

TABLE 99 **FORMULATIONS OF LEVODOPA**

Drug name	Dosing (mg)
Carbidopa/levodopa (Sinemet)	10/100, 25/100, 25/250
Carbidopa/levodopa CR (Sinemet CR)	25/100, 50/200
Benserazide/levodopa	12.5/50, 25/100, 50/200
Carbidopa/levodopa ODT (Parcopa, orally disintegrating)	10/100, 25/100, 25/250
Carbidopa/levodopa/entacapone (Stalevo)	12.5/50/200, 18.75/75/200, 25/100/200, 31.25/125/200, 37.5/150/200, 50/200/200

Anticholinergics

Anticholinergics pimarily have a role in young patients with early PD and prominent or refractory resting (alternating) tremor, although benefit may be modest. Available drugs include benztropine and trihexyphenidyl. Adverse effects include dry mouth, mental confusion, hallucinations, blurred vision, and difficulty initiating micturition and urinary retention.

Anticholinergics are contraindicated in glaucoma, and should be avoided, or used with caution, in the elderly because of the high incidence of confusion and only modest antiparkinsonian benefit. Acute withdrawal of anticholinergics may be associated with dramatic worsening of parkinsonism, so the drugs should be discontinued gradually.

Amantadine

Amantadine is approved as an antiviral agent, and has unclear but likely multifactorial mechanisms of action including:

- Anticholinergic (antimuscarinic) effects.
- Weak dopamine agonist activity: releases dopamine from body stores.
- Glutamate receptor antagonist effect.

Amantadine may have a mild and temporary antiparkinsonian effect in early stages of the disease and may reduce dyskinesias in patients with motor fluctuations. Doses should begin with 100 mg capsule in the morning and, if necessary, another added at midday, with a maximal dose of 300–400 mg daily. A lower dose should be used in renal impairment, as its elimination depends on renal clearance.

Adverse effects include skin mottling (livedo reticularis) in one-half of patients, inflamed, swollen legs (erythromelalgia), and anticholinergic effects.

Dopamine receptor agonists

These are synthetic agents that act directly on dopamine receptors, and can be used as a sole treatment agent or in conjunction with other antiparkinsonian drugs. Possible advantages over levodopa include:

- Do not require biologic conversion to an active agent and therefore are not dependent on the presence of residual dopaminergic neurons or a pool of decarboxylase enzyme.
- Long half-life which helps to smooth out motor fluctuations and reduce 'on–off' phenomena.
- Less likely to cause dyskinesias.
- Lack of competition for absorption into the brain.
- Potential to stimulate selectively a subset of dopamine receptors.
- Fewer long-term adverse motor effects (motor fluctuations, dyskinesias).

Disadvantages over levodopa:

- Less potent and therefore less antiparkinsonian effect.
- More likely to cause confusion, hallucinations, peripheral edema, or autonomic symptoms than levodopa, particularly in the elderly.
- Associated with development of impulse control disorders in up to 17% of patients on this class of drugs, e.g. inability to resist excessive involvement in normally pleasurable activities such as gambling, eating, sex, shopping, or other hobbies, potentially resulting in devastating personal and social consequences.

Ergot-derived dopamine agonists

These are now less commonly used in clinical practice, as they may have more severe side-effects such as valvular heart disease, vasospasm, pulmonary edema, and (rarely) pleuropulmonary or retroperitoneal fibrosis. Monitoring requires yearly echocardiograms and chest X-ray before starting treatment.

- Bromocriptine:
  - A D2 dopamine receptor agonist with weak D1 antagonistic effects.
  - Half life 3–5 hours.
  - Available as 2.5 mg tablets, or 5 mg and 10 mg capsules.
  - Adverse effects similar to levodopa can occur, but it is more likely to cause confusion and commonly causes initial nausea because it acts centrally as well as peripherally, and stimulates dopamine receptors in the vomiting center in the medulla.
- Pergolide:
  - A combined D1 and D2 dopamine receptor agonist.
  - Has a long motor benefit (more than hours).
- Lisuride: a D2 dopamine receptor agonist.
- Cabergoline: for patients with motor fluctuations, carbergoline is comparable to bromocriptine and pergolide and increases 'on' time by about 10%, reduces 'off' time by about 17%, increases motor scores by about 37%.

Nonergot dopamine agonists

- Pramipexole:
  - Dose: up to 3–4.5 mg/day.
  - For patients with early untreated PD, monotherapy improves motor scores by 20–30% compared with placebo.
  - For patients with motor fluctuations, pramipexole increases motor and ADL scores by 20–25%, and reduces 'off' time by about 30% compared with placebo; and increases motor scores by 12% and ADL scores by 4% compared to bromocriptine.

- Ropinirole:
  - Dose: up to 24 mg/day.
  - For patients with early untreated PD, monotherapy increases motor scores by 24% compared with placebo, and controls symptoms in about 30% of patients. After 5 years' monotherapy, patients have fewer dyskinesias than if taking levodopa.
  - For patients with motor fluctuations, ropinirole reduces 'off' time by 20%, and enables the levodopa dose to be reduced by about 30%.
- Rotigitine:
  - Dose 2–8 mg daily.
  - Designed as a daily transdermal patch with slow release.
  - Limitations with patch technology and faulty drug delivery resulted in temporary removal from the US drug market, but it was re-released in 2012.
- Apomorphine:
  - A combined D1 and D2 dopamine receptor agonist.
  - Used in patients with motor fluctuations for rapid relief from sudden 'off' periods.
  - Given by subcutaneous injection intermittently.
  - The only other dopaminergic drug with equivalent potency to levodopa.
  - Fast onset: benefit occurs within 5–15 min, lasting 40–90 min.
  - Adverse effects similar to those from levodopa can occur, with the addition of yawning, drowsiness, and local skin reactions or abscesses at injection sites.
  - Requires careful initial titration, usually in a monitored setting, to avoid significant side-effects; oral domperidone, ondansetron, or trimethobenzamide are often given before each dose to prevent nausea. Patient should be started with low dose and titrated up under observation and monitoring of vital signs including blood pressure.

Catechol-O-methyltransferase (COMT) inhibition

COMT inhibition increases availability of levodopa for transport across the blood–brain barrier by reducing levodopa metabolism, thus extending the duration of action of each levodopa dose by about 30–50 minutes, irrespective of whether a standard or slow release form of levodopa is used. It is indicated for PD with motor fluctuations, not for early untreated PD, and must be used in conjunction with levodopa and a peripheral decarboxylase inhibitor.

Adverse effects include an increase in dyskinesias and other dopaminergic adverse effects, which may require a reduction in levodopa dose; diarrhea (usually in 4–12 weeks); orange/brown discoloration of urine, saliva, or sweat.

- Entacapone: extends levodopa half-life by acting as a peripheral COMT inhibitor.
- Tolcapone: extends levodopa half-life more than entacapone by acting as a central and peripheral COMT inhibitor, but is associated with the potentially serious side-effect of hepatic failure, requiring monitoring of liver enzymes, which limits its wide clinical application.

Monoamine oxidase Type B (MAO-B) inhibitors

These drugs selectively and irreversibly inhibit MAO-B, one of the enzymes that catabolizes dopamine in the brain, thereby retarding the breakdown of dopamine and increasing its duration of action. They have mild symptomatic benefit as monotherapy in early PD. There is argument as to whether they protect dopaminergic neurons and slow the progression of PD, but this has never been conclusively shown in human trials. The presumed mechanism is that oxygen free radical formation generated by the MAO-B oxidation of dopamine is reduced and the activation of exogenous neurotoxins is prevented.

MAO-B inhibitors should be used with caution in conjunction with antidepressants, due to theoretical risk of serotonin syndrome. When taken with levodopa, MAO-B inhibitors can slightly improve the duration of the levodopa effect and can smooth out early wearing off, but can also provoke or worsen dyskinesias and psychiatric adverse effects.

- Selegiline HCl:
  - Metabolized to desmethyldeprenyl, methylamphetamine, and amphetamine; these metabolites may have a theoretical effect on fatigue.
  - 5 mg tablets, taken in the morning and, if necessary, at midday to a maximum of 10 mg daily. Avoid evening doses as this may cause insomnia.
  - Adverse effects include nausea, insomnia, musculoskeletal injuries, nonthreatening cardiac arrhythmias, and elevations in liver enzyme levels.
  - Controversy exists as to whether it may be associated with excess mortality.
- Zydis selegiline: wafer formulation that dissolves in the mouth, bypassing hepatic first-pass metabolism.
- Rasagiline:
  - Once daily MAO-B inhibitor, up to 1 mg daily.
  - Free of amphetamine metabolites.
  - Initial US Food and Drug Adminstration (FDA) warning of avoiding high tyramine foods (red wine, aged cheeses, aged meats) was removed after further safety monitoring.

Tip

▶ *Levodopa still remains the gold-standard pharmacologic treatment for PD. Patient disease characteristics (both motor and non-motor symptoms), medical comorbidities, general health, and concomitant medications should be reviewed before determining an individual patient's antiparkinsonian medication regimen.*

Complications of medical therapy and treatment strategies

Motor fluctuations[9]

(See *Table 100.*)

After about 5 years of treatment, 30–80% of patients develop motor fluctuations. Motor fluctuations consist of variations in response to a single dose of levodopa, i.e. swings between parkinsonism and dyskinesias, with a variety of manifestations. This is due to shortening of the striatal half-life of levodopa, resulting in a shortened response from each dose of levodopa and a narrower therapeutic window (570).

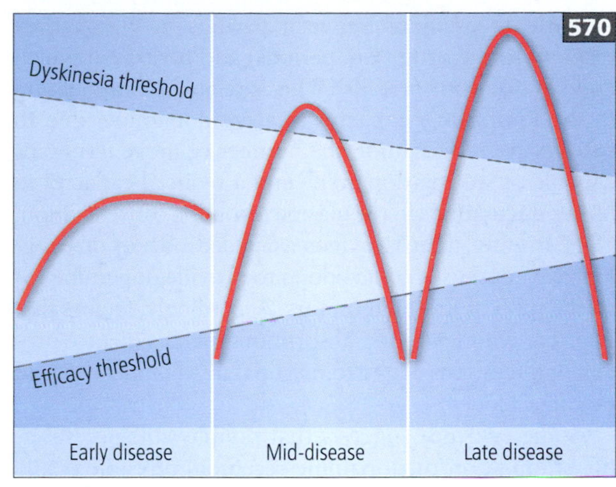

570 **The therapeutic window of Parkinson's disease narrows with progression of the disease, paralleling the progressively shorter striatal half-life of levodopa. In addition, peak-dose dyskinesias may develop, with threshold to the development of dyskinesias lowering over time.**

TABLE 100 **MEDICAL MANAGEMENT OF MOTOR FLUCTUATIONS AND DYSKINESIAS**

Motor fluctuations	**Dyskinesias**
WEARING OFF, END-OF-DOSE DETERIORATION Take levodopa 30 minutes before meals Smaller, more frequent doses of levodopa Add dopamine agonist Add COMT inhibitor Add MAO-B inhibitor	PEAK-DOSE DYSKINESIA Reduce total levodopa dose Add dopamine agonist to maintain motor response EARLY MORNING DYSTONIA Slow-release levodopa at night Long-acting dopamine agonist at night Antispasmodic (e.g. baclofen)
DELAYED 'ON' RESPONSE Take levodopa apart from meals (at least 30 minutes) Low protein diet Antacids, gastric prokinetic agents	EARLY MORNING DYSTONIA Slow-release levodopa at night Long-acting dopamine agonist at night Antispasmodic (e.g. baclofen)
DELAYED 'ON' RESPONSE Take levodopa apart from meals (at least 30 minutes) Low protein diet Antacids, gastric prokinetic agents	END-OF-DOSE DYSTONIA Slow-release levodopa Long-acting dopamine agonist
SUDDEN 'OFF' PERIODS Liquid levodopa Subcutaneuous apomorphine Low protein diet	'OFF' PERIOD DYSTONIA Liquid levodopa Subcutaneous apomorphine
'ON–OFF' PHENOMENA ('yo-yo-ing') Higher, less frequent doses of levodopa Add dopamine agonist Apomorphine infusion	DIPHASIC DYSKINESIAS (beginning and end of dose) Higher, less frequent doses of levodopa (?)

COMT: catechol-O-methyltransferase; MAO: monoamine oxidase.

Patients oscillate between periods in which they respond to the drug ('on' periods) and periods in which they do not ('off' periods). This is related to a reduction in the PD brain's capacity to store dopamine, due to progressive reduction in the number of nerve terminals capable of storing dopamine and a reduced capacity to buffer fluctuations in the plasma levodopa concentration. Concurrently, there is an increasing dependency on exogenously administered levodopa to provide dopamine for stimulation of striatal receptors. Accordingly, factors that interfere with levodopa absorption, such as dietary protein or alterations in gastrointestinal transit time, can lead to 'off' episodes.

Some evidence suggests that nonphysiologic, pulsatile stimulation of dopamine receptors physiologically induces the development of motor fluctuations and dyskinesias. Other mechanisms may include changes in neurotransmitters, cellular signaling pathways, or dopamine receptor expression.

Motor fluctuations can be controlled in the early stages by:

- Strategies that enhance levodopa absorption in the brain (e.g. reschedule protein intake, low protein diet [to avoid competition of neutral amino acids with L-dopa absorption and entry into the brain]).
- Manipulation of the levodopa dose or use of the sustained release formulations of levodopa.
- Inhibiting levodopa catabolism (COMT or MAO-B inhibitors) and prolonging plasma half-life of levodopa.
- Adding dopamine agonists to treatment regime.

In advanced stages of the disease, fluctuations are difficult to treat and patients frequently cycle between 'on' periods complicated by dyskinesia and 'off' periods in which they are frozen and akinetic. Liquid levodopa or surgical approaches should be considered for such patients.

Dyskinesias

Dyskinesias are abnormal involuntary movements occurring as a complication of dopaminergic therapy. The cause is unclear, but may be related to:

- Upregulation of dopamine receptors.
- Post-synaptic changes associated with both PD and exposure to levodopa.
- Influences of glutamatergic projections and other transmitter systems including serotonergic, alpha-2 adrenergic, histaminergic, and cannabinoid pathways.

Dyskinesias tend to develop earlier and more severely in younger PD patients. They are usually choreiform (dance-like), but also may be may be dystonic (sustained and often painful muscle contractions) or myoclonic (sudden jerks) in character. While milder dyskinesias are typically not disabling, severe dyskinesias may be more disabling than the parkinsonism itself.

Dyskinesias may be monophasic, occurring at the time of maximal clinical improvement (peak-dose dyskinesias), or biphasic, occurring at time of disappearance and reappearance of parkinsonian symptoms (onset- and end-of-dose dyskinesias).

Monophasic dyskinesias can be reduced by decreasing and spreading the daily doses of antiparkinsonian medication, but this may preclude a satisfactory antiparkinsonian response and lead to the emergence of motor fluctuations in the form of end-of-dose akinesia and 'on–off' phenomena. Diphasic dyskinesias can be alleviated by increasing the daily dose of antiparkinsonian medication to maintain constant high plasma levels of medication (e.g. levodopa), but this may produce chaotic dyskinesias and severe psychiatric disorders.

The only antidyskinetic agent with evidence-based efficacy is amantadine. Various agents such as anticholinergics, benzodiazepines, serotonin antagonists (e.g. fluoxetine), beta-blockers, low-dose clozapine (50 mg) (a dibenzodiazepine derivative that blocks D1, D2, and D4 dopamine receptors), and riluzole (an inhibitor of glutamatergic transmission in the CNS) have been tried for antidyskinetic effects, but are not commonly used or recommended in clinical practice.

Surgical treatment of PD with advanced motor fluctuations may allow reductions in dyskinesias by allowing reduction in required medication doses and by modulating the abnormal circuitry predisposing to dyskinesias.

Non-motor symptoms

Neuropsychiatric symptoms[10]

These include confusion, hallucinations, delusions, and psychosis. They are more frequent in older patients and more common with longer disease duration. Hallucinations may occur in up to one-third of patients on chronic dopaminergic treatment, usually comprising visual images of people or animals.

Neuropsychiatric symptoms may be induced by all antiparkinsonian drugs, but more commonly with anticholinergics or dopamine agonists. In patients with dementia, it may be difficult to control parkinsonism without adversely affecting mental function. Symptoms can be minimized or treated by:

- Eliminating unnecessary psychoactive or sedative medications.
- Ruling out other medical and neurologic causes of altered mental status (i.e. infections, strokes, mass lesions, medications).
- Withdrawing anticholinergics, dopamine agonists, amantadine and MAO-B inhibitors as tolerated, restricting antiparkinsonian therapy to levodopa monotherapy.
- Using the lowest dose of antiparkinsonian medication that will provide a satisfactory motor response.

While many antipsychotics are labeled as atypical, only two have more consistently been demonstrated not to worsen parkinsonism significantly:

- Clozapine: given in smaller doses than needed for psychosis (starting at 12.5 mg daily and seldom increasing above 100 mg daily), may help to control the psychotic features and permit higher doses of levodopa–carbidopa to be used. Disadvantages are that weekly blood counts are required because of the risk of agranulocytosis, and it also causes sedation, hypotension, or rarely myocarditis.
- Quetiapine: while appearing clinically efficacious, three randomized, controlled trials do not support its efficacy over placebo. Regardless, it is commonly used as first-line therapy in low doses (12.5–150 mg daily), preferably at night as it may also cause sedation and therefore improve any coexistent insomnia.

Acetylcholinesterase inhibitors (donepezil, rivastigmine, and galantamine) were developed as symptomatic treatment of cognition and behavior in mild to moderate dementia of Alzheimer's type, but have been extended to use in PD dementia. They inhibit acetylcholinesterase and thus decrease acetylcholine breakdown in the synaptic cleft. All have broadly similar efficacy, although only rivastigmine has been demonstrated to show improvement in a randomized, controlled trial.

Two randomized, double-blind trials suggest that memantine (an NMDA receptor antagonist) may lead to global improvement of cognitive function or at least in some cognitive subdomains, such as speed on attention tasks.

Mood disorders: PD patients may have coexisting depression (20–40% prevalence) and anxiety (5-40% prevalence). These may be an inherent component of parkinsonism (given degeneration of noradrenergic, serotonergic, and cholinergic nuclei and disruption of mesocortical, limbic, and frontal pathways) or a reaction to having a chronic progressive neurodegenerative disorder.

In depression, treatment for PD should be the first consideration and may itself improve the depression. Tricyclic antidepressants (amitriptyline, nortriptyline, imipramine) have anticholinergic properties that may improve PD features in the early stages but may aggravate mental function in patients with more advanced disease. SSRIs (fluoxetine, paroxetine, citalopram, or sertraline) are probably preferable. While earlier reports suggest that this class of drugs may worsen parkinsonism, they do not appear to do so on average, and may even improve symptoms. Other non-SSRI agents used in practice but not studied specifically in PD include venlafaxine, mirtazapine, duloxetine, and buproprion. Class IV studies suggest that ECT may be effective.

In anxiety, there are no clinical trials to support PD-specific therapies. Nonpharmacologic therapies include psychotherapy, relaxation therapy, and biofeedback, while pharmacologic therpies include benzodiazepines, SSRIs, buspirone, and adjusting PD medication if symptoms are 'off' related.

Impulse control disorders: Prevention, education, and screening for abnormal behaviors by physician and families are important. Behaviors usually resolve/improve with dopamine agonist dose reduction or discontinuing agonist treatment entirely, with increase in levodopa to counter any motor decline.

Dysautonomia

- Nausea: may be a side-effect of dopaminergic medications:
  - Start treatment slowly with low doses of levodopa/dopamine agonists, i.e. one-half of a tablet of the smallest dose, and increase by one-half of a tablet every third day. Initial tolerance may be poor, but may improve with slow titration.
  - Take the medication 30 minutes after food.

- If nausea persists, options include:
  - Supplemental carbidopa 25 mg tablets with each dose.
  - Administering the peripherally acting antiemetic drug domperidone 10 mg, taken 30 minutes before each dose of antiparkinsonian medication (i.e. with food, followed by antiparkinsonian drug 30 minutes later).
  - Avoid other dopamine-receptor blocking antiemetics such as metoclopramide and prochlorperazine, which may worsen parkinsonism.
- Constipation: standard measures such as dietary modifications with high fiber, increase fluid intake, laxative medications (colace, senna, bisacodyl, magnesium sulfate, polyethylene glycol), suppositories, enemas.
- Sialorrhea: anticholinergic drugs, botulinum toxin.
- Urinary dysfunction:
  - Urodynamic testing, urologic evaluation.
  - Standard agents for neurogenic bladder dysfunction (no validation in PD population), such as the anticholinergics oxybutynin and tolterodine; cholinergic side-effects are possible (orthostatic hypotension, cognitive dysfunction, urinary retention).
  - Muscarinic agonists (bethanechol).
  - Intermittent self-catheterization or indwelling catheter.
  - Pelvic floor physical therapy.
  - Botulinum toxin.
- Orthostatic hypotension:
  - Minimize dose of nonlevodopa antiparkinsonian drugs (particularly dopamine agonists, selegiline).
  - Take antiparkinsonian drugs after meals.
  - Increase fluid consumption.
  - Adequate salt intake.
  - Elastic support/compression stockings (typically poorly tolerated).
  - Small frequent meals to minimize post-prandial hypotension.
  - Head-up tilt of the bed at night.
  - Conditioning exercises.
  - Medications:
    - Volume expanders (fludrocortisone).
    - Vasoconstictors (midodrine: peripherally acting alpha-1 agonist).
    - Other: caffeine, pseudoephedrine, indomethacin, domperidone, desmopressin (DDAVP), subcutaneous octreotide (inhibits release of vasodilator peptides).
- Hyperhydrosis: adjustment of PD medications, propranolol.

Sleep disorders

- Obstructive sleep apnea (OSA): detection by sleep study, positive pressure ventilation, weight loss.
- REM behavioral disorder: clonazepam, melatonin.
- Excessive daytime sleepiness: eliminate sedating medications, minimize dopaminergic medications, identify and treat underling sleep disorders, consider stimulants such as modafinil, methylphenidate, or caffeine (no clear evidence, may worsen tremor or neuropsychiatric symptoms).

Impotence

- Impotence may be treated with sildenafil, yohimbine, intracavernosal injections of papaverine, prostaglandin E, or implantation of a penile prosthesis.

Tip

▶ *Both motor and non-motor side-effects can occur at any point during treatment with antiparkinsonian medications, and should be screened for regularly during follow-up visits.*

Surgical therapies

Surgical treatments for PD are now standard treatment options after the development of models of basal ganglia circuitry, refinements of stereotactic surgery (due to better stereotactic frames, imaging by high resolution brain CT and MRI, and intraoperative electrophysiologic microelectrode assessment), and continued long-term evidence of overall safe and effective outcomes with positive impact on quality of life in select patients. The main surgical targets are the internal (medial or posteroventral) globus pallidus and the subthalamic nucleus. The most common surgical strategy is reversible, unilateral or bilateral, high-frequency deep-brain stimulation (DBS) via stimulating electrodes, while lesional surgery has become less favorable due to its irreversible effects, usual limitation to a unilateral procedure, and higher incidence of side-effects.

Deep brain stimulation[11]

High frequency DBS (about 150 cycles per second) functionally inhibits neuronal activity in specific brain targets without the need to make a lesion. By connecting an implanted stimulating electrode to a subcutaneous pacemaker, target sites can be continuously stimulated by adjustable parameters. Proper patient selection is critical, with the ideal patient showing the following characteristics:

- Diagnosis of idiopathic PD.
- Significant clinical improvement or motor symptoms with levodopa therapy.
- Presence of motor fluctuations and dyskinesia that are not fully managed by medications; or, medication refractory tremor.
- Absence of significant dementia, psychosis, or depression.
- Age under 75 and general good medical health, although select older patients may benefit.
- Appropriate understanding of risks and outcomes of surgery.
- Supportive caregivers and family.

Chronic bilateral stimulation of the subthalamic nucleus may dramatically improve all cardinal features of PD and medication requirements but ballism may emerge. DBL was first used in PD patients in 1993, and is currently the preferred surgical treatment for PD. Mechanism of action is unclear and likely complex, but stimulation appears to mimic the effects of an ablative lesion.

Studies show significant post-operative reduction of off-state UPRDRS scores (by ~50%) and dyskinesias (by ~69%), and reduction of anti-parkinsonian medications (by ~56%). Quality of life is improved in comparison to medical management alone. Speech, gait, and cognitive symptoms may be less improved than other cardinal features, and in some cases can worsen post-operatively.

Stimulation of the GPi may also improve the cardinal features of PD, and is effective for treating severe dyskinesias. Stimulation of ventralis intermediate nucleus of the thalamus may effectively and safely suppresses tremor in >80% of patients, but has no effect on the other cardinal symptoms of PD.

The advantages of DBS over thermolytic lesioning are that it is reversible and causes minimal or no damage to the brain. However, it requires two surgical procedures (one for targeting and another for definitive electrode internalization), the life of the battery is limited to a few years, and it does not combat continued progression of underlying disease.

Complications of DBS may include: hardware or electrode-related difficulties, side-effects of stimulation (dysarthria, visual symptoms, paresthesias, dyskinesias), cognitive deficits (particularly decreased word fluency), apathy, mood or psychiatric disorders (depression, mania), tissue infection, weight gain, or stroke.

Newer DBS targets include the pedunculopontine nucleus, median parafasicular complex of the thalamus, or caudal zona incerta.

Lesional surgery

- Pallidotomy:
  - Lesions in the posteroventral portion of the GPi presumably reduce the inhibitory output from the medial globus pallidus and thereby improve many of the 'off' period symptoms of PD (tremor, rigidity, and bradykinesia on the side contralateral to the surgery and some elements of gait). Lesions may also reduce levodopa-induced dyskinesias by up to 75%.
  - However, they do not improve the patient's level of function when 'on' except for elimination of peak-dose levodopa-induced dyskinesias. Midline symptoms, such as postural instability and abnormal gait, also improve less. Any improvements are immediate and sustained for at least 6 months.
  - Complications include homonymous hemianopia (up to 14%), facial paresis (up to 51%), and hemiparesis (up to 4%).
- Subthalamotomy: lesions may improve motor signs but at present carry an unacceptable risk of inducing hemiballismus or causing midbrain hemorrhage due to its high vascularity.
- Thalamotomy:
  - Effective predominantly for medically intractable tremor.
  - A thermally induced lesion of the ventro-intermediate nucleus of the thalamus improves contralateral tremor in about 90% of patients.
  - Recurrence of tremor occurs in about 5–10% of cases, usually within the first 3 months.
  - Lesioning the ventralis oralis anterior/posterior (rostral to the ventrointermediate nucleus) may improve rigidity of the contralateral limbs.
  - Risks of this procedure are intracerebral hemorrhage and lesioning of structures adjacent to the target site. Mortality varies from 0.4 to 6%.

Dopaminergic transplantation strategies

While strategies based on the notion that dopaminergic cells transplanted to the striatum may compensate for degenerating nigral neurons have been pursued, none has yet been demonstrated as effective in double-blind trials. Transplantation of fetal porcine nigral cells, fetal nigral cells, and retinal pigmented epithelial cells has not demonstrated significant benefit over placebo, with some patients experiencing disabling forms of dyskinesias ('off-medication dyskinesias'), some requiring treatment with DBS surgery, likely related to nonphysiologic dopaminergic stimulation. Additionally, autopsy examination of implanted dopamine neurons has been noted to contain Lewy bodies, suggesting that the PD pathologic process may overwhelm transplanted cells[12]. Stem cell transplantation, growth factor infusion, and gene therapies are currently in investigational stages.

Prognosis

Symptoms progress slowly over several years. About one-half of patients experience significant complications of therapy after 5 years. Unless there is an intercurrent cause of death, patients may eventually succumb to secondary complications of the disease, with pneumonia as the most common. The average duration of the disease from diagnosis to death is about 15 years, with a mortality ratio of 2:1.

The longest prospective study in PD (Sydney Multicenter study)[13] showed:

- Non-motor features predominate after 15 years of disease in the one-third of surviving cohort: cognitive decline (83%), falls (81%), daytime sleepiness (79%), depression (50%), incontinence (41%) in survivors after 20 years.
- Mean duration from diagnosis to death was 9.1 years.

Prognostic factors include:

- Gait disturbance or postural instability at presentation (PIGD phenotype) are associated with more severe disease including faster rate of progression and higher incidence of dementia.
- Tremor-dominant parkinsonism tends to have a more favorable course with slower progression.
- Onset of PD after the age of 60 years is associated with a greater likelihood of developing dementia, while younger patients have a greater risk of developing adverse effects associated with using levodopa long term (i.e. dyskinesias, motor fluctuations).

MULTISYSTEM DEGENERATIONS ('PARKINSONISM PLUS' OR ATYPICAL PARKINSONISM)

MULTIPLE SYSTEM ATROPHY

Definition and epidemiology

Multiple system atrophy (MSA) is a sporadic, adult onset, progressive, neurodegenerative disease of unknown etiology, characterized by autonomic dysfunction combined with parkinsonism and/or ataxia. While clinically protean, different manifestations of the disease are unified by common cellular pathology featuring glial cytoplasmic inclusions.

The term MSA was coined in 1969 by Graham and Oppenheimer. They reported a patient who developed autonomic failure followed by cerebellar and pyramidal signs, dying at age 62 years only 4 months after disease onset. Autopsy revealed cell loss and gliosis (without Lewy bodies) in the substantia nigra, striatum, olives, pons, cerebellum, and intermediolateral cell columns of the spinal cord. The term was proposed as shorthand to cover many cases described under different titles that overlapped with each other, including:

- Sporadic olivopontocerebellar atrophy (OPCA): cerebellar signs, dysautonomia, later development of parkinsonism, pyramidal signs.
- Shy–Drager syndrome (SDS), described in 1960 by Shy and Drager: progressive, primary orthostatic hypotension due to autonomic failure owing to loss of cells in the intermediolateral column of the spinal cord, and neurologic signs of extrapyramidal, pyramidal, and cerebellar dysfunction. Autopsy showed cell loss and gliosis in the striatum, substantia nigra, cerebellum, pons, olives, and intermediolateral cell columns.
- Striatonigral degeneration (SND), described in 1964 by Adams *et al.*: with parkinsonism, brisk reflexes, autonomic failure, late cerebellar signs. Autopsy showed evidence of striatal neuronal loss, demyelination, and gliosis, principally in the putamen and substantia nigra, but also in the olives and the cerebellum (and the pons in one case). Incidental nigral Lewy bodies were found in one patient.

MSA is now considered a well defined clinicopathologic entity with protean manifestations, rather than three different diseases with several clinical features in common.

- Prevalence: 1.9–4.9 per 100,000.
- Age: mean age of onset: 60 years (range 34–83 years).
- A predominantly parkinsonian phenotype (MSA-P) accounts for 80% of patients in western countries, although Japanese series report a higher cerebellar phenotype (MSA-C) predominance.
- Gender: M=F.

- Risk factors: unclear. Rare familial cases have been reported, although spinocerebellar ataxia may present with MSA-like features and may be hard to differentiate. Variants in the alpha-synuclein gene (*SNCA*) appear to convey risk of developing MSA, particularly the MSA-C subtype.

Etiology and pathophysiology

Complex and not well understood.

Clinical features[14]

Clinical diagnosis has been revised in 2008 by a group of experts via a consensus conference[15]. Any combination of symptoms and signs of documented autonomic dysfunction, which, like PD, may pre-date the motor features[16]:

- Orthostatic hypotension.
- Impotence.
- Urinary incontinence.

Plus one of the following:

- Predominantly cerebellar signs: dysarthria, gait ataxia, oculomotor dysfunction (termed MSA-C).
- Predominantly parkinsonism, with poor, mild, or transient response to levodopa therapy (termed MSA-P).

The following signs may be present and are considered 'red flags' of supportive features for the diagnosis of MSA:

- Pyramidal signs: brisk reflexes, Babinski sign, spastic quadriparesis (about 50% of patients).
- Stridor, inspiratory sighs, dysphonia, new or increased snoring.
- Rapidly progressive parkinsonism.
- Dysphagia within 5 years of motor onset.
- Orofacial dystonia[17].
- Disproportionate antecollis (**571**).
- Camptocormia (severe anterior spine flexion) and/or Pisa syndrome (severe lateral spine flexion).
- Contractures of hands/feet.
- Pathologic laughter or crying.
- Myoclonic, jerky action and postural tremor.

The following features are not supportive of MSA and may suggest an alternative diagnosis:

- Classic pill-rolling rest tremor (more common with PD).
- Clinically significant neuropathy.
- Family history of ataxia or parkinsonism (as MSA is sporadic).
- Dementia or hallucinations not induced by drugs.
- White matter lesions on brain MRI.
- Onset after age 75.

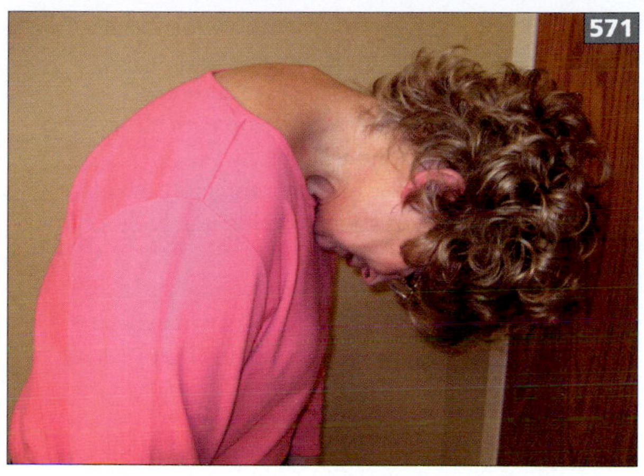

571 **A patient with multiple system atrophy-parkinsonism displaying early presentation of severe, disproportionate antecollis before the insidious development of dysautonomia and parkinsonism. Dystonic symptoms were helped mildly by botulinum toxin injections, but total dose and therapeutic effect were limited by risk of dysphagia related to anterior neck injections.**

Differential diagnosis

Parkinsonism

- Idiopathic PD:
  - Most MSA patients are initially diagnosed as having idiopathic PD, and one-third retain this erroneous diagnosis until they die.
  - A small subset of PD patients may present with earlier dysautonomia, making the early distinction between the two diseases difficult.
  - Between 4% and 22% (mean 8%) of brains in parkinsonian brain banks are found to have MSA.
  - Unlike MSA, idiopathic PD will not give rise to pyramidal or cerebellar signs.
  - PD and MSA may be distinguished by nuclear imaging tests:
    - ^{123}I-MIBG cardiac scans: MSA involves preganglionic/central sympathetic degeneration (showing normal or only mildly reduced MIBG uptake), as opposed to the loss of integrity of post-ganglionic noradrenergic neurons in PD (showing reduced MIBG uptake).
    - PET scans show more widespread hypometabolism, including the putamen, brainstem, and cerebellum in MSA compared to PD.

- DLB can also cause parkinsonism with autonomic failure, but not pyramidal or cerebellar signs.
- PSP: autonomic features are rare, although urinary incontinence may develop with pathologic involvement of the spinal cord.
- CBD: autonomic features are rare, more asymmetric, signs of cortical involvement in addition to extrapyramidal features.
- Other heredodegenerative or secondary parkinsonism disorders (see later sections): manganese intoxication symptoms and imaging may overlap with MSA.

Autonomic failure

- Primary: pure autonomic failure (PAF) (isolated) is a syndrome that has several causes. It may be due to the rare dopamine-beta-hydroxylase deficiency or may persist in isolated form and be revealed at autopsy to be related to the pathology of DLBD or MSA. So, with the passage of time, an initial syndrome of pure autonomic failure may mature into clinical idiopathic PD, DLBD, or MSA. Helpful distinguishing tests are plasma norepinephrine concentrations in the supine resting position (normal in MSA, low in PAF), and plasma arginine vasopressin in upright tilt (very little increase in patients with MSA for the degree of hypotension, marked rise in patients with PAF for the same degree of hypotension).
- Secondary:
  - Addison's disease.
  - Amyloidosis.
  - Diabetes.
  - Drugs.

Cerebellar ataxia

- Inherited spinocerebellar ataxia (SCA).
- Multiple sclerosis.
- Posterior fossa/diencephalic arteriovenous malformation/tumor.
- Drug toxicity.
- Fragile X-associated tremor ataxia syndrome (FXTAS).

Pyramidal signs

- Parasagittal meningioma.
- Multi-infarct state.
- NPH.
- Cervical spondylitic myelopathy.
- Amyotrophic lateral sclerosis.

Investigations

CT brain scan

CT is used to exclude some of the differential diagnoses and to identify atrophy of the cerebellum and brainstem, particularly the pons, inferior olives, vermis, and cerebellar peduncles; however, MRI has a much higher resolution for these structures.

MRI brain

Several MRI findings may be detected in MSA, with varying degrees of sensitivity and specificity, including putaminal atrophy or hypointensity, a hyperintense rim bordering the putamen, or focal atrophy of the brain, particularly the pons, inferior olives, vermis, dentate nuclei and cerebellar peduncles[18]. The 'hot cross bun' sign (**572**) in the pontine basis accompanies this atrophy and is a sign of selective loss of transverse pontocerebellar fibers and neurons in the pontine raphe, with sparing of the pontine tegmentum and corticospinal tracts.

- Abnormally low signal intensity may be noted in the putamen compared with the globus pallidus on T2-weighted images due to the excess iron deposition.
- Linear signal changes along the outer/lateral margin of the dorsolateral putamen, manifesting as slit-like hyperintensities (on T2-weighted and proton density sequences and hypodensities on T1-weighted sequences): a useful MRI feature to help differentiate between PD and MSA predominantly affecting the extrapyramidal system.
- Regional apparent diffusion coefficient (rADC) in the middle cerebellar peduncle and rostral pons may be a sensitive and specific sign in MSA.

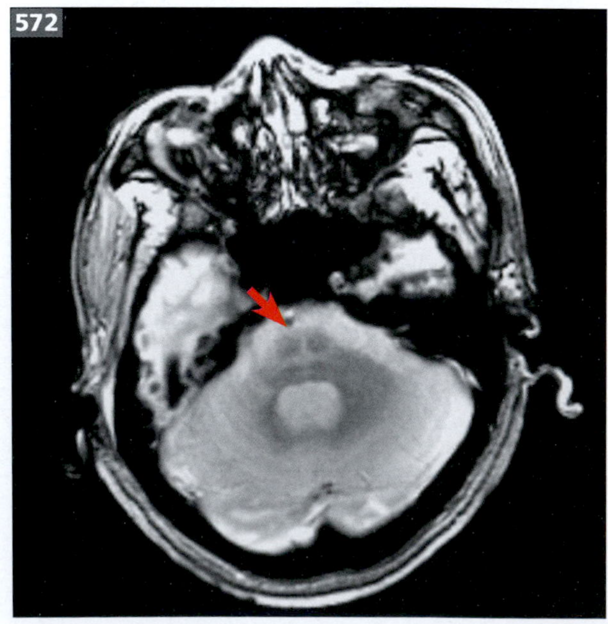

572 Axial T2-weighted image from a patient with multiple system atrophy of the cerebellar type (MSA-C), demonstrating the 'hot cross bun' sign (arrow).

PET

- ^{18}F-fluorodeoxyglucose PET: decreased glucose metabolism is found in cerebellum, thalamus, putamen, and cortex (i.e. forebrain glucose metabolic defects as well as cerebellar).
- ^{11}C-diprenorphine: decreased putamenal uptake.
- ^{18}F-fluorodopa: decreased putamenal uptake (as in all parkinsonian syndromes).

Cardiovascular autonomic function tests

- Plasma norepinephrine concentrations are normal or slightly raised.
- ^{123}I MIBG cardiac scintigraphy could be helpful to differentiate PD from MSA, demonstrating that there is a myocardial postganglionic sympathetic dysfunction in PD with autonomic failure but not in MSA.

Sphincter electromyogram

At least 80% of MSA patients may have signs of neuronal degeneration in Onuf's nucleus with spontaneous activity and increased polyphasia. Anal sphincter EMG test may help to distinguish MSA from early PD, pure autonomic failure, or cerebellar ataxias, in the absence of other causes for sphincter denervation.

Diagnosis

According to the second consensus statement on the diagnosis of MSA, the following categories of diagnostic certainty have been outlined:

- Definite MSA: pathologically confirmed on autopsy.
- Probable MSA: autonomic failure: urinary incontinence with erectile dysfunction in males, or orthostatic decrease in blood pressure within 3 minutes of standing by at least 30 mmHg systolic or 15 mmHg diastolic and either:
  - Poorly levodopa-responsive parkinsonism, or
  - A cerebellar syndrome.
- Possible MSA: at least one feature suggesting autonomic dysfunction (urinary urgency, erectile dysfunction, frequent or incomplete bladder emptying, orthostatic blood pressure drop that does not meet the probable criteria) and:
  - Parkinsonism, or
  - A cerebellar syndrome, and
  - At least one additional feature listed above in the 'red flags' for MSA.

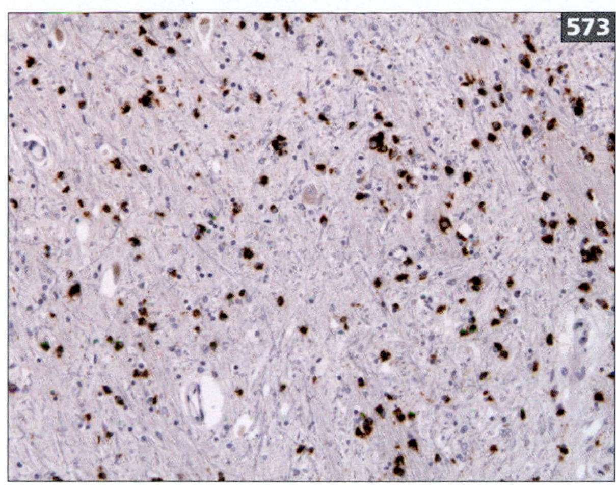

573 Alpha-synuclein immunostaining reveals glial cytoplasmic inclusions in subcortical white matter, often seen in MSA (hyperpigmented inclusions staining positive for alpha-synuclein). *Jensflorian/Wikimedia Commons.*

Pathology[19]

Cell loss and gliosis of varying degrees and proportions occurs without Lewy bodies (unless incidental), in the striatum (particularly the putamen), substantia nigra, locus ceruleus, inferior olives, pontine nuclei, cerebellar Purkinje cells, intermediolateral cell columns, and Onuf's nucleus of the spinal cord; other, more widespread, pathologic changes may also be present.

Five cellular features are present:

- Glial cytoplasmic inclusions (GCIs) containing alpha-synuclein filaments in oligodendroglia: the most characteristic cellular pathology (573)[20].
  - Widely distributed, more common in white matter than gray matter, more common in motor fibers than sensory fibers, and may be flame- or sickle-shaped.
  - Ultrastructurally, they are randomly arranged tubules or filaments, of diameter 20–40 nm, and associated with granular material.
  - They are present in the brains of all cases of MSA (i.e. 100% sensitivity) but not all brains containing GCIs are from patients with MSA (i.e. <100% specificity).
  - They are also found in CBD, PSP, SCA1, and chromosome 17-linked dementia.
- Neuronal cytoplasmic inclusions.
- Neuronal nuclear inclusions.
- Glial nuclear inclusions.
- Neuropil threads.

Treatment[21]

- Parkinsonism: dopaminergic agents: similar strategies to PD with the following caveats:
  - The response to levodopa is usually transient, poor, waning, or absent, due to striatal pathology; however efficacy has been documented in up to 40% for up to a few years of therapy. Up to 1000 mg of levodopa daily may be tried if necessary and tolerated. In contrast, in idiopathic PD, the substantia nigra degenerates but the striatum is normal, which is the reason that dopamine replacement therapy is so effective. The minimal responsiveness (or lack of) to levodopa is therefore a clinical clue to the diagnosis of MSA.
  - Levodopa may induce dyskinesias (predominantly dystonic) of the head and neck in 50% of MSA-P patients.
  - Dopamine agonists or other agents such as MAO inhibitors and amantadine are second- and third-line therapies due to side-effect profiles and decreased efficacy.
- Dysautonomia: similar to PD, as features of dysautonomia are otherwise indistinguishable between the two diseases.
- Ataxia: no known effective treatments.
- Palliative therapies:
  - Continuous positive airway pressure (CPAP) for prominent stridor; tracheostomy rarely needed and may fatally exacerbate sleep disordered breathing[22].
  - Botulinum toxin for drooling, dystonia, or contractures.
  - Percutaneous endoscopic gastrostomy (PEG) for severe dysphagia.
  - Physical, occupational, and speech therapies.

Prognosis

MSA has a more aggressive course than idiopathic PD, and in most cases significantly shortens life, with median survival about 6–9 years (range 0.5–15 years)[23]. Poor prognostic factors include:

- Older age of onset.
- Female sex.
- Early-onset autonomic failure or respiratory symptoms (stridor, respiratory insufficiency).
- Earlier development of disability milestones (falls, dysphagia, dysarthria, and so on).

DEMENTIA WITH LEWY BODIES (DLB)

Definition and epidemiology[24]

A dementia and motor syndrome associated with the widespread presence of Lewy bodies, characterized clinically by fluctuating visual hallucinations and delusions, parkinsonism (muscle rigidity and bradykinesia), progressive dementia, and a poor tolerance of neuroleptic drugs. Please see the Dementia section of this chapter, p. 552, for the full summary of DLB.

PROGRESSIVE SUPRANUCLEAR PALSY (PSP)

Definition and epidemiology

PSP is a multisystem neurodegenerative disease of the basal ganglia and brainstem, also known as the Steele–Richardson–Olszewski syndrome, which presents with a disturbance of balance, impaired downward gaze, subcortical FLD, and levodopa-unresponsive parkinsonism, first described in 1963 by Steele and colleagues. Patients suffer from progressive dysphagia and dysarthria. Death typically occurs from complications of immobility, aspiration, or falls.

- Second most common form of parkinsonism after PD.
- Estimated prevalence: 6.4 per 100,000.
- Age of onset: 40–60 years of age, mean onset 60–65.
- Gender: M=F.

Etiology and pathophysiology

Complex and poorly understood, PSP is considered a sporadic disorder but a few cases show autosomal dominant inheritance, and recent studies suggest some genetic influences. A genetically determined alteration in the microtubule-binding protein τ (tau) may be a risk factor for neuronal degeneration (MAPT H1 haplotype), and may account for an increase in 4-repeat tau, which is found in both PSP and CBD as the predominant component of tau inclusions.

Clinical features[25]

Typical findings include[26]:

- Insidious onset of a progressive, symmetric (but may be asymmetric) parkinsonian syndrome, unresponsive to levodopa, characterized by:
  - Staring, nonblinking, wide eyed (lid retracted) facies, described as worried or surprised, with suggestion of the term 'procerus sign' to describe the often seen characteristic forehead wrinkling.
  - Axial (neck and trunk) dystonia and rigidity and symmetric bradykinesia.
  - Retrocollis or dystonic arm.
  - Unsteady gait (wide-based, shuffling, the patient moves 'en bloc').
  - Postural instability.
  - Sudden falls.

- Supranuclear ophthalmoparesis, initially involving vertical (particularly downgaze) and subsequently horizontal eye movements. The disproportionate hypometria of vertical compared with horizontal saccades produces a curved course of oblique saccades. In some patients in whom full vertical excursions are present, vertical saccades can only be accomplished by moving the eyes in a lateral arc instead of strictly vertically, in the mid-line. The slowing of vertical saccades probably reflects impaired function of burst neurons in the rostral interstitial nucleus of the medial longitudinal fasciculus (riMLF). As a consequence of the downgaze paresis, patients have difficulty reading and walking downstairs.
- Mild subcortical dementia, characterized by slowness of central processing time.
- Pseudobulbar palsy.
- Dysarthria (spastic: voice has a strained, harsh quality).
- Dysphagia.
- Spasticity of lower and (less so) upper limbs, with hyper-reflexia and extensor plantar responses.
- Bladder and bowel dysfunction in end-stage disease.
- Frontal lobe signs (bradyphrenia, perseveration, primitive reflexes: forced grasping, pout and palmomental reflex; imitation and utilization behavior).
- Stuttering speech, torticollis, and blepharospasm may occur.
- Segmental dystonia or myoclonus may occur.
- Nocturnal disturbances: prolonged latency of sleep onset, prolonged wakefulness, frequent early morning awakenings, reduced total sleep time.
- No family history.

Atypical findings, that do not exclude the diagnosis, but are less common, include:
- Appendicular (limb) more than axial rigidity.
- Narrow-based gait.
- Mild rest tremor.
- Upper limb apraxia.
- Upper limb ataxia.
- Myoclonus.
- Chorea.
- Respiratory disturbance.

Absence of:
- Unilateral presentation or pronounced asymmetry.
- Early and prominent dysautonomia, particularly postural hypotension.
- Prominent polyneuropathy.
- Pronounced rest tremor.
- Discriminative ('cortical') sensory loss.
- Alien limb sign.

Atypical presentations of PSP
- PSP-parkinsonism (PSP-P): recent clinicopathological studies indicate that as many as 32% of patients with a retrospective pathologic diagnosis of PSP may have not shown the typical features of the classically described syndrome during life, but instead mimic a more aggressive form of Parkinson's disease, including features of asymmetric onset, tremor, and a moderate initial response to levodopa. This clinical manifestation of PSP has been termed 'PSP-P' (as opposed to the originally described 'Richardson syndrome'). The PSP-P phenotype has a slightly more benign clinical course and may have a different pattern of tau isoform deposition[27].
- Pure akinesia with gait freezing (PAGF):
  - Longer disease duration.
  - Highly predictive of PSP pathology.
  - Features of gait disturbance (freezing, start hesitation) and freezing of writing and speech, with late, if any, dementia or eye movement abnormalities and no evidence of significant cerebrovascular disease.

Differential diagnosis
This is broad, given the more detailed clinicopathologic reports of patients with PSP pathology (**574**, next page).

Supranuclear vertical gaze paresis[28]
- Normal aging (typically affects upgaze more prominently).
- Idiopathic PD, distinguished from PSP by[29]:
  - More commonly asymmetric onset.
  - Less immobile facies without lid retraction.
  - Blink rate not so reduced until advanced disease.
  - Absence of supranuclear ophthalmoparesis, particularly downgaze.
  - Absence of early pronounced gait imbalance.
  - Absence of signs of pseudobulbar palsy (such as harsh, strained voice quality of spastic dysarthria) until late, if at all.
  - More appendicular than axial rigidity and bradykinesia.
  - Tremor is usually present; PSP tremor may occur in 5–10% of cases but is either absent, not pronounced, or of low amplitude.
  - Responsiveness to levodopa.
- DLB.
- Hydrocephalus.
- FTD with parkinsonism linked to chromosome 17.
- Prion diseases (CJD, familial progressive subcortical gliosis).

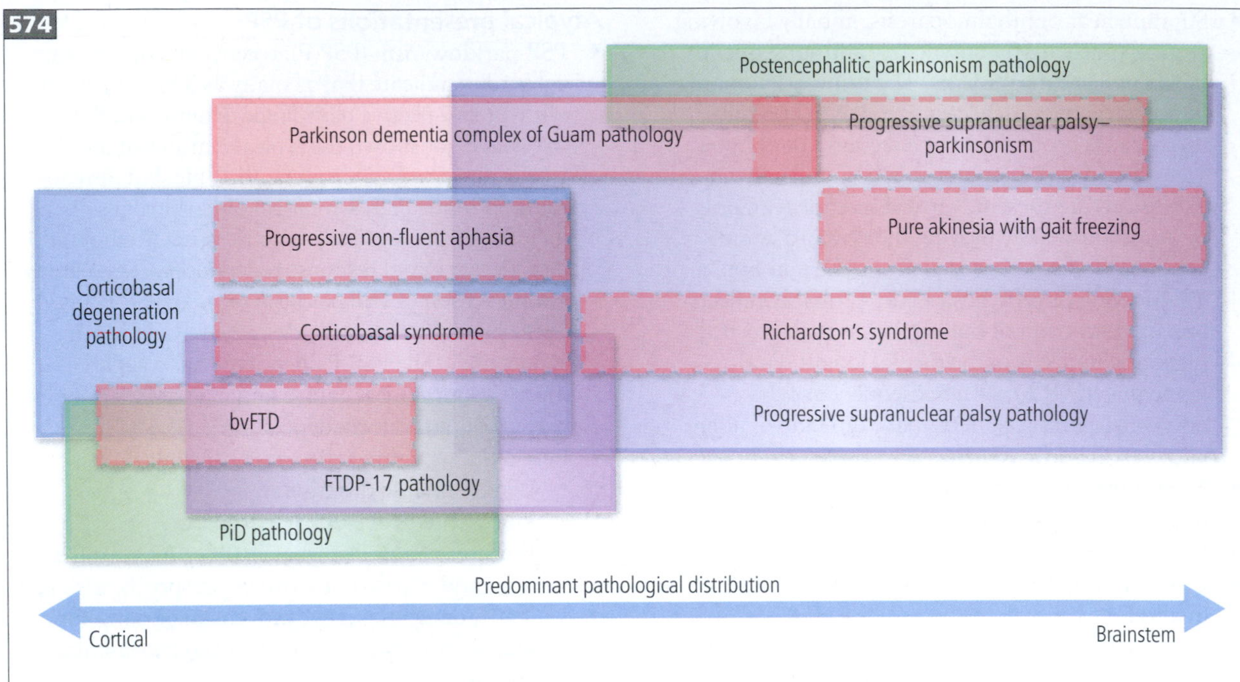

574 Distribution of tau pathology in clinical and pathological nosological syndromes of progressive supranuclear palsy. Dashed boxes: clinical syndromes; solid boxes: pathologically defined diseases. PiD: Pick's disease; FTDP-17: frontotemporal dementia with parkinsonism-17; bvFTD: behavioral variant of frontotemporal dementia. *Adapted from Williams 2009, with permission.*

- Infectious disease: Whipple's disease, brucellosis, neurosyphilis:
  - Whipple's disease[30]: multisystem disorder caused by infection with *Tropheryma whippelii*, typically associated with weight loss, diarrhea, fevers, polyarthritis, and lymphadenopathy, but rarely manifesting in the CNS alone.
  - Main neurologic signs: supranuclear ophthalmoplegia, dementia, parkinsonism, myoclonus; oculomasticatory myorhythmia is considered pathognomonic, but is rare.
  - Detected by CSF PCR for *Tropheryma whippelii* or tissue (bowel, brain) biopsy.
  - Rare treatable cause of a parkinsonian syndrome.
- Niemann–Pick disease type C.
- Cerebrovascular disease ('vascular PSP' or 'multi-infarct PSP').
- Compressive midbrain syndromes (Parinaud syndrome), e.g. pinealoma, glioma.
- CBD.
- Multiple sclerosis.
- Syndrome resembling PSP after surgical repair of ascending aorta dissection or aneurysm.
- Paraneoplastic: cases associated with bronchial carcinoma and B-cell lymphoma.

Other akinetic–rigid syndromes with parkinsonian features[31]

- Idiopathic PD.
- MSA.
- CBD.
- Pallidal, pallidoluysian, and pallidoluysonigral degenerations; dentato-rubro-pallido-luysian atrophy.
- Neurodegeneration with brain iron accumulation diseases (NBIA).
- HD.
- Wilson's disease.
- Cerebrovascular disease[32]:
  - Top of the basilar syndrome causing midbrain and diencephalic infarction.
  - Multiple infarcts in brainstem and basal ganglia.
- Prion diseases.
- Progressive subcortical gliosis.

Subcortical dementia

- DLBD.
- AD.
- VaD.

Investigations

Cranial CT scan may show enlargement of the third ventricle and interpeduncular cistern due to atrophy of the midbrain; however, MRI is more sensitive imaging for brainstem pathology. CT is performed to exclude structural lesions, hydrocephalus, and multi-infarct states which may produce clinical findings similar to PSP.

MRI brain[33] can show various signs of brainstem atrophy such as reduction in size of part of the substantia nigra (as in PD). Reduced diameter of the midbrain on sagittal imaging has been termed the 'hummingbird sign' (575). A high signal in the periaqueductal gray matter is present, and signal hypointensity within the putamen (as in other parkinsonian syndromes) is seen.

Diagnosis

Several proposed criteria exists but the following NINDS/SPSP criteria capture the common core features:

- Definite PSP:
  - A history of probable or possible PSP.
  - Histopathologic evidence of typical PSP.
- Probable PSP:
  - Gradually progressive disorder with onset of symptoms at 40 years of age or later.
  - Vertical supranuclear gaze palsy and prominent postural instability with falls in the first year of disease onset.
  - No evidence of other diseases that could explain the symptoms.
- Possible PSP:
  - Gradually progressive disorder with onset of symptoms at 40 years of age or later.
  - Either vertical supranuclear gaze palsy or slowing of vertical saccades and prominent postural instability with falls in the first year of symptoms
  - No evidence of other diseases that could explain the symptoms.
- Other features of possible PSP or supportive criteria:
  - Frontal/subcortical cognitive dysfunction.
  - Axial rigidity.
  - Pseudobulbar dysphagia and dysarthria.
  - Blepharospasm/apraxia of eyelid opening.

Exclusion criteria for possible or probable PSP

- Recent history of encephalitis or oculogyric crisis, suggesting postencephalitic parkinsonism.
- Severe asymmetry or asymmetric onset of parkinsonian symptoms (bradykinesia) and/or tremor-dominant disease, and/or marked and prolonged levodopa benefit, suggesting PD.
- Hallucinations, especially early-onset or unrelated to dopaminergic therapy, or delusions unrelated to therapy, suggesting Lewy body dementia.
- Cortical dementia of Alzheimer's type (amnesia and aphasia or agnosia).
- Prominent cerebellar symptoms or unexplained dysautonomia (early, prominent urinary incontinence or marked postural hypotension), suggesting MSA.
- Alien hand syndrome, cortical sensory deficits, severe limb apraxia, severe asymmetric bradykinesia, or focal frontal or temporoparietal atrophy, suggesting CBD.
- Neuroradiologic evidence of relevant structural abnormality (infarcts in basal ganglia or brainstem, lobar atrophy).
- Oculomasticatory myorhythmia, suggesting Whipple's disease. However, this is a rare manifestation of Whipple's disease.
- Disease course of <1 year or EEG abnormalities suggestive of CJD.

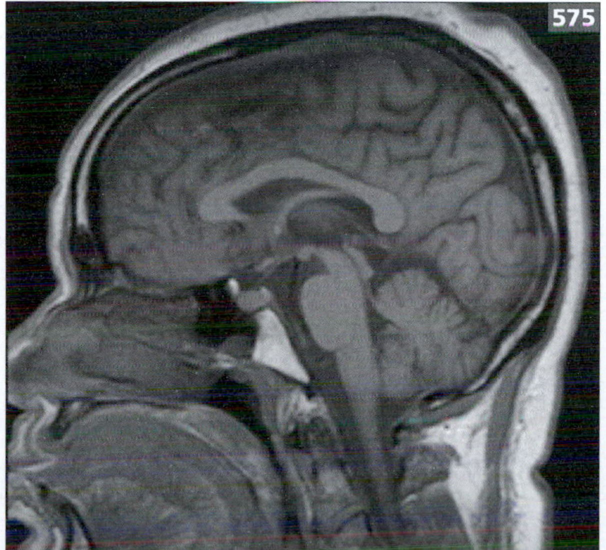

575 A helpful radiographic sign for the diagnosis of progressive supranuclear palsy (PSP), best seen on midsagittal MRI images, is the 'hummingbird' sign. Here, the shape of the midbrain tegmentum represents the bird's head, and the pons the bird's body. Recognition of this sign should strongly raise suspicion for the diagnosis of PSP.

Pathology[34]

Gross pathology includes:

- Atrophy of frontal, parasagittal, or paracentral lobes.
- Atrophy of the brainstem occurs causing dilatation of the third ventricle and cerebral aqueduct, thinning of the midbrain tegmentum (midbrain diameter <17 mm [<0.7 in]), and dilatation of the fourth ventricle (576).
- Decreased pigment in the substantia nigra and locus ceruleus.

Microscopic changes include[35]:

- Neurofibrillary pathology (the cellular hallmark of the disease), with globose and flame-shaped NFT deposition in the striatum, globus pallidus, basal nucleus, subthalamic nucleus, substantia nigra, oculomotor nuclei, raphe nuclei, locus ceruleus, pontine nucleus, tegmental gray matter, and inferior olive. Both PSP and the related tau-deposition disease have similar but distinct patterns of tau deposition (577–579).
- Neuronal loss and gliosis in: substantia nigra, periaqueductal gray matter, superior colliculus, subthalamic nucleus of Luys, red nucleus, pallidum, dentate nucleus, pretectal and vestibular nuclei and to some extent in the oculomotor nucleus.
  - Surviving neurons in these areas contain NFTs.
  - The cerebral and cerebellar cortices are usually spared.
- Sparse-to-many neuropil threads in basal ganglia, internal capsule, thalamic fasciculus.
- Grumose degeneration of cerebellar dentate nucleus.
- Pick body-like tau inclusions in dentate fascia.
- Tufted astrocytes in glia, coiled bodies.

Neuronal degeneration is associated with deposition of hyperphosphorylated tau protein as NFTs. Tau NFTs appear on light microscopy most commonly as globose tangles and on electron microscopy as straight filaments with a diameter of 15–18 nm.

Treatment

Treatment is symptomatic.

- Parkinsonism:
  - Dopaminergic drugs:
    - In order of effectiveness and lower risk/benefit ratio: levodopa, dopamine agonists (bromocriptine > pergolide > lisuride in older literature) may reduce the symptoms in some cases but a sustained response is rare.
    - Amantadine may cause temporary improvement in a small subset of patients.
    - Higher doses of levodopa may be needed for clinical response (up to 1 g daily).
    - Levodopa-induced dyskinesias are rare, but dystonia may occur (dysarthria, apraxia of eyelid closure).
  - Case reports of improvement in some patients with: zolpidem, anticholinergics, idazoxan, tricyclic antidepressants, L-threo-3,4-dihydroxyphenylserine (L-DOPS), methysergide.
- Visual disturbances:
  - Artificial tears (for decreased blink rate).
  - Prisms, talking books.
- Palliative therapies:
  - Speech and swallowing assessment and management (dietary changes, gastrostomy tube).
  - Physical and occupational therapy.
  - Patient and family support: lay associations, supportive psychotherapy.

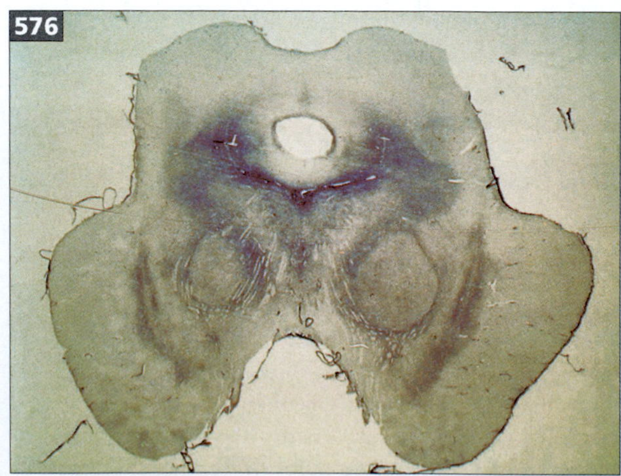

576 Gross pathology: axial section through the midbrain of a patient with progressive supranuclear palsy, showing midbrain atrophy with dilation of the cerebral aqueduct due to loss of neurons and gliosis in the periaqueductal gray matter, the superior colliculus, substantia nigra, subthalamic nucleus of Luys, red nucleus, and to some extent in the oculomotor nucleus.

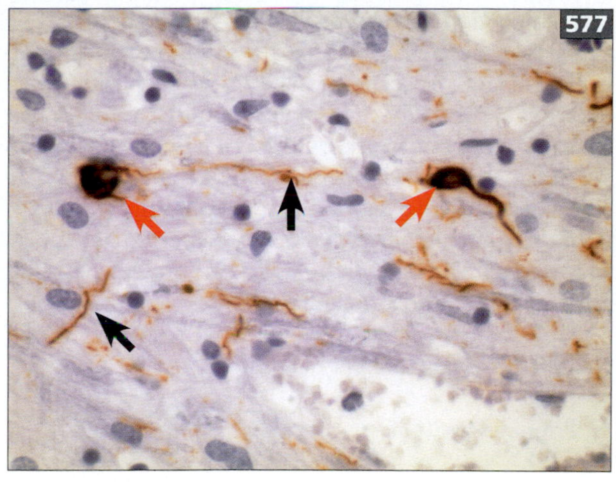

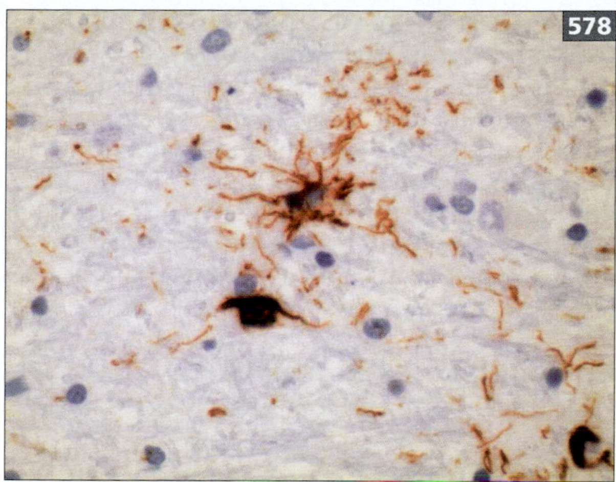

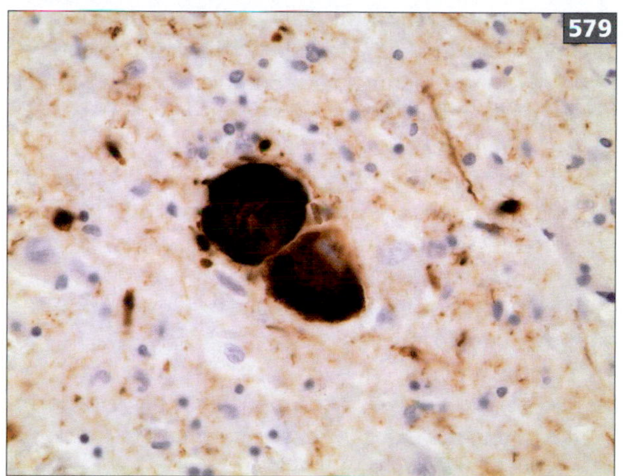

577–579 Tau immunohistochemistry in a patient with pathologically confirmed progressive supranuclear palsy (PSP) demonstrates (577) neuropil threads (black arrows) in the substantia nigra, midbrain, and medullary tegmentum, locus ceruleus, inferior olivary nuclei, thalamus, and subthalamic nucleus; glial fibrillary tangles (red arrows); (578) tufted astrocytes; (579) globose neurofibrillary tangles in the midbrain tegmentum. Similar tau pathology may be found in corticobasal degeneration (CBD) but with a different distribution in the brain, including more numerous neuropil threads in the cortex, cerebral white matter, internal capsule, striatum, thalamic fasciculus, cerebral peduncle, and pons; this different distribution, as well as other features such as numerous ballooned neurons (not pictured) pathologically differentiate PSP from CBD.

- Other:
  - Drooling: botulinum toxin, anticholinergics.
  - Depression/anxiety/emotional incontinence: antidepressants, anxiolytics, dextromethorphan/quinidine.
  - Dystonia (fisted hand, neck extension): botulinum toxin.
  - Apraxia of eyelid opening: botulinum toxin.

Prognosis

PSP has a progressive clinical course leading to immobility and anarthria. Pneumonia is the most common immediate cause of death. Average disease duration is 5.6 (range 2–17) years.

Predictors of a shorter survival time include onset of falls during the first year, early dysphagia, and incontinence.

Tip

▶ *PSP, CBD, and most forms of FTD dementia are related to deposition of tau protein in the brain and are therefore sometimes called 'tauopathies'. The symptoms of these disorders have significant overlap, and they are often hard to differentiate from one another clinically*[36].

CORTICOBASAL DEGENERATION (CBD)

Definition and epidemiology

CBD is a rare, sporadic, progressive extrapyramidal degenerative disease of unknown etiology, characterized by co-occurrence of cortical and basal ganglia signs and symptoms. CBD was first described in 1967 by Rebeiz.

True prevalence rates are difficult to estimate given the continued refinement of the pathologic and clinical manifestations of the disease. It is probably less common than PSP.

Etiology and pathophysiology

Complex and poorly characterized.

Clinical features[37]

Clinical presentation of CBD varies widely, making the disease one of the most misdiagnosed neurodegenerative disorders. Patients may present with either dementia or primarily motor features with relatively preserved intellect until late in the disease. Symptoms may include:

- An asymmetric akinetic–rigid syndrome with dystonic posturing of the hand, with the wrist flexed and the thumb flexed across the palm (580, 581). This may spread to the ipsilateral foot followed by the contralateral limbs[38]. The hand often becomes functionally useless due to a severe apraxia rather than to any weakness.
- Tremor: attempted movement of an affected limb may evoke episodes of fine myoclonus in the forearm flexor muscles that can be misinterpreted as an action tremor.
- Gait disorder/postural instability: with parkinsonian, apraxic, dystonic, or spastic features.
- Choreoathetosis.
- Focal stimulus-sensitive myoclonus and action tremor.
- Cortical sensory loss.
- Some overlap with PSP, including supranuclear gaze palsy.
- Corticospinal tract signs: Babinski signs, spasticity.
- Pseudobulbar palsy.
- Cortical sensory loss, altered visuospatial function.
- Behavioral manifestations: frontal lobe-type behavior and language disturbances.
- Dysarthria is a relatively late sign.

Differential diagnosis[39]

Clinicopathologic correlations have demonstrated poor clinical diagnostic accuracy in CBD, with a positive predictive value of 33.3%. This poor diagnostic accuracy has led some authors to reserve CBD as a pathologic diagnosis, designating the clinic presentation of mixed cortical and basal ganglia signs as 'corticobasal syndrome' (CBS)[40]. Approximately 55% of CBS cases have CBD. Many other alternate pathologies can present with the same clinical features, including[41,42]:

- DLBD.
- AD: increasing number of reports[43].
- PSP.
- Prion disease (CJD).
- FTD.
- Pick's disease

Conversely, CBD pathology may clinically mimic clinical presentation of other pathologies including:

- PSP: significant clinical overlap between clinical features of PSP and CBD is recognized.
- FTD.
- Primary progressive aphasia.
- Progressive speech and oral apraxia.
- Posterior cortical atrophy (early and prominent visuospatial/visuoperceptive deficits).
- AD.

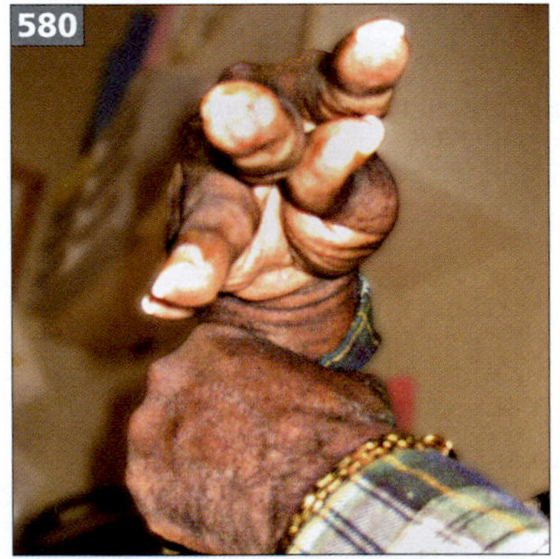

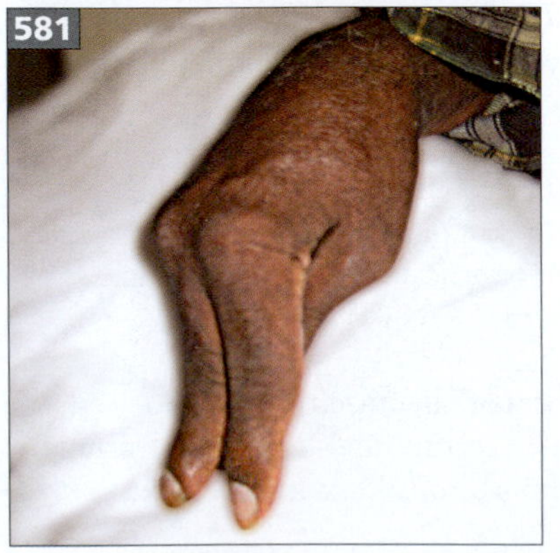

580, 581 Illustration of a painful, dystonic arm (580) and hand (581) in a patient with clinically diagnosed corticobasal syndrome. Note the deformities of the fingers, wrist flexion, and thumb flexion into the palm. Painful spasms were partially relieved by botulinum toxin therapy.

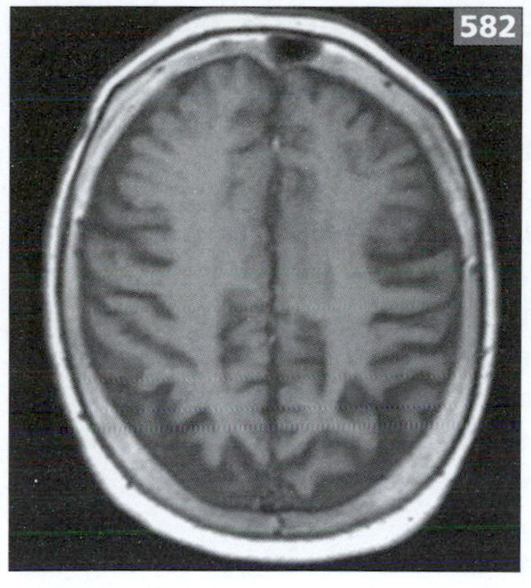

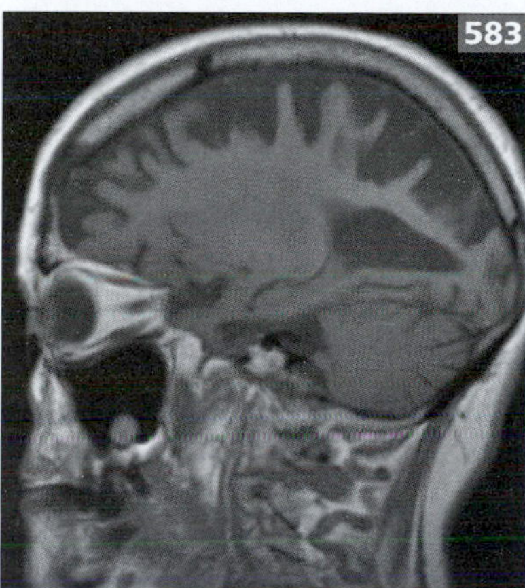

582, 583 Axial (582) and sagittal (583) images from patients with clinically diagnosed corticobasal syndrome, with T1-weighted MRI imaging of the brain showing asymmetric parietofrontal atrophy.

Other conditions that could cause CBS include:

- Paraneoplastic disorders.
- Intracerebral mass lesion.
- Multi-infarct state.
- Prion disease.
- Other heredodegenerative and secondary forms of parkinsonism (see later section).

Investigations

MRI may be normal or nonspecific, or may demonstrate: asymmetric atrophy in posterior frontal and parietal regions contralateral to the most affected side (582, 583); atrophy of the cerebral peduncle; FLAIR sequences show hyperintensity in the subcortical white matter.

PET/SPECT show focal/asymmetric hypoperfusion on functional imaging, maximal in the frontoparietal cortex.

Diagnosis

Definitive diagnosis is established at autopsy. Research criteria have been proposed for the CBS presentation of CBD:

- Insidious onset and progressive development of:
  - Cortical dysfunction – at least one of: asymmetric ideomotor apraxia, alien limb phenomenon, cortical sensory loss, visual or sensory hemi-neglect, constructional apraxia, focal or segmental myoclonus, apraxia of speech/nonfluent aphasia[44].
  - Basal ganglia dysfunction – at least one of: focal or asymmetric appendicular rigidity lacking predominant or sustained levodopa response and/or focal or asymmetric appendicular dystonia.
- Supportive features:
  - Imaging studies.
  - Evidence of focal or lateralized cognitive dysfunction with relative preservation of learning and memory on neuropsychometric testing.

Pathology[45]

Gross pathology includes:

- Lobar neocortical atrophy: asymmetric, paracentral, or frontoparietal, most severe in pre- and post-central regions.
- Mild atrophy of midbrain tegmentum and enlargement of aqueduct.

Microscopic pathology shows:

- Numerous, large pale (achromatic) ballooned neurons in the basal ganglia and the motor and pre-motor cortex (layers III, V, VI). These are intensely neurofilament protein positive (NFP+). These are not specific for CBD, but are found less prominently in PSP, Pick's disease, frontotemporal dementia with parkinsonism linked to chromosome 17 (FTDP-17), and AD.
- Neuropil threads: numerous and widespread thread-like processes in gray and white matter in the cortex, cerebral white matter, internal capsule, striatum, thalamic fasciculus, cerebral peduncle, and pons (see 577–579).
- Globose NFTs in the substantia nigra, locus ceruleus, and raphe nuclei.
- Pick body-like tau inclusions in the cortex (layers II and III).
- Astrocytic plaques in focal atrophic cortices.
- Coiled bodies in oligodendrocytes (tau-positive fibers coiled around nucleus).
- Corticospinal tract degeneration.

Molecular pathology is as for PSP.

Treatment[46]

Symptomatic therapy only, as there is no cure or neuroprotective agent. Given the wide variation in presentation, treatment is highly invidividualized. Severe and widespread pathology typically prohibits any consistently effective or prolonged response to a single treatment method.

The following treatments may be considered based on predominant symptoms, with the caveat that pharmacologic therapy is largely ineffective in the management of the disease:

- Parkinsonism:
  - Dopaminergic agents; relative reported effectiveness in a review of pooled data: levodopa > amantadine > selegiline > dopamine agonists.
  - Anticholinergics.
- Myoclonus/tremor: benzodiazepines (most notably clonazepam), anticonvulsants, propranolol.
- Dystonia: botulinum toxin, anticholinergics, baclofen, benzodiazepines.
- Other:
  - Eyelid movement disorders: botulinum toxin.
  - Behavioral abnormalities: antidepressants, anxiolytics, neuroleptics.
- Palliative therapies: physical, occupational, speech therapies. Apraxia usually compromises benefit.

Prognosis

Prognosis is poor, given the lack of effective treatments and diffuse nature of the disease. Mean survival of 7 years after symptom onset. Death is typically due to secondary complications of generalized immobility.

FRONTOTEMPORAL DEMENTIA (FTD)

Definition

Frontotemporal dementia is a term used to describe patients with one of three major clinical syndromes: frontal variant FTD (dementia of frontal type), semantic dementia (progressive fluent aphasia), and progressive nonfluent aphasia. FTD causes progressive focal atrophy of the frontal and/or temporal lobes, leading to behavioral and personality changes, cognitive impairment, and various motor symptoms including parkinsonism. Please see the Dementia section of this chapter, p. 547, for the full summary of FTD.

HEREDODEGENERATIVE AND SECONDARY PARKINSONISM

Definition and epidemiology

Parkinsonism not related primarily to a multifocal neurodegenerative process or occurring as a variable, secondary or minor feature of another nervous system disease. It is associated with a diverse number of underlying metabolic, traumatic, vascular, pharmacologic, structural, neurodegenerative, autoimmune, or toxic causes. Epidemiology varies widely by subtype, but is generally not well characterized.

Etiology and pathophysiology

Any disease process affecting the nuclei of the basal ganglia and their cortical/subcortical connections may cause parkinsonism, with features determined by combination and degree of involvement of different neuroanotomical structures.

Clinical features

In general, motor signs in secondary causes of parkinsonism more commonly have the following features:

- Rare occurrence of rest tremor.
- More symmetric motor findings.
- Earlier postural instability with falls.
- Signs of other systemic diseases, other concomitant movement disorders, or other neurologic deficits out of the realm of typical idiopathic PD, as reviewed below in the individual pathologic processes.
- Pathology varies according to the underlying disorder.

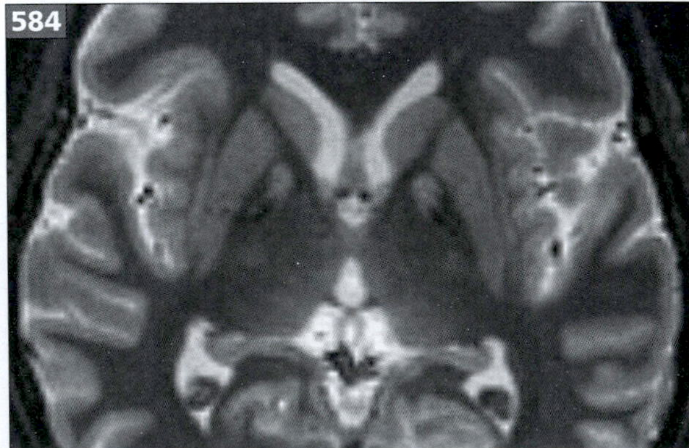

584 T2-weighted MRI imaging demonstrates the 'eye of the tiger' sign in pantothenate kinase-associated neurodegeneration, with low signal intensity in the globus pallidus circumscribing a central region of high signal intensity.

Differential diagnosis

Heredodegenerative parkinsonism

- Inherited:
  - Dopamine-responsive parkinsonism/dystonia: DYT5: levodopa-responsive dystonia-parkinsonism (typically manifests in childhood).
- NBIA[47]: a heterogeneous group of genetic disorders characterized by brain iron accumulation and neuronal death. Subtypes may be recognized by pattern of iron deposition on T2* and fast spin echo MRI sequences:
  - PKAN:
    - Rare, sometimes familial, condition of progressive rigidity, bradykinesia, dystonia, dysarthria, and dementia in childhood, or occasionally adulthood.
    - Epileptic seizures, chorea, cerebellar ataxia, muscle atrophy, and retinitis pigmentosa may also occur.
    - Iron-containing pigment deposited in the substantia nigra and globus pallidus ('eye of the tiger sign') can be imaged by MRI (**584**).
  - Neuroferritopathy: more prominent chorea and dystonia; MRI demonstrates more involvement of dentate nuclei, globus pallidus, and putamen, along with confluent areas of hyperintensity.
  - Aceruloplasminemia: occurs with ataxia, dystonia, and chorea, as well as retinal degeneration and diabetes mellitus; MRI demonstrates low intensity in the striatum, thalamus, and dentate nucleus.
  - Infantile neuroaxonal dystrophy.
- Neuroacanthocytosis.
- Familial progressive subcortical gliosis.
- Hereditary hemochromatosis (controversial).
- Dentato-rubral-pallido-luysian atrophy (DRPLA).
- HD: particularly with early onset (Westphal variant), characterized by:
  - Onset in childhood and adolescence.
  - Usually associated with paternally inherited mutations with large numbers of trinucleotide repeats.
  - Rigidity develops in the trunk and proximal limb muscles and spreads to involve all muscle groups.
  - More parkinsonian features and minimal chorea.
  - Progressive dementia, mask-like facies, and bilateral increased reflexes and extensor plantar responses.
  - Seizures.
  - Death within a few years of onset.
- Spinocerebellar ataxia (particularly types 2, 3, 17).
- FXTAS[48]:
  - Core features of action tremor and ataxia, frequently associated with parkinsonism, executive function deficits/dementia, neuropathy, and dysautonomia.
  - Caused by moderate expansions of the *FMR1* gene.
  - MRI demonstrates middle cerebellar peduncle (MCP) sign: increased T2 signal in the middle cerebellar peduncles.
  - Though recently discovered, may be one of the most common single-gene disorders causing a neurodegenerative syndrome in males. Key to diagnosis in history is obtaining a history of children or grandchildren with mental retardation, autism, or learning disorders or female relatives with premature menopause or early infertility.
- Wilson's disease (hepatocerebral degeneration): rare but potentially treatable cause of parkinsonism[49].
- Ceroid lipofuscinosis.
- Gaucher's disease: mutations in the GBA gene (encoding beta-glucocerebrosidase) have been recently found to be a common risk factor for PD, even in absence of other signs of the disease.
- GM1 gangliosidosis.
- Chediak–Higashi disease.
- Perry syndrome: parkinsonism, depression, weight loss, and central hypoventilation.

Secondary parkinsonism[50,51]

- Drug-induced parkinsonism (*Table 101*)[52]: special note on dopamine receptor antagonists:
  - History of exposure may not be offered and should be sought out.
  - Parkinsonism typically improves after withdrawal, but may take months.
- Toxins (*Table 102*).
- Cerebrovascular disease/vascular parkinsonism (VP)/ vascular 'pseudoparkinsonism'[53]:
  - Controversial diagnosis with no universally used diagnostic criteria, but estimated to account for 3–12% of all cases of parkinsonism.
  - Many patients with true PD have incidental or concurrent cerebrovascular disease, and some patients with VP have some response to levodopa.
  - Attributed to ischemic or hemorrhagic strokes (usually multiple) in the subcortical white matter, striatum, or substantia nigra.

- Most commonly described lesions: bilateral multiple basal ganglia lacunes or 'Binswanger type' confluent white matter lesions (585).
- Heterogeneous syndrome with several possible clinical features:
  - By history: sudden onset, stepwise progression, history of strokes, early gait disturbance with postural instability, vascular risk factors, minimal or no benefit from levodopa, later age at onset.
  - On examination: pyramidal signs, clasp-knife spasticity as opposed to parkinsonian-like cogwheeling rigidity, flexor spasms, concurrent dementia, pseudobulbar palsy, incontinence, absence of rest tremor, lack of true akinesia (i.e. decrement or fatiguing with rapid movements). As opposed to the narrow-based gait of PD, there is predominantly a 'lower-body parkinsonism', including standing more erect in a 'stiff' military posture, with the shoulders back, arms extended, with a wide stance base, and a short shuffling stepping pattern, often with frequent freezing and gait initiation failure.
- May also appear similar to NPH or mimic atypical parkinsonian syndromes such as PSP or CBD (*Table 103*).
- Functional imaging studies have not consistently differentiated VP from PD.

TABLE 101 **DRUGS CAUSING SECONDARY PARKINSONISM**

Neuroleptic drugs	
Typical	Haloperidol, pimozide, chlorpromazine, fluphenazine
Atypical	Ziprasidone, olanzapine, risperidonel, aripiprazole
Antiemetic agents	Metoclopromide, prochlorperazine, promethazine
Dopamine storage/ transport inhibitors	Reserpine, tetrabenazine
Immunosuppressants/ chemotherapeutic agents	Cyclosporin, busulfan, vincristine, adriamycin
Antiepileptics	Sodium valproate, phenytoin
Other	Methyldopa, amiodarone, calcium channel blockers (cinnarazine, flunarizine), alpha-methyldopa, chloroquine

TABLE 102 **TOXIC EXPOSURES ASSOCIATED WITH PARKINSONISM**

- Aliphatic hydrocarbons
- Carbon disulfide
- Carbon monoxide
- Cyanide
- Kava (*Piper methysticum*)
- Manganese poisoning
- Mercury
- Methanol
- Methcathinone (ephedrine) abuse
- Methyl bromide
- N-methyl-4-phenyl-1,2,3,6,-tetrahydropyridine (MPTP)
- Organophosphates
- *Rauwolfia serpentina*
- Street drugs (heroin, toluene, ecstasy)

- Autoimmune[54]:
  - Post-streptococcal, associated with anti-basal ganglia antibodies.
  - SLE.
  - Nonvasculitic autoimmune inflammatory meningoencephalitis.
  - Antiphospholipid antibody syndrome.
- Paraneoplastic: rare.
- Trauma: recurrent head trauma (dementia pugilistica/ pugilistic encephalopathy).
- Metabolic:
  - Calcifications[55]: Fahr's disease or other disturbances of calcium metabolism (hypo- and hyperparathyroidism, pseudohypoparathyroidism).
  - Mitochondrial disease:
    - Leigh's disease (subacute necrotizing encephalopathy).
    - Mitochondrial cytopathies with striatal necrosis.
  - Thyroid disease: hypothyroidism-related slowness.
  - Central pontine or extrapontine myelinolysis
  - Liver disease: Nonwilsonian hepatocerebral degeneration (586, 587)[56]; often associated with bilateral, symmetric bilateral basal ganglian hyperintensities on T1-weighted imaging, presumed secondary to manganese deposition.

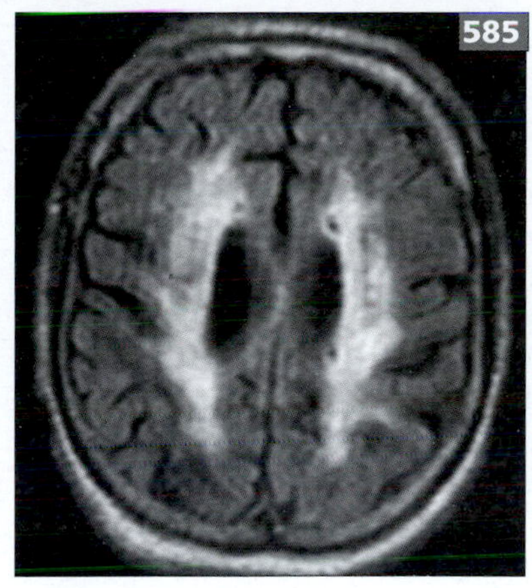

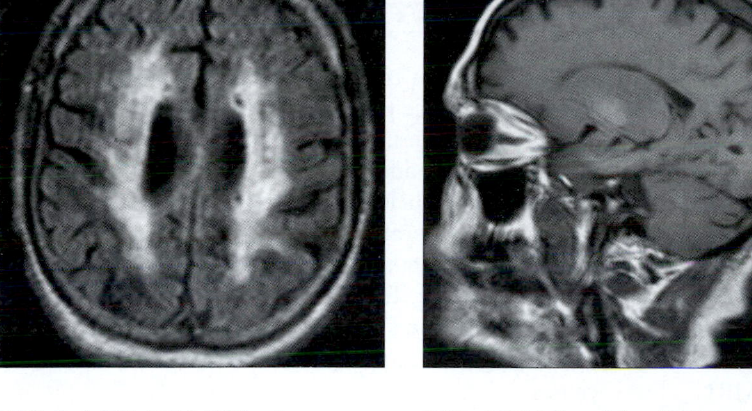

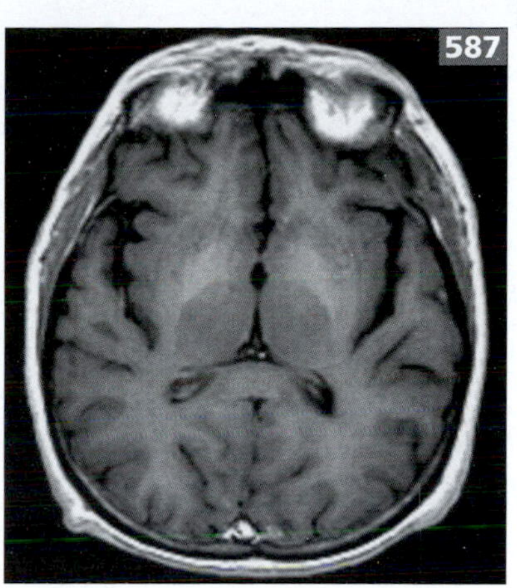

585 Axial FLAIR MRI brain images from a patient with clinically diagnosed vascular parkinsonism, showing confluent white matter subcortical hyperintensities with a frontal predominance and multiple subcortical lacunar infarcts.

586, 587 T1-weighted MRI of the brain in a patient with chronic cirrhosis and tremor-predominant parkinsonism (with tremor limiting the resolution of many images). Bilateral, symmetric hyperintensities of the globus pallidus are seen on sagittal (586) and axial (587) images.

TABLE 103 **CLINICAL FEATURES DIFFERENTIATING MAJOR PARKINSONIAN DISORDERS**

Feature	PSP	PD	MSA-P	CBD	MIP
Motor symmetry	+++	+	+++	–	+/–
Axial rigidity	+++	++	++	++	–
Limb dystonia	+	+	+	+++	+/–
Pyramidal signs	+	–	++	+++	++
Apraxia	+	–	–	+++	+
Postural instability	+++	++	++	+	++
Vertical supranuclear gaze palsy	+++	+	++	++	+
Frontal behavior	+++	+	+	++	+
Dysautonomia	–	+	++	–	–
Levodopa response early in course	+	+++	+	–	–
Levodopa response late in course	–	++	+	–	–
Asymmetric cortical atrophy on MRI	–	–	–	++	+/–

CBD: corticobasal degeneration; MIP: multi-infarct parkinsonism; MRI: magnetic resonance imaging; MSA-P: multiple system atrophy of the parkinsonian type; PD: Parkinson's disease; –: absent or rare; +: occasional, mild, or late; ++: usual, moderate; +++: usual, severe, or early.

Adapted from Golbe 2007, with permission.

- Infection[57]:
  - Primary infection invading basal ganglia structures (i.e. toxoplasmosis, viral encephalitis).
  - Post-encephalitic parkinsonism; now rare, mainly reported as encephalitis lethargica followed a worldwide flu epidemic in 1918.
  - HIV infection/AIDS.
  - Prion disease (CJD, GSS).
  - Whipple's disease.
  - SSPE.
- Hemiparkinsonism/hemiatrophy:
  - Younger age, associated with early-onset dystonia, slow progression, and poor levodopa response, often with a history of perinatal asphyxia.
  - Contralateral cortical hemiatrophy on MRI.
- Tumor involving the basal ganglia and cortical–subcortical connections.
- NPH, noncommunicating hydrocephalus:
  - Greater involvement of the legs than arms ('lower-half parkinsonism').
  - Early dementia.
  - Urinary incontinence.
- Psychogenic[58]:
  - Parkinsonism, outside tremor, is a rare manifestation of a psychogenic movement disorder.
  - Clinical features:
    - Sudden onset.
    - Precipitating factor(s) such as traumatic events.
    - Tremor at rest and with action.
    - No cogwheeling.
    - No fatiguing (decrementing amplitude of movements).
    - Distractibility/entrainment of motor features.
    - Other psychogenic examination findings (giveaway weakness, patterns of false sensory loss, excessive fatigue and effort).
- Depression: common.

Tip

▶ *As there are many causes of parkinsonism, some of which are treatable, every patient presenting with signs and symptoms of parkinsonism should have a thorough history and examination, with ancillary testing as indicated for the conditions listed in this chapter.*

HEREDITARY ATAXIAS

INTRODUCTION

Cerebellar ataxia is a frequent finding among patients seen in neurologic practice and may result from a wide variety of etiologies, both acquired and genetic. Inherited ataxia is a large and important subgroup of the ataxic disorders, and includes metabolic ataxias, autosomal recessive degenerative ataxias, autosomal dominant spinocerebellar ataxias (SCAs), X-linked, and maternally inherited ataxias. This chapter discusses predominantly the inherited causes of cerebellar ataxia, with more limited coverage of acquired and nonsyndromic congenital causes.

Hereditary conditions account for the majority of ataxic syndromes in children and one-third to one-half of patients with adult onset ataxic syndromes. Classification by mode of inheritance is a useful way of organizing the hereditary ataxias for both clinical and research purposes, and this approach will be used here.

CONGENITAL ATAXIAS

This category includes cerebellar aplasia and hypoplasia as well as congenital structural abnormalities such as Chiari malformations, Joubert's syndrome and Dandy–Walker syndrome[1]. These conditions are present at birth and are generally static in nature. Some of these defects are amenable to surgical intervention. For a number of these disorders, the condition affects multiple organ systems.

JOUBERT'S SYNDROME AND RELATED DISORDERS

Definition and epidemiology

- A congenital onset disorder of the cerebellum, with specific involvement of the cerebellar vermis.
- A static and nonprogressive disorder, present from birth.
- Estimated at 1:100,000 in the US.

Joubert's syndrome and related disorders are defined by their typical MRI findings of a 'molar tooth sign', which on axial images at the level of the superior cerebellar peduncles shows enlargement of the interpeduncular fossa and 4th ventricle, hypoplasia or aplasia of the cerebellar vermis, and thickened and elongated superior cerebellar peduncles (588)[2].

Etiology and pathophysiology

There are now at least nine known genetic mutations that can lead to Joubert's syndrome[3]. All these disorders are inherited in an autosomal recessive pattern, suggesting that loss of function of the various genes is critical to pathogenesis. Most of these mutations interfere with either the structure or function of the primary cilia, which are critical for cellular migration during hindbrain development[4].

Clinical features

- Static cerebellar ataxia.
- Developmental delay/intellectual impairment (mild to moderate).
- Hypotonia in infancy.
- Characteristic facial appearance in a majority of cases (broad forehead, arched eyebrows, strabismus, ptosis, and tenting of the mouth consistent with facial hypotonia).
- Abnormal eye movements, including strabismus, nystagmus, and oculomotor apraxia.
- Abnormal breathing patterns, including episodic apnea and tachypnea.

The above symptoms and signs are sometimes complicated by other CNS and non-CNS organ system involvement. Other CNS changes include occipital encephalocele, agenesis of the corpus callosum, and variable brainstem anomalies. Non-CNS involvement can include:

- Ocular disorders: colobomas and blindness secondary to Leber's congenital amaurosis; a later onset degenerative pigmentary retinopathy has also been reported in AHI1 patients[5].
- Up to 30% of cases of Joubert's syndrome are associated with renal involvement. Typical renal involvement includes either cystic dysplasia or juvenile nephronophthisis (NPHP)[6].
- A subset of patients has involvement of cerebellum, eyes, and renal system (so called cerebello-oculo-renal syndrome, CORS).
- Joubert's syndrome can also occur as a component of COACH syndrome (cerebellar vermis hypo/aplasia, oligophrenia, ataxia congenital, coloboma, and hepatic fibrosis)[7]. These patients can also have renal failure as in CORS.

Tip

▶ *Young patients with a 'molar tooth' sign should be evaluated for non-CNS involvement, particularly the renal system.*

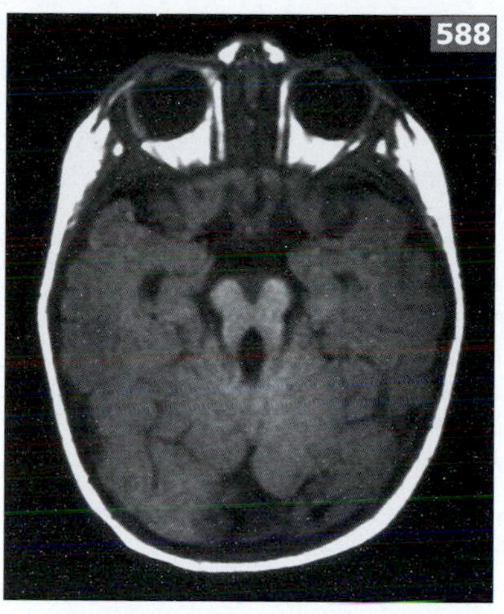

588 Joubert's syndrome. T1 axial image demonstrating the 'molar tooth' sign that results from vermian atrophy and enlargement of the interpeduncular fossa and 4th ventricle, hypoplasia or aplasia of the cerebellar vermis, and thickened and elongated superior cerebellar peduncles. *Courtesy of William Dobyns, University of Chicago.*

Differential diagnosis

A complete differential diagnosis for cerebellar ataxias is included in *Table 104*.

- COACH and CORS syndromes, as described above. The molar tooth sign and ataxia may not be recognized until later in the course of the disorder if not explicitly evaluated.
- Bardet–Biedl syndrome (BBS) can present clinically with many features of Joubert's syndrome-related disorders, including renal involvement, retinal dystrophy, cognitive delay, and ataxia, but it is not typically associated with the presence of the molar tooth sign or other structural abnormalities on MRI[8].
- Dandy–Walker malformation is a congenital brain malformation that can include cerebellar hypoplasia and vermian aplasia/hypoplasia, and a retrocerebellar fluid collection. It is typically also associated with agenesis of the corpus callosum and hydrocephalus. It can be differentiated clinically based on MRI imaging.
- Congenital disorders of glycosylation can present with ataxia, hypotonia, and strabismus, but other typical features on MRI are not usually seen. These can be differentiated based on transferrin isoelectric focusing, which is normal in Joubert's syndrome-related disorders.
- Congenital cerebellar hypoplasia/aplasia can occur as a component of a heterogeneous group of brain malformations[9]. A typical molar tooth sign is not usually seen and these disorders are usually sporadic.

TABLE 104 **DIFFERENTIAL DIAGNOSIS FOR CEREBELLAR ATAXIA**

CONGENITAL DISORDERS

1. Arnold–Chiari malformations
2. Congenital cerebellar hypoplasia/aplasia
3. X-linked cerebella hypoplasia
4. Pontocerebellar hypoplasia
5. Dandy–Walker cyst
6. Joubert's syndrome and its variants (congenital absence or hypoplasia of the cerebellar vermis)
7. Gillespie's syndrome
8. Hydrocephalus

Dominant inheritance

9. The spinocerebellar ataxias (see *Table 105*)
10. Dentato-rubro-pallido-luysian atrophy (DRPLA, Haw river syndrome)
11. Episodic ataxias EA-1, EA-2, EA-3, and EA-4
12. Myelocerebellar disorder
13. Adult onset leukodystrophy

Autosomal recessive inheritance

14. Freidreich's ataxia
15. Ataxia telangectasia
16. Ataxia telangectasia like disorder
17. Nijmegen breakage syndrome
18. Ataxia with oculomotor apraxia I
19. Ataxia with oculomotor apraxia II
20. Ataxia with isolated vitamin E deficiency
21. Bassen–Kornzweig disease (Abetalipoproteinemia)
22. Wilson's disease
23. Aceruloplasminemia
24. Refsum's disease (phytanoyl-CoA hydroxylase deficiency)
25. Aminoacidurias:
   - Hartnup disease
   - Isovaleric acidemia
   - Maple syrup urine disease
26. Hyperammonemias:
   - Biotin-responsive multiple carboxylase deficiency
   - Hypoornithinemia
   - Argininosuccinase deficiency
   - Arginosuccinic synthase deficiency
27. Lysosomal storage diseases:
   - Neimann–Pick type C
   - Neuronal ceroid lipofuscinosis
   - Adult onset hexominadase-A or hexominadase-B deficiency
28. Leukodystrophies:
   - Metachromic leukodystrophy
   - Adrenoleukodystrophy
   - Krabbe's disease
29. Unverricht–Lundborg disease (myoclonic epilepsy and progressive ataxia due to a cystatin B deficiency)
30. Autosomal recessive ataxia type I
31. Spastic ataxia of Charlevoix–Saguenay
32. Ataxia with hypogonadism (Holmes ataxia)
33. Pantothenate kinase associated neurodegeneration (formerly Hallervorden–Spatz syndrome)
34. Cerebrotendinous xanthomatosis (cholestanolosis)
35. Cockayne syndrome
36. Marinesco–Sjögren's syndrome

X-linked inheritance

37. Fragile X tremor ataxia syndrome
38. X-linked sideroblastic anemia with ataxia
39. Adrenomyeloneuropathy
40. X-linked adrenoleukodystrophy
41. Ornithine transcarbamylase defiency
42. Pyruvate dehydrogenase deficiency

Maternal inheritance

43. Mitochondrial disorders:
   - MELAS
   - MERRF
   - NARP
   - Kearns–Sayre syndrome
   - MIRAS
   - Leigh syndrome
   - Coenzyme Q10 deficiency

TOXIC/METABOLIC DISORDERS

44. Alcoholic cerebellar degeneration
45. Drugs (antiepileptic medications, chemotherapy)
46. Toxins:
   - Mercury
   - Arsenic
   - Lead
   - Thallium
   - Toluene
   - Benzene
   - Carbon disulfide
   - Carbon monoxide
47. Insecticides
48. Hyperthermia
49. Hypomagnesemia
50. Hypothyroidism
51. Hypoparathyroidism
52. Extrapontine myelinolysis
53. Hepatocerebral degeneration
54. Portal-systemic encephalopathy

TABLE 104 continued

INFECTIOUS ETIOLOGIES

55. HIV encephalitis/AIDS
56. HSV encephalitis
57. Cerebellar abscess
58. Progressive multifocal leukoencephalopathy
59. Neurocystercercosis (rarely)
60. Lyme disease
61. Tuberculosis
62. Malaria
63. *Legionella*
64. *Mycoplasma*
65. *Streptococcus pneumoniae*
66. Fungal meningioencephalitis
67. Congenital rubella panencephalitis
68. Subacute sclerosing panencephalitis (classically measles, rubella)
69. Viral cerebellitis (including West Nile virus, St Louis encephalitis, eastern equine encephalitis and coxsackie A/B, echovirus, CMV, VZV, mumps, EBV, polio)
70. Toxoplasmosis (rare as only manifestation)
71. Syphilis (rare as only manifestation)
72. Whipple's disease
73. Prion diseases: Creutzfeldt–Jakob disease (CJD), variant CJD, and Gerstmann–Straussler–Scheinker syndrome

VASCULAR ETIOLOGIES

74. Vertebrobasilar insufficiency, including vertebral artery stenosis, basilar stenosis, vertebral artery dissection, and subclavian steal phenomenon
75. Cerebellar stroke, either alone or with associated brainstem signs as in Wallenberg's (lateral medulla) syndrome
76. Cerebellar hemorrhage (secondary to many causes)
77. Superficial siderosis

VITAMIN DEFICIENCIES

78. Wernicke's encephalopathy/thiamine defeciency
79. Vitamin E deficiency
80. B12 deficiency
81. Zinc defeciency

NEOPLASTIC PROCESSES

82. Primary malignant tumors: medulloblastoma, glioma, hemangioblastoma (associated with von Hippel–Landau syndrome), ependymoma
83. Benign tumors: vestibular schwannoma and meningioma
84. Cowden's syndrome/Lhermitte–Duclos disease (PTEN mutations leading to hemartomas in cerebellum and elsewhere)
85. Metastatic cancer: lung, breast, colon, melanoma, renal cell carcinoma most common in adults
86. Lymphoma

AUTOIMMUNE DISEASES

87. Post-infectious cerebellitis (post-VZV, EBV)
88. Multiple sclerosis (note overlap with post-infectious cerebellitis as initial presenting symptom)
89. Acute disseminated encephalomyelitis
90. Miller Fisher variant of Guillain–Barré syndrome
91. Hashimoto's thyroiditis/encephalopathy
92. Vasculitis (Behçet's disease, temporal arteritis, polyarteritis nodosa, among others)
93. Celiac disease (gluten enteropathy with ataxia)
94. GAD antibody-associated ataxia
95. Neurosarcoidosis
96. Histiocytosis X

SPORADIC CEREBELLAR NEURODEGENERATIVE DISEASES

97. Multiple system atrophy/OPCA
98. Progressive supranuclear palsy
99. PKAN (sporadic form)
100. Neuroacanthocytosis

CEREBELLAR ATAXIA MIMICS

101. Obstructive hydrocephalus
102. Normal pressure hydrocephalus
103. Large fiber sensory neuropathy
104. Migraine headache with ataxia
105. Psychogenic conversion disorder

CMV: cytomegalovirus; EBV: Epstein–Barr virus; HIV: human immunodeficiency virus; HSV: herpes simplex virus; MELAS: mitochondrial encephalomyopathy, lactic acidosis, and stroke-like episodes; MERRF: myoclonic epilepsy with ragged red fibers; MIRAS: mitochondrial recessive ataxia syndrome; NARP: neurogenic weakness with ataxia and retinitis pigmentosa; OPCA: olivopontocerebellar atrophy; PTEN: phosphatase and tensin homolog; VZV: varicella zoster virus.

Investigations and diagnosis

In most cases, MRI of the brain reveals the classic 'molar tooth sign'. Genetic testing is currently clinically available for four genes: NPHP1, AHI1, CEP290, and TME067. Together, however, these account for only about 30–40% of cases. Targeted exome-based panels are becoming available that target upwards of 94 ciliopathy genes and are thus close to definitive.

Testing for involvement of systems other than the CNS is critical, including ophthalmologic evaluation with visual evoked responses, liver function tests, and monitoring of renal function. Abdominal ultrasound should be performed to evaluate for renal or hepatic abnormalities.

A sleep evaluation with monitoring for apnea should be considered, as some patients require supplemental oxygen, or, rarely, bilevel positive airways pressure (BPAP) or tracheostomy.

Treatment and prognosis

Supportive. Most children survive to adulthood unless their extra-CNS symptoms are overwhelming.

AUTOSOMAL DOMINANT CEREBELLAR ATAXIAS

Definition and epidemiology

Autosomal dominant cerebellar ataxias (ADCAs) are a heterogeneous group of dominantly inherited late-onset clinical phenotypes that include cerebellar ataxia, nystagmus, dysarthria, dysmetria, intention tremor, and ophthalmoparesis, resulting from neuronal degeneration in the cerebellum and cranial nerve nuclei. There may also be varying degrees of dysfunction of the basal ganglia, brainstem, spinal cord, optic nerves, retinas, and peripheral nerves, resulting in parkinsonism, hyper-reflexia, spasticity, and visual loss.

- Prevalence: about 1 per 100,000 throughout the world.
- Age: adult onset, after age 20 years.

Classification

Classification is clinical, pathologic, and genotypic. The first widely accepted systematic classification of the dominantly inherited ataxias was proposed by Harding in 1993. This classification scheme included:

- ADCA type I: cerebellar ataxia is variably associated with other neurologic features, including involvement of the central and/or peripheral nervous system.
- ADCA type II: cerebellar ataxia is associated with the presence of a pigmentary maculopathy and striking anticipation (a tendency toward earlier onset in successive generations).
- ADCA type III is characterized by a pure cerebellar syndrome.

Due to the large number of genes associated with the dominantly inherited ataxias, this classification scheme has limited clinical utility. SCA7 is the only dominantly inherited ataxia belonging to the class of ADCA type II. It is nevertheless useful to classify the ataxias into those that present as relatively pure cerebellar syndromes (ADCA type III) and those that are cerebellar 'plus' syndromes (ADCA type I).

There are currently at least 29 genetic loci associated with ataxia syndromes that are dominantly inherited (*Table 105*). The most common inherited ataxias (SCA1, SCA2, SCA3, and SCA6) are associated with an expansion of a glutamine encoding trinucleotide (CAG) repeat in the respective disease-causing genes[10].

Disorders of trinucleotide repeats

Five of the eight neurologic disorders caused by an increase in the number of CAG repeats result in spinocerebellar ataxia (*Table 106*). The other three are spinal and bulbar muscular atrophy (Kennedy's disease), HD, and DRPLA. These disorders are characterized by autosomal dominant or X-linked inheritance, onset in midlife, a progressive course, anticipation, preponderance of unstable repeats from the paternal chromosome, and correlation of increased CAG repeats with earlier age at symptom onset. The abnormal proteins in each disorder are expressed in a wide range of tissues and are not limited to the affected brain regions.

Etiology and pathophysiology

Autosomal dominant inheritance. Multiple gene mutations have been identified to date (*Table 105*). The most common of these result from glutamine-encoding CAG repeats in the causative genes. Larger sizes of CAG repeats correlate directly with earlier ages of onset (anticipation). The repeat number increases with paternal transmission of disease (imprinting). The pathogenesis of these disorders is as diverse as the causative genes. The most common autosomal dominant ataxias result from glutamine-encoding CAG repeats. The resulting proteins are not homologous. The mechanism for pathogenesis of these proteins is diverse and includes altered gene transcription, RNA splicing, and intracellular calcium handling. The mechanism for the preferential loss of neurons primarily in the cerebellum and brainstem from these widely expressed proteins remains unexplained.

TABLE 105 **GENETIC LOCI ASSOCIATED WITH DOMINANTLY INHERITED ATAXIA SYNDROMES**

Name	Locus/gene	Protein/mutation	Pathology	Symptoms/signs
SCA1	6p22–p23/ *ATXN1*	Ataxin 1, CAG repeats 41–81 (normal 25–36)	Purkinje cells; pontine nuclei; inferior olivary nuclei	Cerebellar ataxia; dysarthria ophthalmoparesis; dysphagia, amyotrophy; pyramidal signs; extrapyramidal signs
SCA2	12q22–24/ *ATXN2*	Ataxin 2, CAG repeats 35–59 (normal 15–24)	Purkinje cells; basis pontis; inferior olivary nuclei	Cerebellar ataxia, *slow saccades, ophthalmoplegia peripheral neuropathy; minimal pyramidal and extrapyramidal signs; dementia (rarely)
SCA3 (Machado–Joseph Disease/MJD)	14q24.3–q31/ *ATXN3*	Ataxin 3, CAG repeats 62–82 (normal 13–36)	Subthalamic nuclei; substantia nigra; pontine nuclei, dentate nuclei; Clarke's columns; spinocerebellar tracts; anterior horn cells; dorsal root ganglia; mild Purkinje neuron loss	Cerebellar ataxia; ophthalmoparesis; *variable pyramidal signs; extrapyramidal amyotrophic signs; exophthalmos
SCA4	16q22			Cerebellar ataxia; *sensory axonal neuropathy; pyramidal signs
SCA5	11p13/*SPTBN2*	β III Spectrin		Pure cerebellar ataxia (late onset); pyramidal signs in young-onset patients
SCA6	19p13.2/ *CACNA1A*	Cav2.1, CAG repeats 21 to 30 (normal 6 to 17)	Severe loss of Purkinje cells	*Pure cerebellar ataxia
SCA7	3p14.1	Ataxin 7, CAG repeats	Extensive loss of Purkinje cells; dentate nuclei; inferior olivary nuclei; cone–rod dystrophy, loss of retinal ganglion cells; mild loss of pontine neurons	Progressive cerebellar ataxia with *pigmentary macular degeneration; variable ophthalmoplegia; pyramidal signs
SCA8	13q21.33/ *ATXN8OS*	Toxic RNA/possible polyglutamine disease	Depigmentation of substantia nigra; severe loss of Purkinje cells	Spastic and ataxic dysarthria, nystagmus; limb and gait ataxia; limb spasticity; diminished vibration perception
SCA9				Cerebellar ataxia; ophthalmoplegia; dysarthria; pyramidal tract signs; weakness; extrapyramidal signs; posterior column signs; central demyelination (in one patient)
SCA10	22q13/*ATXN10*		Intronic ATTCT repeats	Ataxia; *seizures; polyneuropathy, pyramidal signs; cognitive and neuropsychiatric impairment

TABLE 105 continued

Name	Locus/gene	Protein/mutation	Pathology	Symptoms/signs
SCA11	15q14–21.3/ *TTBK2*	Tau tubulin kinase-2		Relatively pure cerebellar ataxia
SCA12	5q32/*PPP2R2B*	Protein phosphatase PP2A, 51–78 CAG repeats (normal 7–32)		*Upper extremity tremor; hyper-reflexia; dysarthria; mild or no gait ataxia
SCA13	19q13.3–13.4/ *KCNC3*	Kv3.3		Gait ataxia; cerebellar dysarthria; mental retardation in French pedigree, pure ataxia in Filipino pedigree
SCA14	3pter–q24.2/ *ITPR1*	Protein kinase C gamma		Pure cerebellar ataxia; rare chorea and cognitive deficits
SCA15/SCA16	6q27/*TBP*	InsP3 receptor		Pure cerebellar ataxia; rare tremor, cognitive impairment
SCA17/Huntington's disease-like 4 (HDL4)	7q22–q32/ *IFRD1*	TATA box-binding protein	Reduction in brain weight; loss of Purkinje cells; neuronal inclusion bodies throughout the brain gray matter	Ataxia; dementia; psychiatric symptoms; extrapyramidal features; *chorea; lower limb hyper-reflexia
SCA18 Sensorimotor neuropathy with ataxia/ SMNA	7q22–q32	Human interferon-related developmental regulator gene-1		Gait difficulty; dysmetria; hyporeflexia; amyotrophy; *decreased vibratory and proprioceptive sense
SCA19/SCA22	1p21–q21			Pure ataxia or ataxia with cognitive impairment; myoclonus; postural tremor
SCA20	11p13–q11			Cerebellar ataxia with *spasmodic dysphonia or *spasmodic coughing
SCA21	7p21.3–p15.1			Cerebellar ataxia; akinesia, dysgraphia; hyporeflexia; postural tremor; rigidity; resting tremor; cognitive impairment
SCA23	20p13–p12.3		Cerebellar vermis; dentate nuclei; inferior olives; thinning of the cerebellopontine tracts; demyelination of spinal cord posterior and lateral columns (1 patient)	Cerebellar ataxia; decreased vibration below the knees
SCA25	2p21–p13			Cerebellar ataxia; lower limb areflexia; peripheral sensory neuropathy
SCA26	19p13.3			Pure cerebellar ataxia
SCA27	13q34/*FGF14*	Fibroblast growth factor 14		Cerebellar ataxia, tremor, *mild orofacial dyskinesias, cognitive impairment

TABLE 105 continued

Name	Locus/gene	Protein/mutation	Pathology	Symptoms/signs
SCA28	18p11.22–q11.2			Cerebellar ataxia; lower limb hyper-reflexia; rare ophthalmo-paresis; ptosis
SCA29	Genetically heterogeneous			*Congenital nonprogressive cerebellar ataxia
SCA30	4q34.3–q35.1			Pure cerebellar ataxia
SCA31	16q21/*BEAN*	TGGAA repeat in intron		Pure cerebellar ataxia; *sensori-neural hearing loss

*These signs can sometimes be used to differentiate this form of SCA from others clinically.

TABLE 106 **CLINICAL FEATURES OF THE DOMINANTLY INHERITED ATAXIAS**

PURE CEREBELLAR SYNDROME

SCA5, SCA6, SCA11, SCA14, SCA15, SCA26, SCA30, SCA31

CEREBELLAR ATAXIA ASSOCIATED WITH OTHER CLINICAL FEATURES

Eye signs	Movement disorders	Pyramidal signs	Cognitive impairment	Seizures	Neuropathy
Slow saccades SCA1, *SCA2, SCA3, SCA7	*Parkinsonism* SCA1, SCA2, SCA3, SCA12, SCA17, SCA21	SCA1, SCA2, *SCA3, SCA4, SCA7, SCA8, SCA11, SCA12, SCA13, SCA15	SCA1, SCA2, SCA3, SCA13, *SCA17, SCA19, SCA21, *SCA27, *DRPLA	*SCA10, SCA17, *DRPLA	SCA1, SCA2, SCA3, *SCA4, SCA6, SCA8, SCA27, SCA12, *SCA18, SCA22, *SCA25
Ophthlamoplegia SCA1, SCA2, SCA3	*Dystonia* SCA3, SCA17				
Pigmentary retinal degeneration *SCA7	*Limb and head tremor:* SCA8, SCA12, SCA16				
	Palatal tremor SCA19, SCA20				
	Dyskinesias *SCA27				
	Myoclonus SCA2, SCA19, DRPLA				
	Chorea SCA1, SCA17, DRPLA				

*These should be considered first when patients exhibit the indicated clinical syndromes.
(Modified from Manto U., *The Cerebellum*, 2005.)

Clinical features

- Family history of similarly affected members.
- Slow, gradual onset.
- Phenotypically heterogeneous (*Table 105*).
- Cerebellar ataxia, dysarthria, dysmetria, and cerebellar tremor ±:
  - Supranuclear ophthalmoplegia.
  - Optic atrophy.
  - Pigmentatory retinopathy.
  - Dementia.
  - Extrapyramidal dysfunction.

The clinical syndrome may vary remarkably, even among members of the same family.

Tip

▶ *The presence of pigmentary retinopathy in a patient with dominantly inherited ataxia strongly suggests a diagnosis of SCA7.*

Differential diagnosis

- Structural cerebellar, brainstem, or spinal cord lesions (tumor, arteriovenous malformation).
- Alcoholic cerebellar degeneration.
- Multiple sclerosis.
- Hypothyroidism.
- Neurosyphilis.
- Subacute combined degeneration of the spinal cord (sensory, not cerebellar ataxia).
- Wilson's disease.
- Mitochondrial cytopathy.
- Paraneoplastic cerebellar degeneration: usually a subacute ataxic syndrome.
- Iatrogenic cadaveric human growth hormone-induced CJD: a drug history of hormonal therapy should be taken from all young well-muscled, or previously well-muscled, patients and top athletes with signs of cerebellar dysfunction.

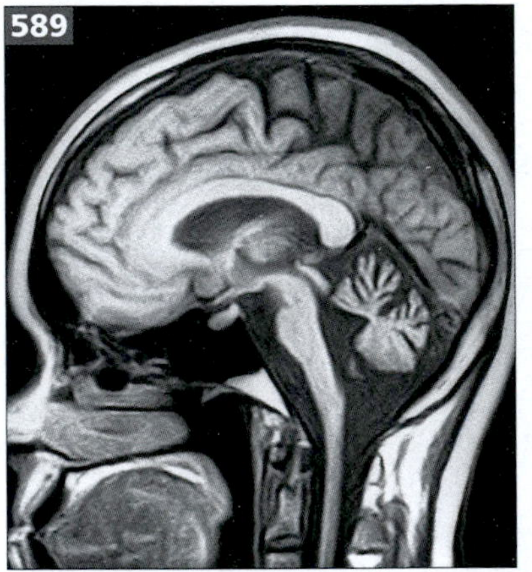

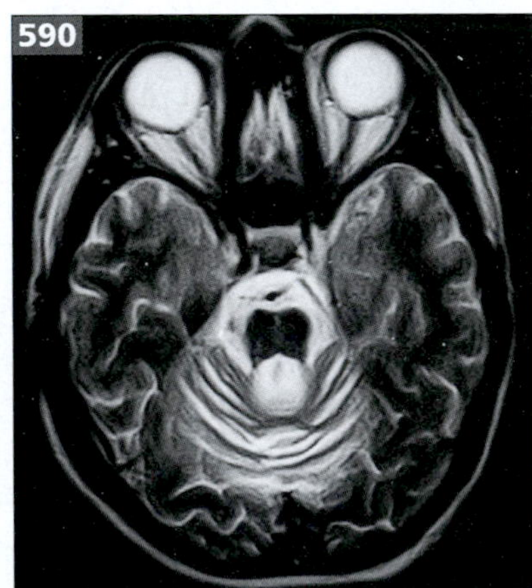

589–591 T1W midline sagittal (589) and T2W axial (590, 591) MRI of the brain in a patient with autosomal dominantly inherited cerebellar ataxia due to a mutation of the gene for spinocerebellar ataxia 1 on chromosome 6 causing expansion of the trinucleotide CAG repeat. Scans show pronounced atrophy of the medulla, pons and cerebellum, particularly affecting the superior vermis.

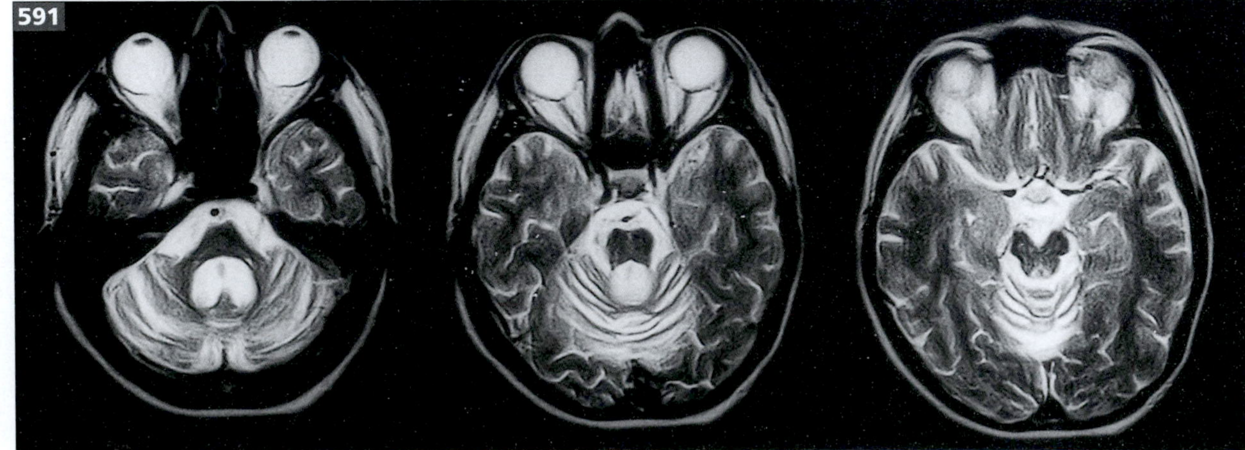

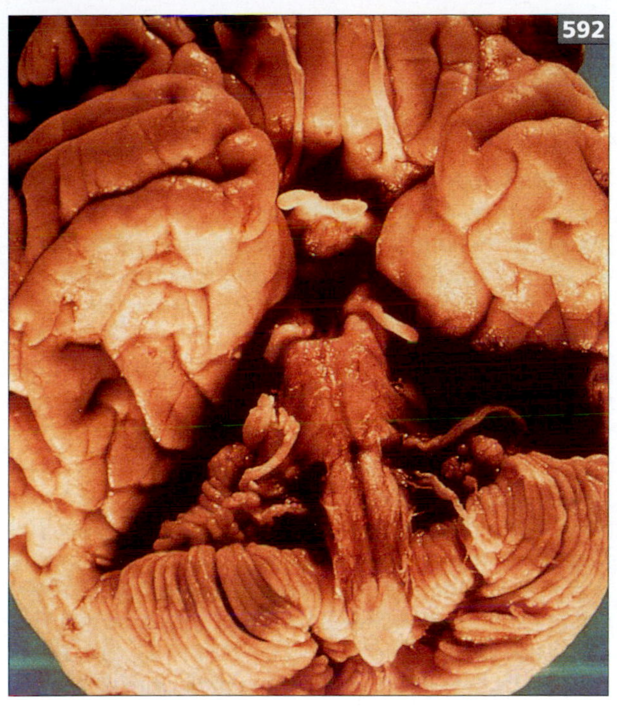

592 Ventral surface of the brain, showing severe atrophy of the medulla, pons and cerebellum.

593 Brainstem from a patient with autosomal dominant cerebellar ataxia (left), showing severe atrophy of the midbrain, pons, and medulla, and a normal brainstem (right). The brainstems have been disconnected from the brains and spinal cords by cuts through the cerebellar peduncles, midbrain, and medulla.

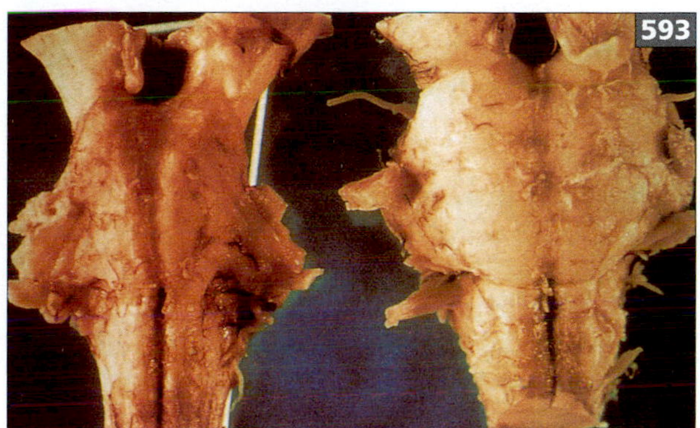

- Sporadic cerebellar degeneration, also known as idiopathic late-onset cerebellar ataxia (ILOCA): age of onset 25–70 years (onset after 55 years: often a relatively pure midline cerebellar syndrome with marked gait ataxia, mild appendicular ataxia).
- MSA of the cerebellar type (MSA-C), with sporadic cerebellar degeneration accompanied by autonomic failure (orthostatic hypotension with bladder incontinence).
- Other inherited cerebellar ataxias including recessively inherited disorders (see Friedreich's ataxia).
- PSP (dementia and supranuclear ophthalmoplegia).

Investigations

- Blood DNA analysis using PCR for gene mutations, commonly CAG repeat expansions, on chromosomes 3, 6, 12, 14, 16.
- Cranial CT or, preferably, MRI scan of the brain and craniocervical junction: pronounced cerebellar atrophy, particularly affecting the superior vermis (**589–591**).
- Complete blood count and sedimentation rate.
- Urea and electrolytes, plasma cortisol, very-long-chain fatty acids (in males, adrenoleukodystrophy).
- Thyroid function tests.
- Liver function tests (alcoholic cerebellar degeneration).
- VDRL, TPHA.
- Vitamin B12 and vitamin E.
- Plasma lactate and pyruvate, mitochondrial DNA analysis (mitochondrial cytopathy).
- Plasma copper, ceruloplasmin (Wilson's disease).
- Alpha fetoprotein (ataxia telangiectasia).
- Antipurkinje cell antibodies (paraneoplastic syndrome).
- ECG, and if abnormal, echocardiography.
- Nerve conduction studies and EMG.
- Visual evoked potentials and somatosensory evoked potentials.
- Autonomic function tests (MSA).
-

Diagnosis

Clinical syndrome of cerebellar ataxia, positive family history, and positive DNA analysis.

Pathology

Macroscopic changes are atrophy of the brainstem and cerebellum (**592**). Microscopically, there is loss of neurons and degenerative changes in various combinations (**593**) of sites that include:

- Pontine and olivary nuclei.
- Cerebellar dentate nuclei.
- Cerebellar Purkinje cells.
- Basal ganglia (substantia nigra, subthalamic nuclei, red nuclei).
- Spinal cord (Clarke's columns, spinocerebellar tracts, anterior horn cells).
- Peripheral nerves (dorsal root ganglia).

Treatment

No effective therapies exist currently for these disorders. Treatment is supportive. Symptomatic medications that have been reported to be of some utility are:

- Cholinergic agents: physostigmine, lecithin, and choline chloride.
- GABAergic drugs: baclofen and sodium valproate.
- Serotonergic compounds: L-5-hydroxytryptophan combined with a peripheral decarboxylase inhibitor, and buspirone hydrochloride.

Prognosis

Gradually progressive.

SCA1

Definition and epidemiology

SCA1 is an autosomal dominant disorder due to a pathologic expansion of glutamine repeats in the *ATXN1* gene. SCA1 is characterized by cerebellar ataxia associated with variable degrees of oculomotor abnormalities, pyramidal and extrapyramidal features, peripheral neuropathy, and cognitive impairment. SCA1 is one of the SCAs that can be classified on clinical grounds as ADCA type I, according to Harding's classification.

The frequency is variable depending on the population studied, and varies from 6% to 27% of dominant ataxias. It is the most frequent dominant ataxia in South Africa (41%)[11] and is also common in Japan, India, Italy, and Australia. SCA1 is less common in Portugal, Brazil, and central Japan.

Etiology and pathophysiology

SCA1 results from expansion of a translated trinucleotide CAG repeat located within exon 8 of the *SCA1* gene. The CAG repeat is highly polymorphic in the normal population and the number varies between 4 and 39 repeats. In SCA1, the CAG repeat is unstable and expands to about 40–83 repeats.

The mechanisms mediating SCA1 pathogenesis are still not completely understood. Transgenic mice expressing a mutant human *SCA1* allele have shown that eventual development of ataxia is not attributable to cell death *per se*, but to neuronal dysfunction and morphological alterations that occur long before the onset of ataxia and cell loss.

The discovery that residues in *ATXN1* outside of the polyglutamine tract are crucial for pathogenesis hints that alterations in the normal function of this protein are linked to its toxicity. Biochemical and genetic studies provide evidence that the polyglutamine expansion enhances interactions that are normally regulated by phosphorylation at the amino acid serine in position 776, and a subsequent alteration in its interaction with other cellular proteins.

ATXN1-interacting proteins are decreased in patients and animal models of the disease, suggesting that the polyglutamine expansion contributes to disease by both a gain-of-function mechanism and partial loss of function.

Clinical features

Age at onset of the disease is usually around the third decade of life, but can occur as early as 4 and as late as 74 years of age. The disease is insidiously progressive and fatal. Typical disease duration is 21–25 years from the age of onset[12].

At onset, the clinical signs consist of cerebellar ataxia, pyramidal signs, which sometimes even precede ataxia, and in most patients, ophthalmoplegia. As the disease progresses, other symptoms occur in variable degrees, such as dysphagia, dysphonia, tongue atrophy, deep sensory loss, peripheral sensory–motor axonal neuropathy, pes cavus, amyotrophy, and fasciculations. Dystonia is the most common extrapyramidal symptom. Rarely, rigidity, tremor, and chorea have also been reported.

At the onset of the disease, ocular movement abnormalities include gaze-evoked nystagmus, impairment of the vestibular ocular reflex, and increased amplitude of saccades with normal velocity. In one-half of the patients, the external ocular movements are full and in the other half there is upgaze or lateral gaze limitation. In later stages of the disease there is severe ophthalmoplegia in all directions with absent nystagmus and slow velocity in saccades.

Neuropsychological features in SCA1 include executive dysfunction.

Differential diagnosis

- Other autosomal dominant spinocerebellar ataxias (see *Table 105*).
- Recessive ataxias (see *Table 104*)

Investigations and diagnosis

The diagnostic test for SCA1 is sequencing of the gene and demonstrating an increase in the CAG repeat size.

Pathology

A characteristic feature of SCA1 pathology is the atrophy and loss of Purkinje cells from the cerebellar cortex. As SCA1 progresses, pathology is noted in other regions of the brain, including the deep cerebellar nuclei, especially the dentate nucleus, inferior olive, pons, and red nuclei. Cranial nerve nuclei III, X, and XII can also show signs of pathology. A pathologic hallmark of SCA1, as well as most of the other polyglutamine disorders, is the presence of the large inclusions containing the mutant polyglutamine protein. Besides containing mutant *ATXN1*, the inclusions are positive for ubiquitin and components of the proteasome and chaperone systems.

Treatment

Treatment is supportive. No definitive treatment exists for SCA1.

SCA2

Definition and epidemiology

SCA2 is an autosomal dominant disorder resulting from a pathologic expansion of glutamine repeats in the *ATXN2* gene. It can manifest either with a cerebellar syndrome or as parkinsonian syndrome. Later stages involve mainly brainstem, spinal cord, and thalamic degeneration.

SCA2 was first recognized in India by Wadia and Swami, who called attention to the early and marked slowing of saccadic eye velocity[13]. A large population of approximately 1000 patients in Cuba facilitated research into SCA2. Worldwide, SCA2 is among the three most frequent types of dominant spinocerebellar ataxias, together with SCA3 and SCA6.

Etiology and pathophysiology

Patients with SCA2 have an expansion of a CAG repeat located in the 5-prime end of the coding region of the *ATXN2* gene. Expansions of 35–64 repeats are found in affected individuals. The normal SCA2 alleles contain 17–29 repeats. There is a strong inverse correlation between the size of the CAG repeat and the age at onset of symptoms.

Ataxin-2 appears to play a role in RNA metabolism, interacts with plasma membrane proteins, and has putative roles in both of these processes.

Clinical features

SCA2 overlaps clinically with other dominantly inherited ataxias and a definitive diagnosis depends on genetic testing. Findings suggesting SCA2 include a combination of a gait ataxia/dysarthria with parkinsonian rigidity/bradykinesia with early and marked saccadic slowing, severe tremor of postural or action type, initial hyperreflexia followed by early hyporeflexia, early myoclonus or fasciculation-like movements, and muscle cramps. In the course of disease, immobility together with distal amyotrophy, dysphagia, opthalmoplegia, incontinence, and mental deficiencies limit the patients' independence. Autonomic problems can be found at late stages, with vasomotor, cardiac, gastrointestinal, urinary, exocrine gland dysfunction, and malnutrition.

Differential diagnosis

Other ADCAs (see *Table 105*).

Investigations and diagnosis

The diagnostic test for SCA2 is sequencing of the gene and demonstrating an increase in CAG repeat size.

Pathology

Macroscopically marked atrophy is seen of the cerebellum, pons, frontal lobe, medulla oblongata, and cranial nerves, as well as pallor of the substantia nigra.

The cerebellar degeneration pattern in SCA2 is characterized by an early and pronounced degeneration of Purkinje neurons throughout both hemispheres and the vermis, with rarefaction of granule cells later in the course of the disease. There is a relative sparing of the dentate nucleus.

Treatment

Treatment is supportive. No definitive treatment exists for SCA2.

SCA3

Definition and epidemiology

SCA3 or Machado–Joseph disease (MJD) is a dominantly inherited ataxia. SCA3 results from expansion of a glutamine-encoding CAG repeat in the *ATXN3* gene.

The disease has a worldwide distribution, including families described in Portugal, the Azores, Spain, Italy, US, Canada, Brazil, China, Taiwan, and Japan. It is most likely the most prevalent dominantly inherited ataxia worldwide[10].

Etiology and pathophysiology

SCA3 belongs to the class of disorders with an abnormal expansion of a glutamine-encoding CAG repeat in the 10th exon of the *ATXN3* gene. In MJD/SCA3, the normal glutamine repeat range of 12–40 is expanded to a disease-causing repeat range of 60–84.

Ataxin-3 is a 42 kDa, widely expressed protein that resides in both the nucleus and the cytoplasm of cells. It has been implicated in many aspects of intracellular protein quality control pathways that rely on ubiquitin, a small modifier protein. Ataxin-3 is a deubiquitinating enzyme (DUB) that cleaves ubiquitin from ubiquitinated substrates or polyubiquitin chains. Another proposed role for ataxin-3 is in the regulation of gene transcription.

The link between the enzymatic action of ataxin-3 as a DUB and its role in gene transcription is unclear. One current hypothesis posits that polyglutamine expansion interferes with ataxin-3 DUB function in some manner that compromises one or more biochemical pathways dependent on ubiquitin, including the ubiquitin–proteasome protein degradation system. A consequence would be misfolding and aggregation of proteins in vulnerable neurons. No direct evidence for altered enzymatic function of glutamine expanded ataxin-3 exists, however.

Clinical features

Even within the same family, persons affected with MJD/SCA3 can have widely varying clinical signs and symptoms.

The first description of MJD occurred in 1972 in a family (the Machado family) of Portuguese immigrants in Massachusetts, who presented a hereditary ataxia characterized by subacute onset of ataxia after age 40, associated with end-gaze nystagmus, mild dysarthria, hyporeflexia, and distal muscle atrophy.

When the clinical syndrome was first described in French and German families, which later was shown to be SCA3, the disease features seemed distinct enough from those experienced by affected families with MJD to assume that it was a separate disease. MJD had already been described and mapped to chromosome 14. Only when the actual MJD mutation was discovered was it demonstrated that SCA3 was in fact the same disease as MJD.

The clinical heterogeneity of the disorder is illustrated by the classification of SCA3 into three distinct phenotypic forms, Types 1–3. Cerebellar ataxia and ophthalmoplegia are common to all types of SCA3. Facial and lingual fasciculations, and staring due to lid retraction are other uncommon but helpful diagnostic features.

Type 1 MJD

- Early symptom onset, typically around 25 years.
- Pyramidal signs.
- Dystonic postures.

Type 2 MJD

- Most common type.
- Middle age symptom onset (40 years, mean).
- Ataxia and ophthalmoplegia with or without pyramidal signs.

Type 3 MJD

- Later onset (47 years, mean).
- Amyotrophy prominent.
- Slow progression.

In addition to these three categories, some patients present with levodopa-responsive parkinsonism that is clinically indistinguishable from idiopathic PD.

Differential diagnosis

Other autosomal dominant spinocerbellar ataxias (see *Table 105*).

Investigations and diagnosis

The diagnostic test for SCA3 is sequencing of the gene and demonstrating an increase in the CAG repeat size.

Pathology

The neuropathology consists of neuronal loss and gliosis in the substantia nigra, motor cranial nuclei, dentate nucleus of the cerebellum, and variable neuronal loss with gliosis in the cerebellar cortex and neostriatum.

The cerebellar cortex is significantly less affected than in SCA1 or SCA2 with typically <30% loss of Purkinje neurons[14]. The inferior olivary nuclei are normal.

Treatment

Treatment is supportive. No definitive treatment exists for SCA3.

Tip

▶ *In patients presenting with a family history of heterogeneous neurologic diagnoses including cerebellar ataxia, parkinsonism, and amyotrophy, consider testing for SCA3.*

SCA6

Definition and epidemiology

SCA6 is a progressive ataxic disorder caused by a CAG repeat expansion in the *CACNA1A* gene encoding the α1 subunit of the neuronal P/Q-type voltage-gated calcium channel (VGCC).

The worldwide prevalence is variable, highest in Japan[10] and moderate in Europe, although accurate absolute numbers are not available. Genetic epidemiologic studies in England have estimated the frequency of the disease-causing mutation at approximately one in every 10,000 individuals.

Etiology and pathophysiology

SCA6 is caused by a mutation in the C-terminus of the α1A subunit of the P/Q-type VGCC. Numerous studies have attempted to determine how the polyglutamine expansion affects the properties of the P/Q-type calcium channel, and ultimately how a small polyglutamine expansion in a VGCC may lead to cell death. Unfortunately, these results appear highly variable and depend on which expression system and auxiliary VGCC subunits are used.

It was recently observed that the endogenous free C-terminal fragment localizes to Purkinje cell nuclei. In addition, C-terminal fragments cleaved from recombinant α1A subunits or expressed as isolated C-termini localize to nuclei in cultured cell lines and primary granule cell cultures. Cleavage and nuclear localization are not however affected by polyglutamine length. The relevance of the cleaved fragment to disease pathogenesis is unclear.

Clinical features

SCA6 is often described as a pure cerebellar ataxia, in comparison to SCAs that are complicated by cortical, subcortical, and/or brainstem dysfunction. It is characterized by gaze-evoked nystagmus, dysarthria, progressive imbalance, and severe limb incoordination. Some patients with SCA6 experience occasional bouts of vertigo, but there is no muscle weakness or cognitive impairment.

SCA6 is a late-onset disorder with an average onset age of 50 years. The disease usually progresses slowly and does not shorten life-span, but most patients do become wheelchair bound by their late 60s.

Differential diagnosis

Other autosomal dominant and recessive spinocerebellar ataxias (see *Tables 104* and *105*).

Investigations and diagnosis

The diagnostic test for SCA6 is sequencing of the gene and demonstrating an increase in the CAG repeat size.

Pathology

Post-mortem analysis of the brains from SCA6 patients demonstrates cerebellar atrophy due to selective Purkinje cell degeneration. These brains display a strikingly selective loss of Purkinje cells, with particularly high losses in the midline vermal region of the cerebellum. The surviving Purkinje cells frequently have decreased dendritic arborizations and decreased cytoplasmic organelles compared with normal controls.

Mild to moderate granule cell loss appears to be secondary to Purkinje cell loss, but basket, stellate, and Golgi cells of the cerebellar cortex appear largely unaffected.

Treatment

Treatment is supportive. No definitive treatment exists for SCA6.

Tips

- *Since SCA1, SCA2, SCA3, and SCA6 account for over 50% of the autosomal dominant ataxias in clinical practice, consider using a tiered approach to genetic testing. Test first for these more common dominant ataxias.*
- *In patients presenting with a mix of familial ataxia and features of HD (chorea, dementia, neuropsychiatric symptoms), consider testing for DRPLA and SCA17.*

AUTOSOMAL RECESSIVE CEREBELLAR ATAXIAS

FRIEDREICH'S ATAXIA

Definition and epidemiology

This is an autosomal recessively inherited disease caused by a large increase in the number of trinucleotide GAA repeats within the first intron of the *FRDA* gene on the proximal long arm of chromosome 9[15]. This results in decreased expression of the target protein frataxin, and dysfunction of the central and peripheral nervous systems and the heart. Clinically, when it presents in classical form, Friedreich's ataxia is characterized by onset before age 25 years of progressive limb and gait ataxia, cerebellar dysarthria, depressed deep tendon reflexes, pyramidal signs, distal vibration and proprioceptive sensory loss, axonal sensory neuropathy, and often skeletal deformities and hypertrophic cardiomyopathy[16]. Now that genetic testing has become available for this disorder, cases with onset in adult life are found commonly, and cases with onset late in life have been reported.

- Prevalence: 2 per 100,000; the most common form of hereditary ataxia[17].
- Carrier frequency: 1 in 120 in European populations.
- Age: adolescence and early adult life. Onset usually occurs at 8–15 years.

Etiology and pathophysiology

Gene mutation

Friedreich's ataxia results from an expanded GAA repeat in the first intron of the *FRDA* gene, which is located on the proximal long arm of chromosome 9 (9q13–q21.1). *FRDA* encodes a novel 210-amino acid protein, frataxin, which is involved in mitochondrial function and iron metabolism. The expanded repeat interferes with *FRDA* transcription, leading to lowered expression of the protein. Complete loss of the protein is incompatible with life. More than 95% of patients with classic Friedreich's ataxia are homozygous for an expansion in their GAA repeat sequence, but a few have a combination of an increase in GAA repeats in one allele and a point mutation in the other allele, confirming that Friedreich's ataxia is a loss-of-function disorder. Larger GAA expansions correlate with lower frataxin expression, earlier age of onset, and shorter times to loss of ambulation.

Gene expression

The GAA repeat represses transcription of frataxin mRNA by altering local chromatin structure[18]. Frataxin appears to be a nuclear encoded mitochondrial protein important for normal production of cellular energy. Reduced frataxin in spinal cord, heart, and pancreas has been postulated to cause neuronal degeneration, cardiomyopathy, and an increased risk of diabetes by altering iron homeostasis in cells and their mitochondria.

Clinical features

The clinical spectrum for Friedreich's ataxia is broader than previously recognized.

History

Symptoms of incoordination and ataxia of the lower limbs begin in the early 'teen' years and progress to involve the upper limbs and cranial musculature, so that by the age of 25 years most patients have some well-established neurologic signs. However, there are cases of patients not diagnosed until their 60s or 70s.

Physical examination

- General:
  - Kyphoscoliosis (may affect posture and pulmonary function).
  - Foot deformity (pes cavus and extension of the metatarsophalangeal joints in about 90% of patients).
  - Hypertrophic cardiomyopathy.
- Cranial nerves:
  - Reduced visual acuity.
  - Optic atrophy.
  - Eye movements:
    - Square wave jerks at fixation.
    - Saccadic intrusion upon smooth ocular pursuits (jerky pursuits).
    - Gaze-evoked nystagmus.
    - Reduced gain of vestibulo-ocular reflex.
  - Speech: slurred, slow, staccato, and explosive (ataxic dysarthria).
- Limbs:
  - Wasting of the intrinsic hand and distal lower leg muscles.
  - Weakness (pyramidal) of the legs (paraparesis).
  - Ataxia of the limbs, speech and eye movements:
    - Bilateral cerebellar tremor.
    - Dysmetria (overshoot).
    - Dysdiadochokinesia (poor coordination of rapid alternating movements).
  - Absent deep tendon reflexes due to axonal degeneration of afferent fibers. This is reflected neurophysiologically by absence of sensory nerve action potential (SNAPs) and loss of the H-reflex. Note that rare patients present with late-onset symptoms, retained reflexes, and spasticity.
  - Extensor plantar responses.
  - Impaired touch, pain, and temperature sensations in the feet and distal lower limbs are unusual, but found in a small fraction of patients.
  - Impaired vibration sense in the feet and hands.
  - Impaired joint position sense in the distal lower limbs and hands.
- Gait: spastic, ataxic (cerebellar and sensory) gait.

Tip

▶ *In adult patients, Friedreich's ataxia can present with both ataxia and concomitant spasticity with retained reflexes.*

Differential diagnosis

The differential for recessively inherited progressive cerebellar ataxias is long and includes many nonhereditary disorders (see *Table 104* for an extensive differential diagnosis list).

Inherited ataxias with known metabolic defects

Ataxia with isolated vitamin E (α-tocopherol) deficiency

- Inherited: autosomal recessive: frame-shift mutations in the gene encoding α-tocopherol-transfer protein (α-TTP) on chromosome 8q (13.1–13.3)[19].
- Acquired fat malabsorption syndromes:
  - Abeta- and hypobeta-lipoproteinemia (Bassen–Kornzweig syndrome).
  - Cholestatic liver disease.
  - Short bowel syndrome.
  - Onset in second to sixth decade of life.

Progressive ataxia, dysarthria, areflexia, extensor plantar responses, and proprioceptive loss ± ophthalmoplegia, dystonic posturing of hands/feet, bradykinesia, tongue fasciculations, and pigmentary retinal degeneration. Low serum vitamin E (11.7 μmol/l [<5 μg/ml]). Low serum lipid concentrations, particularly cholesterol.

Oral vitamin E (800–3500 mg/day [800–3500 IU]) may cause improvement or retard progression.

Hexosaminidase A deficiency (GM2 gangliosidosis)

- Onset in adolescence or early adult life.
- Ataxia, tremor, supranuclear ophthalmoplegia, facial grimacing, dystonia, and proximal neurogenic muscle weakness.

Cholestanolosis (cerebrotendinous xanthomatosis).

- Autosomal recessive inheritance.
- Defective bile salt metabolism.
- Onset in second decade of life.
- Ataxia, dementia, spasticity, peripheral neuropathy, cataracts, tendon xanthomata.
- Chenodeoxycholic acid treatment may improve neurologic function[20].

Leukodystrophies

- Metachromatic leukodystrophy (arylsulfatase A deficiency).
- Late-onset globoid cell leukodystrophy.
- Adrenoleukomyeloneuropathy: a phenotypic variant of adrenoleukodystrophy.

Refsum's disease

- Peroxisomal disorder characterized by retinitis pigmentosa, sensorimotor polyneuropathy, and cerebellar ataxia. ECG changes, sensorineural hearing loss, and ichthyosis are also seen[21].
- The disease usually presents in childhood but can present in early adulthood.
- Results from a mutation in phytanoyl-CoA hydroxylase, an enzyme that acts as a phytanic acid oxidase. In the absence of the enzyme, phytanic acid accumulates in the tissues, resulting in toxicity.
- Testing involves measuring phytanic acid levels in blood or tissue.
- A diet low in phytanic acid can reduce symptoms and potentially be curative[22].

Niemann–Pick disease type C (juvenile dystonic lipidosis)

- Ataxia, supranuclear gaze palsy and psychosis.
- Sphingomyelinase activity is normal.
- Foamy storage cells in bone marrow.

Early-onset cerebellar ataxia with retained tendon reflexes (Holmes ataxia)

- Optic atrophy, severe skeletal deformity, and cardiac involvement do not occur.
- Deep tendon reflexes are normal or increased.
- Gait may have a spastic component.
- Prognosis is worse than Friedreich's ataxia.
- Associated features include:
  - Hypogonadism.
  - Myoclonus.
  - Pigmentary retinopathy.
  - Optic atrophy ± mental retardation (including Behr's optic atrophy syndrome).
  - Cataract and mental retardation (Marinesco–Sjögren syndrome).
  - Childhood deafness.
  - Congenital deafness; extrapyramidal features.

Multiple sclerosis

- Relapsing and remitting course is common in young-onset cases.
- Bladder involvement is common.
- Sensory loss is usually patchy.
- CSF usually shows elevated protein and IgG and oligoclonal bands.
- MRI brain usually shows multiple lesions in periventricular white matter, corpus callosum, and adjacent to the temporal horn of the lateral ventricles.

Structural spinal cord lesion (spinal cord tumor or arteriovenous malformation)

- Pain, particularly nerve root pain, is common.
- Progressive spasticity below the level of the lesion.
- Progressive urgency of micturition.
- Sensory level.
- MRI (± spinal angiography) of spinal cord discloses a focal lesion.

Syphilitic pachymeningitis

- Rare.
- CSF pleocytosis, raised protein and positive VDRL, TPHA, fluorescent treponemal antibody.

Subacute combined degeneration of the spinal cord

- Ataxia is predominantly sensory rather than cerebellar.
- Low serum vitamin B12 level.
- Antibodies to intrinsic factor and gastric parietal cell may be present.

Other

- Mitochondrial cytopathy.
- Wilson's disease.
- Ceroid lipofuscinosis.
- Sialidosis.
- Ataxia telangiectasia, ATLD (see below).
- Ataxia with oculomotor apraxia I and II (see below).

Investigations

- ECG and echocardiography: many have obstructive hypertrophic cardiomyopathy.
- Pulmonary function tests: may deteriorate due to kyphoscoliosis.
- Nerve conduction studies:
  - Absent sensory nerve action potentials.
  - Prolonged sensory conduction velocities.
  - Loss of H-reflex indicative of afferent axonal neuropathy.
- Somatosensory evoked potentials: absence or abnormalities of cortical responses to peroneal or tibial nerve stimulation.
- Electronystagmography: fixational instability with square wave jerks.

- MRI scan of brain and craniocervical junction: non-specific, mild atrophy of the cerebellum (594, 595), the cervicomedullary junction, and upper cervical spinal cord may be present.
- Molecular DNA analysis for point mutation in *FRDA*, or GAA trinucleotide expansion in the first *FRDA* intron, on the proximal long arm of chromosome 9 (9q13–q21.1): useful for diagnosis, determination of prognosis, and genetic counseling.

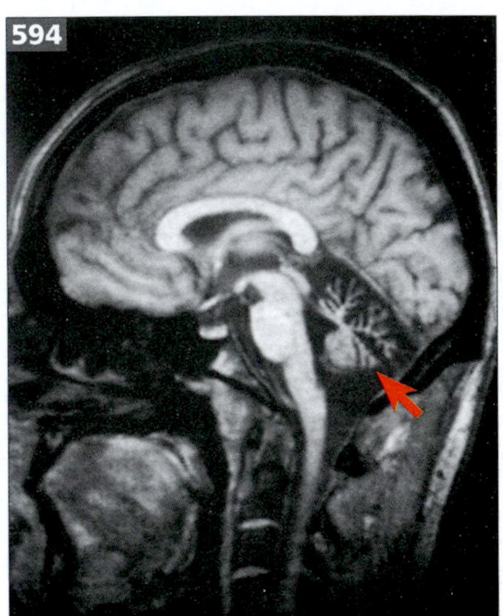

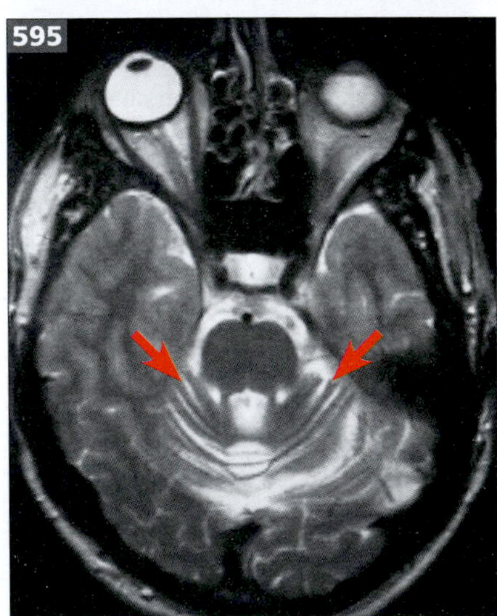

594, 595 T1W midline sagittal (594) and T2W axial (595) MRI of the brain in a patient with Freidreich's ataxia. Note the marked cerebellar atrophy (arrows), but that the rest of the brain, including the brainstem, is normal.

Tests for other disorders on differential diagnosis for recessive ataxias

- Full blood count with peripheral smear for acanthocytes or sideroblasts.
- Serum glucose.
- Serum lipids.
- RPR or VDRL, TPHA.
- Thyroid function tests and antithyroglobulin antibodies.
- Vitamins B12 and E.
- Copper, ceruloplasmin (Wilson's disease, copper deficiency).
- Cortisol and long-chain fatty acids (L C26:C22, C24:C22 ratio) if spastic paraparesis, axonal neuropathy, male (adrenoleukodystrophy).
- Alpha fetoprotein (ataxia telangiectasia and ataxia with oculomotor apraxia type II).
- Antigliadin, antitissue transglutaminase and anti-endomysial antibodies (celiac disease).
- Anti GAD-65 antibodies (autoimmune ataxia).
- Paraneoplastic antibodies, including Anti-HU, YO, and RI if subacute course (paraneoplastic).
- Hexosaminidase: if vertical gaze palsy, dystonia, neurogenic weakness.
- Arylsulfatase A (metachromatic leukodystrophy).
- Galactocerebrosidase: if dementia, psychiatric problems, optic atrophy, demyelinating neuropathy, radiologic evidence of white matter disease.
- Plasma lactate and pyruvate, muscle biopsy and blood for mitochondrial DNA analysis: if short stature, myoclonus, retinopathy, dementia, stroke-like episodes, and fatiguable weakness.
- Cholestanol: if cataract, tendinous swellings.
- Gonadotrophins: if hypogonadism.
- Ammonia/amino acids: if fluctuating course, mental retardation.
- Bone marrow examination for sea blue histiocytes (Niemann–Pick disease type C): if vertical gaze palsy, epileptic seizures, extrapyramidal signs, dementia.
- Phytanic acid levels (Refsum's disease): if retinitis pigmentosa, sensorimotor polyneuropathy, hearing loss, or ichthyosis (excessive dry scaly skin).

Tip

► *A number of forms of ataxia related to metabolic disorders are treatable if identified early. Thus, measuring cholestanol (cerebrotendinous xanthomatosis), phytanic acid and other long-chain fatty acids (Refsum's disease), vitamin E (AVED, Bassen–Kornzweig syndrome), and ceruloplasmin (Wilson's disease), should all be considered early in the work-up of patients with the correct clinical context.*

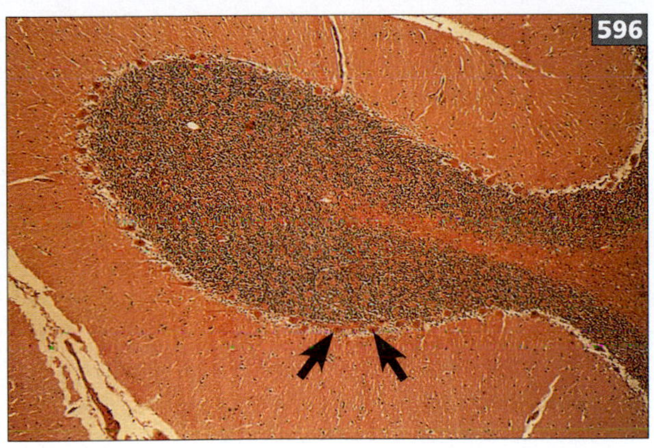

596 Normal cerebellar cortex, H&E stain, with plentiful Purkinje cells (two arrowed).

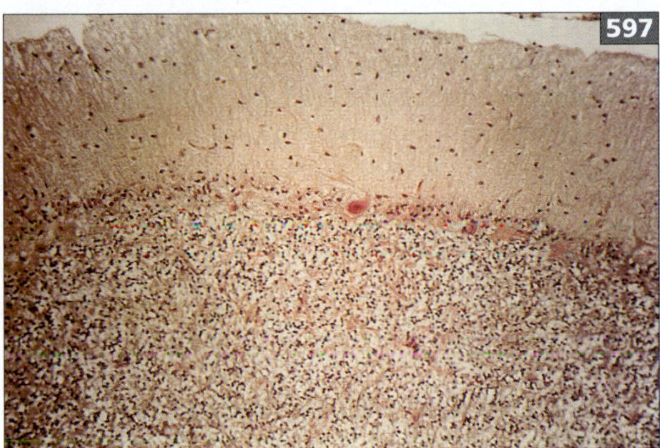

597 Higher magnification view of the cerebellar cortex of a patient with Freidreich's ataxia, showing Purkinje cell loss.

Diagnosis

- Progressive limb and gait ataxia developing before the age of 25 years.
- Absent deep tendon reflexes in most cases.
- Electrophysiologic evidence of axonal sensory neuropathy.
- Point mutation in *FRDA* or unstable GAA trinucleotide expansion in the first *FRDA* intron, on the proximal long arm of chromosome 9 (9q13–q21.1).

Pathology

- Nervous system:
  - Dorsal root ganglia: degeneration/loss of large sensory neurons.
  - Dying back of axons in:
    - Large myelinated sensory nerve fibers in peripheral nerves.
    - Posterior columns of the spinal cord.
    - Nucleus gracilis and cuneatus, and the medial lemniscus.
    - Dorsal and ventral spinocerebellar tracts.
  - Corticospinal tracts: demyelination, with increasing involvement caudally.
  - Cerebellum:
    - Loss of Purkinje cells (**596**, **597**).
    - Degeneration of dentate nucleus.
    - Axonal loss and demyelination of superior cerebellar peduncles.
- Heart: degeneration leading to hypertrophy and diffuse fibrosis.
- Pancreas: degeneration, giving rise to:
  - Diabetes mellitus in about 10% of patients.
  - Carbohydrate intolerance in an additional 20%.
  - Reduced insulin response to arginine stimulation in all patients.

Treatment

Clinical trials with idebenone have demonstrated some benefit for cardiac hypertrophy in Friedreich's patients[23,24]. There was a suggestion of possible benefit for neurologic symptoms at higher doses, especially in patients not yet wheelchair bound[25]. Clinical trials are currently underway to assess this prospectively. Symptomatic treatment of:

- Spasticity medication (e.g. baclofen, botulinum toxin).
- Physiotherapy.
- Occupational therapy.
- Podiatry.
- Speech therapy.
- Social work.
- Cardiology consultation: for hypertrophic cardiomyopathy.
- Pulmonary function.
- Orthopedic spinal surgery (Harrington rod); for scoliosis.

Prognosis

Progressive deterioration. Most patients are unable to walk independently and safely >5–10 years after the onset of symptoms, so almost all are confined to a wheelchair by their late 20s. Death usually occurs 10–25 years after symptoms onset (in 40s and 50s), usually due to cardiopulmonary complications.

ATAXIA TELANGIECTASIA

(LOUIS–BAR SYNDROME)

Definition and epidemiology

A rare autosomal recessive disorder characterized by onset of ataxia in early childhood and subsequent progressive neuromotor degeneration, usually resulting in dependence on a wheelchair by 10 years of age[26].

- Incidence: rare.
- Age: early childhood.
- Gender: M=F.

Etiology and pathophysiology

- Autosomal recessive inheritance.
- Defective gene: *ATM*, mapped to chromosome 11q22–23, which encodes a protein belonging to the superfamily of phosphatidylinositol-3′ kinases.
- Breaks in chromosome 14 and translocations.
- Decreased synthesis of immunoglobulins.
- Defective repair of DNA.
- *ATM* homozygotes are hypersensitive to ionizing radiation and radiomimetic drugs.

Clinical features

- 1–2 years of age: onset with the acquisition of walking; ataxic–dyskinetic syndrome: awkward, unsteady gait.
- 4–5 years of age:
  - Telangiectases: subpapillary venous plexuses, most evident in the outer parts of the bulbar conjunctivae (**598, 599**), over the ears, on exposed parts of the neck (**600, 601**), on the bridge of the nose and cheeks in a butterfly pattern, and in the flexor creases of the forearms (**602, 603**).
  - Ocular pursuit: jerky due to interruption by saccadic intrusions.
  - Saccades: slow and long latency.
  - Apraxia for voluntary horizontal gaze (the head, not the eyes, turn on attempting to look to the side).
  - Loss of optokinetic nystagmus.
  - Limb ataxia and dysarthric speech.
  - Choreoathetosis.
  - Grimacing.
- 9–10 years of age:
  - Mild intellectual decline.
  - Mild polyneuropathy: hyporeflexia.
  - Growth retardation.
- 10–20 years of age:
  - Progressive decline.
  - Premature aging.
  - Recurrent pulmonary and sinus infections due to immunologic abnormalities.
  - Death due to intercurrent bronchopulmonary infection or neoplasia, usually lymphoma, less often glioma.

Differential diagnosis

Ataxia telangiectasia-like diseases

- MUR-11 deficiency and Nijmegen breakage syndrome:
  - Present with later onset and slower progression. No telangictasias.
  - Result from deficiencies of other proteins (MUR11 and NBS1, respectively) that are involved in the same DNA repair pathway as *ATM*.
  - Alpha fetoprotein (AFP) levels may be normal or slightly elevated.
- Xeroderma pigmentosum (XP) is a rare, genetically heterogeneous group of disorders caused by mutations in DNA excision repair enzymes. Presents with ataxia, cognitive decline, peripheral neuropathy, sensorineural hearing loss, and choreathetosis in addition to a variety of cutaneous lesions.
- Cockayne syndrome is a rare disorder with ataxia and deafness similar to XP, but also characterized by retinal degeneration and accelerated aging without an increased incidence of malignancies. It is caused by a defect in transcription-related DNA repair.

Ataxia with oculomotor apraxia Type 1 (AOA1)

- Early-onset cerebellar ataxia with oculomotor apraxia, chorea, facial and limb dystonias, sensorimotor polyneuropathy, and cognitive impairment.
- Usually presents in the first decade of life, although symptom onset has been reported as late as age 25.
- Associated with hypercholesterolemia and hypoalbuminemia.
- Results from a mutation in the *APTX* gene. *APTX* encodes a protein, aprataxin, that is involved in repair of single-stranded DNA breaks.
- A subset of patients with AOA1 have been found to have a deficiency in coenzyme Q10 and may respond to dietary supplementation.

Ataxia with oculomotor apraxia type 2 (AOA2)

- More common than AOA1 and has a later age of onset, in the 20s to 50s. (AOA1 and AOA2 together represent ~20% of autosomal recessive cerebellar ataxia cases.)
- Cognitive impairment and oculomotor apraxia are only features in approximately 50% of cases.
- Also with elevated AFP.
- Results from mutations in the gene *SETX* which encodes a protein, senataxin, of unknown function.

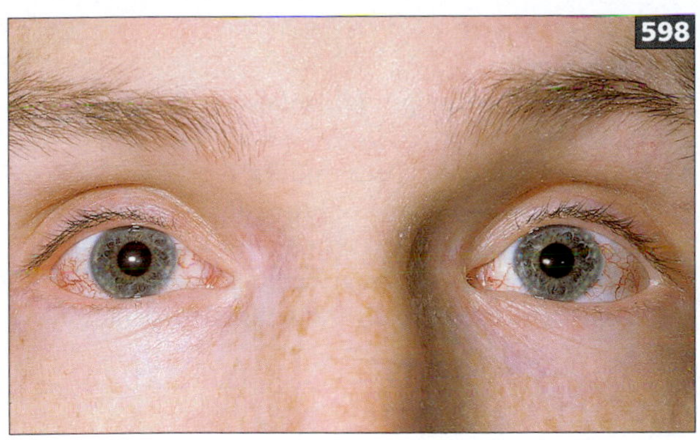

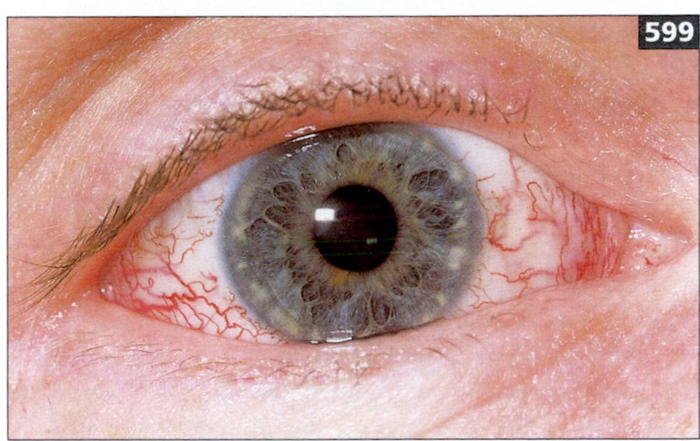

598, 599 Conjunctival telangiectases, most evident in the outer parts of the bulbar conjunctivae, in a young man with ataxia telangiectasia.

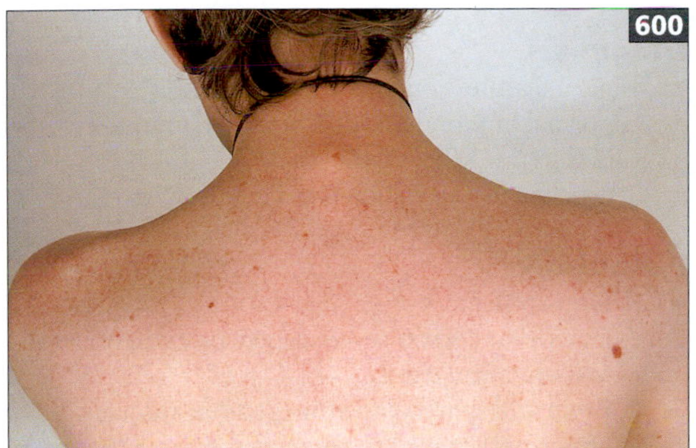

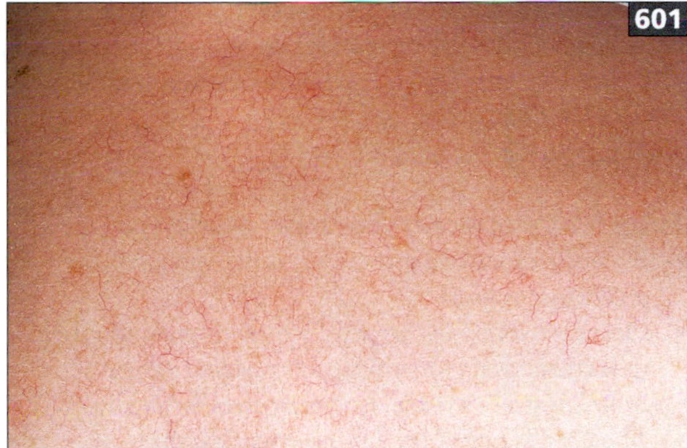

600, 601 Telangiectases on exposed parts of the neck and back.

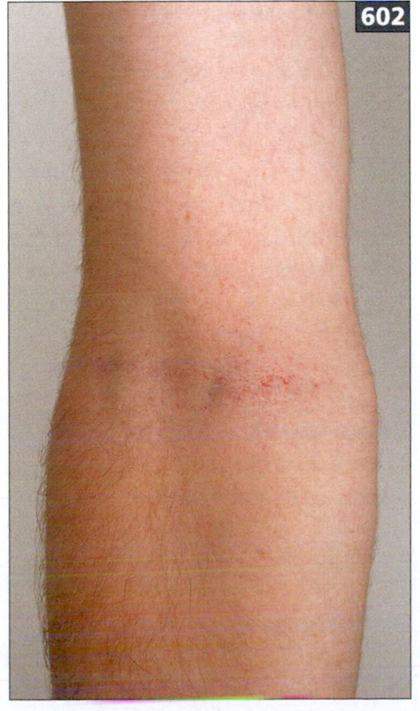

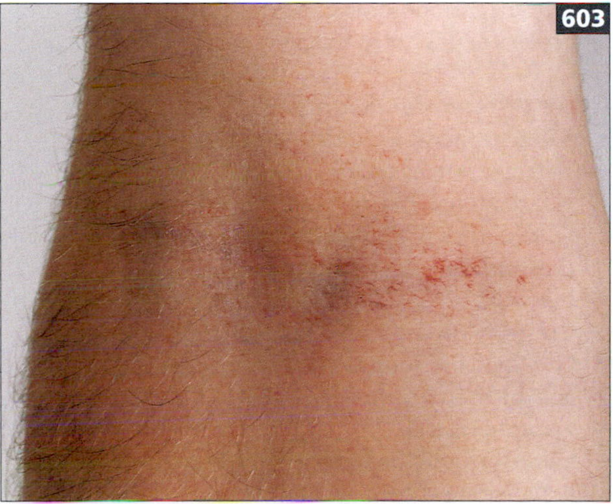

602, 603 Telangiectases in the flexor crease of the right forearm.

Autosomal recessive spastic ataxia (of Charlevoix–Saguenay [ARSACS])

- Rare, early-onset disorder with early spasticity, peripheral neuropathy, finger and foot deformities and hypermyelination of retinal nerve fibers. Most patients have normal intelligence until late in the disease course.
- Initially described in families from Quebec, but cases in Europe and Japan have now been described.
- Children are usually symptomatic by 1 year of age.
- Slowly progressive with most people able to ambulate into their 20s or 30s before becoming wheelchair bound in later life.
- Pathologically, patients have cerebellar vermis atrophy and an almost complete absence of Purkinje cells.
- ARSACS results from a mutation in the *SACS* gene which encodes the protein sacsin, whose function is unknown, although it has homology to a number of heat-shock proteins.
- Treatment is supportive.

Autosomal recessive cerebellar ataxia type 1

- Recently described late-onset, slowly progressive cerebellar ataxia.
- Onset is usually in the early 30s, with prominent dysarthria as the only other consistent finding.
- Imaging studies reveal isolated cerebellar atrophy.
- The prevalence of the disorder worldwide is unknown, but it appears to be the most common inherited cause of cerebellar ataxia in Quebec where it was first identified.
- Results from truncation mutations in the *SYNE1* gene on chromosome 6, which encodes a large protein of unknown function.

Other differential diagnoses

- Metachromatic leukodystrophy: reduced arylsulfatase A in urine.
- Neuroaxonal dystrophy (degeneration): characteristic spheroids within axons on electron microscopy of skin and conjunctival nerves.
- Niemann–Pick disease: reduced sphingomyelinase in leukocytes and cultured fibroblasts.
- GM1 gangliosidosis: deficiency of β-galactosidase activity in leukocytes and cultured fibroblasts.
- Neuronal ceroid lipofuscinosis: inclusions (translucent vacuoles) in lymphocytes and azurophilic granules in neutrophils.
- Abeta-lipoproteinemia (Bassen–Kornzweig acanthocytosis): thorny red blood cells (acanthocytes), reduced serum low density lipoproteins.
- Friedreich's ataxia.

Investigations

- Lymphopenia.
- Immunoglobulins: IgA, IgE and isotypes, IgG2, IgG4: reduced or absent.
- Failure of delayed hypersensitivity reactions.
- Abnormal humoral and cell-mediated immunity.
- AFP: elevated serum levels in almost all patients.
- CT or MRI brain scan may demonstrate cerebellar atrophy and occasionally intracranial vascular malformations may be present.

Tip

► *AFP can be used as a screening test for ataxia telangiectasia and ataxia with oculomotor apraxia Type II prior to formal genetic testing.*

Diagnosis

- Clinical features consistent with diagnosis.
- Abnormal humoral and cell-mediated immunity.
- Raised serum AFP.
- Genetic testing is available on a research basis only.

Pathology

- Nervous system:
  - Cerebellar cortex: severe degeneration; extensive loss of Purkinje cells.
  - Brain and spinal cord white matter: vascular abnormalities, like the mucocutaneous ones, are scattered diffusely in a few cases.
  - Substantia nigra and locus ceruleus: there may be loss of pigmented cells, with cytoplasmic inclusions (Lewy bodies) in the cells that remain.
  - Anterior horn cells: loss at all levels of the spinal cord.
  - Posterior columns: loss of myelinated fibers.
  - Spinocerebellar tracts: loss of myelinated fibers.
  - Sympathetic ganglia cells: degeneration.
  - Dorsal nerve root ganglion neurons: intranuclear inclusions and bizarre nuclear formations may be found in the satellite cells (amphicytes).
  - Posterior nerve roots: degeneration.
  - Peripheral nerves: loss of myelinated fibers.
- Thymus: hypoplasia.
- Lymph nodes: loss of follicles.

Treatment

Treatment is supportive. Case report level data suggest responses in some patients to betamethasone[27]. Prophylaxis of recurrent infections due to immune defect is recommended.

Prognosis

Prognosis is poor. Median age at death is 20 years.

X-LINKED CAUSES OF ATAXIA

FRAGILE X-ASSOCIATED TREMOR ATAXIA SYNDROME (FXTAS)

Definition and epidemiology

- Late onset (almost always after 50, often not until 70s or 80s) progressive neurodegenerative disorder[28].
- Potentially very common. The causative mutation of FXTAS is present in ~1:813 men and ~1:250 women[29].
- The causative mutation shows incomplete penetrance. The disorder is estimated to affect up to 40% of males with pre-mutation alleles (55–200 CGG repeats) of the fragile X mental retardation 1 (*FMR1*) gene who are older than 50 years[30].
- Penetrance is higher in patients with longer repeats (greater than 80 CGGs) and increases with age, such that penetrance of longer repeats in men over 80 years of age is ~75%[31].
- Clinically affected females have been reported, but their frequency remains unclear.
- Most commonly seen in the grandfathers or mothers of children with fragile X syndrome.

Etiology and pathophysiology

FXTAS is caused by an expanded CGG repeat in the 5′ untranslated region of the *FMR1* gene on the X chromosome[32]. Normally, the sequence is less than 45 CGG repeats. Expansion to greater than 200 CGG repeats (a 'full' mutation) leads to transcriptional silencing of the *FMR1* gene and causes fragile X syndrome, the most common inherited cause of mental retardation. Patients with FXTAS have a repeat between 50 and 200 CGG repeats (a 'pre-mutation' range repeat).

The *FMR1* gene in pre-mutation carriers is transcribed efficiently and there is near-normal expression of the fragile X mental retardation protein, FMRP. However, there is a 5–8-fold increase in *FMR1* mRNA levels[33].

Pathologically, it is associated with diffuse brain atrophy with loss of cerebellar Purkinje cells. Microscopically, degenerating areas of the brain demonstrate large ubiquitin positive intranuclear inclusions in glia and neurons[34]. The *FMR1* mRNA containing the expanded CGG repeat is thought to elicit neurodegeneration directly via a gain of function mechanism. The hypothesis is that the expanded CGG repeat binds to, and sequesters, certain RNA-binding proteins involved in RNA splicing, leading to aberrant splicing of other mRNAs[35].

Clinical features

- Most patients have an action tremor and cerebellar gait disorder greater than appendicular cerebellar ataxia.
- Some patients have parkinsonism, which can be levodopa responsive.
- Some patients have cognitive decline, including frank dementia characterized by prominent executive dysfunction.
- Some patients have a sensory or sensory and motor axonal polyneuropoathy.
- Some patients have dysautonomia and can present with a syndrome similar to MSA.
- There are reports of increased anxiety, disinhibition, depression, and apathy in FXTAS patients, but the frequency of these symptoms is unclear.

Tip

▸ *Ask older patients about a history of autism, mental retardation, and early menopause in their children and grandchildren as a hint to a diagnosis of FXTAS.*

Differential diagnosis

Multwiple system atrophy of the cerebellar type or parkinsonian type (MSA-C or MSA-P, also known as olivo-ponto-cerebellar atrophy, nigrostriatal degeneration, or Shy–Drager syndrome)

MSA is a sporadic neurodegenerative disorder affecting the brainstem, cerebellum, and basal ganglia that usually begins in the fifth or sixth decade of life. It is the most common cause of progressive cerebellar degeneration in adults, representing 29% of cases in one large published series[36].

Clinically, it is characterized by a variety of symptoms including parkinsonism, cerebellar signs including ataxia, autonomic dysfunction, pyramidal dysfunction, and, in a subset, dementia[37]. Autonomic symptoms are often prominent with urinary incontinence and orthostatic hypotension leading to recurrent syncope and presyncopal events.

Pathologically it is an alpha-synucleinopathy akin to PD or Lewy body dementia, but the pathology and inclusions are seen in oligodendroglia and are often most predominant in the brainstem, basal ganglia, cerebellum, and spinal cord[38].

MSA-C is a subtype of MSA in which the cerebellar signs are paramount with few other clinical findings early in the course of the disease. The diagnosis (prior to autopsy) is based on history and imaging and the exclusion of other causes discussed above.

Parkinson's disease and other atypical parkinsonian syndromes

- PSP: vertical gaze palsy uncommon in FXTAS; tremor uncommon in PSP.
- Vascular parkinsonism: MRI imaging is typically different, stepwise progression.

Essential tremor

Ataxia and dementia are more severe in FXTAS.

Investigations and diagnosis

- MRI typically reveals multiple white matter lesions, volume loss, and T2-hyperintensities in the bilateral middle cerebellar peduncles ('MCP' sign) in 60% of males with FXTAS (**604**)[28].
- A diagnosis of definite FXTAS requires an action tremor *or* ataxia and an MCP sign on MRI and an expanded CGG repeat.
- Probable FXTAS requires ataxia *and* action tremor without MCP sign *or* MCP sign with some minor symptom of FXTAS (parkinsonism or dementia) in the presence of an expanded CGG repeat.
- Possible FXTAS is defined as action tremor *or* ataxia without MCP sign and with an expanded CGG repeat.

Tips

▶ *The 'MCP' sign is very common in FXTAS, but can also be seen in MSA and some mitochondrial conditions.*
▶ *In patients with sporadic cerebellar degeneration of undetermined cause, inquire in the history about sweating, urinary function, and orthostatic symptoms. A history of absence of sweating; urinary urgency, incomplete bladder emptying or incontinence; or symptomatic orthostatic hypotension raises suspicion for MSA.*

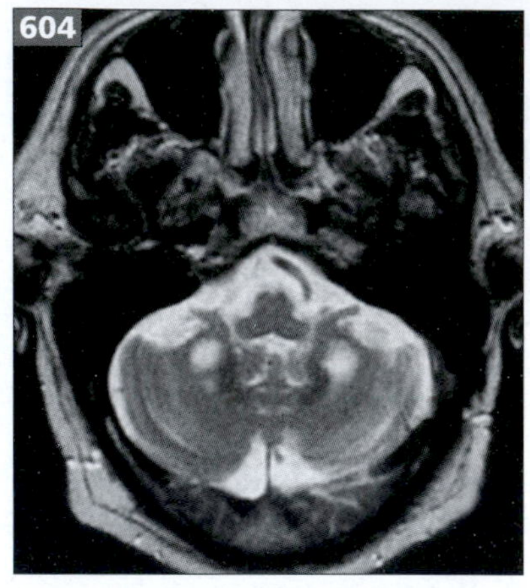

604 **The middle cerebellar peduncle ('MCP') sign, seen in a patient with fragile X-associated tremor ataxia syndrome (FXTAS). Axial T2 image through the cerebellum demonstrating bilateral middle cerebellar peduncle hyperintensities, seen classically in patients with FXTAS. Also note cerebellar and pontine atrophy.** *Courtesy of Deborah Hall, Rush University.*

Treatment

There is no known cure for FXTAS; treatment is symptomatic only. Symptomatic treatment of tremor with primidone or propranolol has been reported. Patients with parkinsonism can respond to levodopa. Treatment of depression and other neuropsychiatric symptoms with SSRIs can be effective. Valproate semisodium (Depakote) should be avoided.

Prognosis

FXTAS is slowly progressive. As it has been described only recently, good longitudinal natural history data are unavailable.

REFERENCES

Dementia

1 Craddock N, Lendon C (1998). New susceptibility gene for Alzheimer's disease on chromosome 12. *Lancet* **352**: 1720–1721.
2 Selkoe DJ (2011). Alzheimer's disease. *Cold Spring Harbor Perspectives in Biology* **3**(7).
3 Petersen RC (2011). Clinical practice. Mild cognitive impairment. *N Engl J Med* **364**(23):2227–2234.
4 Dufouil C, Clayton D, Brayne C, *et al.* (2000). Population norms for the MMSE in the very old: estimates based on longitudinal data. *Neurology* **55**:1609–1619.
5 McKhann GM, Knopman DS, Chertkow H, *et al.* (2011). The diagnosis of dementia due to Alzheimer's disease: Recommendations from the National Institute on Aging-Alzheimer's Association workgroups on diagnostic guidelines for Alzheimer's disease. *Alzheimers Dement* **7**(3):263–269.
6 Okonkwo OC, Alosco ML, Griffith HR, *et al.*; Alzheimer's Disease Neuroimaging Initiative (2010). Cerebrospinal fluid abnormalities and rate of decline in everyday function across the dementia spectrum: normal aging, mild cognitive impairment, and Alzheimer disease. *Arch Neurol* **67**(6):688–696.
7 Schenk D, Basi GS, Pangalos MN (2012). Treatment strategies targeting amyloid β-protein. *Cold Spring Harbor Perspectives in Medicine* **2**(9).
8 Flicker L (1999). Acetylcholinesterase inhibitors for Alzheimer's disease. *BMJ* **318**:615–616.
9 Mayeux R, Sano M (1999). Treatment of Alzheimer's disease. *N Engl J Med* **341**:1670–1679.
10 Rösler M, Anand R, Cicin-Sain A, *et al.* (1999). Efficacy and safety of rivastigmine in patients with Alzheimer's disease: international randomized controlled trial. *BMJ* **318**:633–640.
11 Wilcock GK, Lilienfeld S, Gaens E, on behalf of the International-1 Study Group (2000). Efficacy and safety of galantamine in patients with mild to moderate Alzheimer's disease. Multicentre randomised controlled trial. *BMJ* **321**:1445–1449.
12 Farimond LE, Roberts E, McShane R (2012). Memantine and cholinesterase inhibitor combination therapy for Alzheimer's disease: a systematic review. *BMJ Open* **2**(3).
13 Mulnard RA, Cotman CW, Kawas C, *et al.* (2000). Estrogen replacement therapy for treatment of mild to moderate Alzheimer disease. A randomized controlled trial. *JAMA* **283**:1007–1015.
14 Feldman HH, Doody RS, Kivipelto M, *et al.*; LEADe Investigators (2010). Randomized controlled trial of atorvastatin in mild to moderate Alzheimer disease: LEADe. *Neurol* **74**(12):956–964.
15 Cairns NJ, Bigio EH, Mackenzie IR, *et al.*; Consortium for Frontotemporal Lobar Degeneration (2007). Neuropathologic diagnostic and nosologic criteria for frontotemporal lobar degeneration: consensus of the Consortium for Frontotemporal Lobar Degeneration. *Acta Neuropathol* **114**(1):5–22.
16 Rabinovici GD, Miller BL (2010). Frontotemporal lobar degeneration: epidemiology, pathophysiology, diagnosis and management. *CNS Drugs* **24**(5):375–398.
17 Gass J, Cannon A, Mackenzie IR, *et al.* (2006). Mutations in progranulin are a major cause of ubiquitin-positive frontotemporal lobar degeneration. *Hum Mol Genet* **15**(20):2988–3001.
18 Hutton M (2000). 'Missing' tau mutation identified. *Ann Neurol* **46**:417–418.
19 Neumann M, Sampathu DM, Kwong LK, *et al.* (2006). Ubiquitinated TDP-43 in frontotemporal lobar degeneration and amyotrophic lateral sclerosis. *Science* **314**(5796):130–133.
20 Renton AE, Majounie E, Waite A, *et al.* (2011). A hexanucleotide repeat expansion in C9ORF72 is the cause of chromosome 9p21-linked ALS-FTD. *Neuron* **72**(2):257–268.
21 Wilhelmsen KC (1997). Frontotemporal dementia is on the MAPt. *Ann Neurol* **41**:139–140.
22 Mathuranath PS, Xuereb JH, Bak T, Hodges J (2000). Corticobasal ganglionic degeneration and/or frontotemporal dementia? A report of two overlap cases and review of the literature. *J Neurol Neurosurg Psychiatry* **68**:304–312.
23 McKeith IG (2006). Consensus guidelines for the clinical and pathologic diagnosis of dementia with Lewy bodies (DLB): report of the Consortium on DLB International Workshop. *J Alzheimers Dis* 9(3 Suppl):417–423.
24 McKeith I, Del Ser T, Spano PF, *et al.* (2000). Efficacy of rivastigmine in dementia with Lewy bodies: a randomised, double-blind, placebo-controlled international study. *Lancet* **356**:2031–2036.
25 Amar K, Wilcock G (1996). Vascular dementia. *BMJ* **312**:227–231.
26 de Groot JC, de Leeuw F-E, Oudkerk M, *et al.* (2000). Cerebral white matter lesions and cognitive function: The Rotterdam scan study. *Ann Neurol* **47**:145–1451.
27 Chui HC, Mack W, Jackson JE, *et al.* (2000). Clinical criteria for the diagnosis of vascular dementia. A multicenter study of comparability and interrater reliability. *Arch Neurol* **57**:191–196.
28 Kirshnir HS (2009). Vascular dementia: a review of recent evidence for prevention and treatment. *Curr Neurol Neurosci Rep* 9(6):437–442.
29 Prusiner SB (1982). Novel proteinaceous infectious particles cause scrapie. *Science* **216**:136–144.
30 Bueler H, Aguzzi A, Sailer A, *et al.* (1993). Mice devoid of PrP are resistant to scrapie. *Cell* **73**:1339–1347.
31 Palmer MS, Dryden AJ, Hughes JT, Collinge J (1991). Homozygous prion protein genotype predisposes to sporadic Creutzfeldt–Jakob disease. *Nature* **352**:340–342.
32 Will RG, Ironside JW, Zeidler M, *et al.* (1996). A new variant of Creutzfeldt–Jakob disease in the UK. *Lancet* **347**:921–925.
33 Mastrianni JA, Nixon R, Layzer R, *et al.* (1999). Prion protein conformation in a patient with sporadic fatal insomnia. *N Engl J Med* **340**(21):1630–1638.
34 Perani D, Cortelli P, Lucignani G, *et al.* (1993). [^{18} F]DG PET in fatal familial insomnia: the functional effects of thalamic lesions. *Neurology* **43**:2565–2569.
35 Geschwind MD, Martindale J, Miller D, *et al.* (2003). Challenging the clinical utility of the 14-3-3 protein for the diagnosis of sporadic Creutzfeldt–Jakob disease. *Arch Neurol* **60**:813–816.
36 Satoh K, Shirabe S, Tsujino A, *et al.* (2007). Total tau protein in cerebrospinal fluid and diffusion-weighted MRI as an early diagnostic marker for Creutzfeldt–Jakob disease. *Dement Geriatr Cogn Disord* **24**:207–212.

Parkinson's disease and parkinsonian disorders

1 Lees AJ, Hardy J, Revesz T (2009). Parkinson's disease. *Lancet* **373**:2055–2066.
2 Klein C, Lohmann-Hedrich K (2007). Impact of recent genetic findings in Parkinson's disease. *Curr Opin Neurol* **20**:453–464.
3 Jankovic J (2008). Parkinson's disease: clinical features and diagnosis. *J Neurol Neurosurg Psychiatry* **79**:368–376.
4 Chaudhuri KR, Healy DG, Schapira AH (2006). Non-motor symptoms of Parkinson's disease: diagnosis and management. *Lancet Neurol* **5**:235–245.
5 Tolosa M, Gaig C, Santamaria J, Compta Y (2009). Diagnosis and the premotor phase of Parkinson disease. *Neurology* 72(Suppl 2):S12–S20.
6 Braak H, Tredici KD, Rub U, *et al.* (2003). Staging of brain pathology related to sporadic Parkinson's disease. *Neurobiol Aging* **24**:197–211.

7 Jankovic J, Poewe W (2012). Therapies in Parkinson's disease. *Curr Opin Neurol* **25**:433–447.
8 Nutt JG (2008). Pharmacokinetics and pharmacodynamics of levodopa. *Mov Disord* **23**(3):S580–S584.
9 Jankovic J (2005). Motor fluctuations and dyskinesias in Parkinson's disease: clinical manifestations. *Mov Disord* **20**(Suppl 11):S11–S16.
10 Ehrt U, Aarsland D (2005). Psychiatric aspects of Parkinson's disease. *Curr Opin Psychiatry* **18**:335–341.
11 Okun MS (2012). Deep-brain stimulation for Parkinson's disease. *N Engl J Med* **367**:1529–1538.
12 Kordower JH, Chu Y, Hauser RA, Freeman TB, Olanow CW (2008). Lewy body-like pathology in long-term embryonic nigral transplants in Parkinson's disease. *Nature* **14**(5):504–506.
13 Hely MA, Morris JG, Wayne R, Trafficante R (2005). Sydney Multicenter Study of Parkinson's disease: non-L-dopa-responsive problems dominate at 15 years. *Mov Disord* **20**(2):190–199.
14 Wenning GK, Colosimo C, Geser F, Poewe W (2004). Multiple system atrophy. *Lancet Neurol* **3**:93–103.
15 Gilman S, Wenning GK, Low PA (2008). Second consensus statement on the diagnosis of multiple system atrophy. *Neurology* **71**:670–676.
16 Jecmenica-Lukic M, Poewe W, Tolosa E, Wenning GK (2012). Premotor signs and symptoms of multiple system atrophy. *Lancet Neurol* **11**:361–368.
17 Boesch SM, Wenning GK, Ransmayr G, Poewe W (2002). Dystonia in multiple system atrophy. *J Neurol Neurosurg Psychiatry* **72**:300–303.
18 Tha KK, Terae S, Tsukahara A (2012). Hyperintense putaminal rim at 1.5 T: prevalence in normal subjects and distinguishing features from multiple system atrophy. *BMC Neurology* **12**(39):1–9.
19 Ahmed Z, Asi YT, Sailer A (2012). Review: the neuropathology, pathophysiology and genetics of multiple system atrophy. *Neuropathol Appl Neurobiol* **38**:4–24.
20 Wakabayashi K, Takahashi H (2006). Cellular pathology in multiple system atrophy. *Neuropathology* **26**:338–345.
21 Wenning GK, Stefanova N (2009). Recent developments in multiple system atrophy. *J Neurol* **256**:1791–1808.
22 Ferini-Strambi L, Marelli S (2012). Sleep dysfunction in multiple system atrophy. *Curr Treat Options Neurol* **14**:464–473.
23 Watanabe H, Saito Y, Terao S, *et al.* (2002). Progression and prognosis of multiple system atrophy: an analysis of 230 Japanese patients. *Brain* **125**:1070–1083.
24 Williams DR, Lees AJ (2009). Progressive supranuclear palsy: clinicopathological concepts and diagnostic challenges. *Lancet Neurol* **8**:270–279.
25 Barsottini OG, Felício AC, Aquino CG, Pedroso JL (2010). Progressive supranuclear palsy: new concepts. *Arq Neuropsiquiatr* **68**(6):938–946.
26 Dickson DW, Ahmed Z, Algom AA, Tsuboi Y, Josephs KA (2010). Neuropathology of variants of progressive supranuclear palsy. *Curr Opin Neurol* **23**:394–400.
27 Armstrong RA (2011). Visual signs and symptoms of progressive supranuclear palsy. *Clin Exp Optom* **94**(2):150–160.
28 Williams DR, Lees AJ (2010). What features improve the accuracy of the clinical diagnosis of progressive supranuclear palsy-parkinsonism (PSP-P)? *Mov Disord* **25**(3):357–362.
29 Amarenco P, Roullet E, Hannoun L, Marteau R (1991). Progressive supranuclear palsy as the sole manifestation of systemic Whipple's disease treated with pefloxacine. *J Neurol Neurosurg Psychiatry* **54**(12):1121–1122.
30 Bouchard M, Suchowersky O (2011). Tauopathies: one disease or many? *Can J Neurol Sci* **38**:547–556.
31 Josephs K, Ishizawa T, Tsuboi Y, Cookson N, Dickson DW (2002). A clinicopathologic study of vascular progressive supranuclear palsy. *Arch Neurol* **59**:1597–1601.
32 Stamelou M, Knake S, Oertel WH, Hoglinger GU (2011). Magnetic resonance imaging in progressive supranuclear palsy. *J Neurol* **258**:549–558.
33 Houghton DJ, Litvan I (2007). Unraveling progressive supranuclear palsy: from the bedside back to the bench. *Parkinsonism Relat Disord* **13**:S341–S346.
34 Dickson DW (1999). Neuropathologic differentiation of progressive supranuclear palsy and corticobasal degeneration. *J Neurol* **246**(Suppl 2):II/6–II/15.
35 Belfor N, Amici S, Boxer AL (2006). Clinical and neuropsychological features of corticobasal degeneration. *Mech Ageing Dev* **127**:203–207.
36 Sha S, Hou C, Viskontas IV, Miller BL (2006). Are frontotemporal lobar degeneration, progressive supranuclear palsy and corticobasal degeneration distinct diseases? *Nat Clin Pract Neurol* **2**(12):658–665.
37 Stamelou M, Alonso-Canovas A, Bhatia KP (2012). Dystonia in corticobasal degeneration: a review of the literature on 404 pathologically proven cases. *Mov Disord* **27**(6):696–702.
38 Shelley BP, Hodges JR, Kipps CM, Xuereb JH, Bak TH (2009). Is the pathology of corticobasal syndrome predictable in life? *Mov Disord* **24**(11):1593–1599.
39 Wadia PM, Lang AE (2007). The many faces of corticobasal degeneration. *Parkinsonism Relat Disord* **13**:S336–S340.
40 Boeve BF (2011). The multiple phenotypes of corticobasal syndrome and corticobasal degeneration: implications for further study. *J Mol Neurosci* **45**:350–353.
41 Boeve BF, Maraganore DM, Parisi JE (1999). Pathologic heterogeneity in clinically diagnosed corticobasal degeneration. *Neurology* **53**:795–800.
42 Hassan A, Whitwell JL, Josephs KA (2011). The corticobasal syndrome–Alzheimer's disease conundrum. *Expert Rev Neurother* **11**(11):1569–1578.
43 Murray R, Neumann M, Forman MS (2007). Cognitive and motor assessment in autopsy-proven corticobasal degeneration. *Neurology* **68**:1274–1283.
44 Kouri N, Whitwell JL, Josephs KA, Rademakers R, Dickson DW (2011). Corticobasal degeneration: a pathologically distinct 4R tauopathy. *Nat Rev Neurol* **7**(5):263–272.
45 Kompoliti K, Goetz CG, Boeve BF, *et al.* (1998). Clinical presentation and pharmacological therapy in corticobasal degeneration. *Arch Neurol* **55**(7):957–961.
46 Sha S, Hou C, Viskontas IV, Miller BL (2006). Are frontotemporal lobar degeneration, progressive supranuclear palsy and corticobasal degeneration distinct diseases? *Nat Clin Pract Neurol* **2**(12):658–665.
47 Schneider SA, Bhatia KP (2012). Syndromes of neurodegeneration with brain iron accumulation. *Semin Pediatr Neurol* **19**:57–66.
48 Berry-Kravis E, Abrams L, Coffey SM, *et al.* (2007). Fragile X-associated tremor/ataxia syndrome: clinical features, genetics, and testing guidelines. *Mov Disord* **22**(14):2018–2130. Quiz 2140.
49 Ala A, Walker AP, Ashkan K, Dooley JS, Schilsky ML (2007). Wilson's disease. *Lancet* **369**(9559):397–408.
50 Netravathi M, Pal PK, Devi BI (2012). A clinical profile of 103 patients with secondary movement disorders: correlation of etiology with phenomenology. *Eur J Neurol* **19**: 226–233.
51 Barton RB, Zauber SE, Goetz CG (2009). Movement disorders caused by medical disease. *Semin Neurol* **29**(2):97–110.
52 Shin H, Chung, SJ (2012). Drug induced parkinsonism. *J Clin Neurol* **8**:15–21.
53 Glass PG, Lees AJ, Bacellar A, Zijlmans J, Katzenschlager R, Silveira-Moriyama L (2012). The clinical features of pathologically confirmed vascular parkinsonism. *J Neurol Neurosurg Psychiatry* **83**:1027e–1029.
54 Baizabal-Carvallo J, Jankovic J (2012). Movement disorders in autoimmune diseases. *Mov Disord* **27**(8):935–946.
55 Manyam BV (2005). What is and what is not 'Fahr's disease'? *Parkinsonism Relat Disord* **11**(2):73–80.
56 Burkhard PR, Delavelle J, Pasquier R, Spahr L (2003). Chronic parkinsonism associated with cirrhosis: a distinct subset of acquired hepatocerebral degeneration. *Arch Neurol* **60**(4):521–528.
57 Alarcon F, Gimenez-Roldan S (2005). Systemic diseases that cause movement disorders. *Parkinsonism Relat Disord* **11**(1):1–18.
58 Lang AE, Koller WC, Fahn S (1995). Psychogenic parkinsonism. *Arch Neurol* **52**(8):802–810.

Hereditary ataxias

1 Ashley CN, Hoang KD, Lynch DR, *et al.* (2012). Childhood ataxia: clinical features, pathogenesis, key unanswered questions, and future directions. *J Child Neurol* **27**(9):1095–1120.

2 Shen WC, Shian WJ, Chen CC, *et al.* (1994). MRI of Joubert's syndrome. *Eur J Radiol* **18**(1):30–33.

3 Parisi MA, Doherty D, Chance PF, Glass IA (2007). Joubert syndrome (and related disorders) (OMIM 213300). *Eur J Hum Genet* **15**(5):511–521.

4 Ware SM, Aygun MG, Hildebrandt F (2011). Spectrum of clinical diseases caused by disorders of primary cilia. *Proc Am Thorac Soc* **8**(5):444–450.

5 Parisi MA, Doherty D, Eckert ML, *et al.* (2006). AHI1 mutations cause both retinal dystrophy and renal cystic disease in Joubert syndrome. *J Med Genet* **43**(4):334–339.

6 Parisi MA, Bennett CL, Eckert ML, *et al.* (2004). The NPHP1 gene deletion associated with juvenile nephronophthisis is present in a subset of individuals with Joubert syndrome. *Am J Hum Genet* **75**(1):82–91.

7 Doherty D, Parisi MA, Finn LS, *et al.* (2010). Mutations in 3 genes (MKS3, CC2D2A and RPGRIP1L) cause COACH syndrome (Joubert syndrome with congenital hepatic fibrosis). *J Med Genet* **47**(1):8–21.

8 Forsythe E, Beales PL (2013). Bardet–Biedl syndrome. *Eur J Hum Genet* **21**(1):8–13.

9 Cassandrini D, Biancheri R, Tessa A, *et al.* (2010). Pontocerebellar hypoplasia: clinical, pathologic, and genetic studies. *Neurology* **75**(16):1459–1464.

10 Schols L, Bauer P, Schmidt T, Schulte T, Riess O (2004). Autosomal dominant cerebellar ataxias: clinical features, genetics, and pathogenesis. *Lancet Neurol* **3**(5):291–304.

11 Bryer, A, Krause A, Bill P, *et al.* (2003). The hereditary adult-onset ataxias in South Africa. *J Neurol Sci* **216**(1):47–54.

12 Klockgether T, Ludtke R, Kramer B, *et al.* (1998). The natural history of degenerative ataxia: a retrospective study in 466 patients. *Brain* **121**(4):589–600.

13 Wadia NH, Swami RK (1971). A new form of heredo-familial spinocerebellar degeneration with slow eye movements (nine families). *Brain* **94**(2):359–374.

14 Durr A, Stevanin G, Cancel G, *et al.* (1996). Spinocerebellar ataxia 3 and Machado–Joseph disease: clinical, molecular, and neuropathological features. *Ann Neurol* 39(4):490–499.

15 Campuzano V, Montermini L, Moltò MD, *et al.* (1996). Friedreich's ataxia: autosomal recessive disease caused by an intronic GAA triplet repeat expansion. *Science* **271**(5254):1423–1427.

16 Pandolfo M (1999). Friedreich's ataxia: clinical aspects and pathogenesis. *Semin Neurol* **19**(3):311–321.

17 Bidichandani SI, Delatycki MB (1993). Friedreich ataxia. In: Pagon RA, Bird TD, Dolan CR, Stephens K, Adam MP (eds). *GeneReviews* (Internet). University of Washington, Seattle, 1993–1998 (updated 2012 Feb 02).

18 Martelli A, Napierala M, Puccio H (2012). Understanding the genetic and molecular pathogenesis of Friedreich's ataxia through animal and cellular models. *Dis Model Mech* **5**(2):165–176.

19 Ouahchi K, Arita M, Kayden H, *et al.* (1995). Ataxia with isolated vitamin E deficiency is caused by mutations in the alpha-tocopherol transfer protein. *Nat Genet* **9**(2):141–145.

20 Donaghy M, King RH, McKeran RO, Schwartz MS, Thomas PK, *et al.* (1990). Cerebrotendinous xanthomatosis: clinical, electrophysiological and nerve biopsy findings, and response to treatment with chenodeoxycholic acid. *J Neurol* **237**(3):216–219.

21 Wanders RJA, Jansen GA, Skjeldal OH (2001). Refsum disease, peroxisomes and phytanic acid oxidation: a review. *J Neuropath Exp Neurol* **60**(11):1021–1031.

22 Baldwin EJ, Gibberd FB, Harley C, Sidey MC, Feher MD, Wierzbicki AS (2010). The effectiveness of long-term dietary therapy in the treatment of adult Refsum disease. *J Neurol Neurosurg Psychiatry* **81**(9):954–957.

23 Velasco-Sanchez D, Aracil A, Montero R, *et al.* (2011). Combined therapy with idebenone and deferiprone in patients with Friedreich's ataxia. *Cerebellum* **10**(1):1–8.

24 Meier T, Perlman SL, Rummey C, Coppard NJ, Lynch DR (2012). Assessment of neurological efficacy of idebenone in pediatric patients with Friedreich's ataxia: data from a 6-month controlled study followed by a 12-month open-label extension study. *J Neurol* **259**(2):284–291.

25 Di Prospero NA, Baker A, Jeffries N, Fischbeck KH (2007). Neurological effects of high-dose idebenone in patients with Friedreich's ataxia: a randomised, placebo-controlled trial. *Lancet Neurol* **6**(10):878–886.

26 Gatti R (1993). Ataxia–telangiectasia. In: Pagon RA, Bird TD, Dolan CR, Stephens K, Adam MP (eds). *GeneReviews* (Internet). University of Washington, Seattle, 1993–1998 (updated 2012 Feb 02).

27 Broccoletti T, Del Giudice E, Cirillo E, *et al.* (2011). Efficacy of very-low-dose betamethasone on neurological symptoms in ataxia-telangiectasia. *Eur J Neurol* **18**(4):564–570.

28 Berry-Kravis E, Abrams L, Coffey SM, *et al.* (2007). Fragile X-associated tremor/ataxia syndrome: clinical features, genetics, and testing guidelines. *Mov Disord* **22**(14):2018–2030, quiz 2140.

29 Rousseau F, Rouillard P, Morel ML, Khandjian EW, Morgan K (1995). Prevalence of carriers of premutation-size alleles of the FMRI gene—and implications for the population genetics of the fragile X syndrome. *Am J Hum Genet* **57**(5):1006–1018.

30 Jacquemont S, Hagerman RJ, Leehey MA, *et al.* (2004). Penetrance of the fragile X-associated tremor/ataxia syndrome in a premutation carrier population. *JAMA* **291**(4):460–469.

31 Jacquemont S, Leehey MA, Hagerman RJ, Beckett LA, Hagerman PJ (2006). Size bias of fragile X premutation alleles in late-onset movement disorders. *J Med Genet* **43**(10):804–809.

32 Hagerman RJ, Leehey M, Heinrichs W, *et al.* (2001). Intention tremor, parkinsonism, and generalized brain atrophy in male carriers of fragile X. *Neurology* **57**(1):127–130.

33 Tassone F, Hagerman RJ, Taylor AK, Gane LW, Godfrey TE, Hagerman PJ (2000). Elevated levels of FMR1 mRNA in carrier males: a new mechanism of involvement in the fragile-X syndrome. *Am J Hum Genet* **66**(1):6–15.

34 Greco CM, Berman RF, Martin RM, *et al.* (2006). Neuropathology of fragile X-associated tremor/ataxia syndrome (FXTAS). *Brain* **129**(Pt 1):243–255.

35 Todd PK, Paulson HL (2010). RNA-mediated neurodegeneration in repeat expansion disorders. *Ann Neurol* **67**(3):291–300.

36 Abele M, Burk K, Schols L, *et al.* (2002). The aetiology of sporadic adult-onset ataxia. *Brain* **125**(5):961–968.

37 Gilman S, Wenning GK, Low PA, *et al.* (2008). Second consensus statement on the diagnosis of multiple system atrophy. *Neurology* **71**(9):670–676.

38 Tu PH, Galvin JE, Baba M, *et al.* (1998). Glial cytoplasmic inclusions in white matter oligodendrocytes of multiple system atrophy brains contain insoluble alpha-synuclein. *Ann Neurol* **44**(3):415–422.

FURTHER READING

Dementia

Alzheimer's disease

Dubinsky RM, Stein AC, Lyons K (2000). Practice parameter: risk of driving and Alzheimer's disease (an evidence-based review). *Neurology* **54**:2205–2211.

Mathuranath PS, Nestor PJ, Berrios GE, *et al.* (2000). A brief cognitive test battery to differentiate Alzheimer's disease and frontotemporal dementia. *Neurology* **55**:1613–1620.

Richards SS, Hendrie HC (1999). Diagnosis, management, and treatment of Alzheimer disease. *Arch Intern Med* **159**:789–798.

Snowden JS (1999). Neuropsychological evaluation and the diagnosis and differential diagnosis of dementia. *Rev Clin Gerontol* **9**:65–72.

Terry RD (2000). Where in the brain does Alzheimer's disease begin? *Ann Neurol* **47**:421.

Frontotemporal dementia

Bigio EH (2008). Update on recent molecular and genetic advances in frontotemporal lobar degeneration. *J Neuropathol Exp Neurol* **67**(7):635–648.

Caycedo AM, Miller B, Kramer J, Rascovsky K (2009). Early features in frontotemporal dementia. *Curr Alzheimer Res* **6**(4): 337–340.

Golbe LI (2000). Progressive supranuclear palsy in the molecular age. *Lancet* **356**:870–871.

Pasquier F, Delacourte A (1998). Non-Alzheimer degenerative dementias. *Curr Opin Neurol* **11**:417–427.

Pickering-Brown S, Baker M, Yen S-H, *et al.* (2000). Pick's disease is associated with mutations in the tau gene. *Ann Neurol* **48**:859–867.

Porkaj P, Bird TD, Wijsman E, *et al.* (1998). Tau is a candidate gene for chromosome 17 frontotemporal dementia. *Ann Neurol* **43**:815–825. (Erratum, *Ann Neurol* 1998;**44**:428.)

Schrag A, Ben-Shlomo Y, Quinn NP (1999). Prevalence of progressive supranuclear palsy and multiple system atrophy: a cross-sectional study. *Lancet* **354**:1771–1775.

Dementia with Lewy bodies

Galasko D (1999). A clinical approach to dementia with Lewy bodies. *Neurologist* **5**:247–257.

Weisman D, McKeith I (2007). Dementia with Lewy bodies. *Semin Neurol* **27**(1):42–47.

Vascular dementia

Bousser MG, Tournier-Lasserve E (2001). Cerebral autosomal dominant arteriopathy with subcortical infarcts and leukoencephalopathy: from stroke to vessel wall physiology. *J Neurol Neurosurg Psychiatry* **70**:285–287.

Chui, HC (2006). Vascular cognitive impairment: today and tomorrow. *Alzheimers Dement* **2**(3):185–194.

Dichgans M, Mayer M, Uttner I, *et al.* (1998). The phenotypic spectrum of CADASIL: clinical findings in 102 cases. *Ann Neurol* **44**:731–739.

Garde E, Mortensen EL, Krabbe K, *et al.* (2000). Relation between age-related decline in intelligence and cerebral white-matter hyperintensities in healthy octogenarians: a longitudinal study. *Lancet* **356**:628–634.

Hebert R, Lindsay J, Verreault R, *et al.* (2000). Vascular dementia. Incidence and risk factors in the Canadian Study of Health and Aging. *Stroke* **31**:1487–1493.

Jagust WJ, Zheng L, Harvey DJ, *et al.* (2008). Neuropathological basis of magnetic resonance images in aging and dementia. *Ann Neurol* **63**(1):72–80.

Pohjasvaara T, Mäntylä R, Ylikoski R, *et al.* (2000). Comparison of different clinical criteria (DSM-III, ADDTC, ICD-10, NINDS-AIREN, DSM-IV) for the diagnosis of vascular dementia. *Stroke* **31**:2952–2957.

Reed BR, Eberling JL, Mungas D, *et al.* (2000). Memory failure has different mechanisms in subcortical stroke and Alzheimer's disease. *Ann Neurol* **48**:275–284.

van Gijn J (1998). Leukoaraiosis and vascular dementia. *Neurology* **51**(Suppl 3): S3–S8.

Prion diseases

Brown K, Mastrianni JA (2010). The prion diseases. *J Geriatr Psychiatry Neurol* **23**(4):277–298.

Brown P, Preece M, Brandel JP, *et al.* (2000). Iatrogenic Creutzfeldt–Jakob disease at the millennium. *Neurology* **55**:1075–1081.

Gambetti P, Cali I, Notari S, Kong Q, Zou WQ, Surewicz WK (2011). Molecular biology and pathology of prion strains in sporadic human prion diseases. *Acta Neuropathol* **121**(1):79–90.

Hewitt PE, Llewelyn CA, Mackenzie J, Will RG (2006). Creutzfeldt–Jakob disease and blood transfusion: results of the UK Transfusion Medicine Epidemiological Review study. *Vox Sang* **91**:221–230.

Hsiao K, Baker HF, Crow TJ, *et al.* (1989). Linkage of a prion protein missense variant to Gerstmann–Sträussler syndrome. *Nature* **338**:342–345.

Monari L, Chen SG, Brown P, *et al.* (1994) Fatal familial insomnia and familial Creutzfeldt–Jakob disease: different prion proteins determined by a DNA polymorphism. *Proc Natl Acad Sci USA* **91**:2839–2842.

Parchi P, Castellani R, Capellari S, *et al.* (1996). Molecular basis of phenotypic variability in sporadic Creutzfeldt–Jakob disease. *Ann Neurol* **39**:767–778.

Peden AH, Head MW, Ritchie DL, *et al.* (2004). Preclinical vCJD after blood transfusion in a PRNP codon 129 heterozygous patient. *Lancet* **364**:527–529.

Saa P, Castilla J, Soto C (2006). Presymptomatic detection of prions in blood. *Science* **313**:92–94.

Sanchez-Juan P, Green A, Ladogana A, *et al.* (2006). CSF tests in the differential diagnosis of Creutzfeldt–Jakob disease **67**(4):637–643.

Telling GC, Scott M, Hsiao KK, *et al.* (1994). Transmission of Creutzfeldt–Jakob disease from humans to transgenic mice expressing chimeric human-mouse prion protein. *Proc Natl Acad Sci USA* **91**:9936–9940.

Willison HJ, Gale AN, McLaughlin JE (1991). Creutzfeldt–Jakob disease following cadaveric dura mater graft. *J Neurol Neurosurg Psychiatry* **54**:940.

Parkinson's disease and parkinsonian disorders

Parkinson's disease

Antonini A, Tolosa E, Mizuno Y, Yamamoto M, Poewe WH (2009). A reassessment of risks and benefits of dopamine agonists in Parkinson's disease. *Lancet Neurol* **8**:929–937.

Barone P, Antonini A, Colosimo C, *et al.* (2009). The Priamo Study: a multicenter assessment of nonmotor symptoms and their impact on quality of life in Parkinson's disease. *Mov Disord* **24**(11):1641–1649.

Benabid AL, Chabardes S, Mitrofanis J, Pollak P (2009). Deep brain stimulation of the subthalamic nucleus for the treatment of Parkinson's disease. *Lancet Neurol* **8**:67–81.

Burke RE, Dauer WT, Vonsattel JPG (2008). A critical evaluation of the Braak staging scheme for Parkinson's disease. *Ann Neurol* **64**(5):485-491.

Comella C (2007). Sleep disorders in Parkinson's disease: an overview. *Mov Disord* **22**:S367–S373.

Dickson DW, Braak H, Duda JE, *et al.* (2009). Neuropathological assessment of Parkinson's disease: refining the diagnostic criteria. *Lancet Neurol* **8**:1150–1157.

Dorsey ER, Constantinescu R, Thompson JP, *et al.* (2007). Projected number of people with Parkinson's disease in the most populous nations, 2005 through 2030. *Neurology* **68**:384–386.

Evans AH, Strafella AP, Weintraub D, Stacy M (2009). Impulsive and compulsive behaviors in Parkinson's disease. *Mov Disord* **24**(11):1561–1570.

Fabbrini G, Brotchie JM, Grandas F, Nomoto M, Goetz CG (2007). Levodopa-inducted dyskinesias. *Mov Disord* **22**(10):1379–1389.

Fahn S, Jankovic J (2007). Parkinsonism: clinical features and differential diagnosis. In: Fahn S, Jankovic J (eds). *Principles and Practice of Movement Disorders*. Elsevier, Philadelphia, Ch. 4, pp. 79–103.

Galpern WR, Lang AE (2006). Interface between tauopathies and synucleinopathies: a tale of two proteins. *Ann Neurol* **59**:449-458.

Gasser T (2007). Update on the genetics of Parkinson's disease. *Mov Disord* **22**:S343–S350.

Gelb DJ, Oliver E, Gilman S (1999). Diagnostic criteria for Parkinson disease. *Arch Neurol* **56**:33–39.

George JL, Mok S, Moses D, *et al*. (2009). Targeting the progression of Parkinson's disease. *Curr Neuropharmacol* **7**:9–36.

Hawkes CH, Tredici KD, Braak H (2009). Parkinson's disease: the dual hit theory revisited. *Ann NY Acad Sci* **1170**:615–622.

Hoehn MM, Yahr MD (1967). Parkinsonism: onset, progression, and mortality. *Neurology* **17**(5):427–442.

Jankovic J, Rajput AH, McDermott MP, *et al.* (2000). The evolution of diagnosis in early Parkinson disease. *Arch Neurol* **5**:369–372.

Korczyn AD, Gurevich T (2010). Parkinson's disease: before the motor symptoms and beyond. *J Neurol Sci* **289**(1–2):2–6.

Lang AE, Obeso JA (2004). Challenges in Parkinson's disease: restoration of the nigrostriatal dopamine system is not enough. *Lancet Neurol* **3**:309–316.

Lang AE, Obeso JA (2004). Time to move beyond nigrostriatal dopamine deficiency in Parkinson's disease. *Ann Neurol* **55**(6):761–765.

Lim SY, Fox SH, Lang AE (2009). Overview of the extranigral aspects of Parkinson's disease. *Arch Neurol* **66**(2):167–172.

Litvan I (2007). Update of atypical parkinsonian disorders. *Curr Opin Neurol* **20**:434–437.

Litvan I, Chesselet MF, Gasser T, *et al.* (2007). The etiopathogenesis of Parkinson's disease and suggestions for future research. Part II. *J Neuropathol Exp Neurol* **l66**(5): 329–336.

Litvan I, Halliday G, Hallett M, *et al.* (2007). The etiopathogenesis of Parkinson's disease and suggestions for future research. Part I. *J Neuropathol Exp Neurol* **66**(4):251–257.

Olanow CW, Kordower JH, Lang AE, Obeso JA (2009). Dopaminergic transplantation for Parkinson's disease: current status and future prospects. *Ann Neurol* **66**:591–596.

Olanow CW, Stern MB, Sethi K (2009). The scientific and clinical basis for the treatment of Parkinson disease. *Neurology* **72**(21):S1–S136.

Parkinson Study Group (1999). Low-dose clozapine for the treatment of drug-induced psychosis in Parkinson's disease. *N Engl J Med* **340**:757–763.

Poewe W (2009). Treatments for Parkinson disease – past achievements and current clinical needs. *Neurology* **72**:S65–S73.

Rajput AH, Voll A, Rajput ML, Robinson CA, Rajput A (2009). Course in Parkinson disease subtypes: a 39-year clinicopathologic study. *Neurology* **73**:206–212.

Schrag A, Ben-Shlomo Y, Quinn NP (2000). Cross sectional prevalence survey of idiopathic Parkinson's disease and parkinsonism in London. *BMJ* **32**:21–22.

Schulz JB (2008). Update on the pathogenesis of Parkinson's disease. *J Neurol* **255**:S3–S7.

Simuni T, Lyons KE, Pahwa R, *et al.* (2009). Treatment of early Parkinson's disease: Part 1. *Eur Neurol* **61**:193–205.

Simuni T, Lyons KE, Pahwa R, *et al.* (2009). Treatment of early Parkinson's disease: Part 2. *Eur Neurol* **61**:206–215.

Simuni T, Sethi K (2008). Nonmotor manifestations of Parkinson's disease. *Ann Neurol* **64**:S65–S80.

Sitburana O, Ondo WG (2009). Brain magnetic resonance imaging (MRI) in parkinsonian disorders. *Parkinsonism Relat Disord* **15**:165–174.

Tanner CM, Ross GW, Jewell SA, *et al.* (2009). Occupation and risk of parkinsonism. *Arch Neurol* **66**(9):1106–1113.

Volkmann J (2007). Deep brain stimulation for Parkinson's disease. *Parkinsonism Relat Disord* **13**:S462–S465.

Weintraub D, Comella CL, Horn S (2008). Parkinson's disease – Part 1: pathophysiology, symptoms, burden, diagnosis, and assessment. *Am J Manag Care* **14**:S40–S48.

Weintraub D, Comella CL, Horn S (2008). Parkinson's disease – Part 2: Treatment of motor symptoms. *Am J Manag Care* **14**:S49–S58.

Weintraub D, Comella CL, Horn S (2008). Parkinson's disease – Part 3: Neuropsychiatric symptoms. *Am J Manag Care* **14**:S59–S69.

Widnell K (2005). Pathophysiology of motor fluctuation in Parkinson's disease. *Mov Disord* **20**:S17–S22.

Yang YX, Wood NW, Latchman DS (2009). Molecular basis of Parkinson's disease. *NeuroReport* **20**:150–156.

Zesiewicz TA, Hauser RA (2007). Medical treatment of motor and nonmotor features of Parkinson's disease. In: Miller AE (ed). *Continuum: Lifelong Learning in Neurology*. Lippincott Williams & Wilkins, Philadephia **3**(1):12–38.

Multiple system atrophy

Adams RD, Van Bogaert L, Van der Eecken H (1964). Striato-nigral degeneration. *J Neuropathol Exp Neurol* **23**:584–608.

Ben-Shlomo Y, Wenning GK, Tison F, Quinn NP (1997). Survival of patients with pathologically proven multiple system atrophy: A meta-analysis. *Neurology* **48**:384–393.

Brooks DJ, Seppi K (2009). Proposed neuroimaging criteria for the diagnosis of multiple system atrophy. *Mov Disord* **24**(7):949–964.

Consensus Committee of the American Autonomic Society and the American Academy of Neurology (1996). Consensus statement on the definition of orthostatic hypotension, pure autonomic failure, and multiple system atrophy. *Neurology* **46**:1470.

Rehman HU (2001). Multiple system atrophy. *Postgrad Med J* **77**:379–382.

Schrag A, Ben-Shlomo Y, Quinn NP (1999). Prevalence of progressive supranuclear palsy and multiple system atrophy: a cross-sectional study. *Lancet* **354**:1771–1775.

Shy GM, Drager GA (1960). A neurologic syndrome associated with orthostatic hypotension. *Arch Neurol* **2**:511–527.

Stefanova N, Bucke P, Wenning GK (2009). Multiple system atrophy: an update. *Lancet Neurol* **8**(12):1172–1178.

Tu PH, Galvin JE, Baba M, *et al.* (1998). Glial cytoplasmic inclusions in white matter oligodendrocytes of multiple system atrophy brains containing insoluble alpha-synuclein. *Ann Neurol* **44**:415–422.

Wenning GK, Geser F, Poewe W (2005). Therapeutic strategies in multiple system atrophy. *Mov Disord* **20**(12):S67–S76.

Diffuse Lewy body disease or dementia with Lewy bodies

Kovari E, Horvath J, Bouras C (2009). Neuropathology of Lewy body disorders. *Brain Res Bull* **80**:203–210.

McKeith I, Del Ser T, Spano PF, *et al.* (2000). Efficacy of rivastigmine in dementia with Lewy bodies: a randomized, double-blind, placebo-controlled international study. *Lancet* **356**:2031–2036.

McKeith IG, Galasko D, Kosaka K, *et al.*, for the Consortium on Dementia with Lewy Bodies (1996). Consensus guidelines for the clinical and pathologic diagnosis of dementia with Lewy bodies: Report of the consortium on DLB international workshop. *Neurology* **47**:1113–1124.

McKeith IG, Mosimann UP (2004). Dementia with Lewy bodies and Parkinson's disease. *Parkinsonism Relat Disord* **10**:S15–S18.

McKeith IG, O'Brien JT, Ballard C (1999). Diagnosing dementia with Lewy bodies. *Lancet* **354**:1227–1228.

McKeith IG, Perry EK, Perry RH, for the Consortium on Dementia with Lewy Bodies (1999). Report of the second dementia with Lewy body international workshop. Diagnosis and treatment. *Neurology* **53**:902–905.

Progressive supranuclear palsy

Averbuch-Heller L, Paulson G, Daroff RB, Leigh RJ (1999). Whipple's disease mimicking progressive supranuclear palsy: the diagnostic value of eye movement recording. *J Neurol Neurosurg Psychiatry* **66**(4):523–535.

Golbe LI (2007). Progressive supranuclear palsy. In: Jankovic J, Tolosa E (eds). *Parkinson's Disease and Movement Disorders*. Lippincott Williams & Wilkins, Philadephia, ch. 13, pp. 161–174.

Lang AE (2005) Treatment of progressive supranuclear palsy and corticobasal degeneration. *Mov Disord* **20**:S83–S91.

Litvan I, Campbell G, Mangane CA, *et al.* (1997). Which clinical features differentiate progressive supranuclear palsy and related disorders? A clinicopathologic study. *Brain* **1**:65–74.

Lubarsky M, Juncos JL (2008). Progressive supranuclear palsy: a current review. *Neurologist* **14**:79–88.

Mokri B, Ahlskog JE, Fulgham JR, Matsumoto JY (2004). Syndrome resembling PSP after surgical repair of ascending aorta dissection or aneurysm. *Neurology* **62**:971–973.

Oba H, Yagishita A, Terada H (2005). New and reliable MRI diagnosis for progressive supranuclear palsy. *Neurology* **64**:2050–2055.

Scaravilli T, Tolosa E, Ferrer I (2005). Progressive supranuclear palsy and corticobasal degeneration: lumping versus splitting. *Mov Disord* **20**:S21–S28.

Schrag A, Ben-Shlomo Y, Quinn NP (1999). Prevalence of progressive supranuclear palsy and multiple system atrophy: a cross-sectional study. *Lancet* **354**:1771–1775.

Williams DR, de Silva R, Pavior DC, *et al.* (2005). Characteristics of two distinct clinical phenotypes in pathologically proven progressive supranuclear palsy: Richardson's syndrome and PSP-parkinsonism. *Brain* **128**:1247–1258.

Corticobasal degeneration

Koyama M, Yagishita A, Nakata Y, Hayashi M, Bandoh M, Mizutani T (2007). Imaging of corticobasal degeneration syndrome. *Neuroradiology* **49**:905–912.

Lang AE (2005). Treatment of progressive supranuclear palsy and corticobasal degeneration. *Mov Disord* **20**:S83–S91.

Ludolph AC, Kassubek J, Landwehrmeyer BG, *et al.* (2009). Tauopathies with parkinsonism: clinical spectrum, neuropathologic basis, biological markers, and treatment options. *Eur J Neurol* **16**:297–309.

Frontotemporal dementia with parkinsonism linked to chromosome 17 (FTDP-17)

Boeve BF, Hutton M (2008). Refining frontotemporal dementia with parkinsonism linked to chromosome 17. *Arch Neurol* **65**(4):460–464.

Delacourte A, Buée L (2000). Tau pathology: a marker of neurodegenerative disorders. *Curr Opin Neurol* **13**:371–376.

Goedert M (2005). Tau gene mutations and their effects. *Mov Disord* **20**:S45–S52.

Josephs KA, Peterson RC, Knopman DS, *et al.* (2006). Clinicopathologic analysis of frontotemporal and corticobasal degenerations and PSP. *Neurology* **66**:41–48.

Kertesz A (2008). Frontotemporal dementia: a topical review. *Cogn Behav Neurol* **21**(3):127–133.

Mathuranath PS, Xuereb JH, Bak T, Hodges J (2000). Corticobasal ganglionic degeneration and/or frontotemporal dementia? A report of two overlap cases and review of the literature. *J Neurol Neurosurg Psychiatry* **68**:304–312.

Porkaj P, Bird TD, Wijsman E, *et al.* (1998). Tau is a candidate gene for chromosome 17 frontotemporal dementia. *Ann Neurol* **44**:428.

Heredodegenerative and secondary parkinsonism

Adler CH (1999). Differential diagnosis of Parkinson's disease. *Med Clin North Am* **83**(2):349–367.

Alarcon F, Gimenez-Roldan S (2005). Systemic diseases that cause movement disorders. *Parkinsonism Relat Disord* **11**:1–18.

Benamer HTS, Grosset DG (2009). Vascular parkinsonism: a clinical review. *Eur Neurol* **61**:11–15.

Jang H, Boltz DA, Webster RG, Smeyne RJ (2009). Viral parkinsonism. *Biochim Biophys Acta* **1792**(7):714–721.

McNeill A, Birchall D, Hayflick SJ, *et al.* (2008). T2* and FSE MRI distinguishes four subtypes of neurodegeneration with brain iron accumulation. *Neurology* **70**:1614–1619.

Sibon I, Fenelon G, Quinn NP, Tison F (2004). Vascular parkinsonism. *J Neurol* **251**:513–524.

Tse W, Cersosimo MG, Gracies JM, *et al.* (2004). Movement disorders and AIDS: a review. *Parkinsonism Relat Disord* **10**:323–334.

ACQUIRED METABOLIC DISEASES OF THE NERVOUS SYSTEM

Fernando D. Testai

THIAMINE DEFICIENCY: WERNICKE–KORSAKOFF SYNDROME

Definition and epidemiology[1]

Wernicke disease (thiamine deficient encephalopathy) is a disorder characterized by rather abrupt onset of any combination of nystagmus, gait ataxia, conjugate gaze palsy, and global confusional state in association with thiamine deficiency.

Korsakoff psychosis is a chronic amnestic disorder, also associated with alcoholism and malnutrition, with both antegrade and retrograde components in an otherwise responsive patient. The Wernicke–Korsakoff syndrome is a symptom complex comprising the manifestations of both Wernicke disease and the Korsakoff amnesic state.

- Prevalence (from autopsy studies): 0.8–2.8% of autopsies; 15% in psychiatric inpatients, 24% in homeless men.
- Age: adults.
- Gender: M>F.

Etiology and pathophysiology[2–4]

- Thiamine deficiency:
  - Chronic alcoholism (due to malnutrition and impaired activity of thiamine-dependent enzymes).
  - Malnutrition.
  - Malabsortion.
  - Deliberate starvation:
    - Anorexia nervosa.
    - Hunger strike.
    - Obesity treatment (vertical banded gastroplasty).
  - Intractable vomiting:
    - Gastric carcinoma.
    - Pyloric obstruction.
    - Hyperemesis gravidarum.
  - Prolonged intravenous feeding.
  - Renal dialysis.
  - Acquired immunodeficiency syndrome (AIDS).
- Magnesium depletion: magnesium is an essential cofactor in the conversion of thiamine into active diphosphate and triphosphate esters. Causes of hypomagnesemia include:
  - Diuretics.
  - Alcohol.
  - Hyperemesis gravidarum.
  - Diarrhea: Crohn's disease, gluten enteropathy.

Thiamine is a cofactor for:

- Transketolase. This enzyme links glycolysis to the hexose monophosphate shunt (**605**). The hexose monophosphate shunt is required for the synthesis of:
  - Pentoses (such as ribose-phosphate).
  - Nicotinamide adenine dinucleotide phosphate (NADP): necessary for the synthesis of fatty acid and steroids.
- Pyruvate dehydrogenase E1. Pyruvate dehydrogenase is a complex formed by three enzymes (E1, E2, and E3) that participates in the decarboxylation of pyruvate to form acetyl coenzyme A. This critical step links glycolysis with the Krebs cycle. The deficiency of the pyruvate dehydrogenase complex is connected to impaired adenosine triphosphate (ATP) production and cellular dysfunction.
- Alpha-ketoglutarate dehydrogenase. This enzyme participates in the Krebs cycle and is involved in the conversion of alpha-ketoglutarate to succinyl-CoA. Its deficiency leads to decreased ATP production and cellular dysfunction.

The absorption of thiamine is impaired by both malnutrition and alcohol. In addition, liver disease has been associated with reduced body stores and impaired metabolism of thiamine. In alcoholics, thiamine deficiency may compound the situation and cause neuronal dysfunction independently or by enhancing the toxic effect of alcohol on the brain. Nevertheless, about one-third of substantial alcohol abusers seem to be resistant to developing the Wernicke–Korsakoff syndrome.

Individual differences in thiamine enzyme systems, such as different levels of affinity between thiamine pyrophosphate, which is the active form of thiamine, and transketolase may predispose certain individuals to the Wernicke–Korsakoff syndrome. If so, they are likely to be extragenetic as there is little evidence of an inborn transketolase abnormality.

Clinical features

Wernicke disease

Subacute onset over hours to days of one or, more often, various combinations of:

- Ataxia of stance and gait.
- Ophthalmoplegia: due to involvement of cranial nerve nuclei III or VI. Patient presents with supranuclear horizontal and/or vertical gaze palsies, internuclear ophthalmoplegia, and/or lateral rectus palsies, often causing diplopia.
- Nystagmus: horizontal and/or vertical.
- Mental state disturbance: global confusional state causing apathy, inattention, disorientation, minimal spontaneous speech, forgetfulness, drowsiness, and even coma.

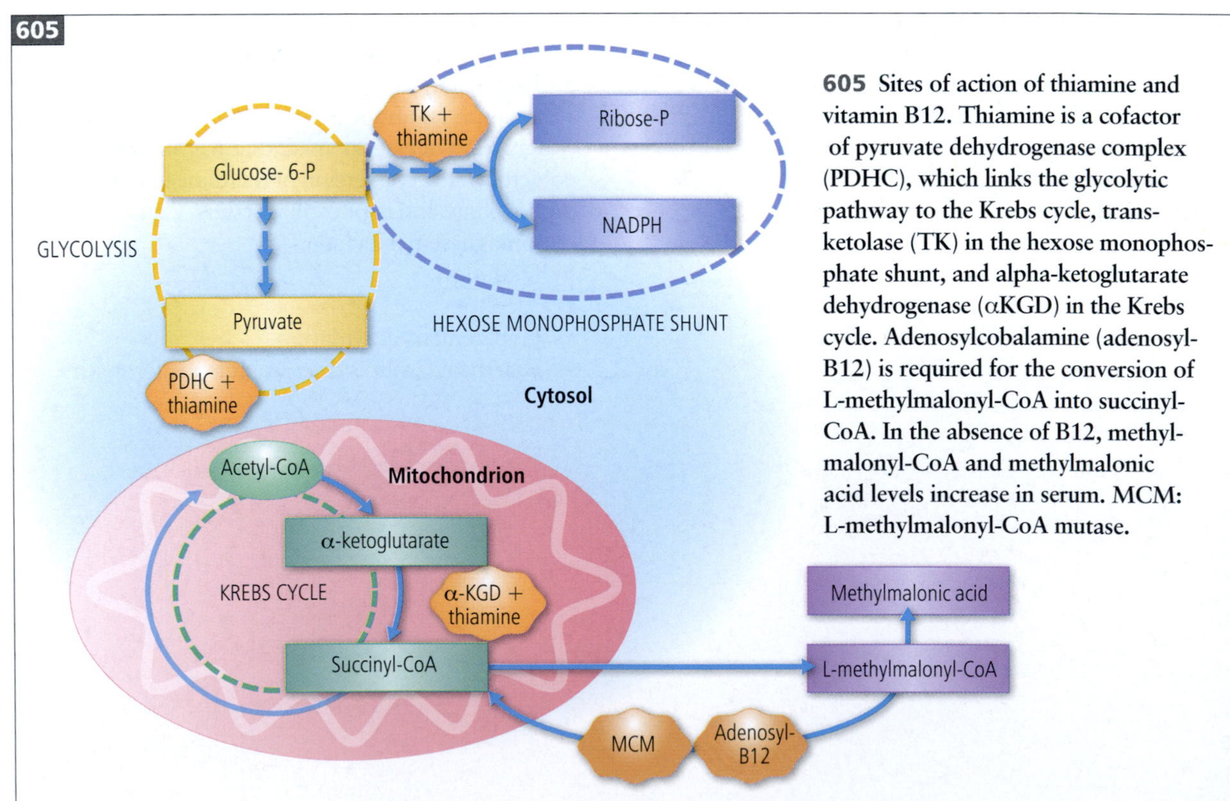

605 Sites of action of thiamine and vitamin B12. Thiamine is a cofactor of pyruvate dehydrogenase complex (PDHC), which links the glycolytic pathway to the Krebs cycle, transketolase (TK) in the hexose monophosphate shunt, and alpha-ketoglutarate dehydrogenase (αKGD) in the Krebs cycle. Adenosylcobalamine (adenosyl-B12) is required for the conversion of L-methylmalonyl-CoA into succinyl-CoA. In the absence of B12, methylmalonyl-CoA and methylmalonic acid levels increase in serum. MCM: L-methylmalonyl-CoA mutase.

Other features may include:

- Stupor or coma as the initial manifestation.
- Signs of alcohol withdrawal: agitation, hallucinations, confusion, and autonomic hyperactivity.
- Hypothermia.
- Postural hypotension (autonomic neuropathy).
- Cardiovascular dysfunction (tachycardia, exertional dyspnea, minor electrocardiogram (ECG) abnormalities.
- Impaired capacity to discriminate between odors (in the chronic stage of the disease due to a lesion of the medial dorsal nucleus of the thalamus).
- Pupil abnormalities: miosis and nonreacting pupils may occur.
- Ptosis.
- Retinal hemorrhages occur occasionally.
- Papilledema, rarely.
- Peripheral neuropathy can been seen in up to 80% of alcoholic patients. Other features seen in this subgroup include dementia, cerebellar ataxia, macrocytosis, and abnormalities of liver function.

Tip

▶ *Beriberi is a neurocardiogenic disease secondary to thiamine deficiency. Dry beriberi is characterized by a length-dependent, axonal, sensorimotor peripheral neuropathy in the absence of cardiac involvement. The term wet beriberi is reserved for individuals with peripheral neuropathy in association with vasodilatation leading to edema, increased arteriovenous shunting, and high-output heart failure (tachycardia).*

Korsakoff amnestic–confabulatory state (Korsakoff psychosis)

Chronic amnestic disorder characterized by:

- Defect in learning (anterograde amnesia), due to defective encoding at the time of original learning rather than exclusively a defect in the retrieval mechanism.
- Loss of short-term verbal and nonverbal memory (retrograde amnesia); immediate memory is preserved and long-term memory appears to be maintained through multifocal networks.
- Confabulation behavior and confusion.

Differential diagnosis

- Wernicke disease:
  - Other causes of confusional states and coma.
    - Hepatic encephalopathy.
    - Alcohol-related encephalopathy.
    - Brainstem/cerebellar/diencephalic stroke.
- Korsakoff amnestic–confabulatory state:
  - Third ventricle tumors.
  - Temporal lobe infarction or surgical resection.
  - Herpes simplex encephalitis.
  - Hypoxic encephalopathy.
  - Alzheimer's disease (AD).

Investigations[5,6]

- Blood:
  - Red cell transketolase (reduced markedly).
  - Thiamine level (reduced).
  - Plasma glucose and magnesium levels.
- CT brain scan: CT may show widening of the third ventricle and interhemispheric fissures, and other features of long-standing alcohol abuse (generalized cerebral atrophy plus more pronounced vermian and cerebellar atrophy).
- MRI brain scan: MRI may show areas of increased signal in the periaqueductal gray matter of the midbrain and medial portions of the thalami, atrophy of the mammillary bodies, and dilatation of the third ventricle. In the chronic stage, the mammillary bodies and the anterior diencephalon may be atrophic.

Diagnosis

Diagnosis is made using clinical diagnostic criteria. Physicians should have a low threshold to suspect this condition, particularly in alcoholics, even in the absence of the complete triad. Supporting data include:

- Red blood cell transketolase assay, with a positive thiamine pyrophosphate effect of >40%.
- Low thiamine level.
- MRI brain: medial thalamic and periaqueductal lesions.
- Clinical response to thiamine.

Tip

▶ *The classic triad of Wernicke's encephalopathy, including delirium, ataxia, and nystagmus or ophthalmoparesis, is seen in only 10% of the cases.*

The diagnosis of Wernicke–Korsakoff syndrome is missed in about 25% of cases. This is commonly because the history of symptom onset may be unclear, due to recent alcohol intoxication or the presence of Korsakoff psychosis, or because the patient is debilitated or elderly. If clinically suspected, however, the diagnosis can be confirmed by showing a marked reduction in blood transketolase activity and a striking restoration toward normal of the transketolase activity and the clinical features, even within hours of the administration of thiamine; completely normal values of transketolase are usually attained within 24 hours. Failure of the ocular palsies to respond to thiamine within a few days should raise doubts about the diagnosis of Wernicke disease. Amnestic recovery is slower and often incomplete.

Pathology

- Wernicke disease:
  - Macroscopic: loss of brain tissue (lower brain weight, increased ventricular volume and pericerebral space) occurs, mainly in white matter.
  - Microscopic: neuronal loss, proliferative symmetric vasculopathy, and gliosis occur in the mammillary bodies (medial mammillary nucleus, diagnostic); thalamus (medial dorsal nucleus); hypothalamus; around the third ventricle, aqueduct in the midbrain, and floor of the fourth ventricle; brainstem and sometimes the cerebellum (606–608). There is little or no specific pathology in the locus ceruleus, hippocampus, and cerebral cortex.

606, 607 Brain, coronal sections, showing petechial hemorrhages in the mammillary bodies (black arrows) and medial dorsal thalamus (blue arrows) of a patient with acute Wernicke's encephalopathy.

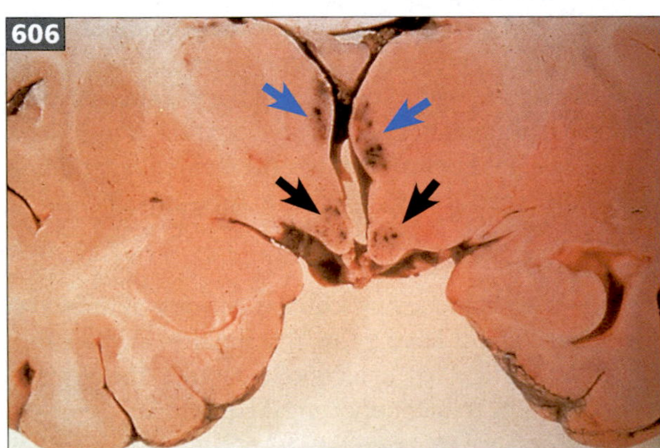

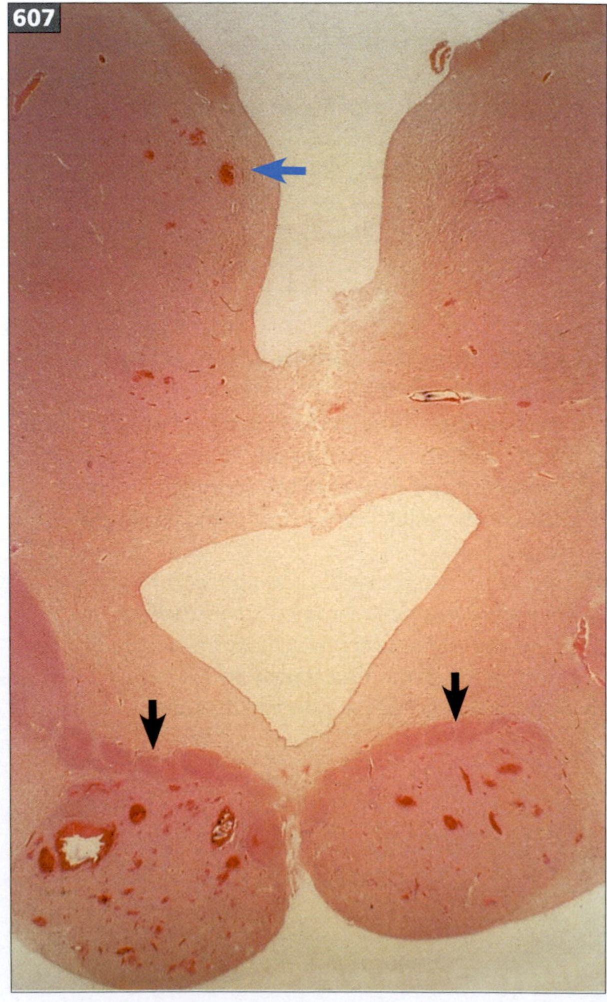

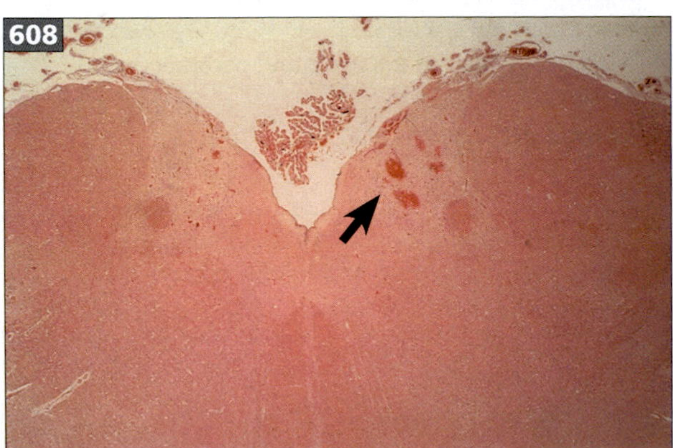

608 Axial section through the medulla, showing a proliferative vasculopathy and petechial hemorrhages (arrow) in the floor of the fourth ventricle of a patient with acute Wernicke's encephalopathy.

- Acute Wernicke's disease is characterized by small areas of petechial hemorrhage and marked vascular endothelial proliferation in the same sites listed above (i.e. mammillary bodies).
- Korsakoff psychosis: cell loss and gliosis occur in the medial mammillary nucleus and medial dorsal nucleus of the thalamus (similar to Wernicke's disease), but there is greater cell loss in the anterior principal nucleus of the thalamus.

Treatment[7,8]

- Thiamine 100 mg intravenously daily for 7 days because intestinal absorption is usually impaired in alcoholics. Thiamine prevents the progression of the disease and reverses the brain abnormalities that have not resulted in fixed structural changes. Hypomagnesemia can compromise the treatment response and replacement therapy should be considered as indicated.
- Oral vitamin maintenance, providing 10–50 mg thiamine daily until the patient is no longer at risk (usually for several months).
- Magnesium replacement (if depleted).
- Balanced diet.
- Alcohol abstinence.
- Psychotherapy and educational efforts: ineffective in arresting the cognitive decline without abstinence.
- Clonidine and fluvoxamine have been reported to be effective in improving function, suggesting dysfunction in noradrenergic and serotonergic systems respectively, but remain experimental.

Prevention

At risk patients should be given vitamin supplements. Comatose patients or those with acute mental status changes should be treated with thiamine, especially if no obvious cause is recognized. At-risk patients should never be given a glucose load (intravenous dextrose, nasogastric feeding) without vitamin supplements because this may consume thiamine and precipitate Wernicke syndrome.

Prognosis

- Depends on the stage of the disease and prompt institution of thiamine treatment.
- Can be fatal if untreated: mortality rate is 10–20%, mainly due to pulmonary infection, septicemia, decompensated liver disease, and an irreversible stage of thiamine deficiency.
- After thiamine treatment, ophthalmoplegia begins to improve within hours to days and nystagmus, ataxia, and confusion within days to weeks. The amnesic symptoms may recover slowly over 1 year or so and incompletely. Recovery of cognitive function depends on age and continuous abstinence from alcohol.
- Residual nystagmus and ataxia in 60% of patients.
- Residual chronic memory disorder in 80% of patients.

VITAMIN B12 DEFICIENCY

Definition and epidemiology

Vitamin B12 deficiency is a nutritional disorder of the nervous system that may be characterized by a symmetric, distal, predominantly sensory peripheral neuropathy due to axonal degeneration, autonomic neuropathy, subacute combined degeneration of the spinal cord, optic neuropathy, dementia, and other disturbances of higher mental function.

- Prevalence:
  - Pernicious anemia (PA): 1–3% over age 65 years.
  - Serum vitamin B12 levels <150 pmol/l (<200 pg/ml): 7–16% of the elderly population.
  - Serum vitamin B12 levels <225 pmol/l (<300 pg/ml) and elevated levels of metabolites of homocysteine and methylmalonic acid: 21% over age 65 years.
- Age: mean age at diagnosis is 60 years.
- Gender: F>M (1.5:1).

Etiology and pathophysiology

The total body store of vitamin B12 is 2–5 mg, half of which is stored in the liver. The body needs about 1–6 µg/day (the average diet contains about 7–30 µg per day).

Vitamin B12 is released from dietary food protein in the stomach and passes into the duodenum and jejunum where it is bound to intrinsic factor, which is produced by gastric parietal cells. The vitamin B12–intrinsic factor complex attaches to specific receptors in the terminal ileal mucosa, where it is internalized and degraded. Vitamin B12 enters the portal circulation, where some binds to transcobalamin II. The vitamin B12–transcobalamin II complex is taken up by cells and degraded in lysosomes, releasing vitamin B12 for conversion to methylcobalamin or adenosylcobalamin.

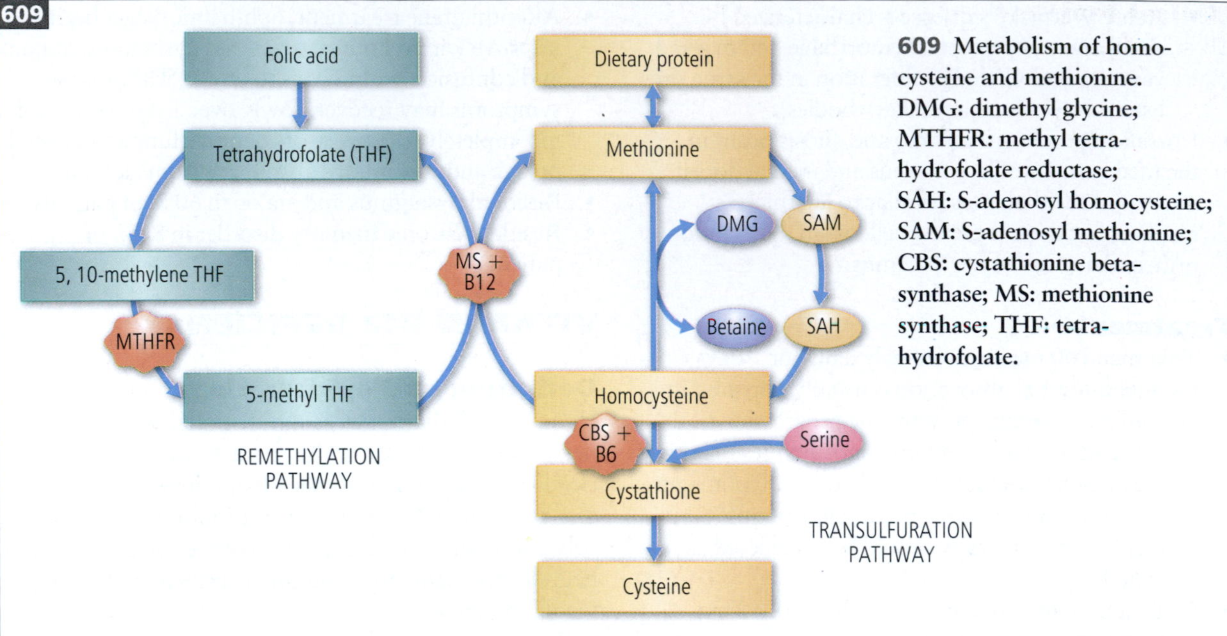

609 Metabolism of homocysteine and methionine. DMG: dimethyl glycine; MTHFR: methyl tetrahydrofolate reductase; SAH: S-adenosyl homocysteine; SAM: S-adenosyl methionine; CBS: cystathionine beta-synthase; MS: methionine synthase; THF: tetrahydrofolate.

Methylcobalamin is a cofactor of methionine synthase, which catalyzes the reaction of homocysteine and methyltetrahydrofolate to produce methionine and tetrahydrofolate. Methionine is further metabolized to S-adenosylmethionine, which is necessary for methylation of myelin sheath products. Tetrahydrofolate is the precursor required for purine and pyrimidine synthesis (**609**). Vitamin B12 is also necessary for the conversion of L-methylmalonyl CoA to succinyl CoA in the mitochondria.

The dietary source of vitamin B12 is from animal sources only. It is highly conserved through the enterohepatic circulation, so it takes 2–5 years to develop vitamin B12 deficiency from malabsorption, and up to 10–20 years for dietary deficiency from strict vegetarianism.

Vitamin B12 deficiency leads to a rise in serum levels of homocysteine and methylmalonic acid. The lack of methionine leads to the decreased production of S-adenosylmethionine, which is required for methylation reactions, including myelin phospholipids. It is puzzling, however, that neurologic complications are rare in folate deficiency, even though methionine synthase also requires folate as a cofactor.

Accumulation of methylmalonic acid and its precursor, propionic acid, may provide abnormal substrates for fatty acid synthesis, resulting in abnormal odd-number carbon and branched-chain fatty acids, which may be incorporated into the myelin sheath.

Nitrous oxide is an oxidizing agent that irreversibly modifies the cobalt core of vitamin B12, rendering methylcobalamin inactive. This inhibits the conversion of homocysteine to methionine, thus reducing the supply of S-adenosylmethionine. In persons with normal stores of vitamin B12, there may be sufficient quantities of unoxidized vitamin B12 to maintain enzyme function for longer periods, but in patients with compromised stores, even brief exposure to nitrous oxide may be sufficient to precipitate a vitamin B12 deficiency syndrome[9,10]. Vitamin B12 deficiency can be:

- Genetic: defect of methylmalonyl CoA mutase.
- Dietary deficiency (low intake): vegetarianism.
- Malabsorption states:
  - PA: lack of intrinsic factor due to autoimmune gastric parietal cell dysfunction.
  - Gastric achlorhydria.
  - Gastric resection.
  - Chronic pancreatic disease.
  - Competition for intraluminal vitamin B12:
    - Bacterial overgrowth in 'blind loops', anastomoses, and diverticula.
    - Cobalamin-metabolizing fish tapeworm (*Diphyllobothrium latum*) infestation.
  - Terminal ileum disease:
    - Crohn's disease.
    - Resection.
- Nitrous oxide exposure (anesthesia).
- Increased requirements: pregnancy.
- Low utilization: enzyme deficiency.

Clinical features

About three-quarters of patients present with neurologic symptoms and about one-quarter with non-neurologic symptoms that result from defective deoxyribonucleic acid (DNA) synthesis in rapidly dividing cells of the bone marrow and gastrointestinal mucosa.

History

- Neurologic symptoms:
  - Paresthesia and numbness in the feet and later the fingers.
  - Lhermitte's symptom occasionally.
  - Impaired memory.
  - Anosmia.
  - Reduced visual acuity.
  - Diminished taste.
  - Impaired manual dexterity.
  - Lower limb weakness (corticospinal tract lesions and peripheral neuropathy).
  - Unsteady gait.
  - Impotence.
  - Incontinence of urine or feces.
- Non-neurologic symptoms:
  - Weakness.
  - Tiredness.
  - Faints (syncope).
  - Palpitations.
  - Headache.
  - Sore tongue.
  - Diarrhea.
  - Bowel disturbances.
- Recent exposure to nitrous oxide.

Physical examination

- General:
  - Pallor of mucous membrane (anemia) (**610**).
  - Lemon-yellow skin.
  - Glossitis (smooth red tongue) (**611**).
  - Premature graying of hair.
  - Orthostatic hypotension.
- Neurologic:
  - Altered higher mental function: depression, hallucinations, frank psychosis (so-called megaloblastic madness), paranoia, violent behavior, personality changes, mental confusion, and dementia occur in about 10% of cases.
  - Optic atrophy, with bilateral centrocecal scotomas and visual failure, is rare.
  - Spastic paraparesis due to corticospinal tract lesions occurs. Lower limb weakness may also be due to accompanying peripheral neuropathy; lower motor neuron signs (e.g. wasting, weakness, areflexia) only become apparent when neuropathy is severe.
  - Reflexes may be increased (with clonus) or decreased depending on the degree of corticospinal tract and peripheral nerve involvement.
  - Plantar responses are often extensor because of corticospinal tract degeneration.
  - Incoordination may be marked because of spinocerebellar degeneration (cerebellar ataxia) or proprioceptive loss (sensory ataxia).
  - Loss of vibration and joint position sense in the feet is due to degeneration of the posterior columns, and loss of pain and temperature sensation distally in the limbs in a 'glove and stocking' distribution due to peripheral neuropathy.

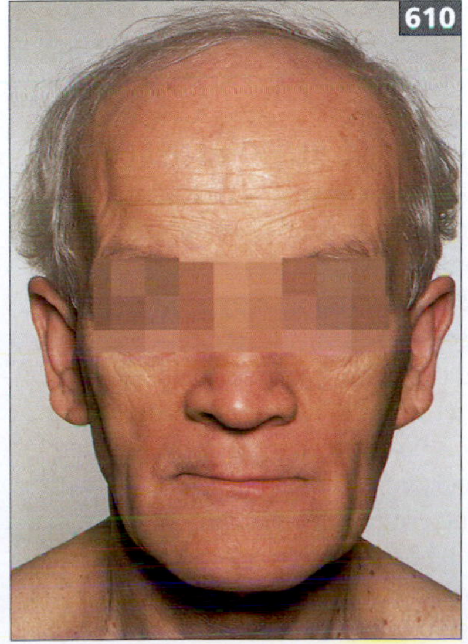

610 Pale appearance of the skin and mucous membranes of a patient with pernicious anemia. *Courtesy of Dr AM Chancellor, Tauranga, New Zealand.*

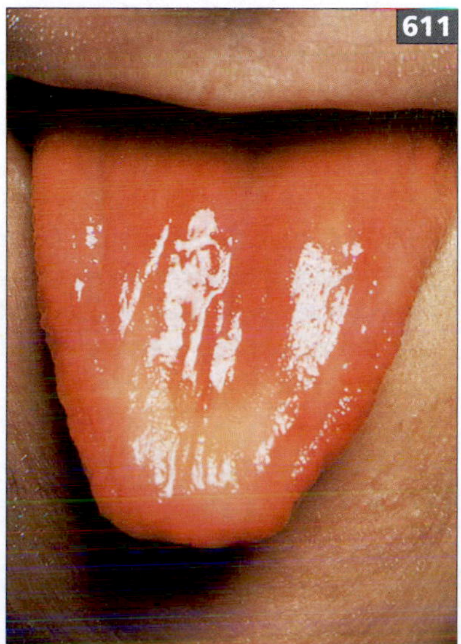

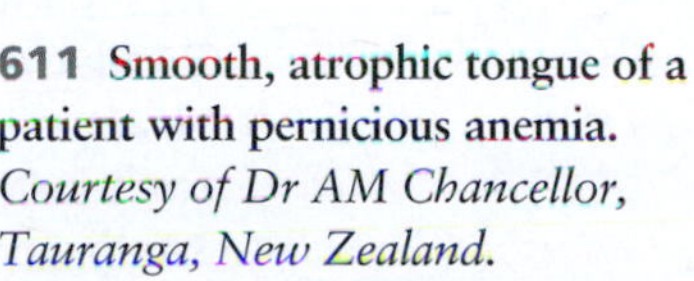

611 Smooth, atrophic tongue of a patient with pernicious anemia. *Courtesy of Dr AM Chancellor, Tauranga, New Zealand.*

- Romberg's sign may be present due to impaired proprioception as a result of degeneration of large diameter fibers in peripheral nerves and posterior columns.
- Broad-based gait.

Neuropathy alone is found in about one-quarter of patients, myelopathy alone in about 12%, and combined myelopathy and neuropathy in about 40%. Paresthesia, vibratory loss, and ataxia may be caused by both neuropathic and myelopathic lesions.

Differential diagnosis

- Myeloneuropathy:
  - Syphilis.
  - Hereditary ataxia.
  - Adrenomyeloneuropathy.
  - Cervical spondylitic myeloradiculopathy.
  - Multiple sclerosis and concurrent peripheral neuropathy (e.g. alcoholic, diabetic).
  - Chronic exposure to nitrous oxide. Nitrous oxide interdicts vitamin B12 metabolism.
  - Acute exposure to nitrous oxide in patients with borderline vitamin B12 levels; these patients may develop an acute vitamin B12 deficiency syndrome after a single exposure to nitrous oxide during a surgical procedure.
  - Celiac disease with vitamin E deficiency: sensory neuropathy, areflexia, confusion, dementia, cerebellar ataxia, myopathy, weight loss, diarrhea, steatorrhea.
- Macrocytosis:
  - Alcoholism.
  - Hypothyroidism.
  - Liver disease.
  - Reticulocytosis.
  - Drugs, cytotoxics.
  - Pregnancy.
  - Myelodysplasia, myeloma, aplastic anemia.
  - Inborn errors of cobalamin metabolism (homocystinuria and methylmalonic aciduria).
- Low serum vitamin B12 level:
  - Vitamin B12 deficiency.
  - Abnormalities of vitamin B12 metabolism: folate deficiency/antagonists.
  - Low serum vitamin B12 level may occur during the second and third trimester of pregnancy; this, however, may not reflect a true tissue deficiency of B12.

Investigations[11]

Diagnosis of vitamin B12 deficiency

- Hematologic work-up:
  - May be normal.
  - Anemia or pancytopenia.
  - Macrocytosis.
  - Neutrophil hypersegmentation (may be a sensitive marker of vitamin B12 deficiency, even in the absence of anemia or macrocytosis).
- Serum vitamin B12 level: <150 pmol/l (<200 pg/ml) (radioassay method) in 90–95%, 150–225 pmol/l (200–300 pg/ml) in 5–10%, and >225 pmol/l (>300 pg/ml) in 0.1–1% of patients.
- Serum homocysteine: raised, but nonspecific: also elevated in chronic renal disease, several inborn errors of metabolism, hypothyroidism, folate deficiency, and pyridoxine deficiency.
- Serum methylmalonic acid level: most sensitive test for B12 deficiency. Levels may be moderately elevated in renal failure and volume depletion.
- Bone marrow: megaloblastic (can be masked by concurrent iron deficiency).

Determine the cause of vitamin B12 deficiency[12]

- Antiparietal cell antibody: sensitive (present in 90% of people with PA) but not specific (also present in 10% of the population over the age of 70).
- Anti-intrinsic factor antibody:
  - Insensitive (present in only 50–60% of people with PA) but highly specific for PA.
  - The presence of anti-intrinsic factor antibody in the setting of serologic evidence of vitamin B12 deficiency (either low vitamin B12 or elevated levels of homocysteine or methylmalonic acid) is diagnostic for PA.
- Serum gastrin level: in the setting of serologic evidence of vitamin B12 deficiency and negative anti-intrinsic factor antibody, serum gastrin levels may help to establish the presence of achlorhydria which is almost invariably associated with PA.
- Schilling test: to determine: 1) if there is vitamin B12 malabsorption in patients with proven B12 deficiency without a known cause (e.g. diet, gastrectomy, drugs); and 2) the cause of the B12 malabsorption:
  - Conducted with and without intrinsic factor (IF).
  - Radioactive B12 alone is given by mouth (part 1). If it is not detected in the urine, the result is abnormal, indicating that radioactive B12 is not absorbed from the gut. The test is repeated with radioactive B12 bound to IF (part 2). Radioactive B12 is now detected in the urine of patients with PA, due to a lack of IF, whereas patients with malabsorption of B12 from the terminal ileum still fail to show any radioactive B12 in the urine.
  - No longer available in many institutions.

Additional investigations[13]

- Nerve conduction studies: reduced or absent sensory potentials (axonal degeneration) and decreased motor conduction velocities (demyelination).
- Electromyography (EMG): spontaneous fibrillations in distal muscles if denervated.
- Sural nerve biopsy: axonal degeneration with or without demyelination.
- Abnormal somatosensory evoked potentials.
- MRI of the brain and spine (**612–614**): may be used to exclude structural causes of the patient's symptoms. In advanced cases, T1 MR images of the spine may show swelling of the upper cervical spinal cord and decreased signal in the posterior columns of the spinal cord, extending up to the brainstem. T2 images may show increased signal in the posterior columns, particularly in the lower cervical and upper thoracic segments. T2 MRI images of the brain may show confluent high density changes in the white matter of the temporo-parieto-occipital lobes bilaterally, corresponding to gliosis and edema with vacuolization of axonal sheath myelin.

Diagnosis[14]

Typical neurologic syndrome (subacute combined degeneration of the spinal cord, neuropathy), macrocytic anemia, low serum vitamin B12 level, and biochemical evidence of vitamin B12 deficiency: elevated methylmalonic acid and homocysteine levels. A normal vitamin B12 assay does not fully exclude vitamin B12 deficiency.

Pathology

- Peripheral nerves: predominantly sensory, distal, symmetric, peripheral neuropathy, characterized by axonal degeneration with or without demyelination.
- Spinal cord: subacute combined degeneration of the spinal cord. Vacuolar myelopathy with myelin loss affecting mainly the posterior columns and lateral corticospinal tracts (**615**).
- Optic neuropathy: white matter degeneration and occasional foci of spongy degeneration in optic nerves and chiasm.
- Brain: white matter degeneration.
- Autonomic neuropathy: degeneration of small unmyelinated axons.

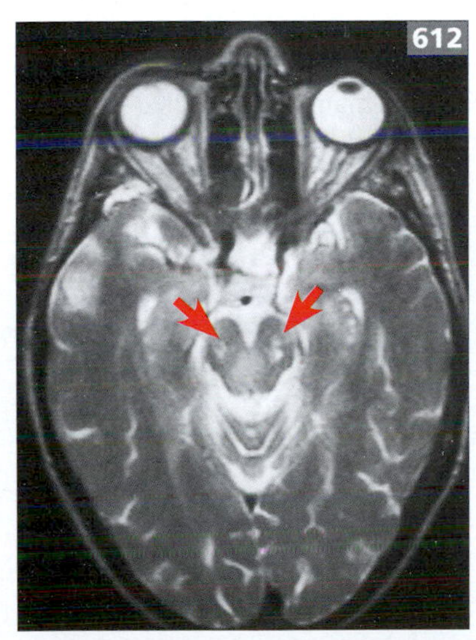

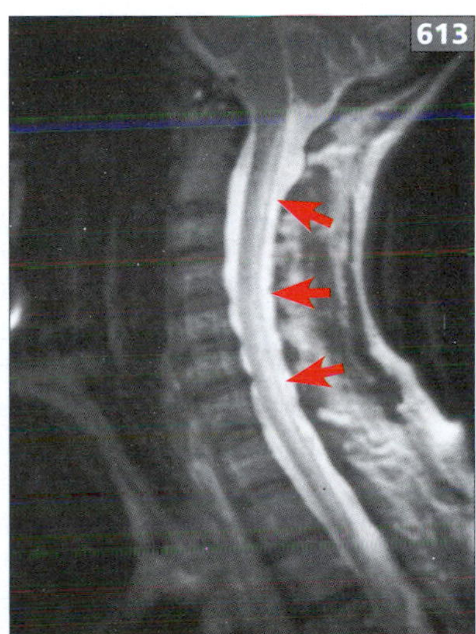

612–614 T2W axial brain (612), T2W midline sagittal cervical spine (613), and T2W axial cervical spine (612) MRI in a patient with pernicious anemia and subacute combined degeneration of the cord. Note the increased signal throughout the sensory long tracts in the brainstem and the posterior columns of the cord.

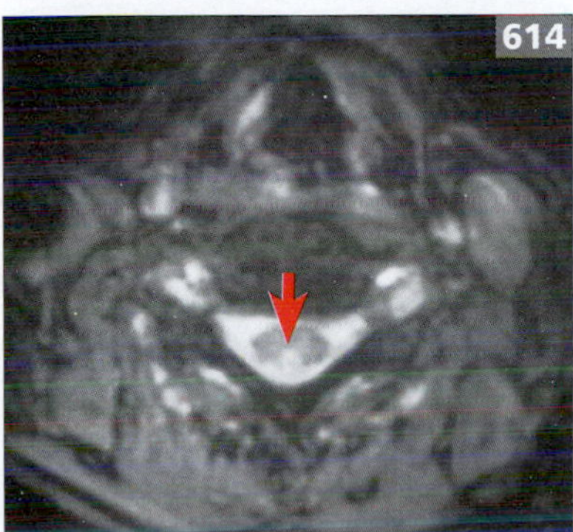

615 Axial section of spinal cord, showing tissue destruction and fibrous gliosis in posterior columns (blue arrows) and anterior (black arrows) corticospinal tracts of a patient with longstanding subacute combined degeneration of the spinal cord. *Courtesy of Professor BA Kakulas, Royal Perth Hospital, Western Australia.*

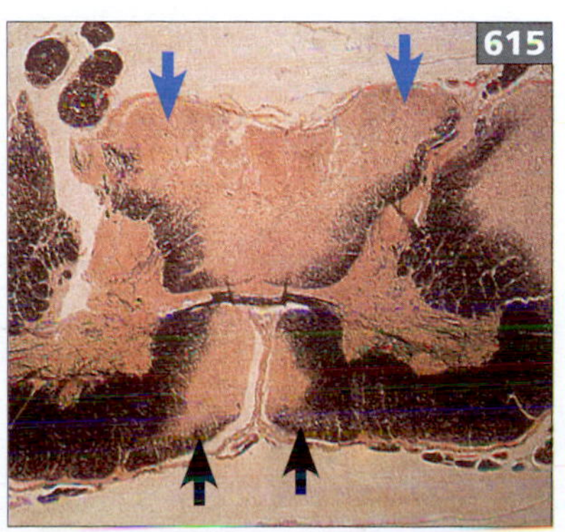

Treatment[15–18]

- Remove/treat the underlying cause.
- Replenish vitamin B12 stores with intramuscular injections of cyanocobalamin 100–1000 μg daily for 5 days, then:
- Maintain vitamin B12 stores with:
  - 100–1000 μg cyanocobalamin intramuscularly each month, or
  - 500–1000 μg cyanocobalamin orally each day, as a supplement, until the underlying cause is removed.

The rationale for oral supplementation (e.g. 1000 μg/day) is that 1% of all ingested vitamin B12 (e.g. 10 μg, more than the average daily requirement [1–6 μg/day]) may be absorbed by passive diffusion. This means that vitamin B12 requirements may be satisfied with oral therapy, even in patients with PA, provided the dose is sufficient.

Tip

▶ *Oral replacement, and even sublingual therapy, are valid alternatives for patients who cannot tolerate intramuscular injections or for whom they are impractical.*

The therapeutic response to B12 should be a reticulocytosis and normalization of the blood count changes (unless concomitant deficiencies or diseases are present). The hemoglobin will rise by 10 g/l per week on average. The bone marrow changes also resolve rapidly, within 48 hours of commencing therapy.

Prognosis

The most important factor influencing the neurologic response to treatment is the duration of symptoms before treatment is started. If treatment is given early enough, it may not only prevent progression but also reverse some neurologic symptoms and signs besides paresthesia in the feet and optic atrophy.

VITAMIN E DEFICIENCY

Definition and epidemiology

Vitamin E deficiency is a nutritional disorder of the nervous system characterized by spinocerebellar syndrome, peripheral neuropathy, acanthocytosis, hemolytic anemia, and retinitis pigmentosa[19].

- Prevalence: unknown, but considered a rare condition.
- Recommended daily allowance of Vitamin E:
  - Age 0.6 months: 3 mg.
  - Age 6–12 months: 4 mg.
  - Age 1–3 years: 6 mg.
  - Age 4–10 years: 7 mg.
  - Adults and elderly: 8–15 mg.

Etiology and pathophysiology[20]

Vitamin E consists of a family of tocopherols (α, β, γ, and δ) and tocoretinols. Alpha-tocopherol is the most biologically active form of vitamin E in humans. Therefore, the terms vitamin E and α-tocopherol are often used as synonyms.

Vitamin E is a fat-soluble vitamin that requires pancreatic esterases and bile salts for its absorption in the gastrointenstinal tract. Due to its liposoluble characteristics, vitamin E circulates in plasma incorporated into lipoproteins (mainly very low-density lipoprotein [VLDL] and chylomicrons) and is stored mainly in the adipose tissue.

Vitamin E is a natural antioxidant and free radical scavenger that protects polyunsaturated fatty acids of cellular membranes from peroxidation. Dietary sources of vitamin E include vegetable oils (sunflower and olive), leafy vegetables, fruits, meats, nuts, and cereals.

Vitamin E has a ubiquitous distribution; therefore, deficiency is almost never a consequence of dietary restriction. Instead, deficiency is usually associated with conditions that cause severe malabsorption:

- Chronic cholestasis.
- Pancreatic insufficiency.
- Celiac disease.
- Crohn disease.
- Cystic fibrosis.
- Bowel resection.

In addition, insufficient supplementation in individuals receiving total parenteral nutrition can cause vitamin E deficiency, and some inherited conditions (*Table 107*):

- α-Tocopherol transfer protein.
- Homozygous hypobetalipoproteinemia.
- Abetalipoproteinemia (Bassen–Kornzweig syndrome).
- Chylomicron retention disease.

Clinical features

Characterized by a spinocerebellar syndrome with peripheral nerve involvement (similar to Friedreich ataxia)[21]:

- Cerebellar ataxia.
- Hyporeflexia.
- Propioception and vibratory sensory loss with sensory ataxia.
- Extensor plantar responses.
- Acanthocytosis.
- Hemolytic anemia (mainly in premature infants).
- Retinitis pigmentosa.
- Specific findings can be seen in association with inherited conditions (*Table 107*).

Differential diagnosis[22,23]

- Tumors in the posterior fossa.
- Paraneoplastic cerebellar degeneration.
- Vitamin B12 deficiency.
- Multiple sclerosis.
- Ataxia associated with antigliadin antibodies (Sprue).
- Alcohol abuse.
- Drug-related cerebellar degeneration (phenytoin use).
- Cerebellar variant of prion disease.
- Multisystem atrophy-C.
- Hereditary cerebellar atrophy.
- Cerebellitis.

TABLE 107 **INHERITED CONDITIONS ASSOCIATED WITH VITAMIN E DEFICIENCY**

	Alpha-tocopherol transfer protein (α-TTP)	Homozygous hypobetalipoproteinemia	Abetalipoproteinemia (Bassen–Kornzweig disease)	Chylomicron retention disease
Defect and transmission	α-TTP gene on chromosome 8; autosomal recessive	Defect in apolipoprotein B gene; autosomal dominant	Microsomal triglyceride transfer protein on chromosome 4; autosomal recessive	Chylomicron synthesis and secretion; gene has not been identified yet, but suspected to be autosomal recessive
Pathophysiology	Impaired incorporation of vitamin E into lipoproteins	Elevated turn-over of apoprotein B-containing lipoproteins (chylomicrons, VLDL, and LDL)	Low levels of apoprotein B-containing lipoprotein	Impaired assembly and secretion of chylomicrons which are retained in the intestinal mucosa
Age of onset	First decade, although adult onset variants have been described	Early childhood	Early childhood	Early childhood
Clinical features	Large-fiber sensory loss with areflexia; ataxia, dysarthria, head titubation and dystonia; retinitis pigmentosa, skeletal deformities, cardiomyopathy, and xanthelasma; fat malabsorption is not usually seen	Ataxia, areflexia, propioceptive sensory loss, and extensor plantar responses; retinitis pigmentosa, acanthocytosis, retarded growth, and malabsorption with steatorrhea		Retarded growth and steatorrhea; ocular and neuromuscular manifestations are less severe; acanthocytes are usually absent
Laboratory findings	Very low serum vitamin E	Low serum fat-soluble vitamin levels (including vitamin E); low to nondetectable apoprotein B, chylomicrons, VLDL, and LDL; serum cholesterol and triglycerides are markedly reduced		Low serum apoprotein B, cholesterol, LDL, and chylomicrons; normal triglycerides

LDL: low-density lipoprotein; VLDL: very low-density lipoprotein.

Investigations[20]

- Blood work-up:
  - Serum vitamin E: this is dependent on the concentration of serum lipids, so it may not reflect accurately tissue levels of vitamin E. For patients with normal serum lipids, serum vitamin E less than 5 mg/l (0.5 mg/dl) is considered deficient.
  - Effective vitamin E concentration: calculated by dividing serum α-tocopherol by the sum of total cholesterol and triglycerides (normal >0.8 mg of α-tocopherol/(cholesterol and triglycerides).
  - Vitamin E level is usually undetectable in individuals with neurologic manifestations.
- Malabsorption work-up.
- Additional investigations:
  - Somatosensory evoked potentials: may show central delay.
  - Nerve conduction studies: axonal neuropathy.
  - MRI of the brain and spine: may be used to exclude structural causes of the patient's symptoms. T2 MR images may show increased signal in the posterior columns, particularly in the cervical spine.

Diagnosis

Typical neurologic syndrome in the setting of low levels of vitamin E.

Pathology

- Loss of myelinated fibers with axonal degeneration noted in peripheral nerves, posterior columns, and sensory roots.
- Swollen dystrophic axons (spheroids) of the gracile and cuneate nuclei.
- Lipofuscin accumulation in the dorsal sensory neurons and peripheral Schwann cells.

Treatment[24]

Treat the underlying cause of vitamin E deficiency. Equivalence is calculated as 1 mg of vitamin E = 1.47 IU 'natural source' vitamin E = 2.2 IU synthetic vitamin E. Replacement dose varies, mainly according to the cause of the deficiency:

- Abetalipoproteinemia: 100–200 IU/kg/d.
- Chronic cholestasis: 15–25 IU/kg/d.
- Cystic fibrosis: 5–10 IU/kg/d.
- Short-bowel syndrome: 200–3600 IU/d.
- Isolated vitamin E deficiency: 800–3600 IU/d.

In severe malabsorption, fat-soluble vitamine E replacement may be ineffective; in these cases, larger oral doses or intramuscular administration of a water miscible form (D-α-tocopherol glycol) may be required.

Vitamin E is used off-label in patients with cancer, cardiovascular disease, stroke, or neurodegenerative disorders (such as Alzhemier's disease and amyotrophic lateral sclerosis). The benefit of vitamin E in treating these conditions as well as the long-term effect and safety of oral supplementation are still unclear. More recently, however, studies of vitamin E supplementation for cardiovascular diseases have not been promising. It has been suggested that vitamin E may increased the risk of bleeding diathesis. Doses of 100–400 IU per day appear to be safe, and the recommended daily upper limit of vitamin E supplementation in the absence of malabsorption is 1000 mg.

Prognosis

Early diagnosis and treatment may result in a dramatic recovery.

NIACIN (NICOTINIC ACID) DEFICIENCY

Definition and epidemiology

Niacin deficiency is a nutritional disorder characterized by the clinical triad of dermatitis, diarrhea, and dementia (pellagra)[25]. Current prevalence is unknown, but it is overall considered a rare condition in developed countries. Recommended daily allowance is:

- Lactation: 17 mg.
- Age 1–3 years: 6 mg.
- Age 4–8 years: 8 mg.
- Age 9–13 years: 12 mg.
- Adults and elderly: 14–16 mg.
- Pregnancy: 18 mg.

Etiology and pathophysiology[26,27]

Niacin (or nicotinic acid) is an end product of tryptophan metabolism. Biotransformation of tryptophan and nicotinic acid requires several vitamins and minerals, such as vitamin B2, vitamin B6, iron, and copper. Nicotinamide is readily deaminated in the body to form nicotinic acid.

Niacin is a precursor of nicotinamide adenine dinucleotide (NAD) and nicotinamide adenine dinucleotide phosphate (NADP). The niacin moiety of these two molecules is involved in electron and hydrogen ion exchange. NAD and NADP are cofactors of enzymes involved in the metabolism of carbohydrates, fatty acids, and proteins, as well as in energy production. Dietary sources of niacin include yeast, cereals, legumes, seeds, meats (especially liver), and milk.

The occurrence of pellagra has decreased significantly with fortification of bread and cereals with niacin. As corn lacks niacin and tryptophan, pellagra may be seen in populations that use this type of food as the primary carbohydrate source. Nonendemic pellagra is usually associated with:

- Alcoholism.
- Malabsorption (such as in anorexia nervosa or after bariatric surgery)[28].
- Secondary deficiency:
  - Seen in cases of vitamin B6 deficiency.
  - Isoniazid treatment (as it depletes body storage of vitamin B6).
- Carcinoid syndrome (niacin deficiency occurs as its precursor, tryptophan, is used in the synthesis of serotonin).
- Bacterial colonization of the small intestine (due to increased metabolism of tryptophan).
- Inherited conditions: Hartnup syndrome – an autosomal recessive disorder characterized by impaired absortion of neutral amino acids (particularly tryptophan).

Clinical features

Characterized by the clinical triad of dermatitis, diarrhea, and dementia[29].

- Dermatologic findings:
  - Extensive hyperkeratotic hyperpigmented dermatitis.
  - Diffuse, but most typically located in sun-exposed areas (face, chest, and dorsum of the hands and feet).
- Gastrointestinal features: stomatitis, diarrhea, abdominal pain, vomiting, and anorexia.
- Neuropsychiatric features:
  - May be seen in the absence of dermatologic and gastrointestinal manifestations (particularly in nonendemic pellagra).
  - Most reported series included alcoholic patients making it difficult to determine what manifestations are directly related to niacin deficiency, and which are due to chronic alcoholism or other concomitant nutritional disorders.
  - Progressive encephalopathy which may progress to coma.
  - Irritability, depression, apathy.
  - Memory loss.
  - Myelopathy, spastic paraparesis, and myoclonus.
  - Peripheral neuropathy (similar to that seen in thiamin deficiency).

Differential diagnosis

- Atopic dermatitis.
- Drug-related photosensitivity.
- Systemic lupus erythematosus.
- Discoid lupus.
- Porphyria.
- Thiamine deficiency.
- Anorexia.
- Alcoholism.
- Vitamin B12 deficiency.

Investigations

Available studies include serum niacin, tryptophan, NAD, and NADP levels. Erythrocyte NAD and niacin plasma metabolites are considered indirect markers of niacin tissue levels. However, none of them is considered sensitive or specific to measure niacin status.

Urinary excretion of niacin metabolites (N-methyl-nitoinamide and N-methyl-2-pyridone-5-carboxamide) may be more sensitive to identify pellagra than blood NAD and NADP. Combined 24-hour urinary excretion of less than 1.5 mg indicates severe niacin deficiency.

Diagnosis

Low niacin levels in the context of clinical manifestations consistent with pellagra. The therapeutic response to niacin supplementation establishes the diagnosis.

Treatment

Treat the underlying cause of niacin deficiency:

- Oral replacement: nicotinic acid 50 mg three times a day.
- Parenteral replacement: nicotinic acid 25 mg three times a day.

Nicotinamide has comparable therapeutic efficacy to nicotinic acid, but it lacks the vasodilatory and lowering-cholesterol properties of niacin. In malnourished patients consider high-protein diet and B-complex supplementation (particularly in alcoholics).

Niacin is used in patients with dyslipidemia and cardiovascular disease. The most common side-effects are flushing, vomiting, pruritus, hives, and transaminitis. Niacin-induced myopathy has also been described.

Prognosis

Excellent if treatment is initiated early. Left untreated, patients develop malabsorption and progressive encephalopathy leading to stupor, coma, and death.

MARCHIAFAVA–BIGNAMI DISEASE

Definition and epidemiology

Progressive neurologic disorder characterized by selective demyelination of the corpus callosum in association with alcohol consumption. Current prevalence is unknown, but it is overall considered a rare condition. The disease was initially described in malnourished Italians who consumed large amounts of red wine. It is not, however, necessarily restricted to individuals of Italian background and, although rarely, may also occur in nonalcoholics.

Etiology and pathophysiology

The exact mechanism of disease is unknown. Histopathologic studies reveal abundant macrophage infiltration of the affected areas with demyelination and cyst formation. Axons are usually preserved, and neuronal degeneration and gliosis of the third and fourth layer of the frontal and temporal cortices (cortical laminar sclerosis) occurs.

Patients present with symmetric demyelination of the central portion of the corpus callosum; other areas and even the entire corpus callosum may be involved. Subsequently, these areas undergo necrosis and cavitation.

Other structures may also be affected, such as the optic chiasm, cerebellar peduncles, pons, anterior and posterior commissures, centrum semiovale, and deep white matter.

Clinical features[30]

Patients usually have a history of alcoholism and poor nutrition.

- Neurologic manifestations:
  - Cognitive decline: patients present with different degrees of cognitive involvement (lethargy, stupor, and coma) and seizures. Symptoms may evolve rapidly (delirium) or have a more protracted course (dementia).
  - Apraxia: ideomotor apraxia may be seen in formal neurocognitive evaluation. The callosal necrosis causes interhemispheric disconnection which manifests clinically by nondominant (usually left-sided) apraxia, alien hand phenomenon, and hemialexia without agraphia.
- Other alcohol-related manifestations, such as behavioral changes, dysconjugate gaze, ataxia, delirium tremens, sensory neuropathy, hyporeflexia, incontinence, and tremors may be seen in patients with Marchiafava–Bignami disease.

Differential diagnosis

- Thiamine deficiency.
- Anorexia.
- Alcoholism.
- Vitamin B12 deficiency.
- Neurodegeneration (AD, corticobasal degeneration [CBD], and frontotemporal dementia [FTD]).
- Encephalitis (infectious or paraneoplastic).
- Central pontine (and/or extrapontine) myelinolysis.
- Seizure disorder.
- Stroke of the corpus callosum.
- Inflammation-mediated demyelination of the corpus callosum (multiple sclerosis).

Investigations

Laboratory investigations are oriented to rule out other medical conditions that may present similarly:

- Metabolic evaluation (including electrolytes, glucose, urea, and liver function tests).
- Toxicology screening.
- Lumbar puncture.
- Electroencephalography (EEG).
- Imaging[31–33]:
  - Head CT: suboptimal sensitivity to assess callosal integrity.
  - Brain MRI:
    - Corpus callosum is usually involved.
    - T2 and fluid attenuated inversion recovery (FLAIR) hyperintensity suggest edema and myelin damage.

- T1 hypodensity is indicative of myelin loss with cyst formation.
- In the chronic phase the corpus callosum becomes atrophic.
- Subcortical U-fibers are usually spared.

Diagnosis

The diagnosis is largely one of exclusion and based mainly on clinical presentation and ancillary studies.

Treatment

There is no specific treatment for this disease, treatment is symptomatic:

- Correct possible metabolic imbalances.
- Seizure control.
- Vitamin B12, folate, and thiamine replacement (particularly in alcoholics, due to risk of Wernicke–Korsakoff syndrome).
- Treatment of alcoholism.

TABLE 108 **PRECIPITATING FACTORS FOR HEPATIC ENCEPHALOPATHY**

Precipitant	Possible mechanism
Dietary protein excess; constipation (anorexia, fluid restriction); gastrointestinal hemorrhage; infection; uremia; hypokalemia	Increased ammonia production
Systemic alkalosis	Increased diffusion of ammonia across blood–brain barrier
Dehydration; hypotension; hypoxemia; anemia	Reduced metabolism of toxins because of hepatic hypoxia
Benzodiazepine use	Activation of central GABA benzodiazepine receptors
Other psychoactive drug use	Compounding of CNS depressant effect
Porto-systemic shunts	Reduced hepatic metabolism of toxins because of diversion of portal blood
Progressive hepatic parenchymal damage; development of hepatoma	Reduced hepatic metabolism of toxins because of reduced functional reserve

CNS: central nervous system; GABA: γ-aminobutyric acid.

Prognosis

No systematic study has been conducted to assess the prognosis of individuals with Marchiafava–Bignami disease. Clinical features at presentation (including severe cognitive impairment and coma) and radiologic findings (such as extension of callosal involvement) have been linked to long-term disability (86%) and mortality (21%).

HEPATIC ENCEPHALOPATHY

Definition and epidemiology

Hepatic encephalopathy (HE) is a clinical neuropsychiatric syndrome characterized by abnormal mental status occurring in patients with severe acute, subacute, or chronic hepatocellular insufficiency[34].

HE is an increasingly common disorder in most major hospitals since the advent of many new hepatotoxic drugs and the increased consumption of alcohol by patients with pre-existing hepatic dysfunction. The prevalence of subclinical HE in cirrhosis patients ranges from 30 to 84%.

- Age: usually middle-aged and elderly.
- Gender: M=F.

Etiology and pathophysioloy

Acute HE in a patient with liver disease (e.g. cirrhosis) is usually associated with a clearly identifiable precipitating factor and usually resolves when the precipitating factor is removed or corrected. Failure to find a precipitating factor may imply a decrease in overall hepatocellular function.

Chronic HE usually occurs in a patient with cirrhosis and substantial porto-systemic shunting, who has hepatic encephalopathy that is persistent or episodic, with or without complete resolution of encephalopathy between episodes.

Porto-systemic venous shunting associated with chronic liver disease

- Predisposing factors: hypoxia, hypokalemia, metabolic alkalosis, electrolyte depletion, excessive diuresis, and use of sedative–hypnotic drugs.
- Precipitating factors (*Table 108*).

Acute liver failure

- Infection:
  - Hepatitis viruses: most commonly hepatitis B virus, but also hepatitis D and E viruses, and rarely hepatitis A, C, and G viruses.
  - Nonhepatotropic viruses: herpes virus, varicella-zoster virus, Epstein–Barr virus, cytomegalovirus, paramyxovirus, and others.
- Drugs and toxins:
  - Acetaminophen (paracetamol) overdose.
  - Poisoning with carbon tetrachloride, natural products such as certain fungi (e.g. *Amanita phalloides*, *Aspergillus flavus*, and *Aspergillus parasiticus*) or medicinal herbs (e.g. kava, ephedra, skullcap), and the recreational drug methylenedioxymethamphetamine ('ecstasy').
  - Hypersensitivity reactions to drugs (e.g. halothane, antidepressants, antithyroid drugs, nonsteroidal anti-inflammatory drugs, and anti-tuberculous drugs).
- Ischemia:
  - Cardiogenic shock.
  - Acute occlusion of suprahepatic veins.
- Miscellaneous:
  - Wilson's disease, sometimes associated with hemolytic anemia.
  - Reye's syndrome.
  - Acute fatty liver of pregnancy.

Pathogenesis is unclear but it is hepatic insufficiency and not the cause of the liver disease which is important in causing the neuropsychiatric clinical features[35].

Possible mechanisms

- Accumulation in brain extracellular fluid of unmetabolized gut-derived neurotoxins (e.g. ammonia, see below) as a result of poor hepatic function and portosystemic shunting.
- Functional disturbance of the blood–brain barrier.
- Alteration in neurotransmission:
  - Decreased neuroexcitation (glutamate, aspartate, dopamine, catecholamines).
  - Increased neuroinhibition (γ-aminobutyric acid [GABA], endogenous benzodiazepines, serotonin).
  - Activation of central GABA-benzodiazepine receptors by ligands of endogenous origin.
  - Production of false neurotransmitters.
- Reduced energy metabolism in the brain:
  - Disturbed activity of Na^+/K^+-ATPase.
  - Decreased activity of urea-cycle enzymes (due to zinc deficiency).
- Deposition of manganese in the basal ganglia.

Neurotoxins

In patients with hepatic failure, ammonia (which is produced in the gut by the action of colonic bacteria and mucosal enzymes on dietary protein) is not completely metabolized to urea through the urea cycle so it enters the systemic circulation and the brain. Ammonia uptake in the brain is increased, where it is normally detoxified in the brain by astrocytes.

Ammonia has a direct post-synaptic effect on excitatory and inhibitory post-synaptic potentials. Expression of the astrocyte glutamate transporter gene, *GLT-1*, is reduced in acute liver failure, resulting in reduced uptake of glutamate into synaptosomes (astrocytes in particular) and a rise in glutamate in the extracellular fluid.

Ammonia also affects cerebral energy metabolism by inhibiting alpha-ketoglutarate dehydrogenase and combining with alpha-ketoglutarate in the Krebs cycle to form glutamic acid, which then combines with more ammonia to form more glutamine. The effect of ammonia on glutamine function also has an effect on tryptophan uptake by the brain.

Excess (2–7-fold) manganese is deposited in the pallidum in patients dying in hepatic coma.

Clinical features

The nature and severity of the symptoms depend on the acuteness and extent of the liver failure and on the development of metabolic or infectious complications[36,37]. Consequently, the clinical manifestations range from subtle abnormalities detectable only on psychometric testing to deep coma (*Table 109*).

Neuropsychiatric findings

Clinically, HE is graded according to the West Haven classification[38]:

- **Grade 0:** Minimal HE (previously known as subclinical HE); lack of detectable changes in personality or behavior; minimal changes in memory, concentration, intellectual function, and coordination; patients may appear normal clinically but perform poorly on psychometric testing; no asterixis.
- **Grade 1:** Shortened attention span; impaired addition or subtraction; hypersomnia, insomnia, or inversion of sleep pattern; euphoria, depression, or irritability; mild confusion; slowing of ability to perform mental tasks (for example, constructional apraxia); handwriting skills impaired; fine postural tremor and poor coordination; asterixis can be detected.

TABLE 109 **WEST HAVEN CLASSIFICATION**[38]

Grade	Level of consciousness	Behavior and orientation	Neurologic signs	EEG
0	Alert	Normal except in psychometric testing	Normal except in psychometric testing	Normal
1	Hypersomnia, insomnia, or inversion of sleep pattern	Forgetfulness, mild confusion, agitation, irritability	Tremor, apraxia, incoordination, impaired handwriting	Triphasic waves
2	Lethargy, slow responses	Intermittent disorientation in time, amnesia, disinhibition, inappropriate behavior	Asterixis, dysarthria, ataxia, hypoactive reflexes	Triphasic waves
3	Somnolent but arousable, confused	Disorientated in place, aggressive behavior	Asterixis, rigidity, hyperactive reflexes, extensor plantar responses	Triphasic waves
4	Coma	None	Decerebration	Delta activity

EEG: electroencephalogram

- **Grade 2:** Lethargy or apathy; disorientation to time; inappropriate behavior; slurred speech; obvious asterixis; drowsiness, lethargy, gross deficits in ability to perform mental tasks, obvious personality changes, inappropriate behavior, and intermittent disorientation, usually regarding time; dysarthria, ataxia, paratonia, and hyporeflexia.
- **Grade 3:** Somnolent but can be aroused, unable to perform mental tasks; disorientation to time and place, with marked confusion, amnesia, and incomprehensible speech; may show aggressive behavior; deep-tendon reflexes become hyperactive, extensor plantar responses; rigidity, paratonia, and hyperventilation; asterixis is present; significant possibility of further progression into grade 4.
- **Grade 4:** Coma and decerebrate posturing with or without response to painful stimuli; represents a medical emergency that requires prophylactic endotracheal intubation for airway protection.

Asterixis

Nonspecific. May be seen in other medical conditions such as uremia, hypokalemia, hypomagnesemia, and nonketotic hyperglycemia. Unilateral asterixis may indicate a structural lesion involving the anterior portion or genu of the internal capsule, thalamus, midbrain, medial-frontal, or parietal cortex.

Signs of advanced liver disease

Jaundice, fetor hepaticus, hepatomegaly (or small liver size), and ascites (**616**).

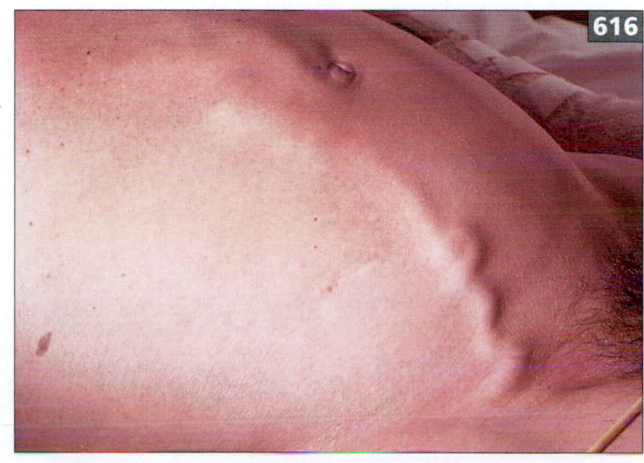

616 Abdomen of a man with hepatic encephalopathy and portal hypertension, showing diminished body hair and dilated superficial abdominal veins shunting blood from the portal to the systemic circulation. Ascites was also present.

Signs of comorbidities

- Comorbidities such as alcoholism, electrolyte disturbance, hypoglycemia, renal failure, hypotension due to gastrointestinal bleeding (e.g. boundary zone infarction), infection, and hemostatic failure may complicate or mask the clinical features of hepatic encephalopathy, and development of metabolic or infectious complications.
- Kayser–Fleischer ring suggests Wilson's disease.
- Bronzed skin and arthropathy is seen in hereditary hemochromatosis.

Differential diagnosis[34,35]

- Metabolic encephalopathy:
  - Hypoglycemia or hyperglycemia.
  - Electrolyte imbalance: hypernatremia, hyponatremia.
  - Hypoxia.
  - Hypercapnia: carbon dioxide narcosis.
  - Uremia: renal failure.
  - Ketoacidosis.
  - Wilson's disease.
  - Liver transplantation may be complicated within the first few weeks by an encephalopathy (headache, confusion, seizures, cortical blindness, coma) due to electrolyte imbalance, hypocalcemia, hypomagnesemia, cyclosporine, air embolism, intracerebral hemorrhage and hypotension. Opportunistic infections may occur later.
  - Hyperammonemia: other causes include ornithine transcarbamylase deficiency, amino and organic acidurias, arginosuccinic aciduria, citrullinemia, argininemia, carbamylphosphate synthetase deficiency, lysinuric protein intolerance, Reye's syndrome, sodium valproate, systemic carnitine deficiency, asparaginase toxicity.
- Toxic encephalopathy:
  - Alcohol:
    - Acute intoxication.
    - Withdrawal syndrome: delirium tremens (rapid postural and action tremor, cortical excitation rather than cortical inhibition).
    - Wernicke–Korsakoff syndrome.
  - Sedative/hypnotic/psychoactive drug intoxication.
  - Salicylates.
  - Heavy metals.
- Intracranial lesions:
  - Intracranial hemorrhage: subdural hematoma.
  - Meningoencephalitis: e.g. herpes simplex encephalitis.
  - Creutzfeldt–Jakob disease.
  - Brain infarction.
  - Brain abscess.
  - Brain tumor.
  - Head trauma.
  - Epilepsy (e.g. nonconvulsive status epilepticus) or postictal encephalopathy.
- Neuropsychiatric disorders: in some patients with an extensive porto-systemic collateral circulation, a disorder of mood (depression), personality, and intellect may be protracted over many months or even years, and be associated with dietary protein intake.

Investigations

Blood

- Liver function tests: hyperbilirubinemia, high aminotransferase levels; in advanced disease transaminases can be normal.
- Plasma ammonia: elevated usually but not consistently. Hyperammonemia is not invariable because blood ammonia levels depend on both the rate of production and metabolism. Arterial blood should be immediately analyzed; venous ammonia level may be artificially elevated due to tourniquet placement which may cause local ischemia of the underlying muscle which releases ammonia to the circulation.
- Prothrombin time: usually prolonged due to decreased synthesis of coagulation factors.
- Viral serology.

Tip

▶ *Hyperammonemia is frequently seen in patients with HE. Clinical assessment, however, is more accurate than ammonia level in assessing treatment response.*

Differential diagnosis investigations

- Urea and electrolytes.
- Glucose: hypoglycemia.
- Alcohol: acute intoxication.
- Erythrocyte transketolase activity: Wernicke–Korsakoff syndrome.
- Toxicology: salicylates, heavy metals, psychoactive drugs.

EEG

Initially the EEG shows nonspecific generalized slowing of the background rhythm. Later, it becomes dominated by trains of high amplitude, bisynchronous, slow waves of delta frequency (1.5–3 Hz) or frontal-dominant, triphasic waves with a phase lag from front to back, before flattening in late coma (**617**). These abnormalities are characteristic of, but not specific for, the disorder, since other metabolic encephalopathies can cause similar abnormalities.

Imaging

- CT brain: to exclude a structural intracranial lesion if suspected (e.g. hemorrhage).
- MRI brain:
  - Increased signal in the basal ganglia (particularly pallidum but midbrain may also be affected) on T1 (**618, 619**).
  - The substances which may cause an increased signal on T1 include manganese, melanin, calcium, and blood. The differential diagnosis of increased signal in the basal ganglia on T1 includes hyper-, hypo-, pseudohypo- and pseudopseudohypoparathyroidism, hyperalimentation, Wilson's disease, pantothenate kinase-associated neurodegeneration ([PKAN] formerly known as Hallevorden–Spatz disease), carbon monoxide poisoning, hemorrhage, and neurofibromatosis.

Cerebrospinal fluid

Cerebrospinal fluid (CSF) is usually normal apart from elevated levels of glutamine, the end product of cerebral ammonia metabolism.

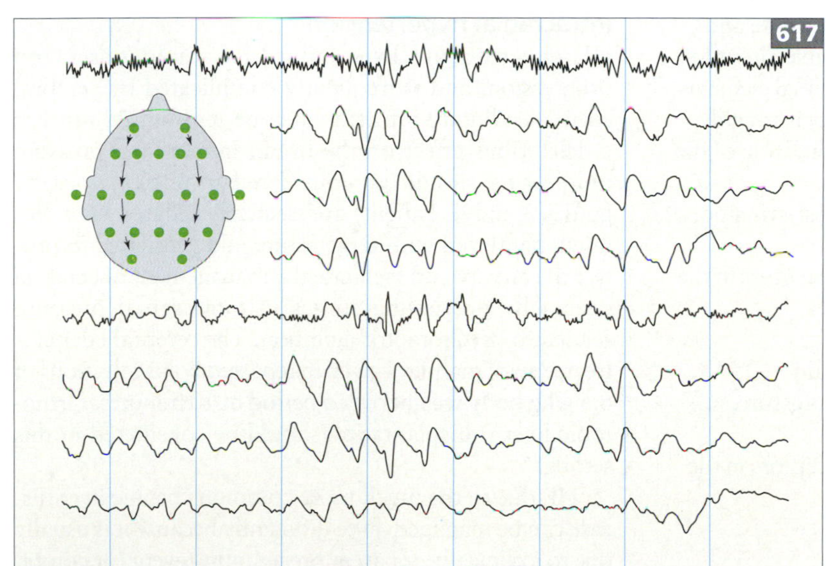

617 EEG, 8 channels, showing trains of medium to high amplitude bisynchronous, frontal-dominant, triphasic waves with a frequency of 1.5–2.5 Hz and phase lag from front to back. Triphasic waves are often seen in patients with an acute deterioration in conscious state due to metabolic disorders such as hepatic or renal failure, or cerebral anoxia. Atypical triphasic waves may rarely be seen in herpes simplex encephalitis, drug withdrawal, Creutzfeldt–Jakob disease, or following head trauma.

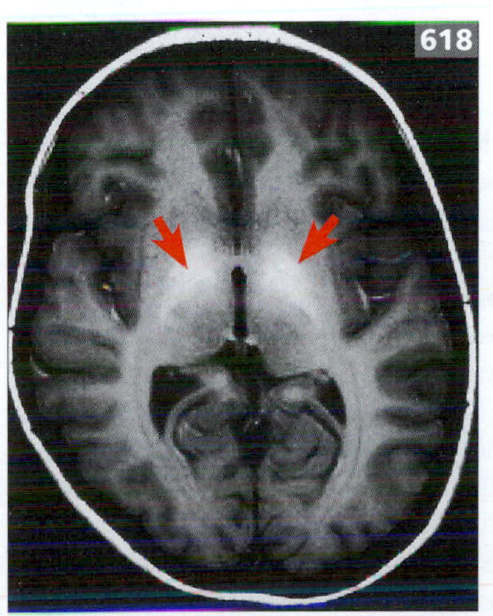

618, 619 T1W axial (618) and T1W sagittal (619) MRI of the brain in a patient with hepatic encephalopathy. Note the increased signal in the basal ganglia (arrows). *Courtesy of Dr R Gibson, Department of Neuroradiology, Western General Hospital, Edinburgh, UK.*

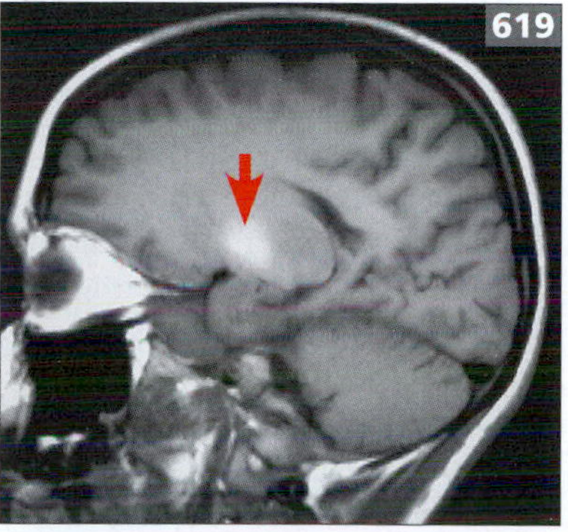

Diagnosis

The diagnosis is based on the history, physical examination, and laboratory findings to:

- Determine the presence of encephalopathy (subclinical or overt).
- Establish hepatocellular insufficiency and increased porto-systemic shunting.

Pathology

- Porto-systemic encephalopathy associated with chronic liver disease.
  - Large Alzheimer type 2 astrocytes (astrocytes containing characteristic glycogen inclusions with periodic acid–Schiff [PAS] staining) are the cardinal neuropathologic feature of porto-systemic encephalopathy.
  - Astrocytic rather than neuronal changes: diffuse increase in the number and size of the protoplasmic astrocytes in the deep layers of the cerebral cortex, lenticular nucleus, thalamus, substantia nigra, cerebellar cortex, and red, dentate, and pontine nuclei, with little or no visible alteration in the nerve cells or other parenchymal elements. The degree of this glial abnormality is roughly proportional to the intensity and duration of the neurologic disorder.
  - Reduced number of pallidal D2 post-synaptic receptors by about 50%.
  - Increased 5-hydroxytryptophan receptors in the hippocampus.
- Acute fulminant liver failure:
  - Cytotoxic brain edema (blood–brain barrier intact), raised intracranial pressure, herniation.
  - Loss of non-NMDA glutamate receptors in the brain.

Treatment

Treatment is determined by the underlying cause[39–41]:

- N-acetylcysteine for early paracetamol overdose.
- Forced diuresis and activated charcoal for mushroom poisoning.
- Acyclovir for herpes virus infection.
- Surgery for acute hepatic vein occlusion.
- Orthotopic liver transplantation: fulminant liver failure, and for severe, refractory HE.

  General measures include:
- Nasogastric tube.
- Central venous line.
- Indwelling urinary catheter.
- Monitor intracranial pressure if encephalopathy grades 3 or 4.
- Avoid maneuvers that increase intracranial pressure (such as sensorial stimuli):
  - Control restlessness.
  - Hydrate carefully.
  - Elevate patient's head 20–30°.
- Avoid (or use with extreme caution) drugs such as sedatives, phenytoin, phenobarbitone (phenobarbital), valproate, and dantrolene, because drug metabolism and protein binding are frequently disturbed in liver disease.
- Avoid/be careful with benzodiazepines, because plasma half-life of benzodiazepines is increased and substantial toxicity may ensue. For patients who have previously been treated with benzodiazepines (e.g. for treatment of behavioral disturbance caused by HE), the administration of a benzodiazepine antagonist, such as flumazenil, may improve conscious level.
- Avoid hypoglycemia (monitor blood glucose).

Intracranial hypertension

HE due to acute liver failure has rapid onset and progression, and is frequently complicated by cerebral edema leading to intracranial hypertension. As this has a deleterious effect on the brain, intracranial pressure monitoring should be considered in encephalopathy grades 3 and 4. Patients are electively sedated with fentanyl, paralyzed with atracurium, and ventilated to protect the airway and facilitate the management of cerebral edema by preventing surges in intracranial pressure related to psychomotor agitation. The cerebral edema is treated with mannitol given in repeated bolus injections of 0.5 g/kg body weight over a period of 10 minutes. Orthotopic liver transplantation should be considered in this setting.

HE due to the much more common chronic liver disease can be managed quite differently because it is usually due to a clinically apparent precipitating event (or combination of events), or to the spontaneous development of porto-systemic shunting, and because cerebral edema is much less frequent.

Blood ammonia levels

Ammonia production should be reduced (restrict intake of dietary protein and inhibit urease-producing colonic bacteria):

- Oral nonabsorbable disaccharides such as lactulose or lactisol (lactose 100 g daily in lactase deficiency): 30–60 g/day to produce 2–4 soft stools daily.
- Oral antibiotics (such as neomycin 6 g daily, metronidazole 800 mg daily, or rifaximin 1200 mg daily) are used against urea-producing organisms. More recently, rifaximin 550 mg twice daily has been shown to be effective, preventing the occurrence of mental status changes in patients with recurrent HE.

Prognosis

The encephalopathy usually evolves over a period of days to weeks. Left untreated, patients usually progress to death. Sometimes the symptoms spontaneously regress completely or partially, and may fluctuate in severity for several weeks or months. Most manifestations are reversible with medical treatment.

Some patients have progressive debilitating neurologic syndromes such as dementia, spastic paraparesis, cerebellar degeneration, and extrapyramidal movement disorders that are associated with structural abnormalities of the central nervous system (CNS) and may be irreversible; the long-term effect of orthotopic liver transplantation on these manifestations is unclear.

UREMIC ENCEPHALOPATHY

Definition and epidemiology

A clinical neuropsychiatric syndrome characterized by abnormal mental status occurring in patients with uremia, which is the final stage of progressive renal insufficiency leading to multi-organ dysfunction.

- Prevalence: not well documented but considered to be an increasingly common disorder given its direct relationship with the prevalence of end-stage renal disease (ESRD), which rate has shown a steady increase over the last decades.
- Age: ESRD may affect individuals of all ages, but is more frequent in the elderly.
- Gender: M=F.

Etiology and pathophysiology

Etiology is complex and likely to be multifactorial[42,43]. Several organic metabolites accumulate in ESRD, including urea, uric acid, and guanidine products (such as guanidine, creatinine, guanidinosuccinic acid, and methylguanidine). Some of these endogenous compounds (mainly those guanidine related) are neurotoxic.

Metabolic changes that affect neuronal function occur in ESRD, such as acidosis, electrolyte imbalances (hyponatremia, hyperkalemia, hypocalcemia, and hypermagnesemia), and dysregulation of fluid management leading to either fluid overload or dehydration.

Amino acid abnormalities (including those related to tryptophan, phenylalanine, and glycine) may also contribute to uremic encephalopathy. There are increased levels of endogenous inhibitors of transketolase, a thiamine-dependent enzyme involved in axon-cylinder myelin sheath maintenance.

Uremic patients also have an imbalance between excitatory and inhibitory (GABA and glycine) neurotransmitters, which contributes to overall cerebral dysfunction. Also, hormonal changes have been reported, such as elevated parathyroid hormone (PTH), which increases the intracellular intake of calcium.

Clinical features

Clinical features are nonspecific of insidious onset. They may progress slowly or rapidly, and include[44]:

- Headache.
- Memory loss.
- Decreased attention and concentration.
- Behavioral changes, such as irritability, agitation, paranoid ideation, and psychosis.
- Malaise.
- Mental status changes, including confusion, stupor, and coma.
- Postural tremors.
- Asterixis.
- Myoclonus or minipolymyoclonus.
- Focal neurologic deficits suggest an alternative diagnosis.
- Uremic polyneuropathy. Usually axonal distal sensorimotor neuropathy (predominantly sensory in the early stages of renal insufficiency).

Differential diagnosis

Dialysis encephalopathy (or dialysis dementia)

- Progressive cognitive decline associated with the use of aluminum in dialysis.
- Myoclonus, dysarthria, tremors, asterixis, and seizures are commonly seen.
- Proximal myopathy.
- Nonfluent aphasia and response to diazepam may be observed; these features are atypical for uremic encephalopathy.

Dialysis disequilibrium syndrome

- Occurs in the setting of institution of dialysis in individuals with chronic renal failure.
- Hemodialysis removes rapidly small molecules (such as urea) from the blood. On the other hand, permeation of these solutes across cellular membranes may take hours. This creates a relative intracellular hyperosmotic state that leads to cytotoxic edema.
- Patients present with neurologic symptoms that start shortly after dialysis, including headache, disorientation, delirium, nausea, vomiting, myoclonus, malaise, seizures, coma and, in severe cases, death.
- Self-limited; usually subsides over several hours.
- In susceptible patients gentle dialysis is warranted.

Complications from renal transplantation

- Primary brain lymphoma.
- Opportunistic infections of the brain.
- Rejection encephalopathy.
- Posterior reversible leukoencephalopathy (see below)

Other conditions

- Neurodegenerative disorders (AD, frontotemporal dementia, dementia with Lewy bodies).
- Vascular dementia.
- Seizure disorder.
- Cerebral hemorrhage (patients are predisposed to suffer hemorrhagic complications due to platelet dysfunction that occurs in renal insufficiency).
- Metabolic abnormalities.
- Nutritional deficiencies.

Investigations[45]

- Laboratory studies:
  - Assess renal function (urea and creatinine).
  - Evaluate for other metabolic abnormalities (glycemia and electrolytes) or concomitant infectious process that may cause mental status changes.
  - CSF is usually normal.
- EEG:
  - Usually shows nonspecific generalized slowing of the background rhythm that becomes more severe as the encephalopathy worsens.
  - Triphasic waves may be seen in advanced cases.
  - Improves with dialysis (as opposed to dialysis disequilibrium syndrome).
- Imaging studies (brain CT and/or MRI): usually done to exclude a structural intracranial lesion if suspected (e.g. hemorrhage).

Diagnosis

Diagnosis is largely one of exclusion and based on the history, physical examination, and laboratory findings.

Pathology[46]

- Meningeal fibrosis, edema, vascular degeneration, neuronal loss, and demyelination of the brain.
- Cerebellar granule cell necrosis.
- Elevated aluminum levels in the cortex and spongiform changes in the outer three cortical layers may be seen in patients with dialysis dementia (see below).

Treatment

Treatment is of concomitant conditions that may contribute to cognitive decline:

- Metabolic abnormalities.
- Electrolyte imbalance.
- Severe anemia.
- Fluid status.
- Infections.
- Acid/base disturbance.
- Intracerebral hemorrhage.
- Subdural hematoma.

Symptoms usually improve as the renal function recovers. Drugs whose metabolism depends on renal function or that may cause cognitive impairment (such as sedatives) should be used with caution. For siezures, anticonvulsants are usually used; however, levels may need to be adjusted by renal function and protein level, and the administration of some anticonvulsants needs to be timed to the dialysis schedule.

Prognosis

Uremic encephalopathy usually responds favorably to medical treatment. Left untreated, it leads to coma and death.

POSTERIOR REVERSIBLE ENCEPHALOPATHY SYNDROME

Definition and epidemiology

Posterior reversible encephalopathy syndrome (PRES) is a clinicoradiologic syndrome characterized by headache, altered mental status, seizures, and blurred vision in association with radiologic evidence of vasogenic edema involving predominantly the brain parenchyma supplied by the posterior circulation. It is also known as 'posterior reversible leukoencephalopahty syndrome'; however, this term may be misleading as PRES is not necessarily restricted to the white matter (**620–623**)[47]. PRES may be seen in the setting of:

- Hypertensive encephalopathy (as seen in hypertensive emergency).
- Preclampsia and eclampsia (hypertensive emergency in pregnancy).
- Hemolysis, elevated liver enzymes, low-platelet count) syndrome (HELLP).
- Acute and chronic renal diseases (e.g. acute glomerulonephritis and uremic encephalopathy).
- Liver failure.
- Endocrine disorders (pheochromocytoma, primary aldosteronism).
- Hypercalcemia/hyperparathyroidism.
- Blood transfusion.
- Thrombotic thrombocytopenic purpura.
- Hemolytic uremic syndrome.
- Collagen vascular diseases.
- Immunosupressive/cytotoxic therapy (calcineurin inhibitors [tacrolimus and cyclosporine], antineoplastic drugs, antiretroviral therapy, and interferon-α)[39].
- Sympathomimetic drugs (cocaine or amphetamines).
- Corticosteroid treatment.
- Withdrawal from antihypertensive agents[48,49].

Prevalence is not well documented but it is an increasingly recognized disorder.

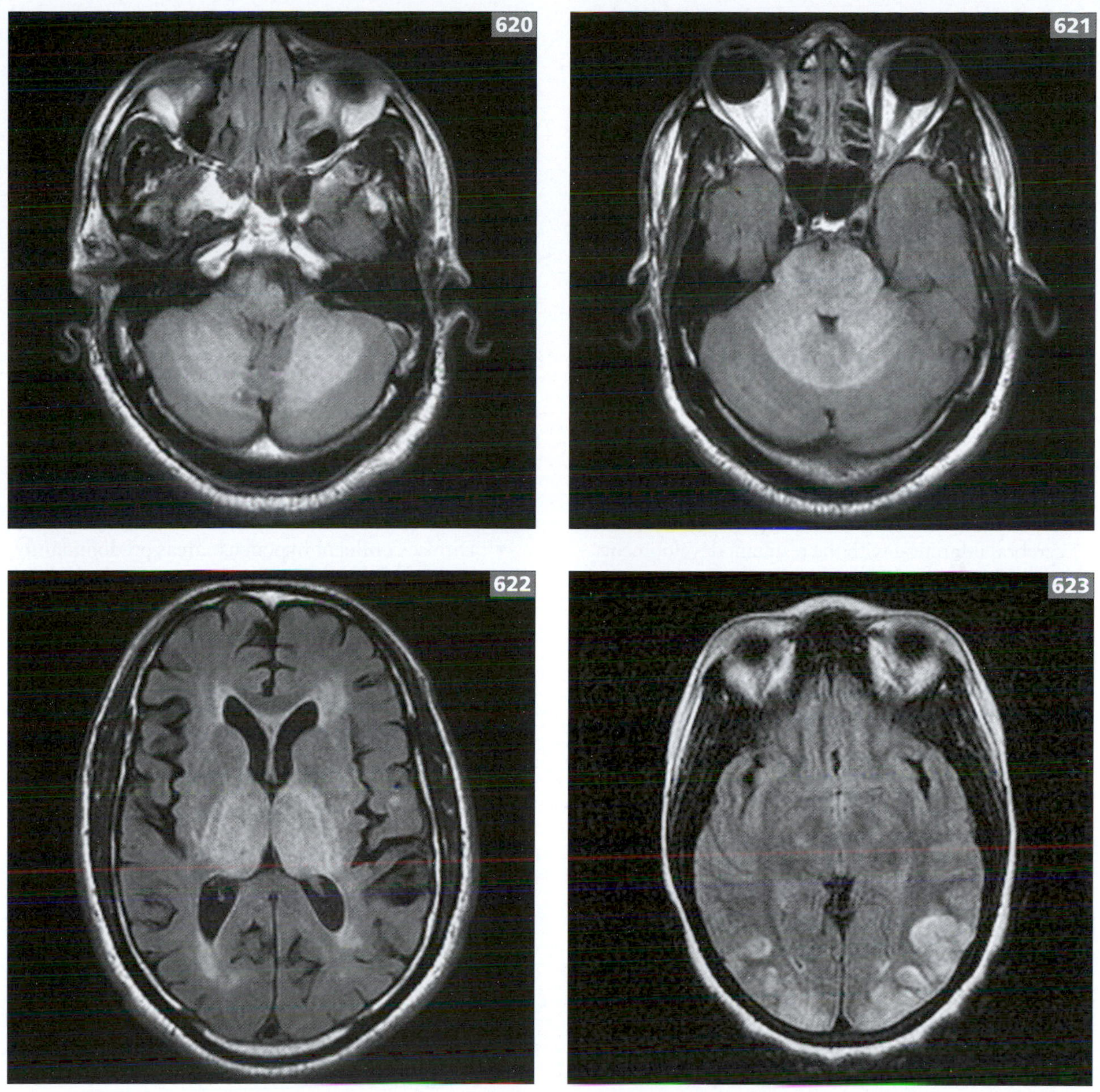

620–623 Posterior reversible encephalopathy syndrome (PRES). Vasogenic edema is noted in the cerebellum (620), pons (621), and thalamus (622) (FLAIR sequence). PRES may, in some cases, involve the gray matter as well (623) (T2 sequence).

Etiology and pathophysiology

Etiology is complex and not completely described[50]:

- Autoregulatory disturbance and endothelial dysfunction have been proposed as key pathogenic mechanisms of PRES.
- Immunosuppressive/cytotoxic agents (e.g. tacrolimus) are toxic to the endothelial cell and cause endothelial dysfunction.
- Blood pressure levels exceeding the upper limit tolerated by vascular autoregulatory mechanisms (as seen in hypertensive encephalopathy) would increase the permeability of the blood–brain barrier allowing the extravasation of fluid into the extravascular space and cause vasogenic edema.
- In an attempt to preserve cerebral blood flow within normal limits, autoregulatory mechanisms induce vasoconstriction. Therefore, areas of vasoconstriction and vasodilation may develop.
- Vasoconstriction may lead to hypoperfusion and cerebral infarction with the resultant development of cytotoxic edema; this occurs more frequently in border zone areas.
- The predilection to affect the posterior circulation has been related to its relatively deficient sympathetic innervation in comparison with that of the anterior circulation.

Tip

▶ *Approximately 15% of PRES cases have intraparenchymal hematoma or sulcal subarachnoid hemorrhage. These have been related to rupture of pial vessels in the face of severe hypertension and impaired cerebral autoregulation and hemorrhagic infarction.*

Clinical features

- Headache, nausea, and vomiting.
- Acute encephalopathy (somnolence, stupor, or coma).
- Behavioral changes (agitation, restlessness, or lethargy).
- Visual impairment (hemianopsia, visual neglect, or cortical blindness).
- Papilledema (which may manifest clinically with visual obscurations).
- Seizures (either focal or generalized).

Differential diagnosis

Broad, as the presentation is nonspecific:

- Stroke (ischemic or hemorrhagic).
- CNS vasculitis.
- Brain tumor.
- Cerebral venous sinus thrombosis.
- Multiple sclerosis.
- Connective tissue diseases with CNS involvement.
- Acute disseminated encephalomyelitis.
- Infective endocarditis.
- Metabolic abnormalities.
- Osmotic disarrangement.
- CNS opportunistic infection (particularly in those individuals treated with immunosuppressive treatment).
- Nutritional deficiencies.

Investigations[51]

- Head CT:
  - Diffuse confluent hypodense areas predominantly of the white matter with effacement of the cortical sulci suggestive of cerebral edema are usually observed in the posterior circulation (e.g. in the occipital or occipital–parietal areas but not necessarily restricted to these hemispheral areas).
  - Suboptimal sensitivity and specificity compared with brain MRI.
- Brain MRI:
  - FLAIR and T2 hyperintense (T1 hypointense) lesions usually affecting the white matter of the occipital and posterior parietal lobes. Changes may also involve the gray matter, frontal lobes, cerebellar hemispheres, brainstem, and basal ganglia (**620**).
  - Increased intensity in apparent diffusion coefficient (ADC) sequence consistent with vasogenic edema.
  - Discrete areas of cytotoxic edema consistent with cerebral infarction (hyperintense in diffusion-weighted imaging [DWI] and hypointense in ADC) may be seen.
  - Hypointense lesions in gradient ECHO ($T2^*$-weighted) or susceptibility-weighted (SWI) sequences denote the presence of blood products.

Diagnosis

Diagnosis is based on the history and findings on neuroimaging studies (mainly brain MRI).

Pathology

- Vascular fibrinoid necrosis.
- Arteriolar and capillary thrombosis.
- Microinfarcts and cerebral edema.

Treatment

Treatment is directed at the cause of PRES[52]:

- Use blood pressure lowering medications in hypertensive encephalopathy.
- Withdraw offending agent in cases of drug-related PRES.
- Delivery in pregnant woman with eclampsia.
- Seizure management.
- Maintain adequate oxygenation.

Hypertensive encephalopathy

- Intravenous agents, particularly beta blockers (e.g. labetalol) or calcium channel blockers (e.g. nicardipine), are usually preferred.
- Vasodilators (such as nitroglycerine, hydralazine, and sodium nitroprusside) have the potential to increase the intracranial pressure and should therefore be avoided, if possible.

In normal individuals, autoregulation holds relatively constant cerebral blood flow across a wide rage of mean arterial blood pressure (approximately 50–150 mmHg). Patients with chronic hypertension may have the autoregulatory curve shifted towards higher blood pressure values (**624**). In these cases abrupt blood pressure lowering may precipitate or worsen ischemia in those areas with hypoperfusion and/or abnormal autoregulation. Therefore, rapid but controlled lowering of blood pressure is recommended.

Blood pressure goal is that at baseline prior to presentation. Lowering the mean arterial pressure by ~25% in the first 8 hours in the absence of acute (ischemic or hemorrhagic) stroke is usually considered safe.

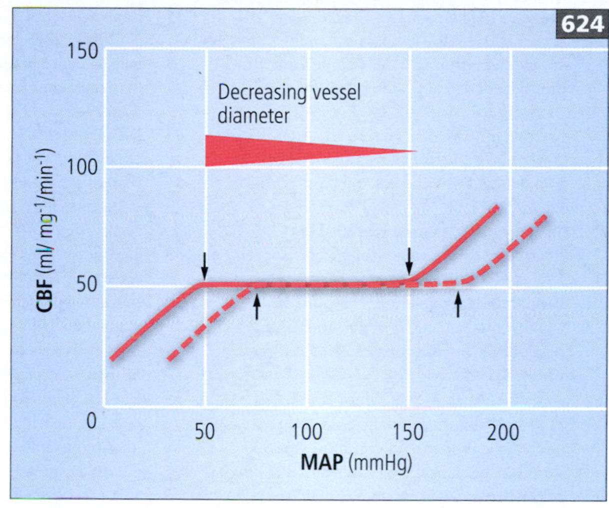

624 Cerebral autoregulation curve. In the normal state (solid line), the cerebral blood flow (CBF) is held constant across a wide range of mean arterial pressures (MAP, 50–150 mmHg). In chronic hypertension (dashed line), the autoregulation curves shifts to the right.

Prognosis

PRES responds favorably to the appropriate medical treatment. The term 'reversible', however, refers mainly to the vasogenic edema evidenced on MRI; persistent neurologic deficits may occur in those cases with stroke. Left untreated, it may lead to coma and death.

REFERENCES

1 Zubaran C, Fernandes JG, Rodnight R (1997). Wernicke–Korsakoff syndrome. *Postgrad Med J* 73:27–31.

2 McLean J, Manchip S (1999). Wernicke's encephalopathy induced by magnesium depletion. *Lancet* 353:1768.

3 Suter PM, Haller J, Hany A, Vetter W (2000). Diuretic use: a risk for subclinical thiamine deficiency in elderly patients. *J Nutr Health Aging* 4:69–71.

4 Zahr NM, Kaufman KL, Harper CG (2011). Clinical and pathological features of alcohol-related brain damage. *Nat Rev Neurol* 7:284–94.

5 Cerase A, Rubenni E, Rufa A, *et al.* (2011). CT and MRI of Wernicke's encephalopathy. *Radiol Med* 116:319–333.

6 Kobayashi M, Kaneko A, Matsunaga T (2011). MRI findings in nonalcoholic Wernicke's encephalopathy. *Intern Med* 50:2245–2246.

7 Day E, Bentham P, Callaghan R, Kuruvilla T, George S (2004). Thiamine for Wernicke–Korsakoff syndrome in people at risk from alcohol abuse. *Cochrane Database Syst Rev* 1: CD004033.

8 Onishi H, Kawanishi C, Onose M, *et al.* (2004). Successful treatment of Wernicke encephalopathy in terminally ill cancer patients: report of 3 cases and review of the literature. *Support Care Cancer* 12:604–608.

9 Amess JA, Burman JF, Rees GM, Nancekievill DG, Mollin DL (1987). Megaloblastic haemopoiesis in patients receiving nitrous oxide. *Lancet* 2:339–342.

10 Mayall M (1999). Vitamin B12 deficiency and nitrous oxide. *Lancet* 353:1529.

11 Thomas PK (1998). Subacute combined degeneration. *J Neurol Neurosurg Psychiatry* 65:807.

12 Andres E, Serraj K (2012). Optimal management of pernicious anemia. *J Blood Med* 3:97–103.

13 Hemmer B, Glocker FX, Schumacher M, *et al.* (1998). Subacute combined degeneration: clinical, electrophysiological, and magnetic resonance imaging findings. *J Neurol Neurosurg Psychiatry* 65:822–827.

14 Green R, Kinsella LJ (1995). Current concepts in the diagnosis of cobalamin deficiency. *Neurology* 45:1435–1440.

15 Delpre G, Stark P, Niv Y (1999). Sublingual therapy for cobalamin deficiency as an alternative to oral and parenteral cobalamin supplementation. *Lancet* 354:740–741.

16 Elia M (1998). Oral or parenteral therapy for vitamin B12 deficiency? *Lancet* 352:1721–1722.

17 Eussen SJ, de Groot LC, Clarke R, *et al.* (2005). Oral cyanocobalamin supplementation in older people with vitamin B12 deficiency: a dose-finding trial. *Arch Intern Med* **165**:1167–1172.
18 Kuzminski AM, Del Giacco EJ, Allen RH, *et al.* (1998). Effective treatment of cobalamin deficiency with oral cobalamin. *Blood* **98**:1191–1198.
19 Stevenson VL, Hardie RJ (2001). Acanthocytosis and neurological disorders. *J Neurol* **248**:87–94.
20 Ricciarelli R, Argellati F, Pronzato MA, Domenicotti C (2007). Vitamin E and neurodegenerative diseases. *Mol Aspects Med* **28**:591–606.
21 Aslam A, Misbah SA, Talbot K, Chapel H (2004). Vitamin E deficiency induced neurological disease in common variable immunodeficiency: two cases and a review of the literature of vitamin E deficiency. *Clin Immunol* **112**:24–29.
22 Huang SH, Schall JI, Zemel BS, Stallings VA (2006). Vitamin E status in children with cystic fibrosis and pancreatic insufficiency. *J Pediatr* **148**:556–559.
23 Jorgensen RA, Lindor KD, Sartin JS, LaRusso NF, Wiesner RH (1995). Serum lipid and fat-soluble vitamin levels in primary sclerosing cholangitis. *J Clin Gastroenterol* **20**:215–219.
24 Gabsi S, Gouider-Khouja N, Belal S, *et al.* (2001). Effect of vitamin E supplementation in patients with ataxia with vitamin E deficiency. *Eur J Neurol* **8**:477–481.
25 Greenberg DM, Lee JW (2001). Psychotic manifestations of alcoholism. *Curr Psychiatry Rep* **3**:314–318.
26 Hegyi J, Schwartz RA, Hegyi V (2004). Pellagra: dermatitis, dementia, and diarrhea. *Int J Dermatol* **43**:1–5.
27 Said HM (2011). Intestinal absorption of water-soluble vitamins in health and disease. *Biochem J* **437**:357–372.
28 Prousky JE (2003). Pellagra may be a rare secondary complication of anorexia nervosa: a systematic review of the literature. *Altern Med Rev* **8**:180–185.
29 Lemoine A, Le Devehat C (1989). Clinical conditions requiring elevated dosages of vitamins. *Int J Vitam Nutr Res Suppl* **30**:129–147.
30 Feuerlein W (1977). Neuropsychiatric disorders of alcoholism. *Nutr Metab* **21**:163–174.
31 Bano S, Mehra S, Yadav SN, Chaudhary V (2009). Marchiafava–Bignami disease: role of neuroimaging in the diagnosis and management of acute disease. *Neurol India* **57**:649–652.
32 Ménégon P, Sibon I, Pachai C, Orgogozo JM, Dousset V (2005). Marchiafava-Bignami disease: diffusion-weighted MRI in corpus callosum and cortical lesions. *Neurology* **65**:475–477.
33 Geibprasert S, Gallucci M, Krings T (2010). Alcohol-induced changes in the brain as assessed by MRI and CT. *Eur Radiol* **20**:1492–1501.
34 Mas A, Rodes J (1997). Fulminant hepatic failure. *Lancet* **349**:1081–1085.
35 Lui HF, Jalan R, Hayes PC (1998). Hepatic encephalopathy: pathogenesis, diagnosis and management. *Proc R Coll Physicians Edinb* **28**:111–118.
36 Jalan R, Hayes PC (1997). Hepatic encephalopathy and ascites. *Lancet* **350**:1309–1315.
37 Jones EA, Weissenborn K (1997). Neurology and the liver. *J Neurol Neurosurg Psychiatry* **63**:279–293.
38 Blei AT, Córdoba J (2001). Hepatic encephalopathy. *Am J Gastroenterol* **96**:1968–1976.
39 Bass NM, Mullen KD, Sanyal A, *et al.* (2010). Rifaximin treatment in hepatic encephalopathy. *N Engl J Med.* **362:1071–1081.**
40 Riordan SM, Williams R (1997). Treatment of hepatic encephalopathy. *N Engl J Med* **337**:473–479.
41 Zafirova Z, O'connor M (2010). Hepatic encephalopathy: current management strategies and treatment, including management and monitoring of cerebral edema and intracranial hypertension in fulminant hepatic failure. *Curr Opin Anaesthesiol* **23**:121–127.
42 De Deyn PP, Vanholder R, D'Hooge R (2003). Nitric oxide in uremia: effects of several potentially toxic guanidino compounds. *Kidney Int Suppl* 2, **84**:S25–S28.
43 Fraser CL, Arieff AI (1988). Nervous system complications in uremia. *Ann Intern Med* **109**:143–153.
44 Lacerda G, Krummel T, Hirsch E (2010). Neurologic presentations of renal diseases. *Neurol Clin* **28**:45–59.
45 Mahoney CA, Arieff AI (1982). Uremic encephalopathies: clinical, biochemical, and experimental features. *Am J Kidney Dis* **2**:324–336.
46 Alfrey AC (1985). Dialysis encephalopathy. *Clin Nephrol Suppl* **1**:S15–S19.
47 Bakshi R, Bates VE, Mechtler LL, Kinkel PR, Kinkel WR (1998). Occipital lobe seizures as the major clinical manifestation of reversible posterior leukoencephalopathy syndrome: magnetic resonance imaging findings. *Epilepsia* **39**:295–299.
48 Erbetta A, Salmaggi A, Sghirlanzoni A, *et al.* (2008). Clinical and radiological features of brain neurotoxicity caused by antitumor and immunosuppressant treatments. *Neurol Sci* **29**: 131–137.
49 Gocmen R, Ozgen B, Oguz KK (2007). Widening the spectrum of PRES: series from a tertiary care center. *Eur J Radiol* **62**:454–459.
50 Lee VH, Wijdicks EF, Manno EM, Rabinstein AA (2008). Clinical spectrum of reversible posterior leukoencephalopathy syndrome. *Arch Neurol* **65**:205–210.
51 Stevens CJ, Heran MK (2012). The many faces of posterior reversible encephalopathy syndrome. *Br J Radiol* **85**:1566–1575.
52 Perez MI, Musini VM (2008). Pharmacological interventions for hypertensive emergencies. *Cochrane Database Syst Rev* **1**:CD003653.

Further reading

Beavers K, Frederick T, Teperman L, *et al.* (2010) Rifaximin treatment in hepatic encephalopathy. *N Engl J Med* **362**:1071–1081.

Rosener M, Dichgans J (1996). Severe combined degeneration of the spinal cord after nitrous oxide anaesthesia in a vegetarian. *J Neurol Neurosurg Psychiatry* **60**:354.

Rusche-Skolarus LE, Lucey BP, Vo KD, Snider BJ (2007). Transient encephalopathy in a postoperative nonalcoholic female with Marchiafava–Bignami disease. *Clin Neurol Neurosurg* **109**:713–715.

Stabler SP (2013). Clinical practice. Vitamin B12 deficiency. *N Engl J Med* **368**:149–160.

DISORDERS OF CIRCULATION OF THE CEREBROSPINAL FLUID

Daniel B. Hier, Edward A. Michals

INTRODUCTION

Cerebrospinal fluid (CSF) is produced by the choroid plexus within the ventricles (mainly residing in the roof of the third ventricle and the floors of the lateral ventricles) at a rate of approximately 0.35 ml/min or 500 ml/24 hr. Total CSF volume is estimated to be approximately 150 ml. It is larger in men than women, and larger in older individuals than younger individuals due to an increase in ventricular size with age. CSF circulates downward from the lateral and third ventricle, through the cerebral aqueduct into the fourth ventricle where it exits into the subarachnoid space around the brain, and communicates with the subarachnoid space around the spinal cord[1]. Spinal CSF volume is estimated to be about 50 ml. CSF is absorbed back into the superior sagittal sinus through the arachnoid villi, via a valve-like one-way mechanism that prevents sinus blood from entering into the subarachnoid space (**625**).

Resorption of CSF at the arachnoid villi requires a positive pressure in the subarachnoid space of at least 60 mm of water. At CSF pressures of less than 60 mmH_2O, resorption probably does not occur at the arachnoid villi.

Normal CSF pressure in the recumbent position is 65–195 mmH_2O. In the recumbent position, CSF pressure is equalized between the ventricles and the brain and spinal subarachnoid spaces. In the erect position, a pressure gradient forms with lower pressures at the vertex (sometimes negative) and higher pressures in the lumbar subarachnoid space.

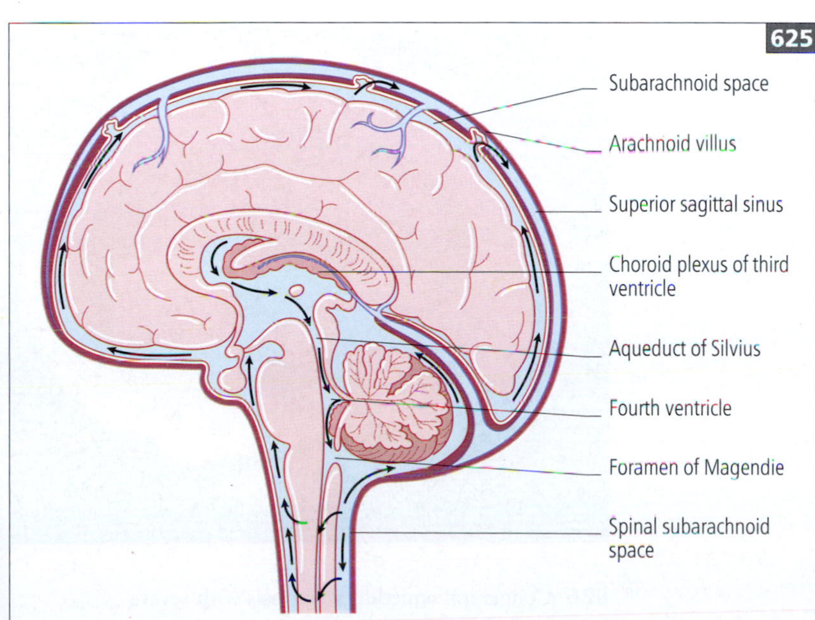

625 CSF is produced at the floor of the lateral ventricles and the roof of the third ventricle by the choroid plexus. It then flows downward through the aqueduct of Sylvius into the fourth ventricle and out into the subarachnoid space through the foramen of Magendie and the paired foramina of Luschka. CSF flows downward into the spinal subarachnoid space and upward around the cerebral convexities, where it is eventually resorbed back into the superior sagittal sinus by the arachnoid villi.

AQUEDUCTAL STENOSIS WITH HYDROCEPHALUS

Definition and epidemiology

Aqueductal stenosis is the most common cause of non-communicating hydrocephalus. In hydrocephalus due to aqueductal stenosis, ventricles are variously enlarged depending on the severity of the stenosis and the compliance (stiffness) of the ventricles. The hydrocephalus of aqueductal stenosis is classified as 'noncommunicating' because there is either incomplete or absent communication between the lumbar subarachnoid space and the lateral ventricles of the brain.

Aqueductal stenosis with hydrocephalus may become apparent either in infancy (shortly after birth) or in adult-hood. The incidence of congenital hydrocephalus at birth is estimated to be 0.2–0.8 children per 1000 live births[2]. Accurate figures of incidence of adult onset aqueductal stenosis are not available.

Etiology and pathophysiology

Since the obstruction in aqueductal stenosis is above the fourth ventricle, the lateral and third ventricles are enlarged whereas the fourth ventricle is small or normal-sized. In many cases, the stenosis at the aqueduct is incomplete causing a decrease in CSF flow through the aqueduct rather than complete blockage. Complete blockage at the aqueduct is generally not compatible with survival in the absence of a CSF diversion procedure (**626**).

Aqueductal stenosis (narrowing of the cerebral aqueduct) may be due a variety of causes:

- Congenital narrowing.
- Midbrain tumors.
- Perinatal intraventricular hemorrhage.
- Meningitis.
- Ventriculitis.

Tip

▶ *In aqueductal stenosis, the lateral and third ventricles are disproportionately enlarged compared to the fourth ventricle.*

Differential diagnosis

The etiology of aqueductal stenosis should be established when possible.

- Meningitis, ventriculitis, peri-aqueductal tumors, and intraventricular hemorrhages as causes should be distinguished from congenital aqueductal stenosis.
- Other causes of hydrocephalus should be considered including communicating hydrocephalus and normal pressure hydrocephalus (NPH).
- Distinguish aqueductal stenosis from macrocephaly (a large head and brain without hydrocephalus).
- Distinguish aqueductal stenosis from hydrocephalus ex vacuo (enlargement of the ventricles due to cortical atrophy).

Clinical features

Adult-onset patients with aqueductal stenosis generally have headache. Other frequent symptoms include:

- Gait disorder.
- Memory impairment.
- Urinary incontinence.

The key symptoms of patients with adult onset aqueductal stenosis closely resemble those of patients with NPH[3]. Less common symptoms include:

- Blurred vision.
- Tremor.
- Parinaud's syndrome (paralysis of upgaze with large pupils).

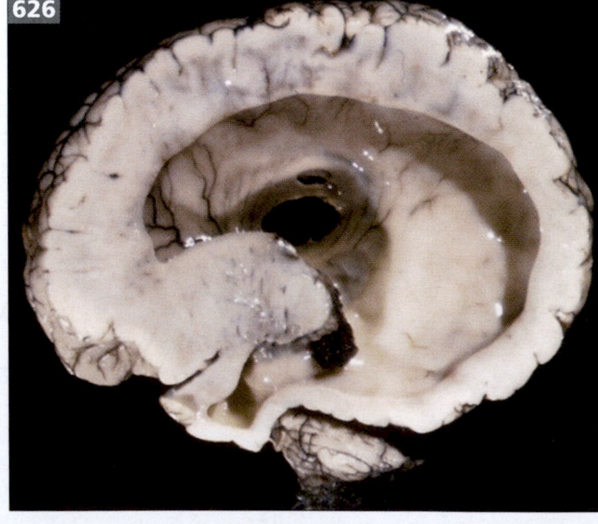

626 Congenital aqueductal stenosis with severe hydrocephalus not compatible with survival.

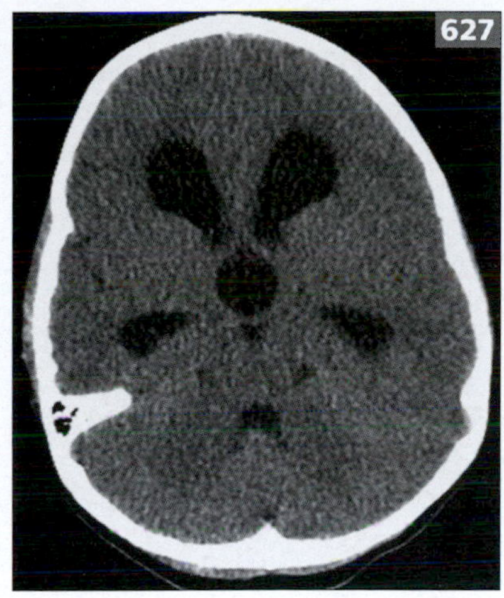

627 Hydrocephalus due to aqueductal stenosis. CT scan shows enlarged lateral and third ventricle. The fourth ventricle is normal in size. The cerebral aqueduct is difficult to visualize on CT.

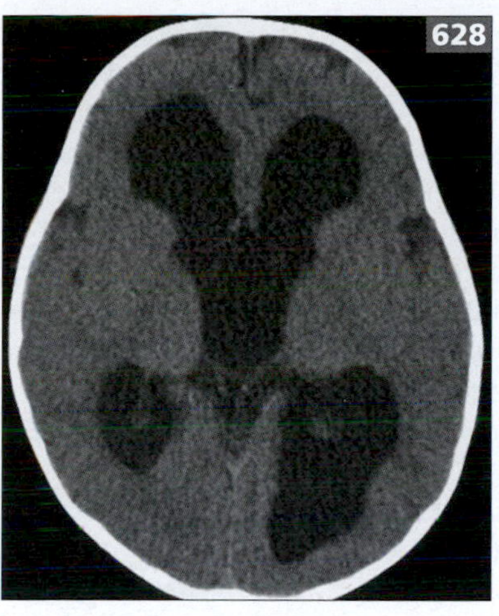

628 CT scan of aqueductal stenosis. Note the massively enlarged lateral and third ventricles

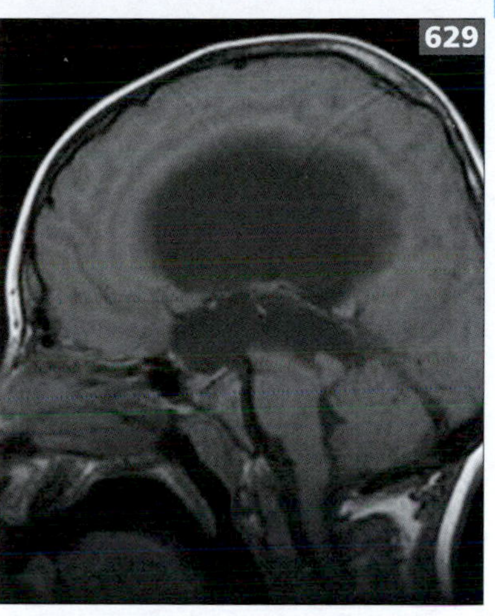

629 Aqueductal stenosis with enlarged lateral and third ventricles. MRI shows narrowed cerebral aqueduct and small fourth ventricle.

Investigations and diagnosis

Magnetic resonance imaging (MRI) and computed tomography (CT) show enlarged lateral and third ventricles with a normal or small fourth ventricle (627–629). Phase contrast MRI is a method for determining if there is flow in the aqueduct. This test can be useful in confirming the diagnosis of aqueductal stenosis and the need for shunting or ventriculostomy of the thirrd ventricle[4].

In cases of aqueductal stenosis, radionuclide cisternography will show no tracer entering the ventricles from the lumbar subarachnoid space.

Treatment

Most patients are treated with ventricular drainage by use of shunt with valves. Current treatment usually involves placement of an adjustable valve (programmable) to allow the amount of drainage to be adjusted:

- Some shunts may under-drain. Under-drainage may be indicated by intracranial pressure (ICP) greater than 200 mmH_2O when lying flat.
- Some shunts may over-drain. Over-drainage is indicated by negative ICP of 100 mmH_2O or more when standing or sitting up.
- Some patients are being treated by ventriculostomy (third ventriculostomy) which obviates the need for a shunt.

Prognosis

The main problem with treatment of aqueductal stenosis by ventriculo-peritoneal shunting is the high complication rate, including:

- Shunt infection.
- Over-drainage.
- Subdural hematoma.
- Subdural hygroma.

At 5 years, the complication rate after shunting can be as high as 50%. Some adult-onset aqueductal stenosis patients with hydrocephalus are asymptomatic and can be followed longitudinally. Symptomatic aqueductal stenosis patients who are not shunted are likely to have continuation of their headache, as well as progressive difficulties with gait, cognition, and sphincter control.

COMMUNICATING HYDROCEPHALUS

Definition and epidemiology

In communicating hydrocephalus the ventricles are enlarged but the ventricles freely communicate with the lumbar subarachnoid space. The usual cause of communicating hydrocephalus is blockage of absorption of the CSF (either in the subarachnoid space around the brain or at the arachnoid villi or pacchionian granulations where resorption occurs). ICP is usually increased except in cases of NPH.

Communicating hydrocephalus in adults is uncommon but not rare[5]. Prevalence rates in the USA are estimated to be between 1 and 2 per 1000 persons. No gender differences in incidence or prevalence of communicating hydrocephalus have been established.

Tip

▶ *In communicating hydrocephalus absorption of CSF is usually impaired, ventricular size is increased, and ICP is increased.*

Etiology and pathophysiology

In most cases of communicating hydrocephalus the flow of CSF is blocked in the subarachnoid space over the convexities of the brain, or resorption of CSF is blocked at the arachnoid villi along the sagittal sinus. In communicating hydrocephalus, the ventricular system communicates freely with the lumbar subarachnoid space. Due to problems in resorption of CSF at the arachnoid villi, intracranial CSF volume and ICP increases. This increase in ICP causes the ventricles to enlarge. With increased ICP, CSF resorption increases and equilibrium between production and resorption is re-established.

Usual causes of communicating hydrocephalus include:

- Infection (meningitis, ventriculitis).
- Inflammation (neurosarcoidosis, lupus cerebritis).
- Hemorrhage (intraventricular hemorrhage, aneurysmal subarachnoid hemorrhage).

Differential diagnosis

Communicating hydrocephalus needs to be distinguished from other causes of ventricular enlargement, such as:

- Hydrocephalus due to aqueductal stenosis.
- Ventricular enlargement due to cortical atrophy (hydrocephalus ex vacuo).

Clinical features

- Headache is common with communicating hydrocephalus. If ventricular enlargement is marked and ICP increased, lethargy, obtundation, or even coma can ensue.
- Frontal lobe dysfunction is common. Mental slowness, cognitive impairment, and abulia are clinical features of communicating hydrocephalus.
- Gait disorders are common with a shuffling slow gait that may be confused with Parkinson's disease.
- Progressive ventricular enlargement with frontal lobe dysfunction can lead to urinary incontinence and sphincter disturbances.

Investigations and diagnosis

MRI and CT will confirm ventricular enlargement that is disproportionate to any cortical atrophy. In communicating hydrocephalus, all ventricles including the fourth ventricle are enlarged.

Lumbar puncture usually shows elevated ICP except in cases of NPH (see below). An examination of the CSF is essential to establishing etiology of the communicating hydrocephalus:

- Cultures for bacteria, such as *M. tuberculosis*, and fungi should be obtained to exclude acute or subacute infection.
- Pleocytosis may point to either an inflammatory or infectious cause for the communicating hydrocephalus.
- Elevated CSF protein with minimal pleocytosis may suggest neurosarcoidosis or other noninfectious inflammatory processes that can produce communicating hydrocephalus.

Treatment

Treatment for communicating hydrocephalus includes treatment of any underlying conditions. Most cases are treated with a ventriculo-peritoneal shunt. Recently third ventriculostomy has emerged as an alternative to ventriculo–peritoneal shunting.

Prognosis

Most patients improve dramatically with ventriculo-peritoneal shunting and treatment of any underlying etiological illnesses. Shunt failures and shunt infections may be common complications. Other problems may include the shunt over-drainage syndrome with headache, subdural hematoma, or subdural hygroma. Shunt revisions are commonly required.

NORMAL PRESSURE HYDROCEPHALUS

Definition and epidemiology

NPH should be considered a special instance of communicating hydrocephalus with normal ICP. NPH is often recognized because of the clinical triad of gait disorder, urinary incontinence, and cognitive impairment.

The exact prevalence of NPH is unknown. In the USA, the total number of cases is estimated to be about 175,000 or 1 per 2000 persons[6]. The prevalence in the elderly is much higher, possibly as high as 1 in 200 persons. Among persons with dementia, the prevalence is at least 1 in 100 or higher. No gender differences in prevalence or incidence have been established.

Tip

▶ *NPH is considered a special case of communicating hydrocephalus with normal ICP.*

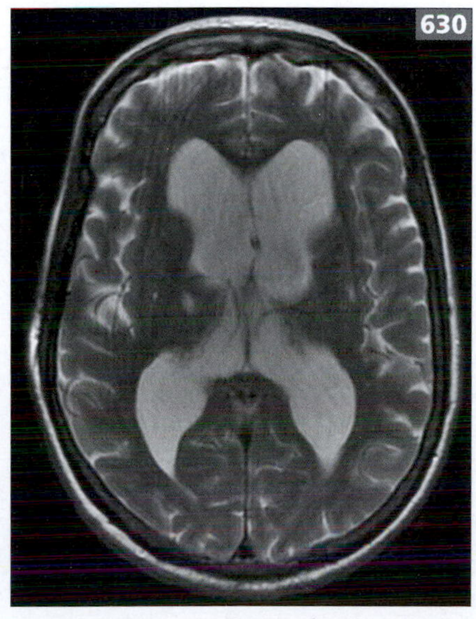

630 MRI (T2-weighted image) shows ventricular enlargement in normal pressure hydrocephalus (NPH). Note the ischemic infarct in the right thalamic area. Ischemic changes are often noted in elderly patients with NPH.

Etiology and pathophysiology

In NPH, ventricular enlargement occurs in the absence of an increase in ICP (630). The degree of ventricular enlargement is disproportionate to any cortical atrophy. The ventricles enlarge due either a block in flow of the CSF in the subarachnoid spaces, or a failure to resorb CSF at the arachnoid villi.

Some cases of NPH appear to be entirely idiopathic with no obvious precipitating cause. Other cases can be related to prior head trauma, brain surgery, subarachnoid hemorrhage, or meningitis. Conditions that can either sclerose the subarachnoid CSF pathways or damage the arachnoid villi seem especially prone to cause NPH.

Differential diagnosis

NPH must be distinguished from hydrocephalus originating in childhood such as aqueductal stenosis or communicating hydrocephalus. If hydrocephalus begins before age 6 years when skull sutures are closing, head circumference will generally be increased (above 59 cm in men and above 57.5 cm in women).

NPH should be distinguished from other neurologic conditions that produce a shuffling gait such as Parkinson's disease, Lewy body dementia, frontotemporal dementia, stroke, and Alzheimer's disease.

Other causes of gait disorder should be considered including cervical spondylosis with myelopathy, lumbar stenosis, cauda equina syndrome, polyneuropathy, and spinocerebellar atrophies.

Clinical features

Patients with NPH often do not have classic features of hydrocephalus associated with increased ICP such as headache, nausea, or vomiting. The diagnosis is usually made when the triad of urinary incontinence, gait disorder, and cognitive impairment is observed in the setting of enlarged ventricles. Because of the many other possible causes for the symptoms of NPH in the elderly that must be ruled out, the existence of NPH as an independent condition has been viewed with skepticism by some.

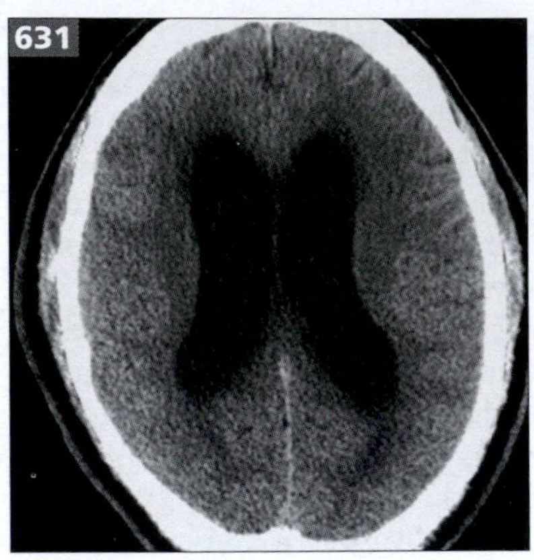

631 CT scan showing ventricular enlargement in normal pressure hydrocephalus. Both lateral ventricles are enlarged. Note the absence of cortical atrophy.

Investigations and diagnosis

Either MR or CT scanning will show enlargement of the ventricles consistent with NPH (**631**). Some enlargement of the subarachnoid space over the convexities of the brain does not definitely rule out NPH but may cast doubt on the diagnosis.

Some patients have coexisting cerebrovascular disease and some patients will remain candidates for shunting for NPH, despite the presence of deep lacunar infarcts on CT or MR. Patients with severe cortical atrophy on CT or MRI are unlikely to be responsive to ventriculo-peritoneal shunting.

A positive response to CSF drainage after 72 hours is a positive predictor of shunt responsiveness in patients with possible NPH. Continuous CSF pressure monitoring has not proven to be predictive of shunt responsiveness.

Treatment

Patients who are felt to be appropriate candidates for ventriculo-peritoneal shunting can be treated with shunts with programmable valves. A programmable valve minimizes the risk of siphoning or over-drainage of the ventricles and may be useful in preventing either subdural hygromas or subdural hematomas[7,8].

Prognosis

Patients with NPH have a higher risk of dying than the general population. One study found that patients with NPH were 3.3 times more likely to die than a comparably aged population[9]. After shunting, gait is improved in 64% at 3 months and 26% are improved at 3 years. Fewer than 10% show sustained improvement on cognitive tests 5 years after shunting.

Nearly one-half of patients who are shunted will require shunt revision within 3 years for shunt malfunction or infection.

CHIARI MALFORMATION

Definition and epidemiology

Chiari Type I malformation is downward herniation of the hindbrain through the foramen magnum. Herniation always involves the cerebellar tonsils. In more severe cases the medulla and fourth ventricle may descend below the foramen magnum (**632**). Chiari Type I has an estimated prevalence of 1 in 1000 persons.

Chiari Type II malformation is a more severe malformation with the cerebellar tonsils herniating below the foramen magnum. Myelomeningocele is always present. About 80% will have hydrocephalus and 40–80% will have syringomyelia of the spinal cord. Elongation and kinking of the medulla may also occur (**633**).

Etiology and pathophysiology

The cause of Chiari Type I malformation is a volume discrepancy between the posterior fossa and the neural components of the posterior fossa (cerebellum, fourth ventricle, and brainstem). Oversized structures in the posterior fossa cause these structures to descend caudally below the foramen magnum.

The exact cause of the Chiari Type I malformation is unknown. No gene abnormality has been identified although familial clustering of cases has been reported.

Differential diagnosis

Chiari Type I malformation must be differentiated from a variety of conditions:

- Neoplasms in the vicinity of the foramen magnum.
- Intrinsic neoplasms of the cerebellum and lower brainstem.
- Low-lying cerebellar tonsils due to intracranial hypotension syndrome.
- Multiple sclerosis.
- Syringomyelia without Chiari malformation.

Clinical features

Patients with Chiari Type I malformation commonly have neck pain and headache. The headaches may be severe and paroxysmal or steady and dull. The Valsalva maneuver may exacerbate the headache.

Compression of the posterior fossa structures can cause lower brainstem symptoms:

- Nystagmus.
- Cerebellar ataxia.
- Dysphagia and aspiration.
- Facial numbness and pain.
- Sleep apnea.
- Hoarseness.
- Tongue atrophy.

Tip

▶*Symptoms with Chiari Type I malformations may vary from just headache and neck pain to more complex symptoms and signs that include nystagmus, ataxia, dysphagia, and facial numbness and pain.*

Investigations and diagnosis

Chiari Type I malformation can be demonstrated on MRI. Gadolinium-enhanced images are needed to exclude a posterior fossa tumor. MRI is adequate to exclude hydrocephalus as a cause of the low-lying tonsils. In questionable cases, phase contrast MRI can determine whether the flow of CSF is impaired across the cranio-cervical junction.

Brainstem auditory evoked responses and somatosensory evoked responses may demonstrate slowing consistent with brainstem or spinal cord compression related to Chiari Type I malformation.

Treatment

No medical treatment is effective for Chiari Type I malformation. Surgical treatment of Chiari I involves decompression of the foramen magnum and restoration of normal CSF flow. Some surgeons open the dura in the posterior fossa and add a graft (duraplasty); others do not manipulate the dura.

Surgical management of Chiari II is complex and involves closure of the myelomeningocele. CSF shunting and decompression of the posterior fossa and upper cervical spinal cord may be needed.

Prognosis

Approximately 65–90% of patients with Chiari Type I malformation show clinical improvement after posterior fossa decompression. Prognosis in Chiari Type II malformation depends upon the severity and complexity of the malformation.

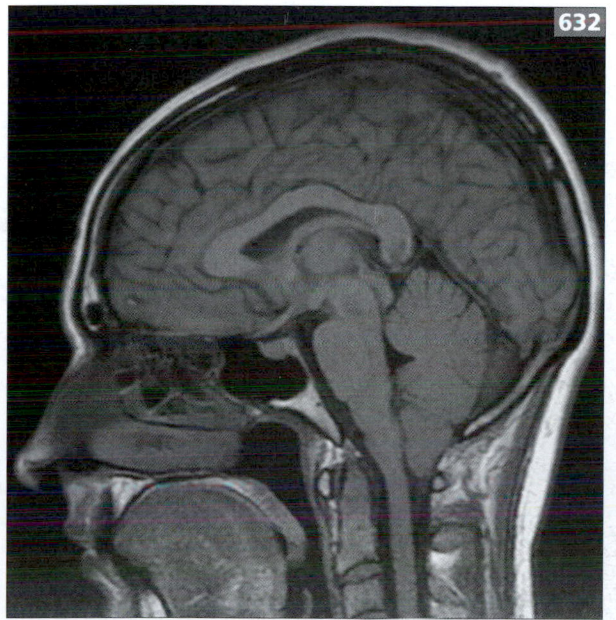

632 MRI (T1-weighted image) shows downward herniation of the cerebellar tonsils below the foramen magnum in a patient with Chiari malformation Type I.

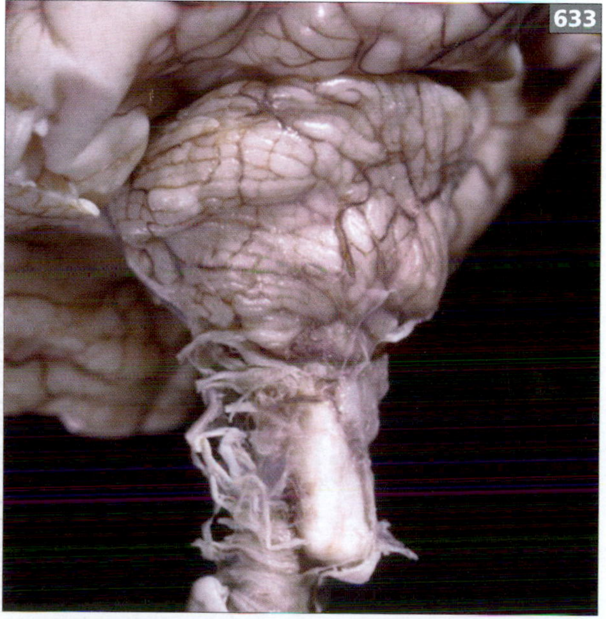

633 Pathologic specimen showing impression of the foramen magnum on the cerebellum in a patient with Chiari malformation Type II. Note the abnormality of lower brainstem and upper spinal cord.

SYRINGOMYELIA
(SYRINGOHYDROMYELIA)

Definition and epidemiology

Syringomyelia (syringohydromyelia) is the presence of a fluid-filled cavity within the spinal cord[10]. It is a rare disorder, and exact incidence and prevalence are unknown.

Etiology and pathophysiology

The cause of syringomyelia is unknown. Low-lying cerebellar tonsils likely play a role in many cases. Normally, during the cardiac cycle CSF flows freely across the foramen magnum (downward during cardiac systole and upward during cardiac diastole). When the cerebellar tonsils are low (as in Chiari I and II malformations) the free flow of CSF is obstructed and backs up into the cranial cavity during diastole. CSF may become trapped in the cervical subarachnoid space, eventually tracking into the substance of the spinal cord causing a syrinx to form.

Syringomyelia may occur due to a variety of disease processes including spinal cord trauma with myelomalacia, Chiari I malformations, Chiari II malformations, spinal cord tumors, communicating hydrocephalus, spinal cord inflammation, and meningitis. An estimated 20–85% of children with Chiari I and 48–88% of children with Chiari II have an associated syringohydromyelia.

Differential diagnosis

Syringomyelia of cervical spinal cord needs to be distinguished from other diseases that affect the cervical spinal cord:

- Sarcoidosis.
- Multiple sclerosis.
- Amyotrophic lateral sclerosis.
- Spinal cord compression by meningioma or neurofibroma.
- Spinal cord compression by metastatic tumors.
- Intrinsic tumors of the spinal cord such as ependymoma or astrocytoma.
- Cervical spondylosis with spinal cord compression, and neurosyphilis.

Tip

▶ *Syringomyelia must be distinguished from other diseases of the spinal cord including multiple sclerosis and amyotrophic sclerosis. MRI of the spinal cord is the test of choice.*

Clinical features

The classic early presentation of syringomyelia is bilateral upper extremity weakness associated with 'cape-like' sensory loss over the shoulders and upper extremities.

There may be a syndrome of 'sensory dissociation' with loss of pain and temperature as the syrinx is located centrally in the spinal cord and in the immediate pathway of the crossing fibers which will become the spinothalamic tracts, but sparing of position and vibration sensation as the syrinx does not yet involve the posterior columns of the spinal cord.

If the syrinx continues to enlarge, increasing myelopathic features can be seen including spasticity, bladder dysfunction, weakness, other sensory loss, and gait disturbance. If the syrinx extends into the brainstem there can be a Horner's syndrome, nystagmus, and lower cranial nerve abnormalities.

Some children with syrinxes will present with scoliosis prior to the development of any motor or sensory symptoms.

Investigations and diagnosis

MRI can detect most syrinxes (**634**). Axial and sagittal images should be reviewed. The syrinx may be confined to the cervical spinal cord or also extend into the thoracic spinal cord.

Somatosensory evoked responses may be delayed due to involvement of the cervical or thoracic spinal cord. When the syrinx extends into the brainstem, brainstem auditory evoked responses may be abnormal.

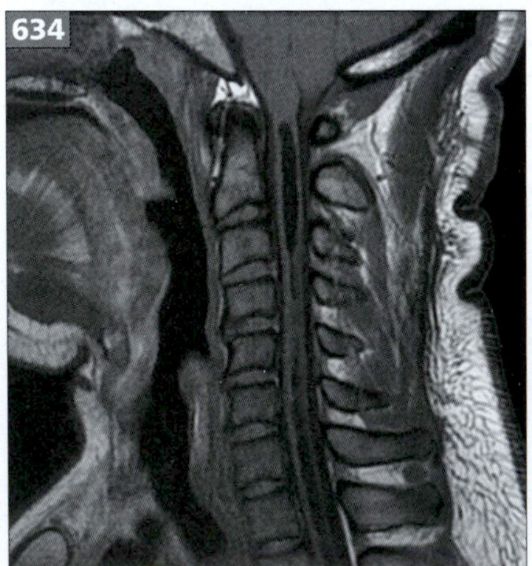

634 MRI shows syrinx involving both the upper and lower cervical spinal cord. The cerebellar tonsils are low-lying, indicating associated Chiari malformation Type I.

Treatment

When the syrinx is associated with Chiari I malformation, the first-line approach to treating syringomyelia is decompression of the posterior fossa. This may correct CSF flow and lead to collapse of the syrinx. Second-line treatment involves shunting or draining the syrinx.

Prognosis

- Posterior fossa decompression leads to clinical and radiological improvement of the syrinx in 50–75% of cases.
- In cases that require shunting of the syrinx, surgery leads to improvement in 30–75% of the patients initially, but failure rates of the shunt at 3 years are high (up to 50%) and complications including infection are frequent.
- Untreated syringomyelia is generally progressive and can lead to bladder dysfunction, increasing weakness and spasticity, and ultimately paraplegia.

IDIOPATHIC INTRACRANIAL HYPERTENSION (PSEUDOTUMOR CEREBRI)

Definition and epidemiology

Idiopathic intracranial hypertension (IIH), also known as pseudotumor cerebri or benign intracranial hypertension, is characterized by increased ICP in the absence of tumors, masses, or hydrocephalus[11]. Diagnostic criteria include:

- Headache.
- Normal brain imaging.
- ICP of 250 mmH_2O or higher on lumbar puncture.
- Normal CSF findings with the possible exception of a low total protein level.
- Normal alertness.
- No identifiable cause of increased ICP.

IIH is more common in women than men (ratio of 4:1 or 8:1). Its prevalence is estimated to be 1 case per 100,000 women. Onset is usually between ages 11 and 58, with a mean age of onset of 30 years. Obesity is a significant risk factor for IIH. Prevalence rises to 13 per 100,000 women 20–44 years of age if they are 10% above ideal body weight and 19 per 100,000 women 20–44 years of age who are more than 20% above ideal body weight.

Etiology and pathophysiology

The precise mechanism causing increased ICP in IIH is unknown; cerebral blood flow and CSF production are normal. Cerebral water and cerebral blood volumes are increased in IIH. Increased ICP in IIH may reflect impaired resorption of CSF at the arachnoid villi due to increased venous pressure at the superior sagittal sinus. Increased venous pressures have been recorded in patients with IIH even in the absence of sinus thrombosis.

The etiology of IIH is unknown. The condition shows a strong association with female gender and obesity. Other known associations include pregnancy, hypothyroidism, as well as the use of corticosteroids, minocycline, cyclosporine, vitamin A, growth hormone, and lithium carbonate.

Clinical features

- Headache is a constant symptom in IIH. The headaches are typically throbbing, generalized, and worse in the morning. The pain may be retro-orbital in location. The Valsalva maneuver may worsen the headache.
- Neck and shoulder pains are common, sometimes with a neuritic component.
- Many patients complain of pulsatile tinnitus and transient visual obscurations that include blurred vision and scotomata.
- Other, less common symptoms include numbness, incoordination, decreased sense of smell, weakness, and dizziness.
- On examination, nearly all patients have papilledema.
- Unilateral or bilateral VIth nerve palsy may be observed due to traction on the VIth nerve.
- A facial palsy may occur uncommonly.
- If there is asymmetric optic neuropathy, an afferent pupillary defect may be detected on the swinging-flashlight test. The papilledema may be unilateral or bilateral.

Tip

▶ *Transient visual obscurations is a key symptom suggesting IIH in patients with headaches.*

Differential diagnosis

IIH should be distinguished from other causes of elevated ICP:

- Lyme disease.
- Bacterial meningitis.
- Viral meningitis.
- Central nervous system (CNS) lupus.
- CNS sarcoidosis.
- Cerebral venous sinus thrombosis.
- Jugular vein thrombosis.
- Primary and metastatic brain tumors.
- Hydrocephalus.
- Subdural hematoma.

Other causes of optic disc swelling or involvement of the optic disc should be considered:

- Optic disc drüsen.
- Optic neuritis.
- Central retinal vein occlusion.
- Temporal arteritis.
- Ischemic optic neuropathy.

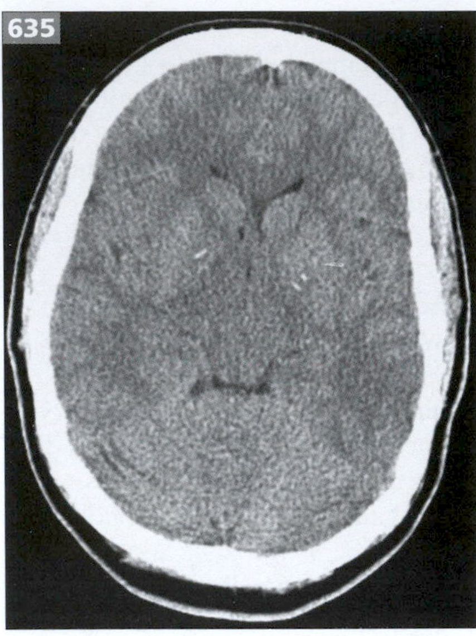

635 CT scan shows small slit-like ventricles in a patient with idiopathic intracranial hypertension.

Investigations and diagnosis

CT of the brain is usually normal. Ventricular size is either normal or decreased (**635**). Only about 11% of patients with IIH have so-called 'slit ventricles', and this finding is not required for diagnosis. Some patients on CT show either enlarged optic sheaths or an empty sella. MRI of the brain is usually normal. Subtle findings on MRI may be noted, including gadolinium enhancement of the optic disc, empty sella, or tortuousity of the optic nerve sheath.

The CSF is normal on lumbar puncture in IIH. CSF opening pressure is usually greater than 250 mmH_2O. However, some patients with IIH and papilledema will have opening pressures less than 250 mmH_2O and some asymptomatic obese women may have opening pressures greater than 250 mmH_2O.

Treatment

- Patients need to be followed closely with repeat ophthalmoscopic examinations, visual acuity testing, and visual field testing.
- Some patients respond to acetazolamide, a carbonic anhydrase inhibitor that reduces the production of CSF. Other patients may respond to furosemide used as a diuretic.
- Weight reduction is useful in obese patients with IIH.
- When headaches are not controlled or in the setting of declining visual function, surgical intervention should be considered which includes optic nerve sheath fenestration and CSF shunting (either ventricular or lumbar shunts).
- Although advocated by some, serial lumbar punctures to reduce ICP are rarely practical, especially in obese patients.
- Current surgical recommendations include using lumbo-peritoneal shunts as an initial therapy for IIH when medical therapy with acetazolamide has failed. Ventriculo-peritoneal shunting or optic nerve sheath fenestration are additional surgical options if lumbo-peritoneal shunting fails or is impractical.

Prognosis

Some patients with IIH remit spontaneously without prolonged medical treatment. However, in the absence of aggressive medical or surgical therapy as many as 17–25% of the patients with IIH will have either permanent visual loss or permanent optic atrophy. The onset of visual loss is usually gradual, but in some patients visual loss may occur precipitously, requiring rapid surgical intervention.

INTRACRANIAL HYPOTENSION SYNDROME

Definition and epidemiology

Idiopathic intracranial hypotension (also known as spontaneous intracranial hypotension) is a syndrome of orthostatic headache, worsening with upright posture, due to reduced intracranial pressure[12].

Idiopathic intracranial hypotension is not rare, but its exact incidence is unknown. There are no known age or gender differences in incidence.

Etiology and pathophysiology

Intracranial hypotension syndrome is caused by reduced ICP, usually 60 mmH_2O or less on lumbar puncture. The usual cause of reduced ICP is a continuing CSF leak. Two theories have been proposed to explain the headache of intracranial hypotension syndrome:

- Traction theory: a decrease in ICP and loss of buoyancy of the CSF causes the brain to sag in the cranium, especially in the erect position. This sagging causes traction on pain-sensitive structures within the head and leads to headache.
- Venous engorgement theory: the drop in ICP leads to a compensatory venous engorgement and this vascular dilation leads to headache.

Most cases of intracranial hypotension are due to a persistent CSF leak, often after a lumbar puncture, spinal anesthesia, or myelogram[13]. CSF leaks may also develop after cranial surgery, head trauma, or after ventriculo-peritoneal shunting. Spontaneous leaks without trauma or surgery may also develop. Spontaneous CSF leaks with CSF hypovolemia can result from trivial trauma such as coughing, lifting, and minor falls.

Other causes of decreased ICP may include dehydration, diabetic coma, hyperpnea, and uremia. Over-drainage by a ventriculo-peritoneal shunt is an important treatable cause of intracranial hypotension syndrome.

Clinical features

The hallmark of intracranial hypotension syndrome is postural headache, made worse on standing and relieved in a recumbent position. The headache may or may not be throbbing, it is usually bilateral, and may be frontal, occipital, or holocephalic in location.

Other, highly variable symptoms include nausea, vomiting, diplopia, altered hearing, dizziness, neck pain, blurred vision, and radicular pain in the upper extremities. Laughing, coughing, or the Valsalva maneuver can exacerbate the headache of intracranial hypotension.

Differential diagnosis

Intracranial hypotension must be differentiated from other causes of headache:

- Migraine.
- Meningitis.
- Subdural hematoma.
- Posterior fossa tumor.
- Hydrocephalus.

Low-lying tonsils in intracranial hypotension syndrome must be differentiated from Chiari malformation Type I.

Investigations

Imaging

A frequent, but not constant, sign of intracranial hypotension syndrome is diffuse pachymeningeal (dural) enhancement with gadolinium without leptomeningeal (pia and arachnoid) enhancement on MRI (**636, 637**). In some symptomatic patients, meningeal enhancement resolves prior to resolution of the headache and other symptoms.

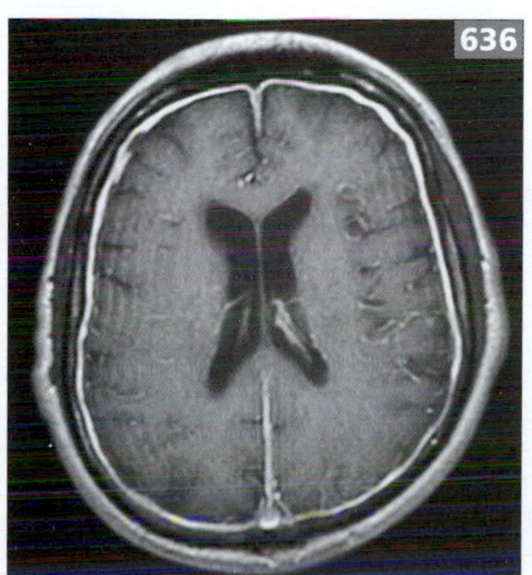

636, 637 Axial (636) and coronal (637) MRI (T1-weighted) gadolinium-enhanced images showing enhancement in dura over the surface of the brain and in the interhemispheric falx in a patient with intracranial hypotension syndrome.

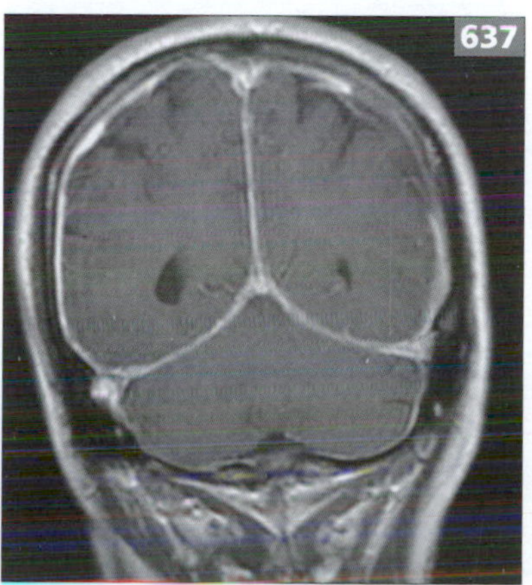

Other findings on MRI include:

- Diffuse thickening of the meninges, engorgement of the venous sinuses, and downward displacement of the brain.
- Subdural fluid collections and enlargement of the pituitary gland may also occur.
- The ventricles may be decreased in size.

It is currently felt that volume depletion due to intracranial hypotension causes a compensatory venous engorgement, thickening of the meninges, and a downward displacement of the brain. The gadolinium enhancement of intracranial hypotension is thick, diffuse, and linear and involves the pachymeninges of both the supra-tentorial and infra-tentorial compartments of the brain. The leptomeninges, including the meninges around the brainstem, are spared.

CT scanning of the brain may show obliteration of the basilar cisterns due to sagging downward of the brain.

If the CSF leak is in the spinal region, CT myelography may be useful in identifying the site of leakage.

Spinal MRI may also be useful in identifying leakage sites in cases of intracranial hypotension syndrome.

Other investigations

Lumbar puncture shows an opening pressure of 60 mmH_2O or less. Analysis of the CSF is usually normal. Cultures are negative for infection. Glucose levels are usually normal. Occasionally pleocytosis, xanthochromia, or mild increases in CSF protein may be noted.

Radioisotope cisternography after injection of radioisotope into the lumbar subarachnoid space may be useful in identifying CSF leaks. Indium-111 is used as a tracer and when a leak is present activity does rise up above the basal cisterns to the cerebral convexities. Due to extravasation of CSF and vascular uptake, radioisotope may appear in the kidneys and bladder in less than 4 hours.

Treatment

Initial treatment consists of bed rest. Presumably a supine position reduces CSF pressure at the site of leakage and allows sealing of the leak to occur. A variety of medical treatments have been proposed for intracranial hypotension syndrome including intravenous or oral caffeine, intravenous or oral theophylline, intravenous hydration, increased salt intake, corticosteroid therapy, and carbon dioxide inhalation. Controlled studies of the efficacy of these remedies are not available and most are of questionable value.

When conservative remedies fail including bed rest, relief can usually be obtained with an epidural blood patch using autologous blood. Blood is injected into the epidural space with immediate and longstanding pain relief obtained in 85–90% of cases, but some patients may require more than one patch.

When a meningeal tear can be demonstrated radiologically, surgical repair may be necessary in some cases.

Prognosis

Prognosis is good in most patients with a simple leak due to puncture of the meninges. When bed rest fails, an epidural blood patch is generally effective. Larger rents in the meninges may need surgical repair. Complete resolution of headache is the rule when ICP is restored to normal.

REFERENCES

1 McLone DG (2004). The anatomy of the ventricular system. *Neurosurg Clin North Am* **15**:33–38.

2 Kulkarni AV (2009). Hydrocephalus. *Continuum* **15**:50–63.

3 Fukuara T, Luciano MG (2001). Clinical features of late-onset idiopathic aqueductal stenosis. *Surg Neurol* **55**:132–137.

4 Stoquart-El Sankari S, Lehman P, Gondry-Jouet C, *et al.* (2009). Phase-contrast MR imaging support for the diagnosis of aqueductal stenosis. *Am J Neuroradiol* **30**:209–214.

5 Beran A, Eide PK (2008). Prevalence of probable idiopathic normal pressure hydrocephalus in a Norwegian population. *Acta Neurol Scand* **118**:48–52.

6 Graff-Radford NR (2007). Normal pressure hydrocephalus. *Continuum* **13**:144–164.

7 Bergsneider M, Black PM, Klinge P, Marmarou A, Relkin N (2005). Surgical management of idiopathic normal-pressure hydrocephalus. *Neurosurgery* **57**: Supplement S2-29–S2-39.

8 Woodworth G, McGirt MJ, Williams M, Rigamonti D (2009). Cerebrospinal fluid drainage and dynamics in the diagnosis of normal pressure hydrocephalus. *Neurosurgery* **64**:919–926.

9 Pujari S, Kharkar S, Metellus P, Shuck J, Williams M, Rigamonti D (2008). Normal pressure hydrocephalus: long-term outcome after shunt surgery. *J Neurol Neurosurg Psychiatry* **79**:1282–1286.

10 Hankinson TC, Klimo P Jr, Feldstein NA, Anderson RCE, Brockmeyer D (2007). Chiari malformations, syringohydromyelia and scoliosis. *Neurosurg Clin North Am* **18**:549–568.

11 Binder DK, Horton J, Lawton MT, McDermott MW (2004). Idiopathic intracranial hypertension. *Neurosurgery* **54**:538–552.

12 Paldino M, Mogilner AY, Tenner MS (2003). Intracranial hypotension syndrome: a comprehensive review. *Neurosurg Focus* **15**(6). Available online at http://thejns.org/toc/foc/15/6.

13 Mokri B (2004). Low cerebrospinal fluid pressure syndrome. *Neurol Clin* **22**:55–74.

CRANIAL NEUROPATHIES
I, V, AND VII–XII

Wilson Cueva, Helene Rubeiz

OLFACTORY NERVE NEUROPATHY (CRANIAL NERVE I)

Definition

Disorder of cranial nerve (CN) I, or olfactory nerve, resulting in a disturbance of smell sensation.

Anatomy and physiology

Nerve fibers subserving the sense of smell have their cells of origin in the mucous membranes of the upper and posterior parts of the nasal cavity. The olfactory mucosa contains three types of cell (**638**):

- Olfactory or receptor cells.
- Sustentacular or supporting cells.
- Basal cells, which are stem cells and the source of both olfactory (receptor) cells and sustentacular cells during regeneration.

The olfactory or receptor cells are bipolar neurons that have a peripheral process (the olfactory rod), from which project 10–30 fine hairs or cilia, and several central processes (or olfactory filia) which are fine unmyelinated fibers that converge to form small fascicles enwrapped by Schwann cells, and pass through openings in the cribriform plate of the ethmoid bone into the olfactory bulb. Collectively, the central processes of the olfactory receptor cells constitute the olfactory nerve.

In the olfactory bulb, the axons of the receptor cells synapse with mitral and tufted cells, the dendrites of which form brush-like terminals or olfactory glomeruli. The axons of the mitral and tufted cells form the olfactory tract, which courses along the olfactory groove on the orbital surface of the frontal lobe.

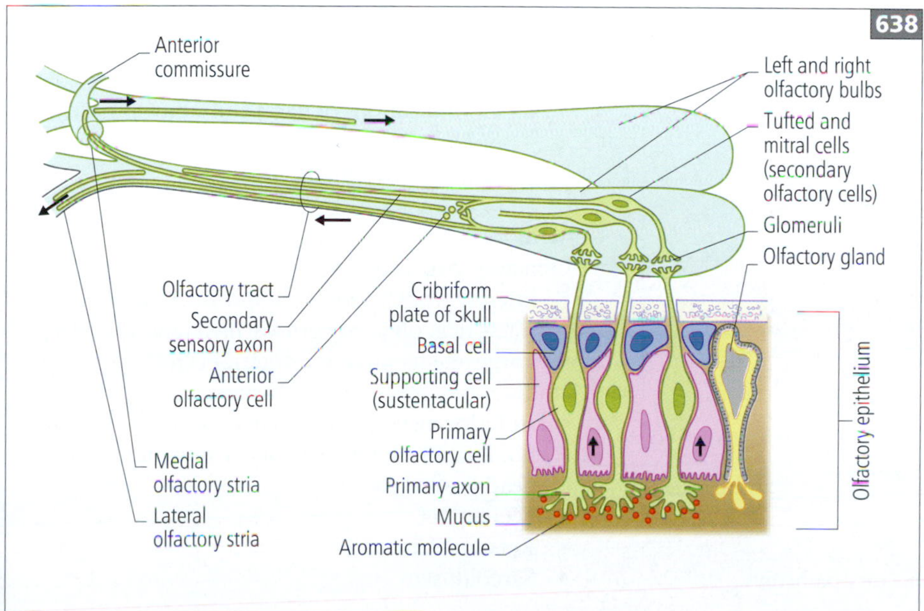

638 Schematic illustration of olfactory epithelium, bulb, and tract. *Adapted from 'Cranial Nerves in Health and Disease' by Linda Wilson-Pauwels.*

The olfactory tract divides into medial and lateral olfactory striae. The medial stria contains fibers from the anterior olfactory nucleus, which pass to the contralateral hemisphere via the anterior commissure. Fibers in the lateral stria give off collaterals to the anterior perforated substance, and terminate in the primary olfactory cortex, which comprises the anterior olfactory nucleus, the piriform cortex, the anterior cortical nucleus of the amygdaloid complex, and the entorhinal cortex[1]. Thus, olfactory impulses reach the cerebral cortex without relay through the thalamus, which is a unique feature among the sensory systems[2].

From the primary olfactory cortex, fibers project to the hypothalamus and to the orbitofrontal cortex (secondary olfactory cortex) via the medial dorsal nucleus of the thalamus (**639**).

During quiet breathing, little of the air entering the nostril reaches the olfactory mucosa; sniffing carries the air into the olfactory crypt. To be perceived as an odor, an inhaled substance must be volatile – i.e. spread in the air as very small particles, and be soluble in water or lipid. The intensity of olfactory sensation is determined by the frequency of firing of afferent neurons. The quality of an odor is probably determined by 'cross-fiber' activation, since the individual receptor cells are responsive to a wide range of odors and exhibit different types of responses to stimulants.

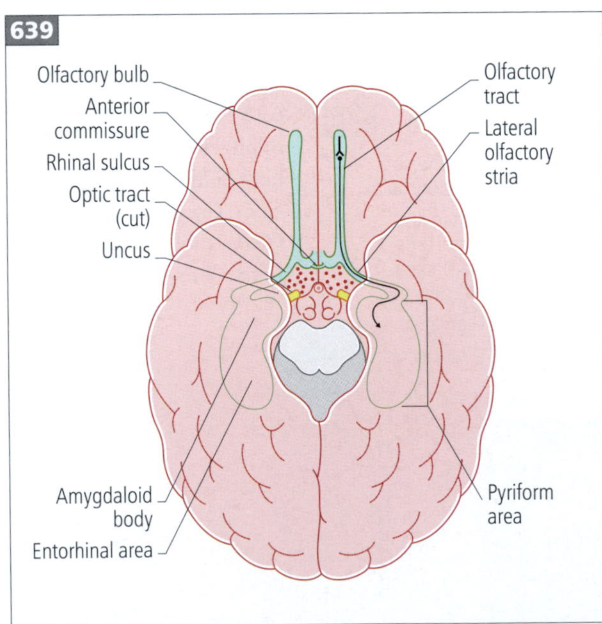

639 **Schematic illustration of olfactory pathways (inferior view).**

Etiology and pathophysiology

Loss of, or reduction of, the sense of smell may be caused by local disease in the nose or by a lesion along the olfactory pathway. A unilateral lesion distal to the decussation of the olfactory fibers is usually asymptomatic due to bilateral cortical representation[3].

Around two-thirds of cases of anosmia and hyposmia are secondary to prior upper respiratory infections, nasal or sinus diseases, or head injury. Other factors include age, smoking habits, presence of a neurodegenerative condition, nasal or intracranial neoplasm, prior nasal surgical procedures, epilepsy, and chemical exposure.

Nasal

- Odorants do not reach the olfactory receptors: upper respiratory infections, nasal obstruction, or inflammation (rhinitis) are by far the most common causes.

Olfactory neuroepithelium

- Damage to olfactory epithelium:
  - Upper respiratory infections.
  - Exposure to chemicals and toxins: herbicides, pesticides, solvents, heavy metals (cadmium, chromium, nickel, manganese).
- Destruction of receptors or their axon filaments:
  - Congenital absence or hypoplasia of primary receptor neurons:
    - Kallman syndrome (congenital anosmia and hypogonadotropic hypogonadism).
    - Albinism.
  - Disruption of the delicate filaments of the receptor cells as they pass through the cribriform plate:
    - Head injury, particularly if severe enough to cause skull fracture but may occur without a fracture. The damage may be unilateral or bilateral. This accounts for 20% of cases of anosmia/hyposmia.
    - Cranial surgery.
    - Complications of nasal and sinus surgery.
    - Subarachnoid hemorrhage.
    - Chronic meningitis.

Central

- Olfactory pathway lesions:
  - Inferior frontal tumor compressing the olfactory tracts (e.g. olfactory groove meningioma, **640**).
  - Large aneurysm of the anterior cerebral or anterior communicating artery.
  - Anterior meningoencephalocele (cerebrospinal fluid [CSF] rhinorrhea may be present in certain head positions).
  - Meningitis.
  - Refsum's disease.
  - Sarcoidosis.

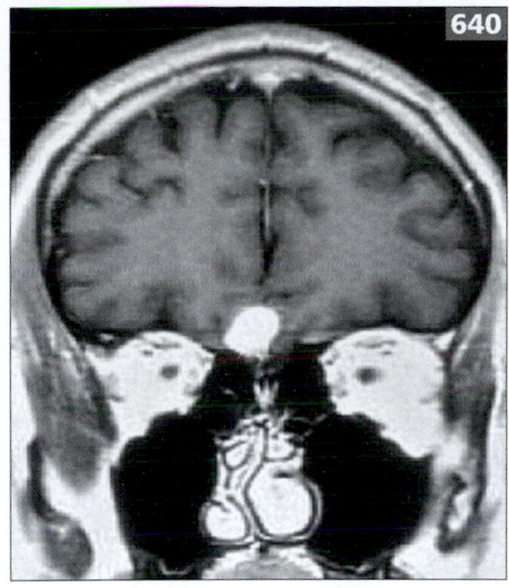

640 Olfactory groove meningioma (coronal view). *From Welge-Luessen A, et al. 'Olfactory function in patients with olfactory groove meningioma' (J Neurol Neurosurg Psychiatry 2001; 70(2); 218–221).*

- Neurodegenerative diseases: olfactory deficit is present in 85–90% of patients with early-stage Parkinson's disease and Alzheimer's disease (AD)[4,5]. Most patients are unaware of the deficit. Anosmia has also been described in Lewy body disease, Huntington's disease, and spinocerebellar ataxias.
- Multiple sclerosis (MS): olfactory dysfunction may wax and wane with disease activity and is related to the presence of plaques in the inferior frontal and temporal regions.
- Temporal lobe epilepsy: patients with complex partial seizures may have olfactory hallucinations. After temporal lobectomy there may be ipsilateral deficits in olfactory discrimination.
- Alcoholic Korsakoff's syndrome: loss of olfactory discrimination has been described in alcoholics with Korsakoff's psychosis due to degeneration of neurons in the higher order olfactory systems of the medial temporal and thalamic regions.
- Migraine: can be associated with olfactory hallucinations or hyperosmia (increased smell sensitivity).

Tip

▶ *Olfactory deficit is present in 85–90% of patients with early-stage Parkinson's disease and AD.*

Psychiatric

- Hysteria: anosmia can be unilateral or bilateral. If unilateral, anosmia may be on the same side as other symptoms such as anesthesia, blindness, or deafness. Hysterical anosmics do not usually complain of loss of taste (whereas true anosmics do) and show normal taste sensation on testing.
- Depression and schizophrenia: patients can have complaints of dysosmia, olfactory hallucinations, or delusions.

Idiopathic

Usually bilateral but can be unilateral.

Clinical features

- Bilateral loss or reduction of the sense of smell (anosmia, hyposmia): this is commonly, but not always, recognized by the patient. It may present as impaired taste, because taste depends largely on the volatile particles in foods and beverages, which reach the olfactory receptors through the nasopharynx; the perception of flavor is a combination of smell and taste. However, these patients are able to distinguish the elementary taste sensations (sweet, sour, bitter, and salty).
- Unilateral loss or reduction of the sense of smell (anosmia, hyposmia): seldom, if ever, recognized by the patient.

Tip

▶ *Olfactory impulses reach the cerebral cortex without relay through the thalamus and this is a unique feature among the sensory systems.*

Dysfunction can be a distortion of smell (dysosmia or parosmia), which may be due to foul odors within the nasal cavity in association with nasal infections, or a spontaneous sensation of smell in the absence of a stimulus (phantosmia).

Associated signs, such as unilateral optic atrophy and contralateral papilledema (Foster–Kennedy syndrome) may be present in conditions such as olfactory groove or sphenoid ridge meningioma which extends posteriorly to involve the ipsilateral optic nerve (resulting in optic atrophy) and also causes raised intracranial pressure (ICP) and contralateral papilledema[6,7].

Investigations and diagnosis

Smell should be tested in each nostril separately with a nonirritating substance, and not with an acrid substance such as ammonia. The reason for olfactory deficit is determined by the clinical findings:

- Computed tomography (CT) or magnetic resonance imaging (MRI) of the brain.
- CSF examination.
- Electroencephalogram (EEG).

Treatment

Treat the underlying cause, if possible.

Prognosis

Prognosis depends on the cause. Anosmia due to head injury is dependent on the severity of the trauma and can occur in the absence of a fracture through the cribriform plate. Anosmia due to closed head injury recovers in about one-quarter of patients[8].

TRIGEMINAL NERVE NEUROPATHY (CRANIAL NERVE V)

Definition and epidemiology

Disorder of the trigeminal (Vth cranial) nerve. It is a common disorder.

Anatomy and physiology

The trigeminal nerve is the largest CN. It is a mixed nerve that provides sensation to the face, mucous membranes of the mouth and nose, cornea, and dura through three sensory branches (V_1, V_2, and V_3), and motor innervation to the muscles of mastication[2]. The motor nucleus is located in the mid pons. The branches of V_1–V_3 have their cell bodies located in the Gasserian or semilunar ganglion, which lies over the apex of the petrous portion of the temporal bone (Meckel's cave). From the ganglion, the sensory fibers enter the pons and terminate on three major sensory nuclei that are located in the brainstem from the mesencephalon to the upper cervical spinal cord. In a rostral to caudal direction, the trigeminal sensory nuclei are distributed as follows (**641**)[1]:

- Mesencephalic nucleus (lower midbrain/upper pons).
- Principal sensory nucleus of CN V (mid-pons).
- Spinal trigeminal nucleus (lower pons/medulla/upper cervical spinal cord).

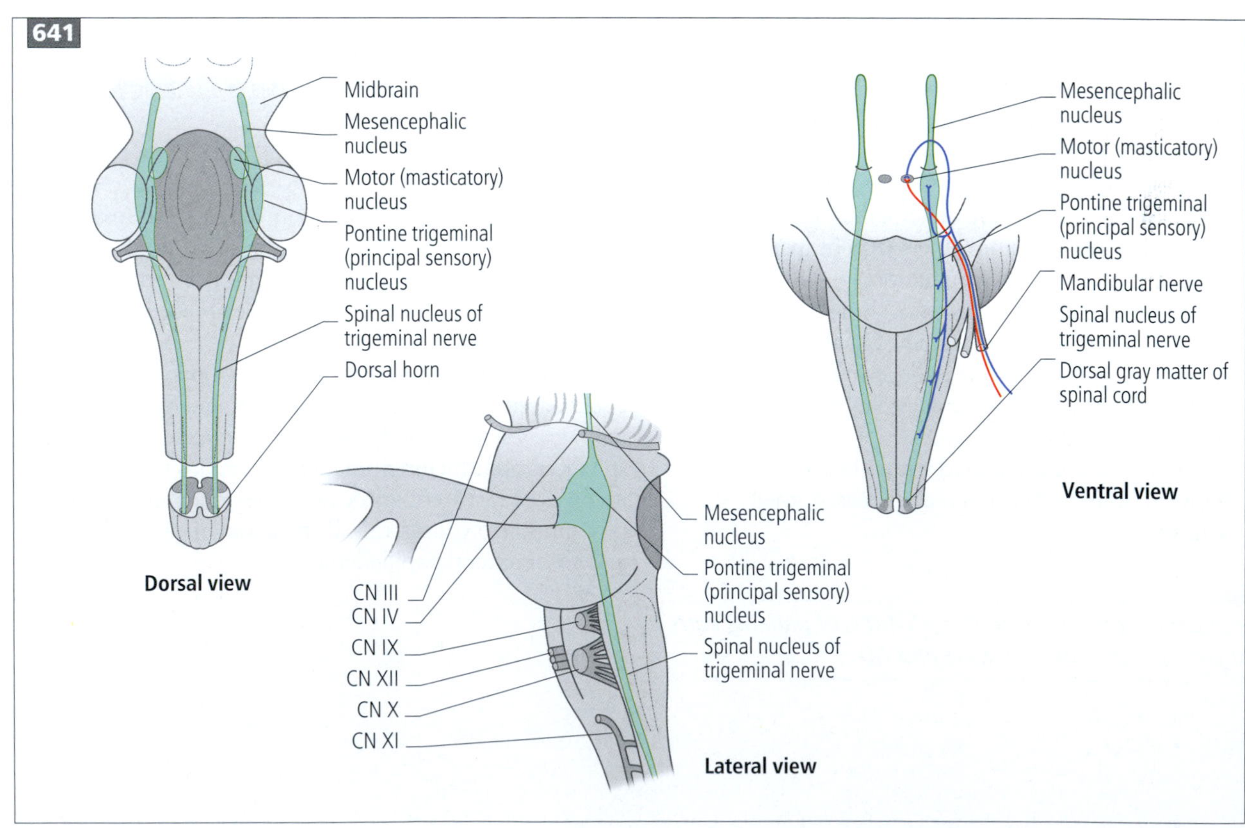

641 Cranial nerve V nuclei. *Adapted from 'Cranial Nerves in Health and Disease' by Linda Wilson-Pauwels.*

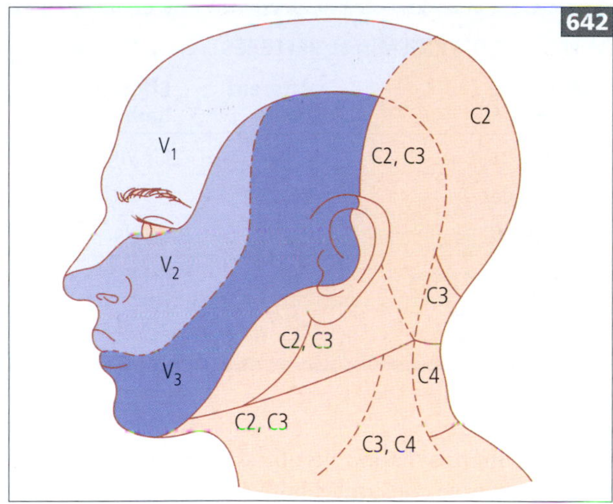

642 **Dermatomal distribution of cranial nerve V branches. V_1: ophthalmic nerve; V_2: maxillary nerve; V_3: mandibular nerve. Spinal nerve roots C2–C4 innervate the skin of the posterior scalp and the neck.**

Sensory and motor peripheral divisions of CN V

Sensory (642)

First (ophthalmic) division or V_1

Innervates the skin of the ipsilateral scalp, forehead, upper eyelid and nose, the upper half of the cornea, conjunctiva, and iris, in addition to the frontal sinuses and dura, via four branches: the lacrimal nerve (skin of lateral eyelid/brow and conjunctiva); the frontal nerve and its branches: the supratrochlear nerve (conjunctiva, medial upper eyelid, forehead, and side of nose) and supraorbital nerve (medial upper eyelid and conjunctiva, forehead and scalp up to vertex, frontal sinuses); the nasociliary nerve (skin of the top of the nose and medial canthus, nasal cavity, conjunctiva, ciliary body, iris, and cornea); the tentorial branch (dura of cavernous sinus, sphenoid wing, anterior fossa, petrous ridge, tentorium, posterior falx, and venous sinuses). The first division carries most of the afferent pathway of the corneal reflex, with perhaps some contribution from the second division for the lower half of the cornea. V_1 enters the orbit and passes through the superior orbital fissure, lateral wall of the cavernous sinus (below the abducens nerve) and eventually reaches the trigeminal sensory ganglion.

Tip

▶ *The ophthalmic (V_1) and maxillary (V_2) nerves are purely sensory. The mandibular (V_3) nerve has both sensory and motor functions.*

Second (maxillary) division or V_2

Innervates the skin of the ipsilateral lower eyelid, lateral nose, upper lip, cheek sparing the skin over the angle of the mandible (which is innervated by the C2/C3 nerve roots), the lower half of the cornea, conjunctiva and iris, the mucous membranes of the maxillary sinus, palate, nasopharynx, upper gum, the upper teeth, and the dura of the middle cranial fossa (via middle meningeal artery). V_2 enters the skull through the foramen rotundum and then passes in the inferolateral wall of the cavernous sinus to the trigeminal sensory ganglion.

Third (mandibular) division or V_3

This division has three main branches: auriculotemporal, lingual, and inferior alveolar nerves. V_3 innervates the skin of the lower lip, chin, lower jaw, upper ear, external auditory canal and tympanic membrane, the mucous membranes of the lower oral cavity, lower gums, anterior two-thirds of tongue (not taste), the teeth of the lower jaw, and the dura of the posterior cranial fossa. V_3 joins the motor root to form the mandibular nerve. V_3 enters the skull through the foramen ovale (with the motor fibers) and passes inferior to the cavernous sinus to the trigeminal sensory ganglion.

Tip

▶ *V_1 enters the skull through the superior orbital fissure, V_2 enters the skull through the foramen rotundum, and V_3 enters the skull through the foramen ovale.*

Motor

The motor nucleus is in the mid pons. The motor root passes through the posterior fossa, enters Meckel's cave, and leaves the base of the skull through the foramen ovale. After leaving the skull, it joins the V_3 division to form the mandibular nerve, which supplies the muscles of mastication: masseter, temporalis, medial and lateral pterygoids, tensor tympani, tensor veli palatini, mylohyoid, and anterior belly of digastric.

Course of sensory fibers: Gasserian ganglion to cortex

From the Gasserian ganglion, sensory fibers enter the pons and terminate on the three sensory nuclei. The principal sensory nucleus mediates pressure and light touch from the face and oral cavity and contains second-order neurons that project to the ipsilateral and contralateral ventral posteromedial (VPM) nuclei of the thalamus via the dorsal trigeminothalamic tract (**643**).

The spinal trigeminal tract and nucleus mediate pain and temperature from V_1–V_3. Fibers in the spinal trigeminal tract descend from the pontomedullary junction to the C2–C4 level of the spinal cord; second-order neurons project to the contralateral VPM nucleus via the ventral trigeminothalamic tract[9].

The mesencephalic nucleus, which is located at the midbrain–pontine junction, contains first-order neurons that receive proprioceptive input from V_3[10]. This nucleus also provides the afferent limb of the jaw jerk reflex. After the trigeminothalamic tracts synapse in the thalamus, third-order neurons from the thalamus project on the somatosensory cortex.

Trigeminal reflexes

The trigeminal nerve constitutes the afferent limb in five monosynaptic reflexes; in one of them it also represents the efferent limb (*Table 110*).

TABLE 110 **TRIGEMINAL REFLEXES**

Reflex	Afferent limb	Efferent limb
Corneal reflex	CN V_1	CN VII
Blink reflex	CN V_1	CN VII
Tearing (lacrimal) reflex	CN V_1	CN VII
Oculocardiac reflex	CN V_1	CN X
Jaw jerk	CN V_3	CN V_3

Jaw jerk

This is a monosynaptic myotatic reflex in which the trigeminal nerve constitutes both the afferent limb (sensory division of V_3) and the efferent limb (motor division of V_3) of the reflex arc. Its first-order neuron is *not* in the Gasserian ganglion but located centrally in the midbrain:

- Afferent limb: Ia fibers in V_3 division that carry proprioceptive sensory information from facial muscles and masseter. Collateral fibers synapse with the motor nucleus of CN V.
- Efferent limb: mandibular fibers that originate in the motor nucleus of CN V. Efferent (motor) fibers are sent to masticatory muscles via the motor division of V_3.

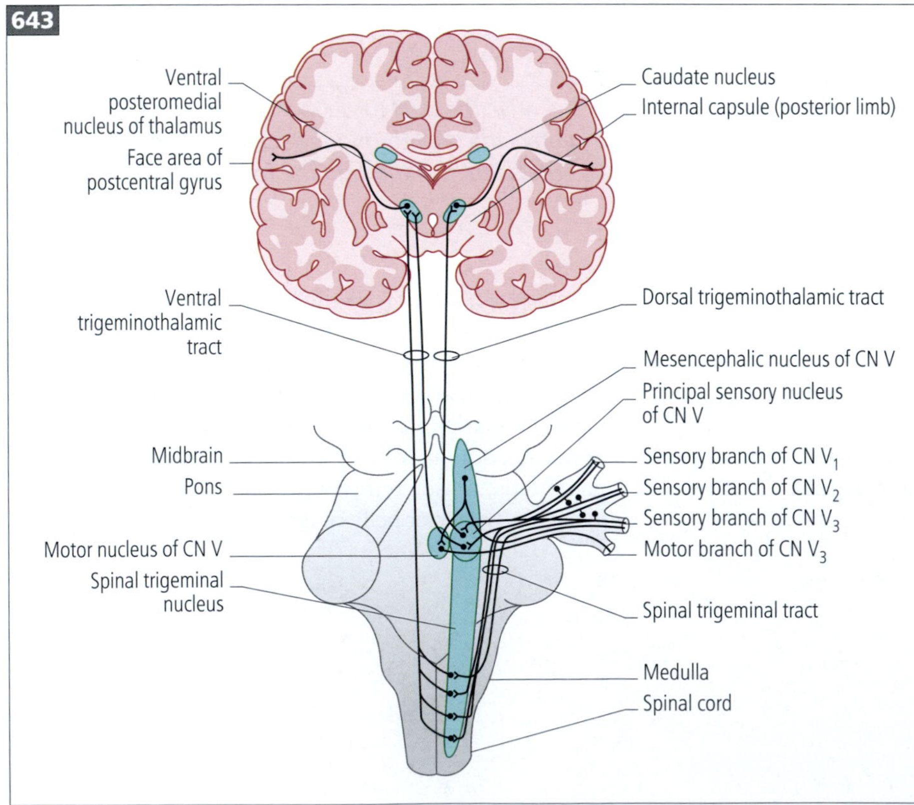

643 Trigeminothalamic pathways. *Adapted from 'High Yield Neuroanatomy, 3rd edition' by James D. Fix.*

Etiology

- Brainstem: lesions are often associated with other CN deficits and long tract involvement:
  - Stroke (lateral medullary syndrome).
  - Multiple sclerosis (MS).
  - Tumor (brainstem glioma, lymphoma, metastases).
  - Syringobulbia.
  - Hemorrhage from hypertension, ruptured vascular anomalies.
  - Inflammatory conditions: sarcoidosis, connective tissue diseases, vasculitis.
  - Infectious conditions.
- Cerebello-pontine angle:
  - Acoustic neuroma compressing CN V (although CN VII is most commonly affected).
  - Trigeminal neuroma (second most common cause of schwannomas affecting CNs).
  - Meningioma (multiple CNs are usually affected).
  - Glossopharyngeal neuroma (rare).
  - Epidermoid/dermoid tumor.
  - Chordoma.
  - Chloroma.
  - Metastases.
  - Aberrant vessels, basilar artery ectasia, or aneurysm.
- Meckel's cave:
  - Schwannoma.
  - Meningioma.
  - Nasopharyngeal cancer and other head and neck malignancies.
  - Sarcoidosis.
  - Petrous apicitis.

Tip

▶ *Trigeminal neuromas are the second most common cause of schwannomas affecting the cranial nerves.*

- Base of the skull:
  - Meningitis (infectious, inflammatory, carcinomatous).
  - Sarcoidosis.
  - Meningovascular syphilis.
  - Chordoma.
  - Metastases to skull base, nasopharyngeal cancer, and other head and neck cancers.
  - Osseous lesions (e.g. Paget's disease).

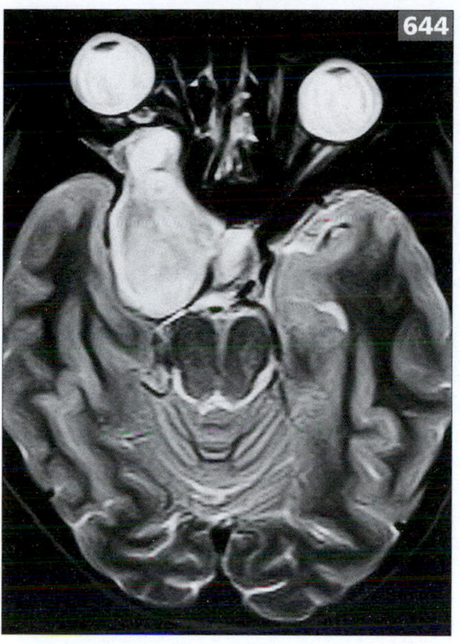

644 Intracavernous schwannoma of V_1. Brain MRI (axial T2 image) showing a large area of increased signal intensity, due to an intracavernous schwannoma of the ophthalmic division of the right trigeminal nerve, extending from the right cavernous sinus into the retro-orbital space (causing proptosis), and compressing the medial right temporal lobe.

- Cavernous sinus (V_1, V_2)/superior orbital fissure (V_1):
  - Aneurysm of carotid siphon or ophthalmic artery.
  - Carotid–cavernous fistula.
  - Cavernous sinus thrombosis.
  - Sarcoidosis.
  - Tolosa–Hunt syndrome: a rare condition that manifests as subacute onset of severe unilateral orbital pain which may be accompanied by a sensory disturbance in V_1 and sometimes V_2 distribution, and ocular motor (III, IV, and VI cranial) nerve palsies. It is caused by a chronic inflammation behind and/or within the orbit.
  - Infectious etiologies.
  - Tumors (**644**).
- Orbit (V_1):
  - Inflammation.
  - Cellulitis.
  - Tumor.

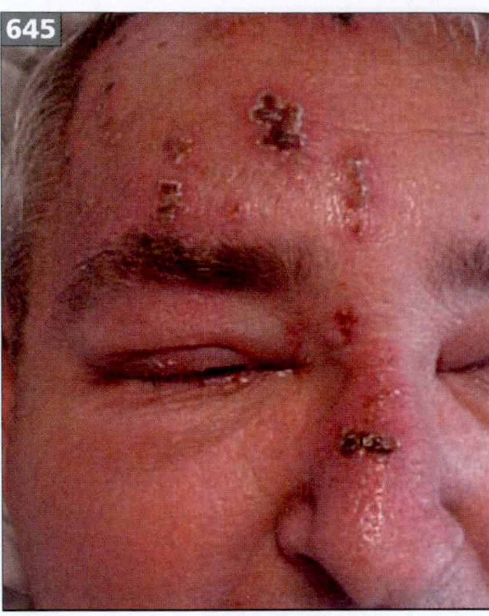

645 Varicella zoster V_1 distribution. *From eMedicine Neurology: Varicella Zoster by Wayne E. Anderson.*

- Mandible (V_3):
  - Inflammation.
  - Tumor: often metastatic.
- Other:
  - Autoimmune trigeminal neuropathy: SLE, Sjögren's syndrome, scleroderma.
  - Guillain–Barré syndrome and other peripheral neuropathies (motor ± sensory).
  - Herpes zoster (usually first sensory division) (**645**).
  - Skull trauma.
  - Trichloroethylene (organic solvent) toxicity: bifacial numbness.
  - Organic mercury poisoning.
  - Isolated trigeminal sensory neuropathy.

Clinical features

Unilateral trigeminal lesions

- Motor involvement:
  - Difficult to detect.
  - Wasting of the ipsilateral temporalis and masseter muscles may be evident.
  - The open jaw deviates to the side of the lesion, due to pterygoid muscle weakness.
- Sensory loss: sensory disturbance in any or all of the three sensory divisions, ipsilateral or contralateral to the lesion, can occur, depending on the location of the lesion (see below).

Lesion in the brainstem

Sensory disturbance in all three sensory divisions can occur, with or without motor loss:

- A lesion in the pons can result in ipsilateral or contralateral facial pain, temperature, touch, and corneal reflex loss, with or without motor loss.
- A lesion in the medulla can cause ipsilateral or contralateral facial pain and temperature loss only.
- Symptoms are usually associated with other brainstem (e.g. lower cranial nerve and long tract) and cerebellar signs.

Cerebello-pontine angle and base of skull

- Ipsilateral facial sensory disturbance (pain [and temperature] and touch [and corneal reflex] loss) in all three sensory divisions and motor loss occurs.
- Symptoms may be associated with other ipsilateral cranial nerve (e.g. VI, VII, VIII, IX), brainstem, and cerebellar signs.

Petrous temporal bone apex (Gradenigo's syndrome)[6]:

- Initially described in children with petrous apex osteitis (mastoiditis) as a complication of otitis media.
- May affect all three divisions of CN V and CN VI (decreased ipsilateral corneal reflex, facial pain, ear pain, double vision from ipsilateral abducens paresis, and motor loss in masticatory muscles).

Cavernous sinus/superior orbital fissure lesion

- Sensory disturbance occurs in the first division of CN V, and sometimes the second division; the third division is spared.
- Symptoms are associated with ocular motor (III, IV, and VI cranial) nerve palsies, Horner's syndrome, optic nerve or chiasm compression, and sometimes pain above and within the orbit.

- Proptosis, eyelid and conjunctival edema (chemosis), episcleral vasodilatation, and papilledema may be present if there is venous obstruction (e.g. cavernous sinus thrombosis). With a carotid–cavernous fistula there is additionally pulsating exophthalmos and an orbital bruit.

Orbital lesion

Sensory disturbance in the first division only, associated with ophthalmoplegia.

Foramen ovale or mandibular lesion

Sensory disturbance in the third division only; sometimes only unilateral numbness of the chin.

Bilateral trigeminal lesions

- Motor involvement: more obvious symptoms are usually evident, with weakness and wasting of the temporalis and masseter muscles bilaterally. If severe, the jaw hangs open.
- Sensory loss:
  - Bilateral facial sensory loss occurs, which may not be complete (e.g. it may be in an 'onion skin' distribution as may occur with syringobulbia).
  - Exposure to trichloroethylene (an organic solvent in glue, paint stripper, and paint) or organic mercury (e.g. methyl mercury).
  - Connective tissue disease such as progressive systemic sclerosis, systemic lupus erythematosus (SLE), and mixed connective tissue disease.

Investigations

These depend on the clinical syndrome and likely location and etiology:

- Direct examination of the nasopharynx and larynx.
- MRI or CT scan of brain, base of skull and orbits (with and without contrast).
- CSF examination (looking for findings suggestive of a possible infectious, malignant or inflammatory process).
- Full blood count and erythrocyte sedimentation rate (ESR).
- Fasting blood glucose.
- Autoantibody screen.
- Chest X-ray (evaluating for primary malignancy or thymoma, sarcoidosis).
- Electrophysiologic testing of the blink reflex may help in lesion localization and in distinguishing classical from symptomatic trigeminal neuralgia.
- Carotid angiography if a carotid–cavernous fistula is suspected.

SELECTED CONDITIONS AFFECTING THE TRIGEMINAL NERVE

ISOLATED TRIGEMINAL SENSORY NEUROPATHY

- Uncommon.
- It may begin as a small numb patch on the face, which spreads to the territory of innervation of the whole division of the nerve and then to the adjacent divisions and even the whole face.
- Severe loss of pain sensation in the face may lead to ulcerative lesions around the nose and in the cornea.
- Known causes need to be excluded, such as a skull base tumor, mixed connective tissue disease, systemic sclerosis, and other connective tissue diseases, but sometimes no cause can be found[11].
- Recovery sometimes occurs after weeks or months.

TRIGEMINAL NEURALGIA (TIC DOULOUREUX)

Definition and epidemiology

Trigeminal neuralgia (TN) is a painful condition caused by processes affecting the trigeminal nerve resulting in demyelination of its fibers. It is characterized by severe, paroxysmal, sharp lancinating pain in the distribution of one or more divisions of the trigeminal nerve (typically affecting $V_2 > V_3$). The condition is known as tic douloureux because of the typical lightning-like jabs of pain that may result in wincing.

- Incidence: 2–8 per 100,000 per year.
- Lifetime prevalence: 0.7% (95% CI: 0.4–1.0%); 4% of MS patients.
- Age: usually starts after the age of 50 years, most commonly in the sixth and seventh decades.
- Gender: F>M (1.5:1).

Etiology and pathophysiology

TN is divided by the International Headache Society into two types:

Classic: idiopathic or presumed to be caused by vascular compression of the trigeminal nerve, most commonly by an aberrant superior cerebellar or anterior inferior cerebellar artery.

Symptomatic: TN due to an underlying cause other than vascular compression. This includes:

- MS due to a plaque of demyelination at the root entry zone in the pons. This accounts for 2–3% of all cases of TN and up to 8% in younger patients.
- A small tumor arising from or compressing the trigeminal nerve (e.g. cerebello-pontine angle [CPA] neurofibroma, meningioma, or angioma).
- Arteriovenous malformations, aneurysms, and herpes zoster may be implicated.

Vascular compression of the trigeminal root appears to be an important contributing factor. At posterior fossa exploration, many patients are found to have a trigeminal root that is compressed or even grooved by a blood vessel, usually the superior cerebellar artery. It is thought that compression results in partial demyelination and axonal damage, rendering the axons hyperexcitable. Damaged axons that are near each other become susceptible to chemical coupling. Under these conditions, normal impulses elicited by light mechanical stimulation can recruit nearby pain fibers, particularly if they have already been made hyperexcitable by axonal damage. This results in synchronous discharge and therefore intense pain.

Differential diagnosis

- Temporomandibular joint (TMJ) disorders.
- Atypical dental pain.
- Phantom tooth pain.
- MS (TN may be bilateral).
- Glossopharyngeal neuralgia: extremely rare. Pain is of a similar nature (i.e. severe, unilateral, lancinating, and episodic) but at a different site: pain arises from the throat, larynx, pharynx, or pinna of the ear (i.e. in the distribution of the glossopharyngeal nerve).

Clinical features

Pain occurs in the face or mouth. It commonly starts in the dermatomal distribution of the second or third division of the trigeminal nerve; only 5% start in the first division. Trigger factors include talking, chewing, swallowing, shaving, brushing the teeth, and wind blowing on the face. Trigger points are areas around the nose, lips, or mouth which, when touched, evoke a paroxysm of pain. When sites are inside the mouth patients become hesitant about eating, drinking, and brushing their teeth.

The pain is described as brief (lasting for seconds) and followed by long pain-free intervals, and as stabbing/lightning or electric shock-like/penetrating jabs of pain or clusters of stabbing pains. The pattern is episodic: pain may recur several times a day for weeks or months, and then may remit for months or years.

Patients may become anxious and withdrawn because of the pain. Oral hygiene may suffer and weight loss may occur as patients attempt to avoid triggering the pain; depression, dehydration, and even suicide can occur in severely afflicted patients.

Investigations and diagnosis

CT may not identify intra-axial demyelination or small extra-axial neurofibroma. Scans should be used particularly if the patient is young (<40 years of age), if bilateral pain is present (more common in MS), or in the presence of neurologic signs (e.g. deafness).

Magnetic resonance angiography may be helpful. In a series of 50 patients with trigeminal neuralgia, neurovascular contact was demonstrated on the affected side in 51 of 55 symptomatic nerves studied and on the contralateral side in only 4 of 45 nerves.

Physical examination is normal in idiopathic TN. If there are abnormalities on examination, such as ipsilateral trigeminal nerve sensory loss, depressed corneal reflex, deafness, or if an aching pain persists between the characteristic stabs, then an underlying cause for the tic-like pains must be searched for.

Diagnosis is clinical. On pathology, focal demyelination and microneuromas are often present at the site of microvascular compression of the trigeminal nerve, but these features may also be found in asymptomatic subjects.

Treatment

Most patients can be managed medically. Carbamazepine, 400–1200 mg daily in divided doses, is the drug of choice for idiopathic TN, being effective initially in about three-quarters of patients[12]. It may control symptoms by suppressing sodium ion currents in the spinal trigeminal nucleus or in the Gasserian ganglion. A small dose of 50–100 mg nightly is the usual starting dose (to avoid drowsiness), escalating the dose as tolerated until pain relief is achieved (or adverse effects occur). A slow release preparation can also be used. The dose is continued for 1 month or so, and can then be tapered slowly, reloading if the pain recurs. Most responders will experience about 6–12 months of respite before recurrence. Up to one-third of patients cannot tolerate carbamazepine in the doses required to alleviate the pain, because of adverse effects such as rash, nausea, drowsiness, and ataxia. Carbamazepine may also cause hyponatremia, megaloblastic anemia (folate interaction), aplastic anemia, agranulocytosis, and hypersensitivity reactions. Oxcarbazepine is usually better tolerated.

Tip

▶ *Brain imaging studies for work-up of TN should be used in young patients (<40 years), if bilateral pain is present, and/or in the presence of neurologic signs/deficits.*

Alternatives include:

- Phenytoin 200–400 mg per day. This is less effective than carbamazepine but can be given intravenously for acute relapses of pain.
- Baclofen, a γ-aminobutyric acid (GABA) B-receptor agonist, 10–20 mg three times daily.
- Gabapentin, or pregabalin.
- Lamotrigine, which is at least as potent as carbamazepine in inactivating sodium ion currents, with fewer adverse effects, is effective in some cases. Lamotrigine is a potent antiglutamatergic agent which may depress excitatory transmission in the spinal trigeminal nucleus. It may cause initial ataxia, diplopia, nausea, vomiting, and blurred vision in 15–35% of patients but these are often dose related. An allergic skin rash is seen in 3–17% of patients.

For patients who fail to respond to medical management, one of several surgical procedures can be undertaken. These are either decompressive or denervating (i.e. permanently damage the trigeminal nerve). However, no clinical trials have established the efficacy of any surgical procedure.

Decompression

Posterior fossa exploration and microvascular decompression (the Jannetta procedure) consists of separating/removing and decompressing the offending artery or vein from the trigeminal nerve root. The majority of patients have immediate relief after microvascular decompression, although some later have recurrent pain. The advantage of this procedure is that facial sensation is preserved. The operation has risks, which include cranial hematomas, CSF leakage, meningitis, ipsilateral facial paresis or hearing loss (1%), brainstem infarction (0.1%), and death (0.2%). Despite its risks, microvascular decompression is currently the best first surgical option, especially late in the course of the disease[13].

Denervation

Percutaneous procedures are less invasive than microvascular decompression and are associated with low rates of mortality and morbidity, but they all create trigeminal nerve lesions, occasionally producing anesthesia dolorosa or keratitis.

- Percutaneous stereotactic radiofrequency thermal rhizotomy of the trigeminal (Gasserian) ganglion: this is a relatively simple procedure in which a probe is inserted into the foramen ovale under local anesthesia without the need for craniotomy. General anesthesia is required for the very painful process of coagulation. This procedure is effective in most cases and preserves some sensation but troublesome dysesthesia develops in about one-sixth of cases.
- Percutaneous glycerol rhizotomy.
- Balloon compression of the trigeminal ganglion.
- Intracranial nerve section of the appropriate divisions of the trigeminal nerve.

Prognosis

Commonly the episodes of pain follow a relapsing and remitting course, with exacerbations lasting weeks to months and spontaneous remissions that become shorter and less frequent over the years. Some patients go into spontaneous remission, and if soon after onset, this may last for years[12].

Ten years after microvascular decompression surgery, 70% of patients are free of pain without medication. Another 4% have occasional pain that does not require long-term medication[13].

The frequency of recurrent pain is similar for both microvascular decompression and percutaneous radiofrequency rhizotomy. Recurrence is more likely and occurs sooner after milder damage to the trigeminal nerve, produced either chemically or by compression with a percutaneously positioned balloon.

Predictors of recurrence after microvascular decompression include:

- Female sex.
- Symptoms lasting >8 years before surgery.
- Venous compression of the trigeminal root entry zone.
- Lack of immediate cessation of pain.

NUMB CHIN SYNDROME

The numb chin syndrome is usually seen in patients with systemic malignancy (lymphoreticular neoplasms, breast, lung, prostate, colon, thyroid cancer), but may be seen with noncancerous etiologies including dental procedures, dental infection, connective tissue disease, or trauma. The mental nerve is a branch of the inferior alveolar nerve, which arises from V_3. It exits through the mental foramen and supplies the chin and lower lip. The nerve may be compressed by a metastasis to bone at the mental foramen or along its course; it may also be infiltrated by tumor. Sensory loss extending beyond the chin and lower lip may indicate a more proximal V_3 lesion or leptomeningeal involvement. Evaluation should include MRI and CSF examination (if needed)[6,14].

FACIAL NERVE NEUROPATHY
(CRANIAL NERVE VII)

Definition and epidemiology

Disorder of the facial (VIIth cranial) nerve.

- Common.
- Age: any.
- Gender: M=F.

Anatomy

The facial nerve has motor, somatosensory, and secretomotor functions. The motor component of the facial nerve innervates the muscles of facial expression; this component represents about 70% of the facial nerve fibers. The remaining 30% are contained in the nervus intermedius and constitute the somatosensory and secretomotor components of the nerve[2].

There are five functional components of the facial nerve (**646**):

- Special visceral efferent: innervates the muscles of facial expression, the stapedius, stylohyoid, and posterior belly of the digastric.
- General visceral efferent: parasympathetic fibers that innervate the lacrimal, submandibular, and sublingual glands in addition to the mucous membranes of the nasopharynx and palate.
- Special visceral afferent: taste sensation from the anterior two-thirds of the tongue.
- General somatic afferent: sensory innervation (touch, temperature and pain) from the auricle, pinna of the ear, and retroauricular region.
- General visceral afferent: light touch, temperature, and pain sensation from the soft palate and surrounding pharyngeal wall.

Motor component

Supranuclear control

- Precentral gyrus: the innervation of the facial muscles begins in the most lateral and inferior aspect of the precentral gyrus, near the Sylvian fissure. This region is supplied by a branch of the middle cerebral artery.
- Corticobulbar fibers course in the corona radiata, the genu of the internal capsule, and the medial aspect of the cerebral peduncle before reaching the pons.
- In the pons, most descending fibers decussate and project on the contralateral facial motor nucleus. The facial motor nucleus is divided into a dorsal and a ventral half. The ventral portion innervates the lower two-thirds of the face and receives crossed supranuclear control. The dorsal portion supplies the upper one-third of the face and has bilateral supranuclear control. As a result, a unilateral hemispheric lesion impairs only the lower facial muscles[6].

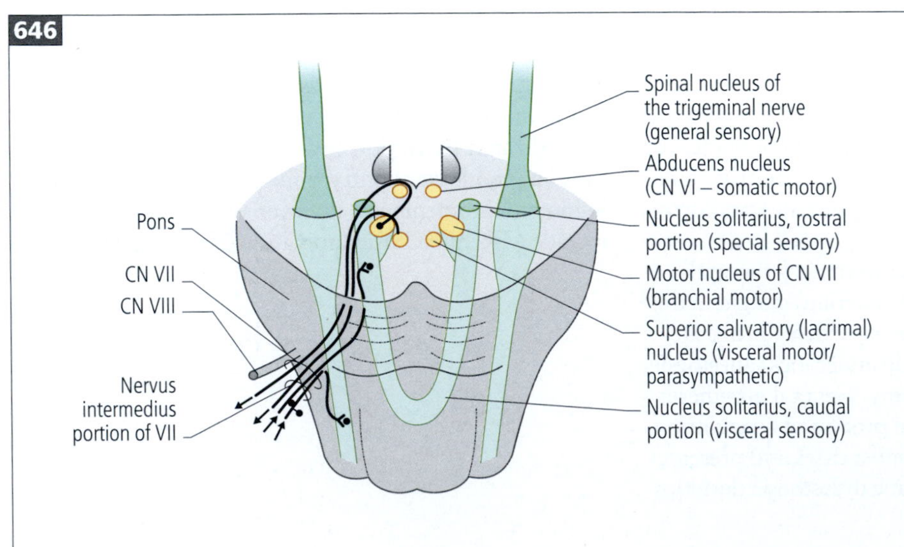

646 Cranial nerve VII brainstem nuclei. *Adapted from 'Cranial Nerves in Health and Disease' by Linda Wilson-Pauwels.*

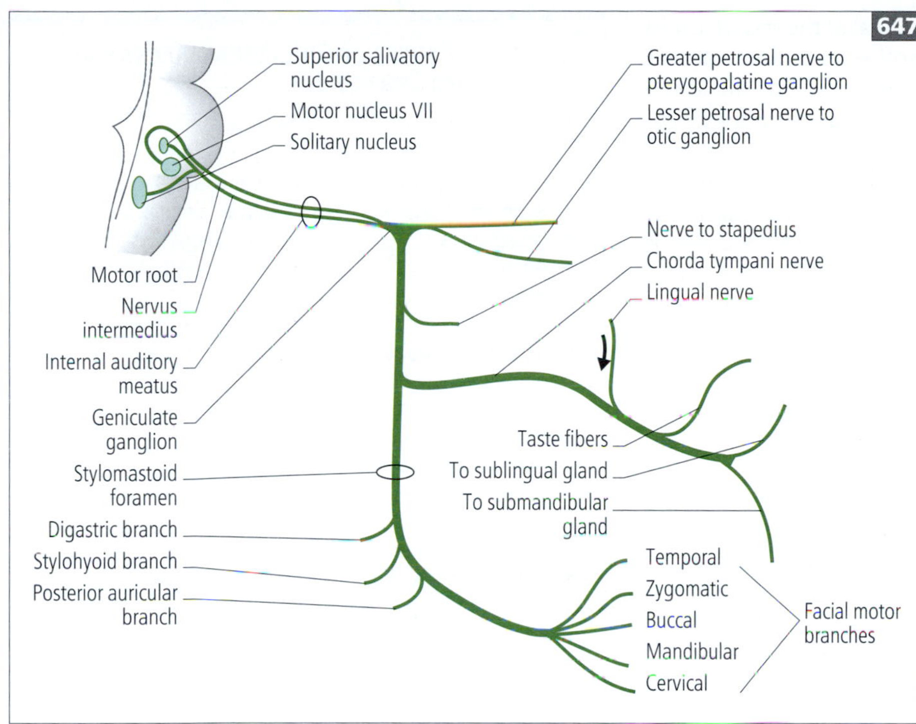

647 Anatomy of cranial nerve VII. *Adapted from Shapiro. EMG.*

Nuclear and infranuclear control (647)

The facial motor nucleus lies ventral and lateral to the abducens nucleus in the lower pons. From the facial nucleus, all the nerve fibers that innervate the ipsilateral facial muscles ascend posteriorly and medially to hook around the abducens nucleus (genu of the facial nerve) before travelling forward through the pons (just lateral to the corticospinal tract), to emerge from the ventro-lateral aspect of the brainstem. The motor division of the facial nerve and the nervus intermedius (see below) then proceed laterally in the CPA along with CN VIII before entering the internal auditory canal of the temporal bone (with CN VIII). The nerve has four segments within the temporal bone:

- Meatal segment: this segment extends from the porus of the internal auditory canal to the meatal foramen. There are no major branches from this facial nerve segment.
- Labyrinthine segment: this segment extends from the meatal foramen to the geniculate ganglion. The labyrinthine segment is the narrowest part of the facial nerve and is susceptible to compression as a result of edema. In this section, which is 3–5 mm in length, the facial nerve changes direction to form the first genu and ends at the geniculate ganglion where the cell bodies of the general somatic and special visceral afferent neurons are located. The greater superficial petrosal nerve, which is the first major branch of the facial nerve, arises from the upper portion of the geniculate ganglion.
- Tympanic segment: this section is 10 mm in length and has no major nerve branches. It extends from the geniculate ganglion to the horizontal semicircular canal. The tympanic segment ends where the facial nerve makes its second genu.
- Mastoid segment: this is the final intracranial portion of the facial canal. The nerve proceeds vertically to the stylomastoid foramen where it exits the cranium. The nerve to the stapedius originates near the upper portion of this segment. The chorda tympani is another branch arising from this segment; it joins the lingual nerve and carries preganglionic parasympathetic fibers (from the superior salivatory nucleus) which innervate the submandibular and sublingual glands and afferent taste fibers from the anterior two-thirds of the tongue. A sensory branch exits the nerve just below the stylomastoid foramen and innervates the posterior wall of the external auditory canal and a portion of the tympanic membrane.

Once it has exited the facial canal at the stylomastoid foramen, the facial nerve gives off several rami before it divides into its main branches. Near the exit site at the stylomastoid foramen, the facial nerve gives off the posterior auricular nerve, which supplies auricular muscles and the occipitalis, the digastric branch, and the stylohyoid branch. The facial nerve then pierces the parotid gland where it divides into five branches that supply muscles of facial expression and the platysma: temporal, zygomatic, buccal, marginal mandibular, and cervical (**648**).

Sensory component

The sensory and parasympathetic component of the facial nerve is the nervus intermedius (of Wrisberg). This division of the facial nerve carries:

- Sensory fibers that carry taste sensation from the anterior two-thirds of the tongue, afferents from the pharyngeal, nasal, and palatal mucosae, and from the skin of the external auditory canal, lateral ear, and post-auricular region. The taste fibers from the anterior two-thirds of the tongue first traverse the lingual nerve (a branch of the mandibular nerve) and then diverge to join the chorda tympani (a branch of CN VII); then they pass through the pars intermedia and geniculate ganglion of the VII nerve to the rostral part of the nucleus of the tractus solitarius in the medulla. Somatic afferent fibers from the external auditory canal and post-auricular region end in the spinal nucleus of cranial nerve V.

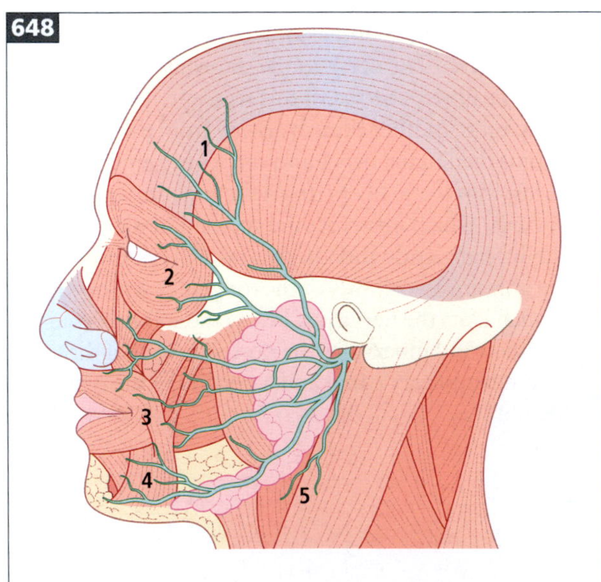

648 Motor branches of the facial nerve. 1: temporal; 2: zygomatic; 3: buccal; 4: mandibular; 5: cervical.

TABLE 111 **CAUSES OF UNILATERAL VII CRANIAL NEUROPATHY**

Pontine
- Infarct
- Multiple sclerosis
- Brainstem tumor
- Encephalitis
- Abscess
- Hemorrhage

Congenital/postnatal
- Möbius syndrome
- Facial neuropathy from forceps/birth trauma
- Hemicranial microsomia
- Congenital lower lip paralysis
- Kawasaki disease
- Albers–Schoenberg disease (osteopetrosis)
- Infantile hypercalcemia
- Cardiofacial syndrome

Tumor
- Acoustic neuroma
- Meningioma
- Cholesteatoma
- Metastatic
- Neurinoma
- Parotid tumor

Meningitis
- Infectious
  - Bacterial
  - Fungal
  - Tuberculous
  - Syphilis
  - Lyme disease/ borreliosis
  - Parasitic (trichinosis, neurocysticercosis)
- Inflammatory
- Sarcoid
- Neoplastic
- Carcinomatous

Lymphomatous
- Leukemia (children)

Infections
- Ramsay Hunt syndrome (HZV)
- Herpes simplex virus
- HIV seroconversion
- Osteomyelitis of skull base
- Otogenic infections
- Parotitis/abscess
- Mastoiditis
- Lyme disease
- Leprosy
- Poliomyelitis
- Mycoplasma
- Influenza

Miscellaneous
- Benign intracranial hypertension
- Trauma
- Melkersson–Rosenthal syndrome
- Amyloidosis
- Wegener's granulomatosis
- Polyarteritis
- Diabetes mellitus
- Sjögren's syndrome
- Pregnancy
- Human T-cell lymphotropic virus type 1
- Hereditary neuropathy with pressure palsies
- Familial Bell's palsy
- Guillain–Barré syndrome
- Chronic inflammatory demyelinating polyneuropathy
- Charcot–Marie–Tooth disease
- Histiocytosis X
- Interferon therapy
- Sclerosteosis
- Ethylene glycol intoxication
- Wernicke–Korsakov syndrome
- Stevens–Johnson syndrome

HIV: human immunodeficiency virus; HZV: herpes zoster virus.

- Parasympathetic fibers to the submandibular and sublingual glands (through the submaxillary ganglion) and to the lacrimal, palatal, and nasal glands (through the pterygopalatine ganglion). The preganglionic parasympathetic fibers originate in the superior salivatory nucleus at the level of the caudal pons; fibers that control lacrimation arise from the adjacent lacrimal nucleus. These fibers exit the brainstem as part of the nervus intermedius and divide into two groups:
  - One group of fibers synapses with the pterygopalatine ganglion through the greater superficial petrosal nerve. Post-ganglionic fibers innervate the lacrimal, palatal, and nasal glands.
  - Another group of fibers will synapse with the submaxillary ganglion through the chorda tympani and branches from the lingual nerve. Post-ganglionic fibers innervate the sublingual and submaxillary glands.

Clinical features

Facial neuropathy can occur at any age and is nearly always unilateral. It is bilateral in 1–2% of cases[15]. Predisposing conditions include diabetes mellitus and pregnancy. Unilateral facial weakness of acute onset may be secondary to a facial neuropathy or a central lesion. A central facial weakness spares the upper face, is not associated with hyperacusis or taste abnormalities, and is often accompanied by other findings referable to the site of the lesion. Most cases of facial neuropathy are caused by Bell's palsy. Other causes of facial neuropathy are listed in *Table 111*.

Bilateral facial neuropathy is most commonly caused by Bell's palsy; other etiologies include (but are not limited to) sarcoidosis, Guillain–Barré syndrome, and Lyme disease (*Table 112*)[15].

TABLE 112 **DISEASES MOST LIKELY TO CAUSE BILATERAL FACIAL NEUROPATHY**

Bell's palsy
Guillain–Barré syndrome
Miller Fisher syndrome
Multiple cranial neuropathies
Brainstem encephalitis
Neoplastic meningitis
Pontine glioma
Prepontine tumors
Syphilis
Leprosy
Infectious meningitis
Lyme disease
Herpes simplex virus, herpes zoster virus
Sarcoidosis
Sclerosteosis
Amyloidosis
Ethylene glycol intoxication
Möbius syndrome
HIV seroconversion
Mononucleosis
Poliomyelitis
Head injury (especially children)

HIV: human immunodeficiency virus.

Supranuclear lesions (upper motor neuron facial palsy)

A supranuclear lesion affecting the corticobulbar tract results in contralateral weakness of the lower facial muscles. The most severely affected muscles are the ones around the mouth and there is occasional involvement of the orbicularis oculi. The muscles of the forehead are spared and there is no hyperacusis, or dysgeusia.

Tip

▶ *Facial paresis from a central lesion spares the upper face and is not associated with hyperacusis or taste abnormalities.*

Nuclear and fascicular lesions

Lesions in the pons affecting the facial motor nucleus or facial nerve fascicles result in an ipsilateral peripheral (or lower motor neuron) facial nerve palsy with lower and upper facial weakness. There is weakness of frowning, eye closure, and of elevation of the eyebrow in addition to involvement of muscles of the lower face. Pontine lesions involving the facial nucleus/fascicles usually affect neighboring structures such as the nucleus or fascicles of CN VI (reduced abduction in ipsilateral eye), the paramedian pontine reticular formation (impaired conjugate horizontal gaze to ipsilateral side), the corticospinal tract (contralateral arm and leg weakness), the spinal tract and nucleus of CN V (ipsilateral facial numbness), and the spinothalamic tract (contralateral hemibody numbness)[10].

Cerebello-pontine angle lesions

A lesion in the CPA may involve the motor fibers of the facial nerve (ipsilateral upper and lower facial weakness), the nervus intermedius (loss of taste over the ipsilateral anterior two-thirds of the tongue), and CN VIII (vertigo, ipsilateral tinnitus, and hearing loss).

Facial canal lesions

- A lesion in the meatal segment has a similar presentation to CPA lesions.
- A lesion between the end of the meatal segment and the take off of the nerve to stapedius results in involvement of the motor division of the facial nerve (ipsilateral peripheral facial weakness and hyperacusis) and the nervus intermedius (loss of taste over the ipsilateral anterior two-thirds of the tongue). Lacrimation is impaired if the lesion is proximal to the greater superficial petrosal nerve.
- A lesion between the nerve to stapedius and the chorda tympani results in ipsilateral peripheral facial weakness and loss of taste over the ipsilateral anterior two-thirds of the tongue, without hyperacusis.
- A lesion distal to the chorda tympani results in ipsilateral peripheral facial weakness without hyperacusis or alteration of taste.
- There is impairment of sensation in the ipsilateral earlobe with lesions proximal to the stylomastoid foramen.

Physical examination

- Drooping of one side of the face with flattening of the forehead creases, widening of the palpebral fissure, flattening of the nasolabial fold, lowering of the corner of the mouth, and impaired smiling and grinning are observed at rest. The patient is unable to elevate the eyebrow, wrinkle the forehead, and close the eye on the affected side.
- The eye may be red and dry as a result of impaired blinking or decreased lacrimation.
- Air escapes between the lips on the affected side when the cheeks are puffed with air.
- Corneal reflex is impaired because the lesion affects the efferent limb of this reflex arc.
- Taste may be impaired if the facial nerve is lesioned proximal to the chorda tympani branch, within the temporal bone.
- Speech may be slurred (flaccid dysarthria).
- Otoscopy of the external auditory canal may reveal findings that could be relevant (e.g. vesicles which may suggest herpetic facial neuropathy [Ramsay Hunt syndrome]).
- Examination of the oral cavity may also reveal vesicles on the ipsilateral palate in patients with Ramsay Hunt syndrome.
- Associated central nervous system (CNS), CN, or peripheral nervous system signs may be present such as contralateral hemisensory loss or gaze palsy ipsilateral to the lower motor neuron facial weakness (suggesting a low pontine lesion), multiple cranial neuropathies (suggesting basilar meningitis or vasculitis), or sensory disturbances in the distal extremities or muscle wasting (which may indicate an underlying neuropathy).

SELECTED CONDITIONS AFFECTING THE FACIAL NERVE

BELL'S PALSY

This condition presents with the acute onset of unilateral facial weakness (**649**) and accounts for up to 70% of cases of facial neuropathy. The incidence is 20–30 per 100,000 persons per year. The incidence of Bell's palsy is higher in diabetics and in pregnant women.

There is evidence supporting reactivation of herpes simplex virus (HSV) infection in the geniculate ganglion as the major cause of Bell's palsy resulting in inflammation and edema of the nerve in the facial canal causing demyelination and in some cases, axonal loss. Other viruses that have been implicated include varicella zoster virus (VZV), cytomegalovirus (CMV), coxsackie, Epstein–Barr virus (EBV), mumps, influenza, and human immunodeficiency virus (HIV)[8].

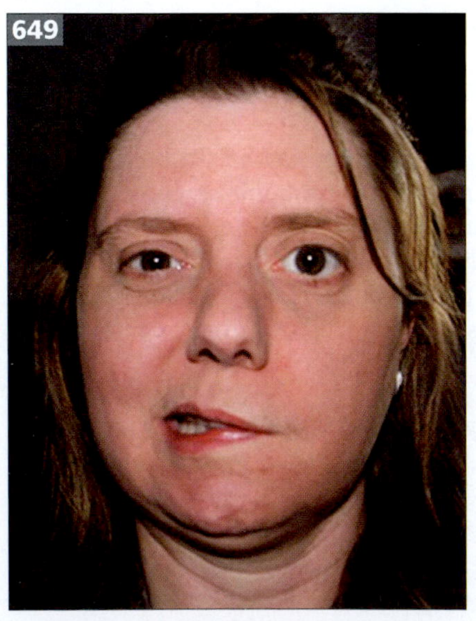

649 Patient with left Bell's palsy.

Clinical features

- A viral prodrome is present in about 60% of patients.
- Pain behind the ear may precede the facial weakness by up to 2 weeks, evolving over about 48 hours before reaching a plateau.
- Unilateral facial weakness of lower motor neuron type follows the pain, and may be associated with excessive tearing due to weakness of the orbicularis oculi (which normally holds the puncta lacrimalia against the conjunctiva) or decreased lacrimation due to impaired innervation of the lacrimal gland.
- Ipsilateral facial numbness is a common symptom, but objective sensory testing is normal.
- Taste may be altered.
- Sensitivity to sound may be increased (hyperacusis), such as when using a telephone.
- The presence of vesicles in the ear canal, behind the ear, or in the palate, is suggestive of Ramsay Hunt (see below).
- Brain imaging is not indicated unless a structural lesion is suspected. A large percentage of patients with Bell's palsy have enhancement of the facial nerve on MRI.

Treatment

A benefit from steroids or acyclovir has not been definitively established; however, available evidence suggests that steroids are probably effective and the combination of steroids and acyclovir is possibly effective in improving functional outcomes. There is insufficient evidence regarding the effectiveness of surgical facial nerve decompression in this condition[16].

- Corticosteroids: controversial, partly because of the good prognosis of the untreated condition and the failure of controlled trials to prove a beneficial effect on long-term outcome[17]. Nevertheless, steroids are used empirically by some neurologists to:
  - Relieve pain that is sometimes an early feature.
  - Prevent progression of incomplete to complete paralysis.
  - Prevent denervation in cases of complete paralysis.
  - Shorten the time to recovery.
  - Retard development of abnormal synkinesis.
  - It is likely that any benefit obtained is due to steroids used early in the course (within 1 week of onset).
- Acyclovir: may be effective if the underlying cause is herpes virus infection. More data are needed from a large, randomized, controlled and blinded trial.
- Other treatments: there is no proven place for adjunctive therapies or surgical decompression of the facial nerve in Bell's palsy.
- Avoid complications: exposure keratitis:
  - Occurs if the cornea is not adequately protected.
  - It can be avoided by using artificial tears, instilling lubricating paraffin ointment, and taping (rather than padding) the eye closed at night.
  - Dark glasses should be worn outdoors.
  - Ophthalmic advice should be sought if the patient reports eye discomfort or the eye becomes irritated despite the above measures.
  - Botulinum toxin injection into the eyelid levator to weaken it may be considered if conservative measures fail.
  - Tarsorrhaphy is rarely necessary in cooperative patients.

Prognosis

Most patients with Bell's palsy have a favorable prognosis. Approximately 60–80% of patients recover completely. In these cases, recovery usually begins within 8 weeks and is complete by 6–12 months. The most favorable prognostic sign is an incomplete rather than complete facial palsy. If weakness is severe or complete, recovery commencing within 3 weeks is a favorable sign. The longer the delay in return of movement, the poorer the recovery. Recurrence occurs in around 7% of patients. If this occurs, alternative causes should be excluded, such as diabetes, sarcoidosis, tumor, or infection[8,14].

From a prognostic standpoint, the amplitude of the facial motor response on electrodiagnostic testing can be helpful in the case of a unilateral facial palsy, by comparing side-to-side amplitude difference 5–7 days after onset of symptoms. On rare occasions, recovery from Bell's palsy may be associated with persistent dysfunction including synkinesis, myokymia, or hemifacial spasm[18].

Predictors of incomplete recovery are:

- Complete facial weakness.
- Pain other than in or around the ear (i.e. back of head, cheek, other).
- Older age.
- Hyperacusis.
- Decreased tearing.

Residual deficits include:

- Facial weakness.
- 'Jaw winking' and other abnormal facial movements (synkinesis) caused by aberrant reinnervation of the muscles of facial expression by regenerating facial nerve fibers.
- 'Crocodile tears' (rare): an excessive flow of tears when eating, caused by aberrant reinnervation of the lacrimal gland by regenerating facial nerve fibers.

RAMSAY HUNT SYNDROME
(HERPES ZOSTER FACIAL PARESIS/
HERPES ZOSTER OTICUS)

- Peripheral facial neuropathy, hyperacusis, ipsilateral taste alteration, and ear pain accompanied by a vesicular rash on the eardrum, external auditory meatus or palate, in addition to erythema of the external ear.
- Reactivation of the varicella zoster virus (VZV) in the geniculate ganglion[19].
- Could be associated with other cranial neuropathies (VIII, IX, or X) resulting in hearing loss, tinnitus, and vertigo.
- Condition can occur in children or adults.
- Seroconversion is common, with an increase in specific antibody to VZV.
- Worse prognosis than Bell's palsy.

There is a lack of prospective, randomized controlled trials in Ramsay Hunt syndrome. Recommended treatment is with prednisone and antiviral agents such as acyclovir, famcyclovir, or valacyclovir.

VESTIBULO-COCHLEAR NERVE NEUROPATHY (CRANIAL NERVE VIII)

Definition and epidemiology

A common disorder of the vestibulo-cochlear (VIIIth cranial) nerve.

Anatomy

The vestibulo-cochlear nerve is a special somatic afferent nerve consisting of two functional divisions: the vestibular nerve, mediating equilibrium and balance information from the vestibular apparatus (semicircular canals, saccule, and utricle), and the cochlear nerve, mediating auditory information from the cochlear apparatus (organ of Corti in the spiral ganglion). Both of these structures are in the inner ear, which is located deep in the temporal bone within a space called the bony labyrinth (**650**). The bony labyrinth contains the so-called membranous labyrinth and is filled with perilymph, a fluid with a chemical content similar to that of CSF and plasma. The membranous labyrinth is filled with endolymph, a highly specialized fluid with high protein content. The membranous labyrinth is further divided in two portions: vestibular and cochlear. The hair cells are the sensory receptors for both the vestibular and the cochlear systems[2].

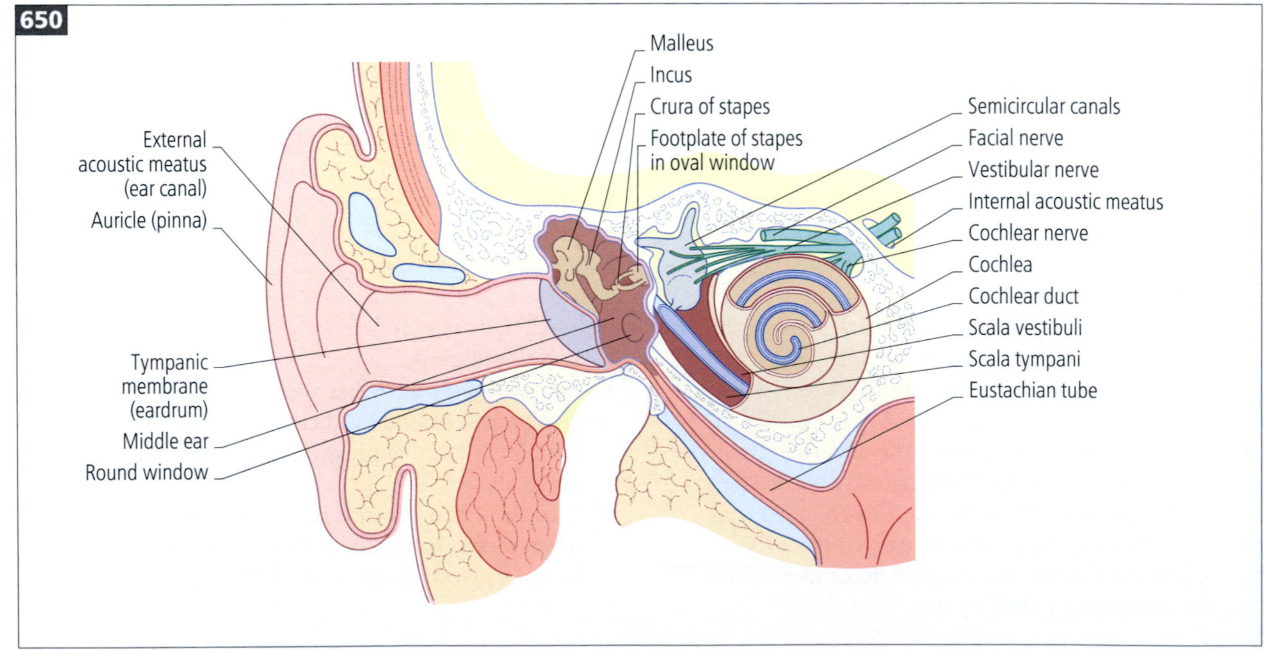

650 Anatomy of the ear.

Vestibular apparatus

The first-order sensory neurons of the vestibular pathway are bipolar cells located in Scarpa's ganglion (vestibular ganglion), in the fundus of the internal auditory meatus. The vestibular portion of the membranous labyrinth is divided into two sections: kinetic labyrinth (formed by the semicircular canals), and the static labyrinth (formed by the saccule and utricle). The vestibular bipolar neurons send peripheral projections to the hair cells in the semicircular canals, saccule, and utricle. Their central projections are to the four vestibular nuclei in the brainstem (lateral, medial, superior, and inferior) located in the caudal pons and rostral medulla. From the vestibular nuclei, central fibers are projected to the nuclei of the CNs responsible for extraocular movements (through the medial longitudinal fasciculus), the spinal cord (via the lateral and medial vestibulospinal tracts), and the flocculonodular lobe of the cerebellum[20].

Semicircular canals

The semicircular canals (SCCs) sense angular acceleration of the head. There are three SCCs in each ear which contain endolymphatic fluid, and are oriented at right angles to each other: lateral (horizontal), posterior, and anterior (superior). Each SSC has an expanded end called the cristae ampullaris, which contains hair cells and the cupula which is a gelatinous structure lying on top of the stereocilia of the hair cells.

During head movement, the endolymph inside the SCCs displaces the cupula, and this in turn causes the stereocilia of the hair cells to bend. The mechanical movement of the hair cells is converted into an electrical signal. Neural activity generated by the canals is transmitted in the vestibular nerve to the vestibular nuclei on the same side of the brainstem.

Otholith organ: utricle and saccule

The utricle and saccule sense linear acceleration of the head. Both are expansions of the membranous labyrinth and contain a macula which consists of hair cells covered by an otolithic membrane (lying on top of the hair cells) and otoconia (composed of calcium carbonate crystals or otoliths) on the surface. The hair cells are deflected by the movement of the otoliths.

Auditory apparatus

The first-order sensory neurons of the cochlear pathway are bipolar cells and their cell bodies are located in the spiral ganglion (lying in Rosenthal's canal). They project peripherally to the hair cells in the organ of Corti and project centrally as the cochlear nerve to the anteroventral, posteroventral, and dorsal cochlear nuclei in the brainstem. Central fibers arising from these nuclei are then projected through the different relays of the auditory pathway before reaching the primary auditory cortex (Brodmann's area 41) located in the transverse temporal gyri of Heschl.

Cochlea

The cochlea has the shape of a tapering helix. Inside, portions of the membranous labyrinth (vestibular and basilar membranes) divide this spiraling tunnel structure into three channels called scalas. The scala vestibuli and tympani are filled with perilymph and are contiguous at the tip of the cochlea by an anatomical portion called helicotrema, whereas the scala media (also known as cochlear duct) lies between the other two scalas, is filled with endolymph and contains the organ of Corti.

Organ of Corti

This contains receptor hair cells which lie on supporting tissue arising from the basilar membrane in the cochlea. The hair cell processes are embedded in a thin membrane that bridges across the organ of Corti, known as the tectorial membrane.

Sound waves are transmitted by the pump-like effect of the stapes in the oval window which creates shock waves that are passed to the round window where the energy dissipates. The pressure wave is transmitted through the perilymph, and leads to vibration of the basilar membrane, depending on the frequency of the sound. When the basilar membrane oscillates, the tectorial membrane has a shearing effect across the hair cells, stimulating the cochlear nerve fibers.

Hair cells located in the tip of the cochlea are stimulated by low-frequency tones and those located at the base are stimulated by high-frequency tones.

Vestibulo-cochlear nerve

The vestibulo-cochlear nerve emerges from the temporal bone to enter the posterior fossa through the internal auditory canal along with the facial nerve. Both nerves pass through the CPA to enter the brainstem at the anterolateral pontomedullary junction.

Brainstem

Vestibular nuclei

These occupy much of the lower lateral pontine tegmentum, with vertical ramifications over the entire brainstem from the midbrain down to the cervical spinal cord. Consequently, vestibular symptoms and signs are almost always present in brainstem disease but are of limited intrinsic localizing value within the brainstem.

Cochlear nuclei

These receive fibers from the cochlear nerve as it enters the pons, and transmit auditory information to the superior olives bilaterally (mainly contralaterally), from which fibers ascend in the lateral lemniscus to the inferior colliculus (midbrain), medial geniculate, and temporal cortex (Heschl's gyrus)[1].

Clinical features

Hearing loss

Abnormalities in the auditory pathways manifest as hearing impairment. Sensorineural hearing loss is a deficit caused by a lesion at the level of the cochlea or CN VIII. Conductive hearing loss is due to a dysfunction in transmission of sound to the cochlea (in the external or middle ear).

Patients with sensorineural hearing loss often have tinnitus. Tinnitus is rarely an isolated symptom of neurologic disease unless it is pulsatile and associated with a bruit that is audible to the examiner. Pulsatile tinnitus may be indicative of a dural arteriovenous fistula, arteriovenous malformation in the neck or head, stenosis of the distal internal carotid artery extra- or intracranially, carotid–cavernous fistula, giant intracranial aneurysm, glomus jugulare tumor, or high cardiac output (e.g. pregnancy, thyrotoxicosis, anemia)[14].

Evaluation of the auditory system includes:

- Examination of the ear.
- Bedside testing of hearing: rubbing fingers or whispering in one ear.
- Differentiating sensorineural from conductive, or mixed hearing loss with bedside testing (Weber's and Rinne's test) and quantitative audiologic testing.
- Sudden sensorineural hearing loss: sudden deafness caused by pathology in the cochlea or CN VIII. This is almost always unilateral. The etiology is often unclear and recovery is variable. Prognosis is poor if hearing loss is profound.
- Stroke: hearing loss can occur with anterior inferior cerebellar artery (AICA) distribution infarcts. The vascular supply of the inner ear comes from the internal auditory artery, which is a branch of the AICA.
- CPA: symptoms include progressive hearing loss, tinnitus, vertigo, and loss of balance. Other symptoms may include facial neuropathy (due to involvement of CN VII) and facial pain (CN V). The most common tumors in this location include acoustic neuroma followed by meningioma.

Vestibular dysfunction

Vestibular dysfunction usually presents with symptoms of vertigo, which is an illusion of motion in the form of a spinning or whirling sensation. It may be associated with nausea, vomiting, oscillopsia, hearing loss, and tinnitus. The presence of associated unilateral hearing loss or fullness in the ear suggests ear pathology. Signs and symptoms referable to the brainstem, CNs, or cerebellum are indicative of a central lesion[20].

Evaluation of the vestibular system includes:

- Neuro-ophthalmological evaluation to assess for the presence of nystagmus in primary gaze and in all directions of gaze. Using Frenzel goggles to remove ocular fixation is often helpful in assessing nystagmus. Peripheral nystagmus usually has horizontal and torsional components; it may be present in primary gaze and becomes more prominent in the direction of the fast phase of the nystagmus, but the direction of the nystagmus does not change. In central vertigo, the nystagmus may have a vertical component and the direction of the nystagmus may change.
- Evaluation of vestibular control of balance: with Romberg testing the patient tends to fall towards the side of vestibular dysfunction. If the patient walks with the eyes closed there is a tendency to veer to the affected side.
- Provocative tests to induce vertigo and nystagmus: Dix–Hallpike test, caloric testing.

Tip

▶ *Peripheral nystagmus usually is horizontal and torsional and the direction of the nystagmus does not change. Central nystagmus can be horizontal and/or vertical and the direction of the nystagmus may change.*

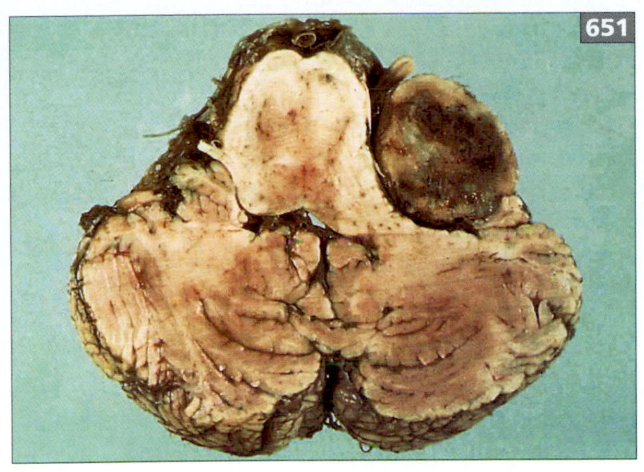

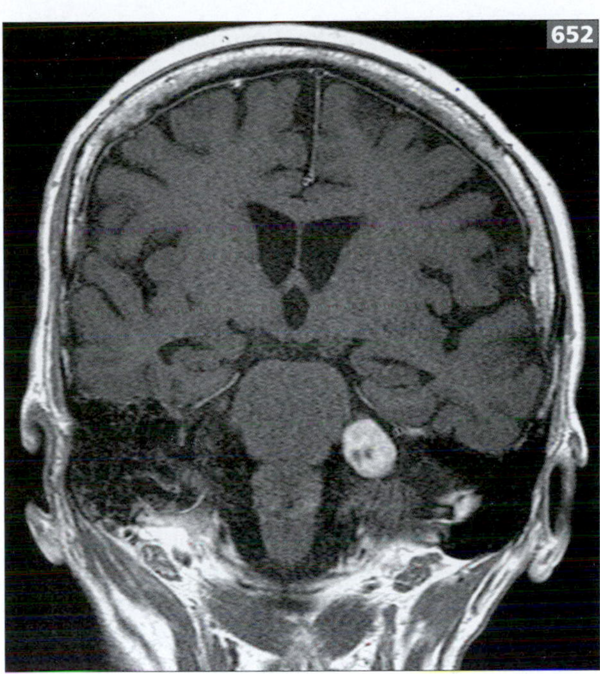

651 Axial section through the pons and cerebellum showing a vestibular schwannoma.

652 Brain MRI, coronal view, showing an acoustic schwannoma. *Courtesy of Dr Laughlin Dawes, University of Sydney.*

Differential diagnosis

Hearing loss

- Brainstem (pontomedullary junction):
  - Infarct or hemorrhage.
  - MS.
  - Tumor.
  - Central pontine myelinolysis.
- CPA:
  - Vestibular schwannoma (**651, 652**).
  - Meningioma.
  - Arachnoid cyst.
  - Epidermoid/dermoid tumor.
  - Chordoma.
  - Metastases.
  - Basilar artery ectasia or aneurysm, AICA aneurysm.
  - Arteriovenous malformation.
- Peripheral nerve lesions:
  - Infectious meningitis: bacterial, viral.
  - Carcinomatous meningitis.
  - Sarcoidosis.
  - Meningovascular syphilis.
  - Herpes zoster oticus.
  - Refsum's disease.
  - Chordoma.
  - Nasopharyngeal carcinoma.
  - Metastases.
  - Paget's disease of the skull: obstruction of foramina.
  - Trauma, base of skull fractures.
- Sensorineural deafness:
  - Ototoxins: aminoglycosides, loop diuretics, quinine, high dose salicylates and nonsteroidal anti-inflammatory drugs (NSAIDs), cis-platinum.
  - Ménière's disease.
  - Cranial radiation.
  - Cogan's syndrome.
  - Susac's syndrome.
- Conductive hearing loss:
  - Middle ear diseases.
  - Cerumen impaction.
  - Otosclerosis.

Vestibular dysfunction

Peripheral causes of vertigo

Peripheral vestibular syndromes usually present with severe vertigo, often associated with tinnitus, hearing loss, and nystagmus. There are no other abnormalities to suggest a central etiology. Nystagmus is unidirectional with the fast phase away from the side of the lesion, usually horizontal with a rotatory component.

- Benign paroxysmal positional vertigo (BPPV): this is a common inner ear disorder characterized by brief attacks of vertigo precipitated by head movement and associated with nystagmus and autonomic symptoms. The vertigo typically lasts less than 30 seconds. Symptoms may occur repeatedly throughout the day. BPPV is due to canalithiasis (otoconia have broken free from the macule of the utricle and become free floating in a SCC) or cupulolithiasis (otoconia become adherent to the matrix gel of the cupula). Most cases of BPPV are due to posterior canalithiasis. The diagnosis of BPPV is confirmed with the Dix–Hallpike maneuver. In posterior canal BPPV, after head tilt toward the affected ear, vertigo develops with concomitant nystagmus with an upbeat and torsional component. The nystagmus develops a few seconds after positioning the patient, fatigues within 30 seconds, and habituates with repeated attempts. Symptoms may last for weeks and may recur[21]. Treatment consists of repositioning maneuvers[22].

- With a central lesion, symptoms develop when the head is turned to either side during the testing maneuver, the vertigo is usually mild and brief, the nystagmus changes direction when the head is turned from one side to the other, and is not fatigable.
- Vestibular neuronitis: this is usually associated with a viral infection or is the result of post-viral inflammation of the vestibular portion of CN VIII. Patients present with severe vertigo that lasts several days, associated with nausea, vomiting, and at times unilateral hearing loss. Examination may show horizontal nystagmus with a torsional component. Treatment is symptomatic with antiemetics and benzodiazepines.
- Other causes of peripheral vertigo: trauma, perilymphatic fistula, Ménière's disease, middle ear disease, syphilis, geniculate zoster, viral and bacterial labyrinthitis.

Central causes of vertigo

Vertigo of central origin is usually less severe than peripheral vertigo and is usually continuous. It is associated with abnormalities referable to the brainstem or cerebellum and hearing impairment is less frequent. Nystagmus can be bidirectional.

- Posterior circulation stroke or transient ischemic attack (TIA) (lateral medullary syndrome, AICA distribution stroke), cerebellar hemorrhage, basilar migraine.
- MS.
- Wernicke's encephalopathy.
- CPA tumors.
- Temporal lobe seizures.

GLOSSOPHARYNGEAL NERVE NEUROPATHY (CRANIAL NERVE IX)

Definition and epidemiology

Disorder of the glossopharyngeal (IXth cranial) nerve. It is a rare disorder, particularly in isolation.

Anatomy

The glossopharyngeal nerve contains sensory, motor, special visceral afferent, and parasympathetic fibers[1].

Medulla (653)

Motor fibers

These arise from the upper part of the nucleus ambiguus in the medulla, and supply the stylopharyngeus muscle (which cannot be tested clinically). The nucleus ambiguus is the main motor nucleus of cranial nerves IX, X, and XI; it receives bilateral supranuclear innervation from corticobulbar fibers[2].

Sensory fibers

- Taste fibers from the posterior third of the tongue and pharynx terminate (via the glossopharyngeal nerve) in the nucleus of the tractus solitarius.
- General somatic afferent fibers (pain, temperature, and tactile sensation) from the posterior one-third of the tongue, tonsils, soft palate, tympanic membrane, and Eustachian tube terminate in the nucleus of the spinal tract of the trigeminal nerve.
- Chemoreceptive (from the carotid body) and baroreceptive (from the carotid sinus) fibers are carried by the glossopharyngeal nerve via the carotid sinus nerve and terminate in the solitary nucleus.

Parasympathetic fibers

These originate in the inferior salivatory nucleus in the medulla and at the petrous ganglion, and travel via Jacobson's nerve and the lesser superficial petrosal nerve to the otic ganglion. Postganglionic fibers supply the parotid gland.

Base of skull (jugular foramen) (654)

The glossopharyngeal nerve emerges from the posterior lateral sulcus of the medulla in line with the vagus and the bulbar fibers of the spinal accessory nerve, and enters the internal part of the jugular foramen lying on the medial side of the sigmoid sinus.

The foramen angles forwards and laterally under the petrous bone, which is excavated by the slight ballooning of the sigmoid sinus as the sinus exits through the skull to become the jugular bulb. The glossopharyngeal, vagus, and accessory nerves exit from the jugular foramen in front of the jugular bulb.

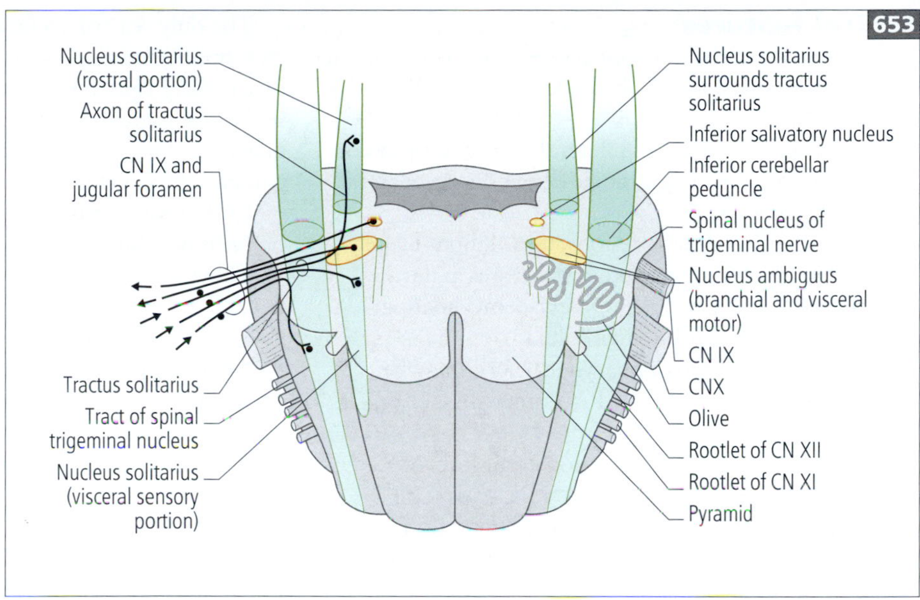

653 Cross-section of medulla at the point of entry of cranial nerve IX. *Adapted from 'Cranial Nerves in Health and Disease' by Linda Wilson-Pauwels.*

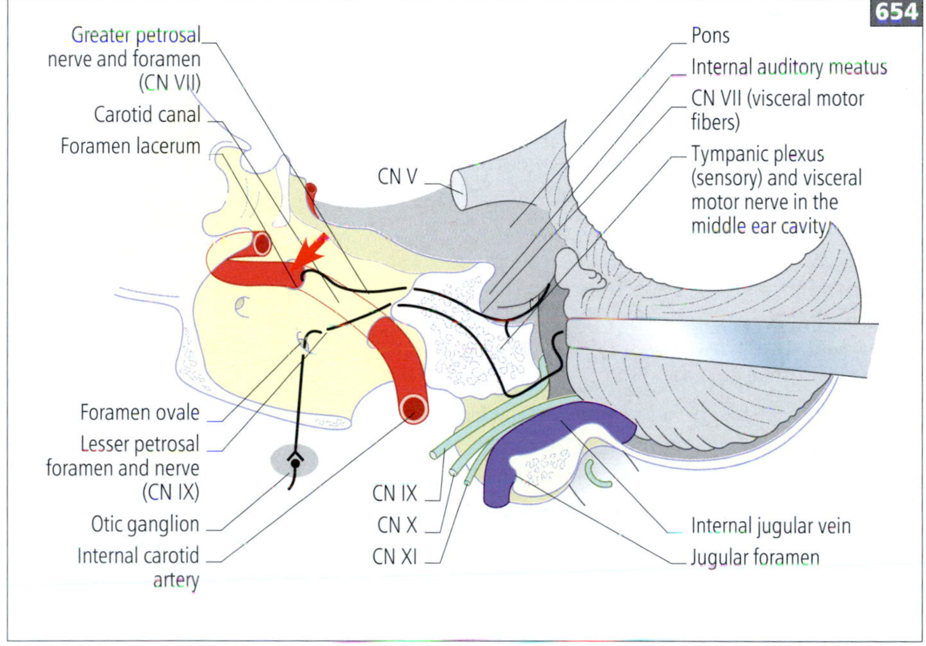

654 Sagittal section through the jugular foramen, showing the relationship of cranial nerves IX, X, and XI with the jugular vein. *Adapted from 'Cranial Nerves in Health and Disease' by Linda Wilson-Pauwels.*

Outside the skull

The glossopharyngeal nerve descends between the jugular vein and internal carotid artery, which ascends to enter the carotid canal just anterior to the jugular vein as it emerges from the jugular foramen. Nearby is the hypoglossal (XII) CN, which exits the skull through the anterior condylar canal posteromedial to the jugular foramen, and comes into close contact with the IXth, Xth, and XIth cranial nerves outside the skull.

The glossopharyngeal nerve then loops forward and medially to reach the soft tissues of the oropharynx, posterior tongue, and palate.

Clinical features

Isolated lesions of the glossopharyngeal nerve are rare. It is more common to see combined lesions of the IX and X cranial nerves[23].

- Supranuclear lesions: a unilateral supranuclear lesion does not result in a neurologic deficit due to bilateral supranuclear input.
- Nuclear and medullary lesions: these lesions usually result in involvement of other structures in the brainstem. These include infarcts, demyelinating lesions, tumors, and syringobulbia.
- CPA lesions: the glossopharyngeal nerve may be involved in lesions of the CPA along with CN V, VII, and VIII.
- Jugular foramen lesions: a lesion at the level of the jugular foramen involves CN IX, X, and XI (Vernet's syndrome). The clinical presentation includes ipsilateral weakness of the trapezius and sternocleidomastoid, ipsilateral anesthesia and paralysis of the pharynx and larynx resulting in dysphonia and dysphagia, palatal droop on the affected side and ipsilateral vocal cord paralysis, and loss of taste from the ipsilateral posterior one-third of the tongue. Lesions at the jugular foramen may result from skull base osteomyelitis, skull base fractures, neoplasms (e.g. glomus jugulare, neurofibroma, metastatic lesions, meningioma, and cholesteatoma), or vascular processes (internal carotid artery dissection)[6,8].
- Retropharyngeal lesions: lesions in the retropharyngeal space may result in symptoms referable to the ipsilateral IXth, Xth, and XIth CNs in addition to the hypoglossal nerve, resulting in ipsilateral tongue weakness and the ascending sympathetic chain resulting in ipsilateral Horner's syndrome (Villaret's syndrome). Causes of lesions in this location include neoplasms, infections/abscesses, surgical procedures, and trauma[6].

Physical examination

The only muscle supplied by the CN IX (stylopharyngeus) cannot be tested clinically. The glossopharyngeal nerve is *not* motor to the palate. When the gag reflex is tested the sensory stimulus is relayed via the glossopharyngeal nerve, and the resulting visible palatal movement is mediated by the vagus nerve. The gag reflex therefore is too gross for accurate clinical diagnosis of a glossopharyngeal lesion.

The only way of accurately testing the integrity of the glossopharyngeal nerve is to test pharyngeal sensation by carefully touching each side of the palate gently, and while the patient is phonating, touching the posterior pharyngeal wall on each side. The patient is then asked to compare these gentle stimuli.

Evaluation of taste sensation over the posterior third of the tongue has no proven value in clinical diagnosis[6,10].

These are clues to the site of involvement (e.g. intracranial *vs.* extracranial):

- Long tract signs indicate an intracranial lesion[6].
- An isolated ipsilateral Horner's syndrome (together with a glossopharyngeal palsy) is suggestive of a lesion outside the skull, as the cervical sympathetic fibers ascend near the area of the jugular foramen.

SELECTED CONDITIONS AFFECTING THE GLOSSOPHARYNGEAL NERVE

GLOSSOPHARYNGEAL NEURALGIA

Glossopharyngeal neuralgia is a rare condition characterized by recurrent brief episodes of unilateral sharp lancinating pain in the throat, ear, base of tongue, or neck, usually in response to chewing, coughing, yawning, or swallowing due to a 'trigger point' in the throat. The pain is stereotyped lasting seconds to minutes. Occasionally, bradycardia and syncope occur (associated with swallowing or coughing), possibly due to cross stimulation of the carotid sinus via the carotid nerve.

This neuralgia is usually idiopathic; however, it may also be a result of a structural lesion along the course of the glossopharyngeal nerve such as tumor, infection, or neuroma. Unlike trigeminal neuralgia, MS is a very rare cause of this syndrome. Symptoms may respond to carbamazepine, gabapentin, or baclofen. In refractory cases, surgical options such as nerve resection, tractotomy, or microvascular decompression may relieve symptoms.

VAGUS NERVE NEUROPATHY (CRANIAL NERVE X)

Definition and epidemiology

An uncommon disorder of the vagus (Xth cranial) nerve.

Anatomy

The vagus nerve is the most widely distributed CN. It carries motor, sensory, and parasympathetic fibers that innervate the head, neck, thorax, and abdomen. The nerve leaves the medulla in the region of the posterior lateral sulcus in close proximity to CN IX. The nerve exits the skull through the jugular foramen (see **654**). In the region of the jugular foramen are two vagal ganglia: the jugular ganglion (superior vagal ganglion) and the nodose ganglion (inferior vagal ganglion) (**655**)[1].

The motor fibers of the vagus nerve arise from the nucleus ambiguus, which receives bilateral supranuclear innervation. These fibers supply all striated muscles of the larynx and pharynx, except the stylopharyngeus (supplied by CN IX) and the tensor veli palatini (supplied by V_3 division of CN V)[2]. Three motor branches arise from the vagus nerve: the pharyngeal nerve, the superior laryngeal nerve, and the recurrent laryngeal nerve. The pharyngeal branch travels between the internal and external carotid arteries, forms the pharyngeal plexus with the glossopharyngeal nerve, and innervates muscles of the pharynx and palate. The superior laryngeal nerve takes off distal to the pharyngeal branch and descends lateral to the pharynx. The external branch of the superior laryngeal nerve supplies the cricothyroid muscle. The third motor branch arising from the vagus nerve is the recurrent laryngeal nerve. The right and left recurrent laryngeal nerves follow different courses. The right recurrent laryngeal nerve descends anterior to the right subclavian artery and turns posteriorly under the artery to ascend in the tracheoesophageal sulcus, whereas the nerve on the left turns posteriorly around the aortic arch and ascends in the same sulcus on the left. Both recurrent branches then enter the larynx and supply all intrinsic muscles of the larynx except the cricothyroid muscle (supplied by the external branch of the superior laryngeal nerve).

Tip

▶ *Motor fibers from vagus nerve supply all striated muscles of the larynx and pharynx except the stylopharyngeus (supplied by the CN IX) and the tensor veli palatini (supplied by the V_3 branch of CN V).*

The sensory fibers carried in the vagus nerve have their cell bodies in the jugular and nodose ganglia. The vagus nerve receives general visceral sensory input from the larynx, pharynx, linings of the trachea, bronchi, heart, aortic arch, and abdominal viscera; these fibers originate in the nodose ganglion and project to the nucleus solitarius. The vagus nerve (through the nodose ganglion) also carries taste sensation from the epiglottis, pharynx, and

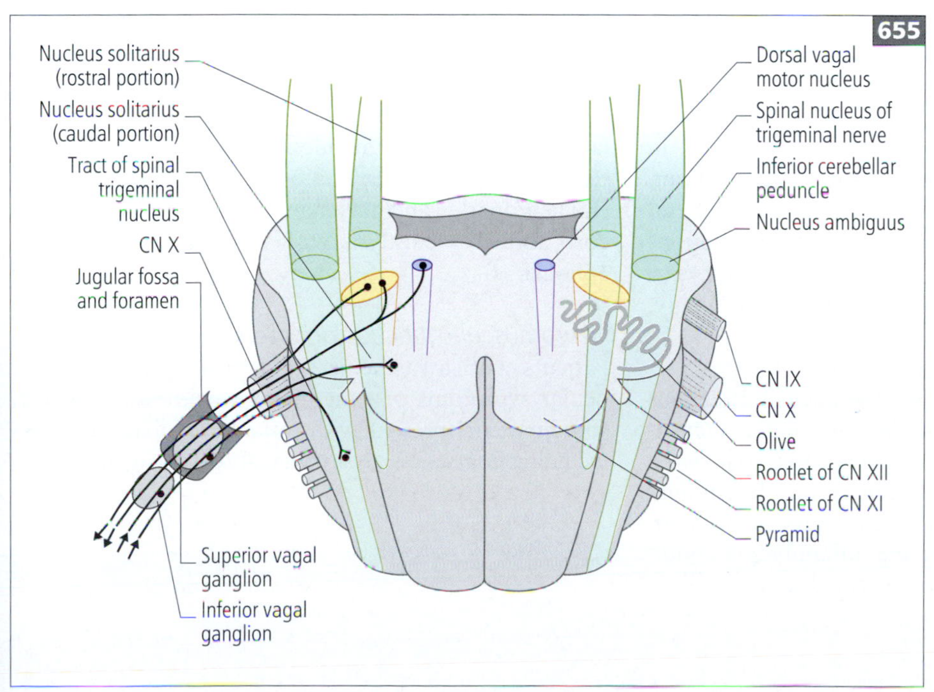

655 Cross-section of the medulla at the point of entry of cranial nerve X. *Adapted from 'Cranial Nerves in Health and Disease' by Linda Wilson-Pauwels.*

palate; these fibers terminate in the nucleus solitarius. The vagus nerve (through the jugular ganglion) also receives sensory input from the concha of the ear and the dura of the posterior fossa; these fibers terminate in the spinal nucleus of CN V.

The vagus nerve supplies parasympathetic innervation to smooth muscle and glands of the pharynx, larynx, and thoracic and abdominal viscera. Pre-ganglionic parasympathetic fibers arise from the dorsal nucleus of the vagus.

Clinical features

Patients with vagal nerve lesions present with symptoms of hoarseness, dysphagia, and dyspnea.

Evaluation of the soft palate and uvula at rest and with phonation

Normally with phonation, there is symmetric palatal elevation without deviation of the uvula. With a unilateral vagus nerve lesion, there is flattening of the ipsilateral palate at rest; with phonation, there is no elevation of the ipsilateral palate and deviation of the uvula to the opposite side. There is also depression of the ipsilateral gag reflex (efferent limb is through the vagus nerve).

With bilateral vagus nerve lesions, there is bilateral drooping of the palate and no palatal movement to phonation[8].

Speech and swallowing

With a unilateral vagal lesion, there may be mild dysphagia and nasal voice quality.

With bilateral lesions, there is severe dysphagia, nasal speech, hoarseness, markedly impaired cough, and dyspnea. An otolaryngological evaluation is essential to assess the larynx/vocal cords.

Localization

Supranuclear lesions

A unilateral supranuclear lesion rarely results in vagal dysfunction due to bilateral supranuclear input. However, dysphagia is not uncommon with a unilateral hemispheric stroke. Bilateral corticobulbar tract lesions result in pseudobulbar palsy. Symptoms include dysarthric speech and dysphagia along with emotional lability.

Nuclear and brainstem lesions

Lesions in the medulla involving the nucleus ambiguus result in ipsilateral weakness of the palate, pharyngeal, and laryngeal muscles. This is often associated with involvement of other CN nuclei and descending/ascending tracts. Etiologies include infarcts, demyelinating lesions, tumors, infectious and inflammatory conditions, syringobulbia, and motor neuron disease.

Posterior fossa, skull base, and jugular foramen

The vagus nerve can be involved in lesions in these anatomical locations along with other cranial nerves (IX, XI). Lesions in the CPA can affect the vagus in addition to causing hearing loss and vertigo (CN VIII), and peripheral facial weakness (CN VII). Lesions at the skull base (infectious, neoplastic, vascular, traumatic) involving the jugular foramen result in symptoms referable to CN IX, X, and XI. Skull base lesions can also affect other contiguous CNs. The vagus nerve can also be affected in the setting of a diffuse leptomeningeal process (infectious, carcinomatous, and inflammatory), trauma, and Guillain–Barré syndrome[14].

Extracranial vagus nerve lesions

The vagus nerve may be involved along its extracranial course by lesions in the neck and chest. Patients with isolated vagus nerve lesions present with hoarseness as their primary symptom. The presence of other associated symptoms is helpful in additional localization. Proximal vagal lesions present with dysphagia and ipsilateral palatal droop in addition to hoarseness. Vagal lesions distal to the pharyngeal branch or lesions of the recurrent laryngeal nerve result in isolated hoarseness.

Lesions of recurrent laryngeal nerve

The recurrent laryngeal nerve is longer on the left than the right and is therefore more susceptible to injury[23]. Both nerves, however, can be damaged due to their course through the upper chest. Etiologies include thoracic malignancies, lymphadenopathy, aneurysms, tumors, and operative injuries. Iatrogenic recurrent laryngeal nerve injury accounts for one-third of cases of vocal cord paralysis (thyroidectomy, carotid endarterectomy, and anterior cervical discectomy). A unilateral recurrent laryngeal lesion results in paralysis of all laryngeal muscles except the cricothyroid (innervated by the superior laryngeal nerve) and manifests as hoarseness. Bilateral recurrent laryngeal nerve lesions (post-operative, peripheral neuropathy, and malignancy) result in bilateral vocal cord abductor paralysis with inspiratory stridor and aphonia.

Neuromuscular junction disorders

Patients with myasthenia gravis usually present with ocular symptoms or generalized weakness. However, some patients present with fatigable bulbar weakness including hoarseness, dysarthria, and dysphagia.

SPINAL ACCESSORY NERVE NEUROPATHY (CRANIAL NERVE XI)

Definition and epidemiology

An uncommon disorder of the spinal accessory (XIth cranial) nerve.

Anatomy

The spinal accessory nerve is a motor nerve arising partly from the nucleus ambiguus in the medulla and partly from upper cervical segments. It supplies two muscles: the sternocleidomastoid and the trapezius (**656**)[24].

Cranial part

- Arises predominantly from the lower part of the nucleus ambiguus.
- The nerve rootlets emerge from the lateral medulla in line with the vagus.
- They are joined by the ascending spinal component, and then run laterally to enter the jugular foramen.
- The cranial portion merges with the vagus nerve to supply the pharynx and larynx.

Spinal part

- Motor to the sternocleidomastoid and trapezius.
- Arises from a column of cells in the ventral horn of the spinal cord extending from C1–C5 (the accessory nucleus).
- The spinal root fibers (C1–C5) emerge from the upper cervical cord laterally between the anterior and posterior spinal nerve roots to form a separate nerve trunk, which ascends into the skull through the foramen magnum.
- Once inside the skull the spinal and cranial roots of CN XI unite and exit by way of the jugular foramen in the same dural sheath as the vagus nerve.
- Upon emerging from the jugular foramen, the spinal part enters the neck between the internal carotid artery and the internal jugular vein. It then penetrates and supplies the ipsilateral sternocleidomastoid, emerges midway through the posterior border of the sternocleidomastoid, and crosses the posterior triangle of the neck to supply the ipsilateral trapezius.
- As the spinal accessory nerve courses through the neck, it receives a contribution from branches of the ventral motor roots of C3 and C4.

Supranuclear innervation

Supranuclear innervation of the sternocleidomastoid is probably ipsilateral, because hemispheric lesions (e.g. stroke) cause weakness of the sternocleidomastoid on the same side as the lesion (i.e. weakness turning head to the side of the hemiparesis); and partial epileptic seizures originating in the frontal lobe cause the head to turn away from the side of the lesion and the epileptic focus, indicating that the ipsilateral sternocleidomastoid is contracting.

Supranuclear innervation of the trapezius is from the contralateral hemisphere.

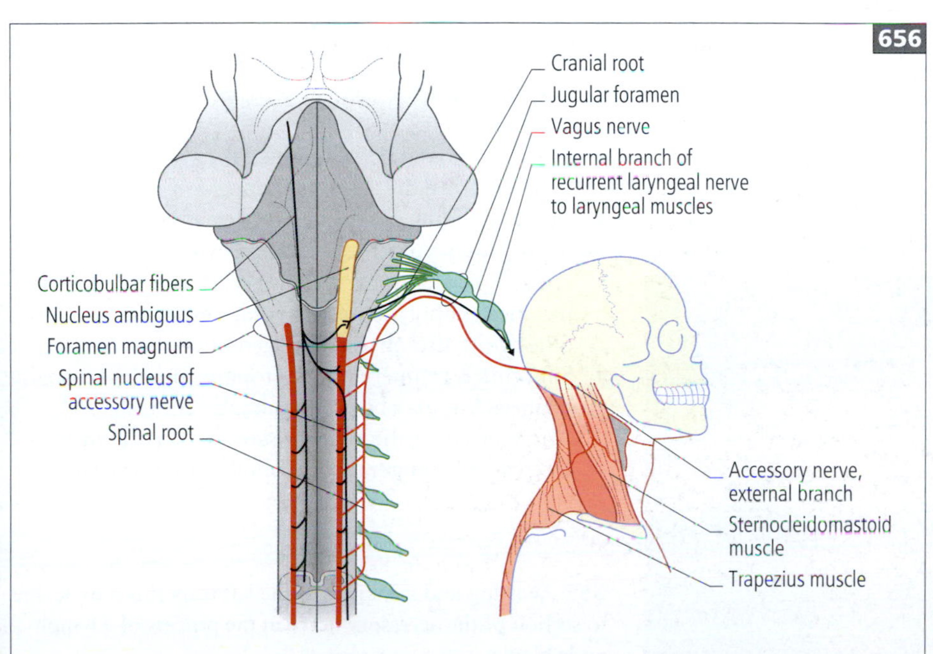

656 Nucleus and course of the spinal accessory nerve. *Adapted from Massey EW 'Spinal Accessory Nerve Lesions' Seminars in Neurology. 2009; 29(1); 82–84. Thieme.*

Clinical features

With unilateral sternocleidomastoid muscle weakness, the patient has difficulty turning the head to the opposite side and with neck flexion there is slight rotation of the head to the unaffected side. If there is weakness of bilateral sternocleidomastoids, there is impairment of neck flexion. When the trapezius is weak, there is drooping of the shoulder at rest and the scapula is displaced downward and laterally with slight winging of the scapular vertebral border. The patient cannot raise the abducted arm above the horizontal.

Proximal spinal accessory nerve lesions result in weakness of the trapezius and sternocleidomastoid. If the nerve is damaged in the posterior triangle of the neck, the sternocleidomastoid is spared. Spinal accessory nerve lesions do not cause a sensory disturbance.

- Nuclear lesions: these are rare and are associated with involvement of other structures in the medulla or upper cervical spinal cord. These can occur with parenchymal lesions, syringomyelia/syringobulbia, and motor neuron disease.
- Skull and foramen magnum lesions: these lesions usually also involve contiguous cranial nerves (IX, X, XI, and XII) and may also affect the medulla or upper cervical cord. Possible etiologies include neoplasms (meningiomas, dermoids), meningeal processes, and traumatic injuries.
- Jugular foramen lesions: see glossopharyngeal nerve section.
- Spinal accessory nerve lesions in the neck: these can result from surgical procedures in the posterior triangle of the neck such as lymph node excision or biopsy (most common cause), jugular vein cannulation, and carotid endarterectomy. Other etiologies include blunt trauma, neuralgic amyotrophy, and radiation therapy (657).

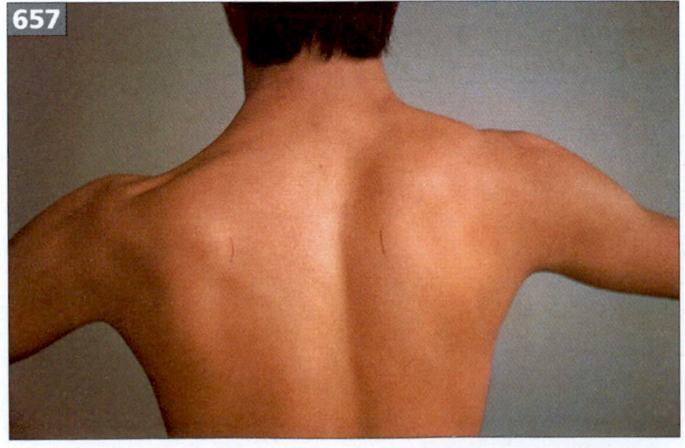

657 Wasting and weakness of the left trapezius muscle due to section of the accessory nerve in the process of a lymph node biopsy.

Investigations

Imaging studies including MRI (to assess the brainstem and craniocervical junction), CT (to assess the skull base), and electromyography to confirm denervation of the sternocleidomastoid and trapezius muscles can be helpful in diagnosis.

HYPOGLOSSAL NERVE NEUROPATHY (CRANIAL NERVE XII)

Definition and epidemiology

A rare disorder of the hypoglossal (XIIth cranial) nerve, which is the motor nerve to the tongue.

Anatomy

- The hypoglossal nerve fibers arise from a nuclear column located under the floor of the fourth ventricle that extends the entire length of the medulla (658).
- Fascicular fibers traverse the full sagittal diameter of the medulla to exit from the ventral surface between the medullary pyramid and the inferior olive.
- Numerous rootlets located medial to cranial nerves IX, X, and XI combine to form two main bundles with their own dural sleeves.
- The two bundles leave the skull through the hypoglossal canal, and unite after passing through the canal. The nerve then descends in the neck in close proximity to the internal carotid artery and the jugular vein, crosses the inferior vagal ganglion, and ascends anteriorly on the hyoglossus muscle, distributing branches to the ipsilateral intrinsic (longitudinal, transverse, and vertical) and extrinsic (styloglossus, hyoglossus, geniohyoid, and genioglossus) muscles of the tongue.
- The hypoglossal nerve receives sympathetic fibers from the superior cervical ganglion and some fibers from the vagus.
- The hypoglossal nerve is joined for a short distance by fibers from the C1 nerve root.
- The descending C1 fibers after branching off from the hypoglossal nerve are joined by fibers from C2 and C3 roots to form the ansa cervicalis; fibers from the ansa supply the sternohyoid, sternothyroid, omohyoid, thyrohyoid, and geniohyoid.
- Supranuclear innervation of tongue muscles is usually bilateral but may be predominantly contralateral. An exception is the genioglossus, which primarily receives contralateral corticobulbar innervation.

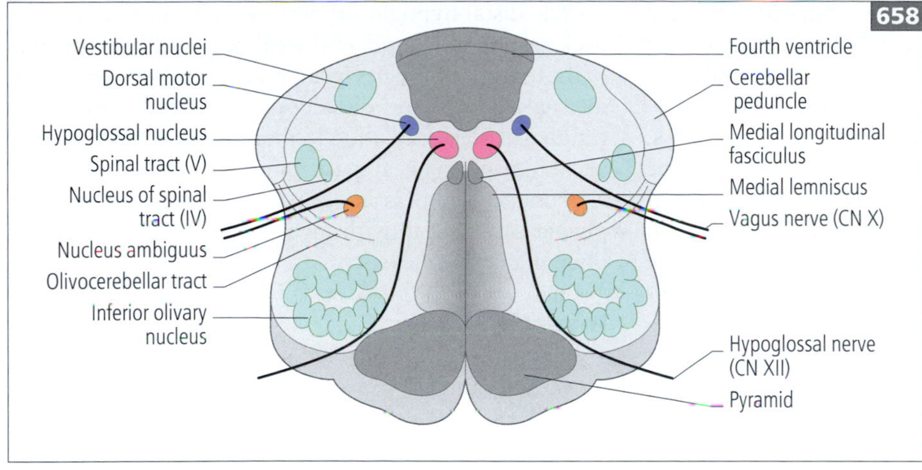

658 Cross-section of medulla showing the hypoglossal nucleus/nerve. *Adapted from 'Localization in Clinical Neurology' 5th edition. Brazis, Biller, et al.*

Clinical features

The tongue needs to be evaluated at rest and with movement.

Unilateral hypoglossal nerve palsy

- Wasting, furrowing, fasciculations, and weakness of one side of the tongue (ipsilateral to the lesion), with deviation of the tongue to the side of the paresis. With tongue protrusion, the normal contralateral muscles force the tongue forward and to the opposite side (which is towards the side of the weak muscle).
- Minimal dysarthria and dysphagia.
- Laryngeal shift to one side on swallowing (contralateral to the lesion) due to failure of the hyoid to elevate on the paralyzed side.

Bilateral hypoglossal nerve palsies

- Bilateral weakness, atrophy, and fasciculations.
- Weakness of tongue protrusion.
- Difficulty manipulating food in the mouth, chewing, and swallowing.
- Difficulty speaking (flaccid dysarthria).
- Difficulty breathing due to the flaccid tongue.

Localization

Supranuclear lesions

These result in deviation of the tongue away from the side of the lesion and toward the hemiparesis (if present). Dysarthria may occur. This is not accompanied by tongue atrophy or fasciculations. With bilateral corticobulbar lesions affecting fibers to the hypoglossal nuclei, the tongue is paretic with slow lateral movements and spastic dysarthria. Other signs of pseudobulbar palsy may be present including emotional lability, brisk jaw jerk (with bilateral lesions above the mid pons), and bilateral corticospinal tract signs[6]. Etiologies include stroke, hemorrhage, tumor, abscess, motor neuron disease, central pontine myelinolysis, and multiple system atrophy[8].

Tip

▶ *Supranuclear lesions of CN XII result in deviation of the tongue away from the side of the lesion and towards the hemiparesis (if present). There is no associated tongue atrophy or fasciculations.*

Nuclear and fascicular lesions

The hypoglossal nuclei in the dorsal medulla may be affected by pathologic processes such as demyelinating disease, motor neuron disease, syringobulbia, Chiari malformation, tumor, arteriovenous malformation, hemorrhage, ischemia, inflammatory, and infectious conditions. A unilateral ischemic lesion in the medulla in the territory of the vertebral or anterior spinal artery (medial medullary syndrome) may result in involvement of the hypoglossal nerve fibers coursing ventrally in the medulla (ipsilateral tongue weakness and atrophy), the pyramid (contralateral arm and leg weakness), and the medial lemniscus (contralateral impairment of position and vibration sense). Lesions in the medulla can also result in involvement of other cranial nerves (CN X and XI)[25].

Peripheral lesions

The hypoglossal nerve may be involved in lesions of the meninges, posterior fossa, the skull base, retropharyngeal space, or neck.

Leptomeningeal processes, which may include infectious, inflammatory (e.g. sarcoidosis), or carcinomatous etiologies, may result in cranial neuropathies.

In the posterior fossa, the hypoglossal nerve is in close proximity to CN IX, X, and XI. The nerve may be involved with meningiomas or neurofibromas.

A skull base lesion involving the jugular foramen and the hypoglossal canal may affect CN IX, X, XI, and XII (Collet–Sicard syndrome)[6]. This presents with ipsilateral deficits including weakness of the trapezius and sternocleidomastoid, vocal cord and pharyngeal weakness, hemi-tongue weakness and atrophy, loss of taste in the posterior third of the tongue, and diminished sensation in the palate, pharynx, and larynx. A skull base lesion may also affect CN XII in isolation. Etiologies include infection, trauma/fracture, malignancies, and Chiari malformation. A lesion at the level of the clivus may involve CN VI and XII; this is seen with malignancy such as nasopharyngeal carcinoma. The occipital condyle may be involved in a neoplastic or inflammatory process, which presents with unilateral occipital pain and ipsilateral hypoglossal neuropathy[8].

A lesion in the retroparotid or retropharyngeal space may involve CN IX, X, XI, and XII and the sympathetic chain resulting in an ipsilateral Horner's syndrome (Villaret's syndrome).

The distal hypoglossal nerve may be involved in the neck resulting in ipsilateral weakness and hemiatrophy of the tongue. Etiologies include: carotid artery aneurysm, internal carotid artery dissection, carotid endarterectomy, trauma, abscess, radiation to the neck, and tumors in the neck, retropharyngeal space, or at the tongue base.

Tongue weakness associated with dysarthria and dysphagia can be seen with myasthenia gravis. Symptoms often fluctuate in severity.

Investigations

- Suspected intracranial lesion:
  - MRI and CT scan of brain and base of skull.
  - CT or MR angiography to evaluate for vascular lesions.
  - CSF examination.
- Suspected extracranial lesion:
  - Direct examination of the nasopharynx/larynx.
  - MRI scan of base of skull.
  - MRI or CT of the soft tissues of the neck.

REFERENCES

1 Carpenter MB (1991). *Core Text of Neuroanatomy*, 4th edn. Williams & Wilkins, Baltimore.

2 Afifi AK, Bergman RA (2005). *Functional Neuroanatomy*, 2nd edn. McGraw-Hill Professional, New York.

3 Doty R (2009). The olfactory system and its disorders. *Semin Neurol* **29**(1):74–81.

4 Doty RL (2003). Odor perception in neurodegenerative diseases. In: *Handbook of Olfaction and Gustation*, 2nd edn. Marcel Dekker, New York, pp. 479–502.

5 Ross GW, Petrovitch H, Abbott RD, *et al.* (2008). Association of olfactory dysfunction with risk for future Parkinson's disease. *Ann Neurol* **63**(2):167–173.

6 Brazis PW, Masdeu JC, Biller J (2007). *Localization in Clinical Neurology*, 5th edn. Lippincott Williams & Wilkins, Philadelphia, pp. 125–130, 271–347, 350.

7 Welge-Luessen A, Temmel A, Quint C, *et al.* (2001). Olfactory function in patients with olfactory groove meningioma. *J Neurol Neurosurg Psychiatry* **70**:218–221.

8 Samii M, Jannetta PJ (1981). *The Cranial Nerves*, 1st edn. Springer-Verlag.

9 Fix JD (2005). High Yield of Neuroanatomy, 3rd edn. Lippincott Williams & Wilkins, Philadelphia, p. 79.

10 Blumenfeld H (2002). *Neuroanatomy through Clinical Cases*, 1st edn. Sinauer Associates.

11 Gonella MC, Fischbein NJ, So YT (2009). Disorders of the trigeminal system. *Semin Neurol* **29**(1):36–44.

12 Bennetto L, Patel NK, Fuller G (2007). Trigeminal neuralgia and its management. *BMJ* **334**:201–205.

13 Barker FG, Jannetta PJ, Bissonette DJ, *et al.* (1996). The long term outcome of microvascular decompression for trigeminal neuralgia. *N Engl J Med* **334**:1077–1083.

14 Ropper A, Samuels M (2009). *Adams and Victor's Principles of Neurology*, 9th edn. McGraw-Hill Professional.

15 Keane JR (1994). Bilateral seventh nerve palsy: analysis of 43 cases and review of the literature. *Neurology* **44**:1198–1202.

16 Grogan PM, Gronseth GS (2001). Practice parameter: steroids, acyclovir, and surgery for Bell's palsy (an evidence-based review). *Neurology* **56**:830–836.

17 Salinas RA, Alvarez G, Ferreira J (2004). Corticosteroids for Bell's palsy (idiopathic facial paralysis). *Cochrane Dat Sys Rev* **4**:CD001942.

18 Preston DC, Shapiro BE (2005). *Electromyography and Neuromuscular Disorders: Clinical-Electrophysiologic Correlations*, 2nd edn. Butterworth-Heinemann.

19 Anderson WE (2011). Varicella Zoster. *eMedicine Neurology*: http://emedicine.medscape.com/article/1166373-overview.

20 Landau ME, Barner KC (2009). Vestibulocochlear nerve. *Semin Neurol* **29**(1):66–73.

21 Froehling DA, Silverstein MD, Mohr DN, *et al.* (1991). Benign positional vertigo: incidence and prognosis in a population-based study in Olmsted County, Minnesota. *Mayo Clin Proc* **66**:596–601.

22 Fife TD, Iverson J, Lempert T, *et al.* (2008). Practice parameter: therapies for benign paroxysmal positional vertigo (an evidence-based review). *Neurology* **70**:2067–2074.

23 Erman AB, Kejner AE, Hogikyan ND, Feldman EL (2009). Disorders of cranial nerves IX and X. *Semin Neurol* **29**(1):85–92.

24 Massey EW (2009). Spinal accessory nerve lesions. *Semin Neurol* **29**(1):82–84.

25 Lin HC, Barkhaus PE (2009). Cranial nerve XII: the hypoglossal nerve. *Semin Neurol* **29**(1):45–52.

Further reading

Dawes L. Acoustic Neuroma. www.radpod.org. http://www.mypacs.net/cgi-bin/repos/mpv3_repo/wrm/repo-view.pl?cx_subject=12028784&cx_repo=mpv4_repo

Finsterer J (2008). Management of peripheral facial nerve palsy. *Eur Arch Otorhinolaryngol* **265**:743–752.

Gilchrist JM (2009). Seventh cranial neuropathy. *Semin Neurol* **29**(1):5–13.

Goldberg C (2005). Peripheral left cranial nerve 7 (Bell's) palsy. *Catalog of Clinical Images*, University of California San Diego. The Regents of the University of California. http://meded.ucsd.edu/clinicalimg/neuro_central_cn7_palsy2.htm.

Hankey GJ, Wardlaw JM (2002). *Colour Handbook of Clinical Neurology*, 1st edn. Manson Publishing, pp. 481–528.

Netter. Anatomy of the inner ear. http://www.netterimages.com/image/40393.htm

Patrick Lynch. http://radiopaedia.org/images/257

Wilson-Pawels L, Stewart PA, Akesson EJ, Spacey SD (2002). *Cranial Nerves in Health and Disease*, 2nd edn. BC Decker Inc.

CRANIAL NEUROPATHIES
II, III, IV, AND VI

Molly E. Gilbert

OPTIC NERVE NEUROPATHY (CRANIAL NERVE II)

Definition

Disorder of the IInd cranial, or optic, nerve resulting in visual disturbance or visual loss.

Although the ganglion cell axons that make up the optic nerve project to the lateral geniculate nucleus, the scope of this section will be limited to optic neuropathies anterior to the chiasm.

Anatomy

The optic nerve consists of approximately 1.2 million ganglion cell axons[1]. The ganglion cells are the innermost neurons of the retina. They receive information from the rods and cones that is modified by amacrine, bipolar and horizontal cells in the outer retina (**659**).

The ganglion cell axons sweep towards the optic nerve head in the ocular fundus following the organization of the retina, a retinotopic pattern. The superior axons enter the optic nerve head superiorly, the inferior axons inferiorly, the nasal fibers nasally, and the macular fibers enter the temporal optic nerve head (**660**)[2]. Within the eye, the size of the optic nerve is 1.5–1.75 mm and it is unmyelinated.

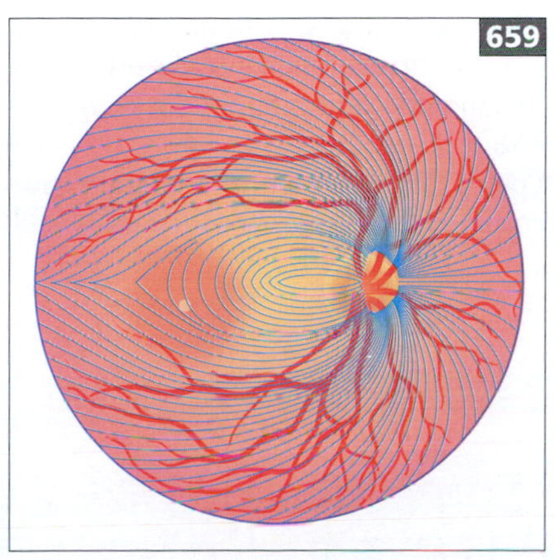

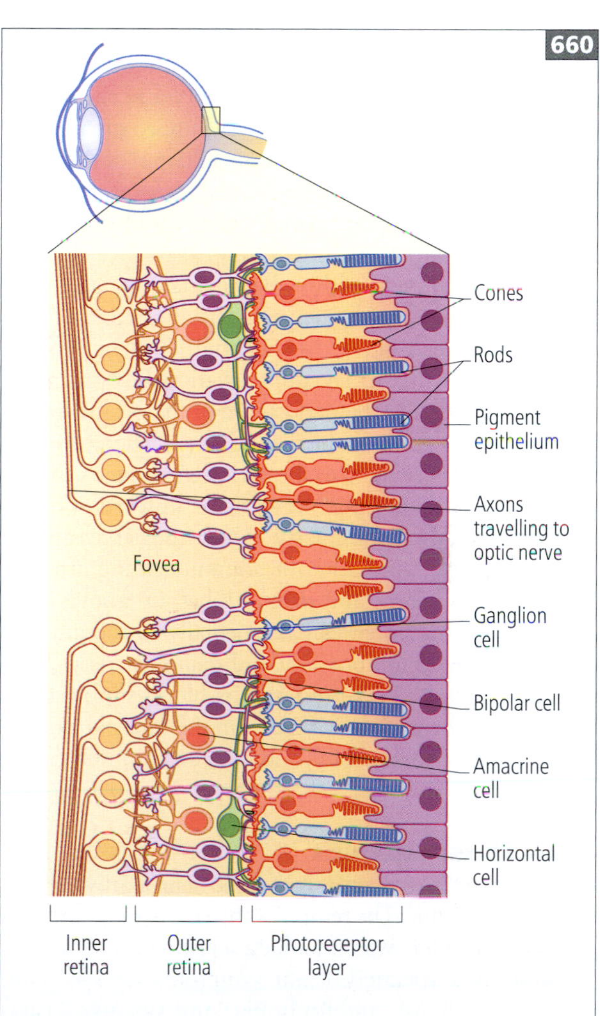

659 Layers of the retina, showing the projection of the photoreceptors to the ganglion cells whose fibers ultimately become the optic nerve.

660 Retinotopic organization of retinal nerve fiber layer with the superior ganglion cell fibers entering the nerve superiorly, the inferior fibers entering inferiorly, and the macular fibers entering the temporal optic nerve head.

The ganglion cell layer of the retina derives its blood supply from the central retinal artery, the optic nerve head is supplied by a circular anastomosis of the posterior ciliary arteries called the circle of Zinn–Haller. These anastomoses are variable and scant, so the optic nerve head can be a watershed area[3]. The posterior ciliary arteries and the central retinal artery are both branches of the ophthalmic artery, which in turn is the first branch of the internal carotid artery.

Behind the globe the size of the optic nerve increases to 2–4 mm because it becomes myelinated and surrounded by dura. The intraorbital length of the optic nerve is approximately 30 mm, longer than the orbit to allow unrestricted movement when the eyes are turned. The intraorbital optic nerve derives its blood supply from anastomoses between pial perforating capillaries that branch from the ophthalmic artery and the central retinal artery which enters the nerve approximately 10 mm behind the globe. The remaining 20 mm of the nerve receives its blood supply from the pial perforating vessels of the ophthalmic artery. Some collateral blood supply from the external carotid artery may exist[4].

The nerve travels within the muscle cone and exits the orbit through the optic canal. The optic canal is situated in the lesser wing of the sphenoid. The length of the canal is about 10 mm. The dura covering the optic nerve becomes invested in the periosteum of the optic canal at the annulus of Zinn at the orbital apex. Therefore, the nerve and dura are fixed to the periosteum in the canal.

The intracranial optic nerve slants upward at a 45° angle to reach the optic chiasm. Above the nerves are the anterior cerebral and anterior communicating arteries. The olfactory nerves and frontal lobes are above these arteries. The optic nerves pass medially to the internal carotid arteries and above the ophthalmic arteries. The intracranial optic nerve receives its blood supply from a pial plexus of vessels arising from the internal carotid artery, the anterior cerebral, and anterior communicating arteries.

Clinical assessment

In order to make a diagnosis of optic neuropathy the history is paramount. The tempo of the visual loss is the first point to consider: was it sudden, episodic, or gradual? In addition, associated ocular symptoms such as pain, proptosis, redness, photophobia, and positive visual phenomena should be inquired about. Other neurologic symptoms such as headache and paresthesias or weakness or incontinence should be sought, as well as underlying systemic illnesses such as rheumatologic or vasculopathic diseases.

The hallmarks of optic neuropathy include reduced visual acuity, color vision loss, afferent pupillary defects, and visual field defects. Each of these components must be covered in the assessment of optic neuropathy; however, each component may be variably affected.

Visual acuity

Visual acuity is the 'ocular vital sign'; however, visual acuity in optic neuropathies is highly variable and sometimes unaffected. Visual acuity testing can be performed at the bedside with handheld cards, provided the patient is wearing their corrective lenses for near vision.

Color vision

More important in diagnosing optic neuropathies is acquired dyschromatopsia. Color perception can be affected by retinal, optic nerve, or cortical lesions. Congenital color blindness occurs in one in eight men and is symmetric and stable during the course of their lives.

Acquired dyschromatopsia, however, may be asymmetric between the two eyes or the hemifields. Kollner's rule states that most retinal lesions will affect the blue–yellow spectrum of color vision, while optic neuropathies tend to affect the green–red spectrum. In truth there is significant cross over between the two types of acquired dyschromatopsia, such as in patients with glaucoma. However, the rule is still useful and easily applicable[5].

Color testing can be done using pseudoisochromatic plates which are widely available. In the hospital setting, dyschromatopsia in optic neuropathies that affect the two eyes differently can be tested by holding up a red bottle top and asking the patient to grade the difference in color saturation subjectively between the two eyes.

Visual field testing

Abnormal visual fields are seen in all optic neuropathies. Three types of defects may be seen with optic neuropathies occurring anterior to the chiasm.

The first is generalized constriction all around the peripheral field. Different conditions can cause this type of defect other than optic neuropathy, including cataract, small pupils, retinal degenerations, or nonorganic visual loss. However, optic neuritis can produce diffuse visual field suppression as can optic neuropathy associated with pseudotumor cerebri.

The second type of defect is central or paracentral scotomas. These occur in many optic neuropathies as well as maculopathies.

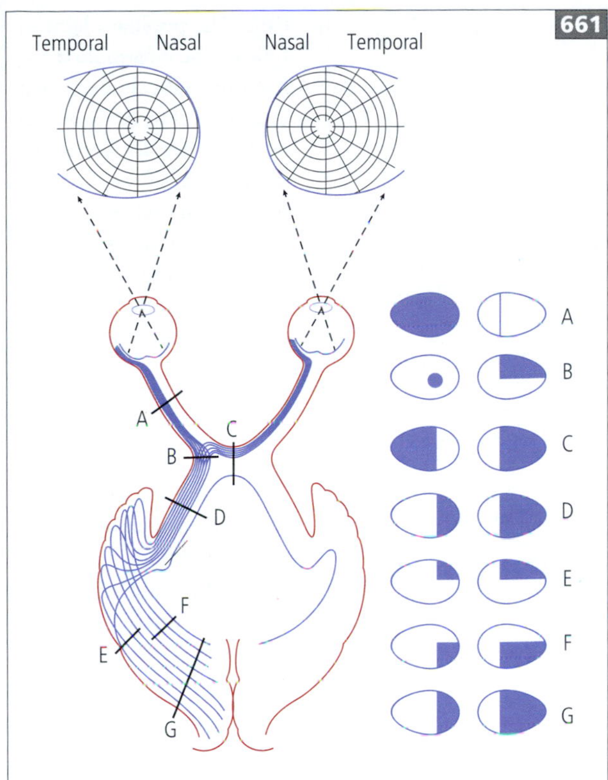

661 Typical visual field defects. Anterior to the chiasm defects are central scotomas or they line up along the horizontal meridian. In most cases these field defects are monocular. At the chiasm the orientation of visual field defects begins to line up along the vertical meridian. Since the nasal retinal fibers, representing the temporal visual fields, cross at the chiasm, field defects here produce a bitemporal defect that affects both eyes. Retrochiasmal defects involve fibers from both eyes, affecting the nasal fibers from the contralateral eye and the temporal fibers from the ipsilateral eye. This produces field defects in both eyes that affect the same side of the visual field and produce homonymous visual field defects.

Finally nerve fiber bundle defects can also be seen. They follow the retinotopic pattern of the nerve fibers as they enter the optic nerve. They respect the horizontal meridian of the visual field and are termed arcuate defects, nasal steps, or altitudinal defects. Visual field defects that occur at the chiasm or further back line up against the vertical meridian (**661**).

Confrontation visual field testing is easily performed at the bedside or in the office. The examiner stands arm's length away from the patient and directs the patient to cover one eye while the examiner closes his/her opposite eye. The examiner asks the patient to look at the examiner's nose, then monitors the fixation by watching the patient for eye movements during the examination. The examiner presents one, two or five fingers in the upper and lower right and left quadrants of the visual field within 30° degrees of fixation and asks the patient to identify the number of fingers displayed. The examination then switches to the other eye. Variations include asking if the patient can see the examiner's entire face while fixated on the nose, or holding a red-topped drops bottle in the upper and lower visual fields to assess for color desaturation across the horizontal meridian.

Tip

► *Tunnel vision is occasionally described by patients with a bitemporal heminanopia, but is also a frequent complaint of patients with functional visual loss. A confrontation visual field that begins with the typical finger counting in each quadrant can be followed by moving 2–2.5 m (6–8 feet) away from the patient and moving the examiner's fist from temporal to nasal into the patient's field. The angle of the visual field should at least double at this distance. If the field does not widen, the visual loss is functional. This can be considered a poor man's version of the tangent screen test.*

Humphrey visual field testing is static automated perimetry that evaluates the central 24–30° of the visual field. It is typically available in ophthalmology offices and is sufficient for assessing the anterior visual pathway. Within the central visual field it presents a standardized, static point of light of varying intensity to establish a threshold of vision. It allows for more information about the size and density of a scotoma to be established.

Goldmann perimetry uses standardized stimulus sizes and intensity to evaluate the entire field of vision. The stimuli are typically presented in a kinetic fashion with the examiner moving the stimulus from a nonseeing part of the field to a seeing part of the field.

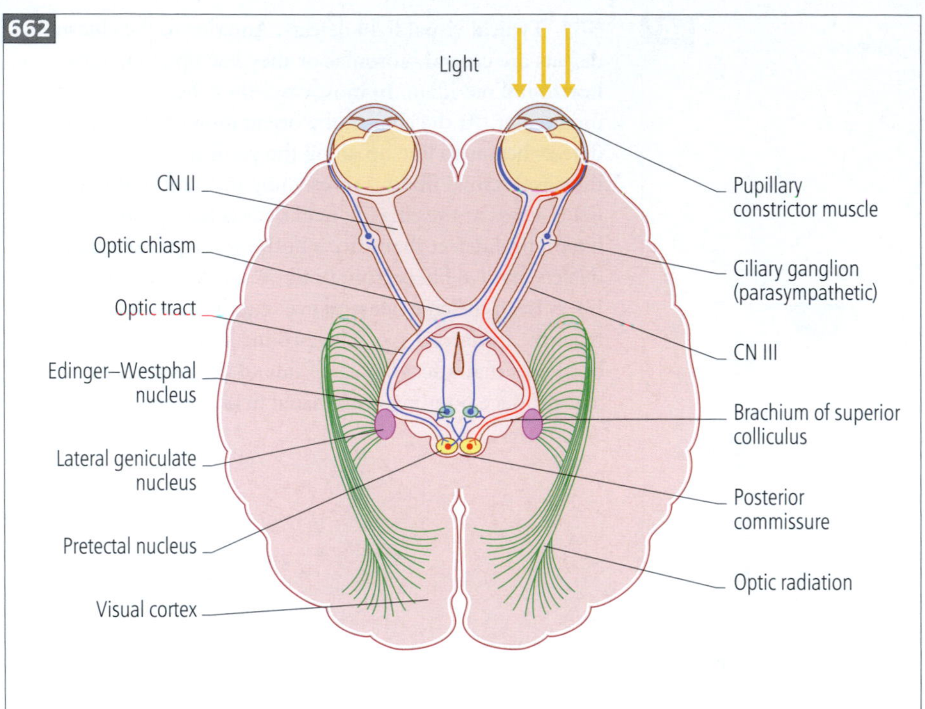

662 The pupillary light reflex. The information from the light shone in one eye projects to the pretectal nuclei bilaterally due to the decussation of the nasal fibers from each eye at the chiasm. In addition, each pretectal nucleus projects to both the right and left Edinger–Westphal nuclei which contain preganglionic parasympathetic neurons. These, via the oculomotor nerves, reach the ciliary ganglia and synapse with the postganglionic parasympathetic neurons which innervate the papillary constrictor muscles.

Afferent pupillary defects (Marcus–Gunn pupil)

Finding an afferent pupillary defect indicates asymmetric disease of the anterior visual pathway. Also called the 'swinging flashlight test', the examiner uses a pen light, Fenhoff light, or indirect ophthalmoscope and moves the light back and forth between the visual axes of each eye. Since the pupillary fibers project bilaterally to the Edinger–Westphal subnuclei of the third nerve, the efferent arc for pupillary constriction is equal between the two eyes regardless of which eye the light is shining in (**662**). If both eyes are normal the amount of pupillary constriction should remain constant, regardless of which eye is stimulated.

If the left eye, for example, has optic nerve damage, the pupils will constrict symmetrically to a light shone in the right eye or the left eye. However, the amount of constriction will be less when the light is shone in the affected eye (in our example the left eye). When the flashlight is passed from the left eye to the right eye both pupils will constrict further and conversely when the light travels from the right eye to the left eye both pupils will dilate. This is a result of poorer conduction of light signal to the Edinger–Westphal subnuclei from the optic nerve of the affected eye. This test can be performed in patients with one fixed pupil or anisocoria because it is the amount of constriction that should remain the same. If the pupils are consistently dilating in response to light shone in one eye that eye has an optic neuropathy (**663**).

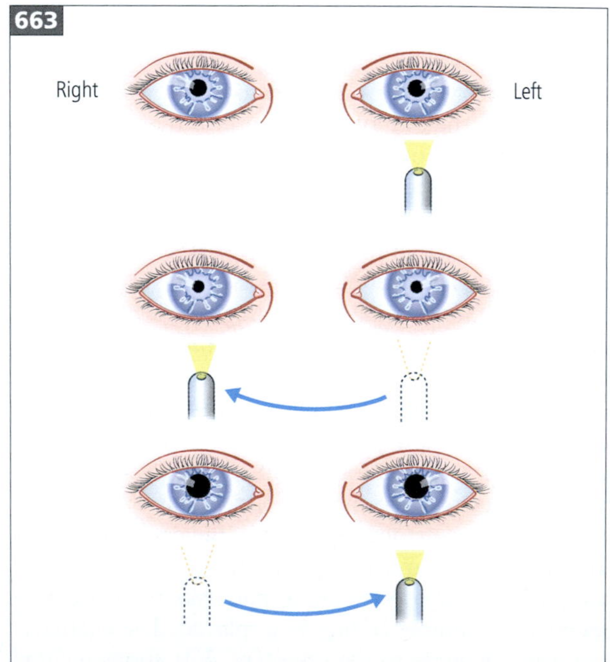

663 Swinging flashlight test to assess for afferent pupillary defect. When the light is moved from the affected (left) eye to the unaffected (right) eye both pupils constrict, and when the direction is reversed both pupils dilate. This is because of reduced signal conduction along the visual pathway by the optic nerve on the affected side.

OPTIC NEUROPATHIES

Optic neuropathies can be inflammatory, ischemic, congenital, hereditary, toxic/metabolic, or traumatic. The predominant features include reduced visual acuity, dyschromatopsia, visual field defects, and afferent papillary defects. Depending on the cause of the optic neuropathy, funduscopic examination of the optic nerves may be normal, swollen, or pale.

Inflammatory optic neuropathies

Typical optic neuritis refers to inflammation of the optic nerve that is either idiopathic or possibly associated with inflammatory demyelinating processes.

Multiple sclerosis

Optic neuritis can be the presenting feature of multiple sclerosis (MS) or it can occur during the course of the disease. The clinical features of optic neuritis are identical in patients with or without MS.

The optic neuritis treatment trial (ONTT)[6] has provided excellent data regarding the clinical presentation, treatment, outcomes, and risk of development of MS of patients diagnosed with optic neuritis but no other history of demyelinating disease. Patients were randomized to treatment with oral steroids, IV steroids followed by an oral taper, or observation.

Clinical features

- Visual acuity loss ranged from 20/20 to no light perception, with the majority of patients (54%) between 20/25 and 20/200.
- Dyschromatopsia was detected by pseudo-isochromatic plates in 88% and was 94% with more rigorous testing.
- Contrast sensitivity was decreased in 98% of the patients.
- Using automated perimetry, 45% of patients had diffuse field loss and 55% had localized defects, the most common of which was an altitudinal defect.
- On fundus examination, one-third of cases had mild disc swelling while in the remainder of the cases the nerve appeared normal (retrobulbar optic neuritis).
- The natural history was rapid loss of vision that could progress for up to 2 weeks.
- Over 90% of patients had an associated globe tenderness and pain on eye movement that disappeared within 5 days.

Tip

▶ *Although patients with demyelinating optic neuritis present with disc swelling one-third of the time, demyelinating disease does not cause severe swelling, optic nerve hemorrhage, or exudates; in addition, the macula should be normal. If any of these other signs are present, other causes of inflammatory optic neuritis must be sought.*

Investigations and diagnosis

No laboratory study, whether blood tests, lumbar puncture (LP), or magnetic resonance imaging (MRI) was useful in the diagnosis of optic neuritis. MRI of the brain was found to be useful in predicting the likelihood of patients developing MS. The 15-year follow-up data showed that patients who had one or more white matter lesions on their initial MRI had a 72% risk of developing MS at 15 years, while those with no lesions on the baseline MRI had a risk of 25%[7].

It should be stressed that these results pertain only to patients with so called 'typical' optic neuritis. For patients that have marked disc swelling with hemorrhage, progressive visual loss beyond 2 weeks, persistent pain, or no recovery at 1 month, other causes of optic nerve inflammation should be sought.

Treatment and prognosis

The visual prognosis was unchanged regardless of no treatment versus treatment with oral or IV steroids. Intravenous steroids increased the rate of recovery but at 1 year all treatment groups had similar visual outcomes. Oral prednisone was found to increase the risk of recurrent optic neuritis for the first 3–5 years after treatment. The cause of this finding is not well understood.

Over 80% of patients experience visual recovery that begins within 1 month of onset. Recovery is nearly complete in most patients, though those with worse vision at onset (20/400 – no light perception) have a poorer prognosis than those with better vision.

Devic's disease/neuromyelitis optica

Neuromyelitis optica (NMO) is a variant of optic neuritis that is typically described as bilateral optic neuritis in association with transverse myelitis. More recently it has been recognized that the optic neuritis associated with NMO can be unilateral and can occur months or years apart from the myelitis[8].

Optic neuritis is the presenting problem in 53.3% of these patients, most with unilateral disease. Recurrent optic neuritis occurs before myelitis in 18.3%. NMO-associated optic neuritis differs from typical demyelinating optic neuritis in that patients are less likely to have preceding pain on eye movement and less likely to experience visual recovery. The ocular morbidity is thus higher than demyelinating optic neuritis, with 53% developing permanent bilateral vision loss over a median of 8 years and 63% blind in one eye. The revised criteria for diagnosis of NMO include two of the following three factors:

- An onset MRI is not specific for MS.
- A longitudinally extensive cord lesion of three or more segments in length.
- Anti-aquaporin-4 IgG seropositivity[9].

It is important to maintain a high index of suspicion for NMO in patients with optic neuritis, since the morbidity and mortality rates are higher in this disease and the treatment options are different than for MS.

Sarcoidosis

Sarcoidosis in a multi-system disorder without a known etiology that is diagnosed pathologically by finding noncaseating epithelioid cell granulomas on biopsy. Ocular involvement is present in 25% of patients with sarcoidosis[10]. The majority of these patients have anterior uveitis. However, optic nerve involvement can present as an optic nerve head granuloma, optic perineuritis (inflammation of the nerve sheath), or retrobulbar optic neuritis.

Typically these patients have less pain and more progressive visual loss than patients with MS or idiopathic optic neuritis. In addition, the visual loss may initially respond immediately to steroid therapy[11]. As noted above, steroid therapy can hasten the recovery of idiopathic/MS-associated optic neuritis but it still takes several weeks. If any of these signs are present, suspicion of sarcoidosis should prompt chest X-ray, testing for angiotensin-converting enzyme, and lysozyme. In addition, a history of rashes, adult onset asthma, joint pain, or arthritis should be inquired about.

Treatment with systemic steroids is needed for long periods of time; therefore, a tissue diagnosis should be sought if possible using skin biopsy, bronchoalveolar lavage, or conjunctival biopsy.

Other causes of optic nerve inflammation

Optic perineuritis typically has bilateral visual loss with swollen optic nerve head and dilated retinal vessels. It resembles papilledema but patients have a normal opening pressure on LP. Causes include:

- Sarcoidosis.
- Syphilis.
- Lyme disease.
- Tuberculosis.
- Idiopathic perineuritis.
- Lupus-associated optic neuropathy (uncommon).
- Autoimmune optic neuropathy: inflammation of the optic nerve in the absence of a connective tissue disease despite extensive rheumatologic or vasculitic work-up.

Ischemic optic neuropathies

Temporal arteritis

Temporal arteritis (TA; also known as giant cell, cranial, granulomatous, or Horton arteritis) is a systemic vasculitis associated with a wide range of symptoms including fatigue, fever, headaches, jaw claudication, loss of vision, scalp tenderness, polymyalgia rheumatica, and aortic arch syndrome[12].

The risk of blindness from TA makes accurate diagnosis and prompt aggressive treatment critically important. It is estimated that visual loss occurs in 7–60% of patients with TA[13], typically from either anterior ischemic optic neuropathy (AION), central retinal artery occlusion or, less frequently, occipital infarction[14].

The visual loss is typically profound with the majority of patients having acuities of 20/200 or less[14,15]. Visual loss is frequently the symptom that brings patients to medical attention. The risk of progressive visual loss despite apparently adequate therapy is high.

Two prospective studies have demonstrated that even with the early institution of high-dose corticosteroids, 13–27% of patients experience progressive loss of vision within the first 5–6 days, making presentation with visual loss an ophthalmic emergency[15,16].

TA involves large and mid-sized arteries which have an elastic lamina. The vasculitis preferentially targets the superficial temporal, vertebral, ophthalmic, and posterior ciliary arteries[17]. This explains the frequency of blindness and neurologic findings seen in these patients. Less commonly involved vessels include the internal carotid, external carotid, and central retinal arteries. Dissection of the aorta and involvement of the coronary arteries have also been reported.

TA is more common in women than men (3:1) and affects patients of northern European descent most frequently. However, patients in other ethnic groups may also be affected. The prevalence increases with increased age. The incidence of TA increased from 2.3 per 100,000 in the sixth decade to 44.7 per 100,000 in the ninth decade and older. It rarely occurs in patients under the age of 50 but there have been individual case reports in the ages from 30–50 years[18–20].

Clinical features

Visual loss may be transient or permanent and may affect one or both eyes. Transient visual loss typically occurs a few days or hours before permanent loss of vision develops. This transient amaurosis is identical to the transient visual loss in patients with carotid artery disease or cardiac valvular disease, although it may alternate between the two eyes[21].

AION is the most common cause of visual loss in patients with TA[22,23]. It is usually unilateral and the second eye may become involved. Involvement of the second eye most commonly occurs within the first 5–6 days after the first eye is involved[24,25]. However, it may occur weeks or months after the first eye is involved, particularly if treatment is tapered too rapidly. The loss of vision with AION in TA is profound, with over 80% of patients having visual acuity of hand motion or worse. The affected optic nerve shows pallid edema that may be associated with intraretinal hemorrhages and/or cotton wool spots (**664**).

Posterior ischemic optic neuropathy (PION) can also occur in TA. It is much less common than AION. These patients have normal appearing fundi with sudden visual loss and afferent pupillary defects[26]. The visual loss may not be as profound as is seen in patients with AION secondary to TA.

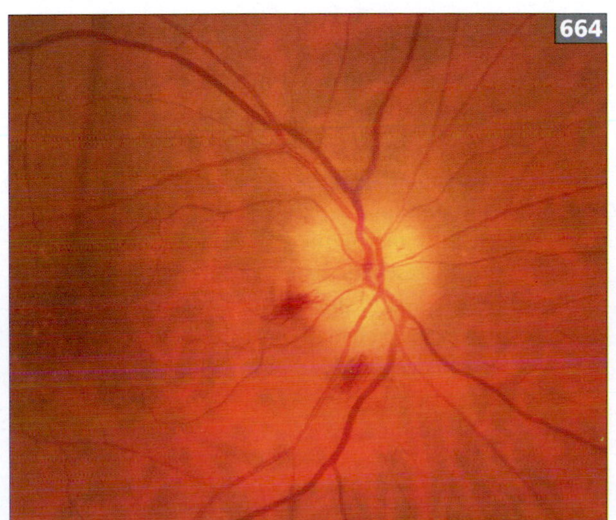

664 **Pallid edema of the optic nerve seen in giant cell arteritis.**

Homonymous visual field defects can occur from damage to the retrochiasmal visual pathway. This usually indicates an occipital lobe infarction from inflammatory thrombosis in the vertebrobasilar arterial system. Cortical blindness can develop from involvement of both occipital lobes[27].

Approximately 25% of patients with TA will present with diplopia. Most frequently, the ocular motor nerve is affected. However, the IVth and VIth cranial nerves can be involved. In addition, diplopia may be a result of brainstem ischemia and a resultant skew deviation or internuclear ophthalmoplegia[28].

Most patients with TA will have premonitory systemic symptoms prior to their visual symptoms. These may include new onset headache, jaw claudication, weight loss, malaise, polymyalgia rheumatica, fever, scalp tenderness, anemia, tongue claudication, tinnitus, or vertigo. Jaw claudication is one of the most specific systemic symptoms associated with TA. It is important to differentiate jaw claudication from temporomandibular joint (TMJ) pain by history. Patients with jaw claudication will describe crescendo pain in the masseter muscles that begins after a period of chewing and abates when chewing ceases. Patients with TMJ report maximal pain when opening the jaw or immediately upon chewing.

Diagnosis

The American College of Rheumatology has published a list of diagnostic criteria for TA[29]. They specify that the diagnosis may be made when patients meet three of the five identified criteria including:

- Age over 50.
- New onset headache.
- Scalp tenderness or decreased temporal artery pulse.
- Erythrocyte sedimentation rate (ESR) greater than 50 mm/hr.
- Positive temporal artery biopsy (TAB).

Other authors have suggested that in the presence of AION or central retinal artery occlusion, any combination of the following factors is sufficient to make the diagnosis[30]:

- Age over 50.
- Ttypical fundus appearance.
- Typical systemic symptoms.
- High ESR or high C-reactive protein (CRP).
- Positive temporal artery biopsy.
- Abnormal fluorescein angiography.

Some patients with TA may have no systemic symptoms, so called occult TA, but these patients will generally have elevated acute phase reactants.

Investigations

Normal ESRs are calculated as[31]: Age (+ 10 if female) divided by 2. However, elevated ESRs are nonspecific and furthermore, up to 22% of patients with TA can have normal ESRs.

Other investigators have shown that elevated CRP (>24.5 mg/l [2.45 mg/dl]) is more sensitive than ESR and that the combination of an elevated ESR and CRP is 97% specific for the diagnosis of TA[13].

Thrombocytosis may have a higher specificity, positive predictive value, and negative predictive value for TA than ESR alone[32]. Thrombocytosis may increase the risk of subsequent visual or neurologic ischemic events[33].

All patients suspected of having TA should undergo a TAB, deemed 95% sensitive and 100% specific for TA. Although the American College of Rheumatology criteria do not mandate a TAB to make the diagnosis, it is prudent medicolegally given the side-effects that can occur from treatment of TA.

There is very little risk from TAB but those that exist include hematoma or brow droop from transection of a branch of the facial nerve. Since the risks are low and the complications of inappropriately treated disease are high, there should be a very low threshold for performing TAB.

Since the pathology of the vasculitis can include skip areas it is important to ensure the biopsy specimen be of sufficient length to reduce the risk of missing the involved portion of the vessel. The recommended specimen length is at least 2 cm, to take into account skip areas as well as artifactual shrinkage of the artery due to processing[34,35].

Disruption of the internal elastic membrane is diagnostic of TA. Obliteration of the lumen and epithelioid giant cells may also be seen but are not necessary for diagnosis.

There is no need to withhold therapy while awaiting a TAB. Attempts should be made to undertake TAB within the first week of starting corticosteroid therapy. However, experienced pathologists can make the diagnosis of 'healed arteritis', characterized by lymphocytic infiltration and scarring, even after several weeks of therapy with corticosteroids.

In patients for whom there is a high suspicion of TA but a negative TAB was obtained, the diagnosis of TA is not eliminated. Therefore, a second TAB should be undertaken in these patients. The yield of a positive second TAB ranges from 5% to 13%[34].

Treatment

When patients present with vision loss, the goal of therapy is to prevent second eye involvement. There is evidence from retrospective studies that corticosteroids retard the progression of visual loss, diminish the risk of fellow eye involvement, and may restore vision in some cases (up to 34%). Furthermore, IV steroids may be more effective than oral steroids in protecting the visual prognosis, due to their higher bioavailability[36,37]. Most neuro-ophthalmologists recommend immediate methylprednisolone 1g/day in patients presenting with visual loss who are suspected of TA. This can be tapered to an oral dose after 3–5 days. The oral steroid dose is tapered after 1 month provided that the ESR remains normal and there is no re-emergence of systemic symptoms. This taper is very slow and may last 6–12 months or longer.

Nonarteritic AION

Nonarteritic AION (NAION) is the most common cause of unilateral optic disc edema and optic neuropathy in patients over 50 years old[38]. These patients describe nonprogressive monocular visual loss of sudden onset, most commonly upon awakening. There are no associated ocular symptoms or systemic symptoms. Typically, the patients describe a painless loss of vision; however, pain has been reported in up to 10% of patients[39].

Most patients are aged 60–70 years old, with a mean age of 66 ± 8.7 years[40]. The annual incidence is 2.3 per 100,000 population per year[38]. The rate is higher in Caucasians than in African-American or Hispanic individuals.

In order to discuss NAION, it is important to review the physiology of blood flow to the optic nerve. Blood flow (BF) to the optic nerve is determined by the perfusion pressure/resistance to flow (BF = PP/RF). PP to the anterior optic nerve is expressed as mean arterial pressure (MAP) minus intraocular pressure (IOP) (PP = MAP − IOP). Therefore, BF = (MAP−IOP)/RF. Any variable that increases the RF or IOP, or decreases the MAP, can compromise the perfusion of the optic nerve head (ONH)[41].

RF is autoregulated so that a constant rate of flow to the ONH is maintained when the MAP and IOP vary[42]. Autoregulation is maintained by endothelially derived vasoactive agents such as thromboxane A2 (vasoconstrictor) or nitric oxide and prostacyclin (vasodilators). Any vascular process which damages the endothelium can therefore lead to disruption of autoregulation.

Patients with microvascular disease such as diabetes mellitus, hypertension, atherosclerosis, or smoking may have poor autoregulation of blood flow[43], although some studies have questioned the role of these diseases in AION[44]. The Ischemic Optic Neuropathy Decompression Trial (IONDT), the largest source of the natural history of the disease, found that 47% of patients with NAION had systemic hypertension and 24% had diabetes[40]. Patients without these systemic risk factors did not have visual loss as severe as that seen in patients with systemic risk factors.

It has been shown that autoregulation only acts over a certain range of PPs. Therefore, very elevated IOP or very low MAP may preclude the normal autoregulatory function of the endothelium. The role of nocturnal hypotension has been suggested as a separate risk factor that may explain the loss of vision upon awakening[45,46]. Patients who take antihypertensive medications before going to bed at night are at particular risk. The peak effectiveness of their medications tends to correspond to the normal dip in MAP that occurs in the very early morning hours. This potentiates the drop in MAP and compromises blood flow to the posterior ciliary vessels in these patients, increasing the risk of NAION. Finally, up to 20% of healthy individuals have abnormal autoregulation of the PP to part or all of their ONHs[47].

Another risk factor for development of NAION is the crowded ONH or so called 'disc at risk'. NAION occurs more often in patients with congenitally small discs. Therefore, the same number of nerve fibers must pass through a smaller lamina leading to crowded nerves. Any insult that leads to swelling of the nerve fibers may then cause a compartment syndrome as the swollen fibers compress the blood supply to surrounding fibers[42]. Furthermore, the posterior ciliary arteries that supply the ONH have variable watershed zones in different individuals, making some people more likely to develop ischemic optic neuropathy (ION) in the setting of predisposing or precipitating factors.

Clinical features

Patients present with decreased visual acuity at any range, although it is typically not as profound as that seen with TA. In the IONDT, 49% of patients had acuity better than 20/64 and 34% had acuity worse than 20/200. In addition, they have dyschromatopsia, an afferent papillary defect, and visual field defects. The most common visual field defect is inferior altitudinal[48]. However, the visual field defect can be any 'optic nerve' type defect, meaning it can be a central scotoma or anything that respects the horizontal meridian (**665**). The disc edema is sectoral in nature, with splinter hemorrhages and dilated capillaries on the surface (**666**). Over time as the edema resolves, the patients are left with sectoral pallor of the ONH.

Investigations

In addition to the atherosclerotic risk factors of diabetes and hypertension, patients with antiphospholipid antibodies have been reported to develop NAION[47]. Therefore, any patient who is younger than 50 should be investigated for this possibility. It is important to note that in general, prothrombotic states are not associated with NAION and therefore do not need to be investigated beyond this particular exception[49].

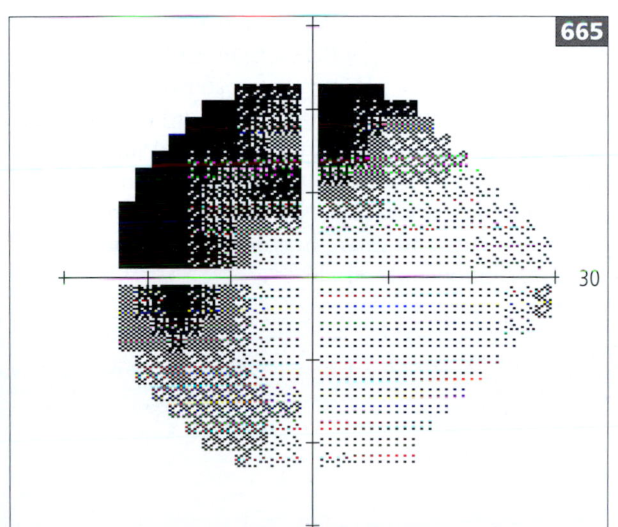

665 Inferior arcuate visual field defect obeying the horizontal meridian as seen in nonarteritic ischemic optic neuropathy.

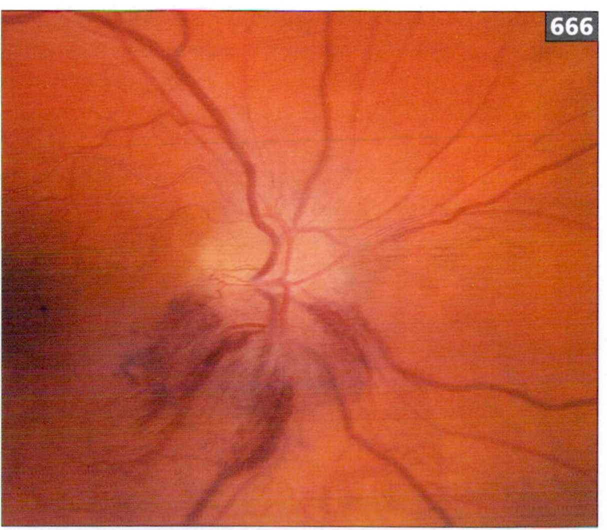

666 Sectoral swelling of the optic nerve head with hemorrhage in nonarteritic ischemic optic neuropathy.

In patients over the age of 50 years, an ESR and CRP should be checked to screen for TA. MRI is generally not necessary except in cases where there is concern for a compressive or infiltrative condition. MRI has been shown to have increased white matter ischemic changes that are reflective of the underlying presence of vasculopathic risk factors[50].

Treatment and prognosis

There is no treatment that reduces or reverses visual loss. The IONDT actually showed a worse outcome in patients treated with optic nerve decompression. In addition, aspirin has not been shown to change the visual outcome, nor does it affect the risk of second eye involvement.

Most patients have a fixed deficit; however, certain subsets of patients were found to have progressive courses or spontaneous recovery in the IONDT. Forty-three percent of nontreated patients recovered three or more lines of vision; this outcome has been supported by other studies as well[51,52]. Approximately 10–15% of patients have a progressive loss of vision over the first month after diagnosis.

There is a lifetime risk of 30–40% of second eye involvement[53]. Pallor of one optic nerve due to previous NAION and acute swelling of the ONH in the second eye has been called pseudo-Foster Kennedy syndrome due to the clinical appearance of the optic nerves (Foster Kennedy syndrome is described below).

There is no demonstrated correlation that the visual outcome in one eye is predictive of the disease course in the second eye. Finally, there is no definitively established increased risk of cerebrovascular or cardiovascular disease in NAION patients.

Postoperative ischemic optic neuropathy

Visual loss after nonocular surgery is a relatively uncommon complication. However, reports of postoperative visual loss (POVL) have been increasing over the last 10–15 years[54–56].

The incidence of ION after nonocular surgery is approximately 1/60,000–1/125,000[57,58]. The incidence of all causes of POVL has been observed to be as high as 4.5% in cardiac surgery[59]. In spine surgery, reported incidences are as high as 0.2%[57]. Determining the actual overall incidence of all causes of POVL is difficult since it is not known what percentage of cases is reported.

A wide variety of surgical interventions have been associated with POVL. The most commonly reported settings include cardiopulmonary bypass[59–61] and lumbar spine surgery[57].

There are several causes of POVL after nonocular surgery. AION and PIONs are most frequently described. PION is a more common presentation than AION[55]. In addition, central retinal artery occlusion (CRAO) and central retinal vein occlusion (CRVO) have been noted, particularly in cases with ocular or orbital compression[62,63]. Cortical blindness is another cause of POVL[57,64].

Surgical factors that influence IOP can lead to abnormal autoregulation of perfusion pressure to the ONH that may result in AION. Two studies have found that IOP rises in prone anesthetized patients[65]. Surgical factors that reduce MAP below the autoregulatory threshold may also precipitate AION in susceptible patients. These factors may include iatrogenic hypotension or acute hemorrhage. Hypotension as may be used to control bleeding during spinal surgery is controversial and has not been definitively associated with POVL. However, a number of case series and retrospective studies have noted that prolonged hypotension is often a factor in POVL[55,56].

Factors that affect the delivery of oxygen to the ONH independent of PP also create a risk of infarction. These include anemia or hemodilution as a result of intravenous fluid replacement but not blood product replacement. Unlike AION, PION very rarely occurs spontaneously. However, the physiology of the blood supply to the posterior optic nerve and certain surgical factors make it a more common cause of POVL than AION.

PION typically affects the posterior optic nerve between the orbital apex and the entry of the central retinal artery[66,67]. It is here that the only blood supply to the optic nerve is the pial vessels that are small branches of the ophthalmic artery. PION is more commonly associated with acute and severe hypotension, low hematocrit or hemodilution and emboli[67,68].

Compressive optic neuropathies

Compressive optic neuropathies have a typical presentation with slowly progressive visual loss and optic nerve atrophy. On occasion, unilateral vision loss may present as 'pseudosudden visual loss' when the good eye is temporally occluded and the patient notices that the affected eye has visual loss. The typical features of optic neuropathy are present including visual loss, dyschromatopsias, visual field loss, and afferent pupillary defects.

Causes of compressive optic neuropathies can be intraorbital, intracanalicular, or intracranial. Intraorbital causes include primary orbital tumors such as cavernous hemangiomas or Schwannomas, secondary tumors such as metastatic or sinus lesions, or enlarged muscles due to thyroid disease or orbital pseudotumor[69,70]. Optic nerve neoplasms such as gliomas, meningiomas, lymphoma, or leukemia can affect the intraorbital, intracanalicular, or intracranial portions of the nerve[71].

Causes of intracranial compressive optic neuropathies include aneurysms, chiasmal lesions or fibrous dysplasia. The classic optic nerve neoplasms including optic nerve gliomas and meningiomas as well as thyroid ophthalmopathy will be discussed in this section.

Direct intracranial compression of one optic nerve due to a space-occupying lesion will produce pallor of that optic nerve. If the lesion becomes large enough to increase the intracranial pressure, the second nerve may be swollen due to papilledema. The pale compressed nerve is atrophic and therefore will not swell in response to increased intracranial pressure. This phenomenon is known as Foster Kennedy syndrome.

Optic nerve gliomas

In children optic gliomas are typically benign and slowly progressive. Most children present before the age of 10 years[72]. About 25% of these children have neurofibromatosis type 1 (NF-1). However, only 15% of patients with NF-1 have optic nerve gliomas[73].

The clinical course is variable. The majority of tumors have only slow growth, but 70% progress within 3 years of diagnosis[74]. Neuroimaging typically shows kinking and a fusiform enlargement of the nerve with enhancement. MRI is the preferred imaging modality because it is better able to assess intracranial extension. The diagnosis can be made radiographically and biopsies are generally not necessary[75].

Treatment and follow-up in children begins with an examination for NF-1 followed by serial MRIs and neurophthalmic examinations. If progression occurs before the age of 6 years, chemotherapy may be necessary. After the age of 6 years radiation may be used since the orbit will be fully formed.

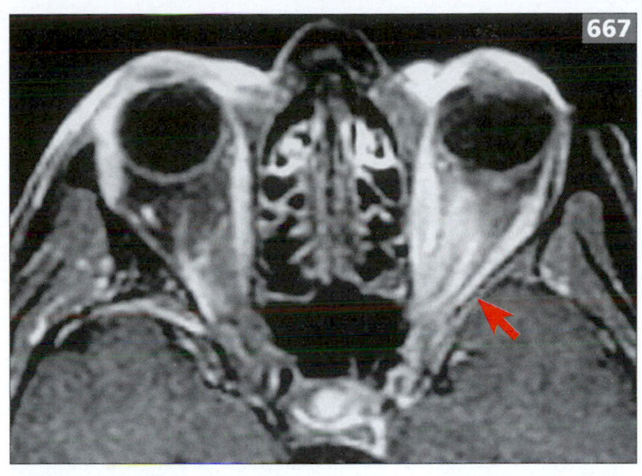

667 Computed tomography of optic nerve meningioma showing calcification – the 'tram track' sign (arrow).

Malignant optic nerve gliomas are much rarer and affect middle-aged and older adults.

Patients have the typical signs of optic neuropathy as well as headache and pain on eye movement[76]. The nerve is often swollen and the retinal vasculature appears engorged. Rapid progression to blindness can occur. There is a high rate of mortality.

Optic nerve meningiomas

Optic nerve sheath menigiomas classically present with insidious visual loss in middle-aged women[77]. The loss of visual acuity is usually in the 20/40 to 20/200 range. The appearance of the optic nerve is atrophic or swollen. Optociliary shunt vessels are present in up to 33% of patients[78]. Most patients also have proptosis.

Neuroimaging is diagnostic as with optic nerve gliomas. The nerve shows calcification on computed tomography (CT) scan that has a so-called 'tram track' appearance because the sheath on either side of the nerve is involved (**667**)[79]. On MRI the tumor is isointense with brain on T1- and T2-weighted images, but enhances with gadolinium[80].

The progression is slow and intracranial extension is very rare[81]. Radiation treatment is reserved for adult patients with visual acuity worse than 20/40. Surgical excision is not recommended, as removal of the arachnoid strips the pial vessel supply to the nerve and visual loss is worsened. Therefore, surgery is reserved for blind and painful or unsightly eyes.

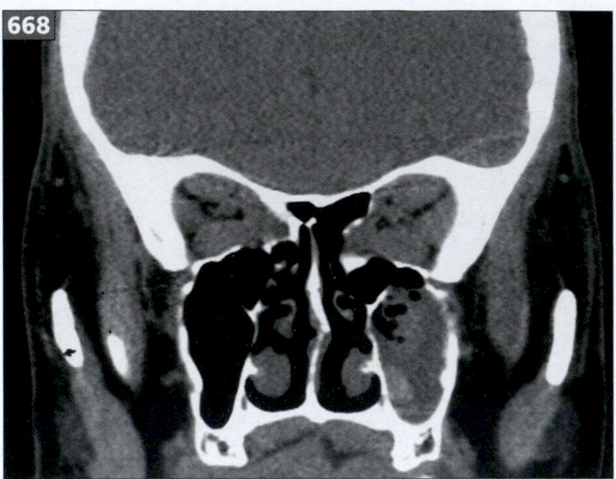

668 Compression of the optic nerve by muscle bellies at the orbital apex in thyroid-associated ophthalmopathy.

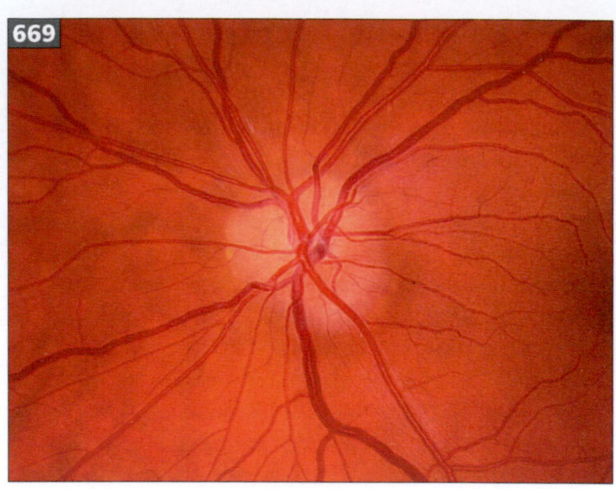

669 Optic nerve head drusen with pseudopapilledema.

Thyroid-associated ophthalmopathy

Graves' disease or thyroid-associated ophthalmopathy (TAO) is the most common orbital disorder in adults, comprising 32–47% of orbital disorders[82]. It may occur in hyperthyroid, euthyroid, or hypothyroid patients[83].

The most common finding is lid retraction; however, proptosis, abnormal eye movements, and optic neuropathy are not uncommon[84]. Optic neuropathy occurs in about 9% of TAO patients[85]. It is a result of the enlarged muscle bellies compressing the nerve at the apex of the orbit (**668**).

Vision loss associated with TAO requires immediate management. If the loss is indolent, radiation to the posterior orbit with concomitant steroid treatment is appropriate. For more rapid visual loss, orbital decompression is necessary.

Congenital optic neuropathies

Congenital optic neuropathies include optic disc drusen, hypoplasia of the optic nerve, colobomas, and tilted nerves. Several of these findings have neurologic associations and will be discussed here.

Optic nerve drusen

Optic disc drusen are seen in 2% of the population. Drusen are calcium deposits below the nerve fiber layer. There are bilateral deposits in 2/3 of cases[86]. They cause an elevation of the ONH that is often confused with papilledema. As patients get older and undergo some involution of the nerve fiber layer the calcific deposits are more visible. Drusen are associated with an abnormal branching pattern of the retinal vessels that can be useful in differentiating from true papilledema (**669**).

Up to 70% of patients will have a visual field defect[87]. The majority of these never progress although progression can occur in some cases. The central visual acuity is never affected in these patients; if central acuity is affected, other causes of visual loss should be pursued even in the presence of disc drusen. Occasionally, because of the crowding of the axons as they pass through the lamina cribrosa into the orbit, ION can occur.

Optic nerve hypoplasia

This is the most common congenital anomaly of the optic nerve. Visual function is widely variable but smaller nerves are associated with worse function[88]. MRI typically reveals thin optic nerves and chiasm.

It may occur in isolation or be associated with other midline abnormalities such as thin or absent corpus callosum, absence of the septum pellucidum, and hypopituitarism. This septo-optic dysplasia or de Morsier's syndrome can also be associated with schizencephaly[89]. Optic nerve hypoplasia can also be seen in association with congenital suprasellar tumors and teratomas[90].

Morning glory discs

Morning glory discs result from a staphyloma or weakness of the posterior globe that allows uveal tissues to protrude through the sclera, in this case involving the optic nerve.

The nerve appears large and vessels radiate in a spoke-like manner from the center of the nerve. The disc itself is filled with white glial tissue[91].

This anomaly can be associated with moya moya disease and/or transphenoidal basal encephaloceles[92].

Colobomas

Colobomas occur when there is incorrect closure of the embryonic fetal fissure that forms the optic cup and stalk. This results in incomplete formation of any part of the eye[88,93]. When the optic nerve is involved the disc appears excavated inferiorly, with normal vessels and a normal superior rim.

These patients need to be investigated radiographically for basal encephaloceles[93].

Hereditary optic neuropathies

Leber's hereditary optic neuropathy

Leber's hereditary optic neuropathy (LHON) is a mitochondrial disorder that occurs more frequently in men. It presents in the second or third decade with sequential painless visual loss in both eyes. The average interval between eye involvement is several months. Visual acuity is typically severely affected to 20/200 or worse in both eyes[94].

Some patients note that they have Uhthoff's phenomenon and a disease resembling MS has been described as occurring with LHON[95]. In addition, cardiac conduction defects including Wolff–Parkinson–White, Q waves, atrial fibrillation, and bundle branch blocks have been described[95,96]. Skeletal abnormalities including hip dislocation, pes cavus, and kyphoscoliosis have also been associated with the disease[95].

Diagnosis is made based on the clinical picture. There are now several mitochondrial mutations that can be tested to make the diagnosis[97–99]. Treatment and prophylaxis have not been effective for LHON. There is a suggestion that smoking and alcohol may contribute to the development of the disease so these should be avoided.

Dominant optic atrophy

Dominant optic atrophy occurs in the first decade of life. Patients usually develop central visual field defects with normal peripheral vision. Visual loss does progress beyond the first decade of life. The visual acuity is 20/60 or better in 40% of the patients[100,101]. The optic nerve develops a wedge-like atrophy with temporal loss of the neuroretinal rim. The disease has been linked to the q arm of chromosome 3[102].

There is no known effective treatment at this time.

Recessive optic atrophy

Recessive optic atrophy presents with severe visual loss in early childhood. Parental consanguinity is often present. In some cases it can be associated with spinocerebellar degeneration (characterized by cerebellar ataxia and pyramidal tract dysfunction) and mental retardation; in these cases it is referred to as Behr's syndrome[103].

There are a number of metabolic and degenerative neurologic diseases associated with optic atrophy such as spinocerebellar degeneration (for example Friedreich's ataxia), Charcot–Marie–Tooth disease, and olivopontocerebellar atrophy[104–106]. Recessive optic atrophy may also be associated with mucopolysaccharidoses (including Hurler, Scheie, Hunter, Sanfilippo, Morquio, and Maroteaux–Lamy variants) and lipidoses (such as Tay–Sachs, adrenoleukodystrophy, metachromatic leukodystrophy, Niemann–Pick and Krabbe's disease).

Nutritional and toxic optic neuropathies

These diseases involve gradual painless loss of vision that is bilateral. In addition, patients typically have bilateral cecocentral visual field loss, normal optic nerve appearance early in the disease, and no metamorphopsias (as associated with maculopathies).

Improvement in vision can be seen with removal of the offending agent or correction of the nutritional deficit. These diseases can be recognized by the patient's exposure history including treatment with chemotherapy, recreational drug use, and antibiotics, or malnutrition.

Vitamin B12 deficiency

Uncommon nutritional cause of optic neuropathy. It can be seen with pernicious anemia, status post resection of the stomach or small intestine, and in very strict vegans. Diagnosis is made in the setting of low B12 or elevated homocysteine or methylmalonic acid. Treatment is with vitamin B12 replacement[107].

Tobacco/alcohol amblyopia

Most common nutritional/toxic optic neuropathy. It is somewhat of a misnomer. Patients often substitute calories from food for calories from alcohol. Although tobacco may be toxic to the optic nerves, ethyl alcohol alone is not toxic to the anterior visual pathway. Therefore, malnutrition may play a large role in the disease process[108,109]. It is important to quantify, as much as possible, the daily alcohol and tobacco intake. Asking the patient to detail a typical daily breakfast, lunch, and dinner can shed light on the potential for malnutrition.

If tobacco alcohol amblyopia is suspected, testing for vitamin B12 and folate levels should be performed[110]. Counseling the patient to reduce alcohol and tobacco use, though frequently unsuccessful, should be documented and the appropriate referrals made.

Supplementation with B vitamins and folate should be instituted even in the absence of documented deficiencies.

Methanol toxicity

Methanol causes a dramatic toxic optic neuropathy characterized by sudden visual loss and disc swelling as well as metabolic acidosis. Very small doses of methanol can lead to optic nerve damage. Exposure tends to occur in suicide attempts or accidental ingestion from contamination of ethyl alcohol[111].

The exact mechanism of optic neuropathy by methanol is not well understood. Methanol is a direct depressant of the central nervous system (CNS) and, on ingestion, it is rapidly absorbed and metabolized in the liver by the alcohol dehydrogenase to formaldehyde, which is then transformed into formic acid; this causes cellular hypoxia via mitochondrial inhibition.

Treatment includes dialysis to control the acidosis and IV ethyl alcohol which competitively inhibits the binding of methanol to alcohol dehydrogenase.

Ethylene glycol toxicity

Found in antifreeze, it causes a similar clinical picture to methanol[112].

Other causes of toxic optic neuropathies

Include ethambutol, carmustine, busulfan, chloramphenicol, cisplatin, disulfiram, fludarabine, interferon, isoniazid, lead, methotrexate, quinine, toluene, and vincristine[113,114].

Traumatic optic neuropathies

Traumatic optic neuropathy can be direct or indirect. Direct injuries are a result of objects penetrating the orbit and lacerating or compressing the optic nerve. The most common cause of traumatic optic neuropathy is retrobulbar hemorrhage leading to compression of the optic nerve[115].

Indirect injuries are a result of forces transmitted to the optic nerve from the orbit or globe[116]. These include optic nerve avulsion, which occurs due to forceful rotation of the eye and leads to separation of the nerve from the globe, and posterior indirect traumatic optic neuropathy (Pi-TON)[116].

Pi-TON is the second most common cause of traumatic optic neuropathy after retrobulbar hemorrhage. It is present in 2% of all closed head injuries and is associated with loss of consciousness and craniofacial fractures[117]. It is typically seen in young men.

Pi-TON is a result of rapid deceleration due to a blow to the forehead or midface. Because the dura covering the nerve is invested in the periosteum of the optic canal, rapid deceleration injuries, which allow the optic nerve to move while the dura stays behind, result in shearing of the dural blood supply to the intracanalicular nerve.

The vision loss associated with Pi-TON occurs immediately following surgery and ranges from 20/20 to no light perception. Patients will initially have no ophthalmoscopic signs of damage to the optic nerve. Pallor of the nerve will develop over weeks to months after the injury.

CT scan with 1 mm slices of the orbits is important to rule out a canalicular fracture. Fractures can be repaired or decompressed with the possibility of visual improvement. There is currently no recommended treatment for Pi-TON and the likelihood of recovery is low[117].

Retinal disease of interest to the neurologist

Susac syndrome

- Microangiopathy of the brain, retina, and inner ear that occurs most often in young women with mean age of onset 30 years.
- It is similar to primary angiitis of the CNS but 90% of patients have retinal arterial occlusions and 66% have sensorineural hearing loss.
- In the patients with retinal arterial occlusions, 60% have bilateral retinal ischemia.
- Autominnune endothelial cell damage has been implicated as the underlying cause although pathogenesis has not been determined.

Mitochondrial diseases

- Typical examples are Kearns–Sayre syndrome and mitochondrial encephalopathy with lactic acidosis and strokelike episodes (MELAS syndrome).
- Are associated with retinal pigmentary changes.
- This type of retinal pigmentary change can also be seen in the mucopolysaccharidoses, spinocerebellar ataxia type 7, and Guacher's disease.

CRANIAL NERVE III, IV, AND VI PALSIES

Definition

Palsies of the nerves that control eye movements lead to diplopia, including IIIrd (oculomotor), IVth (trochlear), and/or VIth (abducens) cranial neuropathies.

Clinical features and investigations

When taking a history from a patient complaining of diplopia the most important historical question is whether the diplopia is present when either eye is closed. If closing either eye relieves the diplopia then it is a binocular process, meaning the muscles in the two eyes are not working together. This is almost always a neurologic process with a few congenital exceptions.

If the diplopia is present when one of the eyes is closed, it is a monocular process. Monocular diplopia is most often related to refractive or intraocular problems such as cataract or macular edema. Usually, if the patient is instructed to view an object through a pinhole, this type of diplopia resolves. Very rarely, patients have monocular diplopia that does not resolve with pinhole viewing, due to occipital lobe lesions causing cerebral polyopia[118].

Other important historical data to obtain are whether the diplopia is horizontal or vertical in nature. This helps narrow down the potential causes. Horizontal diplopia can be caused by VIth nerve palsies, IIIrd nerve palsies, internuclear ophthalmoplegia, convergence insufficiency, or myasthenia gravis.

Central causes of horizontal diplopia include internuclear ophthalmoplegia, one and a half syndrome, and cortical lesions. Horizontal saccades are generated from projections from the frontal eye fields that decussate to the contralateral paramedian pontine reticular formation (PPRF). The PPRF projects to the VIth nerve nucleus which projects to the ipsilateral lateral rectus and sends interneurons through the medial longitudinal fasciculus (MLF) to the contralateral medial rectus subnucleus.

Internuclear ophthalmoplegia (INO) results from damage to the MLF and causes an adduction deficit on the ipsilateral side with a contralateral abducting nystagmus. Stroke and MS are the most common causes. The differential diagnosis includes myasthenia gravis (**670**).

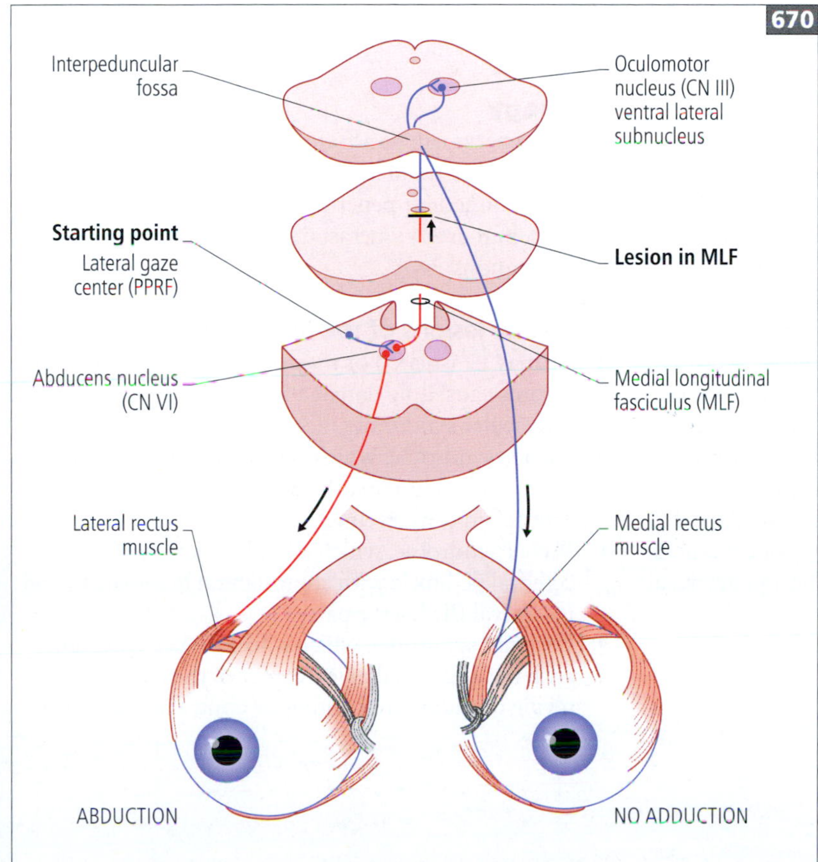

670 **A lesion of the medial longitudinal fasciculus on the left leads to a defect in conjugate eye movement to the right. PPRF: paramedian pontine reticular formation.**

One-and-a-half syndrome causes a gaze palsy to one side with an ipsilateral INO on gaze to the other side. It is also known as paralytic pontine exotropia. It results from a lesion of the PPRF or VIth nerve nucleus causing a gaze palsy with concomitant damage to the MLF leading to the ipsilateral INO.

Vertical diplopia is associated with IVth nerve palsies, IIIrd nerve palsies, skew deviations, thyroid disease, or myasthenia gravis.

Examination of ocular motility should begin with observing the patient for obvious misalignment of the eyes, also called a manifest tropia.

The ductions should be tested. Ductions are the movements of both eyes in all the directions of gaze. Limitations of motility of any of the muscles may be noted during this examination. Vergences are the result of the eyes moving in opposite directions such as convergence and divergence; this should also be examined.

The oculocephalic maneuver can be performed to determine whether the diplopia is due to a peripheral cranial nerve palsy or a lesion of the supranuclear pathways controlling eye movements. If the limitation of eye movements is overcome by the oculocephalic maneuver, the lesion is supranuclear in nature.

In some cases it will be necessary to do more subtle measurement of misalignment of the eyes using Maddox rods or the Krimsky technique. For example, these techniques can elucidate whether the misalignment varies with the direction of the gaze (incomitant deviation) or remains the same in all directions of gaze (comitant deviation). This is important because comitant deviations are often longstanding strabismic problems and not neurologic in nature. Both of these types of measurements can easily be performed by most ophthalmologists.

Any patients complaining of diplopia should be closely examined for signs of pupillary involvement or ptosis, as can be seen with IIIrd nerve palsies or Horner's syndrome. It should be stressed that although management of each of these palsies in isolation will be discussed, if a combination of cranial nerve palsies is seen or if one cranial nerve palsy occurs in the presence of other neurologic signs or symptoms, neuroimaging and further investigation is warranted. Causes of combined IIIrd, IVth and VIth nerve palsies include Wernicke's encephalopathy, Miller Fisher syndrome, skull base lesions, or cavernous sinus disease due to parasellar lesions, nasopharyngeal lesions, vascular lesions, or thrombosis[119–123].

CRANIAL NERVE III

Anatomy (671, 672)

The IIIrd nerve nucleus lies in the midbrain, anterior to the cerebral aqueduct. There is a specific subnucleus for each muscle innervated by the IIIrd nerve. Most of the subnuclei subserve the ipsilateral muscles; however, there are several anatomic tricks to the IIIrd nerve nuclei:

- One subnucleus that is shared between the right and left IIIrd nerve nuclei subserves both levator palpebrae muscles.
- Each superior rectus subnucleus crosses over to innervate the contralateral superior rectus.
- The Edinger–Westphal nuclei, which ultimately innervate sphincter of the pupil, send projections to the sphincter bilaterally[124,125].

The fascicles of the IIIrd nerve nuclei pass through the red nuclei and the cerebral peduncles before entering the interpeduncular fossa[125]. Once in the subarachnoid space, the fascicles pass between the superior cerebellar artery and posterior communicating artery. The IIIrd nerves enter the cavernous sinus just posterior to the clinoid processes and travel to the orbit in the wall of the cavernous sinus. At the orbital apex the IIIrd nerve enters via the superior orbital fissure. At this point it splits into a superior division which innervates the levator and the superior rectus. The inferior division innervates the inferior and medial recti, the inferior oblique, and the pupillary sphincter[126].

Etiology

The IIIrd nerve can be affected by lesions anywhere along its length. Intra-axial lesions usually consist of infarction of the paramedian penetrating vessels from the posterior cerebral artery, metastatic tumors, MS, or vascular malformations[127–129].

Fascicular lesions of the IIIrd nerve

These may be isolated or may occur in conjunction with symptoms caused by damage to surrounding structures. The fascicular syndromes include:

- Claude syndrome, which is ipsilateral IIIrd nerve palsy with contralateral ataxia due to dentatorubrothalamic involvement.
- Weber syndrome, which includes a lesion of the cerebral peduncle with contralateral hemiparesis and ipsilateral IIIrd nerve palsy.
- Benedikt syndrome, which is like Weber syndrome with the additional involvement of the red nucleus, giving the additional finding of contralateral tremor.

671

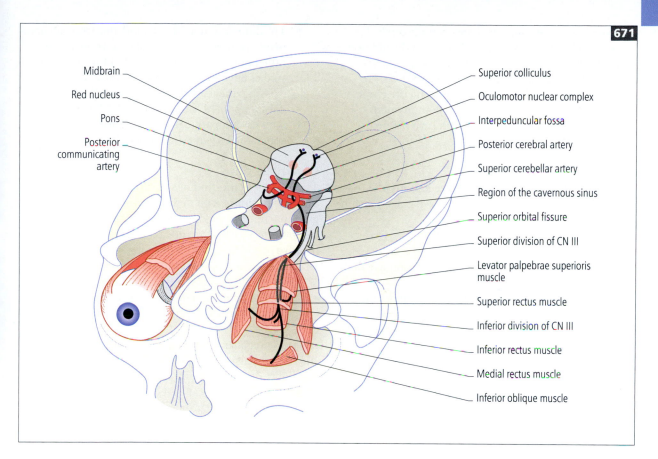

Midbrain
Red nucleus
Pons
Posterior communicating artery
Superior colliculus
Oculomotor nuclear complex
Interpeduncular fossa
Posterior cerebral artery
Superior cerebellar artery
Region of the cavernous sinus
Superior orbital fissure
Superior division of CN III
Levator palpebrae superioris muscle
Superior rectus muscle
Inferior division of CN III
Inferior rectus muscle
Medial rectus muscle
Inferior oblique muscle

672

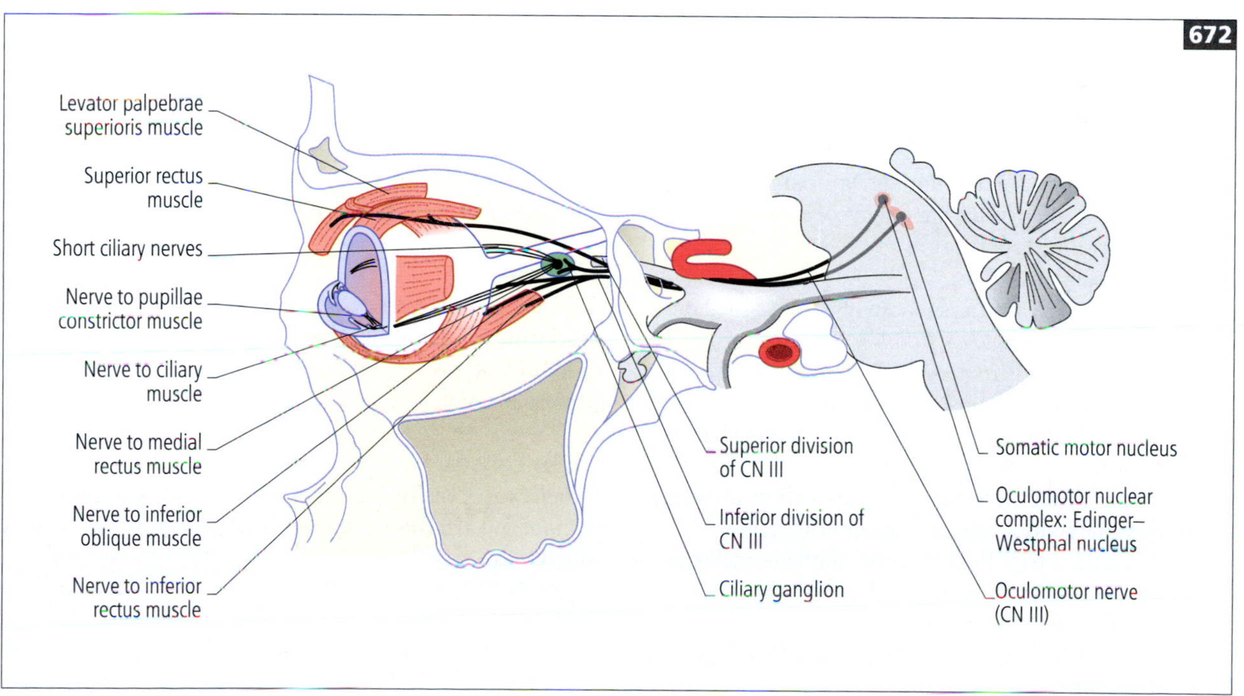

671, 672 Course of the IIIrd cranial nerve. Somatic motor efferents (red) provide innervation of muscles of the eye; visceral motor parasympathetic efferents (blue) for constrictor pupillae and ciliary muscles.

- Nothnagel syndrome which involves the cerebellar peduncle and results in cerebellar ataxia. In addition, the IIIrd nerve fascicles may be involved in dorsal midbrain syndrome with vertical gaze paresis, lid retraction, skew deviation, and convergence retraction nystagmus with or without a homonymous hemianopia if the posterior cerebral arteries are involved[130].

Subarachnoid processes

These may also affect the IIIrd nerve and are the most 'unnerving' potential cause of IIIrd nerve palsy to many clinicians:

- Uncal herniation:
  - Begins with ipsilateral pupil dilation and altered mental status before progressing to complete IIIrd nerve palsy.
  - Caused by compression of the nerve under the tentorial edge, compression by the posterior cerebral artery, or compression of the nerve over the clivus[131].
- Posterior communicating artery (PCom) aneurysms:
  - PCom aneurysms may compress the IIIrd nerve.
  - In this case the pupil is almost always involved.
  - Typically the patients complain of pain and complete or incomplete IIIrd nerve palsy with pupil dilation.
  - The pupil is involved in these cases because the position of the pupillary fibers is dorsomedial at this point in the course of the nerve, making them prone to compression from aneurysms.
  - IIIrd nerve palsies related to aneurysm are important to identify early as greater than 90% of patients with subarachnoid hemorrhage as a result of PCom aneurysms have signs of a IIIrd nerve palsy prior to rupture[132].
- Other aneurysms:
  - Basilar artery aneurysms can also cause IIIrd or IVth nerve palsies.
  - Usually these IIIrd nerve palsies involve the pupil.
  - Other signs of brainstem compression can be seen, such as hemiparesis, homonymous hemianopias, or obstructive hydrocephalus[132].
- Vasculopathic IIIrd nerve palsies also affect the nerve in the subarachnoid space or cavernous sinus.
  - Associated with hypertension, diabetes mellitus, advanced age, smoking, and hyperlipidemia.
  - Usually spare the pupil.
  - Frequently painful with the pain localized around the orbit.
  - The differentiation of vasculopathic from aneurysmal third nerve palsies is not based on pain but rather pupillary involvement[133]. However, some studies have suggested that mild anisocoria may exist in patients with vasculopathic IIIrd nerve palsies up to 40% of the time[134]. Most patients with vasculopathic IIIrd nerve palsies recover spontaneously in 8–12 weeks.

Cavernous sinus

There are specific findings in IIIrd nerve palsy that is caused by compression in the cavernous sinus from slow growing tumors or aneurysms of the intracavernous carotid artery. These are due to aberrant regeneration of the IIIrd nerve. Findings on examination may include:

- Lid retraction during adduction or depression of the eye.
- Miosis on adduction or retraction of the globe on attempted vertical deviation[135].

Aberrant regeneration is not seen after vasculopathic IIIrd nerve palsies and should alert the examiner to the possibility of a compressive lesion in the cavernous sinus. Other causes of aberrant regeneration include trauma, ophthalmoplegic migraine, inflammation, or pituitary apoplexy[136,137].

Tumors

Tumors of the oculomotor nerve include neurinomas and Schwannomas. These typically appear on neuroimaging with thickening of the nerve and enhancement in the subarachnoid space or cavernous sinus. They are slow growing and benign and can be observed in most cases[138]. Other neoplasms of the nerve include malignant meningioma or glioblastoma multiforme[139].

Trauma

Trauma leading to a IIIrd nerve palsy is usually severe head trauma. Typically there is intracranial hemorrhage or skull fractures present. Trauma can lead to aberrant regeneration[137].

Other causes

Other causes of IIIrd nerve palsies include vasculitis due to giant cell arteritis or herpes zoster, infections, and sinus mucoceles.

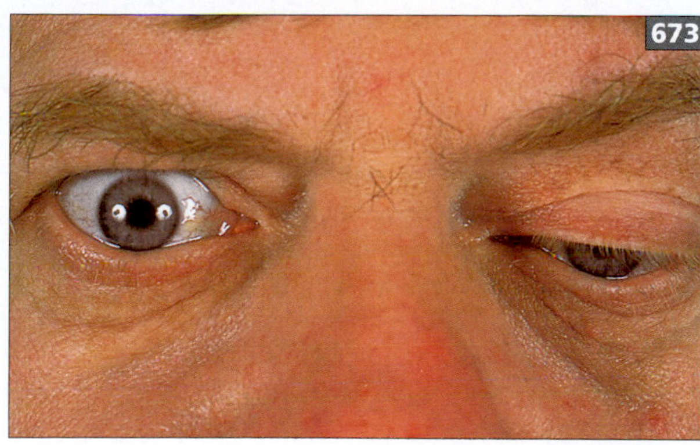

673 IIIrd nerve palsy in primary gaze. There is complete ptosis of the left eye and the eye is in the 'down and out' position.

Clinical features

The IIIrd nerve innervates the medial, inferior, and superior recti muscles as well as the inferior oblique, the levator muscle of the eyelid, and the pupillary sphincter. Therefore, a complete IIIrd nerve palsy causes ipsilateral elevation, adduction, and depression weakness. The eye appears 'down and out', with ptosis and mydriasis (673).

Nuclear palsies of the IIIrd nerve result in bilateral ptosis, worse on the ipsilateral side, and bilateral superior rectus weakness, with all the other typical features of IIIrd nerve palsy outlined above[140].

Investigations

When evaluating patients with IIIrd nerve palsies, the key examination points to pay attention to are whether the palsy is complete or partial, whether the pupil is involved or spared, whether the superior or inferior division is involved in an isolated fashion, and whether aberrant regeneration is present.

Patients with partial involvement of the IIIrd nerve may be evolving a compressive aneurysmal lesion and must have this excluded, especially if the pupil is involved at diagnosis.

If the pupil is spared and the palsy is partial they may be observed for 3–5 days for the IIIrd nerve palsy to become complete and the pupil to remain uninvolved. If no pupil involvement is seen after 5 days, the patient can be managed as a vasculopathic IIIrd nerve palsy with less urgency for imaging or angiography. They should be seen again in 6–8 weeks and improvement in the ptosis and/or motility should be expected at that time. If no improvement is seen after 8 weeks, neuroimaging should be done even in the absence of pupil involvement.

Patients with pupil involvement should also be imaged or undergo angiography to look for aneurysms. Patients with isolated superior division palsies may have a compressive lesion and should undergo neuroimaging. Patients with aberrant regeneration should have neuroimaging to evaluate the cavernous sinus and surrounding structures.

Pediatric IIIrd nerve palsies

In children IIIrd nerve palsies can be congenital or acquired.

- Acquired:
  - The most frequent cause of acquired IIIrd nerve palsies is trauma.
  - PCom aneurysms are unusual in children.
- Congenital:
  - Often associated with neurologic damage.
  - Aberrant regeneration of the IIIrd nerve is often seen in congenital palsies.
  - Aplasia of the nucleus of the IIIrd nerve with malformation of the midbrain may be seen on MRI[141].
  - Infections such as with *Haemophilus influenzae* or pneumococcal meningitis can result in IIIrd nerve palsy.
  - Posterior fossa tumors such as astrocytomas or gliomas can cause IIIrd nerve palsies.
  - Tumor of the orbital apex such as rhabdomyosarcoma may also cause IIIrd nerve palsies in children[142].
- Ophthalmoplegic migraines:
  - Unusual form of migraine that begins in childhood.
  - The IIIrd, IVth, or VIth nerves may be involved but most commonly affected is the IIIrd nerve.
  - The first attack usually occurs before the age of 10 years.
  - There is ipsilateral headache or retrobulbar pain associated with the palsy, although the pain may occur days before the ophthalmoparesis appears.
  - The diagnosis is made by exclusion after normal neuroimaging and LP, as well as multiple attacks with no problems between attacks[143].
  - Children with IIIrd nerve palsies should undergo a neurologic examination to look for associated signs.
  - In addition, MRI should be performed and possibly LP.

Although aneurysms are unusual in children, if there is no family history of migraine and the child is older than 10 years at onset, angiography should be considered.

CRANIAL NERVE IV

Anatomy (674)

The IVth nerve nucleus is located in the pontomidbrain junction, caudal to the IIIrd nerve nucleus. The axons from the nuclei decussate near the roof of the aqueduct and exit the brainstem on the dorsal side below the inferior colliculi. The IVth nerve has the longest course of all the cranial nerves through the subarachnoid space. In addition, it is the smallest of the cranial nerves, containing only 1500 axons. As a result, it is very prone to shearing injuries and trauma.

Etiology

Trauma

- Often bilateral in nature.
- This is due to damage to the decussation of the fibers near the tentorium resulting in contunsion injuries.
- Bilateral IVth nerve palsies can be identified by measuring the excyclotorsion of the eyes.
- If greater than 10° of excyclotorsion is present, bilateral involvement should be suspected.
- In addition, the eyes may be esotropic.
- Traumatic IVth nerve palsies often resolve with time[144].
- If no resolution is seen and measurements remain stable for at least 6 months, surgery to correct the deviation can be considered.

674 Course of the IVth cranial nerve.

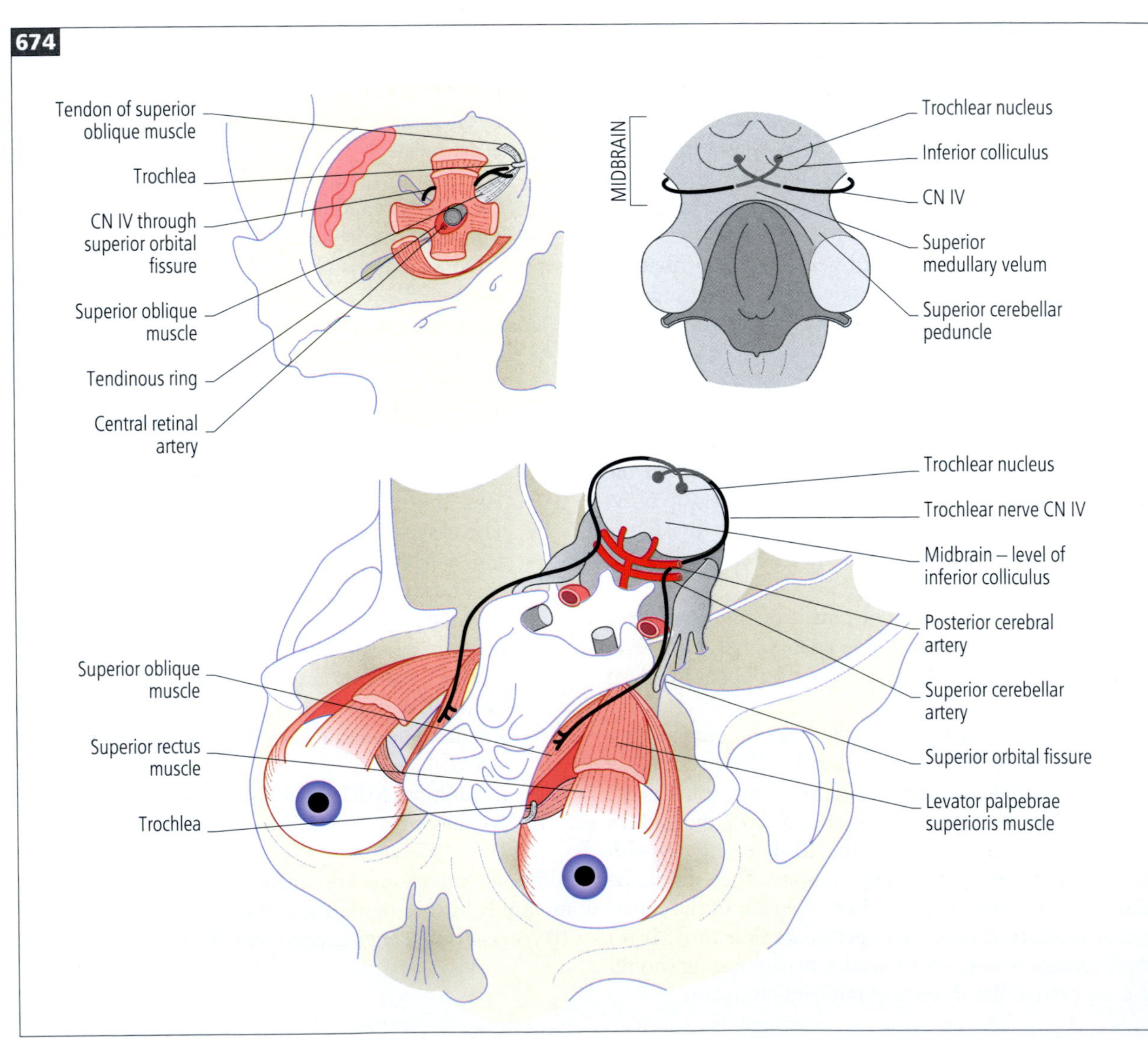

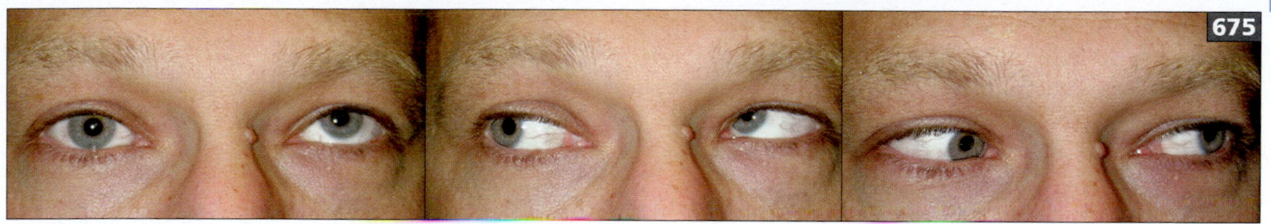

675 **Left IVth nerve palsy. The left eye is elevated and hypertropic. In gaze away from the left side the hypertropia is more pronounced, since the superior oblique has its greatest action in adduction of the eye. In addition, the other depressor of the eye, the inferior rectus, is not active in adduction.**

Vasculopathy

- This occurs in patients aged over 50, and with hypertension, hyperlipidemia, diabetes, a history of smoking, or other vasculopathies.
- Patients often begin with periorbital pain and then develop vertical diplopia.
- Typically, spontaneous resolution is seen within 8–12 weeks.
- Patients with the appropriate demographic and historical background for vasculopathic IVth nerve palsies can therefore be observed for recovery.
- If no resolution is seen after 8–12 weeks, MRI imaging is recommended.

Other conditions

IVth nerve palsies may occur with other neurologic findings that mandate further investigation. For example:

- Patients with a contralateral dysmetria may have a lesion involving the superior cerebellar peduncle.
- Patients with a contralateral INO should be evaluated for lesions of the MLF.
- In those with a contralateral Horner's syndrome, lesions may be found at the dorsal pons[145].

Clinical features

The IVth cranial nerve innervates the contralateral superior oblique muscle of each eye.

The superior oblique is a depressor, abductor, and intorter of the eye. Palsies of the IVth nerve result in a vertical diplopia with a hypertropia on the side with the affected superior oblique (675)[146].

The hypertropia and diplopia worsen when the patient attempts to look away from the affected side. This is because when the eye is adducted, the superior oblique has its greatest vertical action. In addition, the other depressor of the eye, the inferior rectus, is not active in adduction.

The diplopia will be worse when the head is tilted to the ipsilateral side. This is called Bielchowsky's head tilt test. The reason the diplopia becomes worse in this gaze is because when the head is tilted to the right, for example, the intorters of the eye must come to action in order to maintain an object on the macula. The intorters are the superior rectus (also an elevator of the eye) and the superior oblique. When the head is tilted the vertical forces balance unless a paretic muscle is present. If the superior oblique is palsied the superior rectus attempts to intort the eye alone but also elevates the eye, increasing the hyperdeviation on the affected side and highlighting the excyclotorsion of the eye.

Pediatric IVth nerve palsy

Pediatric palsy of the IVth nerve is usually congenital. Patients with congenital IVth nerve palsies may have 'decompensation' of the palsy as they get older, become ill, or are under the influence of alcohol or drugs. These patients develop vertical diplopia. Decompensation of the palsy leading to diplopia is not a result of progressive weakness of the nerve, but rather reduced ability to fuse the vertically dissociated images on the retina. These patients can be identified by several factors including:

- Longstanding head tilt to the contralateral side seen in photographs or by history.
- No inciting event.
- Comitance of measurements (see above).
- Increased vertical fusional amplitudes.

The average individual without congenital IVth nerve palsy can only fuse about 2–3 prism diopters of vertical misalignment; this can be difficult to see on normal duction testing for the examiner. Patients with congenital IVth nerve palsies can typically fuse more vertical deviation, upward of 20 prism diopters in some cases. This results in obvious shifting of the eyes when the eyes are covered alternately by the examiner. Although the examiner can see the large shift that takes place in the eye position, the patient will often report no diplopia with both eyes open. This is very suggestive of congenital IVth nerve palsies.

Other causes include trauma or posterior fossa neoplasms[147].

CRANIAL NERVE VI

Anatomy (676, 677)

- The nucleus of the VIth nerve is located in the dorsal pons.
- The genu of the VIIth nerve fascicle wraps around the VIth nerve.
- The fascicles travel through the body of the pons ventrally, passing through the cortical spinal tracts.
- The fascicles enter the subarachoid space and pass under Gruber's ligament to ascend the clivus through Dorello's canal to cavernous sinus.
- The VIth nerve travels in the body of the cavernous sinus. While in the cavernous sinus, the postganglionic sympathetic fibers to the pupil join the VIth nerve for a short distance[148].
- Cranial nerve VI (abducens nerve) innervates the ipsilateral lateral rectus muscle in each eye.
- In addition, the nucleus of the VIth nerve contains the interneurons that ascend through the MLF to innervate the contralateral medial rectus muscles[146].

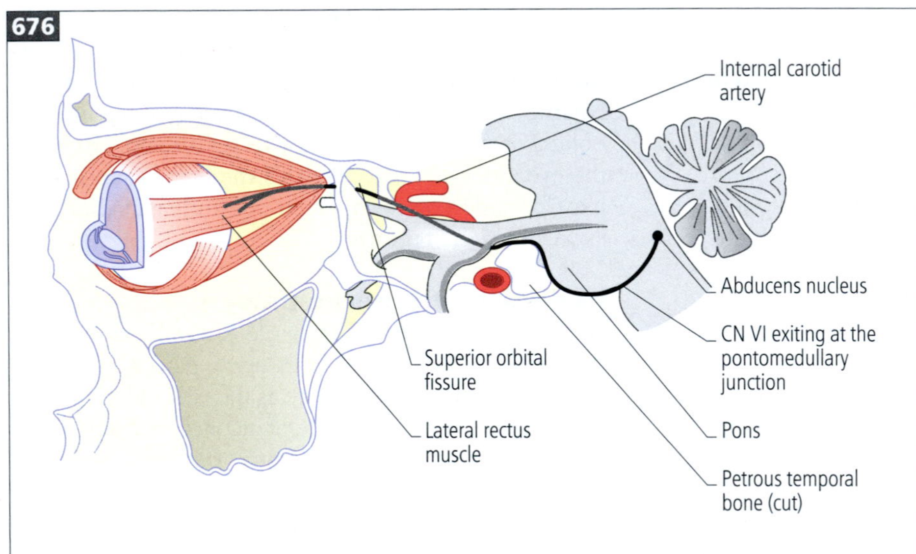

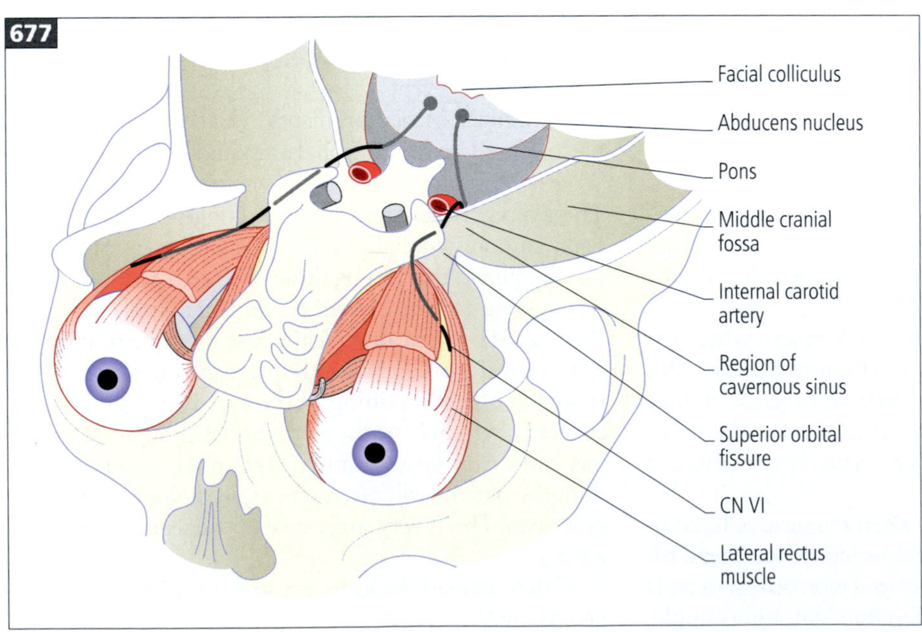

676, 677 Course of the VIth cranial nerve.

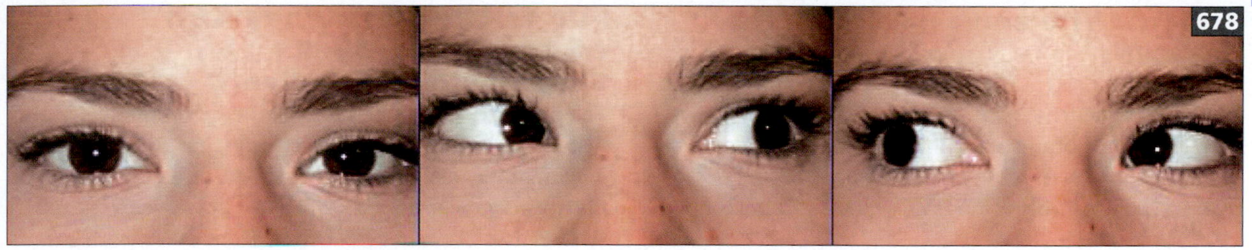

678 Left VIth nerve palsy. In primary gaze the eyes are very slightly esotropic. In gaze to the left the left eye does not fully abduct. There is normal adduction of the left eye in right gaze and full abduction of the right eye in right gaze. Notice how the sclera is buried in abduction of the right eye, whereas in abduction of the left eye the sclera is still visible.

Clinical features

The VIth cranial nerve is responsible for abduction of each eye. Nuclear lesions of the VIth nerve result in a gaze palsy to the affected side (678)[149]. This is due to the anatomy described above, with the interneurons to the medial recti muscles also being affected in a nuclear lesion. In pontine lesions, there may be associated facial weakness if the fibers from the VIIth nerve are affected as they wrap around the VIth nerve nucleus.

Fascicular lesions of the sixth nerve often affect surrounding structures resulting in several syndromes:

- Gasperini's syndrome involves the paramedian pontine reticular formation, cranial nerves VI and VII, the spinothalamic tract, and vestibular neurons.
- Raymond's syndrome involves the cerebellar peduncles and the corticospinal tract with the VIth nerve, resulting in contralateral hemiparesis.
- Millard Gubler syndrome is similar to Raymond's syndrome in that the corticospinal tract and the VIth cranial nerve are involved but it also involves a VIIth nerve palsy.
- Foville's syndrome includes the VIth and VIIth nerves, the corticospinal tract, and the ciliospinal tract, resulting in the addition of Horner's syndrome[150].

Etiology

Subarachnoid lesions

Subarachnoid lesions can cause VIth nerve palsies in isolation. The VIth nerve is fixed along the clivus and over the petrous apex; any increased pressure in the cranial vault, whether pseudotumor cerebri, supratentorial masses, or hydrocephalus, can lead to stretch on the nerve resulting in unilateral or bilateral VIth nerve palsies that are nonlocalizing. Low intracranial pressure can also result in downward pressure on the brain leading to nonlocalizing VIth nerve palsies in the subarachnoid space. Therefore, when seeing a patient with a VIth nerve palsy it is important to ask about other symptoms of increased or decreased intracranial pressure, as well as carefully examining the fundus for papilledema.

Tumors

Skull base neoplasms such as meningiomas and chordomas can also cause isolated VIth nerve palsies. In these cases, the palsies tend to be chronic and are sometimes associated with ipsilateral dry eye due to involvement of the fibers to the lacrimal gland[151].

Vasculopathy

Isolated VIth nerve palsies can be a result of vasculopathic risk factors. These resolve on their own without treatment, typically in 8–12 weeks. No resolution after that time frame mandates imaging to rule out a mass lesion.

Trauma

Traumatic VIth nerve palsies typically occur in the setting of severe head trauma[152–154].

Other causes

- Myasthenia gravis.
- Demyelinating disease.
- Miller Fisher syndrome.
- Temporal arteritis.
- Gradenigo syndrome:
  - Usually seen as a complication of middle ear infection or mastoiditis.
  - Results from involvement of the apex of the petrous temporal bone.
  - Characterized by:
    - Otorrhea.
    - Retro-orbital pain (Vth cranial nerve involvement).
    - Ipsilateral abduscens palsy (VIth cranial nerve involvement).

Pediatric VIth nerve palsies

Congenital

- Rare.
- Duane's syndrome:
  - Result of brainstem abnormalities and absence or hypoplasia of the VIth nerve nucleus.
  - This leads to aberrant innervation of the lateral rectus.
  - Duane's syndrome can be distinguished from an acquired VIth nerve or lateral palsy in that the patients are not esotropic in primary gaze.
  - Patients typically have reduced abduction, adduction, or both[155].
- Mobius syndrome:
  - Much rarer than Duane's syndrome.
  - Bilateral facial diplegia and bilateral abducens weakness with an esotropia.
  - A significant proportion of the time, children with Mobius syndrome have total external ophthalmoplegia[156].

Acquired

Acquired VIth nerve palsies in children are most frequently associated with posterior fossa tumors. These lesions affect the midline structures in the pons and may also present with gaze palsies. If the fourth ventricle is obstructed there may be associated papilledema. If the cerebellar pathways are associated, ataxia and/or nystagmus may be seen.

Acquired comitant esotropia

This is sometimes mistaken for bilateral VIth nerve palsies. Although not technically a VIth nerve palsy, it merits discussion because of its associations. Misalignment of the eyes occurs that is comitant in all directions of gaze; it is a benign condition most of the time. However, there have been several reports of medulloblastomas, pontine gliomas, or astrocytomas causing acquired comitant esotropia in children.

There are usually signs of increased intracranial pressure or cerebellar or brainstem involvement in these children and they must be looked for in all children presenting with new onset acquired esotropias.

All children with acquired VIth nerve palsies must be evaluated with imaging of the posterior fossa and LP to rule out potentially fatal causes of VIth nerve palsy[157].

PUPILLARY PATHWAYS AND COMMON DISORDERS

Sympathetic dysfunction

The pupillary pathway is part of the sympathetic nervous system and is divided into central (first-order) neuron, preganglionic (second-order) neuron, and postganglionic (third-order) neuron (**679**):

- The first-order neuron travels from the hypothalamus to the intermediolateral cell column of the spinal cord at C8–T2.
- The second-order neuron leaves the spinal cord and joins the internal carotid artery to synapse at the superior cervical ganglion.
- The third-order neuron follows the internal carotid into the cavernous sinus, where it briefly joins the VIth (trigeminal) nerve, then passes through the nasociliary branch into the orbit. This neuron releases norepinephrine (noradrenaline) at the iris dilator muscle.

Etiology and clinical features

- Iritis.
- Chronic tonic pupil.
- Pharmacologic miosis (such as pilocarpine).
- Horner's syndrome.

Damage to any of the neurons results in anisocoria with the smaller pupil being the affected pupil, greatest in the dark. This is accompanied by a small ptosis of the lid on the ipsilateral side due to sympathetic innervation to Muller's muscle, a minor lid elevator, and ipsilateral anhydrosis.

Investigations

In suspected Horner's syndrome cocaine testing is used to confirm the presence of Horner's syndrome. Since cocaine blocks the reuptake of norepinephrine at the last synapse in the pathway, a lesion anywhere in the pathway will result in a positive cocaine test, or lack of pupillary dilation on the affected side in response to cocaine. At this point most patients will be referred for MRI/magnetic resonance angiography of the head and neck to rule out a carotid dissection, followed by CT of the chest to look for apical lung lesions.

Further localization of the level of the lesion can be done with hydroxyamphetamine, which enhances the release of norephinephrine at the third neuron. Therefore, if the third neuron is intact, the pupil will dilate in response to hydroxyamphetamine suggesting that the lesion is preganglionic. If the pupil does not dilate, the lesion involves the third neuron in the pathway. This testing cannot be performed until 48 hours after the cocaine test, and clinically is not frequently used.

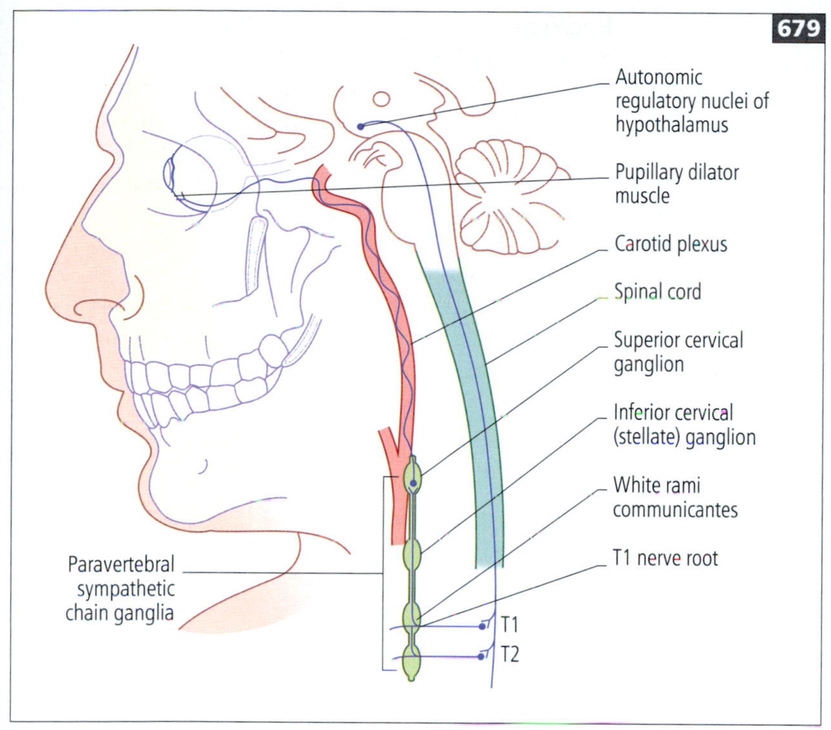

679 **Three-neuron sympathetic pupillary pathway. The first-order neuron is located in the hypothalamus; it travels in the lateral brainstem and synapses in the C8–T1 region of the spinal cord in the ciliospinal center of Budge. The second-order neuron (preganglionic sympathetic neuron) exits the cord via ventral roots of T1 and T2 and skirts the apex of the lung and the subclavian artery before joining the paravertebral sympathetic chain. The second-order neuron ascends and synapses with the third-order neuron (postganglionic sympathetic neuron) in the superior cervical ganglion; this travels through the carotid plexus along the internal carotid artery wall into the orbit and synapses at the iris dilator muscle.**

Tip

► *In testing for Horner's syndrome, most neuro-ophthalmologists will consider a positive cocaine test or a positive apraclonidine test to be sufficient to warrant neuroimaging. Further testing with hydroxyamphetamine is rarely done.*

Etiology of Horner's syndrome

- First-order neuronal dysfunction:
  - Brainstem infarction (lateral medullary syndrome), hemorrhage, or demyelination.
  - Cervical lesions interrupting the descending sympathetic projections such as tumors, demyelination, or syrinx.
- Second-order neuronal dysfunction:
  - Radiculopathy.
  - Pancoast's tumor.
  - Brachial plexus injury (most common cause of congenital Horner's syndrome).
  - Cervical rib.
- Third-order neuronal dysfunction (anhydrosis is usually not seen as the fibers involved in the sudomotor innervation of the face travel with external carotid artery):
  - Ipsilateral carotid artery dissection.
  - Cavernous sinus disease (carotid–cavernous fistula, carotid artery aneurysm, cavernous sinus thrombosis, or inflammation [Tolosa–Hunt syndrome]).
  - Base of skull tumors.

Parasympathetic dysfunction

Retinal ganglion cells ultimately project bilaterally to the Edinger–Westphal subnucleus of the IIIrd cranial nerve (see **662**). The Edinger–Westphal nuclei then issue parasympathetic fibers that travel within the IIIrd nerve and enter the orbit via the inferior division of the nerve; these fibers terminate at the ciliary ganglion in the orbit. The ciliary ganglion then projects to the pupillary sphincter muscles resulting in miosis.

Clinical features and investigations

Anisocoria is greater in the light (the larger pupil is the abnormal). Anisocoria due to IIIrd nerve palsy rarely occurs in isolation; lid height and ocular motility must be checked in any patient with anisocoria. Anisocoria due to pharmacologically dilated pupils leads to a very large pupil (7–8 mm) that is unresponsive to light, near, or 1% pilocarpine.

Tonic pupils

These are painless, more common in women, and patients are generally otherwise healthy. Complaints include photophobia and difficulty reading. Evaluation of tonic pupils includes:

- Larger pupil that appears more anisocoric in bright light (though chronic tonic pupils can be miotic); light-near dissociation, tonic redilation; sectoral constriction of the iris, loss of the pupillary ruff.
- Pharmacologic testing: the iris sphincter develops denervation hypersensitivity causing dilation to dilute (0.125%) pilocarpine (cholinergic agent) which should not have an effect on normal pupils. The test is positive when the presumed tonic pupil constricts more than the normal pupil.

Etiology

- Adie's syndrome:
  - Tonic pupil and absent deep tendon reflexes.
  - Ophthalmologic findings are usually unilateral.
  - Occurs due to aberrant reinnervation after damage to ciliary ganglion or postganglionic short ciliary nerves.
- Argyll Robertson pupil:
  - Pathognomonic of neurosyphilis.
  - Pupils are irregular and miotic; poor pupil response to light but preserved constriction to near reaction (light-near dissociation).
  - Variable iris atrophy.
- Local ocular processes:
  - Trauma.
  - Varicella.
  - Ischemia.
  - Strabismus surgery.
  - Retinal laser.
- Autonomic dysfunction:
  - Shy–Drager syndrome
  - Guillain–Barré syndrome.
- Pharmacologic mydriasis:
  - Scopolamine.
  - Atropine.
  - Phenylephrine.

REFERENCES

1 Kupfer C, Chumbley L, Downer JC (1967). Quantitative histology of optic nerve, optic tract and lateral geniculate nucleus of man. *J Anat* **101**:393–401.

2 Ogden TE (1983). Nerve fiber layer of the macaque retina: retinotopic organization. *Invest Ophthalmol Vis Sci* **24**:85–89.

3 Hayreh SS (2001). The blood supply of the optic nerve head and the evaluation of it – myth and reality. *Prog Retinal Eye Res* **20**:563–593.

4 Hayreh SS (1973). Proceedings: Anatomy and pathophysiology of ocular circulation. *Exp Eye Res* **17**:387–388.

5 Schneck ME, Haegerstrom-Portnoy G (1997). Color vision defect type and spatial vision in the optic neuritis treatment trial. *Invest Ophthalmol Vis Sci* **38**:2278–2289.

6 Beck RW, Cleary PA, Anderson MM, *et al.* (1992). A randomized, controlled trial of corticosteroids in the treatment of acute optic neuritis. *N Engl J Med* **326**:581–588.

7 The Optic Neuritis Study Group (2008). Multiple sclerosis risk after optic neuritis: Final optic neuritis treatment trial follow up. *Arch Neurol* **65**:727–732.

8 Papis-Alveranga RM, Carellos SC, Alvarenga MP, Holander C, Bichara RP, Thuler LC (2008). Clinical course of optic neuritis in patients with relapsing neuromyelitis optica. *Arch Ophthalmol* **126**:12–16.

9 Matiello M, Lennon VA, Jacob A, *et al.* (2008). NMO-IgG predicts the outcome of recurrent optic neuritis. *Neurology* **70**:197–200.

10 Stern BJ, Krumholz A, Johns C (1985). Sarcoidosis and its neurological manifestations. *Arch Neurol* **42**:909–917.

11 Galetta SL, Schatz NJ, Glaser JS (1989). Acute sarcoid optic neuropathy with spontaneous recovery. *J Clin Neuro-ophthalmol* **9**:27–32.

12 Machado E, Michet C, Ballard D, *et al.* (1988). Trends in incidence and clinical presentation of temporal arteritis in Olmsted County, Minnesota, 1950–1985. *Arthritis Rheum* **31**:745–749.

13 Hayreh SS, Podhajsky PA, Raman R, Zimmerman B (1997). Giant cell arteritis: validity and reliability of various diagnostic criteria. *Am J Ophthalmol* **123**:285–296.

14 Chlemeski W, McKnight K, Agudelo C, Wise C (1992). Presenting features and outcome in patients undergoing temporal artery biopsy: a review of 98 patients. *Arch Intern Med* **152**:1690–1695.

15 Danesh-Meyer H, Savino PJ, Gamble GG (2005). Poor prognosis of visual outcome after visual loss from giant cell arteritis. *Ophthalmology* **112**:1098–1103.

16 Hayreh SS, Zimmerman B (2003). Visual deterioration in giant cell arteritis patients while on high doses of corticosteroid therapy. *Ophthalmology* **110**:1204–1215.

17 Wilkinson IMS, Russell RWR (1972). Arteries of the head and neck in giant cell arteritis. A pathological study to show the pattern of arterial involvemtn. *Arch Neurol* **27**:378–391.

18 Hunder GG (2001). Giant cell arteritis and polymyalgia rheumatica. In: Ruddy S, Harris ED, Sledge CB (eds). *Kelley's Textbook of Rheumatology*, 6th edn. WB Saunders, Philadelphia, pp. 1155–1164.

19 Lie JU, Gordon LP, Titus JL (1975). Juvenile temporal arteritis: biopsy study of four cases. *JAMA* **234**:572–577.

20 Biler J, Asconape J, Weinblatt ME (1982). Temporal arteritis associated with a normal sedimentation rate. *JAMA* **247**:486–487.

21 Finelli PF (1997). Alternating amaurosis fugaz and temporal arteritis. *Am J Ophthalmol* **123**:850–851.

22 Keltner JL (1982). Giant cell arteritis. Signs and symptoms. *Ophthalmology* **89**:1101–1110.

23 Jonason F, Cullen JF, Elton PA (1979). Temporal arteritis. *Scott Med J* **24**: 111–117.

24 Liu GT, Glaser JS, Schatz NJ (1994). Visual morbidity in giant cell arteritis: clinical characteristics and prognosis for vision. *Ophthalmology* **101**:1779–1785.

25 Aiello PD, Trautmann JC, McPhee TJ (1993). Visual prognosis in giant cell arteritis. *Ophthalmology* **100**:550–555.

26 Isayama Y, Takahashi T, Inoue M (1983). Posterior ischemic optic neuropathy. III: Clinical diagnosis. *Ophthlamologica* **187**:141–147.

27 Hollenhorst RW, Brown JR, Wagener HP (1960). Neurologic aspects of temporal arteritis. *Neurology* **10**:490–498.

28 Barricks ME, Traviesa DB, Glaser JS (1977). Ophlamoplegia in cranial arteritis. *Brain* **100**:209–221.

29 Hunder GG, Block DA, Michel BA, *et al.* (1990). The American College of Rheumatology 1990 criteria for the classification of giant cell arteritis. *Arthritis Rheum* **33**:1122–1128.

30 Liu GT, Volpe NJ, Galetta Sl (2001). Visual loss: optic neuropathies. In: *Neuro-Ophthalmology*. WB Saunders Philadelphia.

31 Miller A, Green M, Robinson D (1983). Simple rule for calculating normal erythrocyte sedimentation rate. *BMJ* **286**:266.

32 Foroozan R, Danesh-Meyer H, Savino PS, Gamble G, Mekari-Abbagh ON, Sergott RC (2002). Thrombocytosis in patients with biopsy proven giant cell arteritis. *Ophthalmology* **109**:1267–1271.

33 Krishna R, Kosmorsky GS (1997). Implication of thrombocytosis in giant cell arteritis. *Am J Ophthalmol* **124**:103.

34 Klein RG, Campbell RJ, Hunder GG (1976). Skip lesions in temporal arteritis. *Mayo Clin Proc* **51**:504–510.

35 Chambers WA, Bernadino VB (1988). Specimen length in temporal artery biopsies. *J Clin Neuro-ophthalmol* **8**:121–125.

36 Rosenfeld SI, Kosmorsky GS, Klingele TG (1986). Treatment of temporal arteritis with ocular involvement. *Am J Med* **80**:143–145.

37 Matzkin DC, Slamovits TL, Sachs R (1992). Visual recovery in two patients after intravenous methylprednisolone treatment of central retinal artery occlusion secondary to giant cell arteritis. *Ophthalmology* **99**:68–71.

38 Johnson LN, Arnold AC (1994). Incidence of nonarteritis and arteritic anterior ischemic optic neuropathy. Population based study in the state of Missouri and Los Angeles County, California. *J Neuro-ophthalmol* **14**:38–44.

39 Swartz NG, Beck RW, Savino PJ (1995). Pain in anterior ischemic optic neuropathy. *J Neuro-ophthalmol* **15**:9–10.

40 Ischemic Optic Neuropathy Decompression Trial Study Group (1996). Characteristics of patients with nonarteritic anterior ischemic optic neuropathy eligible for the Ischemic Optic Neuropathy Decompression Trial. *Arch Ophthalmol* **114**:1366–1374.

41 Roth S, Pietrzyk Z (1994). Blood flow after retinal ischemia in cats. *Invest Ophtahlmol Vis Sci* **35**:209–217.

42 Hayreh SS (1997). Anterior ischemic optic neuropathy. *Clin Neurosci* **4**:383–417.

43 Hayreh SS (1997). Factors influencing blood flow in the optic nerve head. *J Glaucoma* **6**:412–415.

44 Jacobson DM, Vierkant RA, Belongia EA (1997). Nonarteritic anterior ischemic optic neuropathy: a case control study of potential risk factors. *Arch Ophthlamol* **115**:1403–1407.

45 Hayreh SS, Podhajsky PA, Zimmerman B (1997). Nonarteritic anterior ischemic optic neuropathy: time of onset of visual loss. *Am J Ophthalmol* **124**:641–647.

46 Hayreh SS, Podhajsky P, Zimmerman MB (1999). Role of nocturnal arterial hypotension in optic nerve head ischemic disorders. *Ophthalmologica* **213**:76–96.

47 Pillunat LE, Anderson DR, Knoghton RW, Joos KM, Feuer WJ (1997). Autoregulation of human optic nerve head circulation in response to increased intraocular pressure. *Exp Eye Res* **64**:737–744.

48 Repka MX, Savino PJ, Schatz NJ (1983). Clinical profile and long term implication of anterior ischemic optic neuropathy. *Am J Ophthalmol* **96**:478–483.

49 Salomon O, Huna-Baron R, Kurtz S (1999). Analysis of prothrombotic and vascular risk factors in patients with nonarteritic anterior ischemic optic neuropathy. *Ophthalmology* **106**:737–742.

50 Arnold AC, Hepler RS, Hamilton DR (1995). Magnetic resonanace imaging of the brain in nonarteritic ischemic optic neuropathy. *J Neuro-ophthalmol* **15**:158–160.

51 Arnold AC, Hepler RS (1994). Natural history of nonarteritic ischemic optic neuropathy. *J Neurophthalmol* **14**:66–69.

52 Barrett DA, Glaser JS, Schatz NJ (1992). Spontaneous recovery of vision in progressive anterior ischaemic optic neuropathy. *J Clin Neuro-ophthalmol* **12**:219–225.

53 Beri M, Klugman MR, Kohler JA (1989). Anterior ischemic optic neuropathy VII. Incidence of bilaterality and various influencing factors. *Ophthalmology* **94**:1020–1026.

54 Delattre O, Thoreux P, Liverneaux P, *et al.* (2007). Spinal surgery and ophthalmic complications: a French survey with review of 17 cases. *J Spinal Disor Tech* **20**:302–307.

55 Lee LA, Roth S, Posner KL, *et al.* (2006). The American Society of Anesthesiologists postoperative visual loss registry: analysis of 93 spine surgery cases with postoperative visual loss. *Anesthesiology* **105**:652–659.

56 Myers MA, Hamilton SR, Bogosian AJ, Smith CH, Wagner TA (1997). Visual loss as a complication of spine surgery: a review of 37 cases. *Spine* **22**:1325–1329.

57 Warner ME, Warner MA, Garrity JA, Mackenzie RA, Warder DO (2001). The frequency of perioperative vision loss. *Anesth Analg* **93**:1417–1421.

58 Roth S, Thisted RA, Erickson JP, Black S, Schreider BD (1996). Eye injuries after nonocular surgery: a study of 60,965 anesthetics from 1988 to 1992. *Anesthesiology* **85**:1020–1027.

59 Shaw PJ, Bates D, Cartlidge NE, *et al.* (1987). Neuro-ophthalmological complications of coronary artery bypass graft surgery. *Acta Neurol Scand* **76**:1–7.

60 Breuer AC, Furlan AJ, Hanson M (1982). Central nervous system complication of coronary bypass graft surgery: a prospective analysis of 421 patients. *Stroke* **14**:682–687.

61 Shaw PH, Bates D, Cartlidege NEF (1985). Early neurological complication of coronary artery bypass surgery. *BMJ* **83**:45–47.

62 Wolfe SW, Lospinuso MR, Burke SW (1993). Unilateral blindness as a complication of patient positioning for spinal surgery. *Spine* **17**:600–605.

63 Shahian DM, Speert PK (1989). Symptomatic visual deficits after open heart operations. *Ann Thorac Surg* **48**:275–279.

64 Aldrich MS, Alessi AG, Beck RW (1986). Cortical blindness: etiology, diagnosis and prognosis. *Ann Neurol* **21**:149–158.

65 Hunt K, Bajekal R, Calder I, Meacher R, Eliahoo J, Acheson JF (2004). Changes in intraocular pressure in anesthetized prone patients. *J Neurosurg Anesthesiol* **16**:287–290.

66 Sadda SR, Nee M, Miller NR 92001). Clinical spectrum of posterior ischemic optic neuropathy. *Am J Ophthalmol* **132**:743–750.

67 Williams EL, Hart WM, Tempelhoff R (1995). Posteroperative ischemic optic neuropathy. *Anesth Analg* **80**:1018–1029.

68 Lee AG (1995). Reversible loss of vision due to posterior ischemic optic neuropathy. *Can J Ophthalmol* **30**:327–329.

69 Hassler W, Zentner J, Wilhelm H (1989). Cavernous angiomas of the visual pathways. *J Clin Neuro-ophthalmol* **9**:160–164.

70 Rootman J, Goldberg C, Roberston W (1982). Primary orbital schwannomas. *Br J Ophthlamol* **66**:194–204.

71 Char DH, Norman D (1982). The use of computed tomography and ultrasonography in the ovaluation of orbital masses. *Surv Ophthalmol* **27**:49–63.

72 Wright JE, McNab AA, McDonald WI (1989). Optic nerve glioma and the management of optic nerve tumors in the young. *Br J Ophthalmol* **73**:967–974.

73 Dutton JJ (1994). Gliomas of the anterior visual pathways. *Surv Ophthalmol* **38**:427–452.

74 Alvord EC, Lofton S (1988). Gliomas of the optic nerve or chiasm: outcome by patients' age, tumor site, and treatment. *J Neurosurg* **68**:85–98.

75 Haik BG, Louis LS, Bierly J (1987). Magnetic resonance imaging in the evaluation of optic nerve gliomas. *Ophthalmology* **94**:709–717.

76 Spoor TC, Kennerdell JS, Martinez AJ (1980). Malignant gliomas of the optic nerve pathways. *Am J Ophthalmol* **89**:284–292.

77 Saeed P, Rootman J, Nugent RA (2003). Optic nerve sheath meningiomas. *Ophthalmology* **110**:2019–2030.

78 Muci-Mendoza R, Arevalo JF, Ramella M (1999). Opticociliary veins in optic nerve sheath meningioma. Indocyanine green videoangiography findings. *Ophthalmology* **106**:311–318.

79 Jakobiec FA, Depot MJ, Kennerdell JS (1984). Combined clinical and computed tomographic diagnosis of orbital glioma and meningioma. *Ophthalmology* **91**:137–155.

80 Mafee MF, Goodwin J, Dorodi S (1999). Optic nerve sheath meningiomas. Role of MR imaging. *Radiol Clin North Am* **37**:37–58.

81 Trobe JD, Glaser JS, Laflamme P (1978). Dysthyroid optic neuropathy. *Arch Ophthalmol* **96**:1199–1209.

82 Dallow RL, Pratt SG (1994). Approach to orbital disorders and frequency of disease occurrence. In: Albert DM, Jakobiec FA (eds). *Principles and Practice of Ophthalmology*. WB Saunders, Philadelphia, pp. 1881–1890.

83 Bartley GB, Fatourechi V, Kadrmas EF (1996). Chronology of Graves' ophthalmopathy in an incidence cohort. *Am J Ophthalmol* **121**:426–434.

84 Bartley GB, Fatourechi V, Kadrmas EF (1996). Clinical features of Graves' ophthalmopathy in an incidence cohort. *Am J Ophthalmol* **121**:284–290.

85 Bartley GB, Fatourechi V, Kadrmas EF (1996). Long-term follow-up of Graves' ophthalmopathy in an incidence cohort. *Ophthalmology* **103**:958–962.

86 Boldt HC, Byrne SF, DiBernardo C (1991). Echographic evaluation of optic disc drusen. *J Clin Neuro-ophthalmol* **11**:85–91.

87 Rosenberg MA, Savino PJ, Glaser JS (1979). A clinical analysis of pseudopapilledema. I: population, laterality, acuity, refractive error, ophthalmoscopic characteristics, and coincident disease. *Arch Ophthalmol* **97**:65–70.

88 Brodsky MC (1994). Congenital optic disk anomalies. *Surv Ophthalmol* **39**:89–112.

89 Morishima A, Aranoff GS (1986). Syndrome of septo-optic dysplasia: the clinical spectrum. *Brain Dev* **8**:233–239.

90 Taylor D (1982). Congenital tumours of the anterior visual system with dysplasia of the optic disc. *Br J Ophthalmol* **66**:455–463.

91 Kinder P (1970). Morning glory syndrome: unusual congenital optic disk anomaly. *Am J Ophthalmol* **69**:376–384.

92 Bakri SJ, Siker D, Masaryk T (1999). Ocular malformations, moyamoya disease, and midline cranial defects: a distinct syndrome. *Am J Ophthalmol* **127**:356–357.

93 Apple DJ, Rabb MF, Walsh PM (1982). Congenital anomalies of the optic disc. *Surv Ophthalmol* **27**:3–41.

94 Lessell S, Gise RL, Krohel GB (1983). Bilateral optic neuropathy with remission in young men: variation on a theme by Leber. *Arch Neurol* **40**:2–6.

95 Newman NJ, Lott MT, Wallace DC (1991). The clinical characteristics of pedigrees of Leber's hereditary optic neuropathy with the 11778 mutation. *Am J Ophthalmol* **111**:750–762.

96 Palan A, Stehouwer A, Went LN (1989). Studies on Leber's optic neuropathy III. *Doc Ophthalmol* **52**:671–674.

97 Singh G, Lott MT, Wallace DC (1989). A mitochondrial DNA mutation as a cause of Leber's hereditary optic neuropathy. *N Engl J Med* **320**:1300–1305.

98 Johns DR, Smith KH, Savino PJ (1993). Leber's hereditary optic neuropathy: clinical characteristic of the 15257 mutation. *Ophthalmology* **100**:981–986.

99 Pezzi PP, De Negri AM, Sadun F (1998). Childhood Leber's hereditary optic neuropathy, (ND1/3460) with visual recovery. *Pediatr Neurol* **19**:308–312.

100 Kjer P (1959). Infantile optic atrophy with dominant mode of inheritance: a clinical and genetic study of 19 Danish families. *Acta Ophthalmol* Suppl **54**:1–46.

101 Votruba M, Fitzke FW, Holder BE (1998). Clinical features in affected individuals from 21 pedigrees with dominant optic atrophy. *Arch Ophthalmol* **116**:793–800.

102 Johnston RL, Burdon MA, Spalton DJ (1997). Dominant optic atrophy, Kjer type. Linkage analysis and clinical features in a large British pedigree. *Arch Ophthalmol* **117**:100–103.

103 Houroupian DS, Zuker DK, Moshe S (1979). Behr syndrome: a clinicopathologic report. *Neurology* **29**:323.

104 Rabiaj PK, Bateman JB, Demer JL (1997). Ophthalmologic findings in patients with ataxia. *Am J Ophthalmol* **123**:108–117.
105 Moseley MI, Benzow KA, Schut LJ (1998). Incidence of dominant spinocerebellar and Friedreich triplet repeats amoung 361 ataxia families. *Neurology* **51**:1666–1671.
106 Koeppen AH, Hans MB (1976). Supranuclear ophthalmoplegia in olivopontocerebellar degeneration. *Neurology* **99**:207–234.
107 Lindenbaum J, Healton EB, Savage DG (1988). Neuropsychiatric disorders caused by cobalamin deficiency in the absence of anemia or macrocytosis. *N Engl J Med* **318**:1720–1728.
108 Rizzo JF, Lessell S (1993). Tobacco amblyopia. *Am J Ophthalmol* **116**:84–87.
109 Samples JR, Younge BR (1981). Tobacco-alcohol amblyopia. *J Clin Neuro-ophthalmol* **1**:213–218.
110 Carroll FD (1966). Nutritional amblyopia. *Arch Ophthalmol* **76**:406–411.
111 Hayreh MS, Hayreh S, Baumbach GL (1977). Methyl alcohol poisoning. III. Ocular toxicity. *Arch Ophthalmol* **95**:1851–1858.
112 Jacobs D, McMartin KE (1986). Methanol and ethylene glycol poisonings: mechanism of toxicity, clinical course, diagnosis, and treatment. *Med Toxicol* **1**:309–334.
113 Tsai RK, Lee YH (1997). Reversibility of ethambutol optic neuropathy. *J Ocul Pharmacol Ther* **13**:473–477.
114 Lessell S (1995). Toxic and deficiency optic neuropathies. In: Miller NR, Newman NJ (eds). *Walsh and Hoyt's Clinical Neuro-ophthalmology*, 5th edn. Williams & Wilkins, Baltimore, pp. 663–680.
115 Polito E, Leccisotti A (1994). Diagnosis and treatment of orbital hemorrhagic lesions. *Ann Ophthalmol* **26**:85–93.
116 Crompton MR (1970). Visual lesion in closed head injury. *Brain* **93**:785–792.
117 Levin LA, Beck RW, Joseph MP (1999). The treatment of traumatic optic neuropathy: The International Optic Nerve Trauma Study. *Ophthalmology* **106**:1268–1277.
118 Lopez JR, Adornato BT, Hoyt WF (1993). Entomopia: a remarkable case of cerebral polyopia. *Neurology* **43**:2145–2146.
119 Sima AAF, Caplan M, D'Amato CJ (1993). Fulminant multiple system atrophy in a young adult presenting as motor neuron disease. *Neurology* **43**:2031–2035.
120 Yuki N (1996). Acute paresis of extra-ocular muscles associated with anti-IgG anti-GQ1b antibody. *Ann Neurol* **39**:668–672.
121 Carrizo A, Basso A (1998). Current surgical treatment for sphenoorbital meningiomas. *Surg Neurol* **50**:574–578.
122 Volpe NJ, Liebsch NJ, Munzenrider JE (1993). Neuro-ophthalmologic findings in chordoma and chondrosarcoma of the skull base. *Am J Ophthalmol* **115**:97–104.
123 Keane JR (1996). Cavernous sinus syndrome. Analysis of 151 cases. *Arch Neurol* **53**:967–971.
124 Donzelli R, Marinkovis S, Brigante L (1998). The oculomotor nuclear complex in humans. Microanatomy and clinical significance. *Surg Radiol Anat* **20**:7–12.
125 Bienfang DC (1975). Crossing axons in the third nerve nucleus. *Invest Ophthalmol* **14**:927–931.
126 Porter JD, Baker RS, Ragusa RJ (1995). Extraocular muscles: basic and clinical aspects of structure and function. *Surv Ophthalmol* **39**:451–484.
127 Bogousslavsky J, Maeder P, Regli F (1994). Pure midbrain infarction: clinical syndromes, MRI and etiologic patterns. *Neurology* **44**:2032–2040.
128 Keane JR (1988). Isolated brainstem third nerve palsy. *Arch Neurol* **45**: 813–814.
129 Newman NJ, Lessell Sl (1990). Isolated pupil sparing third nerve palsy as the presenting sign of multiple sclerosis. *Arch Neurol* **47**:817–818.
130 Caplan LR (1980). Top of the basilar syndrome. *Neurology* **30**:72–79.
131 Ropper AH, Cole D, Louis DN (1991). Clinicopathologic correlation in a case of papillary dilation from cerebral hemorrhage. *Arch Neurol* **48**:1166–1169.
132 Kupersmith MJ (1993). *Neuro-vascular Neuro-ophthlamology*. Springer-Verlag, Berlin.
133 Keane JR, Ahmadi J (1998). Most diabetic third nerve palsies are peripheral. *Neurology* **51**:1510–1523.
134 Jacobson DM (1998). Pupil involvement in patients with diabetes-associated oculomotor nerve palsy. *Arch Ophthalmol* **116**:723–727.
135 Landau K (1997). Discovering a dys-covering lid. *Surv Ophthalmol* **42**:87–91.
136 Lepore FE, Glaser JS (1980). Misdirection revisited. A critical appraisal of acquired oculomotor nerve synkinesis. *Arch Ophthalmol* **98**:2206–2209.
137 Sibony PA, Lessell S, Gittinger JS, Jr (1984). Acquired oculomotor synkinesis. *Surv Ophthalmol* **28**:382–390.
138 Kaye-Wilson LG, Gibson R, Bell JE (1994). Oculomotor nerve neurinoma. *Neuro-ophthalmology* **4**:69–72.
139 Hart AJ, Allibone J, Casey AT (1998). Malignant meningioma of the oculomotor nerve without dural attachment. Case report and review of the literature. *J Neurosurg* **88**:1104–1106.
140 Bogousslavsky J, Regli F (1983). Nuclear and prenuclear syndromes of the oculomotor nerve. *Neuro-ophthalmology* **3**:211–216.
141 Ing EB, Sullivan TJ, Clarke MP (1992). Oculomotor nerve palsies in children. *J Pediatr Ophthalmol Strabismus* **29**:331–336.
142 Schumacher-Feero LA, Yoo KW, Solari FM (1999). Third cranial nerve palsy in children. *Am J Ophthalmol* **128**:216–221.
143 Ostergard JR, Moller HU, Christensen T (1996). Recurrent ophthalmolplegia in childhood: diagnostic and etiologic considerations. *Cephalalgia* **16**:276–279.
144 Lepore FE (1995). Disorders of ocular motility following head trauma. *Arch Neurol* **52**:924–926.
145 Brazis PW (1993). Localization of lesions of the trochlear nerve: diagnosis and localization – recent concepts. *Mayo Clin Proc* **68**:501–509.
146 Sacks JG (1983). Peripheral innervation of extraocular muscles. *Am J Ophthalmol* **95**:520–527.
147 Harley RD (1980). Paralytic strabismus in children. Etiologic incidence and management of the third, fourth and sixth nerve palsies. *Ophthalmology* **87**:24–43.
148 Usmansky F, Nathan H (1982). The lateral wall of the cavernous sinus with special reference to the nerves related to it. *J Neurosurg* **20**:205–210.
149 Muri RM, Chermann JF, Cohen L (1996). Ocular motor consequences of damage to the abducens nucleus area in humans. *J Neuro-ophthalmol* **16**:191–195.
150 Bajandas FJ (1977). The six syndromes of the sixth nerve. In: Smith JL (ed). *Neuro-ophthalmology Update*. Masson, New York, pp. 49–68.
151 Volpe NJ, Lessell S (1993). Remitting sixth nerve palsy in skull base tumors. *Arch Ophthalmol* **111**:1391–1395.
152 Mutyala S, Holmes JM, Hodge DO (1996). Spontaneous recovery rate in traumatic sixth nerve palsy. *Am J Ophthalmol* **122**:898–899.
153 Dave AV, Diaz-Marchan PJ, Lee AG (1997). Clinical and magnetic resonance imaging freatures of Gradenigo syndrome. *Am J Ophthalmol* **124**:568–570.
154 Lotery A, Best J, Houston S, *et al*. (1998). Occult giant cell arteritis presenting with bilateral sixth and unilateral fourth nerve palsies. *Eye* **12**:1014–1016.
155 Isenberg S, Urist MJ (1977). Clinical observations in 101 consecutive patients with Duane's retraction syndrome. *Am J Ophthalmol* **84**:419–425.
156 Verzijl HT, Van Der Zwaag B, Cruysberg JR, *et al*. (2003). Mobius syndrome redefined: a syndrome of rhombencephalic maldevelopment. *Neurology* **61**:327–333.
157 Gilbert ME, Meira D, Forozoon R, Edwards J, Phillip P (2006). Double vision worth a double take. *Surv Opthalmol* **51**:587–91.

Further reading

Galetta SL, Plock GL, Kushner MJ (1991). Ocular thrombosis associated with anti-phospholipid antibodies. *Ann Ophthlamol* **23**:207–212.

SPINAL CORD DISEASE

Octavia Kincaid

INTRODUCTION TO MYELOPATHY

Definition

Myelopathy is a disorder of the spinal cord of any etiology.

Etiology

Correctly identifying a spinal cord disorder requires recognition of the clinical syndromes which manifest from damage to spinal cord structures, which, in turn, necessitates an understanding of spinal cord anatomy (680). Critical neurologic functions potentially affected by a lesion in the spinal cord include:

- Ascending sensation:
  - Pain, temperature, light touch via the contralateral spinothalamic tracts.
  - Proprioceptive, vibratory, and discriminatory touch senses via the ipsilateral spinal leminiscal pathway (dorsal columns).
- Descending motor control; limb and bulbar control via the ipsilateral corticospinal and corticobulbar tracts.
- Autonomic control; gastrointestinal and urinary control via the lateral reticulospinal tract.

The somatotopic organization of the spinal cord further assists in identification of a clinical spinal cord syndrome (681). For example, lesions extrinsic to the cord can exert pressure on the superficial fibers, leading to motor deficits in lumbosacral myotomes and proprioceptive deficits in cervical dermatomes.

A spinal cord lesion should be suspected in the following situations:

- Limb weakness:
  - May be flaccid in acute presentations.
  - Typically symmetric.
  - Upper motor neuron (UMN) features (spasticity, hyper-reflexia).
  - Rostral to spastic weakness may be lower motor neuron (LMN) features (atrophy, fasciculations, hyporeflexia).

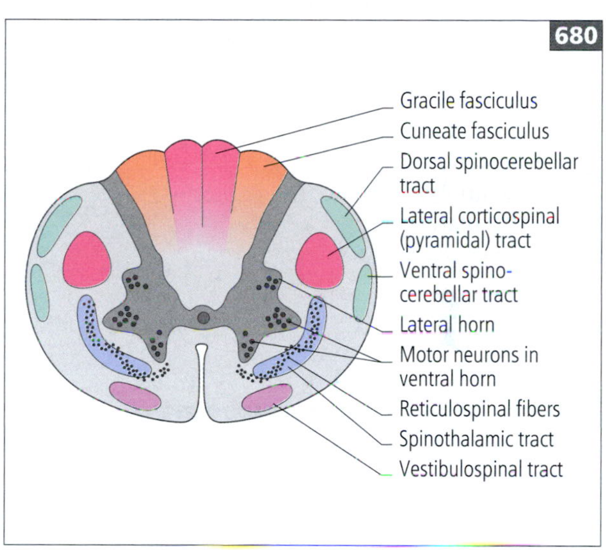

680 Cross-section of the spinal cord, illustrating major fiber tracts.

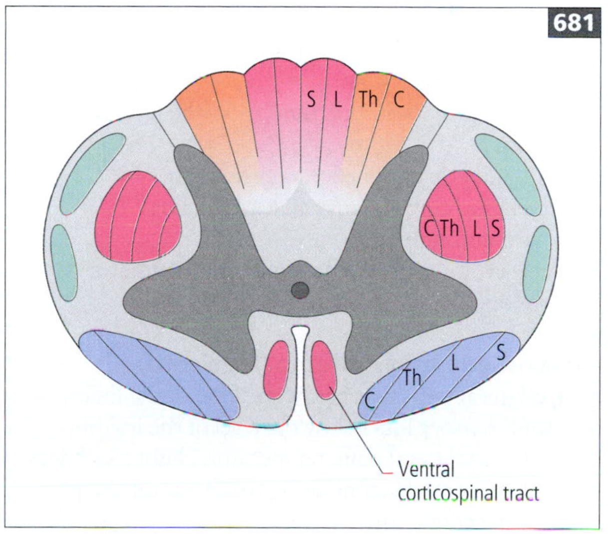

681 Somatotopic organization of major spinal cord tracts, illustrating tract lamination. S: sacral segments; L: lumbar segments; Th: thoracic segments: C: cervical segments.

- Sensory loss:
  - Typically symmetric.
  - Sensory level or symptoms of band-like quality at level of sensory loss.
- Autonomic dysfunction:
  - Urinary incontinence, urgency.
  - Constipation > bowel incontinence.

Classification of spinal cord lesions

- Extramedullary (includes extradural and intradural):
  - Degenerative spine disease.
  - Epidural collection (hematoma, abscess).
  - Neoplastic (metastatic *vs.* primary).
- Intramedullary:
  - Inflammatory.
  - Infectious.
  - Metabolic/toxic.
  - Vascular.
  - Genetic/hereditary.
  - Structural.
  - Neoplastic.
  - Heredodegenerative.

Clinical myelopathy syndromes

Clinical myopathy syndromes may be due to intrinsic or extrinsic processes.

Complete cord transection or transverse myelopathy

- Weakness below the level of the lesion:
  - UMN signs below the lesion and, possibly, LMN signs at the level of the lesion (anterior horn cells affected).
- Complete anesthesia to all sensory modalities below the level of the lesion.
- Loss of autonomic function below the level of the lesion:
  - Bladder incontinence, constipation.
  - Higher cord lesions can lead to spinal dysautonomia.
- Prototypical disorder: trauma or inflammatory myelopathy.

Brown–Sequard syndrome (hemicord)

- Ipsilateral weakness below the level of the lesion.
- 'Split' sensory loss below the level of the lesion:
  - Contralateral pain, temperature, light touch loss.
  - Ipsilateral discriminating touch, vibration, proprioception loss.
- Autonomic function may be spared, depending on the etiology of the lesion.
- Prototypical disorder: trauma or inflammatory myelopathy.

Myelo-radiculopathy syndrome

- Weakness:
  - LMN pattern in one or more myotomes (distribution of motor nerve).
  - UMN pattern below the level of the lesion.
- Pain and sensory changes in one or more dermatomes.
- Prototypical disorder: extradural spinal tumor.

Central cord syndrome (cervical cord)

- Weakness:
  - Distal > proximal upper extremities.
  - Lower extremities less severely affected or normal.
- 'Dissociated' sensory loss below the level of the lesion:
  - Pain, temperature, light touch loss.
  - Discriminating touch, vibration, proprioception preserved.
- Autonomic function may be affected (urinary dysfunction).
- Prototypical disorder: syringomyelia.

Posterolateral column degeneration

- Weakness due to corticospinal tract dysfunction below the level of the lesion:
  - Although weakness may be in UMN pattern with spasticity and hyper-reflexia, some manifestations of this syndrome are associated with peripheral neuropathy, leading to depressed deep tendon reflexes.
- Sensory loss below the level of the lesion:
  - Posterior columns: discriminating touch, vibration, proprioception loss.
  - Spinothalamic tracts (pain, temperature, light touch): spared.
- Prototypical disorder: B12 deficiency ('subacute combined degeneration').

Posterior column syndrome

- Loss of discriminating touch, vibration, proprioception only.
- Prototypical disorder: syphilis ('tabes dorsalis').

Anterior horn cell syndrome

- Weakness only in LMN pattern:
  - May be diffuse or segmental (e.g. 'monomelic' or one limb).
  - May involve cranial nerve nuclei (motor only).
- Prototypical disorder: spinal muscular atrophy (SMA).

Combined anterior horn cell and corticospinal tract syndrome

- Weakness only with both UMN and LMN features: may involve cranial nerve nuclei (motor only).
- Prototypical disorder: amyotrophic lateral sclerosis (ALS).

Anterior spinal artery syndrome

- Weakness below the level of the lesion: flaccid/areflexic acutely, progressing to spastic weakness.
- Sensory loss below the level of the lesion:
  - Loss of pain, temperature, light touch.
  - Preserved discriminating touch, vibration, proprioception.
- Prototypical disorder: anterior spinal artery occlusion.

EXTRAMEDULLARY SPINAL CORD LESIONS (EXTRINSIC MYELOPATHY)

Definition

Any spinal cord syndrome caused by compression of the cord rather than pathology within the cord itself.

Etiology and pathophysiology

Extradural

- Degenerative spine disease:
  - Herniated disc.
  - Vertebral bone spurs.
  - Acquired central spinal stenosis.
- Nondegenerative process:
  - Congenital central spinal stenosis.
  - Hypertrophic ligamentum flavum.
  - Posterior longitudinal ligament ossification.
  - Epidural lipomatosis.
- Trauma: vertebral fracture.
- Vertebral body infiltration:
  - Osteomyelitis (bacteria, tuberculosis [Pott's disease of the vertebral body]).
  - Malignancy (plasmacytoma, primary bone tumor, metastatic lesions – most common to metastasize to vertebral body: prostate, breast).

Intradural

- Epidural abscess.
- Epidural hematoma.
- Spinal arachnoiditis.
- Spinal arteriovenous malformation (AVM).

Clinical features

Clinical features of an extrinsic cord lesion depend on both the level of the spinal cord involved and the etiology of the compression.

Tip

▶ *Due to the somatotopic organization of the spinal cord tracts, compression can lead to lumbosacral motor fiber dysfunction prior to the onset of arm weakness. Dorsal column organization, however, is opposite, and cervical fibers are most superficial, leading to loss of discriminating touch, vibration, or proprioception prior to similar findings in the lower body. Pain and temperature loss is expected to be contralateral to the site of compression and affecting sacral fibers earlier.*

Clues to an extrinsic lesion include:

- Early loss of sacral sensation.
- Early involvement of bowel and bladder function.
- Pain in a radicular pattern (due to nerve root involvement).

Clinical findings depend on the cord level and tracts affected (see syndromes described above):

- Brown–Sequard (hemicord).
- Complete transection.
- Anterior spinal artery or posterior column – if ventral or dorsal compression, respectively.

Differential diagnosis

Cervical spondylotic myeloradiculopathy

Definition and epidemiology

The most common type of extrinsic myelopathy in which the spinal cord (myelopathy) and/or nerve roots (radiculopathy) are damaged, either directly by traumatic compression and abnormal movement, or indirectly by ischemia due to arterial compression, venous stasis, or other consequences of the proliferative changes that characterize spondylosis, such as ligamentum flavum hypertrophy with associated canal narrowing.

Most people older than 50 years have cervical spondylosis. Most have no symptoms apart from reduced mobility of the cervical spine.

- Age: middle-aged and elderly; peak incidence in the age group 50–54 years.
- Gender: M>F (3:2 ratio).

Etiology and pathophysiology

Predisposing factors include:

- Narrowing of the spinal canal in the sagittal (anteroposterior) plane: <11–12 mm (<0.4–0.5 in) results in deformation of the cord, the degree of which correlates with the clinical severity of myelopathy. The salient static measurement is, however, the cross-sectional area of the cord. Reduction in cross-sectional area of the cord by 30% or more, to a value of about 60 mm^2 or less, results in symptoms and signs.

- In patients with cervical spondylotic myelopathy caused by an ossified posterior longitudinal ligament, the dentate ligaments fix the cord against the anterior part of the canal. Sectioning of the dentate ligaments may spread the tension in the cord over a greater area.
- Hypertrophic facet and uncovertebral joints occupy space in the root canal.
- Neck motion: predisposes to spur formation and activates symptoms and signs of cervical spondylotic myelopathy (e.g. patients with athetoid cerebral palsy).

Causes include:
- Bulging or herniated disc (**682**).
- Hypertrophic ligamentum flavum.
- Congenital central spinal stenosis.
- A fixed subluxation due to disc degeneration.
- Microtrauma.

The mechanism can be direct or indirect compression:
- Direct: traumatic compression and abnormal movement. Acute trauma is likely to exacerbate any pre-existing myelopathy in a chronically distorted, narrowly confined cord.
- Indirect: the role of ischemia is uncertain. There is no correlation with atherosclerosis of major vessels or with obstruction of blood flow in the anterior spinal artery. Distortion and compression of small vessels in the cord may have a pathogenetic influence. The influence of venous stasis is uncertain.

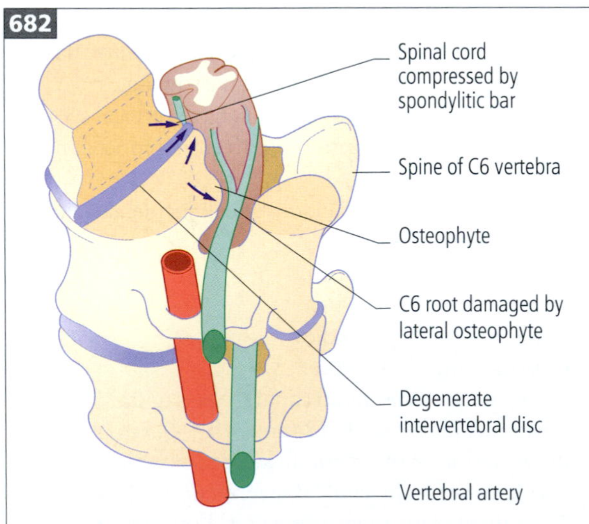

682 The effect of a cervical spondylitic bar, osteophyte, or degenerate intervertebral disc at the C5/6 level, compressing the cervical spinal cord (causing a cervical myelopathy) and/or left C6 nerve root (causing a left C6 radiculopathy).

Clinical features

Clinical myelopathy syndrome with or without symptoms and signs of cervical radiculopathy:
- Neck and arm pain in some.
- Paresthesiae, pain, and cutaneous sensory loss in a radicular distribution.
- Wasting and weakness of proximal arm muscles or in the hands.
- Fasciculations in a segmental distribution in the hands and arms.

Cervical spondylosis alone will not result in cervical spondylotic myeloradiculopathy unless foraminal or spinal canal stenosis is present.

Investigations

MRI cervical spine is the imaging modality of choice. Sagittal T1 and T2 images show the cord and level of any compression (**683**). Axial views at those levels further define the degree of cord and root involvement (**684**).

Cervical disc protrusions are seen in about 30% of neurologically asymptomatic people over 40 years old. Spinal cord impingement (a concave defect in the spinal cord adjacent to a site of disc bulging, without obliteration of the subarachnoid space posterior to the cord) is seen in about one-sixth of neurologically asymptomatic people under 65 years and one-quarter over 65 years.

Cord compression (with obliteration of the posterior subarachnoid space) may also be neurologically asymptomatic but usually the percentage reduction in cord area in asymptomatic people is well below 30% (usually below 15%). Thinning of the cord opposite a disc protrusion is indicative of compression, worse if there is increased signal in the cord at that point on T2. Increased signal intensity on T2 images of a compressed cord reflects myelomalacia, demyelination, gliosis, or microcavities.

Nerve root compression can occur without significant cord compression in which case axial views targeted to the level of the patient's symptoms (plus the level immediately above and below) are required. Absence of the fat signal from within the root canal, in addition to obvious abnormal structural defect (e.g. disc or bone) and displacement or obliteration of the nerve, is suggestive of clinically relevant compression.

Plain films of the cervical spine are useful because they demonstrate narrowing of the spinal canal, osteophytes arising from the posterior surfaces of degenerate discs and at the neurocentral joints, and the alignment of the vertebral bodies. Flexion and extension views may be done to look for instability with movement. They do not, however, give any information on the degree of cord or root compression or the soft tissue abnormalities around the spine.

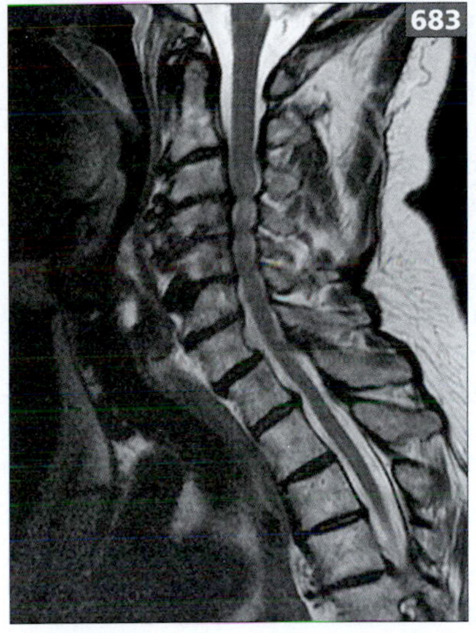

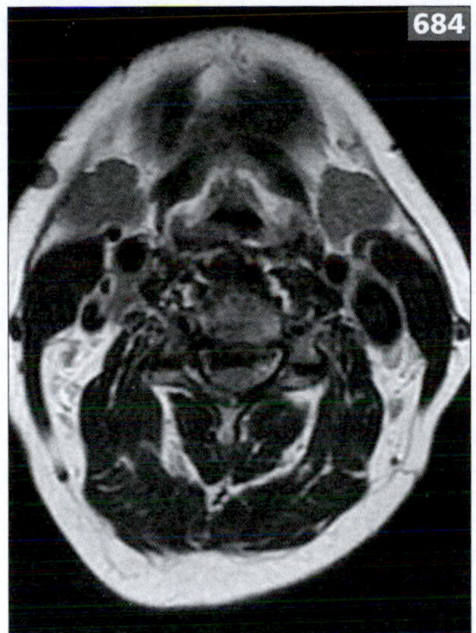

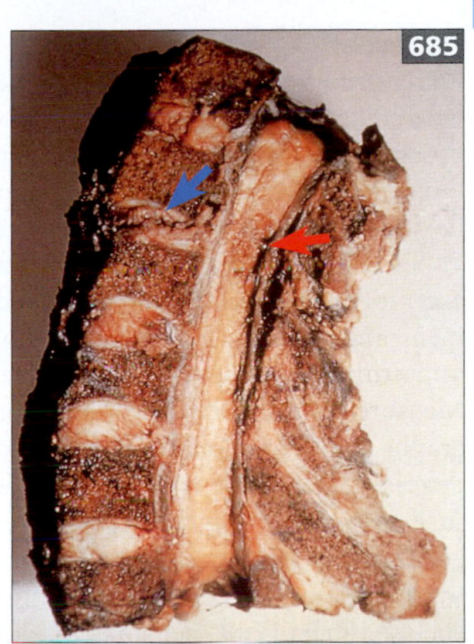

683, 684 Cervical spondylotic myelopathy. Sagittal T2W MRI of cervical spine, showing multilevel disc herniations with signal change within the spinal cord (683). Axial T2W MRI of cervical spine with loss of cerebrospinal fluid signal surrounding the cord (684).

685 Autopsy specimen of the cervical spine in the sagittal plane, showing a degenerate cervical intervertebral disc (blue arrow) compressing the cervical spinal cord and causing a necrosis of the spinal cord at that level (red arrow).

Plain CT has a limited role; it images osteophytes and calcified discs, and accurately measures the dimensions of the bony spinal canal, but the cervical cord and roots cannot be assessed.

Computer assisted myelography (CAM) is useful if the MRI quality is suboptimal or the patient is unable to have an MRI. It is useful for delineating the bone and soft tissue abnormalities but it is an invasive procedure.

Diagnosis

Diagnosis is based on clinical symptoms and signs of spinal cord (± nerve root) compression (i.e. spastic paraparesis) with unequivocal radiologic evidence of spinal cord compression that correlates precisely with the clinical findings.

Pathology

Macroscopic changes in spondylosis of the vertebral column include:

- Transverse bars occur which may extend across the posterior aspect of the vertebrae and compress the spinal cord. The lateral end of the transverse bars may encroach on an intervertebral foramen and compress the nerve root.
- Localized bosses occur centrally or laterally, which may compress the spinal cord.
- Intervertebral disc protrusions are commonly associated with the bars and bosses.
- Frequently these lesions are found at more than one vertebral level.

Spinal cord/root compression involves:

- Indentation, flattening, and distortion of the spinal cord corresponding to the spondylotic protrusions (685).
- The C6 or C7 nerve roots are affected in two-thirds of cases of cervical radiculopathy.

Microscopically, multiple pathologic findings occur at the site of the compression, including demyelination of the lateral columns, ischemic changes with neuronal damage in the central gray matter, and cavitation.

- Degeneration of the dorsal columns occurs rostral to the lesions.
- Degeneration of the lateral columns occurs caudal to the lesions.

Treatment

Patients without major neurologic deficits or signs of worsening are probably best treated conservatively and observed closely over time. A restraining collar may help limit the mobility of the cervical spine, and particularly flexion of the neck which increases dural tension.

Surgical decompression is considered in patients who are moderately or severely disabled on initial assessment and who, on close follow-up, have progressive impairment of function without sustained remission. Measurement of cervical mobility on functional radiographs may help to select patients who are more likely to deteriorate and thus more likely to benefit from surgery, such as those with spinal hypermobility. The aim of surgical therapy is to arrest the progression of myelopathy by elimination of mechanical compression of the dura-enclosed spinal cord, but small randomized trials suggest that conservative treatment (symptom control with medication and physical therapy) may have the same long-term outcome for moderately affected patients.

Prognosis

The natural history is variable and two types of outcome are reported: stabilization of deficit without further decline in function and slow, step-wise deterioration. Spontaneous regression and complete remission are unusual[1].

If spondylitic myelopathy is unlikely (e.g. young age) and/or ruled out with appropriate imaging, alternative etiologies of compressive myelopathy may need to be investigated:

- Malignant infiltration of vertebral body or malignant mass. Consider if:
  - Known primary tumor.
  - Paraproteinemia (risk of multiple myeloma).
- Infectious process (vertebral infiltration or epidural abscess). Consider if:
  - Subacute onset.
  - Fever, weight loss, endocarditis (septicemia seeding bone).
  - Superficial wound at area of suspected compression.
  - Local pain.
  - Recent spinal intervention (spinal surgery, spinal anesthesia, lumbar puncture [LP]).
- Epidural hematoma. Consider if:
  - Acute onset.
  - Recent trauma or intervention (e.g. LP).
  - Known primary tumor (epidural metastases).
  - Bleeding diathesis.
  - Anticoagulant therapy.
  - Arteritis.
  - Known spinal AVM.

Additional investigations to consider based on the above differential diagnosis:

- Spinal angiogram for vascular malformation.
- Serology for arteritis (e.g. antinuclear antibody titer).
- Coagulation profile.
- Erythrocyte sedimentation rate (ESR) for infectious etiologies.
- Blood cultures.
- Cerebrospinal fluid (CSF):
  - Normal in spondylitic myelopathy, but severe obstruction of CSF flow may yield mildly elevated protein.
  - Pleocytosis and elevated protein in epidural abscess.
  - No blood or xanthochromia is present in epidural hematoma unless there is involvement of the subarachnoid space.

INTRAMEDULLARY SPINAL CORD LESIONS (INTRINSIC MYELOPATHY)

Intramedullary causes of spinal cord dysfunction must be considered when extrinsic, or compressive, causes of myelopathy are excluded.

INFLAMMATORY MYELOPATHY (e.g. MYELITIS)

Definition and epidemiology

This category of diseases includes autoimmune or non-infectious etiologies of myelopathies. They range from common (1 million cases of multiple sclerosis [MS] worldwide) to uncommon (1–3% of patients with systemic lupus erythematosus [SLE]) or rare (single-digit case reports of paraneoplastic myelopathy associated with CRMP-5 antibodies).

Etiology and pathophysiology

- MS (see Chapter 12).
- Clinically isolated syndrome (CIS) (as precursor to MS).
- Neuromyelitis optica (NMO).
- Acute disseminated encephalomyelitis (ADEM):
  - May be preceded by systemic viral infection or vaccine, but not required.
  - More common in children (mean age 5–8 years).
- Inflammatory disorders:
  - SLE.
  - Sjögren's syndrome.
  - Behçet's disease.
  - Mixed connective tissue disease (MCTD).
  - Scleroderma.
  - Neurosarcoidosis.
  - Idiopathic transverse myelitis.

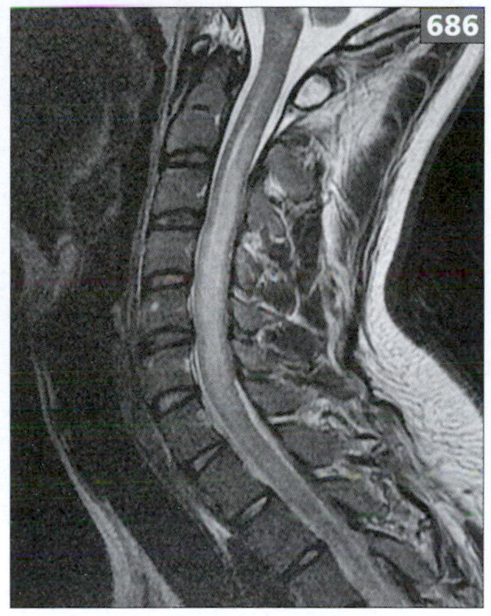
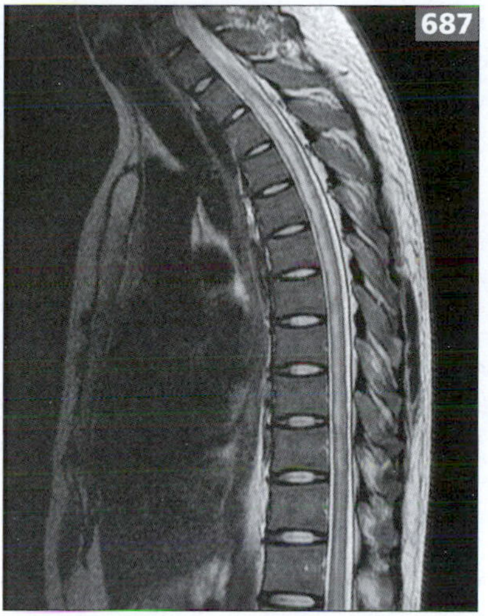

686, 687 Acute transverse myelitis. T2-weighted MRI of the cervical (686) and thoracic (687) spinal cord with longitudinally extensive signal hyperintensity and cord swelling. The patient developed a spinal cord syndrome shortly after a self-limited viral illness.

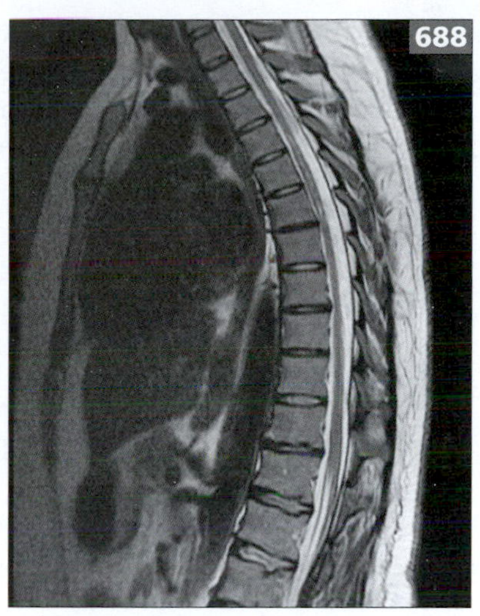

688 Neuromyelitis optica. T2-weighted MRI of the thoracic spinal cord with multifocal hyperintensity within the cord extending across multiple vertebral levels.

- Paraneoplastic myelitis: stiff person syndrome.
- Infectious disorders:
  - Neurosyphilis.
  - HTLV-1 associated myelopathy/tropical spastic paraparesis.
  - Human immunodeficiency virus (HIV)-associated myelopathy.
- Heredodegenerative disorders:
  - Hereditary spastic paraparesis.
  - ALS.

Clinical features

While inflammatory myelopathy can theoretically present with any of the previously described clinical myelopathy syndromes, most common presentations are:

- Brown–Sequard hemicord syndrome.
- Transverse myelopathy.
- Central myelopathy.
- Stiff person syndrome: an unusual presentation of spinal cord inflammation. It is a disorder of motor pathway inhibition which can be seen as an isolated autoimmune entity or as a paraneoplastic syndrome.

Onset of symptoms can range from days to 1 week, although myelopathy associated with systemic disease may have more indolent presentations. Symptoms may range from pure sensory to pure motor (weakness and/or spasticity). Bowel and/or bladder dysfunction is an important clue to localization but is not specific to inflammatory etiology.

Investigations

Neurologic examination should focus on confirmation of localization to the spinal cord. Special attention may be needed to reveal the systemic nature of the etiology[2]:

- SLE: rash, photosensitivity, arthritis, other neurologic dysfunction (e.g. seizures, encephalopathy).
- Sjögren's syndrome: dry eyes or mouth (sicca syndrome).
- MCTD: distal edema, synovitis, Raynaud's phenomenon.
- Scleroderma: skin changes, sclerodactyly, pulmonary fibrosis, digital pitting.
- Neurosarcoidosis: pulmonary or skin changes (may not be evidence of systemic sarcoidosis).
- Behçet's disease: recurrent oral and genital ulcers, uveitis, skin lesions.

Imaging

MRI spine (686–688) is the imaging modality of choice. MRI shows focal cord swelling with one or more areas of increased T2 signal, possible contrast enhancement. MRI may be normal, and mild MRI changes may not correlate with clinical severity.

MRI brain, including orbits, should be obtained in all cases to evaluate more widespread central nervous system (CNS) inflammatory diseases (e.g. MS, NMO, ADEM). Although the original definition of NMO required an absence of brain lesions, patients positive for NMO antibodies are now known to exhibit a spectrum of brain involvement based on MRI, ranging from a couple of small, scattered, white matter abnormalities to more numerous and diffuse lesions[3]. Large, asymmetric and/or poorly defined lesions on T2 or fluid attenuated inversion recovery (FLAIR) sequences, with post-contrast enhancement, point to ADEM with involvement of both gray and white matter.

Blood and CSF

- CSF analysis:
  - Cell count – may be normal or pleocytosis (typically lymphocytic predominant).
  - Elevated protein, especially in the setting of cord edema and CSF block.
  - CSF angiotensin-converting enzyme (ACE) level for suspected neurosarcoidosis.
- Specific serum studies (as directed by clinical presentation and physical examination findings):
  - Rheumatologic work-up:
    - Antinuclear antibodies, anti-DNA antibodies, anti-Smith antibodies, Sjögren's antibodies (SS-A, SS-B), rheumatoid factor, anti-U1 RNP antibodies, ESR.
  - ACE: sarcoidosis.
  - NMO antibody to aquaporin-4 for NMO.
  - Paraneoplastic antibodies:
    - Amphiphysin.
    - CRMP-5.
    - Glutamic acid decarboxylase (GAD) (stiff person syndrome: can be positive in either paraneoplastic or primary autoimmune presentations).

Other diagnostic testing

- Chest imaging, gallium scan, perihilar lymph node biopsy: sarcoidosis.
- Skin biopsy: SLE, Behçet's disease.
- Ophthalmologic evaluation: Sjögren's syndrome, Behçet's disease, sarcoidosis.
- Salivary gland biopsy: Sjögren's syndrome.

Treatment

The majority of treatments are directed at immunomodulation, with few clear guidelines to dictate one modality over another. Acute therapies can be expected to yield positive results (stop progression of symptoms with or without improvement in presenting syndrome) within days to weeks. Chronic therapies may be indicated for certain disorders for months to years. (See Chapter 12 for a full discussion of the treatment of MS and CIS.)
Acute therapies include:

- Corticosteroids (IV methylprednisolone, dosage varies).
- Intravenous immune globulin (IVIG).
- Plasmapheresis (PLEX).

Chronic or maintenance therapies include:

- Corticosteroids.
- Azathioprine.
- Mycophenolate.
- Cyclosporine.
- Cyclophosphamide.
- Monoclonal antibodies (e.g. rituximab).

Prognosis

Depends on the underlying etiology, and ranges from complete remission (most cases of ADEM) to irreversible or recurrent deficit. Successful immunomodulation may lead to gradual recovery from the initial presentation, as well as prevention of recurrence in the spinal cord and elsewhere in the nervous system.

INFECTIOUS MYELOPATHY

Definition and epidemiology

Inflammation of the spinal cord due to bacterial, viral or fungal pathogens. Epidemiology varies, depending on the infectious agent in question. The most common infection of the spinal cord is viral, with chronic infection more prevalent than acute viral infection.

Etiology and pathophysiology

Bacterial myelitis

This is uncommon, and causative pathogens include:

- *Treponema pallidum* (syphilis):
  - Spinal cord involvement of neurosyphilis (late stage of infection): tabes dorsalis.
  - Progressive posterior column dysfunction causes sensory ataxia.
  - Spinothalamic and autonomic functions are also impaired.
  - Ophthalmologic findings are common (Argyll Robertson pupil).
  - Complication: Charcot's (neurogenic) arthropathy.
- *Borrelia burgdorferi* (Lyme disease).
- *Mycobacterium tuberculosis.*
- *Mycoplasma pneumoniae* (more often seen in pediatric populations).
- *Escherichia coli, Staphylococcus aureus, Streptococcus* spp.:
  - Predisposing risk factor – neuro-ectodermal pathology in children. Typically present as intramedullary abscess.

There have been single case reports in the literature involving:

- *Campylobacter jejuni.*
- *Tropheryma whipplei* (Whipple's disease).
- *Orientia tsutsugamushi* (scrub typhus).

Diagnosis
- Isolation of causative bacteria.
- Neurosyphilis:
  - CSF pleocytosis.
  - Positive CSF Venereal Disease Research Laboratory test (VDRL): low sensitivity, false positive when CSF is contaminated by blood.
  - Positive serum fluorescent treponemal antibody (FTA): use as a confirmatory test after positive VDRL or in HIV-positive patients. High sensitivity, positive despite treatment in most patients, and risk of false-positive results (including pregnancy, lupus, other treponemal infections).

Viral acute myelitis
- A wide variety of viruses are associated with acute myelitis (*Table 113*).
- Part of clinicopathologic spectrum of encephalomyelitis.
- Most pathogens are seasonal (warm months) and vector-borne (arthropods: arboviruses).
- Two distinct phenotypes:
  - Acute transverse myelitis:
    - Intramedullary infection and associated inflammation.
    - Not specific to cord tracts or cell types.
    - Acute onset of fever with any combination of neurologic deficits attributable to the spinal cord (sensory disturbance, autonomic dysfunction, weakness with hyper- or hyporeflexia (the latter reflecting either anterior horn involvement or spinal shock).
  - Acute flaccid paralysis:
    - Viral affinity for anterior horn cell (poliovirus model).
    - Prodromal illness with fever and mental status changes.
    - Acute onset of pure LMN pattern of weakness in one or more limbs without sensory or autonomic dysfunction.

TABLE 113 **VIRUSES CAUSING ACUTE MYELITIS**

Pathogen	Associated clinical findings
HERPESVIRUSES	Acute transverse myelitis more common
Herpes simplex virus-2	
Varicella zoster virus	Prodromal (weeks) dermatomal rash
Cytomegalovirus	Immunosuppressed patient
Human herpesvirus 6 and 7	
Epstein–Barr virus	Prodromal pharyngitis with mononucleosis
FLAVIVIRUSES Dengue virus Japanese encephalitis virus Tick-borne encephalitis virus West Nile virus	Acute flaccid myelitis more common
ORTHOMYXOVIRUSES Influenza A virus	Including H1N1 (swine) strain
PARAMYXOVIRUSES	
Measles virus	Rash (skin and oral mucosa)
Mumps virus	Parotitis
PICORNAVIRUSES	Acute flaccid myelitis more common
Coxsackieviruses A and B	Herpangina, cardiac involvement
Echoviruses	Hepatic and cardiac involvement
Enterovirus-70 and -71	Prodromal hand/foot/ mouth vesicular rash
Hepatitis A virus	Clinical hepatitis
Poliovirus types 1, 2, and 3	

Investigations and diagnosis

MRI spine

- Acute transvere myelitis:
  - T2 signal change with or without enhancement, possible cord swelling associated with signal change, typically covering more than one spinal level.
- Acute flaccid paralysis:
  - May be normal or may find signal changes and/or enhancement in the anterior horns and ventral nerve roots (**689**).

MRI brain

This is recommended to identify encephalomyelitis, and may assist with identification of the virus as well as aid supportive care and prognosis.

CSF

- Lymphocytic predominant pleocytosis, elevated protein: nonspecific result.
- Polymerase chain reaction (PCR)/RT-PCR for specific suspected virus(es): highest yield if performed within days of clinical presentation.
- CSF immunoglobulin (Ig) M antibody testing for specific virus(es): indicates intrathecal antibody production.
- Serial serum antibody titers (acute and convalescent phases) can support suspected infection.

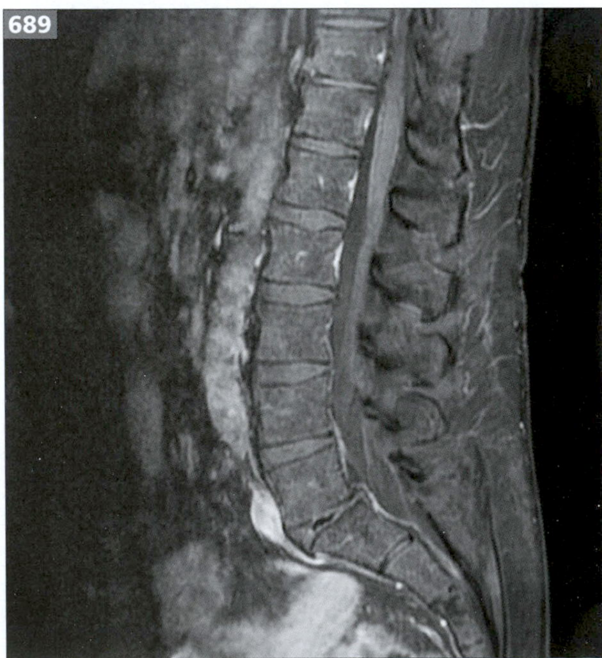

689 T1-weighted MRI with contrast, showing diffuse enhancement of the conus medullaris secondary to infection with West Nile virus.

Electromyography

In acute flaccid paralysis, electromyography (EMG) can document anterior horn cell involvement. If performed serially after acute illness, it may inform prognosis for recovery of strength.

Treatment

- Antiviral agents:
  - Herpesviruses:
    - Acyclovir (and prodrug, valacyclovir): most effective against herpes simplex virus and varicella zoster virus.
    - Gancyclovir and/or foscarnet: for cytomegalovirus infection.
  - Nonherpesvirus infections: supportive care, may involve mechanical ventilation due to associated encephalitis and/or neuromuscular respiratory failure in acute flaccid paralysis.

Prognosis

For both presentations of acute viral myelitis, fatal infection is rare, unless associated with more widespread neurologic deficit (encephalomyelitis) or multi-organ involvement.

- Acute transverse myelitis: guarded with risk of permanent disability.
- Acute flaccid paralysis: permanent disability likely with variable improvement over first 1–2 years after onset.

Viral chronic myelitis

Epidemiology and etiology

Human T-lymphotropic virus (HTLV-1)

- 20–40 million people are infected worldwide.
- Endemic areas occur in the Caribbean, Japan, Central and South American, Middle East, parts of Asia, and Africa.
- Approximately 3% of symptomatic HTLV-infected individuals develop clinical syndrome of HTLV-associated myelopathy/tropical spastic paraparesis (HAM/TSP); given the widespread prevalence of infection, this translates into as many as 1 million cases of HAM/TSP worldwide.
- Based on statistics of countries that screen for HTLV, the lifetime risk of developing myelopathy due to the HTLV infection ranges from less than 1% to as high as 10%, depending on the geographic origins of the individual.

HTLV is transmitted via breast milk (vertical transmission), sexual contact, and contaminated blood products. The virus directly promotes an inflammatory response in the CNS. There is possible molecular mimicry leading to secondary autoimmune-mediated tissue damage. Clinical features include:

- Indolent spastic weakness.
- Transverse myelopathy syndrome with lower extremity sensory loss (both dorsal columns and spinothalamic tracts), prominent bowel/bladder dysfunction.
- Progression over years:
  - Thoracic spine is most commonly affected.
  - First few years of clinical symptoms can be more rapidly progressive with a plateau or gradual progression in subsequent years.

There are guidelines for the diagnosis of HTLV:

- MRI spinal cord may show edema in early disease with eventual thinning (atrophy) most commonly seen in thoracic cord.
- MRI brain may show white matter hyperintensities on T2 or FLAIR sequences in subcortical regions.
- CSF: pleocytosis (mild–moderate) and elevated protein: can regress later in the disease course.
- Testing specific to HTLV-1 virus in the combinations below can increase specificity and sensitivity of the diagnosis:
  - Serum HTLV-1 antibodies.
  - Oligoclonal IgG bands in the CSF.
  - PCR for HTLV-1 deoxyribonucleic acid (DNA) in the CSF.
  - Evidence of intrathecal HTLV-1 antibody production.

The serum viral load and/or ratio of CSF to serum viral load can be checked. When the ratio is high, this supports the diagnosis in suspected cases.

No proven therapy is recommended, but limited uncontrolled reports suggest a possible role for a variety of immunomodulating agents (corticosteroids, plasmapheresis, IVIG, daclizumab, interferon alpha and beta). Attenuation of long-term disability remains elusive and determination of optimal effective dosages and treatment regimes will require further research. Antiretroviral agents have not been shown to be beneficial.

Once symptomatic, the course is slowly progressive over years to decades. Most patients ultimately require assistance to ambulate.

HIV

There are two clinical entities, vacuolar myelopathy and HIV-associated myelitis[4]. Vacuolar myelopathy is the most common primary HIV-related spinal cord syndrome. It is still a relatively rare clinical scenario, although autopsy studies indicated a common pathologic process within the cord prior to the highly-active antiretroviral therapy (HAART) era.

The pathology mimics subacute combined degeneration (SCD) seen in B12 deficiency:

- Posterior and lateral columns with vacuolar changes.
- No direct infection of neural tissues with HIV.
- Sparse macrophage infiltrate.

Clinical features follow from the tracts affected: spastic paraplegia with sensory loss leading to ataxia as well as bladder dysfunction. Concomitant HIV-associated neurologic disorders include neuropathy and dementia.

Diagnosis is largely of exclusion. The MRI is unremarkable and CD4 count and HIV viral load (serum or CSF) do not correlate with disease presence or severity. S-adenosyl-methionine (SAM) levels are low in serum and CSF, analogous to B12-deficiency myelopathy.

Differential diagnosis includes:

- HTLV-1 myelopathy.
- Metabolic myelopathy (vitamin B12 deficiency, copper deficiency, nitrous oxide [NO] exposure).
- Syphilis.
- Cytomegalovirus myeloradiculopathy.

Treatment of HIV does not impact on the clinical syndrome associated with vacuolar myelopathy. L-methionine supplementation was found effective in a small, open trial, but a follow-up randomized, blinded study failed to find benefit.

HIV-associated myelitis is a rare acute inflammatory myelopathy akin to those discussed above (e.g. ADEM, CIS, and so on).

Fungal myelitis

Intramedullary fungal infection is extremely rare:

- Histoplasmosis.
- Aspergillosis.
- Cryptococcal granuloma in the cord (rare case reports).

METABOLIC AND TOXIC MYELOPATHIES

Definition

Clinical and pathologic entity caused by toxic exposure or metabolic derangement resultant from:

- Deficiency of vitamin B12 (i.e. cobalamin), folate, copper.
- Exposure to NO.
- Deficiency of Vitamin E (i.e. alpha-tocopherol).

Subacute combined degeneration

Etiology and pathophysiology

Subacute combined degeneration (SCD) may occur due to deficiency of vitamin B12, folate, or copper[5].

SAM is used for methylation in the nervous system and is essential for, among other things, the production of myelin basic protein. SAM is produced from methionine by methionine synthetase, which requires vitamin B12 and folate as co-factors. The exact mechanism by which the co-factor deficiency produces neuropathologic changes in myelinated fibers has not been definitively determined.

In cases of NO exposure, conversion of homocysteine to methionine is disrupted, mimicking 'true' vitamin B12 deficiency. Chronic exposure to NO (e.g. recreational abuse) can lead to myelopathy, but acute exposure, typically in setting of surgical anesthesia, can precipitate SCD in patients with previously unrecognized pre-exposure deficiencies of vitamin B12.

Copper acts as a required co-factor of innumerable biochemical processes in the human body. The exact contribution of copper to the pathogenesis of SCD remains incompletely elucidated, but the methylation pathway outlined above requires both copper and vitamin B12. Low levels may be caused by excessive exposure to zinc (supplementation, denture creams) or by malabsorption (e.g. gastric bypass surgery).

Clinical features

- Subacute or chronic progressive spastic weakness with sensory ataxia.
- Typically starts with distal extremity parasthesias, but gait abnormalities herald a central process.
- Simultaneous peripheral neuropathy common with all etiologies. Severe neuropathy may lead to depressed deep tendon reflexes. Thus, hypo- or areflexia with bilateral Babinski reflexes is the classical presentation of SCD.
- Cognitive dysfunction: subtle memory or executive dysfunction or frank dementia is possible but not described in copper deficiency.
- Optic neuropathy is described in all etiologies.

Diagnosis

- MRI spine:
  - Non-enhancing T2W signal changes in cervical and/or upper thoracic cord are most common, but contrast enhancement and focal cord swelling have both been described.
  - Axial images may show sparing of the anterior cord.
- Serum:
  - Vitamin B12 level:
    - Low in primary deficiency as well in copper deficiency.
    - Accuracy of screen for total level limited by protein binding.
    - Use with caution in pregnancy, use of oral contraceptives, or hepatic dysfunction.
    - At lower levels of normal, consider adjunctive use of fasting homocysteine and methylmalonic acid levels, which should be elevated in the setting of B12 deficiency, but may also be elevated in unrelated medical conditions (hypothyroidism, renal disease).
    - If suspecting pernicious anemia as the underlying etiology of B12 deficiency, check antibodies against parietal cells and intrinsic factor.
  - Copper:
    - Low (undetectable in some) in all patients with copper deficiency myelopathy.
    - Folate deficiency may be the primary etiology independent of other vitamins and minerals.
    - Zinc is elevated in some cases of copper deficiency.
    - Iron elevation may be associated with copper deficiency.
  - Cell counts:
    - Megaloblastic anemia is seen in vitamin B12 and copper deficiency.
    - Leukopenia is also common in copper deficiency and may precede the neurologic manifestations.
- EMG: axonal sensorimotor neuropathy may be found on nerve conduction studies in all etiologies.

Pathology

Posterior and lateral columns of the spinal cord (mediating functions of discriminating touch and motor control, respectively) are preferentially involved. Predominantly there is axonal damage with some areas of demyelination and spongiform (vacuolar) changes. SCD most often affects cervical and thoracic segments.

Treatment and prognosis

- Replacement of deficient element or cofactor (e.g. vitamin B12 in the case of NO toxicity).
- Goal of therapy is prevention of progressive neurologic deficit.
- Expectation for improvement of existing deficit is variable: better outcome in younger patients with less severe disease at onset of treatment.
- MRI abnormalities are reversible with treatment.

Vitamin E deficiency

Etiology and pathophysiology

Deficiency may be acquired (malabsorption syndromes) or genetic (defects causing impaired vitamin E absorption or transport). Vitamin E is a cellular protectant, scavenging free radicals and preventing oxidative damage. Deficiency of this vitamin leads to demyelinating changes both within the spinal cord and in the peripheral nerves.

Clinical features

- Rarely reported to cause isolated myelopathic syndrome; primarily associated with spinocerebellar syndrome akin to Freidreich's ataxia (see Chapter 14).
- Associated symptoms may include neuropathy, ocular dysmotility, retinopathy, and ataxia.
- Axonopathy occurs due to deficiency of vitamin E with loss of myelinated fibers in peripheral nerves, spinal cord, and brainstem.

VASCULAR MYELOPATHIES

Definition and epidemiology

Infarction of the spinal cord caused by arterial occlusion, or less often, venous occlusion.

- 10 in 100,000 or 5–8% of all acute myelopathies.
- Age: any age; mean 59 years.

Pathophysiology

The blood supply to the spinal cord is illustrated in **690**.

Anterior spinal artery

The gray and inner white matter of the anterior two-thirds of the spinal cord (anterior and lateral columns on either side) receives blood supply via the left and right sulcocommissural arterial branches of the anterior spinal artery, which originates in its most rostral portion from the union of paired branches of the vertebral arteries at the ventral surface of the medulla oblongata and passes down the anterior surface of the cord in the midline, narrowing near the upper fourth thoracic segment.

Along its discontinuous course below T4, it receives segmental input from six to nine intercostal radicular arteries arising from the aorta. The major radicular artery, the great ventral radicular artery or artery of Adamkiewicz, arises usually on the left, variably from T9 to T12, or less commonly anywhere from T5 to L2, and supplies the lumbar cord and conus medullaris. At the lumbosacral level, radicular arteries are derived from larger regional vessels, the largest of which enters the intervertebral foramen at L2 to form the lowermost portion of the anterior spinal artery (the terminal artery) which runs along the filum terminale.

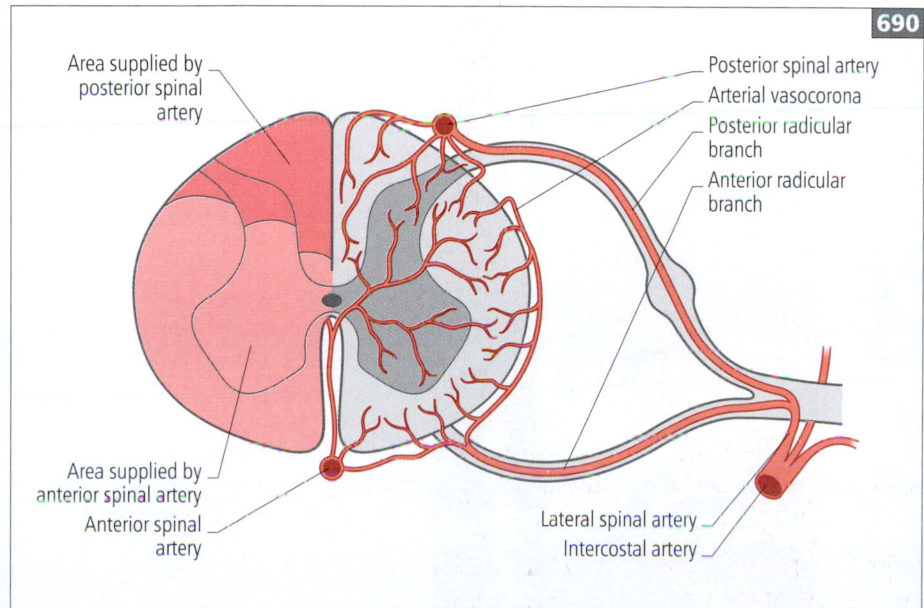

690 Blood supply to the spinal cord.

Posterior spinal arteries

The posterior one-third of the spinal cord (posterior white columns and part of the posterior gray columns) receives its blood supply from the posterior spinal arteries which are paired and considerably smaller than the anterior spinal artery. They receive branches from the posterolateral plexus at various levels.

The surface of the spinal cord is richly interwoven with circumflex anastamoses arising from the anterior and posterior spinal arteries. A relative hypovascularity exists in the mid thoracic region from about T4 to T8, which is the most vulnerable part of the spinal cord to ischemia. Venous drainage occurs via the median posterior and the anterior spinal veins. The lack of venous valves may permit retrograde spreading of abdominal infectious and malignant processes to the spinal cord.

Etiology

- Embolism:
  - Embolism from the heart.
  - Atherothromboembolism from the aorta or origin of the intercostal and lumbar arteries.
  - Air embolism: nitrogen bubbles lodge in spinal veins (decompression sickness).
  - Fibrocartilaginous embolism from intervertebral disc rupture.
  - Therapeutic renal artery embolization.
- Primary vascular disease (**691, 692**):
  - Atherosclerosis and atherothrombosis.
  - Aortic dissection or rupture.
  - Thoracic or abdominal aortic aneurysm.
  - Aortic instrumentation (radiologic or surgical).
  - Descending aortic aneurysm.
  - Intra-aortic balloon pump counterpulsation.
  - Arteritis (syphilis, sarcoidosis, tuberculosis, polyarteritis nodosa, and other connective tissue disease, drugs: cocaine, amphetamine) (**693**).
  - Thoracoplasty.
  - Pneumonectomy.
  - Porto-caval shunt placement.
  - Radicular artery ligation.
  - AVM of the spinal arteries (**694**).
- Venous thrombophlebitis.
- Extradural process:
  - Trauma to the spine.
  - Acute compression of the spinal cord:
    - Vertebral body and disc disease.
    - Extradural masses: hematoma, abscess, tumor, fat (**695**).
    - Subdural masses.
  - Infection within the spine.
- Hematologic:
  - Sickle cell disease.
  - Procoagulant states: thrombocytosis, malignancy.
- Hypoxic–ischemic process:
  - Respiratory or cardiac arrest.
  - Severe hypotension.
  - Severe anemia.
- Cryptogenic (20–50%, depending on series reported).

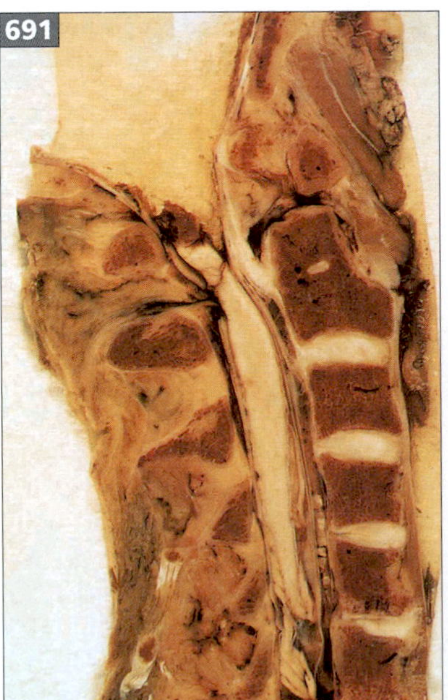

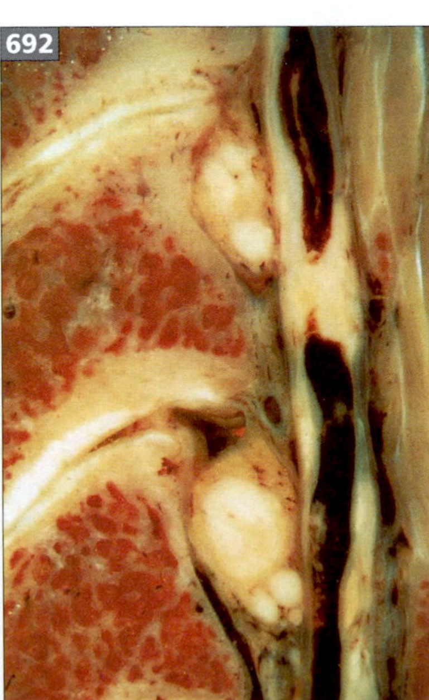

691, 692 Sagittal section of the spine at autopsy, showing dissection of the vertebral artery with secondary vertebral artery thrombosis.

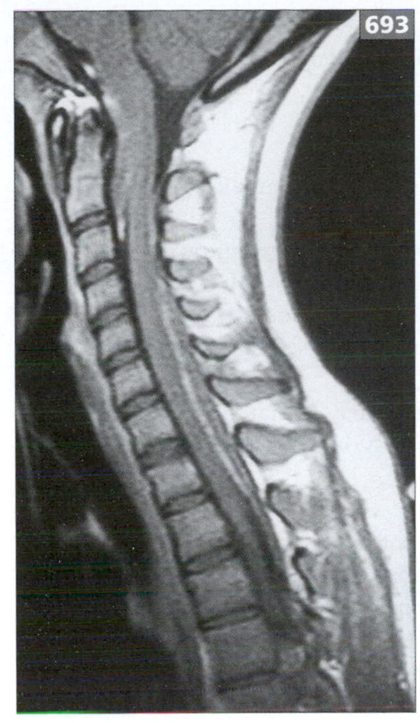

693 MRI cervical and upper thoracic spine, T1W image, sagittal plane, showing a linear streak of high intensity due to hemorrhage in the spinal subarachnoid space, in a patient with arteritis due to Churg–Strauss syndrome (allergic angiitis and granulomatosis).

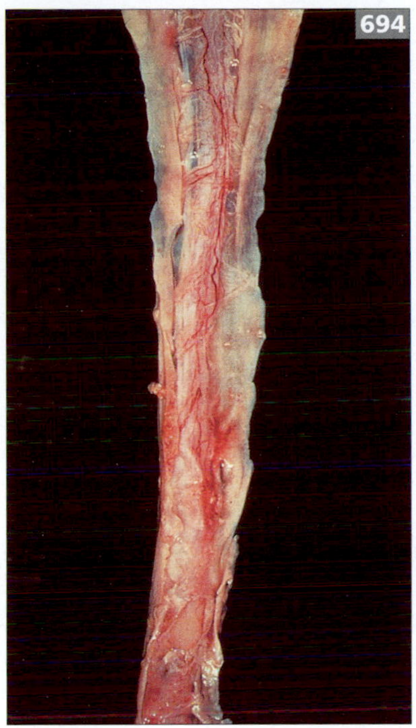

694 Autopsy specimen of a spinal cord arteriovenous malformation.

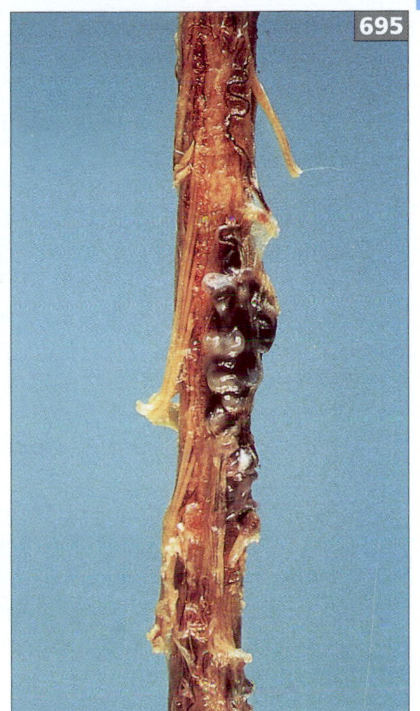

695 Autopsy specimen of spinal cord, showing an epidural spinal arteriovenous malformation (a common cause of spinal epidural hematoma), containing dark clotted blood. *Courtesy of Professor BA Kakulas, Royal Perth Hospital, Western Australia.*

Clinical features

- Anterior spinal artery syndrome
  - Weakness below the level of the lesion.
  - Flaccid/areflexic acutely, progressing to spastic weakness:
    - Sensory loss below the level of the lesion.
    - Loss of pain, temperature, light touch.
    - Preserved discriminating touch, vibration, proprioception.
  - Hyperacute onset (minutes/hours).
- Sulcocommissural artery syndrome: ipsilateral paralysis and contralateral loss of pain and temperature sensation below the level of the lesion.
- Posterior spinal artery syndrome:
  - Rare.
  - Dorsal column (discriminating touch) impairment with sparing of strength (corticospinal tracts), pain/temperature sensation (spinothalamic tracts), and deep tendon reflexes (anterior horn cells unaffected).
- Spinal venous infarction syndrome (part of Foix–Alajouanine syndrome of congestive myelopathy due to spinal dural ateriovenous fistula [AVM]):
  - Subacute onset.
  - Chronic progressive myelopathy due to ischemia (steal phenomenon), venous congestion, focal compression due to vascular malformation.
  - Men >50 years.
  - Months to years of progressive weakness, sensory loss, pain in the legs due to the typical location in the thoracic spinal cord.
  - Intermittent worsening triggered by exertion, trauma and so on.
- Spinal transient ischemic attacks:
  - Painless paraparesis or quadriparesis without loss of consciousness.
  - Sporadic, or precipitated by postural changes in patients with foramenal stenosis during cervical or lumbar extension, which maximally compromises the intervertebral foramina through which pass spinal radicular arteries.

Differential diagnosis

- Acute cord compression:
  - Intervertebral disc prolapse.
  - Vertebral body collapse/fracture (spinal angulation: tuberculosis, tumor).
  - Trauma.
  - Epidural hemorrhage.
- Intramedullary:
  - Hemorrhage.
  - Inflammatory or infectious myelopathy.

Investigations

- MRI spine:
  - To be performed urgently to rule out spinal cord compression.
  - When repeated after several days, MRI is more likely to reveal focal cord swelling, and may reveal increased signal in the cord on T2 (**696, 697**), and gadolinium enhancement of the lesion on T1, a similar appearance to that of inflammatory transverse myelitis.
  - Diffusion-weighted MRI spine may be helpful, although technical limitations exist due to spinal cord size and location.
  - Hemorrhage may be identified by the typical changes (see hemorrhagic brain lesions section).
  - If performed months or years later, MRI shows focal cord atrophy.
  - MRI may be nondiagnostic in >50% of cases of suspected spinal cord infarct.
- CSF:
  - Cells: normal or moderate leukocytosis (<100 mononuclear cells/cm^3).
  - Protein: mild elevation (<1 g/l [100 mg/dl]).
- Other:
  - Myelography: prone and supine, if an AVM is suspected.
  - Spinal arteriography: if myelogram suggests an AVM.
  - Somatosensory evoked potentials: abnormal only if the double perfused posterior columns are infarcted.
  - EMG: abnormal only if infarction involves anterior horn cells or nerve roots.

Pathology

- Infarction of the anterior two-thirds of the spinal cord with occlusion of the anterior spinal artery or a spinal radicular artery.
- Infarction of one dorsal column with unilateral posterior spinal artery occlusion.
- Ischemic or hemorrhagic infarction with venous occlusion.

Treatment

- Treat the underlying cause, if possible, including vascular risk factors.
- Investigate for, and treat, embolic sources as appropriate.
- Embolization or excision of vascular malformations should be considered.

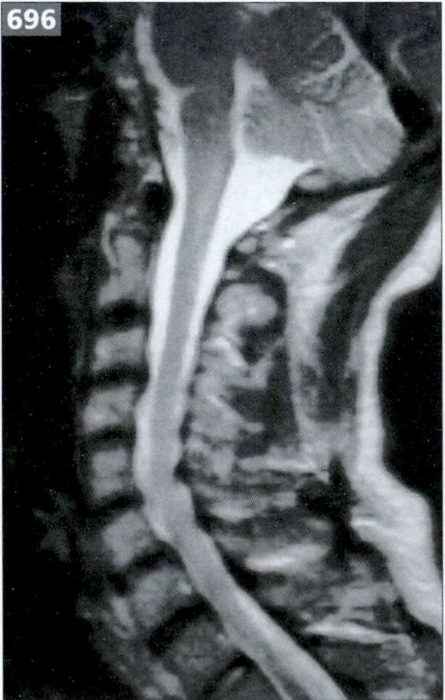

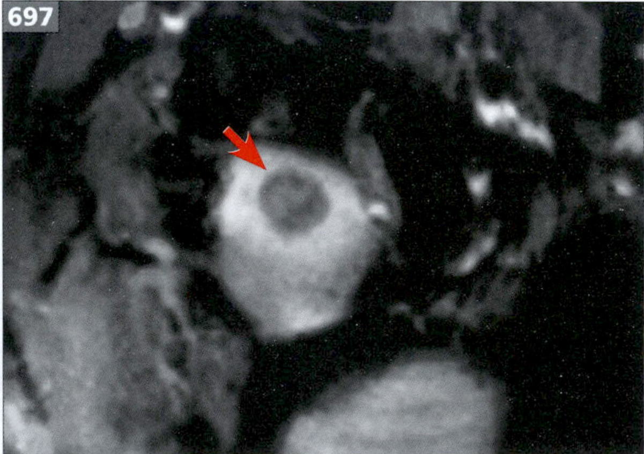

696, 697 T2W sagittal (696) and T2W axial (697) MRI of the cervical spine in a patient with sudden onset of right-sided neck pain followed by a lateral medullary syndrome, showing an infarct in the upper cervical cord/lower medulla. The right vertebral artery was partially occluded, thought to be dissected. Note the increased signal in the upper right side of the cord (arrow).

- Symptomatic control of pain, paresthesia, depression, and autonomic and bladder dysfunction.
- Avoid complications of immobility: regular turning to avoid pressure sores, graduated compression stockings, aspirin or subcutaneous heparin to prevent deep venous thrombosis, and regular bladder emptying.
- Rehabilitation: physiotherapy, occupational therapy, psychologic support, social work.

Prognosis[6]

- Improvement: 25–50%: greater chance for recovery if there is preservation of some degree of neurologic function below the level of the lesion.
- No improvement: 50%: predictors include a more severe deficit at onset, less recovery of motor function at 1 month.
- Death: uncommon (<15%).

STRUCTURAL MYELOPATHIES

SYRINGOMYELIA

Definition

A syringomelia is a fluid-filled cavity within the spinal cord tissue. Syringobulbia is a fluid-filled cavity within the brainstem. A dilation of the central spinal canal alone is termed hydromyelia.

Classification

- Type I: syringomyelia with obstruction of the foramen magnum and with dilation of the central spinal canal. May be with Chiari I malformation (congenital herniation of the cerebellum and brainstem into the foramen magnum) or with another lesion causing obstruction of the foramen magnum.
- Type II: idiopathic syringomyelia (no obstruction of the foramen magnum).
- Type III: acquired syringomyelia with associated disorders:
    - Spinal cord tumor (intramedullary most common).
    - Traumatic myelopathy.
    - Spinal arachnoiditis and pachymeningitis.
    - Myelomalacia secondary to previous cord injury (compression, infarct, inflammation, and so on).
- Type IV: pure dilation of the central canal (hydromyelia), may be associated with hydrocephalus.

Epidemiology

Variable reports, 4–8 cases per 100,000. The majority of patients with syringomyelia have Chiari malformation and about one-half of all patients with Chiari I malformations have concomitant syringomyelia. This association is presumed due to disruption of CSF hemodynamics.

Etiology and pathophysiology[7]

The exact mechanism of origin and maintenance of fluid in the cavity is elusive. Conventional thinking is that the CSF fills the cavity from the subarachnoid space. However, there are inconsistencies with this theory, in that the syrinx is at a higher pressure than surrounding tissue, implying the fluid is moving up a pressure gradient. Fluid pushing on an empty cavity will compress, rather than fill, that cavity.

Emerging theories include that there is increased CSF pulse pressure, causing increased CSF pressure within the spinal cord tissue relative to the surrounding CSF pressure in the subarachnoid space; fluid within the syrinx is made up of extracellular fluid, not CSF; and the increase in cytosolic pressure may be due to partial or complete obstruction of subarachnoid CSF flow in the neighboring subarachnoid space (e.g. from Chiari or other structural abnormality at the foramen magnum).

Clinical features

The classic presentation is of a central cord syndrome. Due to the propensity for cervical segments, a distinctive 'shawl' distribution of sensory findings is reported: numbness and painful parasthesias over the shoulders and upper extremities. Pain is prominent and can also mimic radiculopathy. Symptoms are transiently exacerbated by Valsalva maneuvers (coughing, sneezing, and so on).

Differential diagnosis

- Classes of disease which can mimic syringomyelia:
    - Inflammatory myelopathy.
    - Chronic infectious myelopathy.
    - Heredodegenerative myelopathies (hereditary spastic paraparesis, ALS, and so on).
    - With predominantly LMN findings:
        - Radiculopathy.
        - Brachial plexopathy.
- Classes of disease commonly associated with syrinx: see disorders listed above under Type III (acquired syringomyelia).
    - Other known associations: spinal dysraphisms, diastematomyelia ('split cord'), tethered cord.

Investigations and diagnosis

- MRI: imaging modality of choice (698, 699). Brainstem, cervical, thoracic and lumbosacral spinal segments should be included to investigate common etiologies (tumors, Chiari malformation, and so on).
- CT myelography: not as sensitive as MRI, but able to detect some syringes.

Treatment and prognosis

Surgical treatment is targeted at cause of partial or complete obstruction of CSF flow (e.g. Chiari malformation, tumor, herniated disc). When the obstruction is unclear, or is diffuse rather than a focal surgical target, syrinx drainage can be performed but requires multiple surgeries and outcomes are more modest (stabilization only, some progression).

Symptomatic treatment of spasticity and neuropathic pain is essential, but does not preclude the need for neurosurgical assessment, once a syrinx is diagnosed, as progressive disability is common in nonsurgically-treated patients.

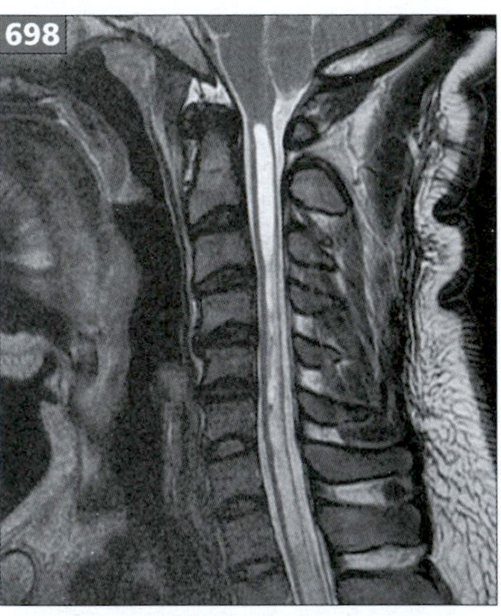

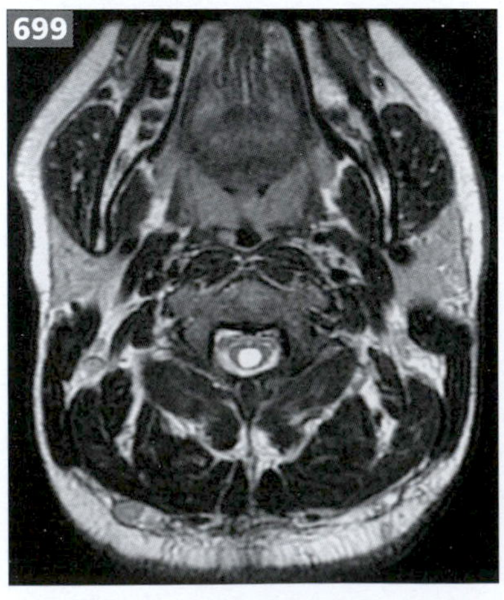

698, 699 Chiari I malformation with cervical syringomyelia. Sagittal (698) and axial (699) T2-weighted MRI of the brainstem and cervical spine. Cerebellar tonsillar herniation below with foramen magnum is associated here with a syrinx in the cervical spinal cord. On axial images, the normal spinal cord tissue is nearly obliterated by the expansive fluid-filled cavity.

HEREDITARY MYELOPATHIES

HEREDITARY SPASTIC PARAPLEGIA

Definition and epidemiology

A group of clinically and genetically diverse disorders characterized by progressive lower limb spasticity and weakness. Hereditary spastic paraparesis (HSP) is also known as familial spastic paraparesis and Strumpell–Lorrain syndrome. The term HSP is more precise because it indicates the genetic basis of this group of disorders; conditions that occur in families (familial) are not necessarily inherited (genetic).

- Uncommon (3–10 cases per 100,000 in Europe).
- Age: age at onset can be difficult to date precisely because incipient disease can go unnoticed unless a clinical examination is performed. Most patients experience symptom onset in the second through fourth decades, but there is a wide range of symptom onset from infancy through to age 85 years.

Classification

- Genetic:
  - Autosomal dominant (70%).
  - Autosomal recessive (30%).
  - X-linked (rare).
- Clinical:
  - Pure (uncomplicated) HSP: most common, and typically autosomal dominant inheritance pattern.
  - Complicated HSP: more likely to be autosomal recessive or X-linked inheritance pattern. Associated with:
    - Cognitive deficit.
    - Optic neuropathy.
    - Retinal pigmentary degeneration.
    - Ophthalmoplegia.
    - Deafness.
    - Extrapyramidal signs.
    - Cerebellar symptoms.
    - Amyotrophy in the upper limbs.
    - Skin disorders (ichthyosis).

Etiology and pathophysiology

There is a heterogeneous pattern of inheritance with over 40 gene loci identified to date[8].

Pure uncomplicated forms

- Autosomal dominant (70%): 50% of autosomal dominant cases can be attributed to two loci:
  - *SPAST* (formerly *SPG4*) on chromosone 2p22 encoding for spastin protein.
  - *SPG3A* on chromosome 14q14–q21 encoding for atlastin protein.
- Many additional genes are identified in families with pure HSP:
  - *NIPA1* (formerly *SPG6*) on chromosome 15q encoding for nonimprinted in Prader–Willi/Angelman syndrome region protein 1.
  - *KIAA0196* (formerly *SPG8*) on chromosome 8q24 encoding for strumpellin protein.
  - *REEP1* (formerly *SPG31*) on chromosome 2p12 encoding for receptor expression-enhancing protein 1.
  - Remaining cases of pure HSP with autosomal dominance are linked to over 15 other loci on more than 10 different genes.
- Autosomal recessive (30%):
  - *CYP7B1* (formerly *SPG5A*) on chromosome 8 encoding cytochrome P450-7B1 (involved in cholesterol metabolism).
  - Other autosomal recessive genes have been linked to pure HSP but only in single families.
- X-linked (rare): mapped to a locus on Xq11.

Complex forms

- Autosomal dominant:
  - *BSCL2* (formerly *SPG17*) on chromosome 11q encoding for seipin protein causes Silver syndrome (HSP with distal amyotrophy).
  - To date, three other loci have been identified for autosomal dominant complex HSP. Protein products have not yet been identified for these genes:
    - *SAX1* (chromosome 12p13) causes spastic ataxia.
    - *SPG9* (chromosome 10q) causes cataracts, motor neuropathy, skeletal abnormalities and gastroesophageal reflux.
    - *SPG29* (chromosome 1) causes sensorineural hearing loss, pes cavus, hiatal hernia, and hyperbilirubinemia.
- Autosomal recessive:
  - At least 14 loci identified to date.
    - *SPG7* on chromosome 16q encoding for paraplegin protein causes cerebellar signs, neuropathy and optic atrophy.
    - *SPG11* on chromosome 15q encoding for spatacsin protein causes thin corpus callosum, cognitive impairment, and neuropathy.
    - Other autosomal recessive loci are found in small numbers of families and most proteins involved have not yet been identified.
- X-linked:
  - Two loci mapped to chromosome Xq28 (*SPG1*) and Xq22 (*SPG2*). Two genes have been identified: L1 cell adhesion molecule and proteolipid protein.

Current theories regarding the pathophysiology postulate that membrane trafficking and axonal transport are deranged in the majority of HSP syndromes, with additional roles for mitochondrial proteins and cholesterol metabolism.

Clinical features

History

- Following normal gestation, delivery, and early childhood development, patients develop leg stiffness and gait disturbance (stumbling and tripping) due to difficulty dorsiflexing the foot and weakness of hip flexion.
- Paresthesias below the knees are quite common.
- Urinary urgency progressing to urinary incontinence is a frequent, although variable, late manifestation.
- A significant minority of patients are asymptomatic and unaware of signs.

Examination

- Cranial nerves:
  - Fundi, and extraocular and facial movements are normal (unless complex HSP: optic neuropathy, retinal pigmentary degeneration, ophthalmoplegia).
  - Jaw jerk may be brisk in older subjects but there is no evidence of frank corticobulbar tract dysfunction.
- Upper limbs: tone and muscle power are normal (unless complex HSP: amyotrophy) but hyperreflexia may be found.

- Lower limbs:
  - Wasting of muscles may occur but is mild and limited to the anterior and posterior tibial compartment in wheelchair-dependent elderly patients.
  - Tone is increased in the hamstrings, quadriceps, and ankles. Ankle clonus is present uniformly.
  - Weakness is most notable of the iliopsoas, tibialis anterior and, to a lesser extent, hamstring muscles.
  - Deep tendon reflexes are pathologically increased (3–4+). Crossed adductor reflexes and extensor plantar responses are present uniformly.
  - Sensation to sharp stimuli is decreased below the knees in occasional patients and vibratory sense is often diminished mildly in the distal lower limbs.
  - Gait: circumduction is present due to difficulty with hip flexion and ankle dorsiflexion.

The clinical phenotypic expression of 'pure' autosomal dominant spastic paraparesis is highly variable. The age of symptom onset, rate of symptom progression, and extent of disability vary within and between HSP kindreds. Phenotype variation is related, at least in part, to symptom duration. However, neurologic dysfunction is disproportionately witnessed in corticospinal and dorsal column tracts innervating the lower limbs.

Tip

▶ *Additional deficits such as visual disturbance, marked amyotrophy, fasciculations, dementia, seizures, or peripheral neuropathy in patients from pure HSP kindreds should not be attributed to variant presentations of pure HSP, but rather, patients should be evaluated thoroughly for concurrent or alternative neurologic disorders.*

Differential diagnosis

- Inherited ataxias:
  - Spinocerebellar ataxias
  - Friedreich's ataxia.
- Inherited leukodystrophies:
  - Adrenoleukodystrophy (ALD)/adrenomyeloneuropathy (AMN).
  - Metachromatic leukodystrophy.
  - Krabbe (globoid cell) leukodystrophy.
- Structural spinal cord abnormality:
  - Arnold–Chiari malformation with or without syringomyelia.
  - Cervical or lumbar spondylosis.
  - Tethered cord syndrome.
  - Tumor of the spinal cord.
  - AVM of the spinal cord.
  - Granuloma (e.g. tuberculous) involving vertebrae and spinal cord.
- Inflammatory myelopathies:
  - Demyelinating disease (MS, NMO, and so on).
  - Rheumatologic disorders.
  - Stiff person syndrome.
- Infectious disease:
  - Tertiary syphilis.
  - Tropical spastic paraparesis.
  - HIV-associated myelopathy.
- Metabolic disorder:
  - SCD of the spinal cord.
  - Mitochondrial encephalomyopathy.
  - Abetalipoproteinemia (Bassen–Kornzweig disease).
- Degenerative disease: motor neuron disease (familial/sporadic).
- Miscellaneous: dopa-responsive dystonia due to tyrosine hydroxylase gene mutations.

Investigations

- MRI brain and spinal cord.
- Serum vitamin B12, copper, folate, vitamin E.
- HTLV-1 and HIV antibodies.
- VDRL/ rapid plasma reagin (RPR), *Treponema pallidum* particle agglutination assay (TPHA).
- Plasma long-chain fatty acid analysis.
- DNA analysis.
- Electrophysiology:
  - Nerve conduction studies: normal unless a complicated form of HSP with associated neuropathy.
  - Somatosensory evoked potentials, after stimulation of peripheral nerves in the lower limbs, shows conduction delay in dorsal column fibers.

Diagnosis

The diagnosis of HSP is straightforward when the family history indicates inheritance of progressive spastic paraparesis as an isolated symptom. In these cases, documenting associated deficits, such as retinitis pigmentosa, extrapyramidal signs, ataxia, amyotrophy, and peripheral neuropathy, is the basis for classifying HSP as pure or complex and helps to distinguish HSP from other neurologic disorders. Otherwise, the diagnosis of HSP is a diagnosis of exclusion, and should only be made after excluding treatable conditions (such as vitamin B12 deficiency, dopa-responsive dystonia, cervical spondylosis) and disorders with a different prognosis (such as familial ALS).

- Definite HSP:
  - Diagnosed when alternative disorders in the differential diagnosis have been excluded.
  - A family history supports inheritance of an X-linked, autosomal recessive, or autosomal dominant disorder (may be confirmed with genetic testing).
  - Progressive gait disturbance is present.

Spastic paraparesis with grade 4 hyper-reflexia and extensor plantar responses: occasionally, evidence of a spastic paraparesis will be found in asymptomatic subjects and, unless serial neurologic examinations have been performed, it is not possible to know whether these signs are static (representing mild spastic cerebral palsy, for example) or represent a progressive gait disorder. Such subjects should be classified as probably affected and examined serially.

Pathology

- Axonal degeneration occurs in the terminal/distal portions of the longest descending and ascending tracts of the spinal cord (700):
  - Corticospinal tract fibers (crossed and uncrossed) from pyramidal neurons in the motor cortex to the legs.
  - Fasciculus gracilis (and cuneatus to a lesser extent) fibers from the dorsal root ganglia neurons.
- Neuronal cell bodies of degenerating fibers are preserved.
- Mild loss of anterior horn cells may occur.
- Dorsal root ganglia, posterior roots and peripheral nerves are normal.
- There is no evidence of primary demyelination.

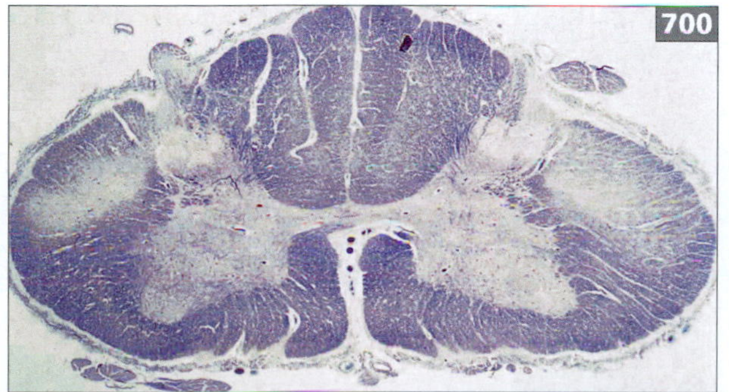

700 Axial section through the spinal cord showing degeneration (pallor) in the corticospinal tracts, spinocerebellar tracts, and dorsal columns.

Treatment

There is no specific treatment to prevent, retard, or reverse the progressive disability. A trial of low-dose levodopa–carbidopa is advised for all patients with childhood onset progressive gait disturbance of uncertain etiology (particularly those with dystonia) because hereditary progressive dystonia with diurnal variation can resemble HSP and is treatable.

For symptomatic treatment, similar treatment approaches are used as for chronic paraplegia from other causes, such as:

- Regular physiotherapy and occupational therapy to minimize contractures and abnormal postures and maximize physical function and independence.
- Oral and intrathecal baclofen.
- Regular local botulinum toxin injections into spastic hip adductors or ankle and toe flexors/invertors (e.g. tibialis posterior).
- Oxybutynin for bladder dysfunction due to detrusor hyper-reflexia.

Genetic counseling must consider that, even within the same family and despite complete genetic penetrance, there may be substantial variation in age of symptom onset, rate of symptom progression, extent of bladder involvement, and functional disability. In some HSP kindreds, the condition begins in childhood and is relatively nonprogressive after about age 10 years.

Prognosis

Gait disturbance progresses insidiously without exacerbations, remissions, or saltatory worsening. The evolution of the disease is similar in patients with early and late onset.

ADRENOMYELONEUROPATHY

Definition and epidemiology

Adrenomyeloneuropathy (AMN) is an adult-onset variant of X-linked childhood degenerative disease, adrenoleukodystrophy (ADL). Both disorders cause toxic accumulation of very-long-chain fatty acids (VLCFAs) leading to axonopathy.

- Incidence 1:40,000.

Classification

- 'Pure' AMN: noninflammatory axonopathy of spinal cord and peripheral nerves without evidence of brain involvement, clinically or radiographically. May involve male patients or 10–15% of female heterozygotes (carriers).
- 'Cerebral' AMN: demyelinating lesions of brain identified on MRI, sometimes associated with cognitive symptoms or behavior disorders. May progress more rapidly than 'pure' form. Affects one-third of AMN patients (male only). Differentiated from classical ADL by later onset and less severe clinical manifestations from cerebral involvement (701, 702).

Etiology and pathophysiology

- *ABCD1* gene encoding for ADL protein (ADLP) is located on chromosome Xp28.
- ADLP is an adenosine triphosphate (ATP) binding cassette (ABC) protein, located in the membrane of perioxisomes; ADLP deficiency leads to toxic accumulation of VLCFAs due to a faulty beta-oxidation process.
- ADLP gene is expressed preferentially in the adrenal glands and neural tissues.

Clinical features

- Progressive spastic paraparesis with autonomic dysfunction (loss of bladder control) and sensory loss (spinothalamic tract and posterior columns affected).
- Onset in 20s and 30s with gait abnormalities.
- Gradual progression to more rostral functions over years.
- Wheelchair bound 5–15 years after onset.
- Specific symptoms of peripheral nerve involvement are not well described.
- Systemic (non-neurologic) features:
  - Adrenal dysfunction in majority of men and none of women:
    - Corticosteroid deficiency: vomiting, hypotension.
    - Hyperpigmentation.
  - Hair loss in men and women (not related to adrenal function).

Differential diagnosis

- Inflammatory myelopathy, including primary progressive variant of MS.
- Chronic infectious myelopathy, including HTLV-1 infection.
- HSP.
- Spinocerebellar ataxia.
- Spinal dural arteriovenous fistula (chronic progressive gait disturbance).
- Metabolic myelopathy (vitamin B12 or copper deficiency).

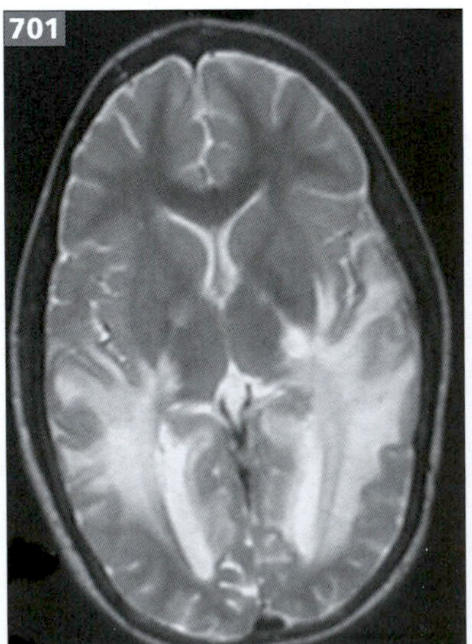

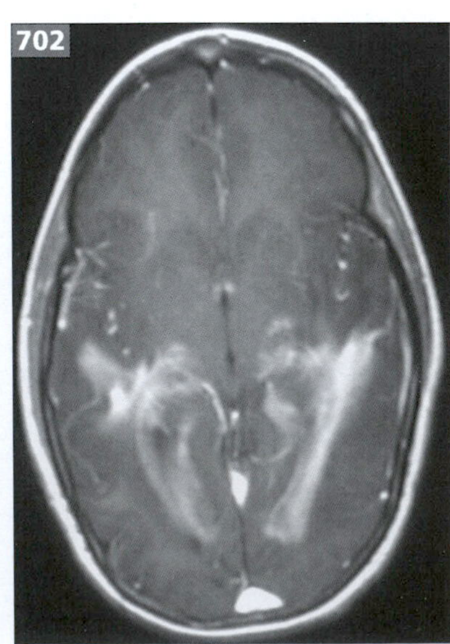

701, 702 Adrenoleukodystrophy. Axial T2-weighted MRI of the brain (701), with characteristic posterior fossa white matter changes and post-contrast enhancement (T1-weighted with gadolinium [702]).

Investigations and diagnosis

- MRI spine: standard sequences only show cord atrophy, due to lack of inflammation within spinal cord tissue.
- MRI brain: when abnormal in AMN, nonenhancing T2W hyperintensities are seen in the splenium and posterior fossa white matter.
- Serum:
  - Elevated levels of VLCFAs in serum (specifically C26).
  - Minority of female carriers will have normal VLCFA levels.
  - Adrenal dysfunction: hyperkalemia, hyponatremia, metabolic acidosis, impaired cortisol response to adrenocorticotropic hormone (ACTH) stimulation.
- EMG shows predominantly axonal sensorimotor neuropathy.
- Sural nerve biopsy demonstrates axon loss with less prominent demyelination and onion bulb formation.
- Genetic testing: *ABCD1* gene testing is commercially available and can detect virtually all affected male patients and a large majority of female carriers (a small percentage may require more extensive genetic analysis).

Treatment

- Adrenal dysfunction:
  - Corticosteroid replacement.
  - No effect on neurologic function.
- Neurologic manifestations: no proven therapy:
  - Early use of Lorenzo's oil (hexacosanoic acid) has been reported to prevent progression to cerebral dysfunction, but this is considered an investigational therapy at this time.
  - Bone marrow transplant: only recommended in childhood and adolescent patients with early manifestations of ADL. Single case reports of transplant in adult disease.

Prognosis

- 'Pure' AMN: 5–15 years to wheelchair dependence with continued slow progression to upper extremity involvement.
- 'Cerebral' AMN: more rapid progression with cognitive and cortical signs and symptoms.

SPINAL CORD TUMORS

Definition and epidemiology

Tumors of the spinal cord.

- Incidence: 10 per 100,000 per year. Primary spinal cord tumors represent about 15% of primary CNS tumors. Metastases to the spine are far more common.
- Age:
  - Young and middle-aged adults predominantly.
  - Intramedullary tumors are more common in children.
  - Extramedullary tumors are more common in adults.
- Gender: M=F.

Etiology

Adult primary tumors of the spine

- Extradural (only 10% in this category are primary tumors with 90% being of metastatic origin):
  - Myeloma (i.e. solitary plasmacytoma).
  - Primary bone tumors.
  - Hemangioma of bone.
  - Osteosarcoma.
  - Chordoma (commonly sacral or clivus).
  - Chondrosarcoma.
- Intradural extramedullary:
  - Nerve sheath tumors (neurofibroma/schwannoma).
  - 30% of intradural tumors in adults.
  - Meningioma (anywhere along the cord, F>M).
  - Myxopapillary ependymoma.
  - Lipoma.
  - Cysts (dermoid/epidermoid: often lumbosacral region).
- Intradural intramedullary (uncommon):
  - Glial cell tumors (80% of intramedullary tumors):
    - Ependymoma (many arise from filum terminale, approximately 50% of intramedullary primary tumors).
    - Astrocytoma (mostly cervical)
    - Oligodendroglioma (rare).
  - Hemangioblastoma (may cause hematomyelia).

Pediatric primary tumors of the spine

- Extradural:
  - Neuroblastoma.
  - Lymphoma/leukemia.
  - Teratoma.
  - Ewing sarcoma and other primary tumors of bone (osteochordoma, and so on).
- Intradural extramedullary:
  - Nerve sheath tumors (neurofibroma/ schwannoma).
  - Meningioma.
  - Myxopapillary ependymoma.
  - Cysts (dermoid/epidermoid).
- Intradural intramedually:
  - Astrocytoma (increased percentage with age, approaching 90% in the youngest age groups).
  - Ependymoma.

Secondary tumors (metastases) of the spine

Most spinal tumors are metastases, rather than primary benign or malignant tumors.

- Extradural is the most common site of metastases (703).
- More than 90% are bony metastases in the vertebral column which involve the spinal canal directly or via the intervertebral foramina.
- The remaining minority represent hematogeous spread to extramedullary, or, very rarely, intramedullary space.
- Primary source:
  - Breast.
  - Bronchus.
  - Prostate.
  - Melanoma.
  - Multiple myeloma.
  - Lymphoma.
  - Renal cell carcinoma.
- Intradural but extramedullary (rare): leptomeningeal metastases of carcinoma or lymphoma causing malignant meningitis (**704**).
- Intramedullary (very rare): small-cell lung cancer (most common).

Clinical features

Clinical features depend on the site and extent of the spinal cord lesion, as well as the rate of growth. There are three typical clinical syndromes:

- Transverse myelopathy.
- Myeloradiculopathy.
- Central cord (syringomyelic).

Features specific to extramedullary tumors

Tumors usually involve a few segments with root compression (usually dorsal) and progressive compression of the cord to cause an incomplete or complete transection syndrome. Pain and local tenderness is the initial symptom of extradural metastases in about 95% of adults. It is a good localizing sign of the level of the lesion. Spinal pain at night or at rest is suggestive of a tumor.

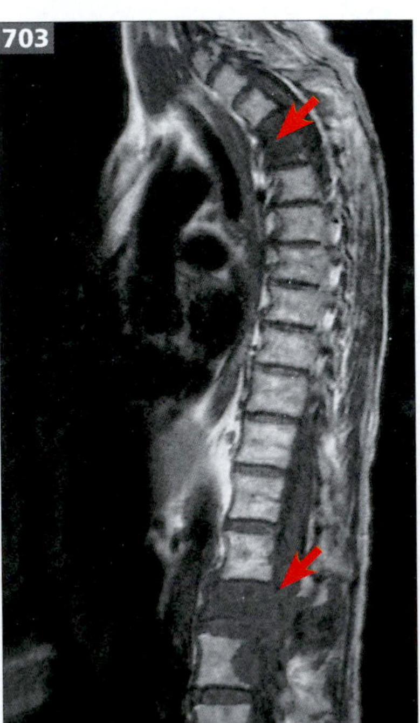

703 T1W midline sagittal MRI showing metastatic extradural lesions in the upper thoracic and upper lumbar regions (arrows). Note the involvement of the vertebral bodies in the malignant process as shown by the altered marrow signal.

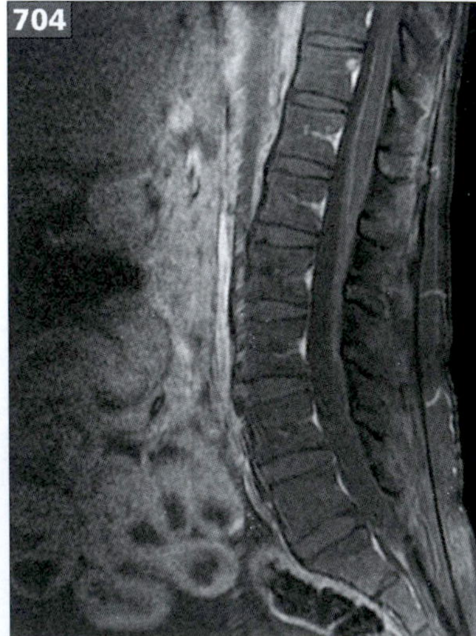

704 Leptomeningeal carcinomatosis. Sagittal T1-weighted MRI with contrast, demonstrates meningeal enhancement at the level of the conus medullaris in a patient with metastatic breast cancer.

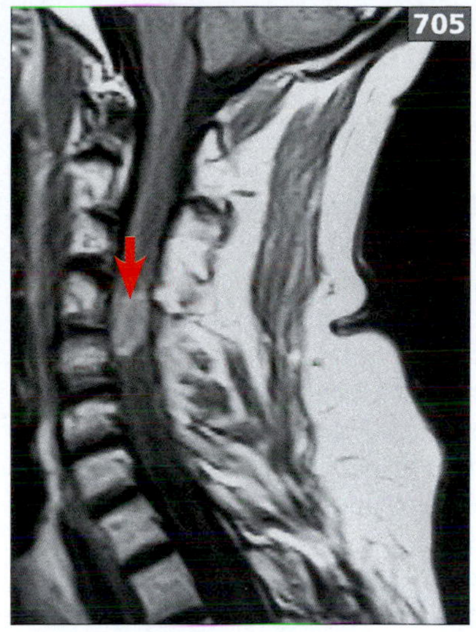

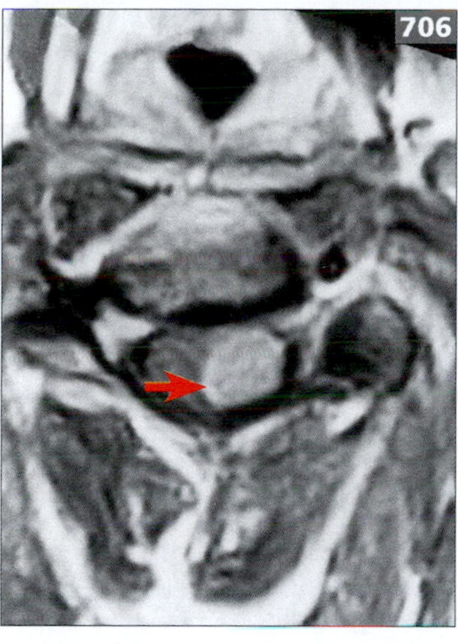

705, 706 MRI cervical spine, sagittal (705) and axial (706) sections, showing a hyperdense mass (arrows) in the left hemicord (causing a Brown–Séquard syndrome) due to metastatic malignant melanoma.

There is a variable pattern of spastic paraparesis and sensory loss below the lesion, as well as bladder (and less commonly bowel) dysfunction, if the cord is compressed. Vascular spinal cord syndromes may occur, and are suggestive of metastases (and abscesses) because they tend to occlude spinal vessels.

Features specific to intramedullary tumors

Tumors may extend over multiple levels and give rise to a clinical picture similar to syringomyelia (see p. 755). Other features suggestive of the cause include:

- Skin lesions, e.g. café-au-lait spots of neurofibromatosis; pigmented melanoma.
- Breast mass or other evidence of primary cancer.
- Weight loss, malaise: metastases.

Differential diagnosis[9]

- Acute onset:
  - Intervertebral disc prolapse.
  - Vertebral body collapse (spinal angulation: tuberculosis, tumor).
  - Trauma.
  - Epidural hemorrhage.
  - Intramedullary hemorrhage: AVM.
  - Spinal cord infarction.
  - Inflammatory or infectious myelopathy.
- Subacute onset:
  - Epidural abscess (e.g. pyogenic, tuberculous, and fungal granulomatous lesions).
  - Paraneoplastic necrotizing myelopathy.
- Slow onset:
  - Spondylosis.
  - Syringomyelia.
  - Tethered cord syndrome.
  - Radiation myelopathy.
  - Meningeal carcinomatosis.

Investigations

- Full blood count and ESR.
- Syphilis serology.
- Urine: hematuria with renal cell carcinoma.
- Chest X-ray:
  - Infection with tuberculosis.
  - Tumor: primary or secondary.
  - Paravertebral shadow (neurofibromatosis, Pott's disease).
- CSF cytology may reveal malignant cells. Repeated LP (>3) may be necessary to increase the yield of cytologic studies.
  - Froin syndrome: discoloration of CSF with rapid clotting and dramatically increased protein levels, due to isolation or loculation of the CSF below the site of the tumor.
  - LP may precipitate acute deterioration if there is cord compression and may damage the spinal cord if it is tethered to the low lumbar or sacral vertebral bodies.
- MRI spine: the imaging method of choice as it displays bones and soft tissues impinging on spinal cord and roots better than myelography and CT, and it images inside the spinal cord and can detect intramedullary tumors and exclude a syrinx, which myelography cannot (705, 706).
- CT scan of the vertebral canal with contrast enhancement may demonstrate tumors and delineate the extraspinal extent of tumors.
- Myelography followed by CT scan: useful if MRI is contraindicated. Widening of the spinal cord in the antero-posterior (AP) view may be due to anterior or posterior cord compression, but widening in the AP and lateral view suggests cord tumor, myelitis, or a syrinx.

- Spine X-ray:
  - Vertebral body collapse (osteoporosis, infection, tumor).
  - Erosion of vertebral bodies or pedicles by tumor.
  - Scalloping of posterior margin of vertebral body (chronic tumor).
  - Vertebral body alignment: subluxation, spondylolisthesis.
  - Intervertebral disc space narrowing (spondylosis) or destruction.
  - Intervertebral exit foramina (in oblique views of neck) are enlarged in neurofibroma, reduced in spondylosis.
  - Spinal canal width, osteophytes.

Diagnosis

MRI spine and tissue biopsy in a patient with appropriate clinical features.

Treatment

Rapidly progressive spinal cord compression by extradural tumor calls for emergency MRI, immediate high-dose corticosteroids, and a tissue diagnosis either by CT-guided percutaneous biopsy or open surgical biopsy. If the tumor is benign it should be removed surgically if technically possible. If the tumor is malignant, the spinal cord and roots should be decompressed by surgery, radiotherapy, chemotherapy or hormonal therapy, depending on tumor type and the clinical circumstances. If a metastatic lesion is found without a known primary source, then further investigation is indicated to identify the underlying malingnancy.

Operative fixation of the vertebral column may be worthwhile in patients with unremitting pain due to spinal instability.

Prognosis

Prognosis depends on the underlying cause and duration and degree of spinal cord and nerve root compression/infiltration. In contrast to brain tumors, many spinal tumors are benign and produce their effects mainly by compression of the spinal cord rather than by invasion.

MYELOPATHY ASSOCIATED WITH MOTOR NEURON DISEASE

AMYOTROPHIC LATERAL SCLEROSIS (ALS)

Definition and epidemiology

Motor neuron diseases (MNDs) are a heterogeneous group of inherited and sporadic disorders of UMNs and LMNs which lead to progressive weakness of bulbar, limb, thoracic, and abdominal muscles with relative sparing of oculomotor muscles and sphincter function.

- Incidence: 1.9 per 100,000 person years, relatively constant throughout the world but higher (5 per 100,000 per year) in the western Pacific (Guam).
- Prevalence: 5/100,000 of the total population.
- Age: 3–99, with less than 5% occurring in patients <25 years old.
  - Sporadic MND: median age of onset: 64 years; M>F (1.5:1).
  - Familial MND (5–10% of all ALS cases): mean age of onset: 50 years; M=F.

Etiology

- Familial ALS (FALS) (5–10% of cases) is almost always in an autosomal-dominant inheritance pattern *(Table 114)*.
- Sporadic ALS (SALS) (90–95% of cases): failure to identify a single environmental or genetic risk factor for the development of SALS has lead to a theorized multifactorial etiology. Factors which have been associated with increased risk:
  - Smoking has been identified as a 'probable' risk factor for development of SALS with relative risks and odds ratios generally less than 2.0.
  - Veterans of the first Gulf War (1990–1991) experienced an increased risk of developing SALS, with a shorter survival compared to nonveteran ALS patients.
  - Other factors identified, but not proven to increase risk include prior electrical injury, increased physical activity or involvement in professional sport, and exposure to environmental toxins (e.g. heavy metals).

TABLE 114 **AUTOSOMAL DOMINANT GENES IN AMYOTROPHIC LATERAL SCLEROSIS**

	Gene locus	Protein	Onset	Proposed mechanism of pathophysiology	Comments
ALS1	21Q21.1	Superoxide dismutase 1 (SOD1)	Adult	Multiple, including reduction of free radicals	20% of FALS, 2% of SALS
ALS3	18q21	Unknown	Adult	Unknown	
ALS4	9Q34	Senataxin (SETX)	Juvenile	RNA processing	
ALS6	16q21	Fused in sarcoma (FUS)	Adult	RNA processing	
ALS7	20p13	Unknown	Adult	Unknown	
ALS8	20q13	VAMP (vesicle-associated membrane protein)-associated protein B (VAPB)	Adult	Intracellular membrane trafficking	
ALS9	14q11	Angiogenin (ANG)	Adult	Unknown	Mutation found in both FALS and SALS
ALS10	1q36.22	TAR DNA-binding protein (TARDBP)	Adult	RNA processing	Protein found in ubiquitinated inclusions in both SALS and FALS (except SOD1 FALS)
ALS	2p13	Dynactin 1 (DCTN1)	Adult	Axonal transport	May be associated with LMN variant of ALS
ALS-FTDP	17q21.1	Microtubule-associated protein tau (MAPT)	Adult	Axonal transport	ALS with frontotemporal dementia
ALS-FTD1	9q21–22	Expanded GGGGCC hexanucleotide repeat in non-coding region	Adult	Unknown	

FALS: familial amyotrophic lateral sclerosis; LMN: lower motor neuron; SALS: sporadic amyotrophic lateral sclerosis.

Pathophysiology

The mechanisms involved in motor neuron cell survival and death are not well known. It is suspected that cellular mechanisms are at play in the motor neuron degeneration:

- Excitotoxicity via overstimulation of postsynaptic glutamate receptors.
- Oxidative stress.
- Protein and neurofilament aggregation.
- Disordered axonal transport and cellular signaling mechanisms.

Although inflammation of neural tissues is thought to play a role in the pathogenesis of ALS, extensive clinical trials of immunomodulating therapies have failed to impact the clinical course of the disease.

Clinical signs

History

- Gradual onset.
- Limb weakness: 70% present with progressive asymmetric weakness of the limbs:
  - Muscle twitches and cramps may be present, which may be severe.
  - Local pain may herald the onset of weakness and wasting by several weeks; pain occurs in the late stages secondary to immobility and contractures.
  - Paresthesia is an occasional symptom but the sensory examination is normal.
- Bulbar symptoms: 25% present with:
  - Slurred speech (dysarthria): spastic (pseudobulbar palsy), flaccid, nasal speech (bulbar palsy), or a combination of the two.
  - Difficulty swallowing (dysphagia), often with drooling of saliva.
  - Alteration in voice quality (dysphonia).
  - Emotional lability (common in pseudobulbar palsy).
- Nocturnal breathlessness due to respiratory failure is a presenting symptom in 3%.
- Family history:
  - 5–10% have a family history, suggesting autosomal dominant inheritance of ALS.
  - 20% of such families have mutations of the Cu, Zn SOD1 gene on chromosome 21.

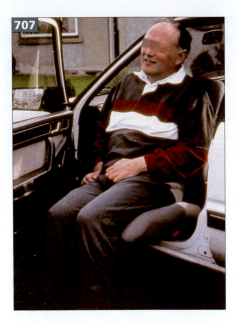

707 A patient with severe limb weakness due to motor neuron disease, in his own environment. Note the severe wasting of the hands. *Courtesy of Dr AM Chancellor, Tauranga, New Zealand.*

Physical examination

Signs may be initially confined to the UMNs or LMNs or to one anatomic area, such as the lumbar segment of limbs, bulbar, or respiratory musculature.

- LMN (nuclear or infranuclear) signs:
  - Muscle wasting (707).
  - Fasciculations.
  - Muscle weakness.
  - Areflexia.
- UMN (supranuclear) signs:
  - Increased (spastic) tone: may be marked, particularly in young patients.
  - Clonus.
  - Hyperactive deep tendon reflexes, including brisk jaw jerk in patients with bilateral corticospinal tract lesions above the mid pons.
  - Weakness in a pyramidal distribution.
  - Extensor plantar responses.
- Combined UMN and LMN signs:
  - Increased tendon reflexes in a corresponding wasted, fasciculating, and weak myotome.
- Bulbar palsy (dysfunction of the muscles of the pharynx, larynx, and tongue innervated by cranial nerves IX–XII originating in the medulla oblongata [the 'spinal bulb']):
  - Flaccid dysarthria: labial sounds are usually affected first; palatal weakness gives the speech a nasal quality and difficulty with palatal sounds such as 'ing', 'egg', and 'ka'.
  - Dysphonia.
  - Dysphagia.
  - Weakness, wasting, and fasciculation of lower facial muscles and tongue.
  - Reduced voluntary and reflex movement of the palate, and also tongue bilaterally.
  - Reduced cough and gag reflexes.
  - Absent jaw jerk.
- Pseudobulbar palsy (dysfunction of the muscles of the pharynx, larynx, and tongue due to bilateral corticobulbar pathway involvement rostral to lower cranial nerve nuclei):

- Spastic dysarthria: slow and forced speech with difficulty enunciating labial and lingual sounds.
- Dysphagia: slow and difficult swallowing.
- Reduced voluntary movement of the palate with the patient saying 'ah'.
- Normal reflex movement of the palate.
- Brisk/exaggerated jaw jerk and facial reflexes.
- Small, contracted tongue which cannot be fully protruded.
- Bilateral spastic quadriparesis.
- Associated emotional lability: inappropriate and excessive laughter or crying.

- Ventilatory failure:
  - Increased respiratory rate, orthopnea.
  - Reduced vital capacity, which is worse on lying flat.
  - Nocturnal hypoventilation causing daytime sleepiness/fatigue, frequent arousal and morning headaches, anorexia.
  - Somnolence or mental status changes due to carbon dioxide retention/hypercapnia.
- Other:
  - Mild cognitive impairment, particularly of frontal lobe function, and less so memory, may be present.
  - Eye movements are normal, besides impaired smooth pursuit by saccadic intrusions.
  - Bladder and bowel function is usually preserved, although urinary urgency can be seen.

Variants of ALS

- Progressive bulbar palsy: about 10% of patients present in this manner and most progress to classical MND. Incidence of bulbar onset disease increases with age (>40% of patients are over the age of 70 years).
- Progressive muscular atrophy: about 10% of patients show only LMN signs but 50% go on to develop UMN signs. Pathologic studies demonstrate UMN pathway involvement.
- Primary lateral sclerosis: progressive symmetric spinobulbar spasticity and weakness of the limbs, more marked in the legs (spastic quadriparesis), and sometimes the bulbar musculature, causing a pseudobulbar palsy. LMN signs are absent and higher cognitive function is preserved. Linked to ALS by pathologic studies.
- Flail arm and leg variants (brachial amyotrophic diplegia or Vulpian–Bernhart syndrome in the arms and polyneuritic ALS in the leg): about 10% of patients present with initially asymmetric flaccid weakness in the arms or legs, with much slower progression to respiratory and swallowing impairment.

Differential diagnosis

Initially diagnosis is incorrect in about 10% of cases; clues are failure to progress, development of atypical features, and the results of radiologic and neurophysiologic investigations.

Brain

- Pseudobulbar palsy:
  - Parasagittal meningioma.
  - Pick's disease.
  - Bilateral corticobulbar vascular lesions (e.g. brainstem and/or capsular).
  - MS.
- Bulbar palsy:
  - Myasthenia gravis.
  - Posterior fossa tumors or aneurysms involving medulla or lower cranial nerves.
  - Syringobulbia.
  - Polyneuritis cranialis: low-grade basal meningitis, vasculitis.
  - X-linked recessive bulbar and spinal muscular atrophy (Kennedy's syndrome).
  - Creutzfeldt–Jakob disease (amyotrophic form).

Spinal cord

- Craniocervical junction abnormality (Chiari malformation).
- Cervical radiculomyelopathy.
- Cervical myelopathy and lumbosacral spondylotic polyradiculopathy.
- Syringomyelia.
- AVM.
- Vasculitis.
- Infection: poliomyelitis, syphilis, HIV, HTLV-1.
- Intramedullary neoplasia: lymphoma, carcinoma.
- Paraneoplastic syndrome: encephalomyelitis with anterior horn cell involvement.
- Post-radiation myeloplexopathy.
- Hereditary spastic paraparesis with distal amyotrophy (ethnic origin [Amish, Tunisian, Lebanese], early age of onset, positive family history, slow progression, pes cavus, vibration sense loss, dementia).
- Late-onset SMA.
- Hexosaminidase A, B deficiency (adult GM2 gangliosidosis) (ethnic origin [Ashkenazi Jews], intellectual impairment, psychiatric disturbances, ataxia, stutter-dysarthria, pyramidal tract signs, dystonia, dyskinesias, supranuclear ophthalmoplegia, white cell/skin fibroblast hexosaminidase A deficiency; electron microscopy of rectal biopsy).

Metabolic and toxic disorders
- SCD.
- Thyrotoxicosis.
- Hyperparathyroidism.
- Diabetic 'amyotrophy'.
- Lead poisoning.
- Mercury poisoning.
- Manganese toxicity.

Neuromuscular
- Monomelic amyotrophy (Hirayama's disease).
- Multifocal motor neuropathy with conduction block (defined electrophysiologically).
- Cramp-fasciculation syndrome due to peripheral nerve hyperexcitability:
  - Benign fasciculations with normal morphology on EMG.
  - Normal muscle strength without progression to weakness over at least 1 year.
- Myasthenia gravis.
- Stiff person syndrome.
- Lambert–Eaton syndrome.
- Myopathy: inclusion body myositis, scapuloperoneal dystrophy.

Investigations
- Serum creatine phosphokinase (may be slightly raised), calcium, lead levels.
- Thyroid function tests.
- Serum vitamin B12, copper, folate levels.
- Serology for syphilis (RPR, TPHA), HIV antibodies, HTLV-1 antibodies, anti-GAD antibodies.
- White blood cell/skin fibroblast hexosaminidase A levels.
- Nerve conduction studies: conduction velocity of sensory fibers is normal, and of motor fibers is normal for nerves of unaffected muscles, and not <70% of average normal value in nerves of affected muscles. Subclinical sensory pathway abnormalities are seen in approximately 10% of patients.
- EMG: active denervation (e.g. increased insertional activity, spontaneous fibrillation potentials and positive sharp waves, fasciculations with abnormal morphology) and chronic partial denervation (reduction in number and increase in amplitude and duration of motor unit action potentials with increased population of polyphasic and unstable potentials, neurogenic recruitment pattern). Clinically unaffected muscles may have the above findings.
- MRI is indicated to exclude other causes of clinical presentation:
  - Brain: increased signal intensity on T2W MRI along the corticospinal tract (brain>brain-stem>spinal cord). May show atrophy of the precentral gyrus.
  - Cervical spinal cord: particularly recommended if a combination of spastic paraparesis and LMN signs in the upper limbs is present, to exclude a compressive lesion in the neck (most commonly cervical spondylosis). May show atrophy and increased signal in the anterolateral parts of the spinal cord due to gliosis.
- CSF: normal or mildly elevated protein (<1 g/l [100 mg/dl]).
- Neuropsychologic testing: may reveal frontal lobe dysfunction.
- Ventilatory muscle strength: forced vital capacity (FVC) is reduced in the setting of diaphragmatic weakness. Pronounced weakness of lower facial muscles may lead to falsely reduced measurement of FVC due to poor lip seal around the testing equipment, so the patient may need to use a mask or other specialized testing equipment.
- Arterial blood gases: abnormalities occur late after the onset of clinically significant ventilatory failure. Hypercapnia is seen in advancing neuromuscular respiratory compromise.

Diagnosis
There is no specific diagnostic test.

Diagnostic criteria (from El Escorial criteria):
- Clinical, electrophysiologic or neuropathologic presence of:
  - LMN degeneration: atrophy, weakness, fasciculation (either in concert with weakness or EMG evidence of active denervation).
  - UMN degeneration: increased tone, hyperreflexia, pathologic reflexes (Babinski, and so on).
  - Progression of the disorder.

Diagnostic categories (Revised El Escorial Research Diagnostic Criteria for ALS):
- Definite ALS: UMN and LMN signs in three regions*.
- Probable ALS: UMN and LMN signs in two regions, with at least some UMN signs rostral to LMN signs (thereby excluding myelopathy, which is characterized by the reverse).
- Probable ALS (laboratory supported): UMN signs in one or more regions and LMN signs (defined by EMG only) in at least two regions.

- Possible ALS:
  - UMN and LMN signs in one region.
  - UMN signs in two or more regions (e.g. monomelic MND, progressive bulbar palsy, and primary lateral sclerosis).
  - UMN and LMN signs in two regions with no UMN signs rostral to LMN signs.

(*Regions are: bulbar, cervical, thoracic, and lumbosacral.)

Absence of:
- Prominent sensory signs.
- Visual disturbances.
- Autonomic dysfunction (excluding spastic bladder, which may be present).
- Parkinson's disease.
- Alzheimer-type dementia.
- ALS 'mimic syndromes' (see Differential diagnosis, above).

Pathology

Macroscopically, brain and spinal cord often appear normal; the precentral gyrus and corticospinal tracts may show atrophy (708–712). Microscopic findings (713, 714) are:
- Loss of Betz cells of the motor cortex.
- Degeneration and gliosis of the corticospinal tracts.
- Degeneration of lower brainstem motor nuclei (not oculomotor nuclei) in most cases.
- Cytoplasmic eosinophilic inclusions (Bunina bodies) and ubiquitin immunoreactive inclusion bodies (containing TAR DNA binding protein 43 [TDP-43]) in degenerating cranial motor nuclei, anterior horn cells, and Betz cells.
- Muscle shows features of denervation.
- Non-motor pathways also demonstrate pathologic changes, including sensory pathways and peripheral sensory nerves.

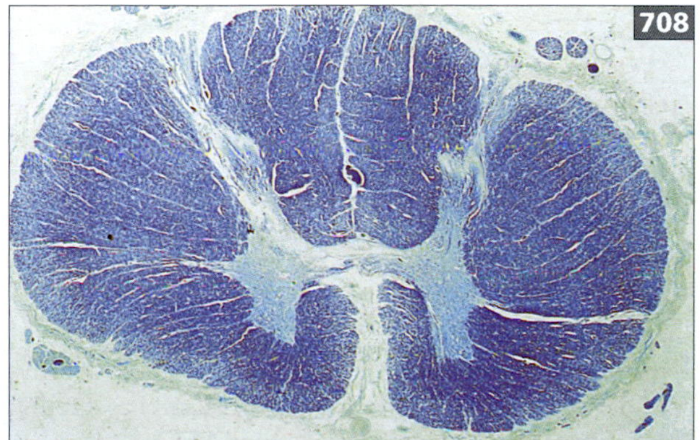

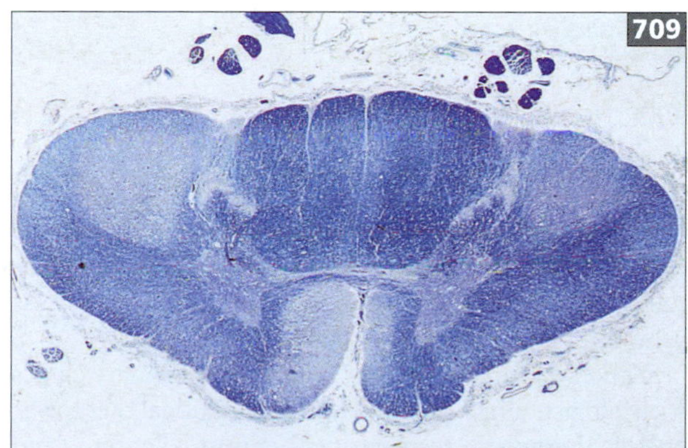

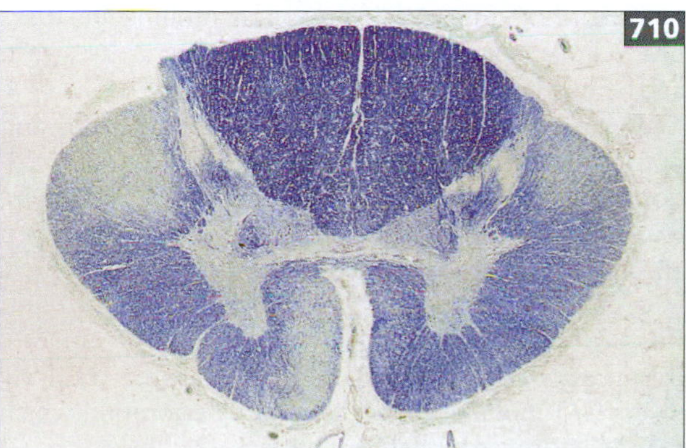

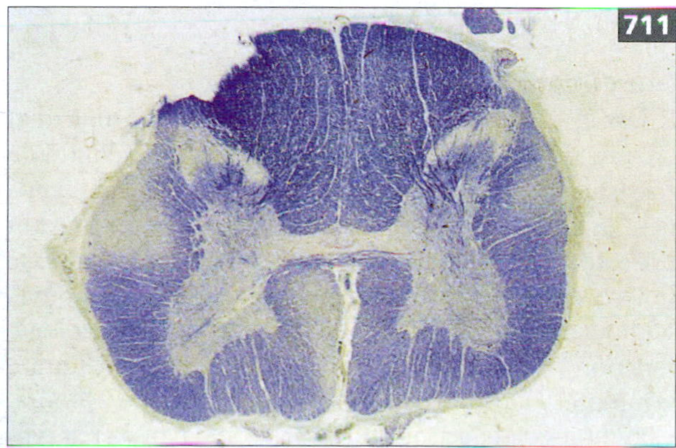

708–711 Axial section through a normal cervical spinal cord (708) and an abnormal spinal cord at the cervical (709), thoracic (710) and lumbar (711) levels, showing degeneration in the anterior and lateral corticospinal tracts, which is more prominent on the right than the left.

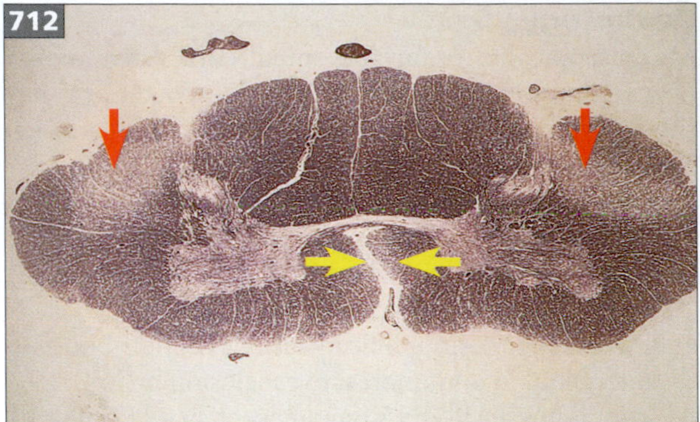

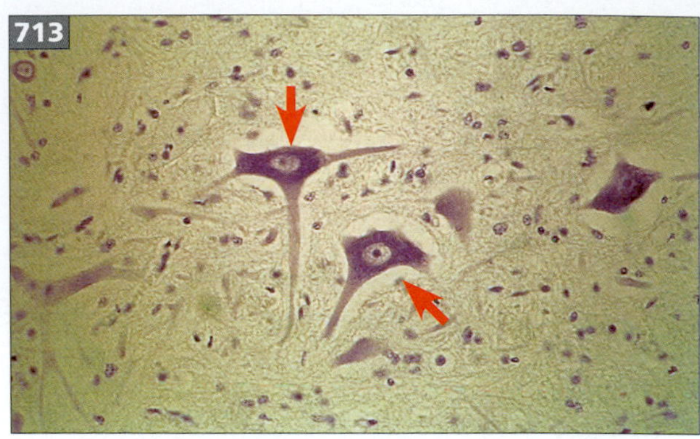

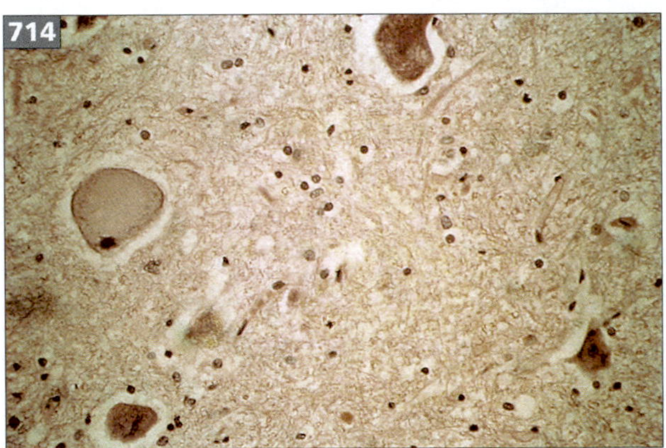

712 Axial section through the spinal cord of another patient with motor neuron disease showing degeneration in the anterior (yellow arrows) and lateral (red arrows) corticospinal tracts.

713 Normal neurons in the anterior horns of the spinal cord (arrows).

714 Chromatolysis of neurons in motor neuron disease.

Treatment

While a cure remains elusive, both FALS and SALS patients can benefit from a combination of specific treatment with riluzole and supportive therapies to address symptoms and progressive disability[10,11].

Patients treated in specialized multidisciplinary clinics (neurologist, nurse, physical and occupational therapists, speech therapists, respiratory therapist, dietitian, and social worker) may experience prolonged survival and improved quality of life.

Drug treatment

Riluzole (2-amino-6-[trifluoromethoxy]benzothiazole) crosses the blood–brain barrier. It inhibits glutamate release, inactivates voltage-dependent sodium channels, and interferes with intracellular events involved in excitotoxicity. Riluzole slows the progression of disease (improves tracheostomy-free survival by about 3 months without any effect on muscle strength and neurologic function) but does not arrest the disease or ameliorate symptoms. Dose is one 50 mg tablet every 12 hours. Common side-effects include fatigue and nausea but typically it is well tolerated. Monitoring of full blood count and liver function tests is required at monthly intervals for the first 3 months of treatment and then every 3 months.

Nutritional support

In early dysphagia, evaluation and counseling by a speech therapist is required, and changes made in dietary consistency with thickening agents, and so on. Placement of a feeding tube (percutaneous endoscopic gastrostomy [PEG] or radiologically inserted gastrostomy) to supplement or replace oral food intake in patients with dysphagia has been shown to stabilize weight and, compared to patients who refuse such intervention, prolong life. Risks of PEG placement include infection, respiratory arrest, and hemorrhage.

Regardless of gastrostomy placement, weight and nutritional status should be monitored closely and nutritional supplements used when indicated. No vitamin, mineral, or herbal supplement has, to date, been shown effective in modifying disease progression.

Respiratory support

Respiratory parameters should be measured regularly (every 2–3 months) to monitor for deterioration which may be improved with intervention:

- FVC (including supine): may influence timing of PEG placement and/or initiation of noninvasive ventilation.

- Maximal inspiratory pressure (MIP).
- Nocturnal pulse oximetry to monitor for nocturnal hypoventilation.
- Noninvasive ventilation (e.g. bilevel positive airways pressure) (**715**).
  - Indicated for FVC < 50% predicted value and/or MIP < –60 cm.
  - Associated with prolonged survival and improved quality of life when used in patients with symptomatic respiratory insufficiency.
- Additional interventions to manage progressive respiratory weakness: cough assist devices, nebulizer treatments to thin secretions.
- End-stage disease can be characterized by 'air hunger' and palliative use of low-dose benzodiazepines may alleviate the anxiety associated with this symptom.
- Tracheostomy with mechanical ventilation will prevent death from respiratory failure, but patients should be extensively counseled regarding the continued progression of weakness to eventual quadriplegia.
- Mechanical ventilation typically results in nursing home placement, as home care with a ventilator requires 24-hour supervision, which is impractical and costly.

Symptomatic management

- Physical therapy: muscle tone and strength, mobility, bracing to improve energy efficiency (e.g. ankle–foot orthoses).
- Occupational therapy: activities of daily living, prompt provision of aids and appliances.
- Dysarthria requires evaluation by a speech pathologist: letter boards, speaking techniques, picture books, voice amplifiers, computerized speech augmentation devices (infrared eye movement detection, light writers, and so on) can be of assistance.
- Excess saliva can be treated with anticholinergic medications (e.g. scopolamine) or tricyclic antidepressants (e.g. amitriptyline). A home suction device can be used.
- Constipation is likely due to poor diet, reduced fluid intake, limited mobility and abdominal wall weakness. Encourage fluid intake and use stool softeners and/or laxatives.
- Muscle cramps: no proven treatment, although anecdotal reports suggest benefit from gabapentin.
- Spasticity: physiotherapy, baclofen, tizanidine, benzodiazepines (especially useful for largyngospasm).
- Immobility: evaluation by a seating and mobility specialist for manual or motorized wheelchair.
- Depression and insomnia are common; antidepressants and hypnotics can be used when appropriate.
- Emotional lability (e.g. in pseudobulbar affective disorder): selective serotonin reuptake inhibitors (SSRIs) are of some benefit in patients bothered by symptoms (not all patients or families find these symptoms problematic enough to warrant medication).
- Referral to a local hospice should be given when appropriate, but patients in multidisciplinary clinics typically remain under the care of a neurologist until death.

Prognosis

ALS is progressive. Median life expectancy is 2.5–3.5 years; about 2 years for patients with bulbar onset and 4 years for patients with onset of limb weakness. 25% survive 5 years from onset of symptoms. Death is usually from respiratory failure due to diaphragmatic weakness, and may be precipitated by aspiration pneumonia.

Cognitive symptoms range from impaired executive (frontal lobe) function (common, >25% of patients) to frontotemporal dementia (5%).

Favorable prognostic factors include:

- Early age of onset (some may survive 20 years).
- Progressive muscular atrophy.
- Primary lateral sclerosis: mean disease duration: 15 years (median: 19 years).

Poor prognostic factors include:

- Bulbar onset.
- Older age.
- Female sex.

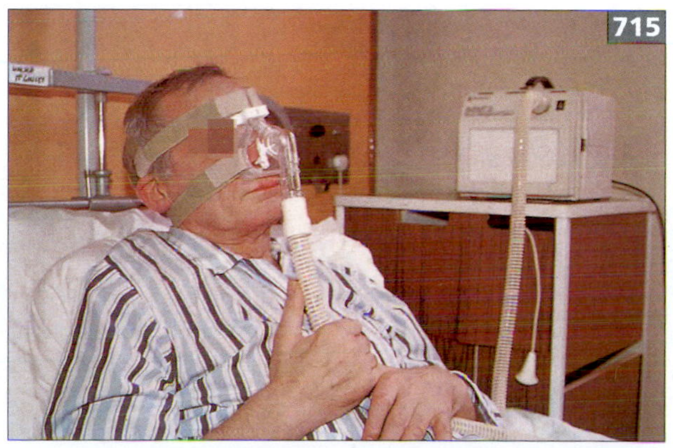

715 A patient with ventilatory failure due to motor neuron disease. Note the severe wasting of the hands. *Courtesy of Dr AM Chancellor, Tauranga, New Zealand.*

SPINAL MUSCULAR ATROPHY (SMA)

Definition and epidemiology

Spinal muscular atrophy (SMA) is a class of inherited diseases characterized by progressive degeneration of anterior horn cells and subsequent muscular atrophy and paralysis. For disease linked to the survival of motor neuron (*SMN*) gene:

- Incidence: infantile and juvenile SMA: 1 per 6000 newborns.
- Incidence of gene carrier status: 1–2% of population.
- Age: onset varies from birth to adulthood.
- Gender: depends on inheritance (males only if X-linked).

Classification

Increasing understanding of the genetic nature of the disease has led to two subgroups of SMA: SMA linked to the *SMN* gene on chromosome 5q, and variants not linked to the *SMN* gene (see below).

SMN gene-linked SMA has a spectrum of clinical presentations divided by age of onset and best motor milestone reached before disease onset:

- Congenital SMA with arthogryposis: diffuse weakness and contractures at birth with facial and extraocular muscle involvement.
- SMA I (Werdnig–Hoffman syndrome): onset from birth to 6 months old; child never sits independently.
- SMA II: onset at 6–18 months old; child sits, but never walks.
- SMA III (Kugelberg–Welander syndrome): onset >18 months old; child walks, but typically not normally.
- SMA IV (adult-onset SMA): onset is in second or third decade; patient walks normally into adulthood.

Etiology and pathophysiology

There is autosomal recessive loss of *SMN1* gene on chromosome 5q13. *SMN* has multiple copies in the normal human genome: one copy of *SMN1* and varying copies of *SMN2*. The product of both *SMN1* and *SMN2* is a protein involved in ribonucleic acid (RNA) processing, which, although ubiquitous, is highly concentrated in motor neurons. *SMN2* is rapidly degraded within the cell, thus the volume of protein produced by *SMN2* is largely determined by the functional status of the *SMN1* copy. SMA patients lose normal *SMN1* function, but the amount of remaining *SMN2* gene function can predict severity of disease phenotype. It is estimated there are 2% *de novo* mutations where only one parent is identified as a carrier.

SMA IV (adult onset) may be autosomal recessive, linked to *SMN*, but a large percentage of cases are autosomal dominant.

Clinical features

Features common to all forms of SMA:

- Progressive symmetric weakness (proximal > distal).
- Preserved sensation.
- Reduced or absent deep tendon reflexes.
- Normal cognitive function.
- Distal tremors of extremities (older patients).

SMA I (Werdnig–Hoffman disease)

- Severe generalized muscle weakness and hypotonia at birth or within the first 6 months of life ('floppy infant' syndrome).
- Death from respiratory failure usually occurs within the first 2 years.
- Paradoxical respirations due to initial sparing of diaphragm strength with weak intercostal muscles (bell-shaped chest).
- Lower cranial nuclei involvement leads to poor suck and swallow, resulting in dependence on tube feeding and tongue weakness with fasciculations.

SMA II (intermediate or childhood onset)

- Children can sit, but cannot stand or walk unaided.
- Survive beyond 2 years.
- Bulbar weakness may compromise nutritional status.
- Scoliosis and joint contractures are common with advancing age.

SMA III (juvenile onset: Kugelberg–Welander disease)

- Onset is in childhood or adolescence (18 months–18 years) with difficult walking due to hip-girdle weakness.
- Bulbar musculature is spared.
- Scoliosis and joint contractures often develop during the course of the disease.
- Variable course of progression with loss of walking in childhood or preservation of ambulation into early adulthood.
- Compatible with a normal life span.

Type IV (adult onset)

- Uncommon (less than 10% of all SMA).
- Proximal leg weakness (difficulty getting out of chair, climbing stairs, and so on) with eventual progression to proximal arm weakness.
- Fasciculations common.
- Preservation of walking (although possibly with assistive devices) for decades.
- Respiratory and bulbar weakness are not common.

Differential diagnosis

- SMA I is included in the differential of 'floppy infant': Pompe disease, congenital myopathy, congenital muscular dystrophy, congenital myotonic dystrophy, congenital myasthenia gravis.
- Non-5q SMA:
  - Spinobulbar muscular atrophy (Kennedy's syndrome) (see p. 774).
  - Spinal muscular atrophy with respiratory distress:
    - Autosomal recessive.
    - Onset within 3 months of birth.
    - Paralysis of hemidiaphragm.
  - Scapuloperoneal SMA (autosomal dominant).
  - Tay–Sachs disease:
    - Autosomal recessive.
    - Motor neuronopathy with cerebellar degeneration and cognitive decline.
  - Fazio–Londe disease ('progressive bulbar paresis of childhood'):
    - Autosomal recessive.
    - Lower cranial nuclei affected only.
    - Onset first and second decade.
  - Distal SMA:
    - Weakness and wasting of distal muscles only (lower extremities followed by gradual upper extremity involvement).
    - May mimic hereditary sensorimotor neuropathies (Charcot –Marie–Tooth disease) but no sensory symptoms.
    - Juvenile or adult onset with variety of genetic syndromes and inheritance patterns described.
  - Monomelic amyotrophy (Hirayama disease):
    - Distal asymmetric upper extremity weakness and atrophy in young adult men.
    - Predominantly affecting C7–T1 myotomes.
    - May have brisk reflexes in a weak limb.
    - Rare progression to generalized disease has been reported.
- ALS(see p. 764).
- Muscular dystrophy:
  - Limb-girdle forms.
  - Dystrophinopathy (Becker muscular dystrophy).
- Inflammatory myopathies (polymyositis, dermatomyositis).
- Neuromuscular disorders (myasthenia gravis, Lambert–Eaton myasthenic syndrome).
- Neuropathy (chronic inflammatory demyelinating polyneuropathy [CIDP], multifocal motor neuropathy, Guillain–Barré syndrome, hereditary motor neuropathy, Charcot–Marie–Tooth disease).

Investigations

- *SMN* gene deletion test:
  - If positive for homozygous *SMN1* deletion, no further testing is required.
  - If negative for deletion, but clinical suspicion remains high, further genetic analysis for a combination of mutation in one copy of *SMN1* with deletion of the second copy.
- Serum creatine kinase: normal in SMA I and SMA II, mildly elevated in later onset disease.
- Nerve conduction studies and EMG: denervation with normal sensory responses and normal motor conduction velocities.
- Muscle biopsy: evidence of skeletal muscle denervation with groups of atrophic and hypertrophic fibers and type grouping (in chronic cases).

Diagnosis

Diagnosis is confirmed by positive genetic testing for homozygous loss of *SMN* (deletion or 'loss of function' mutation).

- Electrophysiology:
  - Nerve conduction studies: normal sensory nerve action potentials, motor nerve conduction velocities >70% normal for age.
  - Needle EMG: abnormal spontaneous activity, e.g. fibrillations, positive sharp waves, and fasciculations. Increased mean duration and amplitude of motor unit potentials by EMG.
- Histopathology of muscle (**716**):
  - Groups of atrophic muscle fibers of both types.
  - Hypertrophic fibers of type 1.
  - Type grouping (chronic cases).

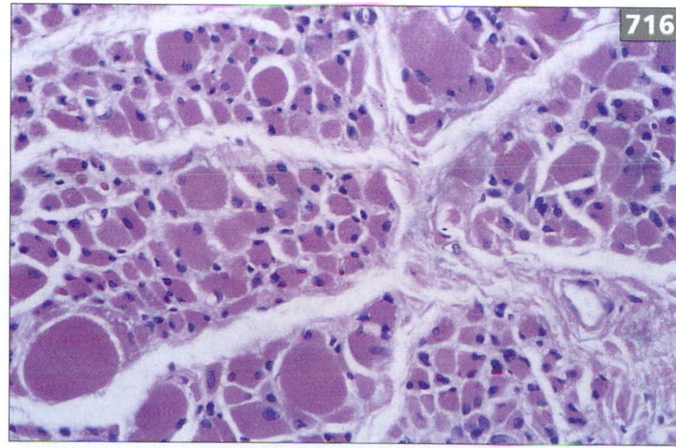

716 Muscle biopsy, H&E stain, showing denervation atrophy. Several fascicles consist of atrophic fibers containing dark pyknotic nuclei, indicating denervation of muscle.

In congenital SMA, these characteristic features may not be present. Instead, there are small fibers of both types. In SMA IV, there may be a concomitant myopathic pattern.

Pathology

Loss of anterior horn cells in the spinal cord and lower cranial nuclei with degeneration of lower motor neurons, typical signs of axonal degeneration (reduction of myelin and dystrophic axons with shrunken and condensed axon structures). Muscle shows grouped atrophy with large type 1 fibers and smaller type 2 fibers.

Treatment

There is no specific therapy for SMA. A multidisciplinary team approach is required involving the neurologist, primary physician, geneticist, physical and occupational therapists, speech/swallowing therapist, respiratory therapist, and social worker[12].

Disease progression leads to the following categories of symptoms and complications:

- Pulmonary decline causing sleep-disordered breathing and ineffective cough/clearance of secretions.
- Gastrointestinal dysfunction characterized by feeding and swallowing problems.
- Orthopedic complications such as spinal deformities, contractures, osteopenia.

Genetic counseling should be given to families for discussion of prenatal genetic testing for carrier status.

Prognosis

The prognosis depends on the age of onset and subtype:

- SMA I: death before age 2.
- SMA II: death after age 2.
- SMA III and SMA IV: normal life span.

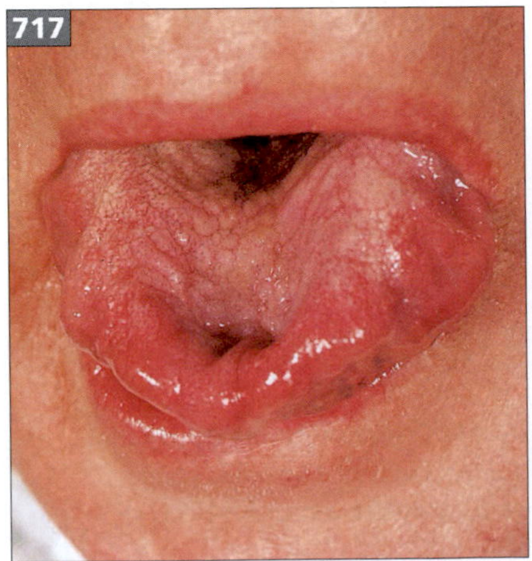

X-LINKED BULBOSPINAL MUSCULAR ATROPHY (KENNEDY'S SYNDROME)

Definition and epidemiology

This syndrome is also known as X-linked spinobulbar neuronopathy, due to the identification of both sensory and motor neuron involvement.

- Incidence 1 in 50,000, but increased in Japanese and Finnish populations.
- Males only due to X-linked inheritance, but female carriers (heterozygotes) can manifest a mild form.
- Age: onset second to seventh decade.

Etiology and pathophysiology

The gene is localized to Xq21–22, where a tandem repeat of CAG in the androgen receptor disrupts the gene:

- Encodes a receptor with abnormal folding which leads to a toxic 'gain of function'.
- Expansion of the CAG zone to greater than 38 repeats (normal <34 repeats) is characteristic of disease.
- Longer CAG repeats are associated with earlier onset of disease and increased severity of symptoms.

Clinical features

Motor findings include:

- Symmetric, slowly progressive weakness affecting the limbs and bulbar muscles.
- Early symptoms may be fatigue, decreased exercise tolerance, myalgias.
- Cramps and tremors.
- Atrophy and muscle twitching are common, especially in face, chin, and tongue (717).
- No UMN findings.
- Reflexes are reduced or absent.

Sensory findings may include subtle or asymptomatic loss of vibration. Endocrinologically, patients may show:

- Gynecomastia (may be asymptomatic).
- Testicular atrophy.
- Oligospermia with reduced fertility.

Differential diagnosis

- MNDs (ALS, adult-onset SMA).
- Neuromuscular junction disorders (myasthenia gravis, Lambert–Eaton myasthenic syndrome).
- Myopathies (inflammatory myopathies, limb-girdle muscular dystrophies).
- Neuropathies (CIDP, multifocal motor neuropathy).

717 Wasting and fasciculations of the tongue in a man with X-linked recessive bulbar and spinal neuronopathy (Kennedy's syndrome).

Investigations

- Nerve conduction studies: reduced amplitude motor and sensory responses with preserved conduction velocities.
- Needle EMG: chronic denervation with prominent fasciculations.
- Genetic testing for abnormal expansion of the trinucleotide (CAG) repeat in the first exon of the androgen receptor gene on the X chromosome confirms diagnosis.

Treatment

There is no known definitive treatment. Supportive therapies should focus on maintenance of ambulation and use of noninvasive ventilation if needed.

Prognosis

Considered to have the 'best' course of all MNDs, normal life span is expected. Loss of ambulation decades after onset of symptoms is possible.

REFERENCES

1 Matz PG, Anderson PA, Holly LT, *et al.* (2009). The natural history of cervical spondylotic myelopathy. *J Neurosurg Spine* **11**(2):104–111.

2 Jacob A, Weinshenker BG (2008). An approach to the diagnosis of acute transverse myelitis. *Semin Neurol* **28**(1):105–120.

3 Wingerchuk DM, Lennon VA, Lucchinetti CF, Pittock SJ, Weinshenker BG (2007). The spectrum of neuromyelitis optica. *Lancet Neurol* **6**(9):805–815.

4 McArthur JC, Brew BJ, Nath A (2005). Neurological complications of HIV infection. *Lancet Neurol* **4**(9):543–555.

5 Kumar N (2006). Copper deficiency myelopathy (human swayback). *Mayo Clin Proc* **81**(10):1371–1384.

6 Novy J, Carruzzo A, Maeder P, Bogousslavsky J (2006). Spinal cord ischemia: clinical and imaging patterns, pathogenesis, and outcomes in 27 patients. *Arch Neurol* **63**(8):1113–1120.

7 Batzdorf U (2005). Primary spinal syringomyelia. *J Neurosurg Spine* **3**(6):429–435.

8 Depienne C, Stevanin G, Brice A, Durr A (2007). Hereditary spastic paraplegias: an update. *Curr Opin Neurol* **20**(6):674–680.

9 Traul DE, Shaffrey ME, Schiff D (2007). Part I: Spinal cord neoplasms–intradural neoplasms. *Lancet Oncol* **8**(1):35–45.

10 Miller RG, Jackson CE, Kasarskis EJ, *et al.* (2009). Practice parameter update: The care of the patient with amyotrophic lateral sclerosis: Drug, nutritional, and respiratory therapies (an evidence-based review): Report of the Quality Standards Subcommittee of the American Academy of Neurology. *Neurology* **73**(15):1218–1226.

11 Miller RG, Jackson CE, Kasarskis EJ, *et al.* (2009). Practice parameter update: The care of the patient with amyotrophic lateral sclerosis: Multidisciplinary care, symptom management, and cognitive/behavioral impairment (an evidence-based review): Report of the Quality Standards Subcommittee of the American Academy of Neurology. *Neurology* **73**(15):1227–1233.

12 Wang CH, Finkel RS, Bertini ES, *et al.* (2007). Consensus statement for standard of care in spinal muscular atrophy. *J Child Neurol* **22**(8):1027–1049.

Further reading

Cervical spondylotic myelopathy

Baron EM, Young WF (2007). Cervical spondylotic myelopathy: a brief review of its pathophysiology, clinical course, and diagnosis. *Neurosurgery* **60**(1 Suppl 1):S35–S41.

Inflammatory myelopathy

Hu W, Lucchinetti CF (2009). The pathological spectrum of CNS inflammatory demyelinating diseases. *Semin Immunopathol* **31**(4):439–53.

Pittock SJ, Lucchinetti CF (2006). Inflammatory transverse myelitis: evolving concepts. *Curr Opin Neurol* **19**(4):362–368.

Tenembaum S, Chitnis T, Ness J, Hahn JS; International Pediatric MS Study Group (2007). Acute disseminated encephalomyelitis. *Neurology* **68**(16 Suppl 2):S23–S36.

Infectious myelopathy

Araujo AQ, Silva MT (2006). The HTLV-1 neurological complex. *Lancet Neurol* **5**(12):1068–1076.

Di Rocco A, Werner P, Bottiglieri T, *et al.* (2004). Treatment of AIDS-associated myelopathy with L-methionine: a placebo-controlled study. *Neurology* **63**(7):1270–1275.

Irani DN (2008). Aseptic meningitis and viral myelitis. *Neurol Clin* **26**(3):635, 655, vii–viii.

Kincaid O, Lipton HL (2006). Viral myelitis: an update. *Curr Neurol Neurosci Rep* **6**(6):469–474.

Oh U, Jacobson S (2008). Treatment of HTLV-I-associated myelopathy/tropical spastic paraparesis: toward rational targeted therapy. *Neurol Clin* **26**(3):781–797, ix–x.

Power C, Boisse L, Rourke S, Gill MJ (2009). NeuroAIDS: an evolving epidemic. *Can J Neurol Sci* **36**(3):285–295.

Puccioni-Sohler M, Rios M, Carvalho SM, *et al.* (2001). Diagnosis of HAM/TSP based on CSF proviral HTLV-I DNA and HTLV-I antibody index. *Neurology* **57**(4):725–727.

Wright EJ, Brew BJ, Wesselingh SL (2008). Pathogenesis and diagnosis of viral infections of the nervous system. *Neurol Clin* **26**(3):617–633, vii.

Metabolic and toxic myelopathies

Singer MA, Lazaridis C, Nations SP, Wolfe GI (2008). Reversible nitrous oxide-induced myeloneuropathy with pernicious anemia: case report and literature review. *Muscle Nerve* **37**(1):125–129.

Winston GP, Jaiser SR (2008). Copper deficiency myelopathy and subacute combined degeneration of the cord – why is the phenotype so similar? *Med Hypotheses* **71**(2):229–236.

Vascular myelopathies

Atkinson JL, Miller GM, Krauss WE, *et al.* (2001). Clinical and radiographic features of dural arteriovenous fistula, a treatable cause of myelopathy. *Mayo Clin Proc* **76**(11):1120–1130.

Masson C, Pruvo JP, Meder JF, *et al.* (2004). Spinal cord infarction: clinical and magnetic resonance imaging findings and short term outcome. *J Neurol Neurosurg Psychiatry* **75**(10):1431–1435.

Nedeltchev K, Loher TJ, Stepper F, *et al.* (2004). Long-term outcome of acute spinal cord ischemia syndrome. *Stroke* **35**(2):560–565.

Shinoyama M, Takahashi T, Shimizu H, Tominaga T, Suzuki M (2005). Spinal cord infarction demonstrated by diffusion-weighted magnetic resonance imaging. *J Clin Neurosci* **12**(4):466–468.

Structural myelopathies

Brodbelt AR, Stoodley MA (2003). Post-traumatic syringomyelia: a review. *J Clin Neurosci* **10**(4):401–408.

Fernandez AA, Guerrero AI, Martinez MI, *et al.* (2009). Malformations of the craniocervical junction (Chiari type I and syringomyelia: classification, diagnosis and treatment). *BMC Musculoskelet Disord* **10**(Suppl 1):S1.

Greitz D (2006). Unraveling the riddle of syringomyelia. *Neurosurg Rev* **29**(4):251–263; discussion 264.

Hereditary myelopathies

Powers JM, DeCiero DP, Ito M, Moser AB, Moser HW (2000). Adrenomyeloneuropathy: a neuropathologic review featuring its noninflammatory myelopathy. *J Neuropathol Exp Neurol* **59**(2):89–102.

Salinas S, Proukakis C, Crosby A, Warner TT (2008). Hereditary spastic paraplegia: clinical features and pathogenetic mechanisms. *Lancet Neurol* **7**(12):1127–1138.

Schiffmann R, van der Knaap MS (2004). The latest on leukodystrophies. *Curr Opin Neurol* **17**(2):187–192.

Spinal cord tumors

Binning M, Klimo P, Jr, Gluf W, Goumnerova L (2007). Spinal tumors in children. *Neurosurg Clin N Am* **18**(4):631–658.

Ecker RD, Endo T, Wetjen NM, Krauss WE (2005). Diagnosis and treatment of vertebral column metastases. *Mayo Clin Proc* **80**(9):1177–1186.

Rossi A, Gandolfo C, Morana G, Tortori-Donati P (2007). Tumors of the spine in children. *Neuroimaging Clin N Am* **17**(1):17–35.

Sansur CA, Pouratian N, Dumont AS, Schiff D, Shaffrey CI, Shaffrey ME (2007). Part II: Spinal-cord neoplasms – primary tumours of the bony spine and adjacent soft tissues. *Lancet Oncol* **8**(2):137–147.

Myelopathies associated with motor neuron disease (amyotrophic lateral sclerosis [ALS])

Armon C (2003). An evidence-based medicine approach to the evaluation of the role of exogenous risk factors in sporadic amyotrophic lateral sclerosis. *Neuroepidemiology* **22**(4):217–228.

de Carvalho M, Dengler R, Eisen A, *et al.* (2008). Electrodiagnostic criteria for diagnosis of ALS. *Clin Neurophysiol* **119**(3):497–503.

Dion PA, Daoud H, Rouleau GA (2009). Genetics of motor neuron disorders: new insights into pathogenic mechanisms. *Nat Rev Genet* **10**(11):769–782.

Gouveia LO, de Carvalho M (2007). Young-onset sporadic amyotrophic lateral sclerosis: a distinct nosological entity? *Amyotroph Lateral Scler* **8**(6):323–327.

Horner RD, Kamins KG, Feussner JR, *et al.* (2003). Occurrence of amyotrophic lateral sclerosis among Gulf War veterans. *Neurology* **61**(6):742–749.

Mackenzie IR, Rademakers R (2008). The role of transactive response DNA-binding protein-43 in amyotrophic lateral sclerosis and frontotemporal dementia. *Curr Opin Neurol* **21**(6):693–700.

Pugdahl K, Fuglsang-Frederiksen A, de Carvalho M, *et al.* (2007). Generalised sensory system abnormalities in amyotrophic lateral sclerosis: a European multicentre study. *J Neurol Neurosurg Psychiatry* **78**(7):746–749.

Radunovic A, Annane D, Jewitt K, Mustfa N (2009). Mechanical ventilation for amyotrophic lateral sclerosis/motor neuron disease. *Cochrane Database Syst Rev* **4**:CD004427.

Tripodoro VA, De Vito EL (2008). Management of dyspnea in advanced motor neuron diseases. *Curr Opin Support Palliat Care* **2**(3):173–179.

Van Damme P, Robberecht W (2009). Recent advances in motor neuron disease. *Curr Opin Neurol* **22**(5):486–492.

Wijesekera LC, Leigh PN (2009). Amyotrophic lateral sclerosis. *Orphanet J Rare Dis* **4**:3.

Wijesekera LC, Mathers S, Talman P, *et al.* (2009). Natural history and clinical features of the flail arm and flail leg ALS variants. *Neurology* **72**(12):1087–1094.

Myelopathies associated with motor neuron disease (non-ALS)

Finsterer J (2009). Bulbar and spinal muscular atrophy (Kennedy's disease): a review. *Eur J Neurol* **16**(5):556–561.

Lunn MR, Wang CH (2008). Spinal muscular atrophy. *Lancet* **371**(9630):2120–2133.

AUTONOMIC NERVOUS SYSTEM DISORDERS

Robert Henderson, Judy Spies

AUTONOMIC NEUROPATHY

Definition

Autonomic neuropathy is a disorder of the autonomic nervous system.

Anatomy

The autonomic nervous system consists of two major divisions that have complementary function: sympathetic and parasympathetic (**718**). There are nicotinic cholinergic receptors for the pre-ganglionic receptors, adrenergic receptors for sympathetic organs, and muscarinic cholinergic end-organ receptors for the parasympathetic organs and sympathetic receptors in the skin.

Sympathetic nervous system

Sympathetic nerve fibers descend from the hypothalamus and other regions of the brain, through the midbrain, pons, and medulla, to the intermediolateral cell columns of the spinal cord. Between T1 and L2, pre-ganglionic sympathetic fibers exit from the spinal cord with the anterior nerve roots of peripheral nerves, before separating to join the sympathetic chain which consists of a series of nerve ganglia in a pre-vertebral or pre-aortic region.

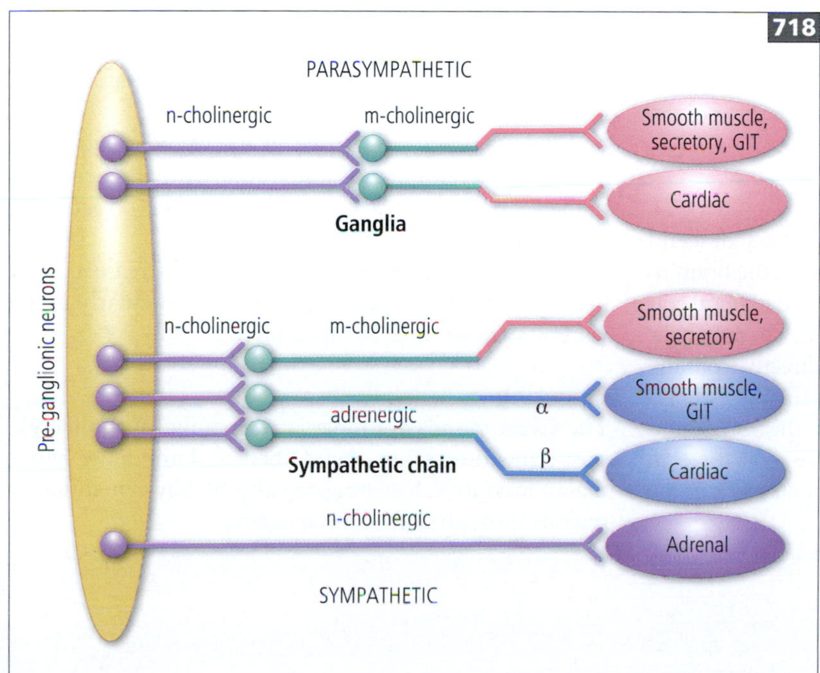

718 Components of the autonomic nervous system, including the main sympathetic and parasympathetic divisions, pre- and post-ganglionic pathways, and messaging systems: n- (nicotinic) cholinergic, m- (muscarinic) cholinergic, and adrenergic. α, β: alpha and beta adrenoreceptors; GIT: gastrointestinal tract.

Pre-ganglionic sympathetic fibers which have nicotinic cholinergic properties enter the sympathetic chain synapsing with ganglia within the chain, or pass through the chain to synapse at more peripheral ganglia such as the celiac or other mesenteric ganglia and the adrenal medulla.

Post-ganglionic sympathetic fibers join the different nerves within the body and are distributed to the different sympathetic organ systems, where alpha and beta adrenoceptors increase or decrease activity and contract or relax muscles to play a role in the control of vasomotor tone and the regulation of regional blood flow in the:

- Blood vessels (vascular smooth muscle particularly eye, salivary and lacrimal glands, sexual and sphincter organs, skin, visceral and endocrine organs, bronchioles, and arteries such as coronary, renal, and cerebral arteries).
- Heart (cardiac muscle, sinoatrial and atrioventricular nodes).

The sympathetic nervous system also influences sweat gland secretions through both adrenergic and cholinergic (muscarinic) receptors. Pre-ganglionic fibers responsible for sweating and vasomotor control in the face synapse in the superior cervical ganglion before joining the trigeminal nerve supplying facial skin.

Pre-ganglionic sympathetic fibers to the bladder travel from the intermediolateral columns in the T11–L2 segments of the spinal cord to the corresponding nerve roots, and hence to the hypogastric plexus. Post-ganglionic fibers join the subserosal plexus on the bladder wall and innervate mainly the trigone and neck of the bladder.

For the cranial nerves, preganglionic sympathetic fibers to the eye leave the spinal cord at T1 to synapse in the superior cervical ganglion. Post-ganglionic fibers travel from the superior cervical ganglion along the carotid artery joining the ophthalmic (first) division of the trigeminal nerve and travel to the pupil.

Parasympathetic nervous system

Parasympathetic pre-ganglionic nerve fibers descend from the hypothalamus and other regions of the brain to the brainstem and then travel in the intermediolateral columns of the spinal cord to the sacral region. The parasympathetic pre-ganglionic nerve fibers exit directly from the brainstem as part of cranial nerves (CN) III, VII, XI, and X, and also from the sacral spinal cord in the S2, S3, and S4 nerve roots. The fibers in the S2–4 nerve roots travel in pelvic nerves to form a diffuse subserosal network in the bladder wall and also in sexual organs.

Pre-ganglionic parasympathetic fibers are long and post-ganglionic fibers are short, because the ganglia lie close to the innervated structures. Parasympathetic fibers innervate the following:

- Pupillary and ciliary muscles (via CN III, the ciliary ganglion, and ciliary nerve).
- Lacrimal, submandibular and sublingual glands (CN VII, and branches of the greater superficial petrosal and chorda tympani nerves).
- Parotid gland (CN IX).
- Thoracic and abdominal viscera (CN X).
- Bladder smooth muscle fibers, large bowel, and genital system (sacral outflow).

Post-ganglionic fibers in the parasympathetic nervous system are muscarinic cholinergic.

Tip

► *The sympathetic nervous system has nicotinic cholinergic pre-ganglionic fibers, and both adrenergic and muscarinic cholinergic post-ganglionic fibers that arise from the sympathetic chain (T1–L2). The parasympathetic nervous system has muscarinic cholinergic post-ganglionic fibers that arise from cranial nerves and sacral nerves.*

Physiology ('fight or flight, rest and digest')

Blood pressure and heart rate

These are controlled by baroreflex pathways. Baroreceptors in the carotid body, aortic arch, and other thoracic regions respond to alterations in blood pressure (BP), and send information from the carotid body (via afferent fibers in the glossopharyngeal nerve) and from the aortic arch and thoracic low pressure receptors (via fibers in the vagus nerve) to the nucleus of the tractus solitarius in the brainstem.

Efferent fibers are carried in the vagus nerve to the heart and visceral organs and in the sympathetic nerves to the heart, mesenteric vascular bed, and blood vessels in the skin and muscles.

A fall in BP results in a compensatory increase in heart rate and peripheral vasoconstriction (particularly in the visceral vascular bed) to maintain BP.

Sweating

The sweat glands are innervated mainly by cholinergic post-ganglionic sympathetic fibers and are under hypothalamic control. Sweating can also be driven in different regions through central mechanisms.

Bladder and bowel

Afferent

- Parasympathetic afferent fibers convey sensations of bladder fullness and pain of overdistension and overcontraction. They also mediate the reflex for bladder contraction through S2–4 segments.
- Sympathetic afferent fibers transmit painful sensation from the trigone area and a sensation of bladder fullness. They play no part in the micturition reflex.
- Somatic fibers in the pudendal nerve convey sensations from the urethra and sphincter of urethral pain and temperature, urine passing, and bladder emptying.

Efferent

- Parasympathetic efferent impulses cause the detrusor muscles of the bladder to contract and the bladder neck to shorten, thus allowing the passage of urine.
- Sympathetic efferents may inhibit the detrusor, but do not play a role in the act of micturition.
- During ejaculation, sympathetic activity causes the bladder neck to contract, preventing retrograde ejaculation.
- Somatic fibers in the pudendal nerve (S2–4) innervate the external sphincter of the bladder and the anal sphincter, causing relaxation of the sphincter during micturition (as the detrusor is contracting). It can also be voluntarily contracted to terminate the act of micturition.

Pupillary reflexes

Light reflex

The normal pupil contracts briskly in the eye to which the light is directed (direct response) and also in the opposite eye (consensual response). The afferent pathway is from the retina, along the optic nerve, to the optic tract, where fibers separate from those destined for the lateral geniculate body and go to the pretectal region and then to part of the cranial nerve III nucleus (Edinger–Westphal nucleus) of both sides.

The efferent pathway is from both Edinger–Westphal nuclei via the IIIrd cranial nerves to the pupils, accounting for both the direct and consensual light reflexes.

Accommodation reflex

- Normal pupils constrict as the eyes converge ('near response').
- Pathways descend from the parieto-occipital cortex to the Edinger–Westphal nucleus in the midbrain, and then as pupilloconstrictor fibers in both IIIrd nerves to the pupil.

Etiology and pathophysiology

Autonomic disorders may be localized (e.g. Horner's syndrome) or generalized (e.g. pure autonomic failure).

Autonomic disorders affecting the central nervous system

- Major component of autonomic failure: autonomic failure with multiple system atrophy (MSA-A) and advanced Parkinson's disease[1].
- Minor component of autonomic failure: miscellaneous disorders such as stroke, multiple sclerosis, spinal cord lesions, and Wernicke's encephalopathy.

Tip

▶ *Autonomic disorders can be subdivided into localized or general, peripheral or central, primary or secondary, and acute or chronic. In many disorders, the autonomic dysfunction is a minor component.*

Disorders affecting the peripheral nervous system

Disorders with no associated large-fiber peripheral neuropathy

- Acute and subacute autonomic neuropathy:
  - Mainly adrenergic manifesting as predominantly orthostatic intolerance.
  - Predominantly cholinergic resulting in gastrointestinal, pupillary, and sweating disorders.
  - Acute pandysautonomia, (equivalent to Guillain–Barré syndrome restricted to the autonomic nervous system)[2].
- Chronic autonomic neuropathy:
  - Cholinergic – chronic anhidrosis manifesting as heat intolerance or a chronic enteric neuropathy.
  - Adrenergic – manifesting as orthostatic hypotension.
  - Pandysautonomia.
- Disorders associated with involvement of acetylcholine receptors:
  - Botulism.
  - Lambert–Eaton myasthenic syndrome.

Disorders associated with peripheral neuropathy

- Major component of autonomic failure:
  - Diabetes.
  - Acute inflammatory polyradiculopathy (Guillain–Barré syndrome).
  - Acute intermittent porphyria.
  - Primary and secondary amyloidosis.
  - Familial dysautonomia (hereditary sensory and autonomic neuropathy).
  - Sjögren's syndrome and, rarely, other connective tissue disorders.
  - Chronic idiopathic sensory and autonomic neuropathy.
- Minor component of autonomic failure:
  - Alcoholism and nutritional diseases.
  - Toxic neuropathies (vincristine and other newer chemotherapeutic agents, acrylamide, heavy metals).
  - Metabolic disorders (vitamin B12 deficiency, chronic renal failure).
  - Malignancy.
  - Chronic inflammatory demyelinating neuropathy.
  - Human immunodeficiency virus (HIV)-associated neuropathy.

Drugs which may affect the autonomic nervous system

- All drugs with anticholinergic effect including antidepressants (especially the tricyclic group).
- Antihypertensive drugs especially vasodilators and sympathetic blocking agents.
- Alpha-adrenergic blocking drugs (e.g. as used in prostatic obstruction).
- Atropine and ciliary blocking drugs.

Clinical features

The most common clinical manifestations of autonomic dysfunction are:

- Postural (orthostatic) hypotension.
- Erectile and ejaculatory dysfunction.
- Bladder dysfunction.
- Abnormalities of sweating.
- Vasomotor disturbances.

Sympathetic adrenergic failure

- Postural hypotension.
- Ejaculatory failure.

Sympathetic cholinergic failure

- Anhidrosis.

Parasympathetic failure

- Fixed heart rate.
- Sluggish urinary bladder and bowel.
- Gastrointestinal motility impairment.
- Erectile failure.

Eye

Pupillary reflexes represent both sympathetic and parasympathetic function.

Light reflex

Lesions of cranial nerve III, which carries efferent parasympathetic fibers, cause ipsilateral pupil dilatation. Shining a light into either eye fails to evoke a direct or consensual response in the affected eye, because of the defect in the efferent arc of the reflex. However, shining a light in the eye ipsilateral to the lesion (the affected eye) evokes a consensual reaction in the eye contralateral to the lesion (the unaffected eye) because of the preserved afferent pathway.

Accommodation reflex

Any lesion involving the pupilloconstrictor muscle fibers will impair the reaction of accommodation. Selective impairment of accommodation may occur in some midbrain lesions such as a craniopharyngioma and its treatment.

Horner's syndrome

- Ptosis.
- Anisocoria.
- Dry eyes, rarely excessive lacrimation.

Sudomotor system

- Sweating abnormalities (anhidrosis, e.g. odorous socks and undergarments, but occasionally gustatory facial sweating; regional hyperhidrosis, e.g. palms and axilla).
- Heat intolerance.

Cardiovascular system

Postural (orthostatic hypotension): symptoms include lightheadedness, dizziness, faintness, visual disturbances, or loss of consciousness (syncope) on standing upright. It is usually defined as a fall in systolic BP of at least 20 mmHg or to <80 mmHg within a minute or two of standing, but such falls are neither sensitive nor specific (e.g. they can occur in the normal asymptomatic elderly or with cardiac failure).

Gastrointestinal system

- Constipation.
- Diarrhea, e.g. nocturnal.
- Post-prandial bloating.
- Abdominal discomfort.

Renal and urinary bladder

- Nocturia.
- Frequency and urgency.
- Incontinence.
- Retention of urine.

Reproductive system

- Erectile and ejaculatory failure.

Involvement of other neurologic systems may help clarify the etiology of the autonomic failure:

- Extrapyramidal, cerebellar or pyramidal dysfunction (MSA).
- Motor and sensory dysfunction (peripheral neuropathy).

Examples of conditions with prominent involvement of the autonomic nervous system

- Pure autonomic failure (PAF)[3]:
  - Degeneration of peripheral autonomic fibers of uncertain cause.
  - Age of onset: 40–60 years.
  - Postural hypotension (dizziness and weakness on standing or walking).
  - Erectile failure.
  - Bowel and bladder disturbances.
  - Loss of sweating.
  - Normal neurologic examination (which separates PAF from MSA where involvement of other CNS systems occurs).
  - Slowly progressive course.
- Small fiber neuropathy[4]:
  - Degeneration of distal small somatic and autonomic nerve fibers.
  - Age of onset: usually greater than 60 years.
  - Painful, burning feet and rarely hands; allodynia.
  - Normal neurologic examination apart from distal loss of temperature and altered sensation.

Diagnosis

The clinical approach to the patient with clinical features of dysautonomia aims to determine:

- Whether autonomic function is affected.
- Which organ systems are affected.
- The site of the lesion (central, pre-ganglionic, or post-ganglionic).
- The cause of the lesion.

Investigations

Is autonomic function normal or abnormal? A number of sources summarize approaches to investigation of autonomic neuropathies[5,6].

Blood pressure

- Change of blood pressure (BP) with posture (postural hypotension) (**719**):
  - Normally, changing from the supine to the standing position does not alter BP, apart from a narrowing of the pulse pressure, i.e. an increase in the diastolic BP.
  - A fall exceeding 20–30 mmHg is abnormal, indicating significant postural hypotension.
  - Autonomic neuropathies involving sympathetic function are associated with postural hypotension.

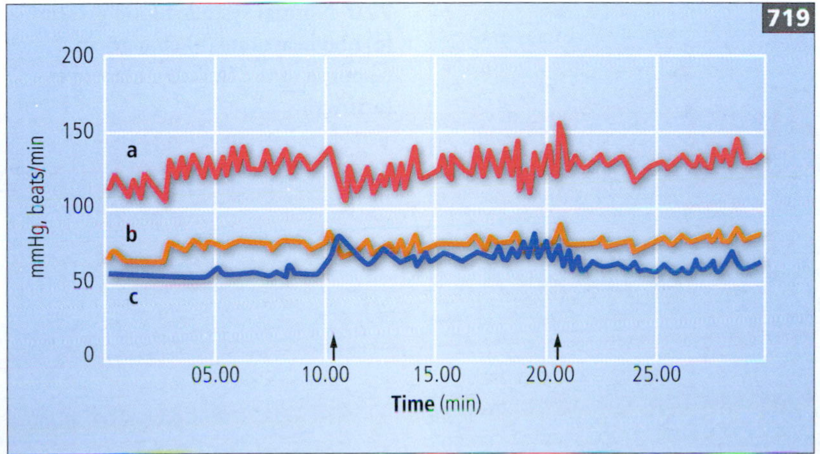

719 Normal systolic blood pressure (a), diastolic blood pressure (b), and heart rate (c) in response to tilting (arrows).

Heart rate

- Change of heart rate (HR) with posture (reflex tachycardia):
  - Normally, changing from the supine to the standing position increases the HR by about 11–29 beats per minute, reaching a maximum after 15 beats, after which a reflex bradycardia may ensue, reaching a maximum at about the 30th beat.
  - The ratio of the R–R interval (heart period) on an electrocardiogram (ECG) corresponding to the 30th and 15th beats, is the 30:15 ratio. The ratio is normally considerably greater than one, but varies with age.
  - Autonomic neuropathies affecting the parasympathetic function reduce the rise in HR associated with a change of posture, and reduce the 30:15 ratio.
- Change of HR with deep breathing (sinus arrhythmia):
  - Normally, inspiration is associated with an increase in HR and expiration with a decrease in HR (sinus arrhythmia). This difference is less pronounced in older individuals.
  - Autonomic neuropathies involving parasympathetic function are associated with impaired variation of the HR with respiration (loss of sinus arrhythmia).
- Valsalva maneuver (720): normally, forced expiration against a closed glottis or mouthpiece (Valsalva maneuver) alters the HR and BP:
  - Phase I: BP rises as the raised intrathoracic pressure associated with the Valsalva causes mechanical compression of the aorta and increased peripheral resistance. A compensatory fall in HR follows, mediated by the parasympathetic fibers in the vagus nerve.
  - Phase II: BP falls due to the fall in venous return (associated with continuously high intrathoracic pressure) and thus fall in stroke volume. A compensatory rise in HR (due to parasympathetic vagal withdrawal) and total peripheral resistance (due to peripheral vasoconstriction) follows.
  - Phase III: forced expiration ceases and venous return increases rapidly, increasing the stroke volume and BP and decreasing the HR.
  - Phase IV: BP rises further and overshoots because the peripheral circulation is still vasoconstricted for up to 30 seconds, because of the increase in peripheral sympathetic vasoconstrictor tone induced by stages II–III. Therefore, stage IV is a measure of sympathetic vascular tone.

The patient assumes the semi-recumbent posture and is asked to expire forcefully, maintaining a column of mercury at 40 mmHg pressure for 10–15 seconds, while the ECG and BP are continuously recorded. The ratio of the longest pulse interval to the shortest pulse interval recorded on the ECG during the maneuver (the Valsalva ratio) normally exceeds about 1.4 in young adults. Increased age and parasympathetic and sympathetic neuropathies are associated with a reduced ratio.

Other tests of autonomic function

Isometric contraction

Normally, sustained isometric contraction (e.g. a firm handgrip) for up to 5 minutes increases the HR (and thus cardiac output) and total peripheral resistance (by peripheral vasoconstriction), leading to an increase in systolic and diastolic BP. Diastolic BP rises by 15 mmHg or more. Autonomic neuropathies affecting sympathetic function are associated with an impaired response.

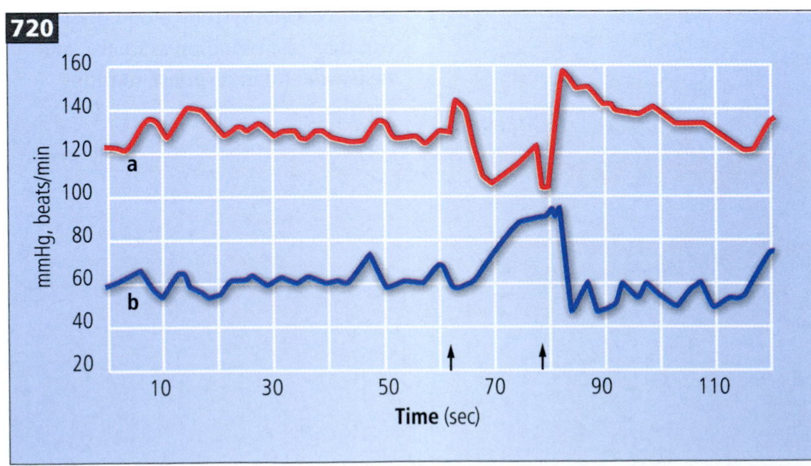

720 Normal systolic blood pressure (a) and heart rate (b) changes in response to the Valsalva maneuver (arrows).

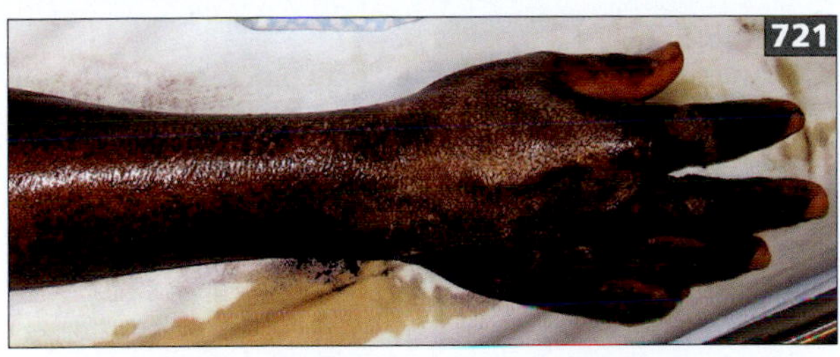

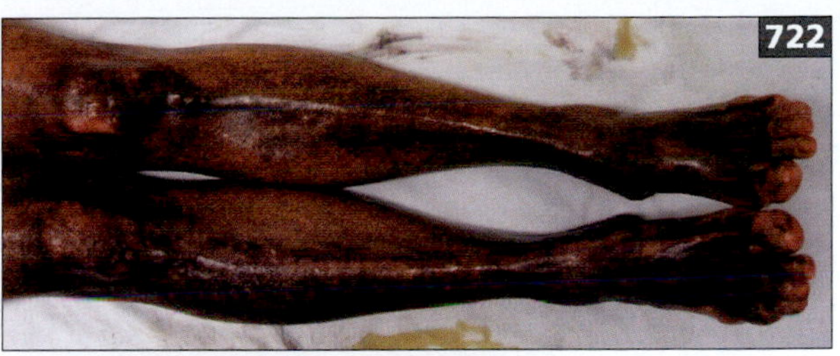

721, 722 Normal sweating of the arm and leg using a starch/iodine preparation.

723, 724 A length-dependent abnormality in sweating. Reduced sweating below the knee in a peripheral neuropathy (723), and reduced sweating following a sympathectomy (724).

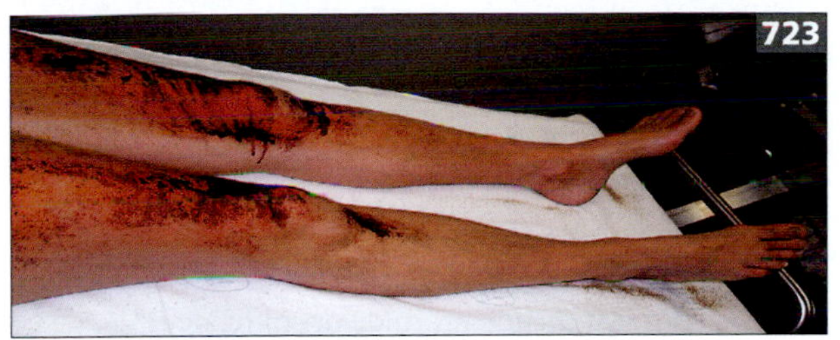

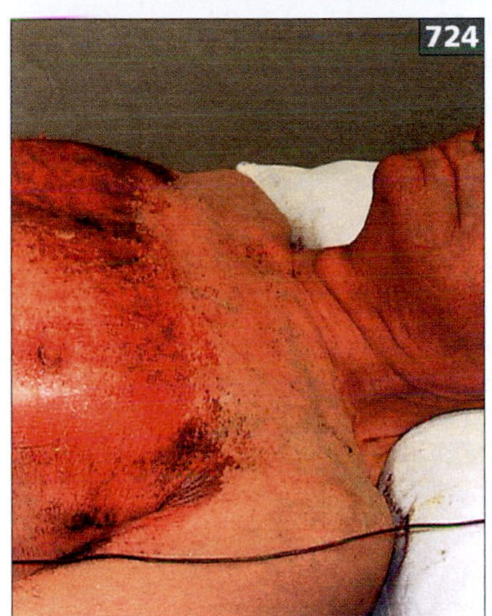

Response to emotional and other stimuli

Normally, mental arithmetic, a loud noise, or cold or painful stimuli usually evoke peripheral vasoconstriction and increase the total peripheral resistance and arterial blood pressure. In some normal people, this response may not be present. Autonomic neuropathies affecting sympathetic efferent fibers are associated with an impaired response.

Sweating

Autonomic neuropathies affecting sympathetic efferent fibers are associated with impaired sweating. The thermoregulatory sweat test (TST) determines the distribution of sweat loss (anhidrosis). The skin is covered with a powder such as alazarine red or a starch/iodine combination that changes color when sweating occurs. The patient is warmed by radiant heat sufficient to raise the body temperature by 1°C (1.8°F) (**721, 722**). Recognition of patterns of response is important (**723, 724**).

Local sweating may also be tested by injection or iontophoresis of acetylcholine, or by application of idioine-based preparations or pilocarpine which stimulates the sweat glands directly. The quantitative sudomotor axon reflex test is a test of post-ganglionic sympathetic sudomotor function. If the TST is abnormal (i.e. anhidrosis) and the quantitative sudomotor test is normal, then the site of the sympathetic lesion is pre-ganglionic, e.g. PAF or MSA.

Skin vasomotor reflexes are measured by laser Doppler flow meters (e.g. on the pulp of index finger) in response to stimuli such as standing, Valsalva, or cold water. This test is limited if the patient is nervous and resting skin blood flow is minimal.

Pupillary responses

- Metacholine (methacholine), instilled into the conjunctival sac, does not affect the size of the normal pupil but it causes pupillary constriction if parasympathetic innervation is impaired. This is because of the denervation supersensitivity of the constrictor muscle of the pupil.
- Epinephrine (adrenaline) has no effect on the normal pupil but causes pupillary dilatation if post-ganglionic sympathetic innervation is impaired, also because of denervation supersensitivity.
- Cocaine eye drops cause dilatation of the normal pupil because cocaine blocks the reuptake of norepinephrine (noradrenaline), but if peripheral sympathetic innervation is impaired, pupillary dilatation does not occur.

In addition to the above tests, a number of other tests of baroreflex sensitivity, vasomotor control, and bladder control exist, but are more difficult to perform.

Tip

▶ *Autonomic function tests are indirect measures that are usually not widely available. There are many possible tests; however, tests of BP and HR, and sweating function are the most commonly available.*

History, examination

Underlying and associated disorders, such as diabetes mellitus and amyloidosis (see above), need to be excluded. Seropositivity for antibodies that bind to, or block, ganglionic acetylcholine receptors identifies patients with various forms of autoimmune autonomic neuropathy and distinguishes these disorders from other types of dysautonomia[7]. However, these tests are not commercially performed in Australia and many other countries.

Tip

▶ *Finding and treating the underlying cause is important; however, many autonomic neuropathies remain idiopathic. Important disorders with prominent primary autonomic involvement include amyloid neuropathy, PAF, and MSA.*

Treatment

Aims to remove the underlying cause if possible, and relieve symptoms.

Postural hypotension[8]

General advice

- Maintain hydration and salt intake (150 mmol/l [150 mEq] salt): urinary sodium excretion can be measured as a guide.
- Avoid dehydration, diuretics, and other hypotensive drugs and deconditioning.
- Rise slowly from the lying and sitting positions, particularly in the morning, after hot baths, and heavy meals.
- Avoid straining and extremes of temperatures.
- Frequent small meals (avoids depletion of the blood volume into the splanchnic circulation).
- Elevate the head of the bed by 10–15 cm (4–6 in) using a block of wood or bricks (reduces renal arterial pressure and thus increases the secretion of renin, resulting in retention of sodium and water, and increased blood volume).
- Elastic stockings with lower abdominal constriction (reduce the volume of the venous capacitance bed).

Medications

- Fludrocortisone, a mineralocorticoid, is the most commonly used drug. It increases circulating effective blood volume and has a mild sympathetic effect. The starting dose is 0.1 mg/day and can be increased, with caution in the elderly. The main adverse effects are supine hypertension, fluid retention (and heart failure), and potassium depletion.
- Ibuprofen and other nonsteroidal anti-inflammatory drugs can be used, e.g. for post-prandial hypotension, but they have side-effects.
- Alpha antagonists: ephedrine and methylphenidate hydrochloride (Ritalin) have been largely replaced by midodrine, an alpha-adrenergic agonist which acts by improving arterial and venous constriction in response to standing[9]. May be limited by supine hypertension which itself may respond to beta blockade.
- Cardiac pacing may be considered in selected patients with syncope.

Bladder dysfunction

- Frequency of micturition:
  - Anticholinergic drugs:
    - Propantheline bromide or solifenacin (once-daily advantage).
    - Tricyclic antidepressant drugs (e.g. amitriptyline 25–100 mg/day).
  - Botulinum toxin injections into the detrusor muscle (2.5 MU of Botox injected per single site, up to 30 injections).
- Distended bladder with incomplete emptying: cholinergic drugs: bethanechol chloride 10 mg three to four times daily.

Gastroparesis

- Metoclopramide 10 mg before meals and at night. Have caution with long-term use, where domperidone up to 10 mg three times per day in adults is preferable.

Tip

▶ *There is a range of pharmacologic and physical treatments for symptomatic management of autonomic neuropathies. Management of postural hypotension is often the most rewarding.*

REFERENCES

1 Kauffmann H (2000). Primary autonomic failure: three clinical presentations of one disease? *Ann Intern Med* **133**:382–384.

2 Klein CM, Vernino S, Lennon VA, *et al.* (2003). The spectrum of autoimmune autonomic neuropathies. *Ann. Neurol* **53**:752–758.

3 Mabuchi N, Mabuchi PN, Hirayama M, *et al.* (2005). Progression and prognosis in pure autonomic failure (PAF): comparison with multiple system atrophy. *JNNP* **76**:947–952.

4 Hoitsma E, Reulen JP, de Baets M, Drent M, Spaans F, Faber CG (2004). Small fiber neuropathy: a common and important clinical disorder. *J Neurol Sci* **227**(1):119–130.

5 Low PA, Bennaroch E (1997). *Clinical Autonomic Disorders*, 2nd edn. Lippincott, Raven, Philadelphia, pp. 130–164.

6 American Academy of Neurology (1998). Assessment: Clinical Autonomic Testing. Report of the Therapeutics and Technology Assessment Subcommittee of the American Academy of Neurology. http://aan.com/professionals/practice/pdfs/pdf_1995_thru_1998/1996.46.873.pdf

7 Vernino S, Low PA, Fealey RD, *et al.* (2000). Autoantibodies to ganglionic acetylcholine receptors in autoimmune autonomic neuropathies. *N Engl J Med* **343**:847–855.

8 Schatz IJ (2001). Treatment of severe autonomic orthostatic hypotension. *Lancet* **357**:1060–1061.

9 Doyle JF, Grocott-Mason R, Hardman T, Malik O, Dubrey SW (2012). Midodrine: use and current status in the treatment of hypotension. *Br J Cardiol* **19**:34–37.

Further reading

Donofrio PD, Caress JB (2001). Autonomic disorders. *Neurologist* **7**:220–233.

Low PA, Bennaroch E (1997). *Clinical Autonomic Disorders*, 2nd edn. Lippincott, Raven, Philadelphia, pp. 130–164.

Mathias CJ (1997). Autonomic disorders and their recognition. *N Engl J Med* **336**: 721–724.

Naumann M, Jost WH, Toyka KV (1999). Botulinum toxin in the treatment of neurological disorders of the autonomic nervous system. *Arch Neurol* **56**:914–916.

Oldenburg O, Mitchell A, Nurnberger J, *et al.* (2001). Ambulatory norepinephrine treatment of severe autonomic orthostatic hypotension. *J Am Coll Cardiol* **37**: 219–223.

DISEASES OF THE PERIPHERAL NERVE AND MONONEUROPATHIES

Andrea Swenson

PERIPHERAL NEUROPATHY

Definition and epidemiology

A disorder of any or all of the peripheral nerves, with pathology occurring at the level of the nerve cell bodies, the axons, or the myelin sheaths.

Anatomy

A peripheral nerve consists of a cell body and about six fascicles, each of which contains many myelinated and unmyelinated axons. Each fascicle has small nutrient blood vessels which are integral to its function (**725**).

A motor unit consists of an anterior horn cell, its axon, the neuromuscular junctions, and all of the muscle fibers innervated by the axon. Three types of connective tissue surround the axons in the nerve trunk:

- Endoneurium. This forms the supporting structure around individual axons within each fascicle.
- Perineurium. Collagenous tissue that binds each fascicle and probably acts as a blood–nerve barrier.
- Epineurium. Collagen tissue, elastic fibers, and fatty tissue that bind individual fascicles together, providing protection from compression. Merges in the dura mater of the spinal cord.

Nerve trunks contain myelinated and unmyelinated fibers. Certain properties of the nerve determine whether myelination will occur.

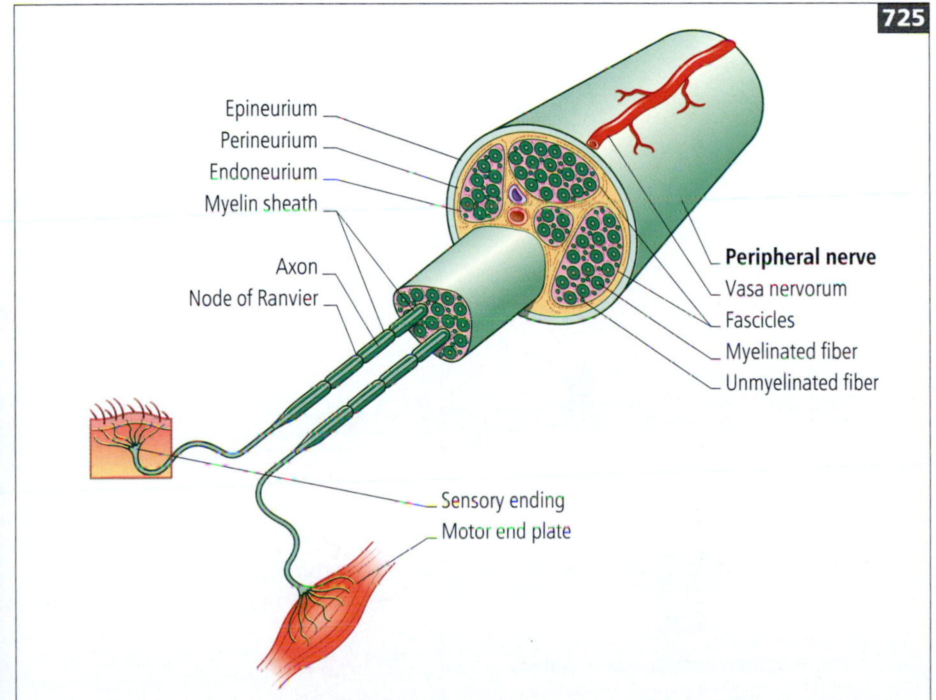

725 Diagrammatic representation of peripheral nerve.

- Myelinated fibers:
  - Schwann cells produce myelin. Their membranes wrap around the axon to form the myelin sheath.
  - Nodes of Ranvier – interruptions in the myelin sheath. Action potentials propagate from one node to the next with the rate proportional to the fiber diameter.
  - >1 μm in diameter.
  - Largest and fastest conducting fibers.
  - Motor and sensory nerves have myelinated fibers. The sensory modalities include proprioception, position sense, and touch sensation.

Unmyelinated fibers:
- 8–15 small axons (0.1–1.3 μm) contained within the infolding of a single Schwann cell. The axons are separated by a constant periaxonal space.
- Responsible for pain and temperature sensation and autonomic functions.

Small arteries located in the epineurium are termed the vasa nervorum. They branch into arterioles that penetrate the perineurium to form capillary anastomoses in the fascicles.

Classification of disease

Polyneuropathy is diffuse dysfunction of multiple nerves, usually creating a 'stocking–glove' pattern of numbness, paresthesias, and weakness (726). The most distal nerves (e.g. in the feet) are affected first. As the symptoms progress and move up the leg, numbness and paresthesias are noticed in the distal fingers. Upper extremity symptoms usually begin when the lower extremity symptoms reach the knees. In most cases, the sensory and motor nerves are both involved (sensorimotor). However, there are certain polyneuropathies that selectively affect only the sensory nerves or the motor nerves.
- Axonal – damage to the axons. Most common type of polyneuropathy.
- Demyelinating – disturbance of the structure and function of the myelin sheath or Schwann cell with sparing of the axons.

Mononeuropathy is dysfunction of an individual peripheral nerve (see below).

Mononeuropathy multiplex is dysfunction of multiple individual peripheral nerves. If many nerves are involved, the neuropathies may coalesce into a pattern that resembles a polyneuropathy. In order to distinguish between these two entities, a thorough history of present illness is essential.

Epidemiology[1] of polyneuropathy is as follows:
- Overall prevalence is approximately 2400 per 100,000 population.
- In individuals >55 years old, the prevalence rises to approximately 8000 per 100,000 population (8%).
- After a polyneuropathy is diagnosed, many patients undergo evaluation for a secondary cause (see Investigation section below). However, in one-third of cases, a cause is not discovered and the polyneuropathy is considered idiopathic.

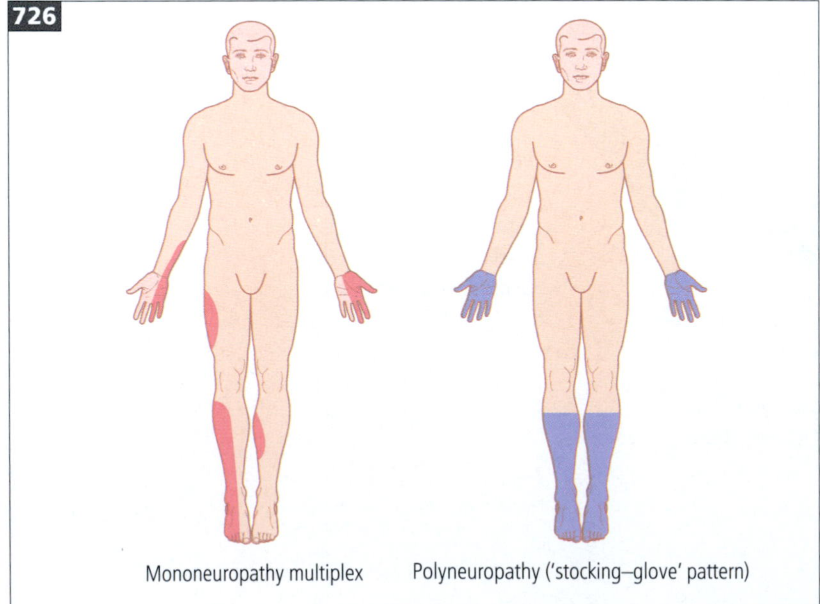

726 Mononeuropathy multiplex *vs.* polyneuropathy, illustrating differing patterns of sensory change and weakness (red/blue areas).

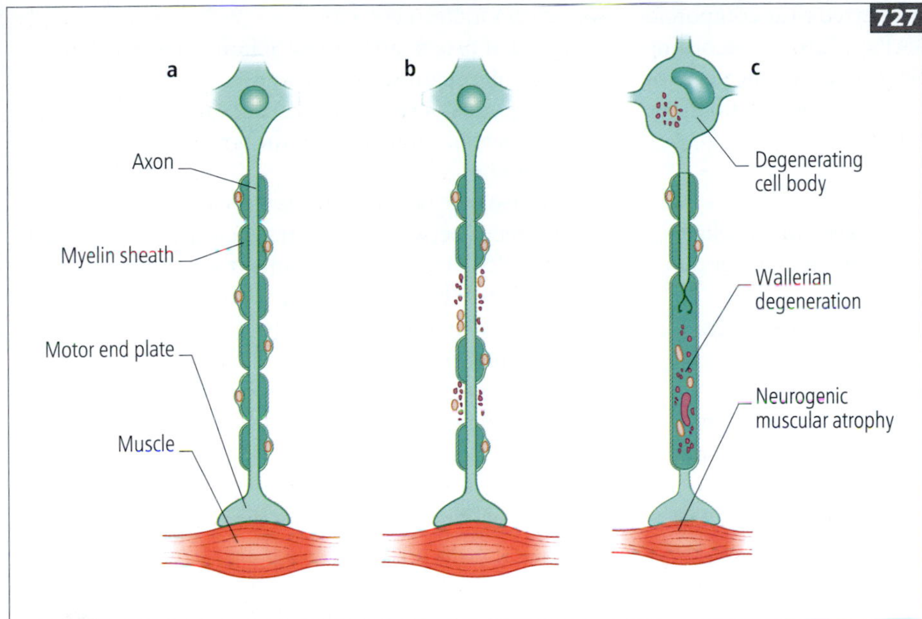

727 **Schematic representation of different types of nerve damage: (a) normal nerve; (b) segmental demyelination; (c) axonal degeneration.**

Etiology and pathophysiology

Types of nerve damage (727) include:

- Neurapraxia:
  - Failure of nerve conduction due to metabolic or microstructural dysfunction.
  - Usually reversible.
  - No damage to the axon.
  - Example: paresthesias after crossing the legs.
- Axonotmesis:
  - Disruption of the axon and myelin sheath.
  - Supporting connective tissue (endoneurium and epineurium) is preserved.
  - Axonal degeneration distal to the injury site.
  - Nerve sprouts regenerate from the proximal stump in attempts to reinnervate muscle or skin.
  - Rate of regrowth is quite slow at 1 mm/day.
  - Functional improvement can take months to a few years, depending on the length of the injured nerve.
- Neurotmesis:
  - Partial or complete severance of a nerve.
  - Disruption of the axons, myelin sheaths, and supporting connective tissue.
  - Degeneration of the axons distal to the injury site.
  - Because the supporting connective tissue is no longer intact, regeneration is difficult and portends a poor prognosis for recovery.
- Wallerian degeneration: structural alterations in the normal nerve distal to injury or transection of the nerve.
- Segmental demyelination:
  - Disturbance of the Schwann cells/myelin associated with significant reduction of nerve conduction velocity.
  - Axonal degeneration cannot create this degree of conduction velocity slowing.

Investigations

Nerve conduction studies

Nerve conduction studies (NCS) involve the recording and analysis of electric waveforms of the peripheral nerves elicited in response to electric or physiologic stimuli. Sensory, motor, and autonomic nerves can be evaluated.

In sensory nerves, waveforms are referred to as sensory nerve action potentials (SNAPs). Recording electrodes are placed on the skin over a sensory or mixed nerve. A stimulus is given at different points along the nerve, in a distal to proximal fashion. Total current flow across the nerve membrane is dependent on the membrane's surface area. Thus, the small myelinated and unmyelinated fibers contribute little to the SNAP.

Although sensory abnormalities may be an initial sign of polyneuropathy, such abnormalities may not be reflected in sensory NCS unless changes occur in the very largest sensory axons. Therefore, a neuropathy involving only the small fibers will have normal NCS.

Tip

► *Nerve conduction studies only assess large nerve fibers. Therefore, a patient with a small fiber neuropathy will have normal nerve conduction studies.*

In motor nerves, waveforms are referred to as compound muscle action potentials (CMAPs) (**728**). A recording electrode is placed over a muscle supplied by the nerve of interest. A stimulus is given at different points along the nerve, in a distal to proximal fashion.

Amplitude

- Maximum voltage difference between the baseline of the action potential and the peak (area under the curve).
- The amplitude is a reflection of the number of functioning axons.
- For the CMAP, the amplitude is an estimate of the number of viable axons and the muscle fibers they innervate. Significant muscular atrophy from a primary muscle disease can cause the CMAP amplitude to be reduced or absent, despite an intact supplying nerve.
- Reduced amplitudes are indicative of axonal loss, most commonly from polyneuropathies.

Distal latency

- Interval between the onset of a stimulus and the onset of the resulting response.
- For the CMAP, the measurement is taken from the onset of the stimulus to the onset or take-off of the response.
- For the SNAP, the measurement is taken from the onset of the stimulus to the peak.
- Delayed distal latency is associated with demyelinating neuropathies and can also occur with marked axonal loss.

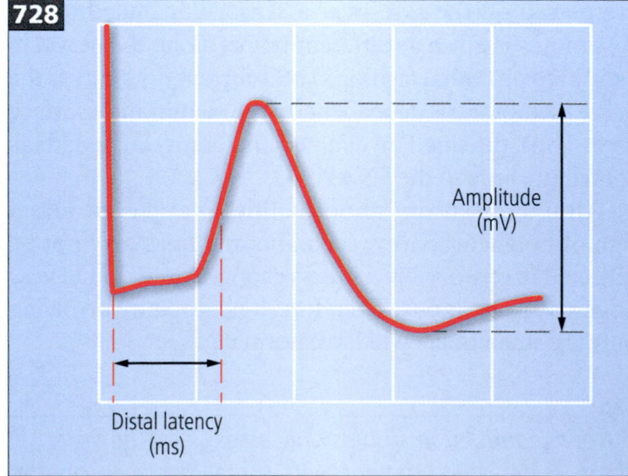

728 **Compound muscle action potential.**

Nerve conduction velocity

- Speed of propagation of an action potential along a particular segment of a nerve.
- Two points of stimulation are obtained (e.g. for the ulnar nerve, stimulation at the wrist and just below the elbow).
- The distance between the two points is divided by the difference between the corresponding distal latencies. The calculated velocity signifies the conduction velocity of the fastest fibers.
- Measured in meters/second (m/s).
- Important measure for demyelination:
  - Prolonged conduction velocities are a hallmark of hereditary demyelinating neuropathies.
  - Can identify nerve damage at compression sites (e.g. slowing of the median nerve response at the carpal tunnel or the ulnar nerve across the elbow).

F-waves

- A supramaximal stimulus is delivered resulting in the primary response, the CMAP.
- The CMAP is derived from orthodromic conduction of the action potential. Additionally, the initial nerve depolarization also produces an antidromic response, which travels toward the spinal cord. When the response reaches the corresponding anterior horn cells, a second action potential is propagated in an orthodromic direction along the entire length of one or more of the same motor axons. This second response is then recorded from the original muscle as the F-wave (**729**).
- With multiple stimulations, the CMAP morphology remains stable due to activation of all responsive muscle fibers. The F-waves, on the other hand, have different latencies and morphologies due to activation of different motor units with subsequent stimulations.
- Prolongation or absence of response may indicate very proximal demyelination (i.e. at the level of the nerve root in polyradiculopathies).

Technical factors

- Decreased temperature of the skin may result in falsely increased amplitude of CMAP and SNAP, reduced conduction velocities, and prolonged F waves. Hand temperature should be >33°C (91.4°F) and foot temperature >31°C (88°F).
- Patient movement during the testing.
- External electrical interference from the room.

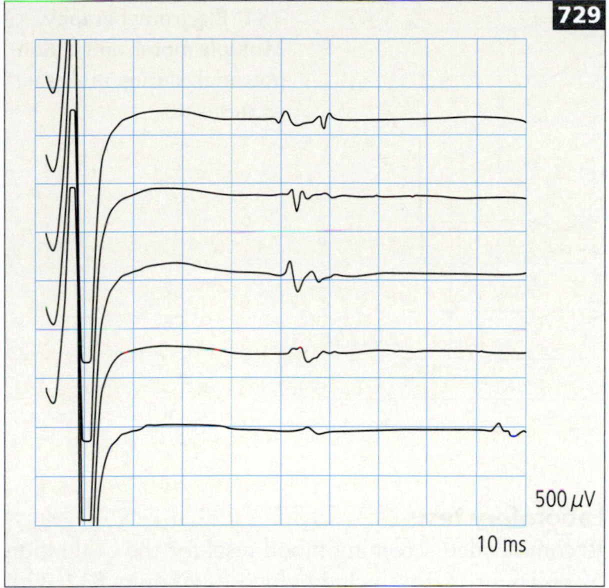

729 **Diagram to demonstrate analysis of a nerve conduction study, showing tibial nerve F-waves.**

Electromyography

Electromyography (EMG) is performed by inserting a needle electrode into a muscle, recording insertion activity, spontaneous activity, and voluntary electric activity of the muscle. Recordings are visualized on a computer screen and heard through a speaker system. EMG determines the type of abnormality within a specific muscle (i.e. neurogenic *vs.* myopathic processes). EMG results are used in conjunction with the NCS results.

Insertion activity

- Transitory burst of electrical activity recorded within the muscle as a result of insertion or movement of the needle electrode.
- Related to disruption of muscle fibers.
- Increased insertion activity (prolonged) can occur in neurogenic disorders and muscle disorders with membrane instability.
- Insertion activity may be decreased (less activity upon insertion) in long-standing muscle disorders, in which cases the muscle is fibrotic or replaced by fat.

Spontaneous activity

Electric activity recorded from muscle at rest after insertion activity has subsided. Normal muscle should be electrically silent, with the exception of needle movement.

Positive sharp waves and fibrillations (denervation potentials) are the most common forms of (abnormal) spontaneous activity. Their presence suggests disruption of the continuity between the muscle fiber and its axon in the acute or chronic phase of the disorder. These occur most commonly in neurogenic disorders involving axon loss (anywhere from the anterior horn cell to the terminal nerve). Positive sharp waves and fibrillations may also be observed in certain primary muscle disorders, presumed to be due to muscle membrane instability (**730**).

Fasciculations are random and spontaneous twitching of a group of muscle fibers or a motor unit that is often grossly visible in a limb or the tongue. A fasciculation potential is a recording often associated with clinical fasciculations. This has the configuration of a motor unit action potential (MUP) but occurs spontaneously. Fasciculation potentials can occur in any nerve disorder, but are most notoriously associated with motor neuron disease.

Complex repetitive discharges are activity that originates from a reverberating circuit that has developed within contiguous myofibers. Its sound is machinery-like with an abrupt onset and cessation. Complex repetitive discharges can occur in chronic nerve and muscle disorders.

Myokymic discharges originate from the peripheral nerve and result from ephaptic transmission between damaged contiguous axons. These can occur in a variety of nerve disorders, but are most commonly associated with radiation-induced nerve injury.

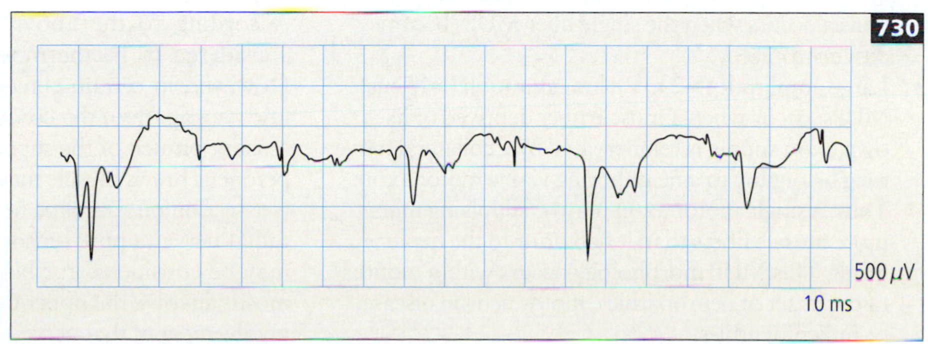

730 **Electromyography. Spontaneous activity: positive sharp waves with a few fibrillations in the first dorsal interosseous.**

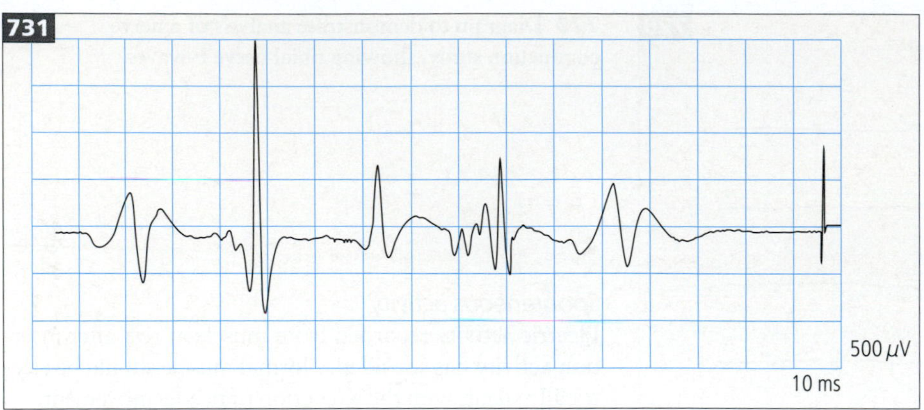

731 Electromyography. Multiple motor unit action potentials during moderate recruitment.

Motor unit action potential recruitment

The electromyographer asks the patient to activate gradually the muscle being tested. This allows for evaluation of the number of MUPs the patient is capable of activating (recruitment). In normal recruitment, as isometric tension in the muscle intensifies, an increasing number of MUPs are seen and heard on the EMG machine display. With minimal effort, the first MUP is recruited and fires at a rate of approximately 5–7 Hz. As the effort in contraction increases, the first MUP begins to fire faster. When the firing rate reaches 10 Hz, the second MUP should appear. With normal recruitment, multiple MUPs are appreciated. Each has its own distinctive sound and configuration due to its relationship with the recording needle (i.e. MUPs that are closer to the recording needle have a crisper sound and sharper rise time in initial deflection) (**731**).

In neurogenic recruitment, with axon loss there is a reduced number of motor units available to recruit. The remaining motor units need to fire at a greater frequency in order to compensate for this loss. During the study, a single MUP may be observed to fire at a rate greater than 15 Hz with no other MUP recruited. Normal MUPs have a triphasic configuration (**731**). In neurogenic MUPs:

- Polyphasia occurs: extra turns and phases are incorporated into an individual MUP. Noticeable within weeks to months of injury and occurs in myopathies, axon loss, and demyelinating nerve disease. Polyphasia occurs when the single fiber MUPs become desynchronized.
- Large amplitude (>2 mV), long duration (>15 ms) MUPs: occur when a muscle fiber deprived of its own axon supply is reinnervated by a collateral nerve twig belonging to a neighboring viable motor axon. Thus, a single motor axon may be supplying many more muscle fibers than it had prior to the nerve insult. This MUP morphology occurs within months of the onset of neuropathies, motor neuron disease, or radiculopathies.

Laboratory tests

Recommended screening blood tests for the evaluation of polyneuropathy include glucose, vitamin B12 with metabolites (methylmalonic acid with or without homocysteine), and serum protein immunofixation electrophoresis. If glucose is normal, testing for impaired glucose tolerance (i.e. glucose tolerance test) should be considered[1].

Cerebrospinal fluid (CSF) analysis should be considered (lumbar puncture) for the assessment of demyelinating polyneuropathies or polyradiculopathies (see section on chronic inflammatory demyelinating polyneuropathy [CIDP], p. 807). Any polyneuropathy may produce a mild elevation in total protein levels.

Nerve biopsy

Nerve biopsy can be used as a diagnostic measure to further delineate the specific form of neuropathy. The biopsy site is chosen based on the following criteria[2]:

- Is affected by the neuropathy, based on clinical and electrophysiological evidence.
- Constant in its location and readily accessible.
- Pure sensory nerve: fewer post-operative complications compared with a pure motor or mixed nerve.
- A nerve that is long enough so that 6–10 cm of the same fascicles can be removed.
- Located away from a common site of compression.

According to the above criteria, the sural nerve is considered to be the most suitable nerve for biopsy. However, in certain clinical circumstances (e.g. vasculitic neuropathy), the combination of biopsies from the sensory branch of the superficial peroneal nerve and the peroneus brevis muscle may have higher diagnostic value (see section on vasculitic neuropathy, p. 811). Superficial radial nerve (a pure sensory branch of the radial nerve) may be considered for biopsy if the clinical symptoms mostly involve the upper extremities and the NCS show involvement of that nerve.

Nerve biopsies should only be performed in carefully selected patients after a thorough clinical work-up, due to high complication rates. The indications for nerve biopsy are mostly confined to evaluation for suspected vasculitic neuropathies, leukemic infiltration, or amyloid. Hereditary neuropathies may be considered, however, and molecular genetic testing is available in most cases.

Muscle biopsy

Muscle biopsy is not indicated for nerve disorders. However, in the event that muscle tissue is obtained, certain muscle patterns occur in the setting of nerve damage. Axonal degeneration of motor nerves results in muscle pathology referred to as neurogenic atrophy. Denervated muscle fibers become atrophic and angulated in appearance. Nerve sprouts reinnervate the surrounding denervated muscle fibers. The muscle fibers then take on the fiber type of the new nerve (i.e. type 1 *vs.* type 2 muscle fibers). This results in fiber type grouping and loss of the muscle's mosaic pattern.

DIABETIC NEUROPATHY

Definition and epidemiology

Neuropathic complications from diabetes mellitus or impaired glucose tolerance. Diabetes mellitus is the most common cause of polyneuropathy in the developed world. In patients with diabetes, the prevalence of polyneuropathy ranges from 28% to 55%[3]. In all forms of diabetes, 66% of patients have objective signs of a neuropathy. However, only 20% are symptomatic. In one study of patients with painful idiopathic sensory neuropathy, 65% had evidence of abnormal glucose metabolism (diabetes or impaired glucose tolerance)[4].

Etiology and pathophysiology

The pathogenesis of neuropathy in the setting of hyperglycemia is unknown. Theories include a metabolic process, microangiopathic ischemia, or an immunologic disorder.

Clinical features

Neuropathy may be the presenting feature of diabetes.

Distal symmetric sensory and sensorimotor polyneuropathy

This is the most common form of diabetic neuropathy (732). It begins with sensory loss in the toes (length dependent) and gradually progresses up the feet, ankles, and legs in a symmetric fashion. The progression occurs over years. When the symptoms roughly reach the knees, the fingertips become involved with numbness and paresthesias. Pain can be a bothersome feature, particularly at night. Patients may comment that they cannot tolerate the bed sheets touching their feet. Pain exacerbation at night may be due to lack of daytime activity distractions. The polyneuropathy associated with impaired glucose tolerance often affects the small fibers resulting in painful paresthesias.

Sensory ataxia occurs in advanced polyneuropathy. Intrinsic foot and hand muscle atrophy may occur, but should prompt investigation for other processes (i.e. median, ulnar, or peroneal compressive mononeuropathies, concurrent inflammatory or hereditary neuropathy). Lower extremity involvement may present as foot dorsiflexion weakness creating a foot drop and steppage gait. Other etiologies such as a superimposed peroneal neuropathy or L5 radiculopathy should be considered.

In NCS, sensory responses are often affected with reduced or absent amplitudes. Motor responses are less frequently affected and may have slowing within a demyelinating range.

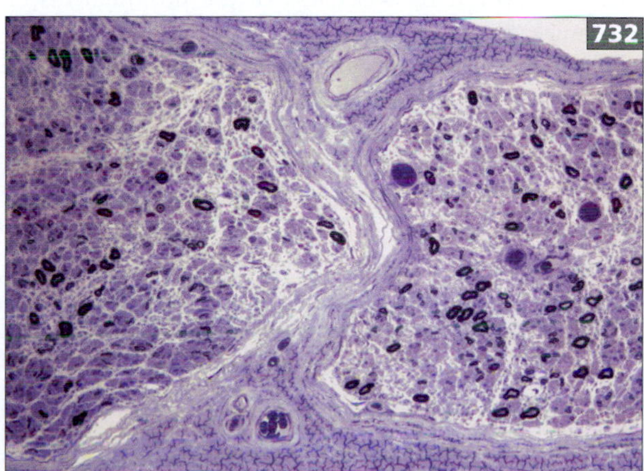

732 Toluidine blue stain of a nerve. Two fascicles are pictured. There is loss of myelinated nerve fibers (dark blue circles). *Courtesy of Tibor Valyi-Nagy, MD, PhD.*

Autonomic neuropathy

Autonomic neuropathy is often associated with distal symmetric sensorimotor polyneuropathy. Features include abnormal sweating, dry eyes and mouth, pupillary abnormalities, cardiac arrhythmias, orthostatic hypotension, gastroparesis, postprandial bloating, erectile dysfunction, urinary incontinence, chronic diarrhea, or constipation.

Treatment includes fludrocortisone or midodrine for orthostatic hypotension, metoclopramide for gastroparesis, and PDE5 inhibitors (sildenafil, vardenafil) for erectile dysfunction.

Mononeuropathy

Patients with diabetic polyneuropathy are at risk of developing mononeuropathies. The most common mononeuropathies and their corresponding sites of compression are as follows:

- Median neuropathy at the wrist.
- Ulnar neuropathy at the elbow.
- Peroneal neuropathy at the fibular head.
- Lateral femoral cutaneous neuropathy (meralgia paresthetica) at the inguinal ligament.
- Cranial nerves:
  - Most common is facial neuropathy, then oculomotor and abducens neuropathy.
  - Less frequently, trochlear neuropathy.
- Multiple mononeuropathies may give the appearance of mononeuropathy multiplex (most commonly associated with vasculitic neuropathy).

Diabetic lumbosacral radiculoplexus neuropathy

Other monikers include diabetic amyotrophy, Bruns–Garland syndrome, or proximal diabetic neuropathy. It predominantly affects individuals with type 2 diabetes. The pathogenesis is believed to be a T-cell mediated microvasculitis involving small epineurial and perineurial vessels[5].

It usually begins with sudden onset of severe aching of the hip and thigh area that may last for days or weeks. This is followed by weakness of the proximal lower extremity that may spread distally to involve the entire lumbosacral plexus. About 50% of patients have spread of symptoms to the contralateral leg. Weight loss without other constitutional symptoms is a common feature.

The natural course is monophasic, but recovery may be slow and some patients may be left with residual deficits. Treatments such as intravenous immunoglobulin (IVIG), IV methylprednisolone, and other immunosuppressants may be helpful in hastening recovery. IV methylprednisolone may be most effective in pain control, allowing for necessary physical therapy. Physical therapy is probably the most important intervention.

Chronic inflammatory demyelinating polyneuropathy

Diabetic patients, particularly type 1, may have a higher risk of developing CIDP than the general population[6]. These cases seem to respond to the standard CIDP treatments. (See section on CIDP.)

Elevated CSF protein and demyelinating features on NCS can be characteristic of diabetic polyneuropathy without CIDP. If conduction block is present on NCS, there is a higher likelihood of CIDP. Conduction block is a rare finding in diabetic polyneuropathy[6].

CIDP with diabetes may not respond as well to treatment. In one study comparing idiopathic CIDP to CIDP with diabetes, those with diabetes presented with a higher frequency of autonomic dysfunction, associated axonal loss, and a poorer outcome at 6 months[7].

Differential diagnosis

Other etiologies for neuropathy, although less likely, should be ruled out. These include:

- Alcoholism.
- Vitamin deficiencies.
- Drug-induced.
- Monoclonal gammopathy.

Investigations

- NCS should be performed to further define the type of neuropathy.
- EMG can assist in determining the degree of axonal involvement.
- Fasting blood glucoses and hemoglobin A1c to evaluate glycemic control. Diabetes is defined as a fasting blood glucose ≥1.26 g/l (126 mg/dl).
- Glucose tolerance test: impaired glucose tolerance is defined as 2-hour glucose between 1.4 g/l (140 mg/dl) and 1.99 g/l (199 mg/dl). Impaired glucose tolerance has been linked to peripheral neuropathy.

Neuropathy may be associated with metabolic syndrome (obesity, hypertriglyceridemia, hypertension, insulin resistance)[8].

TABLE 115 **TREATMENT OPTIONS FOR NEUROPATHIC PAIN**

Medication	Dosing	Side-effects
FIRST LINE		
Tricyclic antidepressant (e.g. amitriptyline, nortriptyline)	10–250 mg qhs	Anticholinergic (i.e. urinary retention, constipation, dry mouth and eyes, sedation)
Gabapentin	100–1200 mg tid	Cognitive abnormalities, sedation, limb edema
Pregabalin	50–100 mg tid	Cognitive abnormalities, sedation, limb edema
Duloxetine	60–120 mg daily	Cognitive abnormalities, sedation, nausea, diarrhea, constipation, diaphoresis
SECOND LINE		
Carbamazepine	200–400 mg tid	Cognitive abnormalities, vertigo, leukopenia, liver dysfunction
Lamotrigine	200–400 mg daily	Stevens–Johnson syndrome (slow titration to prevent)
Tramadol	25–50 mg every 4–6 hours as needed	Cognitive abnormalities, gastrointestinal upset
Venlafaxine	150–225 mg daily	Sedation, nausea
THIRD LINE		
Topiramate	200–400 mg bid	Cognitive abnormalities (particularly memory and language impairment), sedation, weight loss, glaucoma, metabolic acidosis, nephrolithiasis
Mexiletine	200–300 mg tid	Arrhythmias
TOPICAL AGENTS		
Capsaicin cream	Apply to feet 3–4 times daily	Warn patients that initial applications may exacerbate neuropathic pain which should improve with subsequent applications
Lidocaine 5% patch or gel	1–3 patches or applications per 12–24 hours	Skin irritation

Treatment

- Adequate blood glucose control is important for prevention of neuropathies or preventing worsening of existing neuropathies.
- Impaired glucose tolerance: diet and exercise intervention with weight loss, low-density lipoprotein and triglyceride reduction, and improved glucose control.
- Small uncontrolled trials suggest light exercise may improve neuropathy symptoms. Symptomatic treatment: burning pain and paresthesias can be a bothersome and debilitating feature of neuropathy. Many medications are available for symptom relief (*Table 115*).

Tip

▶ *Polyneuropathy may improve with better glycemic control, but it is generally not reversible.*

TOXIC NEUROPATHY

Definition

Neuropathic complications from the toxic effects of drug or environmental exposures.

Tip

▶ *Neuropathies tend to improve when offending agents/exposures are removed, but this is not always the case. Some neuropathies may worsen over time.*

Etiology and pathophysiology

Alcohol

Alcoholics can develop a generalized axonal sensorimotor polyneuropathy or rarely a more acute demyelinating polyneuropathy (similar to Guillain–Barré syndrome [GBS]). The more acute neuropathy typically has normal or only slightly elevated CSF total protein.

The pathogenesis of nerve injury is not known. It may be related to nutritional deficiency or a direct toxic effect to the nerves. Treatment involves abstaining from alcohol and maintaining a balanced diet. Recovery depends on initial severity of the polyneuropathy.

Chemotherapeutic agents

The risk of developing a neuropathy increases with higher doses and concomitant use of other potentially neurotoxic drugs. Neuropathies are usually an axonal polyneuropathy that is length-dependent with greater sensory involvement or a sensory neuronopathy.

Medication withdrawal or dose reduction at an early stage of the neuropathy can prevent progression to a more severe grade and may result in functional resolution. However, if treatment is continued and high cumulative doses are received, residual neuropathic deficits are inevitable.

ARA-C (cytosine arabinoside)

- An antimetabolite used for treatment of leukemia and lymphoma.
- Sensory neuropathy and severe sensorimotor polyneuropathy resembling GBS may begin within hours–weeks after treatment initiation.
- Pathogenesis is unknown. Hypotheses include inhibition of proteins involved in myelin production, axonal structure, or axonal transport or the immunomodulating effects of the medication predisposing peripheral nerves to immune attack.

Bortezomib

- A selective, reversible inhibitor of the proteasome that has been approved for multiple myeloma.
- New onset neuropathy or symptomatic worsening of a neuropathy occurred in 35% of patients in treatment trials.
- NCS usually reveal a length-dependent axonal sensory polyneuropathy.
- The neuropathy usually improves with dose reduction or drug discontinuation.
- Pathogenesis is possibly related to a build-up of proteins that impairs neuronal function in the dorsal root ganglia, leading to a retrograde axonopathy of small nerve fibers followed by larger nerve fibers.

Etoposide

- Semisynthetic derivative of podophyllotoxin used to treat lymphoma, leukemia, small-cell lung cancer, and testicular carcinoma.
- Mechanism of action is inhibition of the deoxyribonucleic acid (DNA)-unwinding enzyme topoisomerase II.
- 4–10% of patients develop a predominantly sensory axonal polyneuropathy.
- The neuropathy resolves several months after drug discontinuation.

Ifosfamide

- An ankylating agent used for treatment of testicular and cervical carcinomas, sarcomas, lymphomas, and lung cancers.
- A sensory neuropathy occurs in 3% of patients taking high-dose therapy with onset 1–2 weeks after treatment. The symptoms gradually resolve, but do tend to recur if re-challenged with the medication.

Misonidazole

- Used as a red blood cell sensitizer before radiation therapy for various malignancies, particularly pharynx, larynx, and lung.
- Painful paresthesias and occasional distal weakness in a length-dependent pattern may occur after 3–5 weeks of drug administration. The neuropathy usually improves after drug discontinuation.

Platinum agents: cisplatin

- Platinum compound used for a wide variety of malignancies, most notably ovarian, testicular, lung, bladder, head and neck, and germ cell cancers. Cisplatin kills malignant cells by disruption of DNA function.
- There is an 85% incidence of neuropathies with doses >300 mg/m^2 of body surface and practically universal with doses >600 mg/m^2. The pathogenesis for neuropathy is not known, but a proposed mechanism involves DNA binding of the drug and impairing axonal transport.
- The induced neuropathy is usually a symmetric sensory neuropathy or neuronopathy, which is related to total cumulative dose. At higher cumulative doses, severe proprioceptive defects may appear such as sensory ataxia and pseudoathetosis (see section on sensory neuronopathy).
- Cisplatin-induced neuropathies have an important characteristic of off-therapy deterioration, known as coasting. The neuropathic symptoms may not appear for up to 8 weeks after therapy has been stopped. In 30% of patients, the neuropathy continues to progress for as long as 6 months after medication withdrawal. With time, the neuropathy may subside. However, long-term follow-up studies reveal 40% of patients noting residual sensory symptoms.

Platinum agents: oxaliplatin

- Platinum chemotherapy agent designed to have fewer side-effects. However, it has actually been associated with a unique, but frequent, sensory neuropathy, which is triggered or exacerbated by cold exposure. The neuropathy is rapidly reversible without persistent impairment of sensory function.

Suramin

- Hexasulfonated naphthylurea that is active against hormone-refractory prostate cancer, malignant thymoma, non-Hodgkin lymphoma, and other solid tumors such as adrenocortical, ovarian, and renal cell carcinoma.
- Peripheral neuropathy, occurring in 25–90% of patients, is a dose-limiting side-effect. There are two distinct types of toxic neuropathy – a dose-dependent, distal, axonal sensorimotor polyneuropathy and a subacute demyelinating polyradiculoneuropathy, which may be immune-mediated. The latter type is less common but can be quite severe, resulting in mechanical ventilation in up to 25% of affected patients. Plasmapheresis has been used, but with mixed results. The neuropathy may progress for 1 month following discontinuation and can take several months to recover.

Taxanes: paclitaxel, docetaxel

- Used in the treatment of ovarian, breast, lung, bladder, cervical, head and neck cancers, and non-Hodgkin lymphoma. Mechanism of action is promotion of microtubule assembly that leads to accumulation of disordered microtubular bundles. Accumulation may also occur in the axons and the dorsal root ganglion neuronal cell body.
- When treatment is combined with granulocyte colony-stimulating factor, peripheral neurotoxicity becomes the dose-limiting factor. Usually, myelosuppression is the dose-limiting factor.
- A dose-dependent, predominantly sensory neuropathy may occur. Most patients improve 1–2 months after chemotherapy cessation, but symptoms have potential to worsen for several months after discontinuation.

Thalidomide

- Older therapy currently being utilized for new therapeutic indications (multiple myeloma, graft-*vs*.-host disease, erythema nodosum leprosum, autoimmune diseases).
- It can be associated with a painful, axonal sensorimotor neuropathy that often persists years after drug discontinuation.

Vinca alkaloids: vincristine, vinblastine, vindesine, vinorelbine

- Mechanism of action involves inhibition of microtubule formation by binding to tubulin, which can also impair axoplasmic transport and leads to cytoskeletal disarray and axonal degeneration.
- Most commonly used to treat leukemia, Hodgkin's disease, and non-Hodgkin lymphoma. It is also utilized for lung cancers, breast carcinomas, and childhood tumors.
- Neurotoxicity is vincristine's dose-limiting side-effect, while myelotoxicity limits the use of vinblastine and vinorelbine.
- The neuropathy is usually a symmetric sensorimotor polyneuropathy that commonly includes autonomic symptoms and less frequently involves cranial nerves.
- The median duration of symptoms after stopping vincristine is approximately 3 months.

Other medications

Amiodarone

- A neuromyopathy may develop after taking the medication for 2–3 years.
- Severe proximal and distal weakness can develop primarily in the legs, combined with distal sensory loss, tingling, and burning pain.
- Presumed mechanism for neuropathy: amphiphilic properties of the medication lead to drug–lipid complexes that result in accumulation of autophagic vacuoles.
- NCS show absent sensory responses and reduced or normal CMAPs. Also, conduction velocities may be significantly prolonged, suggesting a demyelinating component. EMG reveals denervation in the distal muscles and myopathic-appearing MUPs in the proximal muscles due to the accompanying toxic myopathy.
- Other clinical features include tremor, optic neuropathy, thyroid dysfunction, keratitis, pigmentary skin changes, hepatitis, pulmonary fibrosis, and parotid gland hypertrophy.

Chloroquine/hydroxychloroquine

- Similar mechanism of action to amiodarone.
- A toxic myopathy or a distal sensorimotor axonal polyneuropathy may develop. The myopathy and neuropathy may occur simultaneously, manifesting as both proximal and distal weakness (neuromyopathy).
- The signs and symptoms are usually reversible with discontinuation of the medication.

Colchicine

- Used to treat gout.
- Mechanism of action involves inhibition of the polymerization of tubulin into microtubules. Axoplasmic flow can be impaired leading to neurotoxicity.
- The neuropathy is length-dependent, involving large fiber modalities.
- A superimposed myopathy may occur, which leads to proximal weakness.
- Muscle biopsies reveal a vacuolar myopathy and sensory nerve biopsies show axonal degeneration.

Dapsone

- Used for the treatment of leprosy and various dermatologic conditions.
- A primarily motor neuropathy can develop 1 week into treatment to up to 5 years after initiation.
- The hands tend to be more affected.
- Discontinuation of the drug results in marked improvement.
- The risk of developing neuropathy is greatest in individuals with a slower acetylation rate of dapsone.

Disulfiram

- Used to aid in the detoxification of patients with chronic alcoholism.
- A neuropathy with distal weakness (i.e. foot drop) and sensory loss may occur at various times throughout the treatment (10 days–18 months after initiation).
- The pathogenesis of the neuropathy may be due to toxicity from carbon disulfide, which is a metabolite of disulfiram.
- Histological feature: axonal swellings caused by accumulation of neurofilaments (see carbon disulfide below).

HMG-CoA reductase inhibitors ('statins')

- Used to treat hyperlipidemia.
- Case reports of axonal sensorimotor neuropathy or purely small fiber neuropathy, with the former improving after withdrawal of the medication. The small fiber neuropathic symptoms may be persistent. Currently, the neuropathy appears to be a rare phenomenon[9].
- Hypothetical mechanisms for nerve injury include inhibition of guanosine triphosphate signaling-related binding proteins, inhibition of the formation of selenoproteins, and reduction of antioxidant defense pathways.

Isoniazid

- Used for the treatment of tuberculosis, peripheral neuropathy is one of the most common side-effects.
- The usual presentation is numbness and paresthesias in hands and feet.
- The neuropathy can develop within a few weeks on higher doses.
- The symptoms resolve after discontinuing the medication.
- The neuropathy is due to pyridoxine deficiency (isoniazid inhibits pyridoxal phosphokinase). Patients with slow acetylation (i.e. elderly or those with the autosomal recessive trait) maintain a higher serum concentration of the drug and are at greater risk for developing neuropathy.
- Prophylactic pyridoxine 100 mg daily can prevent neuropathy.

Metronidazole

- Used to treat protozoan infections (trichomoniasis, giardiasis, amebiasis) and anaerobic infections (*Clostridium difficile*). Also used in higher doses for Crohn's disease.
- There are several reports of a sensory neuropathy or neuronopathy that developed on high doses. Doses of $<$12 g over 5 days are unlikely to cause a neuropathy.

Nitrofurantoin

- Used to treat a wide range of Gram-positive and Gram-negative organisms, most frequently for urinary tract infections.
- An acute, severe sensorimotor polyneuropathy may develop. Paresthesias are painful. Occasionally, quadriparesis occurs.
- Elderly and patients with renal insufficiency are at greatest risk for neuropathy.
- There is slow improvement after drug discontinuation.

Phenytoin

- Used to treat several types of epilepsy.
- A rare side-effect is a mild sensory neuropathy, which improves after drug discontinuation.

Tacrolimus

- An immunosuppressive agent used to prevent solid-organ transplant rejection, treat graft- *vs.*-host disease and various autoimmune diseases.
- Mechanism of action involves modulation of T-cell function.
- Although neuropathy is a rarely reported side-effect, the best-characterized peripheral nerve disorder is a chronic demyelinating neuropathy, which may resemble CIDP with NCS demonstrating demyelinating features.
- Patients do improve with plasmapheresis or IVIG.
- Another syndrome is an acute, severe, motor-predominant, axonal polyneuropathy that commences 1–2 weeks into the treatment regimen. Onset is abrupt with progression to flaccid quadriparesis occurring in a few days. Other features include ptosis, bilateral facial weakness, lethargy, and foot pain. Symptoms should improve with discontinuation of the drug, but may require additional treatment with plasmapheresis or IVIG. The neuropathy may relapse if re-challenged with tacrolimus.
- The pathogenesis of neuropathy may be mediated by a dysimmune process. Tacrolimus may enhance autoreactive T cells directed against peripheral nerve myelin.

Human immunodeficiency virus (HIV) medications

See section on Infectious neuropathy (p. 816).

Industrial agents

Acrylamide

- A vinyl monomer used in soil grouting for stabilization, in waterproofing, and as a flocculator.
- Oral, dermal, and respiratory absorption.
- Accumulates distally in the nerves. Acrylamide has been used in animal models of distal axonal neurotoxic injury.
- Chronic exposure may lead to an axonal polyneuropathy; potential recovery when exposure is eliminated.

Carbon disulfide

- Used to make rayon and cellophane.
- Dermal or respiratory absorption.
- Chronic exposure can result in a length-dependent axonal polyneuropathy.
- Histological feature: giant axonal swellings (neurofilamentous debris within axons).

Ethylene oxide

- Used to sterilize heat-sensitive materials.
- Absorbed across respiratory membranes.
- Sensorimotor polyneuropathy is the most common neurotoxic effect, which can occur at exposure levels that do not affect other tissues.

Hexacarbons

- Water-insoluble organic solvents, used in industrial and household glues.
- Dermal absorption or through inhalation (i.e. glue sniffing).
- A subacute sensorimotor polyneuropathy may progress over 4–6 weeks, leading to quite extensive weakness with sparing of respiratory muscles.
- Pathogenesis of neuropathy is hypothesized to involve cross-linking between axonal neurofilaments, resulting in aggregation, impaired axonal transport, swelling of the axons, and axonal degeneration (similar to carbon disulfide).
- Histological feature: loss of large myelinated fibers and swollen axons filled with neurofilaments.

Nitrous oxide

- Used as an inhaled dental anesthetic.
- Interferes with vitamin B12 metabolism and may produce a syndrome similar to the subacute combined degeneration associated with vitamin B12 deficiency. In these cases, the vitamin B12 concentrations are normal.
- Toxicity can produce a myeloneuropathy. Reported cases with both recreational abuse and professional exposure.

Organophosphates

- Used in insecticides/pesticides, flame retardants, war gases, and suicide attempts.
- Dermal, respiratory, and gastrointestinal tract absorption.
- Clinical features include organophosphate-induced delayed neurotoxicity:
  - Rapidly progressive axonal sensorimotor polyneuropathy developing a few weeks after acute exposure to a large quantity.
  - Pathogenesis of the neuropathy stems from phosphorylation of neurotoxic esterase.
  - Reduced erythrocyte acetylcholinesterase activity.
  - Neuropathy may slowly improve with no further exposure.

Heavy metals

Arsenic

- Exposure can occur from intentional poisoning or from industry such as smelting.
- Toxicity may result in a sensorimotor polyneuropathy with onset within 5–10 days of ingestion. The neuropathy may progress for several weeks and can mimic GBS. Severe intoxication can involve the proximal muscles and cranial nerves.
- Respiratory muscles may be affected necessitating mechanical ventilation.
- Skin examination may reveal Mee's lines (transverse lines at the base of fingernails and toenails that appear after 1–2 months of exposure). Mee's lines can also be a feature of exposure to thallium (733).
- NCS reveal an axonal pattern with demyelinating features.
- CSF studies may show elevated protein with normal cell count. These features, in addition to the clinical presentation, may lead to the misdiagnosis of GBS.
- Slow recovery of the neuropathy with removal of the exposure. British anti-Lewisite (BAL) chelation therapy has yielded inconsistent results.

Lead

- Intoxication from accidental ingestion (e.g. children eating lead-based paint chips) and industrial exposure of lead-containing products.
- Most common presentation of lead poisoning is encephalopathy.
- A motor neuropathy can occur, which often presents with a wrist drop (i.e. radial neuropathy). Foot drop (i.e. peroneal neuropathy) may also occur. Bluish discoloration of the gums is an associated feature.
- Other investigations reveal a microcytic anemia with basophilic stippling of erythrocytes and an elevated serum coproporphyrin level.
- Treatment requires removal of the exposure source. Chelation therapy with calcium disodium ethylenediamine tetraacetate, BAL, and penicillamine has shown some efficacy in neuropathy improvement.

Mercury

- Elemental mercury can be found in older thermometers.
- Organic:
  - Contaminated fish.
  - Paresthesias in hands and feet and may involve the face and tongue. Encephalopathy, hearing loss, and vision loss may also occur.
  - Due to its water-solubility, it remains in the body and may have limited urinary excretion and difficult to measure.
- Inorganic:
  - Found in batteries, procedures (plating processes, felt manufacturing).
  - Primary symptoms include gastrointestinal symptoms and nephritic syndrome. Encephalopathy and a sensorimotor polyneuropathy may also develop.
  - Measured in 24-hour urine sample.
- Remove the source of exposure. Chelation treatment has been tried, but with variable success.

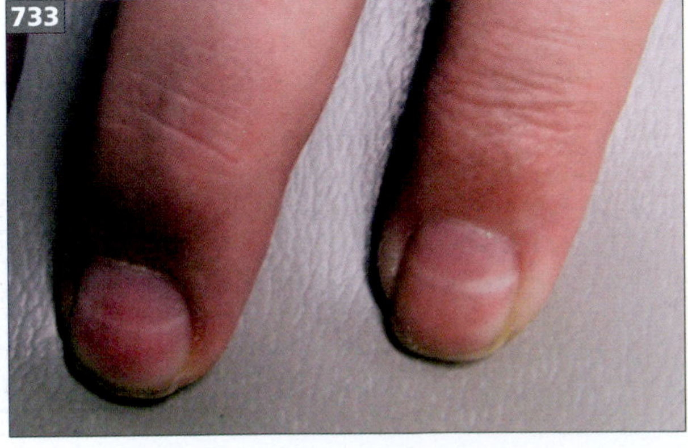

733 Mee's lines on the fingernails after exposure to arsenic.

Thallium[10]

- Used in the manufacture of glass and optical lenses, semiconductors, cardiac scanners, fireworks, insecticides, and rodenticides. Toxicity usually occurs with accidental or intentional ingestion of rat poison.
- After a few weeks of exposure, clinical features include diffuse alopecia, hepatic dysfunction, and Mee's lines. Distal muscle atrophy and weakness occurs. With severe intoxication, proximal weakness and cranial nerve involvement may be observed. Respiratory muscles may be affected. Death can occur within 48 hours after a significantly high dose.
- As blood and urine thallium concentrations decrease, the neuropathy slowly improves, but may leave a residual sensory neuropathy. Acute toxicity may respond to hemodialysis.

NUTRITION-RELATED NEUROPATHY

Definition and epidemiology

Neuropathic disorders due to nutritional deficiency or toxicity. Patients at risk include those with impaired gastrointestinal absorption (status-post gastric bypass surgery or partial gastrectomy) or decreased nutritional intake (alcoholics, chronic illness, extreme diets, anorexia).

Etiology and pathophysiology

Vitamin B12 (cobalamin) deficiency

Etiology

- Pernicious anemia is the most common cause.
- Gastrectomy, disease of the terminal ileum.
- Vegan diet (no meat, dairy products, or eggs).
- Nitrous oxide exposure can produce a B12 deficiency in those with marginal stores.

Clinical features

- May present as a myeloneuropathy (involvement of both the posterior columns of the spinal cord and the peripheral nerves).
- Symptoms include numbness, sensory ataxia, spastic weakness, reduced vibratory sense and proprioception, abnormal Romberg sign, and absent ankle jerks with hyper-reflexia elsewhere.
- Hand numbness may be more severe than the leg numbness due to the myelopathy.

Investigations

- Measure serum vitamin B12 levels.
- For low normal levels of B12 (<300 pg/ml), check methylmalonic acid and homocysteine levels to improve diagnostic sensitivity.

Treatment

- B12 1000 μg intramuscularly per week for 1 month, followed by monthly treatments.
- Oral replacement may be just as effective at a dose of 2000 mg daily.
- Improvement in the neuropathy depends on duration of symptoms.

Folate deficiency

Etiology

- Poor diet.
- Partial gastrectomy, duodenojejunal resections.
- Celiac disease.
- Medications that interfere with utilization of folic acid (phenytoin, phenobarbital, sulfasalazine, colchicine).

Clinical features

- Similar to vitamin B12 deficiency.

Investigations

- Check serum folate and vitamin B12.

Treatment

- Supplementation usually results in good clinical recovery.

Vitamin B6 (pyridoxine) deficiency or toxicity

Etiology

- Deficiency: malnutrition, chronic peritoneal dialysis, medications such as isoniazid or hydralazine.
- Toxicity: high-dose supplementation (recommended daily dose for adults is 2–4 mg).

Clinical features

- Deficiency: axonal sensorimotor polyneuropathy with more prominent sensory symptoms.
- Toxicity:
  - Sensory neuropathy with paresthesias and sensory ataxia resulting in a wide-based gait.
  - Sensory loss may be more pronounced in the upper extremities.
  - Normal muscle strength.
  - Absent or reduced reflexes.

Investigations

- Serum vitamin B6 level.
- Toxicity: NCS show reduced or absent sensory responses and preserved motor responses.

Treatment

- Deficiency: 50–100 mg daily of vitamin B6, which should be given prophylactically with isoniazid and hydralazine.
- Toxicity: stop B6 supplementation.

Vitamin B1 (thiamine) deficiency

Etiology

- Decreased intake or abnormal absorption:
  - Poor nutrition in alcoholism.
  - Chronic vomiting (e.g. hyperemesis gravidarum).
  - Total parental nutrition.
  - Gastric bypass surgery.
  - Restrictive diets.
  - Hyperthyroidism: increased metabolism and utilization of thiamine may result in a relative deficiency.

Clinical features

- Sensorimotor polyneuropathy.

Investigations

- Thiamine level may not be reliable for the diagnosis.
- Measure erythrocyte transketolase activity and the percentage increase in activity after adding thiamine pyrophosphate.

Treatment

- Intravenous thiamine 100 mg daily for 3 days, then 50 mg oral daily thereafter.
- Slow recovery is expected, but deficits persist with severe neuropathy.

Copper deficiency

Etiology

- Gastric surgery.
- Excessive zinc intake (from supplementation or certain denture creams) may cause copper deficiency by decreasing copper absorption[11].

Clinical features

- Myeloneuropathy similar to vitamin B12 deficiency. Numbness and paresthesias in the lower extremities with brisk reflexes and gait abnormalities.
- Copper deficiency may also cause neutropenia or pancytopenia.

Investigations

- Low serum copper levels.
- Microcytic anemia, neutropenia, or pancytopenia. Bone marrow biopsy may show a myelodysplastic syndrome.
- Magnetic resonance imaging (MRI) of the cervical spine may show abnormal T2-weighted signal in the dorsal columns.

Treatment

- Intravenous or oral copper supplementation:
  - Oral: 8 mg of elemental copper daily for 1 week, 6 mg daily for the second week, 4 mg daily for the third week, and 2 mg daily thereafter.
  - IV: 2 mg daily for 5 days and then periodically if necessary.
- Discontinue zinc source.
- Hematological and bone marrow abnormalities respond promptly to treatment. Neurologic symptoms may not improve, but symptom progression may be halted.

NEUROPATHY IN SYSTEMIC DISEASE

Definition

Untreated systemic disease that is causative of a neuropathic disorder.

Etiology, pathophysiology, and clinical features

Hypothyroidism

- Mononeuropathy at the wrist (carpal tunnel syndrome): occurs in 2–20%, possibly due to weight gain, edema compressing the carpal tunnel, or joint effusions. Usually resolves with thyroid replacement therapy.
- Rarely, a sensory polyneuropathy with painful paresthesias and numbness may occur and improves with treatment.

Hepatic disease

- Length-dependent axonal sensorimotor polyneuropathy, with sensory complaints prevailing.
- The exact mechanism for neuropathy is not known, but possibly related to accumulation of toxins secondary to liver disease that damage the nerve. Also, alcoholism or viral hepatitis may coexist as an etiology.

Renal insufficiency

Polyneuropathy

- Approximately 60% of patients with renal failure (glomeruler filtration rate <12 ml/min) develop a length-dependent axonal sensorimotor polyneuropathy. The pathogenesis may be related to accumulation of medium-sized proteins, which may be toxic to the nerves.

Mononeuropathy

- Median mononeuropathy at the wrist (carpal tunnel syndrome): most often associated with hemodialysis and deposition of β2-microglobulin in the transverse carpal ligament.
- Ischemic monomelic neuropathy: complication of arteriovenous shunt placed in the forearm for dialysis, affecting the median, ulnar, or radial nerves.

Celiac disease (gluten-induced enteropathy)

- Intolerance to gluten, in that gluten exposure results in a malabsorption syndrome.
- About 10% of patients develop neurologic complications, most commonly ataxia and neuropathy. The neuropathy usually presents with distal sensory loss, paresthesias, and unsteadiness. A small fiber neuropathy or autonomic neuropathy may also occur. The neuropathy may be the presenting feature of celiac disease.
- Serum antigliadin and endomysial antibodies are often positive.
- The pathogenesis of the neuropathy may be due to vitamin malabsorption or immune mediated.
- A gluten-free diet does not necessarily result in neuropathy improvement.
- Vitamin B12 and vitamin E supplementation should be considered.

Inflammatory bowel disease (ulcerative colitis and Crohn disease)

- This may be associated with a variety of neuropathies such as acute or chronic demyelinating polyneuropathy, axonal sensory or sensorimotor polyneuropathy, small fiber neuropathy, or brachial plexopathy.

Paraneoplastic neuropathy

- This refers to neuropathic complications preceding the diagnosis of an underlying malignancy.
- Most malignancies are detected within 4–12 months of symptom onset. However, there have been reports of malignances discovered after 8 years or more.
- Paraneoplastic neurologic syndromes are rare and occur in <1% of patients with cancer[12]. Small-cell lung carcinoma (SCLC) is the most common malignancy associated with a paraneoplastic syndrome. Other associated malignancies include carcinoma of the esophagus, breast, ovaries, kidney, and lymphoma.

Sensory neuronopathy/ganglionopathy

- Patients present with acute–subacute numbness and paresthesias in the distal extremities, often beginning in the hands (to be distinguished from a length-dependent polyneuropathy). On neurologic examination, all sensory modalities are affected and reflexes are depressed. Sensory ataxia and pseudoathetosis may be present.

Autonomic neuropathy

- Patients present with severe gastrointestinal dysmotility. Often associated with another neurologic syndrome such as limbic encephalitis or sensory ganglionopathy.
- Associated antibodies include anti-Hu and CRMP-5. However, negative antibody tests do not exclude the diagnosis of a paraneoplastic neuropathy[13]. It is believed that there is antigenic similarity between proteins expressed in the tumor cells and the neuron cells, resulting in an immune response directed against both types of cells.

Paraproteinemia

- There is an association between immunoglobulin (Ig)M, IgG, and IgA monoclonal proteins and polyneuropathy. Most cases are a benign form called monoclonal gammopathy of unknown significance. Other syndromes include primary systemic amyloidosis, osteosclerotic myeloma, multiple myeloma, Waldenstrom's macroglobulinemia, and cryoglobulinemia.
- The neuropathy is usually a slowly progressing sensorimotor polyradiculopathy or polyneuropathy that resembles CIDP. The sensory deficit appears earlier and is more prominent than the motor deficit. CSF total protein is elevated, often >1g/l (100 mg/dl).
- Treatment: plasmapheresis, corticosteroids, and chemotherapy have been used with variable success.

POEMS

(Polyneuropathy, organomegaly, endocrinopathies, M-protein, skin changes, including thickening and hyperpigmentation, and clubbing of the fingers.)

- A syndrome that presents with a slowly progressive, mainly motor demyelinating neuropathy.
- Most common endocrinopathies include hypogonadism, diabetes, and hypothyroidism.
- Usually IgG or IgA monoclonal protein. Serum vascular endothelial growth factor is elevated.

GUILLAIN–BARRÉ SYNDROME (GBS)/ACUTE INFLAMMATORY DEMYELINATING POLYRADICULONEUROPATHY (AIDP)

Definition and epidemiology

Acute onset of extremity paresthesias, numbness, and progressive weakness, with potential risk of respiratory insufficiency due to a demyelinating process involving the nerve roots and peripheral nerves (polyradiculoneuropathy).

- Worldwide incidence of 0.6–4 cases per 100,000.
- AIDP (demyelinating form) accounts for about 90% of North American and European cases; 5–10% of cases constitute an axonal subtype, acute motor axonal neuropathy (AMAN).
- Two-thirds of cases have an antecedent infection within 6 weeks of symptom onset, most commonly an upper respiratory infection or gastroenteritis. Usual infections include Epstein–Barr virus, *Mycoplasma pneumoniae*, *Campylobacter jejuni*, and cytomegalovirus (CMV).
- Reports of GBS occurring after vaccinations, surgery, and head trauma.

Pathophysiology[14]

Caused by an aberrant immune response that damages peripheral nerves.

- Activated macrophages invade intact myelin sheaths resulting in myelin damage and demyelination. Mechanisms may be explained by the following:
- Activated helper T cells react against antigens on the surface of Schwann cells and direct activated macrophages to this region.
- Humoral immunity: antibodies bind to epitopes on the surface of Schwann cells inducing complement activation and subsequent myelin destruction.
- In severe cases, inflammatory mediators may induce axonal damage in addition to the demyelination.
- In AMAN, the macrophages are believed to invade the space between the Schwann cell and axon, leaving the myelin sheath intact.

Clinical features

- Initial symptoms are pain, numbness, paresthesias, or weakness in the limbs. The severity of symptoms varies greatly among individuals.
- The main feature of GBS is rapidly progressive bilateral and relatively symmetric weakness of the limbs, usually affecting the lower extremities first. Classically, both proximal and distal muscles are involved simultaneously. This may also be accompanied by respiratory and/or cranial nerve involvement.

- The facial nerve is the most common cranial nerve affected. Facial neuropathy occurs in 50% of cases and is frequently bilateral[14].
- About 25% of patients have severe respiratory involvement warranting mechanical ventilation.
- Dysautonomia (cardiac arrhythmia, hypertension or hypotension, ileus, urinary retention) occurs in up to 15% of patients.
- Reflexes are almost always depressed or absent.
- Many patients have back pain during the course of the disease.

Variants

- AMAN presents similarly to AIDP, but has a more rapid and severe course, often resulting in mechanical ventilation. Autonomic involvement is mild.
- Miller–Fisher syndrome (MFS):
  - Clinical triad of ophthalmologic abnormalities, ataxia, areflexia.
  - Ophthalmologic abnormalities include acute ophthalmoplegia, internuclear ophthalmoplegia, Parinaud's syndrome, convergence failure, divergence paralysis, optic neuritis, ptosis, isolated abducens nerve palsy.
  - Rare respiratory failure.
  - Generally, recovery is good. There are no randomized controlled trials for IVIG or plasmapheresis in the treatment of MFS. However, if symptoms are severe (limb weakness, autonomic symptoms, respiratory involvement, dysphagia), patients may benefit from a course of IVIG[15].
- Bickerstaff brainstem encephalitis: similar syndrome that presents with cranial or peripheral nerve involvement and may evolve to altered consciousness and even coma. Plasmapheresis should be considered.

Differential diagnosis

- Vasculitic neuropathy.
- Acute intermittent porphyria.
- Heavy metal intoxication (arsenic poisoning).
- Acute onset of chronic inflammatory demyelinating polyneuropathy (CIDP).
- Tick paralysis.
- Vitamin B1 deficiency.

Investigations

NCS

Motor NCS determine diagnostic criteria. Sensory NCS help to differentiate various forms of axonal GBS, for example AMAN, from acute motor and sensory axonal neuropathy (AMSAN)[14].

Neurophysiological criteria for AIDP

- CMAP amplitude (measured in mV) may be normal or reduced, depending on the degree of axonal involvement.
- Conduction block; must occur at a noncompression site, such as between the wrist and below elbow when testing the ulnar nerve (**734**):
  - Definite conduction block is defined by >50% reduction in the proximal CMAP amplitude compared with the distal CMAP amplitude.
  - Probable conduction block is >30% reduction.
  - Conduction block cannot be diagnosed if CMAP amplitude is <1 mV.
  - Temporal dispersion is diagnosed by >30% increase in proximal negative peak CMAP duration.
  - Motor conduction velocity, measured in m/s, is <70% of the lower limit of normal.
  - Distal motor latency, measured in ms, is >150% of the upper limit of normal.
  - F-wave latency, measured in ms, is >120% of the upper limit of normal.

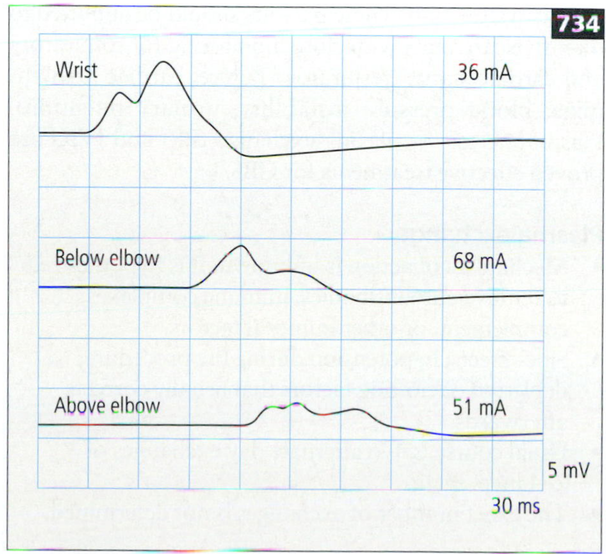

734 Nerve conduction study in acute inflammatory demyelinating polyradiculoneuropathy. Conduction block at a noncompression site (between the wrist and below elbow stimulation sites) and temporal dispersion noted in the left ulnar nerve. Wrist CMAP amplitude: 7.5 mV; below elbow CMAP amplitude: 4 mV; above elbow CMAP amplitude: 4 mV.

At least 85% of patients with AIDP have evidence of demyelination on NCS. For patients with normal NCS, repeat studies in 1–2 weeks may be required for diagnosis confirmation[14]. Since AIDP initially affects the very proximal (nerve roots) and very distal nerve fibers, the first abnormalities noted on NCS may be prolonged F responses and normal sural responses. The latter finding is termed sural sparing. As the disease progresses, the sural response becomes reduced or absent.

Other tests

- EMG: used to assess the degree of axonal loss, which is primary in AMAN or secondary in AIDP.
- CSF studies:
  - In 80% of cases, CSF studies reveal increased total protein with a normal white blood cell count. This finding is referred to as albuminocytologic dissociation. If white blood cells are present in the CSF, there should be <50 cells/mm. If there are >50 cells/mm in the CSF, other diagnoses such as HIV polyradiculopathy should be considered[14].
  - CSF studies are often normal 1 week after disease onset. However, by the end of the second week, 90% of patients will have elevated total protein.
- Serum antibodies[15]: in about 50% of patients with GBS, serum antibodies to various gangliosides have been found:
  - Pure motor or axonal variants are associated with GM1, GM1b, GD1a, and GalNAc-GD1a.
  - MFS and GBS overlapping syndromes (Bickerstaff brainstem encephalitis) are associated with GQ1b, GD3, and GT1a.
  - The antibodies associated with AIDP are not known.

Treatment

Severe cases can lead to respiratory distress and autonomic dysfunction. These patients should be admitted to intensive care units with close monitoring for respiratory and cardiac status (respiratory failure, cardiac arrhythmias, blood pressure instability, urinary retention). Plasmapheresis or plasma exchange (PE) and IVIG are proven effective treatments for GBS.

Plasma exchange

- Mechanism of action is unknown. It is hypothesized to remove autoantibodies, immune complexes, complement, or other humoral factors.
- Side-effects: hypotension during the procedure, depletion of clotting factors that usually corrects afterwards.
- Usual course is 4–6 alternate day exchanges of 2–4 liters each.
- The exact number of exchanges is not determined.

Intravenous immunoglobulin

- Proven to be as effective as PE. IVIG is readily available at most centers, while PE may only be available at tertiary care centers.
- IVIG may inhibit the binding of ganglioside antibodies to their respective antigens, preventing complement activation.
- Common side-effects include headaches and flu-like symptoms that can occur during the infusion or within the next few days following treatment. Renal failure is a risk with preparations containing sucrose. Rare side-effects include strokes and myocardial infarctions, but this risk is significantly reduced with slower rates of infusion (should never exceed 300 ml per hour).
- IVIG dosing is 2 g/kg body weight infused over 2–5 days. Younger patients in good health usually tolerate 2-day treatment. Patients who are older, have other comorbidities (e.g. cardiovascular disease), or are intolerant of side-effects may do better with 4- or 5-day treatment.

Treatment with either IVIG or PE should be initiated within the first 7–10 days of symptoms. Improvement can be delayed 1 week to 1 month. About 10% of responders have a limited relapse after either treatment. At the time, it is not known which of these patients will go on to develop CIDP. An additional course of IVIG or PE should be given. Treating patients who are mildly affected (defined by being able to walk with or without assistance) is somewhat controversial. There is some evidence that treating these patients with PE may hasten motor recovery[15].

Corticosteroids do not appear to be beneficial and some patients actually notice worsening of their symptoms.

Prognosis

- Nadir should be around 2–4 weeks, followed by progressive recovery over weeks to months. GBS is usually a monophasic illness, although 7–16% of patients have a recurrence in symptoms[14].
- During recovery, 10–20% of patients experience disabling motor deficits. Up to 15% of patients die by 1 year after onset.
- Adverse prognostic factors include older age at onset (>50 years old), severe disease at nadir (bed bound or on mechanical ventilation), rapid onset of disease, infection with *Campylobacter jejuni* or CMV, and evidence of axonal loss on neurophysiologic studies[14].

Tip

► *If symptoms continue to worsen after 8 weeks, consider the acute onset of CIDP rather than GBS.*

CHRONIC ACQUIRED DEMYELINATING POLYNEUROPATHY

A group of demyelinating peripheral nerve disorders that share common clinical and pathologic features. These polyneuropathies often respond to immunomodulatory therapy[16].

CHRONIC INFLAMMATORY DEMYELINATING POLYNEUROPATHY (CIDP)

Definition

- Immune-mediated neuropathy with a relapsing or progressive course that is characterized by both proximal and distal weakness.
- Considered to be the 'chronic variation' of AIDP.
- Most common of the chronic acquired demyelinating polyneuropathies.

Epidemiology

- 2 per 100,000.
- Usual onset 40–60 years of age.
- Slight male predominance.

Etiology and pathophysiology

- Immune-mediated process for which the specific antigens are not known.
- Certain comorbidities may make people more susceptible to acquiring CIDP, including Charcot–Marie–Tooth disease (CMT), hepatitis C, diabetes, or a paraproteinemia.

Clinical features

- Most cases present with progressive, symmetric proximal and distal weakness of arms and legs.
- Up to 80% of cases have both motor and sensory symptoms.
- Sensory abnormalities on examination are predominantly the large fiber modalities (i.e. vibration, position sense, and touch). Sensory ataxia and unsteady gait may be a presenting symptom.
- Diffuse areflexia or hyporeflexia.
- Symptoms must be present for at least 2 months to distinguish from AIDP.
- Infection and pregnancy may trigger an exacerbation.

Tip

▶ *CIDP presents with both proximal and distal weakness.*

Differential diagnosis

- Diabetic CIDP.
- Toxic (cyclosporine, tacrolimus, tumor necrosis alpha blockers).
- HIV neuropathy.

Investigations

Motor NCS

The American Academy of Neurology (AAN) has developed research criteria for the diagnosis of CIDP, which involve mandatory and supportive findings on electrophysiologic studies[17].

Mandatory

There must be three of the following four criteria, which indicate acquired, segmental demyelination of the nerves.

- Reduction in conduction velocity in two or more motor nerves:
  - <80% of lower limit of normal (LLN) if amplitude >80% of LLN (indicating disruption of the myelin with intact and functioning axons).
  - <70% of LLN if amplitude <80% of LLN (both demyelinating and axonal features).
- Partial conduction block or abnormal temporal dispersion occurring at a noncompression site in one or more motor nerves (i.e. peroneal nerve between ankle and below fibular head, median nerve between wrist and elbow, ulnar nerve between wrist and below elbow):
  - Partial conduction block is defined by >20% amplitude drop between proximal and distal stimulation sites.
  - Temporal dispersion is defined by >15% increase in duration after proximal stimulation. This occurs from desynchronization of components of the CMAP due to different rates of conduction.
- Prolonged distal latencies in two or more motor nerves:
  - >125% of upper limit of normal (ULN) if amplitude >80% of LLN.
  - >150% of ULN if amplitude <80% of LLN.
- Absent F-waves or prolonged minimum F-wave latencies (10–15 trials) in two or more nerves:
  - >120% of ULN if amplitude >80% of LLN.
  - >150% of ULN if amplitude <80% of LLN.

Supportive

- Reduction in sensory conduction velocity <80% of LLN.
- Absent H reflexes.

Sensory NCS

- Low amplitude or absent SNAPs in both upper and lower extremities.
- If SNAPs are obtained, distal latencies may be prolonged and conduction velocities slowed.
- Median, ulnar, and radial SNAPs may be abnormally low amplitude compared with the sural SNAP, which suggests a nonlength-dependent process. If this phenomenon does occur, the differential diagnosis should include a demyelinating neuropathy or sensory neuronopathy.

EMG

- Spontaneous activity such as fibrillations may be noted if secondary axonal degeneration has occurred.
- Myokymic discharges (cross-talk between demyelinated nerve fibers) may be noted.
- MUPs appear morphologically normal, but have reduced recruitment with rapid firing. This may be one of the earliest abnormalities.

CSF studies

- 85–90% of cases have an elevated protein with a mean of 1.35 g/l (135 mg/dl).
- Cell count is usually normal (up to 10% may have pleocytosis with greater than 5 lymphocytes/mm^3).
- Oligoclonal bands may be present.

Other tests

- Lumbar spine MRI. Enhancement of the nerve roots may be observed (735–737).
- Nerve biopsy (not essential for the diagnosis):
  - Segmental demyelination and remyelination. However, because of the multifocal process, this finding may be missed on biopsy.
  - Onion bulbs:
    - Formed from proliferation of the surrounding Schwann cells, due to chronic demyelination and remyelination.
    - Usually not a prominent feature on biopsy.
  - Inflammatory cell infiltrate may be evident in the epineurium, perineurium, or endoneurium, but is usually subtle or absent.
  - Teased fiber preparations may demonstrate segmental demyelination, remyelination, and/or axonal degeneration (738, 739).

Treatment

Corticosteroids, IVIG, and PE are acceptable first-line treatments for CIDP.

Corticosteroids

- Usually start with 60–100 mg daily for up to 4 weeks. When strength has improved, a slow taper can be initiated (5 mg every 2–3 weeks).
- Most patients require some type of immunosuppressive therapy to prevent relapses. A steroid-sparing agent such as azathioprine, mycophenolate mofetil, cyclophosphamide, cyclosporine, or methotrexate (*Table 116*) may be necessary if symptoms flare during the taper.

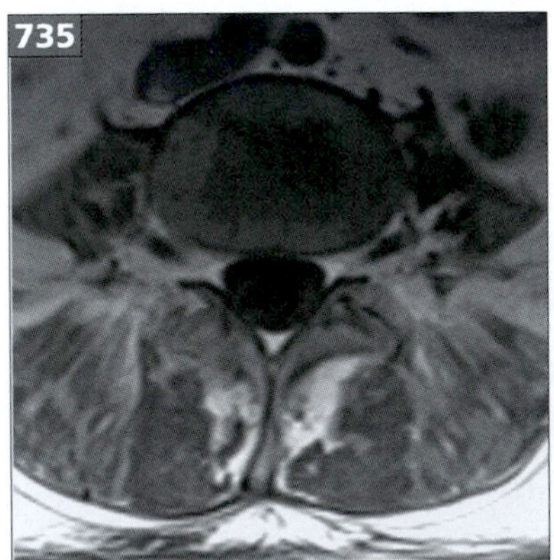

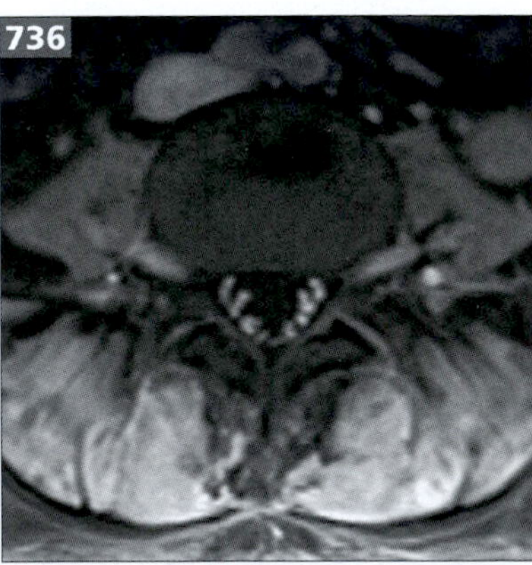

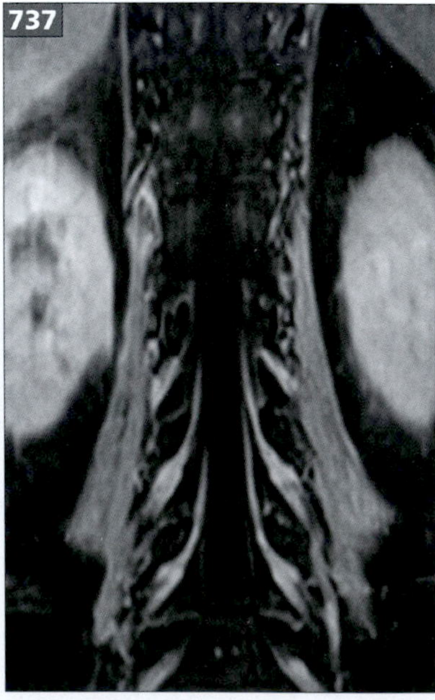

735–737 Lumbar spine MRI in chronic inflammatory demyelinating polyneuropathy (CIDP). (735) Noncontrasted T1-weighted image; (736, 737) contrasted T1-weighted images which show enhancement of the nerve roots in a case of CIDP.

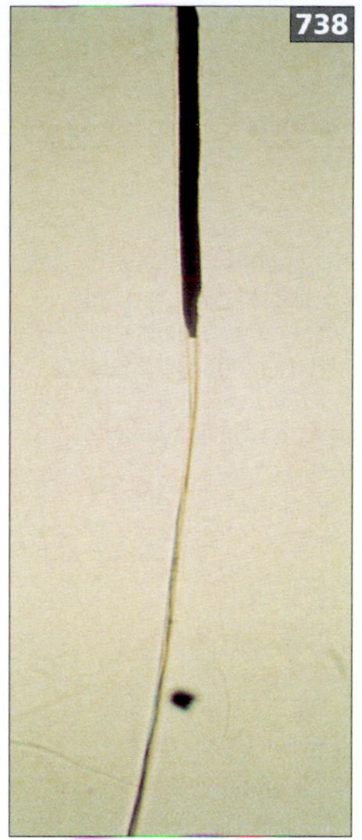

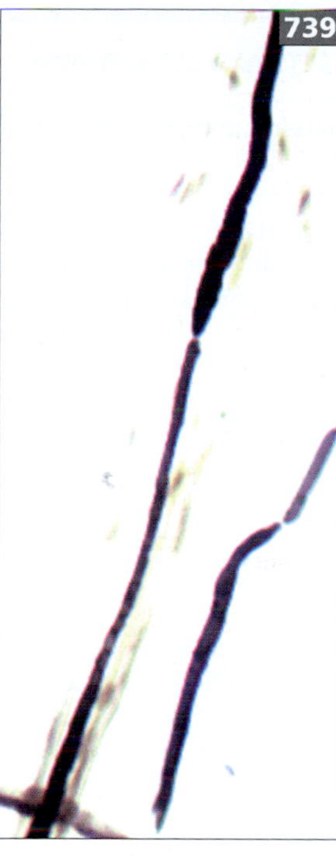

738, 739 **Teased nerve fiber preparation showing segmental demyelination; (738) in a case of chronic inflammatory demyelinating polyneuropathy; (739) in the lower half of the image.** *739 courtesy of Tibor Valyi-Nagy, MD, PhD.*

IVIG

- After an initiation dose of 2 g/kg, dosing is usually 1 g/kg monthly. However, dosing can range from every 2 weeks to every 8 weeks, depending on symptoms.

PE

- Use may be limited by availability.
- Because the effect of PE only lasts for a few weeks, it is difficult to use as a chronic therapy. Can be helpful during disease flares.

MULTIFOCAL MOTOR NEUROPATHY (MMN)

Definition

- An immune-mediated neuropathy only affecting the motor nerves.

Epidemiology

- 1 per 100,000 with predilection for young adults.

Etiology and pathophysiology

- Immune-mediated process that is a distinct entity from CIDP.
- Presumed antigens to be specific to the motor nerve.

Clinical features

- Painless asymmetric limb weakness usually in the distribution of an individual nerve with normal or diminished reflexes.
- Muscle fasciculations may be present, a finding that can lead to a misdiagnosis of motor neuron disease.
- Radial neuropathy is the most common presentation.

Differential diagnosis

- Vasculitic neuropathy, although pain is usually a prominent feature.
- Immune-mediated brachial plexus neuropathy.
- Amyotrophic lateral sclerosis; usually presents with hyper-reflexia in the affected limbs. In MMN cases, reflexes are usually normal or diminished in the affected limbs.

Investigations

Motor nerve conduction studies

Conduction block at a noncompression site is the electrophysiologic hallmark of MMN. However, it does not need to be present to make the diagnosis.

In one series, 31% of patients with MMN had conduction block, while 94% had other electrophysiologic features of demyelination (prolonged distal latencies, temporal dispersion, slowed conduction velocity, prolonged or absent F responses)[16].

- Normal sensory responses on NCS.
- EMG: denervation may be present if secondary axonal loss has occurred.
- CSF studies: total protein is normal in most cases (as opposed to CIDP).
- Serum antibodies[16]:
  - 40–80% of MMN cases have polyclonal IgM antibodies directed against GM1.
  - Very high titers of anti-GM1 are specific for MMN, but low titers can be present in other disorders such as GBS, CIDP, or motor neuron disease.

TABLE 116 **IMMUNOSUPPRESSANT MEDICATIONS SIDE-EFFECTS AND MANAGEMENT**

Potential side-effects	**Management/monitoring of side-effects**
AZATHIOPRINE	
• Nausea, vomiting • Pancytopenia • Hepatic toxicity • Increased risk of infection and malignancy • Hypersensitivity reaction occurring within the first several weeks (nausea, vomiting, rash, fever, malaise, myalgias, elevation of liver transaminases)	• Less nausea if taken in divided doses • Baseline complete blood count with platelets and liver transaminases, then weekly the first month, twice monthly the next 2 months, then monthly while on treatment • Discontinue drug or reduce dose if white blood cell count <3000/ml • Measure thiopurine methyltransferase: low activity may lead to bone marrow toxicity • Warn patients of allergic reaction, which requires drug discontinuation
CYCLOPHOSPHAMIDE	
• Hemorrhagic cystitis, risk of transitional cell carcinoma of bladder • Dose-related bone marrow suppression • Increased risk of infection associated with leukopenia • Gonadal toxicity, permanent infertility • Teratogenicity	• Routine urinalysis to evaluate for hematuria (may indicate bladder carcinoma) • Ample fluids following dosing • Complete blood counts with platelets weekly for the first month and then monthly while on treatment; total leukocyte counts <3500/ml mandates taper or suspension of the medication • Birth-control measures
METHOTREXATE	
• Bone marrow toxicity • Hepatic fibrosis and cirrhosis, elevated liver function tests • Increased risk for opportunistic infections • Stevens–Johnson syndrome, toxic epidermal necrolysis • Pulmonary fibrosis	• Baseline complete blood count with platelets and liver function tests, then repeated every 3 months; should be checked if fever develops • Prophylactic trimethoprim/ sulfamethoxazole twice weekly • Discontinue medication if rash develops • Baseline pulmonary function tests
MYCOPHENOLATE MOFETIL	
• Pancytopenia • Malignant epithelial neoplasm of the skin (nonmelanoma) • Diarrhea	• Complete blood count with platelets weekly during first month, twice monthly for next 2 months, then monthly through the first year on medication
PREDNISONE	
• Increased susceptibility to infections • Increased appetite, weight gain • Hyperglycemia, hypertension • Insomnia • Avascular necrosis of femoral heads • Osteoporosis • Peptic ulcer disease • Cataracts	• Monitor diet and weight, regular exercise program • Periodic serum glucose and blood pressure monitoring • Supplemental calcium with vitamin D, may require bisphosphonates if abnormal bone density testing • Proton pump inhibitor • Ophthalmology evaluation
RITUXIMAB	
• Bone marrow suppression • Severe infusion reactions • Arrhythmia, cardiogenic shock • Angioedema • Flu-like symptoms	• Baseline complete blood count, repeat at 2 and 4 weeks, then monthly • Caution in patients with a history of coronary artery disease or arrhythmias • Discontinue in cases of severe reactions

Treatment[16]

Typically, patients have a good response to IVIG, which begins within several days and lasts several weeks. Serial IVIG (administered approximately monthly) is the mainstay treatment for MMN. If a patient is going to respond to IVIG, it is often apparent after the first treatment. Nonresponders to the first treatment generally will not respond to subsequent doses. For nonresponders to IVIG, other treatments such as cyclophosphamide, rituximab, or mycophenolate mofetil are less studied options.

OTHER VARIANTS

Distal acquired demyelinating symmetric neuropathy (DADS)

Predominantly sensory symptoms and signs including gait ataxia and occasional tremor.

Despite mostly sensory findings on examination, the motor NCS are abnormal. Distal latencies are significantly prolonged resulting in a short terminal latency index. This indicates the conduction velocity slowing is most prominent in the distal nerve segments.

There is a strong association with antibodies against myelin associated glycoprotein (anti-MAG). This is often discovered after finding an elevated IgM level on serum immunofixation electrophoresis. Patients respond poorly to immunomodulatory therapy.

Multifocal acquired demyelinating sensory and motor neuropathy (MADSAM)

Insidious onset of motor and sensory loss in the distribution of individual nerves with accompanying pain and paresthesias. Arms are usually involved initially with eventual spread to the legs. Reflexes are diminished or absent in accordance with the involved nerves. As the disease progresses, diffuse areflexia may develop.

Similarly to MMN, motor NCS may reveal conduction block, temporal dispersion, prolonged distal latencies, slowed conduction velocities, and prolonged F responses. Unlike MMN, sensory responses may also be abnormal.

CSF total protein is elevated in a majority of cases. There may be improvement with IVIG or corticosteroid treatment.

VASCULITIC NEUROPATHY

Definition and epidemiology

Ischemia and infarction of one or more peripheral nerves due to vasculitis (destruction of the blood vessel wall from inflammatory cell infiltration) of the vasa nervorum.

- Peripheral nerve involvement can occur in up to 30% of systemic vasculitidies[5].
- Of all cases of vasculitic neuropathy, approximately 30% have no other organ involvement (nonsystemic vasculitic neuropathy)[18].

Etiology

Systemic vasculitic neuropathy

The vasculitidies most commonly associated with vasculitic neuropathy are those affecting small- to medium-sized vessels. The vasa vasorum contains vessels ranging from 50–400 µm in diameter.

- Primary systemic vasculitic neuropathy occurs in the setting of a disorder with mainly vasculitic manifestations:
  - Churg–Strauss syndrome: neuropathy is common, occurring in 65–80% of cases.
  - Microscopic polyangiitis occurs in >50% of cases.
  - Polyarteritis nodosa: up to 75% of patients.
  - Wegener granulomatosis: 14–40% of patients.
- Secondary systemic vasculitic neuropathy occurs in the setting of a disorder with nonvasculitic manifestations such as systemic lupus erythematosus (SLE), rheumatoid arthritis, and Sjögren's syndrome. Vasculitic neuropathy is uncommon in SLE and rheumatoid arthritis, but is a relatively common occurrence in Sjögren's syndrome.

Other vasculitic neuropathies

- In nonsystemic vasculitic neuropathy, vasculitis is isolated to the peripheral nerves with no other systemic manifestations. However, in 6–37% of these cases, systemic vasculitis is discovered later on in the course of the disease.
- Hypersensitivity and infectious vasculitic syndromes with associated neuropathy are rare:
  - Infectious: hepatitis C (often associated with cryoglobulinemia), HIV, CMV, herpes zoster, Lyme disease, syphilis, tuberculosis, beta-hemolytic streptococci.
  - Drug-induced: sulfonamides, amphetamines, cocaine.
- Paraneoplastic vasculitic neuropathy from an underlying malignancy (rare etiology).

Pathophysiology

- An inflammatory process with unknown triggering events. Altered expression and function of adhesion molecules and leukocyte and endothelial cell activation appear to play a role in pathogenesis[19].
- Drug-induced: most likely related to a complement-mediated leukocytoclastic reaction.

Clinical features

Mononeuropathy multiplex is the classic presentation of peripheral nerve involvement.

Symptoms occur in multiple individual nerve distributions. The first symptom is often the sudden onset of severe, throbbing pain localized to the region of acute nerve infarction, which usually occurs in the upper arm or thigh due to watershed areas of the vasa nervorum. The absence of pain is rare and should raise concern for an alternative diagnosis. The pain is followed by sensory abnormalities and weakness in the distribution of the affected nerves.

Nerves that are particularly susceptible to injury include the peroneal nerve (90%), tibial nerve (38%), ulnar nerve (35%), and median nerve (26%)[5].

Mononeuropathies may occur within days or weeks of each other. However, in the event that only one nerve is clinically symptomatic, vasculitic neuropathy should be included in the differential diagnosis if the mononeuropathy was preceded by severe limb pain.

In clinical practice, the majority of patients have a confluence of multiple mononeuropathies, which appears as a generalized and asymmetric polyneuropathy at the time of presentation. It is important to ask the patient direct questions regarding the onset and progression of symptoms. They may describe a stepwise progression of individual nerve involvement coalescing into a diffuse pattern (e.g. right foot drop followed by left foot drop later on). Again, pain should be a prominent feature.

Occasionally, symptoms may worsen rapidly over days and evolve into a painful quadriparesis.

Tip

▶ *Mononeuropathy multiplex – think vasculitis.*

Signs and symptoms associated with systemic vasculitis

- Weight loss, malaise, fevers/chills, and night sweats.
- Signs of other end organ dysfunction (skin, lung, bowel, kidney, joints, central nervous system [CNS]).
- Churg–Strauss syndrome usually presents with asthma, pulmonary infiltrates, fevers, and eosinophilia. However, an initial presentation of vasculitic neuropathy occurs in more than 20% of cases.
- Most common pattern of nerve involvement in polyarteritis nodosa is mononeuropathy multiplex. Cranial neuropathies and CNS involvement occur in <2% of patients. The neuropathy is commonly associated with hepatitis B, which portends a more aggressive disease course.
- Wegener granulomatosis is a necrotizing vasculitis of the respiratory tract and kidneys. Early symptoms include nasal discharge, coughing, and hemoptysis. Neuropathy usually occurs in the setting of severe renal involvement. Cranial neuropathies occur in 5–10% of cases as a result of extension of nasal granulomas rather than vasculitis.
- Skin rash of erythematous macules or purpuric papules associated with cryoglobulinemia (**740**).

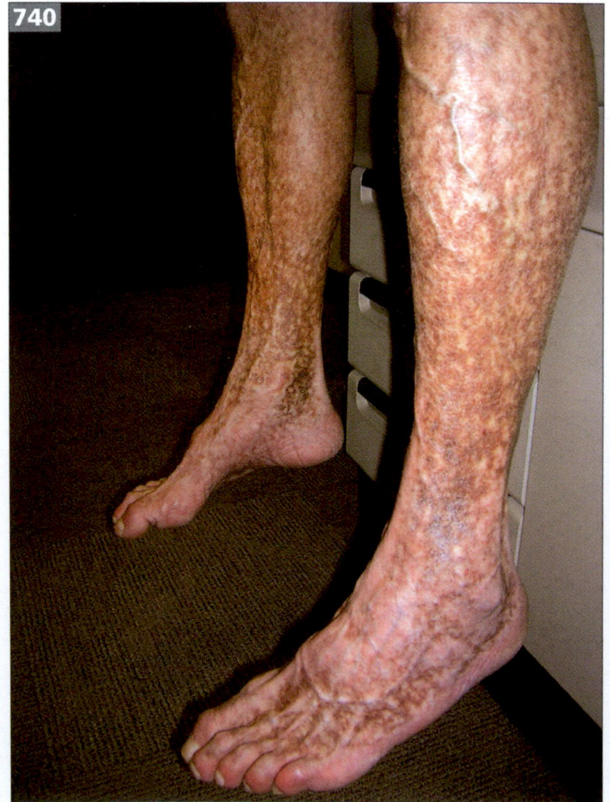

740 Skin rash associated with cryoglobulinemia.

- Sicca symptoms (dry mouth, dry eyes) associated with Sjögren's syndrome. Sjögren's syndrome may present with a sensory neuronopathy (dorsal root ganglionopathy) or distal sensory neuropathy. Cranial neuropathies, such as trigeminal neuropathy, can occur.
- Rheumatoid vasculitis occurs as a late manifestation of severe seropositive disease. With advancements in effective treatment, this is declining in incidence. Many patients with rheumatoid arthritis develop a mild, symmetrical polyneuropathy, which is distinct from vasculitic neuropathy. Median mononeuropathy at the wrist (carpal tunnel syndrome) and other compressive neuropathies are quite common.
- Nonsystemic vasculitic neuropathy usually presents with mononeuropathy multiplex. Individual attacks of mononeuropathy are less frequent than systemic vasculitic neuropathy. Most affected nerves recover gradually.
- When considering drug-induced vasculitic neuropathy, there should be a temporal relationship with drug ingestion.

Differential diagnosis

- Compression or entrapment neuropathies; however, conduction block in vasculitic neuropathy is not located at common compression sites.
- Multifocal motor neuropathy: usually not painful.
- Malignant infiltration of individual nerves.
- Diabetic lumbosacral radiculoplexus neuropathy may present with similar clinical features.

Investigations

NCS

- Sensory and motor responses are absent or have reduced amplitudes (axonal degeneration). Pattern of nerve involvement is often multifocal and asymmetric and can be nonlength dependent.
- Usually demyelination features are not present. However, conduction blocks (not at common compression sites) can be identified if the NCS are performed within a few days after nerve infarction and prior to Wallerian degeneration. This phenomenon has been labeled pseudoconduction block due to the 'disappearance' of the conduction block on follow-up studies performed after 1 week or more. At that time, the motor responses have reduced amplitude due to the axon loss.

Blood and CSF

- CSF studies are often not helpful other than ruling out other etiologies (infections, inflammatory, carcinomatous)[19].
- Routine blood and urine tests: complete blood count, metabolic panel (electrolytes, glucose, blood urea nitrogen, creatinine), erythrocyte sedimentation rate, C-reactive protein, antinuclear antibody, urinanalysis.
- Other blood tests that should be included in the work-up for a systemic vasculitis:
  - Rheumatoid factor, anti-cyclic citrullinated peptide antibody (rheumatoid arthritis). Rheumatoid factor can be positive in other autoimmune diseases, infections (hepatitis C), and following chemotherapy and radiation treatment for cancer. However, anti-CCP antibody has a high specificity for rheumatoid arthritis[20].
  - Antineutrophil cytoplasmic antibodies (positive in 90% of Wegener granulomatosis and 50% of Churg–Strauss syndrome).
  - Serum complement levels, anti-double stranded DNA antibodies (SLE).
  - Anti-SSA, anti-SSB (Sjögren's syndrome).
  - Hepatitis B and C panel.
  - Cryoglobulins.

Nerve biopsy

Evaluating for vasculitic neuropathy is an important indication for nerve biopsy. In most cases, the diagnosis of vasculitic neuropathy is established by nerve biopsy, although the onset of neuropathy following a diagnostic biopsy of another affected organ (e.g. kidney, lung) can practically secure the diagnosis (systemic vasculitic neuropathy).

Nerve biopsy is mandatory to confirm the diagnosis of nonsystemic vasculitic neuropathy. Combined nerve and muscle biopsy is recommended as this improves the diagnostic yield (e.g. sensory branch of the superficial peroneal nerve and peroneus brevis muscle). The frequency of a diagnostic nerve biopsy or combined nerve/muscle biopsy (with a mandatory finding of vessel wall disruption) is approximately 60%.

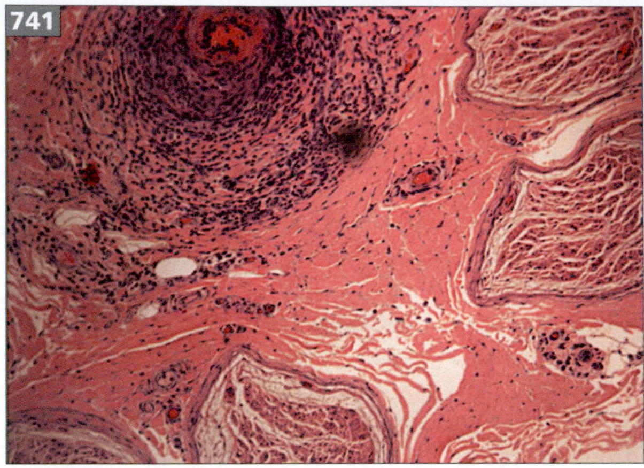

741 **Sural nerve biopsy showing inflammation of a blood vessel wall and surrounding epineurial connective tissue and fascicles.** *Courtesy of Tibor Valyi-Nagy, MD, PhD.*

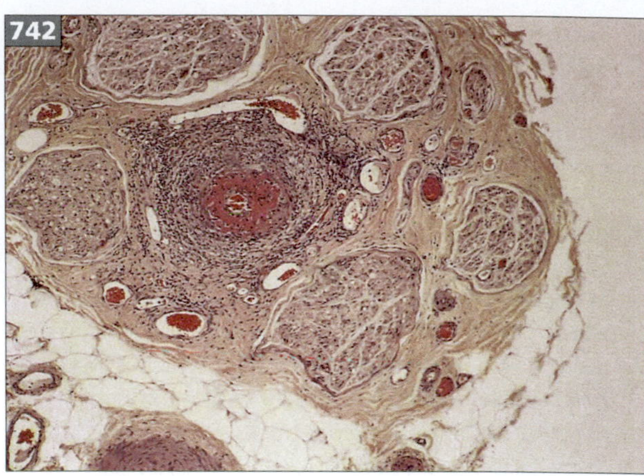

742 **Sural nerve biopsy from a patient with ischemic neuropathy due to polyarteritis nodosa, showing infiltration by neutrophils and fibrinoid necrosis of the vessel wall.**

Characteristic histopathological findings include:

- Inflammatory cell infiltration of blood vessels: T cells and macrophages invading epineurial arteries (**741, 742**).
- Necrosis of the vessel wall leading to structural damage.

Immunohistochemically, immunoglobulin (IgM, IgG), complement, membrane attack, and complex deposition on blood vessels is seen. A supportive feature is multifocal, asymmetric nerve fiber loss with variable degrees of axon degeneration among different nerve fascicles[5].

EMG shows denervation in muscles supplied by affected nerves.

Treatment

Systemic vasculitic neuropathy

There are currently no controlled treatment trials. Thus, treatment regimens are derived from studies in patients with systemic vasculitis without neuropathy.

Initial treatment includes prednisone 1 mg/kg/day and oral or IV pulse cyclophosphamide with doses of 1–2 mg/kg/day and 1 g/m^2, respectively. In severe cases, IV methylprednisolone can be used instead of oral prednisone. Cyclophosphamide seems to be the most effective medication for induction of remission. Most patients require 3–12 months of cyclophosphamide before transitioning to a maintenance immunosuppressant (i.e. azathioprine, methotrexate, rituximab, mycophenolate mofetil).

After 1–2 months a slow prednisone taper can be started. The daily dose can be reduced by 5–10 mg every month with an even slower taper when doses reach <20 mg daily.

Nonsystemic vasculitic neuropathy

The neurological deficits often spontaneously resolve over time. The disease may remit for many years before returning. Therefore, the risks of immunosuppressive therapies should be thoroughly weighed against the potential benefits prior to initiation.

Prednisone monotherapy is often adequate, at a dose of 40–60 mg daily for 2–3 months. If there is an adequate clinical response, a slow taper can be initiated with transition to alternate day dosing[19].

A retrospective study indicated that combination therapy of prednisone and cyclophosphamide had a superior response after 6 months and fewer relapses compared with patients taking prednisone alone. However, the patients treated with cyclophosphamide had a greater incidence of pneumonia, herpes zoster, and sepsis[5].

Other options for corticosteroid nonresponders or those with tapering difficulties include azathioprine or methotrexate.

Prognosis

If left untreated, systemic vasculitic neuropathy may be fatal. Thus, therapeutic intervention is almost always indicated.

Unlike systemic vasculitic neuropathy, untreated nonsystemic vasculitic neuropathy is not usually fatal. Long-term follow-up studies have shown that most patients with nonsystemic vasculitic neuropathy can walk without assistance.

IMMUNE-MEDIATED BRACHIAL PLEXUS NEUROPATHY (IBPN)

Definition and epidemiology

Acute to subacute injury to the brachial plexus or individual nerves of the upper extremity resulting in severe arm pain, weakness, and sensory changes. Other terminologies include Parsonage–Turner syndrome, acute brachial plexitis, and neuralgic amyotrophy.

- Annual incidence: 1.64 per 100,000 population.
- Male to female ratio: 2:1.
- Age: Any age group, but most commonly occurs in ages 20–50 years[21].

Etiology and pathophysiology

- Unknown. Possibly an autoimmune reaction to a preceding trigger such as immunizations, infections, or surgery (not occurring near the affected arm).
- Most cases occur in healthy individuals.
- Some reports hypothesize the production of antibodies against the peripheral nerve.

Clinical features

Usually presents with an acute onset of severe pain in the shoulder, which is often described as a 'hot poker' jabbed into the shoulder. Movement of the shoulder or arm exacerbates the pain. The pain lasts for several days to a few weeks, but a dull ache can last for years. When the pain somewhat subsides, weakness and sensory changes are noted. Because the pain is so severe initially, arm weakness may go unnoticed, as arm movement may not even be attempted.

Weakness and sensory changes depend on the distribution of nerve involvement (i.e. upper or lower trunk, specific cords, or terminal nerves). The most common pattern involves the upper trunk or a single mononeuropathy or multiple mononeuropathies, primarily the suprascapular, long thoracic, or axillary nerves. Less likely, the phrenic nerve or anterior interosseous nerve may be affected.

In cases involving individual nerves, it has been proposed that the pathology is probably within the corresponding fascicle of the brachial plexus rather than a separate trunk of the respective nerve. Most cases are unilateral, but up to 10% can have bilateral involvement.

Hereditary neuralgic amyotrophy

- Inherited as an autosomal dominant trait.
- Associated with a mutation in the gene septin 9.
- Genetically distinct from hereditary neuropathy with liability to pressure palsies.
- Episodes consist of pain, weakness, and sensory loss in the distribution of the brachial plexus and may be precipitated by pregnancy, infection, and other physical stressors and tend to recur.
- Congenital anomalies, such as syndactyly and hypotelorism, are common associated features.

Differential diagnosis

- Multifocal motor neuropathy: nerve conduction studies may show conduction block and other demyelinating features. IBPN is usually axonal.
- Vasculitic neuropathy.
- Nerve sheath tumors.
- Radiation-induced brachial plexopathy *vs.* tumor invasion of the brachial plexus (neoplastic plexopathy):
  - Radiation-induced brachial plexopathy:
    - Malignancies such as breast cancer, lung carcinoma, and lymphoma are often treated with radiation therapy to the chest. The brachial plexus often falls within this radiation plane.
    - Radiation results in direct toxic effects on axons and on the vasa nervorum (secondary microinfarction of the nerve). Fibrosis of the surroundings tissues may also affect the nerves.
    - Risk of injury is dose-dependent. Pathologic changes of the Schwann cells, endoneurial fibroblasts, and vascular and perineural cells are noted with doses above 1000 cGy.
    - Overall frequency of radiation-induced brachial plexopathy in treated patients is 1.8–4.9%[22].
    - Can occur months to years following therapy.
    - Usually affects the upper trunk and is painless.
    - Strongly associated with myokymic discharges on EMG.
  - Neoplastic plexopathy:
    - Less common than radiation-induced.
    - Painful and usually affects the lower trunk. May have associated Horner's syndrome.
    - MRI appears to be more sensitive than computed tomography (CT) in detecting tumor invasion. The presence of a mass compressing a portion of the brachial plexus is the most helpful feature distinguishing tumor invasion from radiation injury[23]. Increased T2 signal may be present in radiation injury. Usually there is no contrast enhancement of the brachial plexus with radiation-induced plexopathies[22].

Investigations

NCS

Abnormalities depend on which sites of the brachial plexus are involved.

In most cases, the upper trunk is affected resulting in abnormal motor responses recorded from the deltoid (axillary nerve) and biceps (musculocutaneous nerve), median and radial sensory responses, and lateral antebrachial cutaneous response. Lower trunk involvement results in abnormal median and ulnar motor responses, ulnar sensory response, and medial antebrachial cutaneous response.

Other tests

- EMG: denervation of the muscles supplied by the affected nerves.
- CSF; occasional abnormalities of elevated protein or pleocytosis.
- MRI with and without contrast of the brachial plexus to evaluate for a mass lesion (i.e. tumor invasion, lymphoma, neurofibroma, schwannoma). In IBPN, there may be increased T2 signal suggestive of inflammation or edema.

Treatment

- Pain can be treated with high-dose prednisone and taper. However, there is limited evidence for efficacy. Physical and occupational therapy are important to initiate immediately to prevent joint contractures (i.e. 'frozen shoulder').

Prognosis

IBPN is usually monophasic, although attacks can occasionally recur. One large study found that 36% of patients recovered most functions within the first year, 75% within the second year, and 89% within the third year[24].

INFECTIOUS NEUROPATHY

LEPROSY

Definition, epidemiology, and etiology

- Leading cause of peripheral neuropathy worldwide.
- 15–20% of affected individuals will develop neuropathy.
- Most prevalent in southeast Asia and other tropical areas.
- In the USA, cases of leprosy have been found in Hawaii, and some southern states.

Pathophysiology

Caused by *Mycobacterium leprae*, an acid-fast organism that reproduces best in cool temperatures, which explains its attraction to cooler areas of the body (skin, superficial nerves, nose, testes, and ears). It is probably spread by the respiratory route.

Clinical features

Primarily affects the skin and nerves. There are two main clinical presentations, which depend on the immunologic status of the patient: tuberculoid and lepromatous.

Variants

Tuberculoid leprosy

- Host with good immune status. Clinical syndrome is due to the intense immune response produced by the bacterial exposure.
- Well-localized disease process that produces sharply demarcated, raised skin lesions with a hypopigmented anesthetic center. Skins lesions occur on the extensor surfaces of the arms, legs, face, and buttocks.
- Good prognosis with lesions often healing spontaneously.

Lepromatous leprosy

- Host with poor immune status.
- Extensive bacterial infiltration of the skin, nerves, and dissemination through the blood.
- Skin lesions include nodules, bullous lesions, ulcers, macules, papules.
- Diffuse, symmetric disease with solitary lesions only occurring in the initial stages.
- Poor prognosis if left untreated.

Borderline leprosy

- Clinical syndrome that lies between tuberculoid and lepromatous.
- If treated, may move toward tuberculoid.
- If left untreated, prognosis is poor and tends to transition into lepromatous.

Neuropathy

- Most common symptom is such severe sensory loss that painless injuries to the skin occur.
- Mononeuropathy can occur if a particular nerve trunk passes through an area of inflammation.
- Frequently involved nerves include the ulnar nerve at the elbow, median nerve in the forearm, peroneal nerve at the fibular head, and facial nerves.
- In tuberculoid, patchy sensory loss occurs, primarily affecting small fiber nerves.
- In lepromatous, diffuse polyneuropathy occurs later on in the disease process (months to years).
- Examination findings:
  - Tender enlargement of one or more peripheral nerves over part of their superficial course (e.g. the superficial radial sensory nerve at the wrist).
  - Hypopigmented areas of skin may be present, but can be difficult to detect in Caucasians. Loss of pain sensation and often anhidrosis in the affected skin areas.
  - Painless ulcerations of the fingers and toes may be present.

Differential diagnosis

Thickening of the nerves may be noted in the following:

- Hypertrophic forms of hereditary neuropathies.
- Neurofibromatosis.
- Phytanic acid deficiency (Refsum disease).
- Amyloidosis.

Investigations and diagnosis

- NCS: Nerves most affected are ulnar nerve at the elbow and median nerve in the distal forearm.
  - May find more diffuse disease when clinical examination only reveals single nerve involvement.
- Diagnosis of leprosy is confirmed by identifying acid-fast organisms in a skin biopsy from affected areas.
- Sensory nerve biopsy can be informative if skin biopsy is indeterminate.
- Serum assay for phenolic glycolipid-1 (PGL-1) antibodies is very sensitive and correlates with bacterial load.

Treatment

Patients are divided into two groups:

- Paucibacillary:
  - Fewer bacilli on biopsy.
  - World Health Organization (WHO) recommendations: rifampicin 600 mg monthly, dapsone 100 mg daily for 6 months; single-lesion paucibacillary: single dose of rifampicin 600 mg, ofloxacin 400 mg, and minocycline 100 mg (ROM).
- Multibacillary:
  - Infiltrating disease, many bacilli on biopsy.
  - WHO recommendations: rifampicin 600 mg and clofazimine 300 mg monthly; dapsone 100 mg and clofazimine 50 mg daily for 12 months.

Prognosis

Risk of relapse is negligible, so post-treatment surveillance is not recommended.

LYME DISEASE

Definition, epidemiology, and etiology

Caused by the spirochete *Borrelia burgdorferi* and transmitted by *Ixodes dammini* (a deer tick endemic in some areas of the USA) as a primary vector. The tick must be attached for about 12–24 hours to transfer the spirochete to the human host.

Pathophysiology

- Target organs are skin, heart, nervous system, and joints.
- Peripheral nerve injury may be due to an indirect immunologic response or a type of vasculopathy.

Clinical features

There are three stages of disease: early, disseminated, and late.

Early infection

- Skin lesion (erythema migrans) appears within a few days to a few weeks of the bite.
- An erythematous circular area appears around the original bite site and gradually expands with a central clearing, creating a 'bull's eye' appearance. This lasts for about 1 month and resolves spontaneously.
- Some patients may not develop erythema migrans.

Disseminated infection

- Spirochetes spread through body and systemic symptoms develop (fever, chills, fatigue, myalgias, headaches).
- Patients may have pericarditis and inflammatory arthritis.
- Neurologic complications can occur including facial neuropathy (bilateral in approximately 50% of cases) and polyradiculoneuropathy similar to GBS.

Late-stage infection

- Arthritis worsens.
- Acrodermatitis chronica atrophicans: bluish discoloration of the skin.
- 40–60% of patients develop a polyneuropathy many years after the original infection.

Investigations

NCS may show an axonal polyneuropathy. If the facial nerve is involved, patients may have reduced facial nerve CMAP and an abnormal blink reflex.

CSF studies show increased protein and lymphocytic pleocytosis if there are cranial neuropathies or polyradiculitis.

Diagnosis

- Detection of antibody to *B. burgdorferi* in serum and/or CSF.
- False-positive antibodies have been identified in rheumatoid arthritis, tuberculous meningitis, mononucleosis, and Rocky Mountain spotted fever.

Treatment

- Early infection without evidence of CSF involvement; oral doxycycline or amoxicillin for 3 weeks.
- Late infection or clinically severe disease: intravenous ceftriaxone or cefotaxime for 2–4 weeks.

DIPHTHERIA

Definition, epidemiology, and etiology

Caused by the bacteria *Corynebacterium diphtheriae*. Diphtheria has been eliminated in most developed countries through childhood immunization programs.

- Children who have not been immunized are at risk (primarily in developing countries).
- Adults who were previously immunized in childhood and now have lost the immune protection are at risk during epidemics.
- 20% of infected patients develop a polyneuropathy.

Pathophysiology

- Inhaled or permeates through the skin (e.g. in warfare).
- Polyneuropathy is caused by a toxin that is released from the bacteria:
  - The toxin disrupts the Schwann cells' production of myelin.
  - The clinical effects of demyelination do not occur until the cells recycle and myelin cannot be produced.

Clinical features

- Initial infection presents with flu-like symptoms including fatigue, headaches, myalgias, and fever within 1 week of exposure. The pharynx may be covered in a white membranous exudate resulting in dysarthria and regurgitation of liquids from palatal paralysis. Within 1 month, development of blurred vision occurs from failure to accommodate. The phrenic nerve may be involved causing respiratory distress.

Polyneuropathy may develop over the next 2–3 months, manifesting as progressive numbness, paresthesias, and weakness of the arms and legs. Weakness may progress to inability to ambulate over the course of weeks.

Differential diagnosis

Distinguish from GBS, which has less severity of bulbar involvement compared with diphtheria.

Investigations and diagnosis

NCS

- Demyelinating polyneuropathy.
- Initially, increased distal latencies and prolonged F responses, normal SNAPs.
- As the weakness progresses, conduction velocity slowing worsens and SNAP amplitude decreases.
- There is a dissociation between electrodiagnostic and clinical findings (i.e. weakness may be improving, but electrodiagnostic abnormalities continue to worsen).

CSF

- Elevated protein with or without lymphocytic pleocytosis.

Diagnosis is from culturing bacteria from throat swabs or elevated serum diphtheria antibody titers.

Treatment

Antitoxin should be administered within 48 hours of symptom onset. Treatment beyond 48 hours does not affect development of polyneuropathy or prevent death.

Prognosis

80% of people will have resolution of the polyneuropathy 1 year following the infection.

HUMAN IMMUNODEFICIENCY VIRUS (HIV)

Epidemiology and pathophysiology

Approximately 20% of HIV patients will develop some type of neuropathy, either due to the virus itself, secondary infections, or toxicity from antiretroviral medications. The pathophysiology is unknown, but does not appear to be due to infection of the nerves. Neuropathies may be immune-mediated and caused by the release of cytokines.

Clinical features[25]

The types of neuropathy include distal symmetric polyneuropathy (DSPN), AIDP or CIDP, mononeuropathy multiplex, motor neuronopathy, and sensory ganglionopathy.

DSPN is the most common type of neuropathy associated with HIV and is often found in patients with aquired immunodeficiency syndrome (AIDS).

AIDP

- Usually occurs at the time of seroconversion.
- Progressive weakness, sometimes evolving to respiratory insufficiency.

CIDP

- Can occur at anytime.
- May follow a progressive or relapsing course.
- Mononeuropathy multiplex due to vasculitis is rare in HIV.
- Motor neuronopathy presentations have been similar to primary lateral sclerosis, amyotrophic lateral sclerosis, and bibrachial diplegia and respond to antiretroviral therapy.
- Sensory ganglionopathy results in abnormalities in all sensory modalities and gait ataxia.

Differential diagnosis

- For mononeuropathy multiplex, consider co-infection with hepatitis C (cryoglobulinemia) or CMV.
- Progressive polyradiculopathy due to CMV-infected cauda equina.
- Neurosyphilis.
- Lymphomatous meningitis.
- Sensory ganglionopathy: Sjögren's syndrome, paraneoplastic.

Investigations

- CD4 lymphocyte count and serum viral load.
- NCS and EMG to further define the specific type of neuropathy.
- Nerve biopsy is indicated if vasculitis or an infiltrative process of the nerve is likely.
- Lumbar spine MRI with and without contrast to evaluate for enhancement of nerve roots.
- CSF to evaluate for pleocytosis, increased protein, and/or viral polymerase chain reaction (PCR) for CMV.

Treatment

Initiation of highly active antiretroviral therapy (HAART) is necessary to suppress viral replication, but the associated neuropathy is usually not responsive to this treatment. Neuropathy (particularly DSPN) has been a disabling side-effect of dideoxynucleoside antiretrovirals (d-drugs), which are suspected to cause a neuropathy through direct toxicity on mitochondrial DNA replication. Elevated lactate levels may help distinguish d-drugs neuropathy from HIV-induced neuropathy with a specificity and sensitivity of 90%[26]. The associated neuropathic pain has limited the use of these medications in the developed world. Protease inhibitors may have a small risk of DSPN, but this should be weighed against the importance of treatment[27].

Medications should be given for neuropathic pain. Treatments for AIDP, CIDP, mononeuropathy multiplex, and sensory ganglionopathy are similar to those used in the HIV-negative population.

CMV infection should be treated with gancyclovir or foscarnet.

Prognosis

- Most neuropathies persist and require symptomatic management.
- Natural course of AIDP and CIDP is similar to that in the HIV-negative population.
- Even with treatment, the prognosis for progressive polyradiculopathy with CMV is poor and most patients die within weeks or months.

HEREDITARY MOTOR AND SENSORY NEUROPATHY (CHARCOT–MARIE–TOOTH DISEASE)

Definition and epidemiology

Genetic disorders resulting in peripheral neuropathies. CMT is the most common type of hereditary neuropathy. Epidemiological studies have reported the prevalence to be approximately 10–20 per 100,000 population, with the majority of cases being CMT type 1[28].

Etiology and pathophysiology

Neuropathies are classified based on pathology (axonal *vs*. demyelinating), inheritance pattern (autosomal dominant, autosomal recessive, or X-linked), and specific gene mutations. There is a classification scheme of the most common subtypes and those with unique clinical features. However, this is an ever-evolving classification process as novel genes are being discovered, and there are more subtypes than are covered in this chapter.

Tip

▶ *Approximately 60% of autosomal dominant neuropathies are CMT type 1A.*

CMT type 1

Autosomal dominant, demyelinating. The mutations disrupt myelin and Schwann cell function leading to segmental demyelination and secondary axonal loss.

CMT type 1A

- 70% of type 1 cases.
- Duplication of the peripheral myelin protein-22 (*PMP22*) gene on chromosome 17 (17p11.2), which theoretically produces a toxic gain of function of the protein.
- The normal function of *PMP22* is not known, but it is believed to help maintain myelin structure and is expressed in compact myelin.

CMT type 1B

- 20% of type 1 cases.
- Mutation of the myelin protein zero (*MPZ*) gene on chromosome 1 (1q22–23).
- *MPZ* maintains linkage between myelin layers and accounts for the majority of myelin protein in the peripheral nervous system.

CMT type 1C

- Rare.
- Mutations in lipopolysaccharide-induced tumor necrosis factor-alpha factor (LITAF) also known as small integral membrane protein of the lysosome/late endosome (SIMPLE) on chromosome 16 (16p13.3–p12).
- LITAF is expressed on Schwann cells and if abnormal may have altered protein degradation.

CMT type 1D

- <1% of type 1 cases.
- Mutations in the early growth response 2 (*ERG2*) gene on chromosome 10 (10q21.1–22.1).
- *ERG2* may play a role in regulating myelin genes in Schwann cells.

CMT type 2

Mostly autosomal dominant, axonal; nerve conduction velocity >38 m/s; much less common than type 1. Disruption of axonal transport is a feature.

CMT type 2A2

- Most common of type 2 cases (33%)[1].
- Mutation of the mitofusin-2 (*MFN2*) gene on chromosome 1 (1p36.2).
- *MFN2* is presumed to function in the maintenance of the mitochondrial network[29].

CMT type 2B1

- Autosomal recessive.
- Usually North African descent.
- Mutation of lamin A/C gene on chromosome 1 (1q21.2).
- Lamin A/C is involved in nuclear stability.

CMT type 3

- Dejerine–Sottas syndrome, severe demyelination or hypomyelination.
- Autosomal dominant: *PMP22*, *MPZ*.
- Autosomal recessive: *ERG2*, periaxin (possibly plays a role in maintaining myelin integrity).

CMT type 4

- Autosomal recessive, axonal or demyelinating.
- Type 4A is due to a mutation of ganglioside-induced differentiation-associated protein-1 (GDAP1) on chromosome 8 (8q13–q21).
- GDAP1 helps regulate the mitochondrial network.

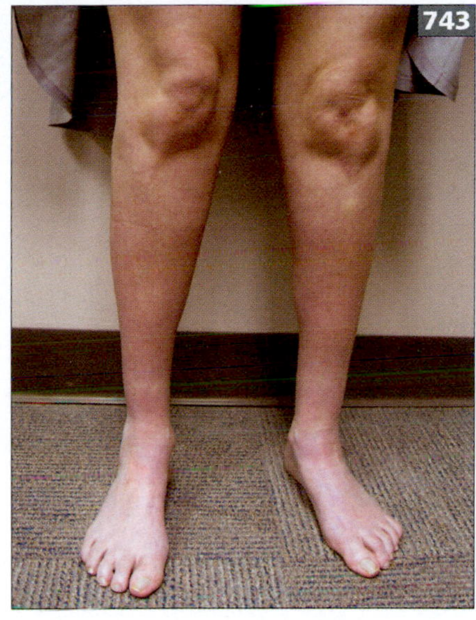

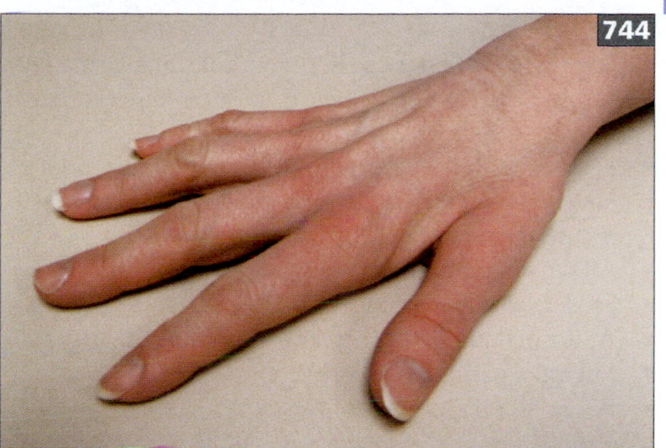

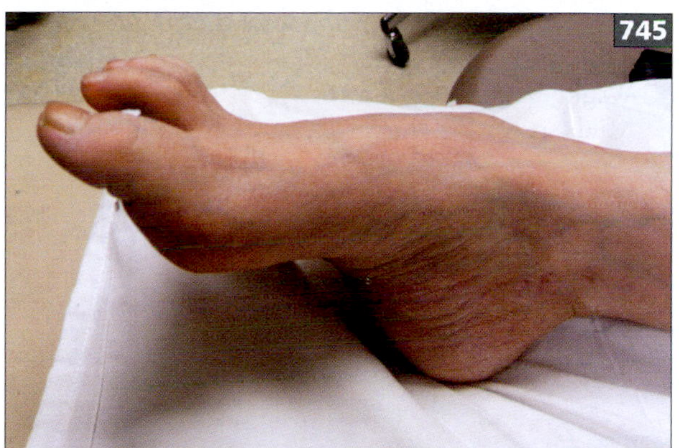

743 Tapering of the legs to the ankles in a case of CMT type 1A.

744 Intrinsic hand muscle atrophy with mild clawing of the fourth and fifth fingers in a case of CMT type 1A.

745 High arch and hammer toes in a case of CMT type 1A.

CMT type 1X

- X-linked dominant.
- Approximately 12% of all CMT cases.
- Mutation of connexin-32 on chromosome X (Xq13).
- Connexin-32 is a gap junction formation in the Schwann cells.

Hereditary neuropathy with liability to pressure palsies (HNPP)

- Autosomal dominant.
- Majority of cases are due to deletion of the PMP-22 gene on chromosome 17 (17p11.2), as opposed to duplication of the gene in CMT type 1A.

Clinical features

CMT type 1

- Usual onset in teens to 40s. Patient may experience frequent ankle sprains prior to diagnosis.
- Patients may not complain of sensory loss (as opposed to acquired neuropathies), but examination of sensory modalities (vibratory sense, proprioception) reveals marked diminishment.
- Anterior compartment of the distal lower extremities is usually affected first resulting in foot drop and 'inverted champagne bottle'-shaped legs (**743**).
- Relative sparing of the proximal extremities, although, over time, proximal weakness may develop.
- Atrophy of the distal upper extremities, formation of claw-hand deformities (**744**).
- Generalized areflexia.
- Upper limb tremor may be present and when prominent is known as Roussy–Levy syndrome.
- Pes cavus and hammer toes are more frequent than in other types (**745**).

CMT type 2

- Presents later in life.
- Patients may not complain of sensory loss, but examination of sensory modalities (vibratory sense, proprioception) reveals marked diminishment.
- Less intrinsic hand involvement and less frequent foot deformities compared with type 1.
- Anterior and posterior compartments of the distal lower extremities tend to be equally affected.
- Generalized areflexia is unusual.
- CMT type 2A2: optic atrophy, hearing loss, pyramidal signs, white matter abnormalities.

CMT type 3

- Usually weakness at birth (hypotonic infant); if severely affected, may have respiratory distress that may lead to death.
- Less severe cases present in early childhood. Children have significant delay in motor milestones, but may eventually ambulate.
- All sensory modalities are affected.
- Sensorineural hearing loss.
- Abnormal pupillary reaction.
- Enlarged peripheral nerves.
- Pes cavus and kyphoscoliosis.

CMT type 4

- Onset in early infancy with motor developmental delay.
- Weakness and muscle atrophy.
- Mild sensory loss, areflexia, may have scoliosis.

CMT type 1X

- Affected men have a similar presentation to CMT type 1.
- Female carriers may present with a mild neuropathy that is usually asymptomatic.
- Rare CNS involvement.

HNPP

- Presentation occurs in second or third decade.
- Some patients present at an earlier age while others may be asymptomatic for their lifetime.
- Painless sensory loss and weakness in a single nerve distribution after light external compression of that nerve (e.g. peroneal neuropathy after briefly crossing the legs). Mononeuropathies usually resolve, but may take weeks or months.
- Most commonly affected nerves include median nerve at the wrist, ulnar nerve at the elbow, radial nerve in the spiral groove, peroneal nerve at the fibular head. Cranial nerves with physiologic entrapment sites, such as the facial and acoustic nerves, may also be involved.
- On examination there is diminished sensation to all modalities, depressed or normal reflexes, pes cavus, hammer toes.

Differential diagnosis

- Other hereditary motor and sensory neuropathies (Refsum disease, Fabry's disease, porphyria, familial amyloid polyneuropathy).
- Hereditary spastic paraparesis if there is clinical examination evidence of pyramidal tract involvement or white matter disease.
- CIDP when proximal weakness is present.
- Distal myopathy: Miyoshi myopathy (dysferlinopathy).
- For HNPP: other causes of mononeuropathy multiplex such as vasculitic neuropathy or diabetes.

Investigations

The various forms of hereditary neuropathies may be difficult to distinguish from one another based on the clinical phenotype. NCS are helpful to determine whether the neuropathy is demyelinating or axonal. Based on these results, appropriate genetic testing can be obtained. Many genetic tests are available commercially. Nerve biopsies are usually not necessary to perform, as the diagnosis is often achieved through less invasive modalities.

CMT type 1

NCS

- May be normal at birth, but severe conduction velocity slowing is evident by age 5 and remains relatively unchanged.
- In most cases, nerve conduction velocities range from 20 m/s to 25 m/s.
- Markedly prolonged distal motor latencies.
- CMAP amplitudes may be reduced when recorded from an atrophic muscle or as a manifestation of axonal loss occurring over time.
- Delayed or absent F-waves.
- Because demyelination is uniform throughout the nerve, most cases do not have conduction blocks or temporal dispersion, which is helpful to distinguish from acquired demyelinating neuropathies.

EMG

- Denervation of the distal lower extremities (i.e. tibialis anterior, gastrocnemius, intrinsic foot muscles) and distal upper extremities (i.e. forearm and intrinsic hand muscles).

Genetic testing

- Obtain testing for CMT type 1A (*PMP22* duplication) first, as this is the most common type of hereditary neuropathy.

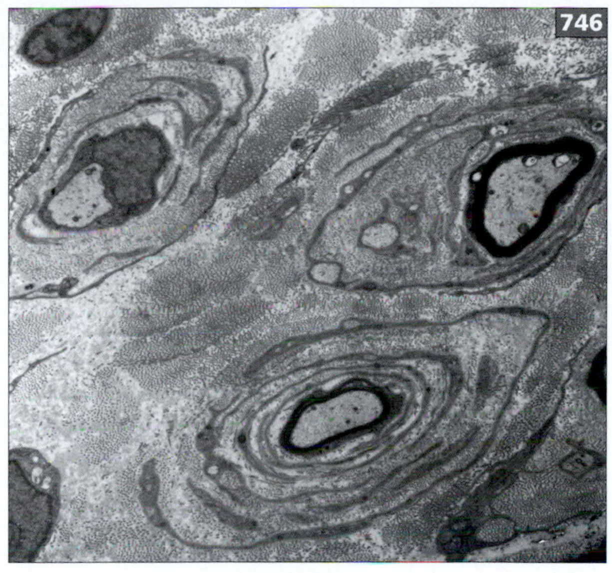

746 'Onion bulb' formation.

Nerve biopsy

- May appear normal in early childhood, but as time goes on the axons become thinly myelinated.
- Recurrent demyelination and remyelination causes shortening of the internodal length.
- 'Onion bulbs', comprising concentrically proliferated Schwann cells surrounding surviving myelinated fibers, are characteristic beyond adolescence (**746**).

CMT type 2

NCS

- Evidence of axonal neuropathy with reduced or absent SNAPs and reduced CMAP amplitudes.
- Distal motor latencies are usually normal or mildly prolonged.
- Nerve conduction velocities are normal or minimally slow, depending on the amount of axonal loss, and are usually >38 m/s.
- The nerve conduction studies may be similar to nonhereditary axonal polyneuropathy. However, in CMT type 2, sensory abnormalities are not a major complaint; patients with axonal polyneuropathy from other etiologies usually present with sensory symptoms.

EMG

- Denervation in distal extremity muscles.

Nerve biopsy

- Reduction in myelinated fibers.
- Axonal atrophy.
- Onion bulbs are not a classic feature.

CMT type 3

NCS

- Motor nerve conduction velocity is usually 5–10 m/s or less, indicating that the myelin was not able to form well.
- Markedly prolonged distal motor latencies.
- Absent SNAPs.

EMG

- Denervation with neurogenic MUPs; severe cases may have less reinnervation resulting in small, myopathic-appearing MUPs.

Nerve biopsy

- Three categories of disease severity:
  - Most common, occurring in infantile onset: hypomyelination with basal lamina onion bulbs.
  - Mild form: classic onion bulbs.
  - Severe form: nerves have virtually no myelin, no onion bulbs; many patients do not survive.

CMT type 4

NCS

- Reduced CMAP amplitudes.
- Absent SNAPs.
- Individual variability in nerve conduction velocity from normal to quite slow (axonal or demyelinating). Both Schwann cells and neurons express GDAP-1, which may explain this variability.

Nerve biopsy

- Hypomyelination with basal lamina onion bulbs.
- Type 4B also has fibers with excessively folded myelin sheaths.

CMT type 1X

NCS

- Both axonal and demyelinating features that are more pronounced in men than in women.
- Nonuniform slowing of motor conduction velocities and dispersion of CMAPs, gives appearance of an acquired demyelinating neuropathy.

EMG

- Denervation in distal extremity muscles.

Nerve biopsy

- Axonal atrophy, loss of myelinated fibers.
- Mild grade onion bulb formation surrounding the thinly myelinated fibers.

HNPP

NCS

- Despite focal clinical symptoms, NCS reveal prolonged distal latencies, slightly slowed conduction velocity, and normal/mildly reduced amplitudes.
- Slowing of nerve conduction velocities and conduction block occur at common entrapment and compression sites.

Nerve biopsy

- Nerve fiber loss with demyelination and remyelination and axonal atrophy, but not as severe as CMT type 1.
- Tomacula: focal, large, sausage-shaped thickening of the myelin sheath (superfluous loops of myelin), which is best viewed on tease fiber preparations. Also found in asymptomatic cases.

Treatment

- Current treatment is symptomatic.
- Ankle–foot orthoses for foot drop.
- Neuropathic pain can be severe in CMT and is usually treated medically.
- Severe foot deformities can be evaluated by orthopedic surgery for potential intervention.
- Genetic counseling.
- For HNPP, patients should avoid sitting with their legs crossed, wearing backpacks, and frequent kneeling. Careful positioning during anesthesia is important.
- Small trials of exercise, creatine, purified brain gangliosides, and orthoses have not shown significant benefit[30].
- Potential minor benefit was noted in a very small trial of neurotrophin-3. However, further trials are advocated[30].

Prognosis

Depending on the type, CMT has the potential to cause significant disability. However, implementing use of splints and compliance with exercise can help reduce heel cord and finger contractures.

If patients are well monitored and aware of their limitations, many can lead active lives. Many do have to modify their activities, such as avoiding jobs involving fine hand movements or constant standing.

SYNDROMIC HEREDITARY PERIPHERAL NEUROPATHIES

REFSUM DISEASE (HEREDOPATHIA ATACTICA POLYNEURITIFORMIS)

- Autosomal recessive.
- Mutation in the phytanoyl-CoA alpha-hydroxylase (PAHX) gene on chromosome 10 (10p13).
- Onset in first or second decade.

Etiology

- Defect in alpha-oxidation of branched-chain fatty acids, which elevates the serum phytanic acid level.
- Phytanic acid accumulates in central and peripheral nervous systems (particularly the olivocerebellar tracts, anterior horn cells, and peripheral nerves).

Clinical features

- Onset in infancy to early adulthood.
- Classic features include retinitis pigmentosa (night blindness, which is often the presenting symptom), peripheral neuropathy causing muscle atrophy and weakness in the distal legs and foot drop, cerebellar ataxia (may be a late manifestation).
- Other features include sensorineural hearing loss, cardiac conduction abnormalities, anosmia, and ichthyosis.

Investigations

- NCS: mild to marked conduction velocity slowing; CMAP amplitudes are normal or reduced.
- Elevated serum phytanic acid levels.
- Elevated CSF protein.
- Nerve biopsy: loss of myelinated fibers, onion bulb formation is associated with the remaining axons.

Treatment

- Low phytanic diet results in considerable improvement in clinical symptoms as well as the findings on NCS.

FABRY'S DISEASE (ANGIOKERATOMA CORPORIS DIFFUSUM)

- Rare, X-linked.
- Age of onset: 10–30 years.
- Primarily affects males.
- Mutation in the alpha-galactosidase gene located on chromosome X (Xq21–22).

Etiology

- Defective alpha-galactosidase activity results in accumulation of ceramide trihexosidase in the skin, blood vessels, cornea, and the dorsal root ganglia.
- Lipid depositions in endothelial cells of the vessel walls.
- Axonal degeneration of the small myelinated and unmyelinated fibers.

Clinical features

- Severe paresthesias/burning of hands and feet.
- Rashes include angiokeratomas (reddish maculopapular lesion usually located around the umbilicus, scrotum, and inguinal region) and angioectasias of the nailbeds, oral mucosa, and conjunctiva.
- Corneal opacities.
- Premature atherosclerosis results in hypertension, renal failure, cardiac disease, and strokes.
- Women may develop a mild painful small fiber neuropathy.

Investigations

- NCS are usually normal.
- Since it affects mainly the small fibers, quantitative sensory testing indicates impaired temperature perception.
- Diminished activity of alpha-galactosidase as measured in leukocytes and cultured fibroblasts.
- Nerve biopsy: reduced small myelinated and unmyelinated fibers.
- Skin biopsy: reduced epidermal nerve fiber density.

Treatment

- Enzyme replacement therapy with alpha-galactosidase beta.
- Early initiation of treatment may help prevent severe axon loss.

PORPHYRIA

- Autosomal dominant with variable degrees of expression.
- Higher incidence in females.

Etiology

- Impaired porphyrin metabolism.
- Three forms associated with neuropathy:
    - Acute intermittent porphyria (AIP): porphobilinogen deaminase deficiency.
    - Hereditary coproporphyria (HCP): defects in coproporphyrin oxidase.
    - Variegate porphyria (VP): impaired protoporphyrinogen oxidase.

Clinical features

- Attacks are triggered by drugs metabolized by the p450 system and hormonal changes such as pregnancy.
- Initial presentation is often acute abdominal pain followed by agitation, hallucinations, and seizures.
- 2–3 days later, a progressive proximally predominant subacute motor neuropathy can develop, as well as severe back and leg pain. Weakness is rapid.
- The neuropathy may be asymmetric and may involve cranial nerves (facial weakness, dysphagia).
- Autonomic dysfunction (dilated pupils, tachycardia, neurogenic bladder).
- HCP and VP may develop photosensitive skin rashes. Brown discoloration of urine due to the presence of porphyrin metabolites.

Investigations and diagnosis

- Diagnosis: accumulation of the precursors of heme (δ-aminolevulinic acid, porphobilinogen, uroporphobilinogen, coproporphyrinogen, protoporphyrinogen) in urine or stool.
- Specific enzyme activities are reduced in erythrocytes and leukocytes.
- NCS: primary abnormality is significantly reduced CMAP amplitude.
- EMG: denervation in the proximal muscles about 14 days after symptom onset.
- Nerve biopsy: axonal degeneration.
- Differential diagnosis: Guillain–Barré syndrome.

Treatment

- Hematin and glucose should be given to reduce accumulation of heme precursors.
- Avoid medications that can precipitate an attack (i.e. barbiturates, carbamezapine, phenytoin, primidone).

FAMILIAL AMYLOID POLYNEUROPATHIES

- Autosomal dominant.
- Variability in age of onset and severity even among family members.
- Mutations in the transthyretin (*TTR*), apolipoprotein A1, or gelsolin genes.
- *TTR* mutations occur in the majority of cases: most common mutation involves a methionine to valine substitution at position 30 (Val30Met).

Etiology

- *TTR* functions as a transport protein and is synthesized in the liver.
- Mutation results in formation of β-pleated sheets of the protein and resistance to protease degradation (amyloidogenic properties).
- Amyloid deposits in the endoneurium and blood vessels in autonomic ganglia and peripheral nerves.
- Other affected organs include heart, tongue, gastrointestinal tract, skeletal muscles, and kidney.

Clinical features

- Insidious onset of painful paresthesias in the distal lower extremities in the third to fourth decade.
- Most common sensory modalities affected are pain and temperature.
- Can have severe autonomic involvement (postural hypotension, constipation or diarrhea, erectile dysfunction, impaired sweating).
- Amyloid can deposit in the flexor retinaculum resulting in carpal tunnel syndrome.
- Death within 7–15 years due to cardiac failure.

Investigations and diagnosis

- Diagnosis:
  - Detection of amyloid deposition in abdominal fat pad, rectal, or nerve biopsies.
  - Genetic testing by DNA sequencing of the *TTR* gene.
- NCS:
  - Abnormal sympathetic skin testing.
  - Predominantly axonal, but occasionally demyelinating sensorimotor polyneuropathy.
- Nerve biopsy:
  - Amyloid deposits within the endoneurium, epineurium, or perineurium, and around blood vessels in autonomic ganglia and peripheral nerves.
  - Loss of small myelinated and unmyelinated fibers.

Treatment

Liver transplantation, which decreases serum *TTR* levels and may improve clinical symptoms and electrophysiologic features.

MONONEUROPATHIES

Definition

Damage to an individual nerve causing weakness and/or sensory changes in that nerve's specific distribution.

UPPER EXTREMITY NEUROPATHY

SPINAL ACCESSORY NEUROPATHY

Definition

- Dysfunction of the spinal accessory nerve (cranial nerve XI) supplying the sternocleidomastoid and trapezius muscles.

Anatomy

- The spinal accessory nerve does not arise from the brachial plexus.
- It is divided into bulbar (accessory) and spinal components:
  - Bulbar component arises from the medulla and supplies the soft palate.
  - Spinal component arises from the anterior horn cells in the cervical cord down to C6.
- Spinal component fibers ascend the spinal canal and enter the cranial cavity through the foramen magnum and then exit via the jugular foramen to terminate in the sternocleidomastoid and trapezius muscles.

Etiology

- Common: surgical procedures in the posterior triangle (lymph node biopsy or dissection, carotid endarterectomy).
- Although the spinal accessory nerve does not arise from the brachial plexus, it may be involved in IBPN (747).

Examination

Shoulder shrug (trapezius), tilting head towards ipsilateral shoulder and rotating head towards contralateral shoulder (sternocleidomastoid).

Clinical features

- Drooping of the ipsilateral shoulder and lateral winging of the scapula.
- Winging accentuated by shoulder abduction to 90°.
- Most lesions are distal to sternocleidomastoid innervation, affecting only the trapezius.

Investigations

- NCS of the spinal accessory nerve recording off of the trapezius and comparing the CMAP from both sides.
- EMG of the trapezius and sternocleidomastoid.

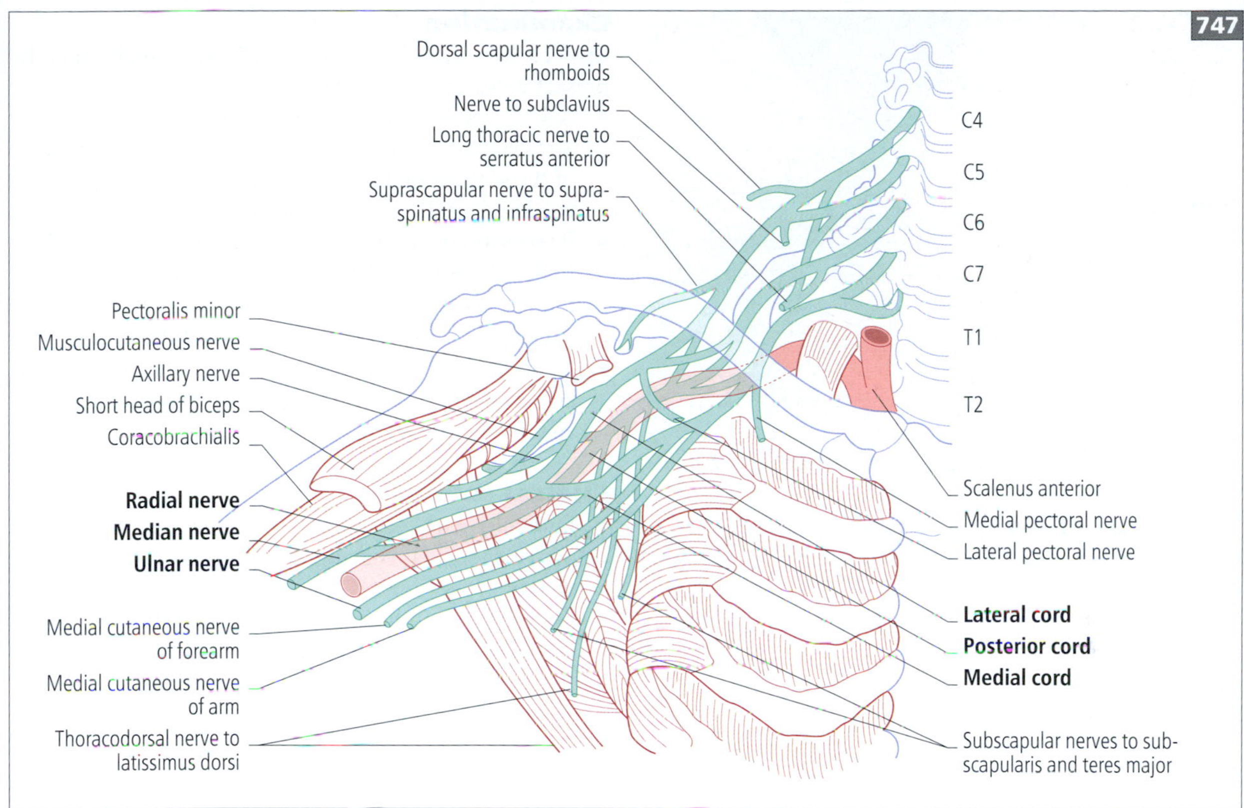

747 Diagram of the brachial plexus.

Treatment and prognosis

- IBPN: see above.
- Surgical injury: recovery depends on degree of nerve injury.

DORSAL SCAPULAR NEUROPATHY

Definition and epidemiology

- Dysfunction of the dorsal scapular nerve supplying the rhomboids and levator scapulae.
- Uncommon in isolation.

Anatomy

- Course of the dorsal scapular nerve:
  - Arises from the upper trunk of the brachial plexus, carrying fibers from the C4 and C5 nerve roots.
  - Pierces the medial scalenus muscle.
  - Innervates the levator scapulae (C4–C5), which elevates the scapula.
  - Courses along the medial border of the scapula to innervate the rhomboids (C5), which adduct the medial border of the scapula.
  - Rhomboids and levator scapulae keep the scapula attached to the posterior chest wall during arm motion.

Etiology

- Whiplash injury: stretching of scalene muscles causing trauma to the nerve[31].
- Entrapment due to hypertrophy of the middle scalene muscle – occupations involving extended overhead work are at risk.
- IBPN may involve the dorsal scapular nerve.

Examination

Stand behind the patient and ask the patient to put their hand behind their back, face the palm of the hand backwards, and ask the patient to push backwards against the resistance of your hand. The muscle bellies can be felt medial to the medial border of the scapula and occasionally visualized. An alternative method involves placing the hand on the hip and pushing the elbow backwards against resistance.

Clinical features

- Scapular winging with the inferior angle rotated laterally.
- Elevation of the arm above the head accentuates the scapular winging.

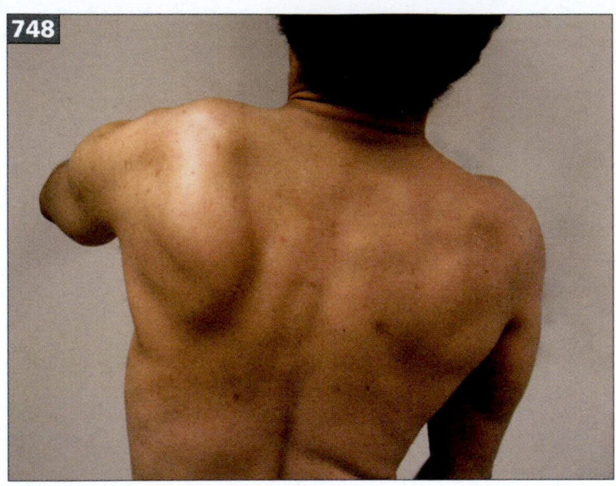

748 Left scapular winging, accentuated by forward abduction of the arm.

Investigations
EMG abnormalities are restricted to the rhomboids and levator scapulae.

Treatment and prognosis
- Sectioning of the middle scalene muscle to relieve compression of the nerve.
- IBPN: see above.

LONG THORACIC NEUROPATHY
Definition and epidemiology
- Dysfunction of the long thoracic nerve to the serratus anterior.
- Uncommon.

Anatomy
- The long thoracic nerve arises from the motor roots of C5, C6, and C7.
- Courses downward through and in front of the medial scalene muscle, descends further dorsal to the brachial plexus along the medial wall of the axilla, and innervates the serratus anterior muscle.

Etiology
- Trauma.
- Surgery to the chest wall: radical mastectomy, axillary node dissection, thoracostomy.
- IBPN: often involves other nerves in addition to the long thoracic nerve.
- Radiation therapy for breast carcinoma.
- Rare: Lyme disease, inherited brachial plexus neuropathy.

Examination
Inspect for scapular winging (**748**), which may be present in the resting position.
- Ask the patient to push against a wall with both arms slightly flexed at the elbow. Look for winging of the scapula on the affected side, which indicates weakness of the serratus anterior.
- If weakness is so severe, the patient may not be able to flex the extended arm at the shoulder and will require assistance from the examiner. Ask the patient to push their fist forward and watch for winging.
- Elevation of the arm may not be possible. This can be achieved if the examiner presses the patient's scapula against the chest wall.

Clinical features
- Difficulty with elevating the upper arm during activities such as shaving, combing hair, eating, and drinking.
- Dull shoulder ache, mainly because of strain on the shoulder muscles and ligaments in the absence of the serratus anterior muscle tightening the scapula against the rib cage.

Investigations
- NCS: record from the serratus anterior and compare bilateral CMAPs.
- EMG: abnormalities noted in the serratus anterior.

Differential diagnosis
- C6 or C7 radiculopathy, but usually there is additional weakness of the extensors of the arms, wrists, or fingers.
- Myopathy: weakness is usually bilateral and involves additional muscles of the shoulder and upper arm.
- Distinguish scapular winging from that of spinal accessory neuropathy and dorsal scapular neuropathy.

Treatment and prognosis
- Physical therapy and occupational therapy.
- Bracing to keep the shoulder abutted against the thorax.
- If shoulder function does not improve, surgery to stabilize the scapula is an option.
- Most recover spontaneously.

Tips

Scapular winging may be due to neuropathy of:

► *The spinal accessory nerve: inferior angle of the scapula is rotated laterally.*

► *The dorsal scapular nerve: inferior angle of the scapula is rotated laterally.*

► *The long thoracic nerve: inferior angle of the scapula is rotated medially.*

SUPRASCAPULAR NEUROPATHY

Definition and epidemiology

- Dysfunction of the suprascapular nerve.
- Uncommon.

Anatomy

- The suprascapular nerve arises from the upper trunk of the brachial plexus, carrying fibers from the C5 and C6 nerve roots.
- Passes under the trapezius muscle and courses from the upper border of the scapula beneath the transverse superior scapular ligament.
- Innervates supraspinatus and infraspinatus muscles.
- Fibers to the infraspinatus pass separately through the spinoglenoid notch, which is covered by the transverse inferior scapular ligament.
- Entrapment sites (**749**):
  - Suprascapular notch.
  - Spinoglenoid notch.
- Supraspinatus muscle abducts the upper arm up to 30° (deltoid takes over abduction at that point).
- Infraspinatus muscle assists in external rotation of the upper arm at the shoulder.

Etiology

- Trauma to shoulder region:
  - Stab wounds above the scapula.
  - Improper use of crutches.
  - Stretching of the nerve that may occur with serving a volleyball or pitching a baseball.
- Ganglion cysts.
- IBPN.
- Lesion at the spinoglenoid notch: isolated weakness and atrophy of the infraspinatus muscle.

Examination

- Test the supraspinatus muscle with the patient abducting the upper arm from resting position against resistance.
- To test the infraspinatus muscle, ask the patient to flex the elbow to 90°. The examiner should stabilize the patient's elbow against the trunk and ask the patient to rotate the upper arm externally against resistance on the dorsum of the patient's hand.

Clinical features

- May have pain at the superior margin of the scapula radiating towards the shoulder.
- Atrophy of the supraspinatus and infraspinatus muscles.

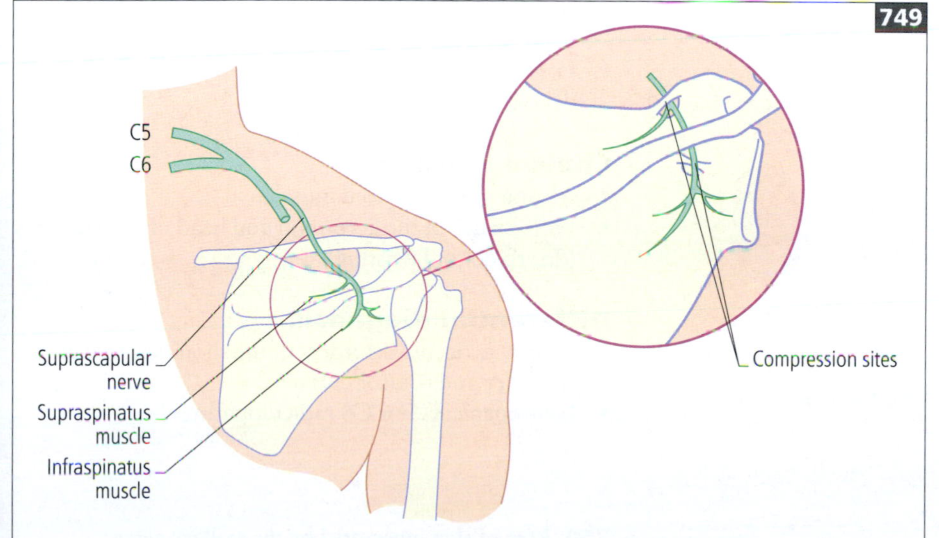

749 Course of the suprascapular nerve and sites of compression.

Differential diagnosis

- Non-neurogenic disorders of the shoulder:
  - Frozen shoulder: pain, inhibited mobility of the shoulder joint, wasting and weakness of the muscles around the shoulder, especially the supraspinatus, deltoid may also be involved.
  - Rotator cuff tear.
  - Tendonitis.
- Neurogenic disorders:
  - C5 or C6 radiculopathy, but usually pain radiates into the arm and the biceps reflex is diminished.

Investigations

- Motor NCS are technically limiting.
- EMG is more helpful:
  - Denervation in both supraspinatus and infraspinatus muscles if the lesion is proximal to the suprascapular notch.
  - Denervation is limited to the infraspinatus muscle if the lesion occurs at the spinoglenoid notch.

Treatment

- Conservative therapy with pain control is recommended.
- Corticosteroid injections to the sites of compression.
- Surgical decompression of the entrapment sites is controversial.

AXILLARY NEUROPATHY

Definition and epidemiology

- Dysfunction of the axillary nerve.
- Uncommon.

Anatomy

- The axillary nerve arises from the posterior cord of the brachial plexus, carrying fibers from the C5 and C6 nerve roots.
- Passes just below the shoulder joint, encircles the humerus until it is under the deltoid muscle and then passes through the quadrilateral space (teres minor, teres major, long head of the triceps, neck of the humerus).
- Innervates the deltoid muscle and teres minor muscle.
- The lateral cutaneous nerve of the upper arm arises from the axillary nerve, follows a short and separate route, and innervates a small area of skin overlying the deltoid muscle.

Etiology

- Trauma:
  - Fracture or dislocation of the head of the humerus.
  - Hyperextension of the shoulder (e.g. during sleep or surgery).
  - Intramuscular injections into the deltoid.
- Soft-tissue or peripheral nerve tumor.
- IBPN.
- Ischemia (e.g. vasculitis).
- Multifocal motor neuropathy.

Examination

- Ask the patient to keep the arm abducted in the horizontal plane against resistance. The supraspinatus muscle initiates the first 30° of arm abduction.
- The teres minor muscle cannot be examined in isolation because it acts together with the infraspinatus muscle in external rotation of the upper arm.
- Loss of sensation in a small area of skin overlying the deltoid muscle (750).

Clinical features

- Atrophy of the deltoid muscle.
- Prominence of the acromion and head of the humerus (due to deltoid wasting).

Differential diagnosis

- Non-neurogenic disorders of the shoulder: frozen shoulder and rotator cuff tear.
- Neurogenic: C5 or C6 radiculopathy.

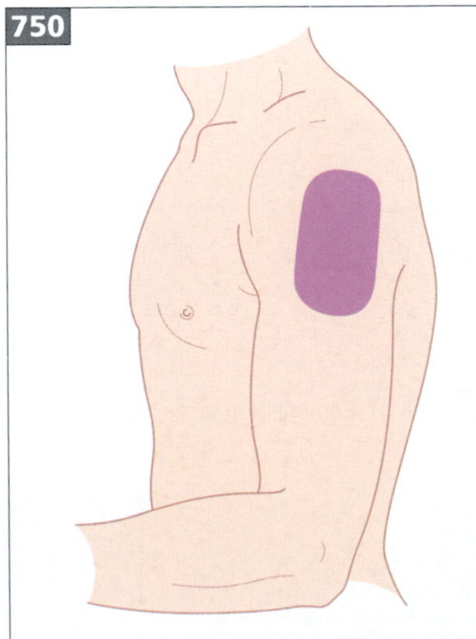

750 Area of skin innervated by the axillary nerve.

Investigations

- NCS:
  - Axillary CMAPs recorded from the deltoid muscle with supraclavicular stimulation of the brachial plexus.
  - Bilateral comparison to identify asymmetric loss of amplitude on the affected side.
  - Superficial radial SNAP can help distinguish a posterior cord lesion from an upper trunk lesion.
- EMG: denervation in deltoid and teres minor muscles (although teres minor is difficult to localize for testing).

Treatment and prognosis

- Conservative treatment with physical therapy and occupational therapy, primarily to prevent a frozen shoulder (the elderly are particularly vulnerable).
- If there is no improvement within 6 months, surgical treatment and nerve grafting should be considered.
- Axillary neuropathy due to penetrating injury should be surgically explored.
- Partial lesions tend to recover spontaneously. Otherwise, recovery occurs very slowly over many months.

MUSCULOCUTANEOUS NEUROPATHY

Definition and epidemiology

- Dysfunction of the musculocutaneous nerve.
- Rare in isolation.

Anatomy

Course of the musculocutaneous nerve:

- Arises from the lateral cord of the brachial plexus, carrying fibers from the C5 and C6 nerve roots.
- Passes through the axilla, pierces the coracobrachialis muscle (giving off branches to it), descends between the biceps and brachialis muscles, giving off branches to both parts of the biceps muscle and the brachialis muscle, and terminates as the lateral antebrachial cutaneous nerve.
- The sensory branch (lateral antebrachial cutaneous nerve) innervates the skin of the lateral aspect of the forearm from the elbow to the wrist.

Etiology

- Trauma:
  - Fractures or dislocations of the shoulder.
  - Clavicle fracture.
- Axillary node dissection.
- Strenuous exercise of the arm (e.g. heavy weight training, repetitive push-ups) resulting in hypertrophy of the biceps muscle compressing the nerve.
- Soft-tissue or peripheral nerve tumor.
- IBPN.
- Ischemia (e.g. vasculitis).
- Multifocal motor neuropathy.

Examination

- With the forearm in full supination, ask the patient to flex the elbow against resistance to test the biceps and brachialis muscles.
- Coracobrachialis weakness results in difficulty with arm elevation.

Clinical features

- Numbness or paresthesias of the lateral forearm.
- May have pain in the elbow or forearm.
- Absent biceps stretch reflex.
- Weakness of elbow flexion with the forearm supinated.

Differential diagnosis

- Nonneurogenic: ruptured biceps tendon, but no sensory loss and on contraction of the biceps muscle, a hardening mass evolves under the insertion of the pectoralis major muscle.
- Neurogenic: C6 radiculopathy, although this is usually accompanied by sensory loss in the hand and weakness of other C6-innervated muscles.

Investigations

NCS

- Lateral antebrachial cutaneous SNAP should be reduced in axonal lesions of the musculocutaneous nerve and upper trunk or lateral cord lesions, but normal in C6 radiculopathy.
- Musculocutaneous CMAP can be obtained with recording from the biceps muscle and stimulating the brachial plexus in the supraclavicular fossa. Comparison of both sides is necessary.

EMG

- Denervation in the biceps, brachialis, and coracobrachialis muscles.

Treatment

- Most cases are treated conservatively.
- Nerve injury from severe trauma may require surgical treatment.

RADIAL NEUROPATHY

Definition and epidemiology

- Dysfunction of the radial nerve.
- Reasonably common.

Anatomy

Course of the radial nerve (751):

- Arises from the posterior cord of the brachial plexus carrying fibers from the C5, C6, C7, C8, and occasionally T1 nerve roots.

Axilla

- Courses through the axilla, giving off branches to the triceps muscle, goes between the medial and lateral heads of the triceps muscle, then enters the spiral groove, winding around the humerus posteriorly from the medial to the lateral side.
- The spiral groove is a common compression site, particularly affecting the motor fibers.

Upper arm

- In the spiral groove, a sensory branch (posterior antebrachial cutaneous nerve) leaves the radial nerve to innervate the skin of the lateral arm and the dorsal forearm.
- As the radial nerve emerges from the spiral groove, it supplies the brachioradialis, which is the only flexor muscle innervated by the radial nerve, and more distally the extensor carpi radialis longus and brevis.
- Lateral to the biceps at the level of the lateral epicondyle, it enters the forearm between the brachialis and brachioradialis.

Forearm

- The radial nerve divides into a motor branch, the posterior interosseous nerve, and a sensory branch, the superficial radial nerve.
- The posterior interosseous nerve innervates the supinator, the abductor pollicis longus, extensor carpi ulnaris, extensor digitorum communis, extensor digiti minimi, extensor pollicis longus and brevis, and extensor indicis.
- The superficial radial nerve branches off the main trunk about 10 cm (4 in) above the wrist to supply the skin over the lateral dorsum of the hand. The sensory fibers originate from the C6 and C7 nerve roots (752).

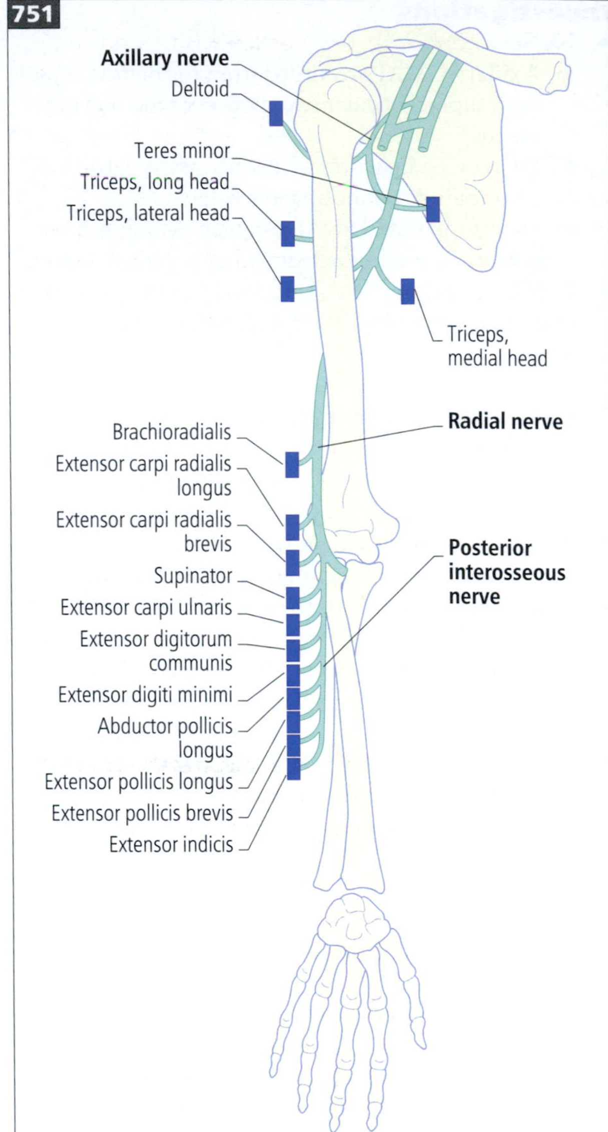

751 Diagram of the axillary and radial nerves and the muscles which they supply.

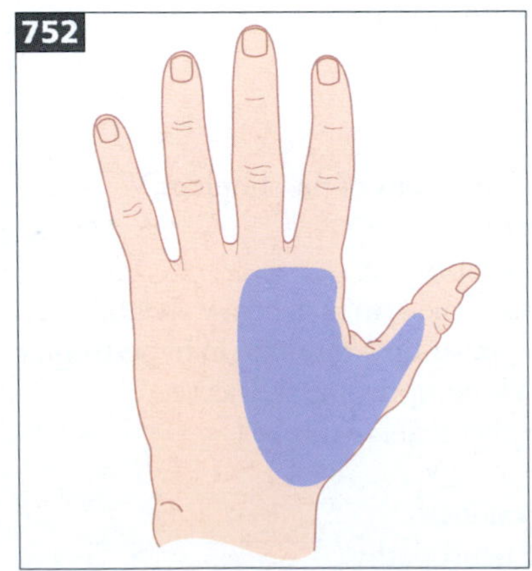

752 Area of skin innervated by the superficial radial sensory nerve.

Wrist

- The superficial terminal branch of the radial nerve passes superficially on the lateral side of the forearm, over the styloid process just proximal to the wrist (where it can be easily compressed) and towards the dorsum of the thumb.
- It ends in five dorsal digital nerves: two supply the dorsum of the thumb, two supply the dorsum of the index finger, and one supplies the first phalanx of the middle finger.

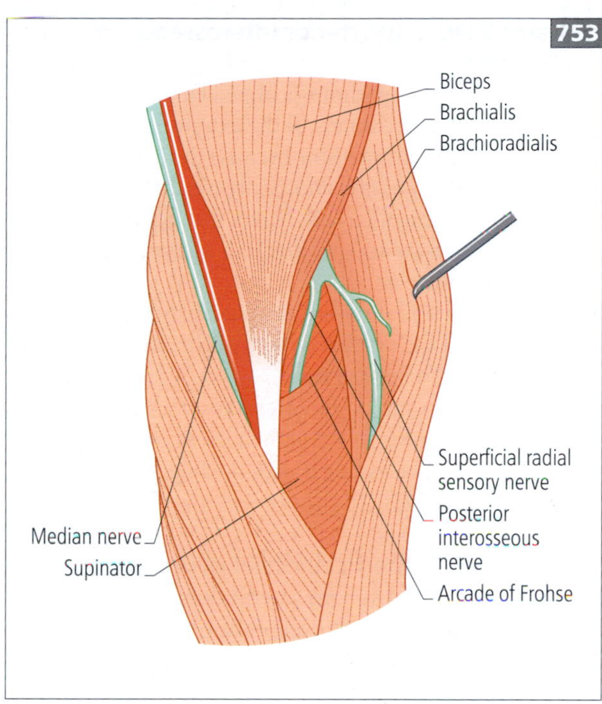

753 Course of the radial nerve through the forearm, showing arcade of Frohse and relationship to the posterior interosseous nerve.

Etiology

Axillary lesions

- Rare in isolation.
- Compression from crutches, but usually involves the median and ulnar nerves as well.

Upper arm lesions

- Fracture of the humerus.
- External compression against the spiral groove:
  - Falling asleep after intoxication, with the arm folded over the back of a chair (Saturday night palsy).
  - Improper positioning during general anesthesia.
  - Stretch injury due to hyperabduction of the arm.
  - HNPP.
  - Traumatic aneurysm of the radial artery.
- Soft-tissue or peripheral nerve tumor.
- IBPN.
- Ischemia (i.e. vasculitis).
- Multifocal motor neuropathy.

Forearm lesions (posterior interosseous neuropathy)

- IBPN.
- Compression by tumors, ganglion cysts, lipoma.
- Compression by the arcade of Frohse (753).
- Dislocation of the elbow.
- Fracture of the ulna with dislocation of the radial head.
- Rheumatoid arthritis of the elbow joint.
- Arteriovenous fistula for dialysis.
- Congenital hemihypertrophy of the supinator muscle.
- Accessory brachioradialis muscle.
- Soft-tissue or peripheral nerve tumor.
- Ischemia (e.g. vasculitis).
- Multifocal motor neuropathy.

Wrist lesions (superficial radial neuropathy)

- External compression (e.g. handcuffs, tight watch bands).
- De Quervain tenosynovitis.
- Soft-tissue or peripheral nerve tumor.
- Transposition of a flexor tendon towards the thumb.

Examination

Axillary lesions

- Weakness of the triceps and all muscles extending the wrist, fingers, and thumb.
- Decreased sensation on the back of the upper arm and forearm, in the web between the index finger and the thumb, and lateral dorsum of the hand.

Upper arm lesions

- Hand and finger drop due to weakness of wrist extensors and metacarpophalangeal joints.
- Sparing of the triceps muscle and sensation in the upper arm.
- May have decreased sensation in the posterior aspect of the forearm and lateral dorsum of the hand.
- Weakness of brachioradialis and supinator.

Forearm lesions (posterior interosseous neuropathy)

- Dropped fingers without dropped hand.
- Despite severe weakness of the extensor carpi ulnaris, wrist extension is possible because the extensor carpi radialis functions normally (the branch to the extensor carpi radialis leaves the radial nerve above the elbow and proximal to innervation of the supinator muscle).
- If extensor carpi ulnaris is weak, a distinct lateral deviation of the extended hand occurs when the patient tries to make a fist.
- The examiner should be careful to check interossei (ulnar nerve) muscle strength appropriately. The interossei can be assessed with the fingers supported on a flat surface.

Wrist lesions (superficial radial neuropathy)

Reduced sensation over the lateral dorsum of the hand, the dorsum of the thumb (except the nail area), the index finger (proximal to the middle phalanx) and the first phalanx of the middle finger.

Clinical features

Axillary lesions

- Pain is not prominent.

Upper arm lesions

- Sudden onset of inability to extend wrist, fingers, and thumb and numbness/paresthesia of the lateral forearm.
- May have pain in the elbow or forearm.

Forearm lesions

- Slowly progressive onset of symptoms.
- Initially, the little finger gets curled up during tasks such as retrieving something from a trouser pocket.
- Later, inability to extend the metacarpophalangeal joint of the little finger and then similar weakness begins in other fingers, one after the other.
- May have difficulty playing the piano, but writing and grip strength remain normal.
- Pain is uncommon.

Wrist lesions

- Shooting pain in the lateral side of the wrist.
- Painful paresthesias in the thumb and index finger evoked by palpating the lateral side of the wrist.
- Reduced sensation on the lateral side of the hand.

Differential diagnosis

- Nonneurogenic:
  - Diseases of extensor tendons.
  - Compartment syndrome of the deep extensor muscles of the forearm.
- Neurogenic:
  - Upper motor neuron lesion.
  - Spinal muscular atrophy: often have weakness in intrinsic hand muscles as well.
  - C7 radiculopathy.

Investigations

NCS

- Decreased or absent superficial radial SNAP.
- Radial nerve CMAP:
  - Recorded from the extensor indicis with stimulation at various locations along the nerve.
  - Important to stimulate below and above the spiral groove to assess for conduction block or conduction velocity slowing across this site, indicating compression of the nerve at the spiral groove.

EMG

- Localize the site and severity of a radial nerve lesion.
- For example, denervation of the extensor carpi ulnaris and not the extensor carpi radialis is consistent with posterior interosseous neuropathy.

Treatment

- Surgical exploration is recommended for mass lesions (i.e. tumor, lipoma, aneurysm of the radial artery) and penetrating trauma with severe axonal injury.
- Closed trauma injury, including humerus fracture, usually recovers spontaneously. Thus, conservative therapy is tried prior to surgery.
- Conservative therapy: finger and wrist splints, pain control, physical therapy, occupational therapy.
- Posterior interosseous neuropathy:
  - Surgery is recommended if a posterior interosseous neuropathy is related to open trauma. If not, it should be managed conservatively.
  - Decompressive surgery is controversial, with rare cases improving with surgery.

MEDIAN NEUROPATHY

Definition and epidemiology

- Dysfunction of the median nerve.
- Common.

Anatomy

The median nerve (754) arises from the lateral and medial cords of the brachial plexus, carrying fibers from the C6–T1 nerve roots.

Axilla

- Emerges from the axilla with the radial and ulnar nerves and the axillary artery and vein, through the inelastic axillary sheath.

Upper arm

- Descends through the upper arm and bicipital sulcus to the elbow, where it lies medial to the brachial artery.
- The median nerve does not innervate any muscles in the upper arm.

Forearm

- Enters the forearm between the two heads of the pronator teres.
- Supplies the pronator teres, flexor carpi radialis, palmaris longus, and flexor digitorum superficialis muscles.
- Distal to the pronator teres, the anterior interosseous nerve arises:
  - Purely motor nerve, which descends anterior to the interosseous membrane (which joins the radius and the ulna) and between the flexor digitorum profundus I and II and flexor pollicis longus.
  - Innervates the flexor digitorum profundus I and II, flexor pollicis longus, and pronator quadratus.

Wrist and hand

- A few centimeters proximal to the wrist, the palmar cutaneous branch leaves the main trunk of the median nerve and travels over the transverse carpal ligament to the thenar eminence and innervates the skin on the lateral side of the palm (thenar eminence).
- Immediately proximal to the wrist, the median nerve becomes more superficial and enters the carpal tunnel formed by the carpal bones with the transverse ligament serving as the roof (nine flexor tendons to the fingers lie within the carpal tunnel).
- Within, or distal to, the carpal tunnel, the recurrent motor branch arises and innervates the abductor pollicis brevis, the opponens pollicis, and the superficial head of the flexor pollicis brevis.

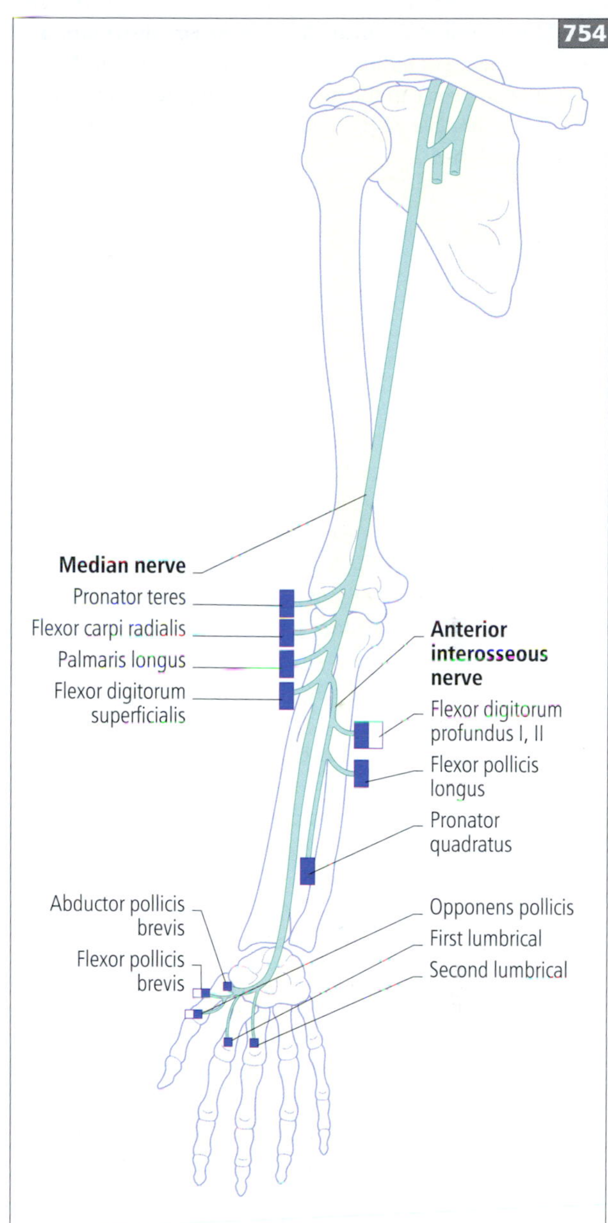

754 Diagram of the median nerve and the muscles which it supplies. Note: the white rectangle signifies that that particular muscle receives part of its nerve supply from another nerve.

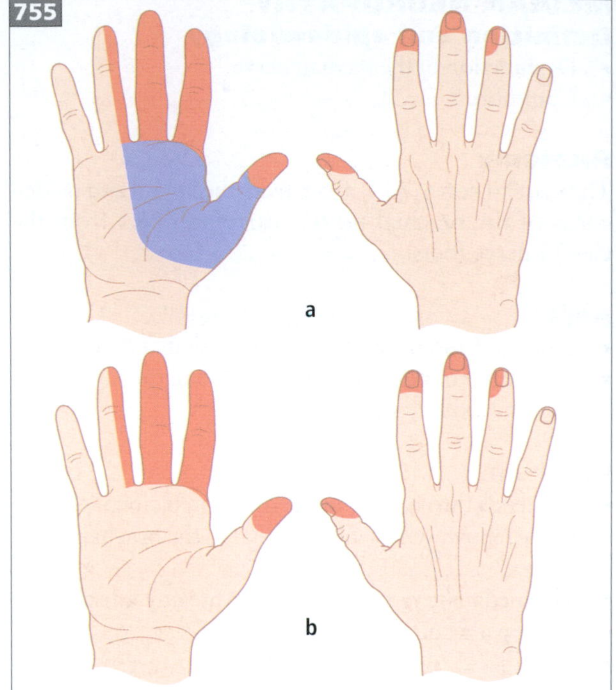

755 Illustration of the median nerve sensory distribution. Red and blue areas indicate the sensory changes with lesions of the median nerve in the forearm (a); red areas indicate the sensory changes with lesions of the median nerve at the carpal tunnel (b).

- Terminal branches of the median nerve supply the first and second lumbrical muscles.
- The digital branches provide sensation to the skin on the palmar aspect of the thumb, index finger, middle finger, and lateral side of the ring finger (755).
- Anomalies:
  - Fibers from the median nerve in the forearm may cross to the ulnar nerve (the Martin–Gruber anastomosis) in 15–30% of the general population and a high frequency in patients with trisomy 21 (756).
  - The most common variation is that fibers of the anterior interosseous nerve anastomose with the ulnar nerve to innervate muscles normally innvervated by the ulnar nerve (usually first dorsal interosseous, adductor pollicis, and abductor digiti minimi).
  - The number of axons taking the anomalous course varies.
- Less common:
  - Median nerve may innervate the hypothenar muscles via an anomalous branch arising from its course in the carpal tunnel.
  - The deep motor branch of the ulnar nerve may communicate with the median nerve in the hand (Riche–Cannieu anastomosis).
  - Any of the intrinsic hand muscles (flexor pollicis brevis in particular) may receive median, ulnar, or dual innervation.

Etiology

Proximal lesions

- Compression in the axilla (improper use of crutches).
- Trauma: shoulder dislocation, humerus fracture, tourniquet paralysis.
- Compression by ligament of Struthers.
- Pronator teres syndrome: controversial syndrome as there is usually no objective evidence of weakness in median-innervated muscles. This is caused by a thickened lacertus fibrosum, fibrous arch of the flexor digitorum superficialis, or tendonous band or hypertrophied pronator teres muscle.
- Ischemia (e.g. vasculitis).
- IBPN.
- Soft-tissue or peripheral nerve tumor.
- Multifocal motor neuropathy.

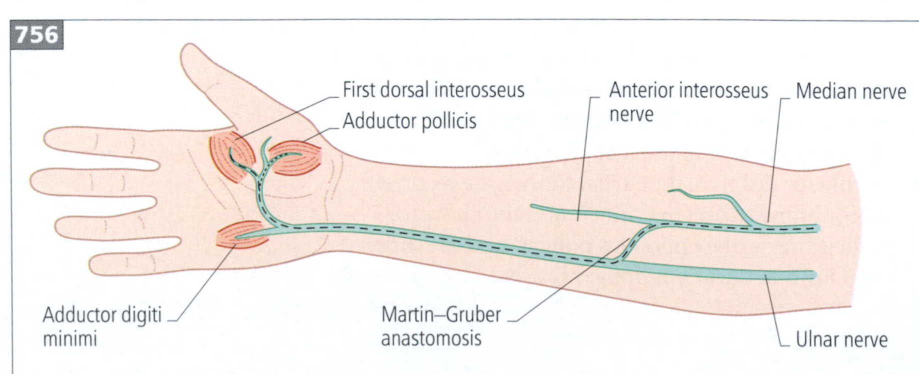

756 Martin–Gruber anastomosis. Note: dotted line indicates fibers from the median nerve and anterior interosseous nerve that cross over into the ulnar nerve and ultimately supply the first dorsal interosseous, adductor pollicis, and abductor digiti minimi muscles.

Anterior interosseous syndrome

- IBPN.
- Compression by a fibrous band between the deep head of the pronator teres muscle and the flexor digitorum superficialis.
- Compartment syndrome.
- Ischemia (e.g. vasculitis).
- Soft-tissue or peripheral nerve tumor.
- Multifocal motor neuropathy.

Wrist lesions (i.e. carpal tunnel syndrome)

- Idiopathic (45% of cases).
- Occurring in the setting of a polyneuropathy (e.g. diabetic).
- Obesity.
- Pregnancy.
- Anatomic predisposition: limited longitudinal sliding of the median nerve under the transverse carpal ligament, a smaller cross-sectional area of the tunnel.
- Degenerative joint disease or rheumatoid arthritis.
- Sarcoidosis or amyloidosis.
- Endocrinopathies (i.e. hypothyroidism, acromegaly, diabetes).
- Structural lesions (i.e. ganglion cysts, lipomas, hemangiomas, osteomas).
- Trauma: fracture of carpal bones, repetitive movement in the workplace.
- HNPP.

Tip

▶ *Median mononeuropathy at the wrist (carpal tunnel syndrome) is the most common mononeuropathy.*

Examination

- Anterior interosseous nerve: test flexion of the interphalangeal joint of the thumb (flexor pollicis longus) and terminal phalanx of the index finger (flexor digitorum profundus I and II). To test the pronatus quadratus the examiner should give resistance against the patient's hand as pronation is attempted with the elbow flexed; this muscle is usually less severely affected. No sensory loss.
- Carpal tunnel syndrome: sensory loss over the thumb, index finger, middle finger and lateral side of ring finger. Test thumb abduction at a right angle to the palm (abductor pollicis brevis), thumb flexion at the interphalangeal joint (flexor pollicis brevis), and opposition of the thumb to little finger (opponens pollicis) (757).

Clinical features

- Proximal lesions should have weakness of median-innervated forearm muscles (pronator teres, flexor carpi radialis, flexor digitorum superficialis) in addition to weakness in hand muscles. Sensory loss of the thumb, index finger, middle finger, and lateral ring finger.
- Anterior interosseous syndrome: ask the patient to form a circle by pinching the terminal phalanx of the thumb and index finger together (the 'OK' sign) (758).

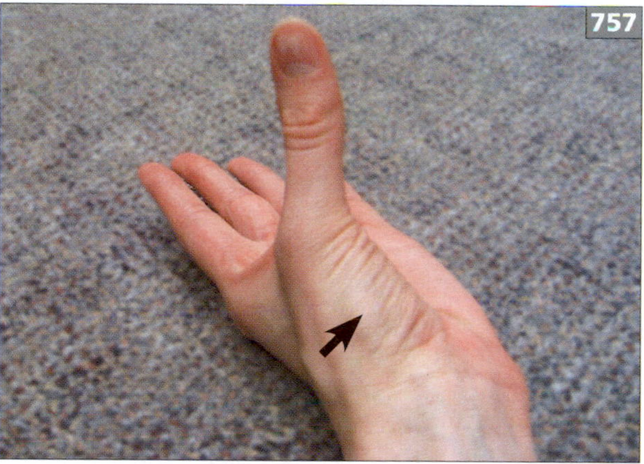

757 Action of the abductor pollicis brevis, displaying the muscle belly (arrow).

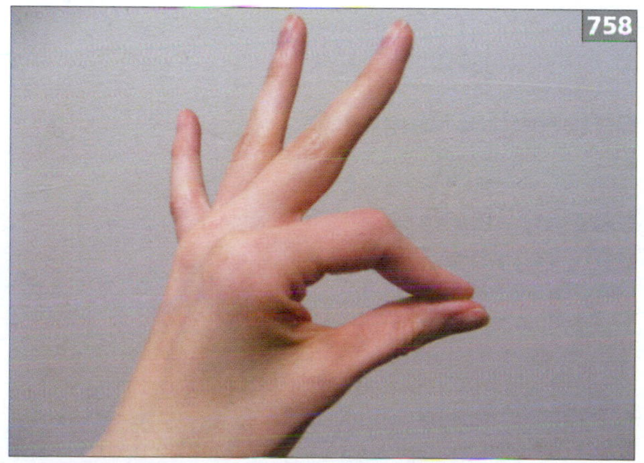

758 The 'OK' sign testing for anterior interosseous neuropathy. The patient is not able to form a circle with the thumb and index finger.

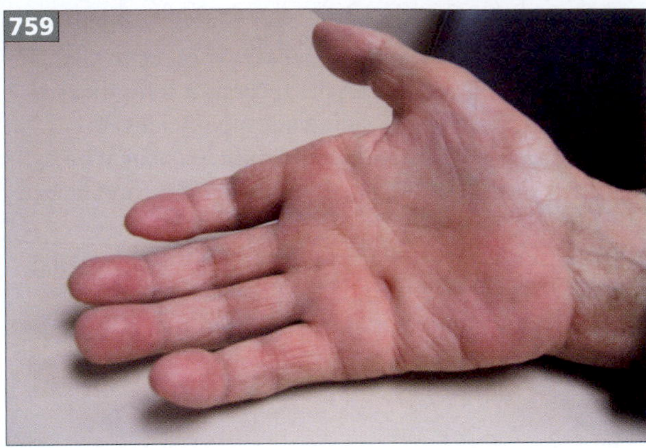

759 Atrophy of the thenar eminence due to chronic compression of the median nerve at the wrist (severe carpal tunnel syndrome).

Carpal tunnel syndrome

- Paresthesias/numbness involving the palmar surface of the hand (particularly thumb, index finger, middle finger, ring finger) and may extend into the forearm and arm.
- Pain frequently wakes the patient from sleep.
- Pain is relieved by rapid shaking of the hands (the 'flick' sign). This may help distinguish from the pain of arthritis and soft-tissue injuries, which may be exacerbated by this movement.
- Median nerve provocative tests (which are often negative):
  - Tinel's sign: percussing over the flexor retinaculum of the carpal tunnel causes paresthesias in the median nerve territory.
  - Phalen's sign: forced flexion of the wrist for 60 seconds produces paresthesias in the median nerve territory.
- If severe axonal damage, atrophy of the abductor pollicis brevis may create a 'scalloped' appearance to the thenar eminence (759).

Differential diagnosis

C6, C7, C8 radiculopathy.

Investigations

NCS

Proximal lesions

- Median SNAP and CMAP (usually recorded from the abductor pollicis brevis) have reduced amplitude depending on the amount of axon loss.
- Distal latency or conduction velocity of the median SNAP is normal or slightly prolonged compared with the loss of amplitude.
- Important to evaluate for conduction velocity slowing, temporal dispersion, or focal conduction block within the upper arm or forearm (i.e. MMN).

Carpal tunnel syndrome

- 10% of cases with histories highly suggestive of carpal tunnel syndrome will have normal NCS.
- Perform studies on median SNAP and CMAP. Include other upper extremity nerves to exclude a more diffuse process such as polyneuropathy.
- Median SNAP is more sensitive than CMAP in detecting carpal tunnel syndrome abnormalities. CMAP amplitude is usually affected much later in the course (as axon loss progresses).
- Earliest abnormality: prolonged distal latencies or slowing of the median SNAP.
- Compare median SNAP distal latency/conduction velocity following wrist stimulation, with recordings following palmar stimulation. This assesses for more focal slowing or conduction block across the wrist and is valuable in those who have polyneuropathy to check for a superimposed carpal tunnel syndrome.

EMG

- Denervation noted in median-innervated muscles. Performed to assist in further lesion localization.

Treatment and prognosis

- Nonsurgical therapy:
  - 20–70% improve to some degree.
  - Wrist splints (particularly while sleeping).
  - Corticosteroid injections into the carpal tunnel.
- Surgical decompression: division of the transverse carpal ligament:
  - Rationale: to create an environment under which the nerve can recover and the symptoms resolve; it does not aim to improve nerve function itself. The capacity of the nerve to recover also depends on patient age, coexisting disease, and severity of the deficit.
  - Usually performed after a trial of conservative therapy.
  - 75% success rate with about 8% worsening.
  - <50% success rate in those with marked thenar atrophy, absent responses on NCS, or denervation on EMG. In these cases, surgery can be considered for pain relief rather than improved strength or sensation.
- Poor prognosis if there is significant axonal degeneration, particularly with proximal lesions, due to the long distance the nerve must grow to completely reinnervate.
- Carpal tunnel syndrome has the best prognosis if there are minimal electrodiagnostic abnormalities and no active denervation on EMG, and conservative therapy is initiated within 3 months.

ULNAR NEUROPATHY

Definition and epidemiology

- Dysfunction of the ulnar nerve.
- Reasonably common.

Anatomy

- The ulnar nerve arises from the lower trunk and medial cord of the brachial plexus, carrying fibers from C8 and T1 (and occasionally C7) nerve roots.
- Travels through the axilla in close proximity to the median nerve and axillary artery.
- Passes between the biceps and triceps.
- Midway down the upper arm, it deviates posteriorly and becomes superficial behind the medial epicondyle (lying in the ulnar groove), where it can be easily injured.
- Supplies no muscles in the upper arm.

Forearm

- Enters the forearm and innervates the flexor carpi ulnaris and flexor digitorum profundus III and IV (ring and little fingers).
- Gives off the dorsal cutaneous branch of the ulnar nerve, supplies the skin over the medial aspect of the dorsum of the hand.
- Just prior to entering Guyon's canal at the wrist, the palmar branch arises to supply sensation to the hypothenar eminence and innervates the palmaris brevis.

Hand

- Passes through Guyon's canal (formed by hook of hamate, pisiform, pisiohamate ligament as the floor, transverse carpal ligament as the roof).
- Just distal to Guyon's canal, the nerve divides into its terminal branches:
  - Superficial terminal branch: supplies sensation to palmar aspect of the little finger and medial side of the ring finger, and distal portion of these digits dorsally.
  - Deep motor branch: innervates the hypothenar muscles (abductor, opponens, and flexor digiti minimi) and then deviates laterally, supplying the third and fourth lumbricals and interossei to reach the lateral aspect of the hand to innervate the adductor pollicis and medial half of the flexor pollicis brevis.

Etiology

Proximal lesions (axilla to upper elbow)

- Trauma: improper crutches, tourniquet paralysis.
- Compression during sleep.
- Soft-tissue or peripheral nerve tumor.
- Ischemia (e.g. vasculitis).
- Multifocal motor neuropathy.

Elbow lesions

- External pressure – compression at the ulnar groove:
  - Resting the elbow against a hard surface.
  - Prolonged bed rest.
  - Malpositioning during general anesthesia.
  - HNPP.
  - Polyneuropathy (e.g. diabetic): possibly more susceptible to neuropathy at compression site.
- Deformities of the elbow joint:
  - Tardy ulnar palsy: deformities of the elbow due to previous fractures of the humerus or other trauma to the joint.
  - Compression by the arcade of Struthers.
  - Arthritis.
  - Ganglion cyst.
  - Rheumatoid synovial cyst.

Wrist and hand lesions

- External compression (e.g. bicyclist, walking cane).
- Structural lesion (i.e. ganglion cyst, lipoma, nerve sheath tumor).
- Osteoarthritis and rheumatoid arthritis.

Examination

Sensation

- Decreased sensation of the little finger and medial side of the ring finger.
- Extent of sensory changes depends on level of the lesion (**760**).
- Sensory abnormalities should be distal to the wrist and not extend into the forearm.

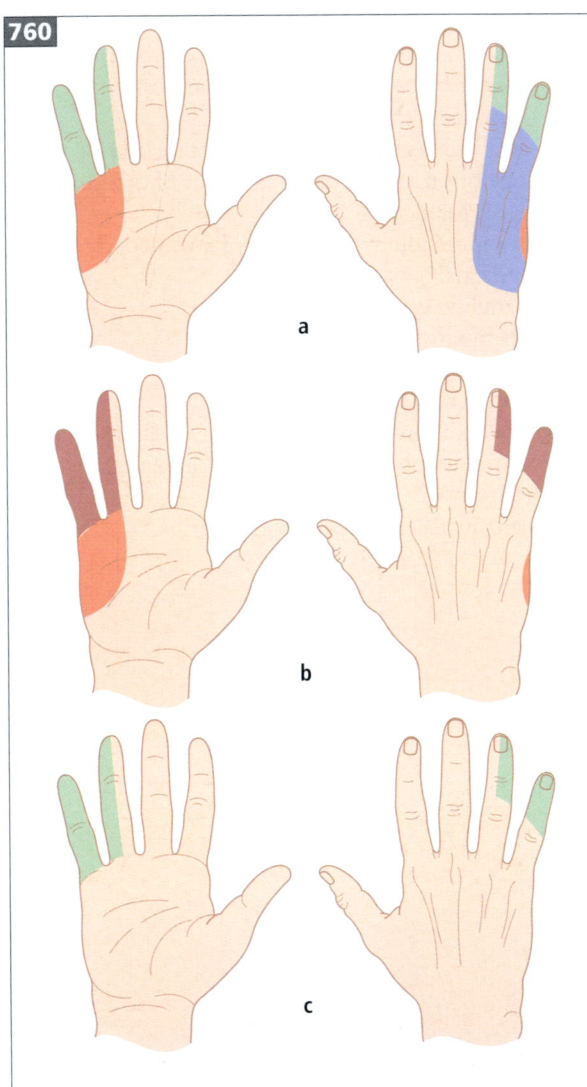

760 Ulnar nerve sensory distribution. Sensory changes with ulnar nerve lesions: above the origin of the dorsal cutaneous branch: green, red, and blue areas (a); below the origin of the dorsal cutaneous branch and above the origin of the palmar branch: green and red areas (b); below the origin of the palmar branch: green areas (c).

Weakness

- Proximal lesions have the same pattern of weakness as compressive lesions at the elbow.
- Early stages of proximal lesions show weakness and wasting of the hypothenar eminence and first dorsal interosseous. Flexor carpi ulnaris and flexor digitorum profundus are rarely weak or wasted initially.
- To test flexor digitorum profundus III and IV, fix the middle phalanx of the ring finger and little finger and ask the patient to flex the distal interphalangeal joint against resistance.
- To test adductor pollicis, ask the patient to squeeze a piece of paper between the base of the thumb and the index finger. If the adductor pollicis is weak, the interphalangeal joint of the thumb flexes due to the use of the median-innervated flexor pollicis longus to hold onto the paper (Froment's sign).

*Wrist and hand lesions (***761***)*

1. Just proximal to or within Guyon's canal:
   - Affects both the superficial sensory and the deep motor branches.
   - Sensory loss of the palmar aspect of the little finger and medial side of the ring finger.
   - Weakness in all ulnar-innervated hand muscles.
   - Dorsal ulnar cutaneous nerve is spared.
2. Compression just outside Guyon's canal:
   - Only superficial sensory branch is affected.
   - Sensation is decreased, but all motor function is spared.
3. Proximal deep motor branch: compression is distal to the take-off of the superficial sensory branch; affects only the deep motor branch including all ulnar-innervated hand muscles.
4. Distal deep motor branch: sensation spared and only the interossei and adductor pollicis muscles are affected.

Clinical features

- Flexor carpi ulnaris often escapes compression at the elbow, but if not, there may be a lateral deviation of the hand on wrist flexion. Wrist flexion is generally not affected due to an intact flexor carpi radialis (median-innervated).
- Severe ulnar neuropathy gives rise to the 'ulnar claw hand' with guttering of the dorsum of the hand from atrophy of the interosseous muscles and the third and fourth lumbricals, hyperextension of the fourth and fifth metacarpophalangeal joints, mild flexion of the interphalangeal joints, and abduction of the little finger.

Differential diagnosis

- C8–T1 radiculopathy (i.e. cervical rib, Pancoast tumor).
- Motor neuron disease: atrophic intrinsic hand muscles.

Investigations

NCS

Proximal lesions

- Reduced amplitude of the ulnar CMAP with no conduction block or slowing across the elbow.

Ulnar neuropathy at the elbow

- Ulnar SNAP and dorsal ulnar cutaneous SNAP may be abnormal.
- Ulnar CMAP is usually recorded from the abductor digiti minimi. However, recording from the first dorsal interosseous can be performed for comparison. Because of the fascicular arrangement of the fibers within the nerve, one muscle may be more affected than the other.
- Compression of the nerve initially creates demyelination at the ulnar groove, which shows slowed conduction velocity between the above-elbow and below-elbow recordings. The segment between the below-elbow and wrist recordings should be normal.

Wrist and hand lesions

- Just proximal to or within Guyon's canal:
  - May have abnormal ulnar SNAP.
  - Normal dorsal ulnar cutaneous SNAP.
  - May have abnormal CMAP when recorded from either first dorsal interosseous or abductor digiti minimi.
- Compression just outside Guyon's canal: only ulnar SNAP may be abnormal.
- Proximal deep motor branch:
  - Normal ulnar SNAP.
  - May have abnormal CMAP when recorded from either first dorsal interosseous or abductor digiti minimi.
- Distal deep motor branch:
  - Ulnar SNAP and CMAP recorded from the abductor digiti minimi should be normal.
  - Only the ulnar CMAP recorded from the first dorsal interosseous would be abnormal.

EMG

Proximal lesions and ulnar neuropathy at the elbow

- Denervation in the flexor carpi ulnaris, flexor digitorum profundus III and IV, and ulnar-innervated hand muscles.
- Not able to distinguish proximal lesions from elbow lesions with EMG.

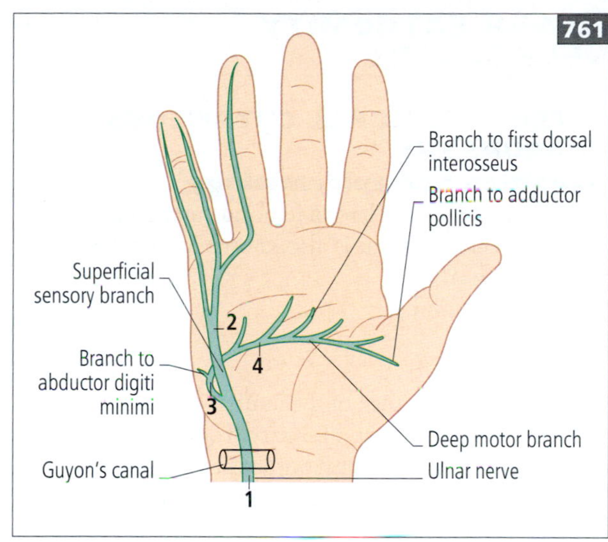

761 **Wrist and hand lesions (numbered as in the text) of the ulnar nerve.**

Wrist and hand lesions

- Just proximal to or within Guyon's canal: denervation in the first dorsal interosseous and abductor digiti minimi with sparing of the flexor carpi ulnaris and flexor digitorum profundus III and IV.
- Compression just outside Guyon's canal: no EMG abnormalities.
- Proximal deep motor branch: denervation in the first dorsal interosseous and the abductor digiti minimi.
- Distal deep motor branch: denervation in the first dorsal interosseous and adductor pollicis with sparing of the abductor digiti minimi.

Treatment

- Prevention: adequate support of the arms of bedridden patients and during surgeries.
- Nonsurgical therapy:
  - Elbow pads, particularly while sleeping.
  - Splinting the elbow in extension at night.
  - Avoidance of leaning on the elbows.
- Surgical approach:
  - Options include simple decompression, medial epicondylectomy, and nerve transposition.
  - Appropriate candidates have failed conservative therapy and have motor signs and symptoms. However, 30% or more patients have persisting symptoms.

LOWER EXTREMITY NEUROPATHY

LATERAL FEMORAL CUTANEOUS NEUROPATHY

Definition and epidemiology

- Dysfunction of the lateral femoral cutaneous nerve. The syndrome is also known as meralgia paresthetica.
- Not uncommon.

Anatomy

The first sensory branch of the lumbar plexus (**762**):

- Arises from the L2 and L3 nerve roots.
- Emerges from the lateral border of the psoas major muscle and courses along the brim of the pelvis to the lateral end of the inguinal ligament.
- Reaches the upper thigh after passing through a tunnel formed by the lateral attachment of the inguinal ligament and the anterior superior iliac spine.
- About 12 cm (4.7 in) below the exit from the tunnel, the nerve gives off an anterior branch, which supplies the skin over the lateral and anterior surface of the thigh, and a posterior branch which innervates the lateral and posterior portion of the thigh.

Etiology

- Idiopathic: diabetes, obesity, and pregnancy appear to be risk factors.
- External compression:
  - Tight trousers.
  - Heavy belts as worn by police officers and construction workers.
  - Seat belt trauma.
- Surgeries: retrocecal appendectomy, hip surgery, Cesarean section, aortobifemoral bypass grafting.
- Trauma:
  - Avulsion fracture of the anterior superior iliac spine.
  - Anterolateral thigh injury.

Clinical features

Paresthesias, numbness, or burning pain of the anterolateral thigh in a 'pants pocket' distribution (**763**). No weakness.

Differential diagnosis

- L2 or L3 radiculopathy.
- Lumbosacral plexopathy.

762 Diagrams of the lumbosacral plexus, with anterior division colored green and posterior divisions colored purple.

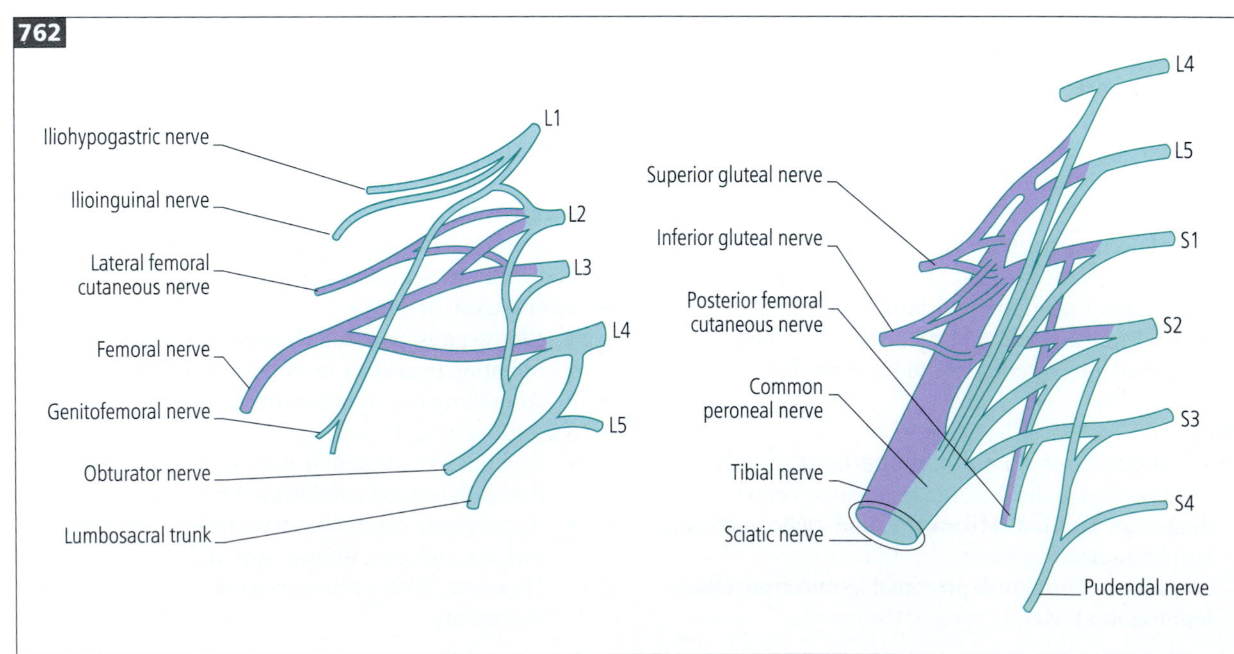

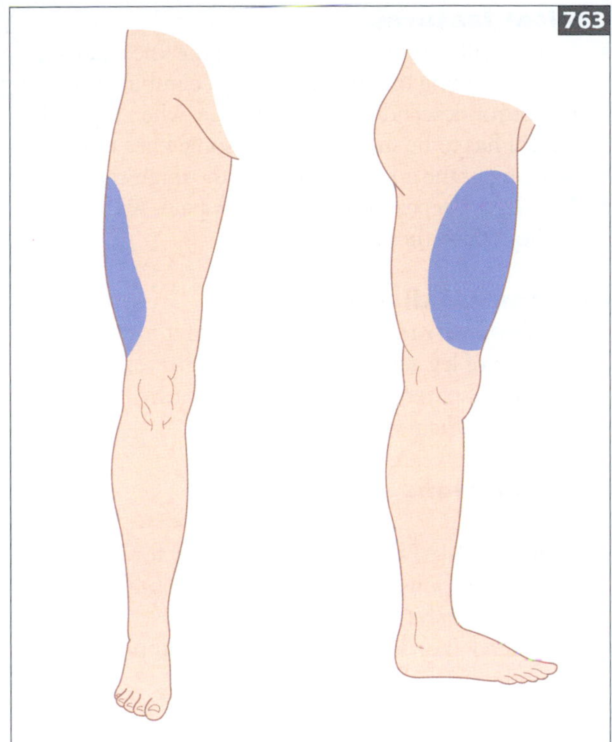

763 Area of sensory change resulting from a lateral femoral cutaneous neuropathy (meralgia paresthetica).

Investigations

NCS

- SNAPs should be performed bilaterally to evaluate for asymmetry.
- Normal individuals may have absent SNAPs bilaterally.
- Some advocate the use of cutaneous somatosensory evoked potentials (SSEP), to distinguish from radiculopathy or plexopathy by comparing to the ilioinguinal SSEP.

EMG

- Should be normal and may help distinguish from radiculopathy and plexopathy.

Treatment

- Nonsurgical therapy:
  - Removal of the external compression.
  - Weight loss.
  - Steroid injection at the suspected trigger point at the inguinal ligament.
- Surgical approach: as a last resort, neurolysis with transposition or sectioning of the nerve.

POSTERIOR FEMORAL CUTANEOUS NEUROPATHY

Definition and epidemiology

- Dysfunction of the posterior femoral cutaneous nerve.
- Uncommon.

Anatomy

- The posterior femoral cutaneous nerve arises from the lower part of the lumbosacral plexus, carrying fibers from the S1, S2, and S3 nerve roots.
- Descends together with the inferior gluteal nerve through the greater sciatic notch, below the piriformis muscle.
- Enters the thigh at the lower border of the gluteus maximus and close to the sciatic nerve, giving off branches to the skin of the perineum.
- Descends superficially over the hamstring muscles to the popliteal fossa, supplying fibers to the skin over the lower part of the buttocks, the dorsal aspect of the thigh, and the proximal third of the calf.

Etiology

- External compression: prolonged sitting, extensive cycling.
- Trauma: wounds to the posterior thigh.
- Structural lesions: colorectal tumors, hemangiopericytoma, venous malformation.

Clinical features

Altered sensation in the skin over the lower part of the buttock and the posterior aspect of the thigh. No weakness.

Differential diagnosis

Sacral radiculopathy.

Diagnosis

- Requires the presence of isolated sensory loss confined to the distribution of the posterior femoral cutaneous nerve.
- No specific electrodiagnostic studies.

Treatment

- Nonsurgical: relieve pressure to the lower buttock and dorsal thigh.
- Surgical approach: removal of the responsible mass lesion.

FEMORAL NEUROPATHY

Definition and epidemiology

- Dysfunction of the femoral nerve.
- Uncommon.

Anatomy

- The femoral nerve arises from the L2, L3, and L4 nerve roots.
- Reaches the front of the leg passing along the lateral edge of the psoas muscle, which it supplies together with the iliacus.
- Exits the pelvis under the inguinal ligament just lateral to the femoral artery and vein.
- Sensory branches supply the skin of the anterior thigh and medial aspect of the calf (**764**).
- Saphenous nerve: largest and longest sensory branch of the femoral nerve:
  - Supplies the skin over the medial aspect of the thigh, leg, and foot.
  - Accompanies the femoral artery in the femoral triangle and then descends medially under the sartorius muscle.
  - Gives off the infrapatellar branch at the lower thigh, supplying the medial portion of the knee.
  - Accompanying the long saphenous vein, the terminal branch passes just anterior to the medial malleolus to supply the medial portion of the foot.
- Muscle branch innervates the pectineus, the sartorius, and the quadriceps femoris (consists of the rectus femoris, vastus lateralis, vastus intermedius, and vastus medialis).

Etiology

- Retroperitoneal hematoma.
- Lithotomy position.
- Retractor blades used during abdominal surgery.
- Hip arthroplasty or dislocation.
- Femoral artery procedures (e.g. catheterizations).
- Femoral artery aneurysms or pseudoaneurysms.
- Radiation to the pelvis for malignancy.

Examination

- Weakness of hip flexion (iliopsoas) and knee extension (quadriceps), which should be tested with the knee flexed to prevent the advantage of a locked knee (subtle weakness could be missed).
- Decreased or absent knee jerk.
- Loss of sensation over the anterior and medial aspect of the thigh and the medial aspect of the lower leg.

Clinical features

- Sudden falls caused by buckling of the knee, particularly if walking on uneven surfaces, climbing up an incline, or descending a staircase (i.e. when the body weight has to be supported with some knee flexion).
- Wasting of the anterior aspect of the thigh can occur.
- May have deep, severe nerve trunk pain, with or without paresthesias.

Differential diagnosis

- Lumbosacral radiculopathy: important to test strength of leg adduction (obturator nerve), as this should be spared in a femoral neuropathy.
- Diabetic radiculoplexus neuropathy.

Investigations

NCS

- Femoral CMAPs performed bilaterally for comparison. The responses may be difficult to obtain with large body habitus.
- Estimated axon loss based on CMAP amplitude is a good measure of prognosis.

EMG

- Denervation noted in iliopsoas and quadriceps.

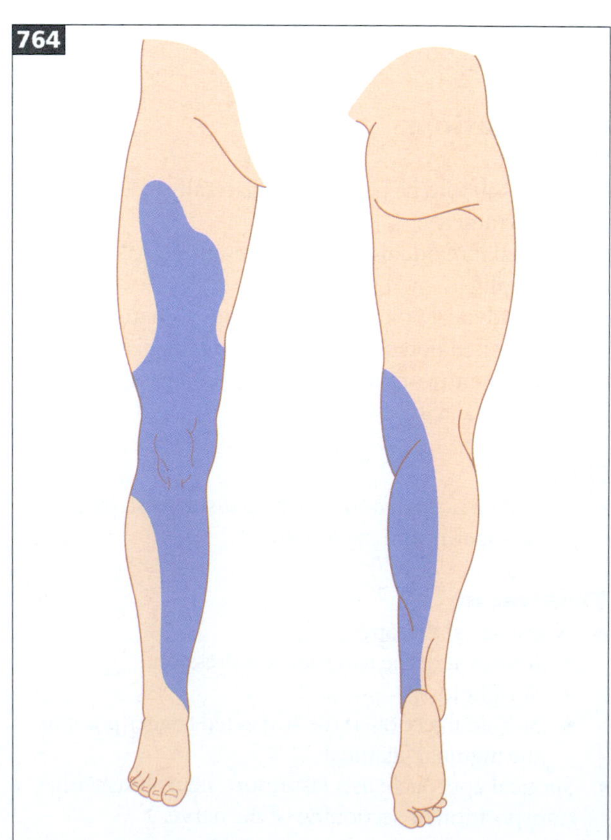

764 Area of skin innervated by the femoral nerve.

Treatment and prognosis

- Conservative treatment with pain management.
- Surgical approach:
- Only if direct penetrating trauma with severe axonal injury or complete interruption of nerve continuity.
- Retroperitoneal hematomas are usually decompressed surgically or aspirated to relieve pain and may not improve nerve recovery.
- Femoral neuropathy after surgery, from stretch injury or compression, tends to recover spontaneously, although this may take months.

OBTURATOR NEUROPATHY

Definition and epidemiology

- Dysfunction of the obturator nerve.
- Rare in isolation.

Anatomy

- The obdurator nerve arises from the anterior divisions of the L2, L3, and L4 nerve roots, formed within the psoas muscle.
- Enters the pelvis immediately anterior to the sacro-iliac joint.
- Passes through the obturator canal and gives off an anterior branch supplying the adductor longus and brevis and gracilis, and a posterior branch supplying the obturator externus and half of the adductor magnus muscle.
- Sensory fibers supply the skin of the medial upper thigh (**765**).

Etiology

- Pressure during normal labor.
- Pelvic fracture.
- Surgical procedures for pelvic cancer.
- Urological surgery with prolonged hip flexion.
- Psoas muscle hematoma.
- Endometriosis.

Examination

- Weakness in hip adduction.
- Normal strength of quadriceps muscle and normal knee jerk.
- Pain in the groin is usually the initial symptom.
- Reduced sensation on the inner aspect of the thigh.
- Broad-based gait may be present.

Differential diagnosis

- Lumbosacral plexopathy or radiculopathy (L2–L4).
- Osteitis or other disorders of the symphysis: pain in the groin and medial thigh is similar to the neuralgic pain of an obturator neuropathy.

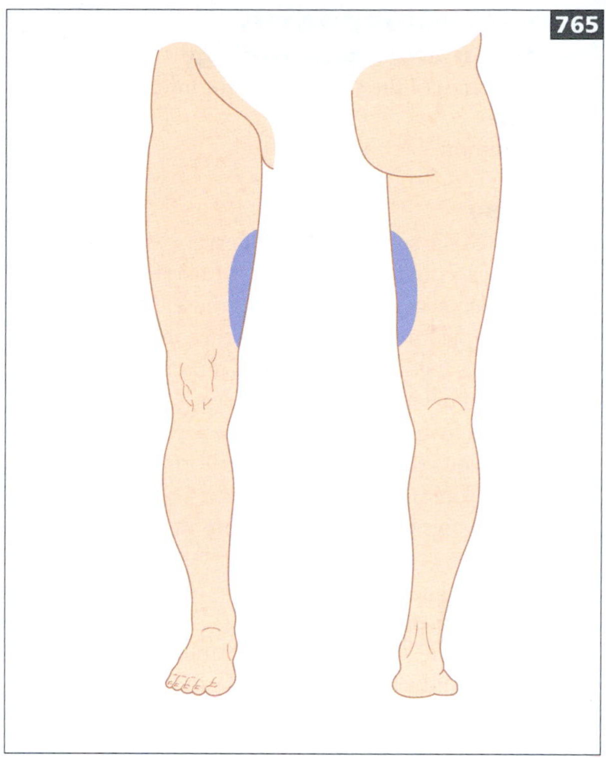

765 **Area of skin innervated by the obturator nerve.**

Investigations

- No NCS technique is described.
- EMG: denervation confined to the hip adductors.

Treatment

Conservative treatment with pain management unless surgical treatment is required based on the etiology (e.g. psoas muscle hematoma drainage).

GLUTEAL NEUROPATHY

Definition and epidemiology

- Dysfunction of the superior and/or inferior gluteal nerves.
- Uncommon.

Anatomy

- Course of the superior gluteal nerve:
  - Arises from the L4, L5, and S1 nerve roots.
  - Descends over the piriformis muscle, through the suprapiriform foramen, and then innervates the gluteus medius and minimus muscles.
- Course of the inferior gluteal nerve:
  - Arises from the L5, S1, and S2 nerve roots.
  - Descends through the infrapiriform foramen, dorsolateral to the sciatic nerve.
  - Innervates the gluteus maximus muscle.

Etiology

- Superior gluteal nerve:
  - Fall on the buttocks with entrapment of the nerve between the piriformis muscle and the major sciatic incisure.
  - Intramuscular injection into the buttocks.
  - Hip surgery via a posterior approach.
- Inferior gluteal nerve: colorectal tumor.
- Bilateral gluteal neuropathy: prolonged labor.

Clinical features

- Pain in buttocks.
- Difficulty walking: weakness of gluteus medius and minimus leads to weakness of hip abduction, which causes defective tilting of the pelvis and difficulty swinging the contralateral leg forward.
- Weakness of hip extension (gluteus maximus) causes difficulty with descending stairs and arising from chairs.

Differential diagnosis

- Proximal myopathy (certain muscular dystrophies, polymyositis).
- Hip joint disorder.

Investigations

EMG of the glutei. No NCS technique is described.

Treatment

Conservative with pain management.

SCIATIC NEUROPATHY

Definition and epidemiology

- Dysfunction of the sciatic nerve.
- Not uncommon.

Anatomy

- The sciatic nerve arises from the L4, L5, S1, and S2 nerve roots.
- Leaves the pelvis through the greater sciatic foramen.
- Consists of a peroneal portion derived from the posterior division of the anterior rami and a tibial portion composed of the anterior divisions.
- The peroneal and tibial components separate in the lower part of the thigh to form the common peroneal nerve and tibial nerve.

Etiology

- External compression: prolonged sitting on toilet seat (stupor from alcohol or drugs).
- Gluteal compartment syndrome from hematoma.
- Misdirected intragluteal injection.
- Hip arthroplasty or fracture.
- Femur fracture.
- Lithotomy positioning.
- Intraoperative thigh tourniquet.
- Compression from intra-abdominal structural lesion:
  - Spread of neoplasm from the genitourinary tract or rectum.
  - Abscess of the pelvic floor.
  - Pressure from pregnancy.
- Neurinoma of the sciatic nerve.
- Ischemia from aortic occlusion.
- Endometriosis ('catamenial sciatica').
- Infiltration by lymphoma.
- 'Piriformis syndrome':
  - Controversial syndrome.
  - Theoretically, it is sciatic nerve compression by the piriformis muscle at the level of the sciatic notch.
  - Symptoms include buttock and posterior thigh pain that is reproduced with maneuvers that stretch the sciatic nerve.
  - No objective clinical, electrodiagnostic, or imaging evidence of nerve injury.

Clinical features

- Wasting and weakness of the muscles innervated by the sciatic nerve: knee flexion ('hamstring muscles' – semitendinosus, semimembranosus, biceps femoris) and all movements of the foot and toes. May be painful.
- Within the buttock and proximal thigh, the two components of the sciatic nerve (tibial and peroneal) have anatomically separated. In sciatic nerve injuries, the peroneal component tends to be more affected than the tibial component, which lends towards a misdiagnosis of an isolated peroneal neuropathy.
- Absent ankle jerk if the tibial component is involved.
- Diminished sensation of the entire foot and the distal lateral leg.

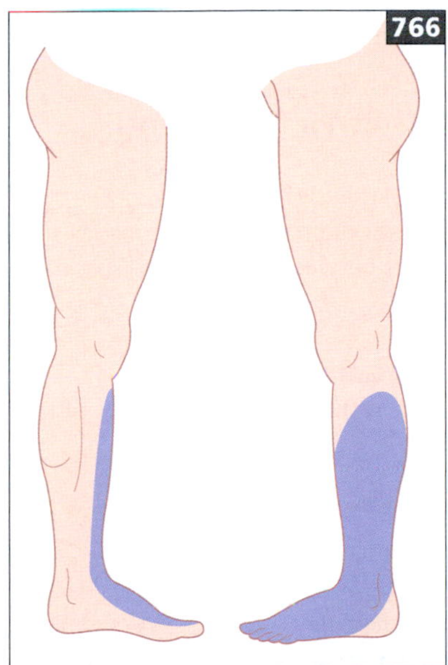

766 Area of skin innervated by the common peroneal nerve.

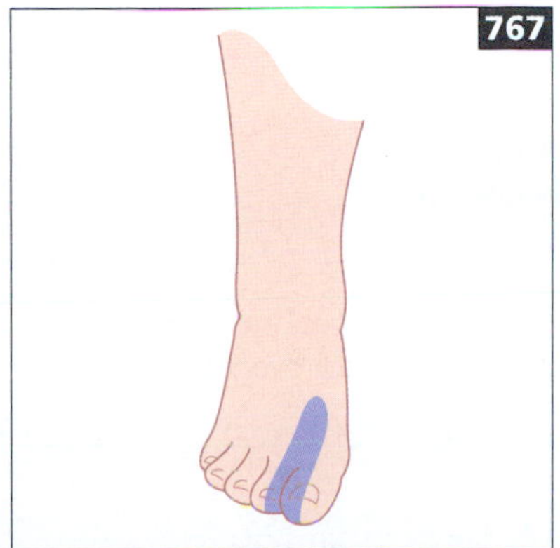

767 Area of skin innervated by the deep peroneal nerve.

Tip

▶ *Peroneal nerve fibers within the sciatic nerve have less connective tissue and are positioned laterally and posteriorly. This makes them more susceptible to injury than the tibial nerve fibers.*

Differential diagnosis

- L5 or S1 radiculopathy.
- Lumbosacral plexopathy.

Investigations

NCS

May have abnormal tibial and peroneal CMAPs and/or sural and superficial peroneal SNAPs.

EMG

Denervation noted in peroneal- and tibial-innervated muscles.

Treatment

- Nonsurgical: pain management, may benefit from epidural steroid injection.
- Surgical approach: resection of compressive lesion, fasciotomy may be indicated if local pressure has caused rhabdomyolysis of the gluteal compartment.

PERONEAL NEUROPATHY

Definition and epidemiology

- Dysfunction of the peroneal nerve.
- One of the most common mononeuropathies.

Anatomy

- The common peroneal nerve (**766**) arises from a division within the sciatic nerve, separating at the level of the popliteal fossa. It carries fibers from the L4, L5, and S1 nerve roots.
- Below the knee, it winds around the head of the fibula, becoming quite superficial and prone to compression or stretch injury.
- Enters the leg and gives off a small recurrent nerve supplying sensation to the patella.
- Bifurcates into the superficial peroneal and deep peroneal nerves:
  - Superficial peroneal nerve innervates the peroneus longus and brevis, then divides into the medial and intermediate dorsal cutaneous nerves, which supply the skin to the lateral lower leg and dorsum of the foot and toes.
  - Deep peroneal nerve supplies the tibialis anterior, extensor digitorum longus and brevis, extensor hallicus longus, peroneus tertius, and an area of skin between the first and second toes (**767**).

- A sural communicating branch joins the medial sural cutaneous branch of the tibial nerve to form the sural nerve, supplying skin over the lateral side of the heel, the sole, and the little toe.

Tip

▶ *The short head of the biceps femoris is innervated by peroneal nerve fibers, making it the only peroneal-innervated muscle above the knee.*

Etiology

Compression at the fibular head

- Prolonged squatting or kneeling.
- Lithotomy position.
- Sitting with legs crossed.
- Bed rest.
- Malpositioning during anesthesia.
- Weight loss from starvation or malignancy.
- Casts or tight stockings.
- Fracture of the femur or fibula.
- Proximal tibia osteotomy.
- Surgery in the popliteal fossa.
- Knee surgery.
- Baker cyst.
- Tumors or cysts of the tibiofibular joint.
- Underlying polyneuropathy: predisposition to compressive neuropathies.
- HNPP.
- Pretibial myxedema.

Lesion between the fibular head and the ankle

- Vasculitis.
- Compartment syndrome: swelling of necrotic muscles from injuries such as trauma or excessive exercise:
    - Anterior compartment syndrome compresses the deep peroneal nerve.
    - Lateral compartment syndrome compresses the superficial peroneal nerve.

Lesion at the ankle

- Anterior tarsal tunnel syndrome: entrapment of the terminal branch of the deep peroneal nerve at the anterior aspect of the ankle:
    - Tight footwear.
    - Ganglion.
    - Local trauma.
    - Talotibial exostoses.
- Compression of terminal branches of the superficial peroneal nerve:
    - Epidermoid cysts.
    - Fascial bands.
    - Cannulation of foot veins.

Clinical features

Lesion above the ankle

- Deep peroneal nerve involvement – motor:
    - Foot drop or dorsiflexion weakness (tibialis anterior muscle innervated by deep peroneal nerve) producing a steppage gait. Family members often report the sound of the patient's foot 'slapping' on the ground.
    - Weakness of toe extension (extensor digitorum longus and brevis and extensor hallucis longus innervated by deep peroneal nerve).
- Weakness of ankle eversion if the superficial peroneal nerve is involved.
- Sensory deficits of the lateral part of the lower leg and dorsum of the foot (superficial peroneal nerve) and/or the area between the first and second toes (deep peroneal nerve).
- Normal ankle jerk, which helps distinguish from a sciatic neuropathy.

Lesion at the ankle (anterior tarsal tunnel syndrome)

- Pain on the dorsum of the foot.
- Atrophy of the extensor digitorum brevis.
- Sensory abnormalities between the first and second toes.

Differential diagnosis

It is important to assess for the different etiologies of foot drop:

- Lower motor neuron:
    - L5 radiculopathy.
    - Lumbosacral plexopathy.
    - Sciatic neuropathy.
    - Anterior horn cell lesion:
        - Spinal muscular atrophy.
        - Motor neuron diseases.
        - Amyotrophic lateral sclerosis (also look for UMN signs).
- Upper motor neuron:
    - Stroke or tumor.
- Distal myopathy:
    - Dysferlinopathy.
    - Myotonic dystrophy.
    - Inclusion body myositis.

Tip

▶ *In addition to foot dorsiflexion weakness, L5 radiculopathy should have both foot eversion and inversion weakness.*

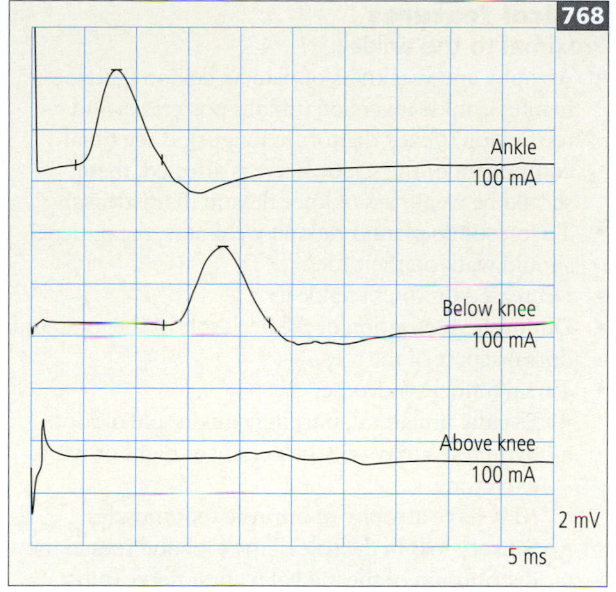

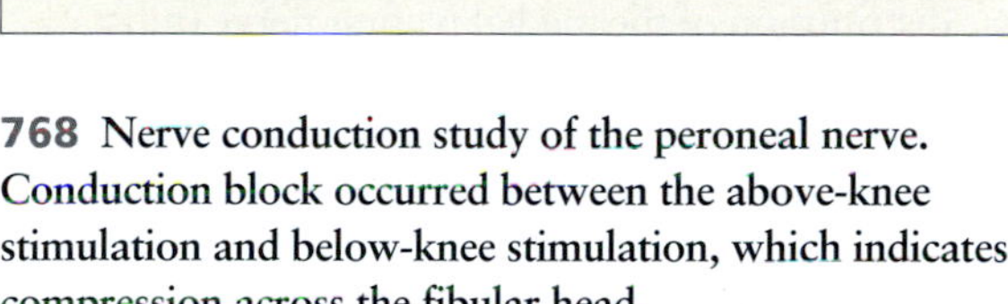

768 Nerve conduction study of the peroneal nerve. Conduction block occurred between the above-knee stimulation and below-knee stimulation, which indicates compression across the fibular head.

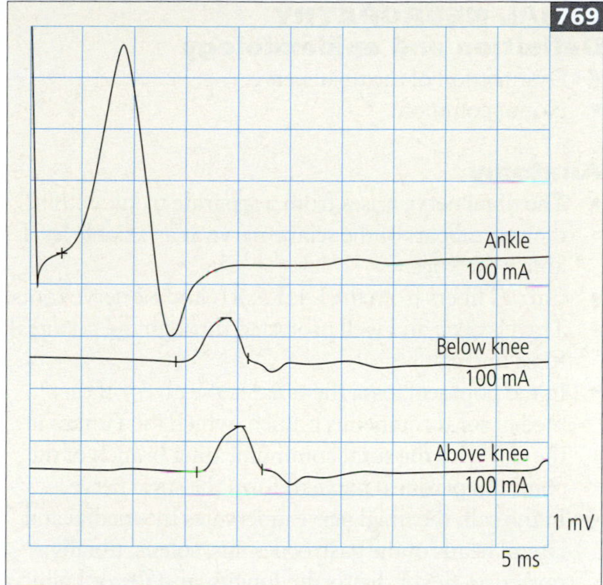

769 Nerve conduction study of the peroneal nerve. Conduction block and temporal dispersion occurring between the below-knee stimulation and ankle stimulation, which indicates an acquired demyelinating neuropathy.

Investigations

NCS

- Usually recorded off of the extensor digitorum brevis.
- Lesions at the fibular head: stimulation below the knee and above the knee may show slowing of conduction velocity and/or conduction block at the fibular head. Recording from the tibialis anterior may increase the chance of detecting a conduction block (768).
- If conduction block is detected in the segment of the nerve above the ankle and below the knee (between stimulation at the ankle and stimulation below the knee, not a common compression site), consider a demyelinating neuropathy such as CIDP (769).
- An accessory deep peroneal nerve (anomalous communicating branch) may be discovered if the distal amplitude is smaller than the proximal amplitude.

EMG

- Helpful in distinguishing L5 radiculopathy: L5-innervated muscles that are not supplied by the peroneal nerve (i.e. gluteus medius, tibialis posterior).
- Rule out motor neuron disease.
- Poor prognosis if there are no recruitable motor units noted when testing the tibialis anterior.

Treatment

- Most cases that are due to external compression recover spontaneously over weeks to months.
- Ankle–foot orthoses to prevent dragging of the toes on the ground and tripping.
- Surgical decompression:
  - Penetrating trauma, which may have disrupted the continuity of the nerve and which necessitates immediate exploration.
  - Local mass lesions such as nerve tumors, lipomas, or ganglions.
  - Fasciotomy for compartment syndromes.

TIBIAL NEUROPATHY

Definition and epidemiology

- Dysfunction of the tibial nerve.
- Not uncommon.

Anatomy

- The tibial nerve arises from a separate trunk within the ventral part of the sciatic nerve at a variable level above the knee.
- Carries fibers from the L4, L5, S1, and S2 nerve roots.
- Travels deep and well protected through the popliteal fossa and calf.
- In the popliteal fossa the tibial nerve gives off the medial sural cutaneous branch, which then unites in the calf with the sural communicating branch of the common peroneal nerve to form the sural nerve.
- In the calf, the tibial nerve innervates the medial and lateral heads of the gastrocnemius, soleus, tibialis posterior, flexor digitorum longus, and flexor hallucis longus muscles.
- Enters the foot, passing between the medial malleolus and the flexor retinaculum (the tarsal tunnel).
  - Splits into medial and lateral plantar nerves after giving off the calcaneal nerve:
  - Medial plantar nerve supplies the abductor hallucis and short flexor digitorum muscles and the skin over the medial anterior two-thirds of the sole and the plantar aspect of the first three toes and medial fourth toe.
  - Lateral plantar nerve supplies the flexor and abductor digiti minimi, abductor hallucis, and the interossei and the skin over the fifth toe, the lateral fourth toe, and the lateral aspect of the sole.

Etiology

Proximal to the ankle

- Compression from casts or tourniquets.
- Penetrating wounds.
- Tibial plateau fractures or dislocations.
- Tumor (i.e. neurofibroma, osteochondroma, lymphoma, lipoma).
- Ruptured Baker cyst.
- Popliteal hemorrhage.

Ankle and foot

- Tarsal tunnel syndrome.
- Ganglion arising from the flexor hallucis longus tendon sheath.
- Fractures of the metatarsals in the foot.
- Poorly fitting footwear.
- Rheumatoid arthritis.

Clinical features

Proximal to the ankle

- Atrophy and weakness of plantar flexion (gastrocnemius), ankle inversion (tibialis posterior), and toe flexion (flexor digitorum longus). If the tibial component of the sciatic nerve is affected, there should be weakness of knee flexion (hamstrings).
- To test subtle plantar flexion weakness, the patient should walk on their toes.
- Decreased or absent ankle jerk.
- Diminished sensation of the heel, sole of the foot, and dorsal aspect of the toes.
- Tarsal tunnel syndrome:
  - Usually unilateral, burning pain in sole of foot.
  - Symptoms may only be present at night or while exercising.
  - May have atrophy of intrinsic foot muscles.
  - Sensory loss in the sole of the foot and toes in the distribution of the medial plantar nerve (most commonly), lateral plantar nerve, or both.
  - Often, idiopathic tarsal tunnel syndrome occurs in the setting of polyneuropathy.

Differential diagnosis

- S1 radiculopathy.
- Lumbosacral plexopathy.
- Tibial neuropathy at the ankle (tarsal tunnel syndrome):
  - Plantar fasciitis.
  - Stress fractures.
  - Polyneuropathy.

Investigations

NCS

Proximal to the ankle

- Reduced amplitude of the tibial CMAP, usually recorded off of the abductor hallicus.
- Depending on the location of the lesion, sural SNAP may or may not be abnormal.

Tarsal tunnel syndrome

- Prolonged motor latencies along the medial or lateral plantar nerve with stimulation proximal to the medial malleolus. Affected side should be compared with the unaffected side.
- Difficult to demonstrate conduction velocity slowing across the flexor retinaculum, unlike in carpal tunnel syndrome.

EMG

- Denervation noted in the muscles innervated by the tibial nerve; most commonly in the gastrocnemius.
- Intrinsic foot muscles may show denervation in the tarsal tunnel syndrome, polyneuropathy, or normal individuals.

Treatment

Proximal to the ankle

- Treat underlying cause.

Tarsal tunnel syndrome

- Conservative therapy includes change in footwear.
- Surgical decompression is an option when conservative management fails.

SURAL NEUROPATHY

Definition and epidemiology

- Dysfunction of the sural nerve.
- Uncommon.

Anatomy

- The sural nerve arises from the confluence of the medial sural cutaneous branch from the tibial nerve and the sural communicating branch from the common peroneal nerve (770).
- Descends the calf more laterally, between the Achilles tendon and the lateral malleolus.
- Curves around the lateral malleolus and terminates at the lateral border of the foot.
- Innervates the skin of the lateral side of the ankle and the lateral border of the dorsum of the foot up to the base of the fifth toe.

Etiology

- At the popliteal fossa:
  - Baker's cyst.
  - Surgery in the popliteal fossa.
- At the level of the calf:
  - High-topped footwear (e.g. ski boots).
  - Calf muscle biopsy.
  - Vasculitis.
- At the ankle:
  - Residual symptoms from a sural nerve biopsy.
  - Prolonged crossing of the ankles.
  - Ganglion.
  - Neuroma.
  - Fifth metatarsal bone fracture.

Clinical features

Pain and/or paresthesias of the lateral ankle or sole of the foot.

Differential diagnosis

- S1 radiculopathy.

Investigations

NCS should be abnormal with sural neuropathy and normal with lesions proximal to the dorsal root ganglion (i.e. S1 radiculopathy).

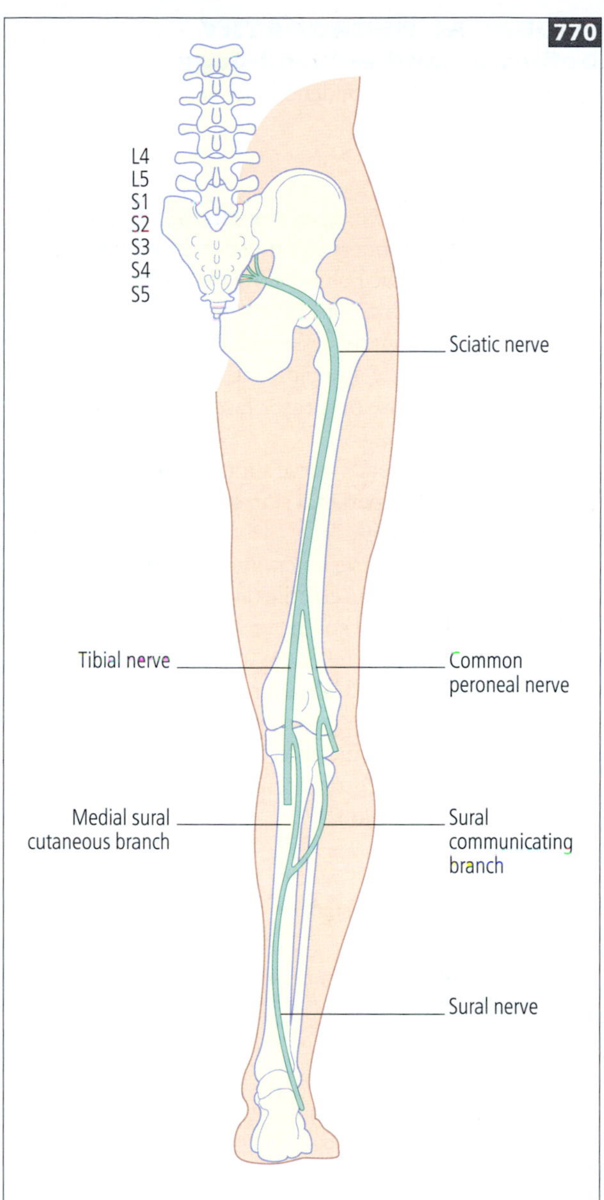

770 Origin and course of the sural nerve.

Treatment

- Avoid external compression if causative factor.
- Neurolysis or nerve section for compression by post-traumatic fibrosis or tumors.

PUDENDAL NEUROPATHY

Definition and epidemiology

- Dysfunction of the pudendal nerve.
- Not uncommon.

Anatomy

- The pudendal nerve arises from the S2, S3, and S4 nerve roots and innervates most of the perineum.
- Descends from the pelvis below the piriformis muscle, crosses the sacrospinous ligament, and enters the perineum through the lesser sciatic notch.
- Courses anteriorly along the intrapelvic wall within a tunnel in the dense obturator fascia and divides into three branches:
  - The inferior rectal nerve supplies the external anal sphincter, the perianal skin and the mucosa of the lower anal canal.
  - The perineal nerve innervates the muscles of the perineum, the erectile tissue of the penis, the external urethral sphincter, the distal part of the mucous membrane of the urethra and the skin of the perineum and labia/scrotum.
  - The dorsal nerve of the clitoris/penis supplies the corpus cavernosum then courses forward on the dorsum of the clitoris/penis to innervate the skin, prepuce, and glans.

Etiology

- Pelvic or hip fractures.
- Childbirth.
- Invasive tumors.
- Prolonged bicycle rides.

Clinical features

- Incontinence of urine or feces.
- Impotence.
- Altered sensation in labia majora/penis and perineum.

Differential diagnosis

- Conus medullaris or cauda equina syndromes.
- Structural abnormalities of the pelvic floor and relevant viscera.
- Polyneuropathy.

Investigations

NCS

- Infrarectal stimulation of the terminal parts of the pudendal nerve, recording from the external anal sphincter.

EMG

- Anal sphincter.

Motor and somatosensory evoked potentials

- Can be used to study central as well as peripheral nerve conduction from the perineal region.

Treatment

Depends on the cause.

REFERENCES

Diseases of the peripheral nerve

1 England JD, Gronseth GS, Franklin G, *et al.* (2009). Practice Parameter: evaluation of distal symmetric polyneuropathy: role of laboratory and genetic testing (an evidence-based review). Report of the American Academy of Neurology, American Association of Neuromuscular and Electrodiagnostic Medicine, and American Academy of Physical Medicine and Rehabilitation. *Neurology* **72**:185–192.

2 Dyck PJ, Lofgren EP (1968). Nerve biopsy. Choice of nerve, method, symptoms, and usefulness. *Med Clin North Am* **52**:885–893.

3 Rutkove SB (2009). A 52-year-old woman with disabling peripheral neuropathy: review of diabetic polyneuropathy. *JAMA* **302**:1451–1458.

4 Novella SP, Inzucchi SE, Goldstein JM (2001). The frequency of undiagnosed diabetes and impaired glucose tolerance in patients with idiopathic sensory neuropathy. *Muscle Nerve* **24**:1229–1231.

5 Gorson KC (2007). Vasculitic neuropathies: an update. *Neurologist* **13**:12–19.

6 Saperstein DS (2008). Chronic acquired demyelinating polyneuropathies. *Semin Neurol* **28**:168–184.

7 Kalita J, Misra UK, Yadav RK (2007). A comparative study of chronic inflammatory demyelinating polyradiculoneuropathy with and without diabetes mellitus. *Eur J Neurol* **14**:638–643.

8 Gordon Smith A, Robinson Singleton J (2006). Idiopathic neuropathy, prediabetes and the metabolic syndrome. *J Neurol Sci* **242**:9–14.

9 Peltier AC, Russell JW (2006). Advances in understanding drug-induced neuropathies. *Drug Saf* **29**:23–30.

10 Zhao G, Ding M, Zhang B, Lv W, Yin H, *et al.* 2008. Clinical manifestations and management of acute thallium poisoning. *Eur Neurol* **60**:292–7.

11 Hedera P, Peltier A, Fink JK, Wilcock S, London Z, Brewer GJ (2009). Myelopolyneuropathy and pancytopenia due to copper deficiency and high zinc levels of unknown origin II. The denture cream is a primary source of excessive zinc. *Neurotoxicology* **30**:996–999.

12 Vedeler CA, Antoine JC, Giometto B, *et al.* (2006). Management of paraneoplastic neurological syndromes: report of an EFNS Task Force. *Eur J Neurol* **13**:682–690.

13 Vernino S (2009). Antibody testing as a diagnostic tool in autonomic disorders. *Clin Auton Res* **19**:13–19.

14 Vucic S, Kiernan MC, Cornblath DR (2009). Guillain–Barré syndrome: an update. *J Clin Neurosci* **16**:733–741.

15 van Doorn PA, Ruts L, Jacobs BC (2008). Clinical features, pathogenesis, and treatment of Guillain–Barré syndrome. *Lancet Neurol* **7**:939–950.

16 Saperstein DS (2008). Chronic acquired demyelinating polyneuropathies. *Semin Neurol* **28**:168–184.

17 Research criteria for diagnosis of chronic inflammatory demyelinating polyneuropathy (CIDP). Report from an Ad Hoc Subcommittee of the American Academy of Neurology AIDS Task Force. *Neurology* **41**(5):617–618.

18 Kararizou E, Davaki P, Karandreas N, Davou R, Vassilopoulos D (2005). Nonsystemic vasculitic neuropathy: a clinicopathological study of 22 cases. *J Rheumatol* **32**:853–858.

19 Schaublin GA, Michet CJ, Jr., Dyck PJ, Burns TM (2005). An update on the classification and treatment of vasculitic neuropathy. *Lancet Neurol* **4**:853–865.

20 Niewold TB, Harrison MJ, Paget SA (2007). Anti-CCP antibody testing as a diagnostic and prognostic tool in rheumatoid arthritis. *QJM* **100**:193–201.

21 Beghi E, Kurland LT, Mulder DW, Nicolosi A (1985). Brachial plexus neuropathy in the population of Rochester, Minnesota, 1970–1981. *Ann Neurol* **18**:320–323.

22 Jaeckle KA (2004). Neurological manifestations of neoplastic and radiation-induced plexopathies. *Semin Neurol* **24**:385–393.

23 Thyagarajan D, Cascino T, Harms G (1995). Magnetic resonance imaging in brachial plexopathy of cancer. *Neurology* **45**:421–427.

24 Tsairis P, Dyck PJ, Mulder DW (1972). Natural history of brachial plexus neuropathy. Report on 99 patients. *Arch Neurol* **27**:109–117.

25 Robinson-Papp J, Simpson DM (2009). Neuromuscular diseases associated with HIV-1 infection. *Muscle Nerve* **40**:1043–1053.

26 Peltier AC, Russell JW (2006). Advances in understanding drug-induced neuropathies. *Drug Saf* **29**:23–30.

27 Ellis RJ, Marquie-Beck J, Delaney P, *et al.* (2008). Human immunodeficiency virus protease inhibitors and risk for peripheral neuropathy. *Ann Neurol* **64**:566–572.

28 Guthmundsson B, Olafsson E, Jakobsson F, Lúthvígsson P (2010). Prevalence of symptomatic Charcot–Marie–Tooth disease in Iceland: a study of a well-defined population. *Neuroepidemiology* **34**(1):13–17.

29 Engelfried K, Vorgerd M, Hagedorn M, *et al.* (2006). Charcot–Marie–Tooth neuropathy type 2A: novel mutations in the mitofusin 2 gene (MFN2). *BMC Med Genet* **7**:53.

30 Young P, De Jonghe P, Stögbauer F, Butterfass-Bahloul T (2008). Treatment for Charcot–Marie–Tooth disease. *Cochrane Database Syst Rev* **1**:CD006052.

Mononeuropathies

31 Akgun K, Aktas I, Terzi Y (2008). Winged scapula caused by a dorsal scapular nerve lesion: a case report. *Arch Phys Med Rehabil* **89**:2017–2020.

Further reading

Amato A, Russell J (2008). *Neuromuscular Disorders*, 1st edn. McGraw-Hill, New York.

Brown W, Aminoff M, Bolton C (2002). *Neuromuscular Function and Disease: Basic, Clinical, and Electrodiagnostic Aspects*, 1st edn. Elsevier Health Sciences, Philadelphia.

Kimura J (2001). *Electrodiagnosis in Diseases of Nerve and Muscle Principles and Practice*, 3rd edn. Oxford University Press, Oxford.

www.who.int/topics/leprosy/en/

www.molgen.ua.ac.be/CMTMutations/Home/IPN.cfm

http://neuromuscular.wustl.edu

NEUROMUSCULAR JUNCTION DISORDERS

Qin Li Jiang, Julie Rowin

MYASTHENIA GRAVIS

Definition

Myasthenia gravis (MG) is an acquired autoimmune disorder characterized by fatigable and fluctuating muscle weakness preferentially affecting certain muscle groups. In most cases it results from serum antibodies targeting the acetylcholine receptors (AChR) on the postsynaptic membrane of the neuromuscular junction (NMJ). Treatment of MG consists of symptomatic control with cholinesterase inhibitors (CIs) and immunotherapies.

Epidemiology

- Estimated prevalence of 20 per 100,000 USA population. Prevalence rate has increased in recent decades.
- Incidence varies according to studied population groups and ranges from 1.7 to 15 per million.
- MG can occur at any age, but peaks at the 2nd decade and 6th–7th decades. Women are three times more likely to be affected than men before age 40. Incidence is nearly equal before puberty and after age 40. Men have a higher incidence after age 50.

Pathophysiology

Anatomy of the NMJ

The NMJ (771) consists of the presynaptic motor nerve terminal, postsynaptic muscle membrane, and the synaptic cleft. Acetylcholine, synthesized from acetyl-CoA and choline catalyzed by the rate-limiting enzyme choline acetyltransferase, is stored in the synaptic vesicles in the presynaptic nerve terminal; acetylcholinesterase breaks acetylcholine into choline and acetate, thus terminating the action of acetylcholine. AChRs are clustered and anchored to the muscle membrane through the actions of rapsyn and muscle-specific receptor tyrosine kinase (MuSK). AChR is a transmembrane glycoprotein receptor that has five subunits: two α, one β, one δ and one ε (γ replaces ε in the fetal form). The α subunit contains the main immunogenic region.

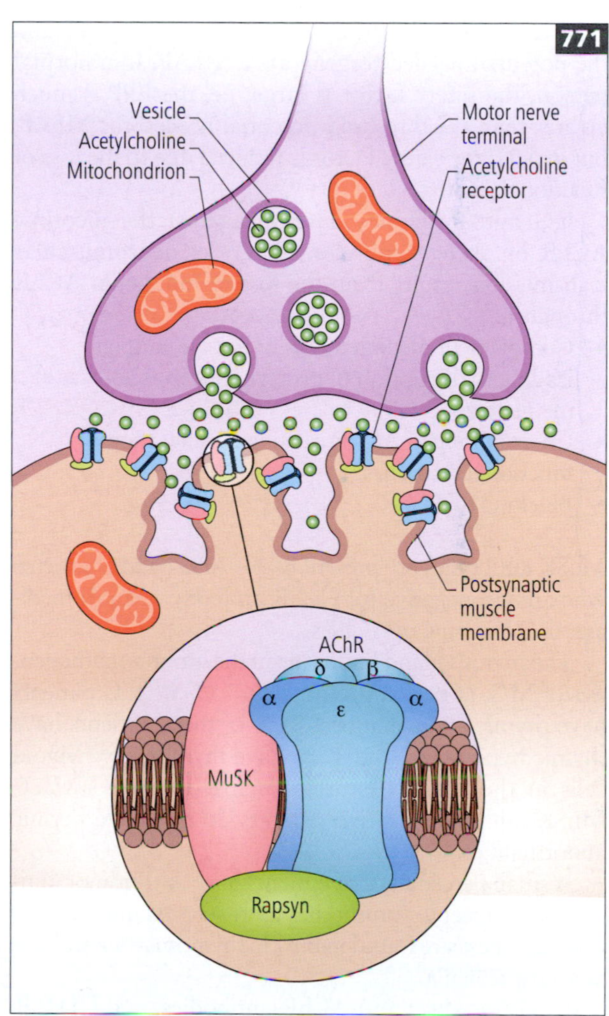

771 Diagrammatic representation of the neuromuscular junction, showing release of the neurotransmitter acetylcholine into the synaptic space and its uptake by receptors on the postsynaptic membrane. AChR: acetylcholine receptor; MuSK: muscle-specific receptor tyrosine kinase.

Acetylcholine is released into the synaptic cleft either spontaneously or triggered by nerve impulse. The release of acetylcholine is dependent on the inward flow of calcium and outflow of potassium ions through voltage-gated ion channels. Binding of acetylcholine to the AChR causes a conformational change of the receptor, which leads to opening of the receptor-operated cation channel and allowing inward flow of ions (mainly sodium ions). The ionic flow eventually leads to the production of an endplate potential (EPP). When the summated EPP reaches a certain threshold, an all-or-none muscle fiber action potential (MFAP) is triggered that propagates around the sarcolemma, causing activation of the muscle contractile mechanism.The safety factor of neuromuscular transmission is the difference between the EPP and the potential needed to generate a MFAP. In a normal person, the safety factor is large, i.e. the EPP is much greater than the threshold potential needed for MFAP, but in MG, the safety factor is reduced due to the loss of functional AChRs.

IgG autoantibodies develop against the nicotinic AChR on skeletal muscles. Failure of neuromuscular transmission results from the loss of functional AChR through[1]:

- Complement mediated lysis of muscle endplate leading to disruption of postsynaptic muscle membrane.
- Cross-linking of AChR causing degeneration of functional receptors.
- Blocking of AChR.

MuSK antibodies are present in 40–70% of MG patients who are seronegative for AChR antibody[2]. MuSK mediates the clustering of AChRs.

The thymus gland has a role in the immunopathogenesis of MG, in that approximately 75% of MG patients have thymic abnormalities; 85% of these patients have thymic hyperplasia and 15% have thymoma[3,4]. Myoid cells in the thymus express AChR on their surface. MuSK antibody-positive patients do not have thymic abnormalities.

A small percentages of patients have anti-titin or anti-ryanodine receptor antibodies (anti-striated muscle antibodies). These are found mainly in thymomatous and late onset myasthenia.

B cells produce anti-AChR antibodies, and $CD4^+$ T cells provide help required for the synthesis of high affinity antibodies. Regulatory T cells appear to be dysfunctional in MG, and may play an important role in the autoimmune reaction.

Clinical features

- The hallmark of MG is fluctuating and fatigable muscle weakness that improves with rest.
- Weakness to varying degrees affects the extraocular, facial, bulbar, limb, and axial muscles. Severe respiratory muscle involvement is seen in myasthenic crisis (see section below).
- Common presenting symptoms: ptosis, diplopia or blurred vision, dysphagia, dysarthria, chewing difficulty, and limb weakness.
- For those presenting with ocular symptoms, slightly more than half will develop generalized disease within 6 months and three-quarters will develop generalized disease within 1 year. After 3 years, the risk of developing generalized disease drops to 6%.
- Only rarely after decades of disease will a patient with ocular myasthenia develop generalized weakness.
- Atypical presentations include neck extensor weakness (head drop), focal limb weakness, limb-girdle phenotype, and selective respiratory muscle weakness.

Ocular muscles

At least one-half of patients present with ocular symptoms including ptosis and diplopia. Ptosis results from weakness in eyelid opening (levator palpebrae superioris). It can be unilateral or bilateral (772), but generally is asymmetric and fluctuating. Almost all patients at some point during the course of their illness develop ocular manifestations.

Diplopia results from extraocular muscle weakness which can be subtle. The medial rectus muscle is preferentially affected. Fatiguing maneuvers, such as sustained upgaze or lateral gaze for 30–60 seconds, can aid in demonstrating weakness and fatigability. The cover–uncover test can help bring out subtle extraocular muscle weakness by causing shifting fixation in the direction of the weak muscle.

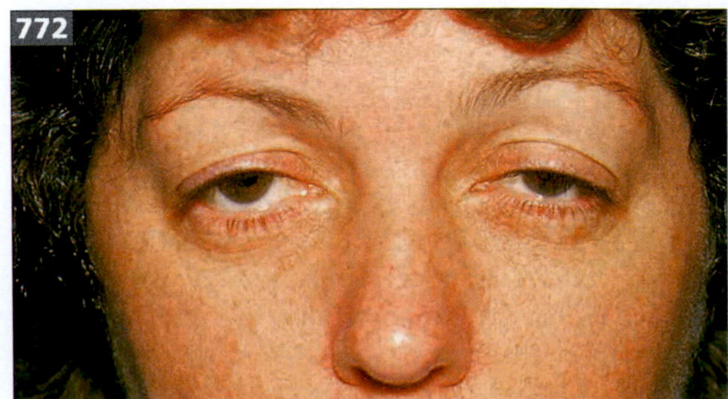

772 Bilateral ptosis in a patient with myasthenia gravis.

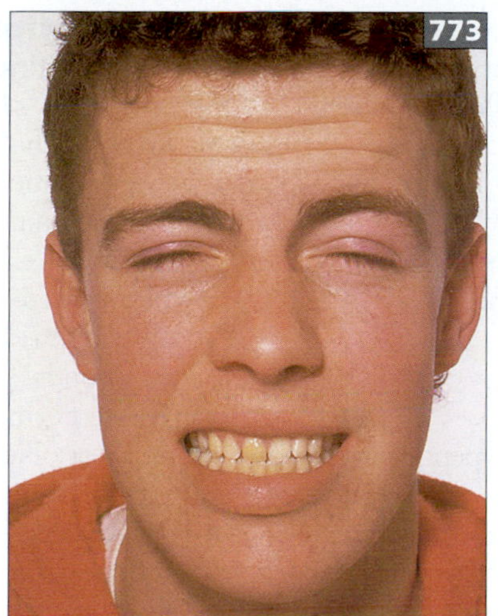

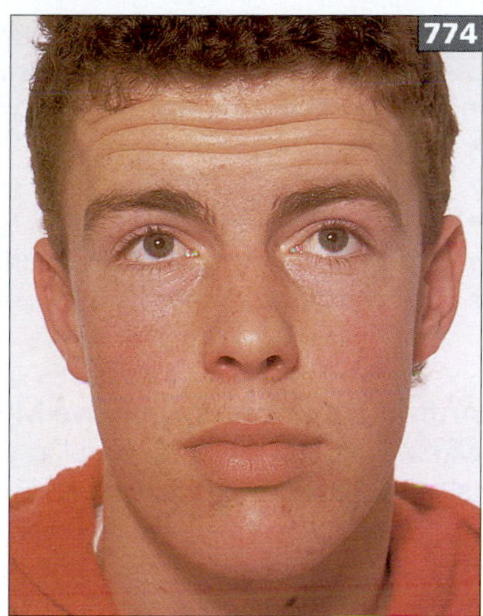

773, 774 **'Myasthenic snarl' as the patient tries to open his eyes, due to facial weakness, before an edrophonium test. Restored muscle power (774) within minutes of injection of edrophonium 5 mg IV.** *Courtesy of Dr AM Chancellor, Neurologist, Tauranga, New Zealand.*

Facial muscles

- Loss of facial expression. 'Myasthenic snarl' results from inability to move the corners of the mouth when the patient attempts to smile (**773, 774**).
- Weakness of eye closure can be tested by asking the patient to close the eyelids forcefully while the examiner attempts to manually open the closed eyelids. A Bell's phenomenon (upward movement of the eyeball) can be seen in a partially closed eye.
- Other signs: inability to fully puff cheeks or whistle.

Bulbar muscles

- Weakness in jaw closure and fatigue with chewing, especially during a prolonged meal or eating large pieces of meat.
- Dysarthria and dysphagia result from oropharyngeal muscle weakness:
  - Nasal regurgitation and nasal quality of speech result from palatal weakness.
  - Weakness in the tongue results in lingual dysarthria, reduced ability to protrude the tongue, and inability to press the tongue against the inside of the cheek.
- 'Dropped head syndrome' can result from neck extensor weakness. Neck flexors can also be affected.

Limb muscles

Proximal muscles are typically more involved than distal and more or less symmetrically, but finger extension and foot dorsiflexion can also be affected. Limb fatigue can be exposed by asking the patient to sustain arm abduction for about 1 minute.

Respiratory muscles

- Weak inspiratory sniff, difficulty clearing throat, blowing nose and weak cough.
- Impending respiratory crisis: initial arterial blood gas may show evidence of respiratory alkalosis (hyperventilation).
- Severe weakness in respiratory muscles can lead to myasthenic crisis (see below).

Tip

▶ *MG patients may have muscle weakness only after exertion; therefore, it is important to perform maneuvers that exercise specific muscle groups to elicit fatigability.*

Myasthenic crisis

Myasthenic crisis is respiratory failure as a result of severe respiratory muscle weakness requiring intubation and mechanical ventilation. Infection (pneumonia or viral upper respiratory tract infection) is the most common precipitant.

Fifteen to twenty percent of patients will experience at least one episode of myasthenic crisis. Median interval from MG symptom onset to first crisis is 8 months, with 75% of cases occurring in the first 2 years of symptom onset. Myasthenic crisis has a higher prevalence in patients with thymoma.

Neck and oropharyngeal muscle weakness is typically associated. Signs of impending respiratory failure include:

- Difficulty clearing secretions or swallowing saliva.
- Severe dysphagia.
- Head drop.
- Rapid and shallow breathing.
- Using accessory muscles for breathing.
- Low forced vital capacity (FVC) or negative inspiratory pressure (NIF).

Anti-MuSK antibody-positive MG

MuSK is a transmembrane endplate polypeptide involved in a signaling pathway that maintains functional integrity of the NMJ. Patients have predominant involvement of bulbar, facial, and respiratory muscles and relative sparing of ocular muscles[5]. Atypical features may include facial and tongue atrophy, paraspinal, and upper esophageal weakness.

- Marked female predominance, age <40 years.
- Respiratory crisis more common.
- Acetylcholinesterase inhibitors may exacerbate symptoms.
- Normal thymus pathology.

MG associated with thymoma

Of patients with thymoma, 40–50% have MG, and 15% of patients with MG have thymoma. The mean age of patients with thymoma is 55 years. One-third of patients with thymoma present with MG symptoms[6]. MG symptoms in thymoma patients are similar to those in nonthymomatous MG; however, the presentation tends to be more severe.

AChR antibodies are present in high titers. Additional antibodies associated with thymomatous MG include anti-striated muscle, AChR-modulating, ryanodine, titin, KCNA4, and other paraneoplastic autoantibodies.

Thymectomy is the treatment of choice. Radiation therapy is needed for invasive cases. Patients typically require chronic immunotherapy in addition to thymectomy. The prognosis in MG with thymoma is similar to nonthymomatous MG.

Investigations and diagnosis

Bedside testing

Edrophonium chloride (Tensilon) test

- An acetylcholinesterase inhibitor with fast onset and short duration that is easy to administer.
- Inject an initial dose of edrophonium 1–2 mg, and observe for response. If no response, give an additional 5–6 mg (to a maximum of 10 mg). A positive response should be observed within 90 seconds (see **774**).
- This test is most useful when resolution of eyelid ptosis or objective improvement in a single paretic extraocular muscle is observed.
- Side-effects result from excessive acetylcholine: abdominal cramps, salivation, bronchial secretions, sweating, nausea, vomiting, and bradycardia. Severe side-effects are rare, but caution should be taken in patients with history of cardiac disease and asthma.
- Atropine should be available and some would also advocate cardiac monitoring.
- Sensitivity ranges from 71.5% to 95% in generalized MG. However, positive tests have been reported in various other disorders.
- Tensilon is no longer available; edrophonium chloride is currently distributed as Enlon®.

Ice pack test

- A bag of ice is placed on the closed eyelid for 2–5 minutes after which ptosis is assessed for improvement.
- Sensitivity of 80%[7].
- May be difficult for patients to tolerate.

Electrophysiologic testing

Repetitive nerve stimulation (RNS)

- RNS at slow rates (2–5 Hz) depletes available stores of acetylcholine and causes failure in neuromuscular transmission. A reproducible decremental response of compound muscle action potential (CMAP) amplitude of at least 10% is characteristic in MG.
- Decrement can occur at baseline or 2–4 minutes after prolonged exercise of 60 seconds (post-exercise exhaustion). Repair of decrement occurs after brief exercise of 10 seconds (post-exercise repair) (**775**).
- RNS is more likely to be positive if performed in a weak muscle. Therefore, sensitivity increases when performed in a proximal or facial muscle.
- Sensitivity ranges from 53% to 100% in generalized MG and is 10–17% in ocular MG.
- RNS may be abnormal in other neuromuscular disorders. Therefore, results must always be interpreted in the context of standard nerve conduction studies (NCS), needle electromyography (EMG) and clinical presentation.

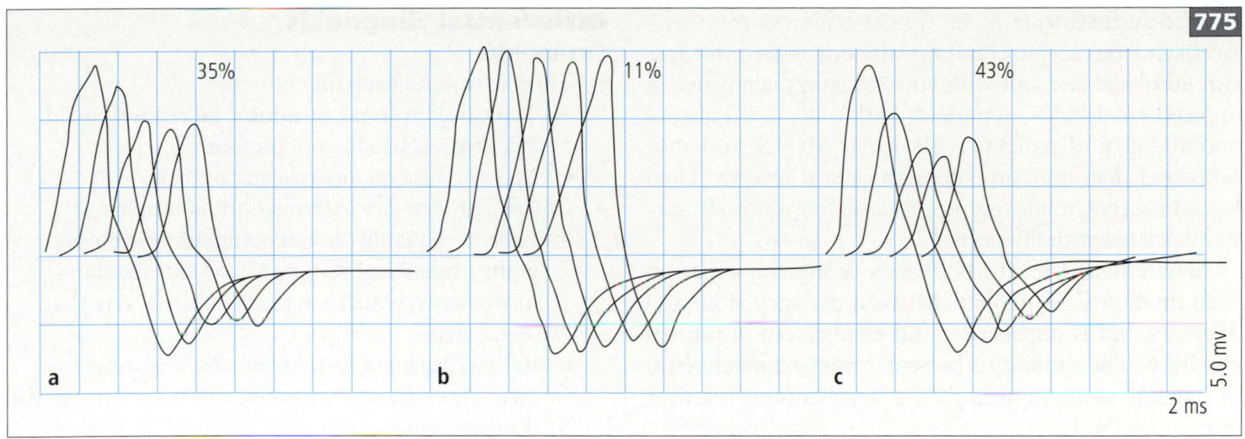

775 Repetitive nerve stimulation (3 Hz) in myasthenia gravis. (a) Baseline; (b) immediately after 10 seconds of exercise (post-exercise repair); (c) 3 minutes after 60 seconds of exercise (post-exercise exhaustion). Percentages indicate the degree of compound muscle action potential amplitude decrement comparing 1st and 4th stimulation.

Single fiber EMG (SFEMG)

- SFEMG needle electrodes are able to record muscle fiber action potentials from individual muscle fibers. Jitter is produced when there is delayed or failed neuromuscular transmission in a pair of muscle fibers supplied by branches of a single motor nerve (776).
- Advantages of SFEMG are that it has a high sensitivity (82–99%) and can show abnormally prolonged jitter in clinically unaffected muscles.
- Disadvantages are that it is not widely available, secondary to the need for specialized training and equipment. It is also limited by its low specificity. Therefore, SFEMG should only be performed in the appropriate clinical setting by an experienced electromyographer when other electrodiagnostic testing is normal.
- SFEMG can also be performed by using conventional disposable electromyography electrodes, and this technique may be comparable.

Tip

▶ *Cholinesterase inhibitors diminish the degree of abnormality seen on repetitive nerve stimulation and single fiber EMG. Therefore, it is recommended to hold this medication prior to performing these tests.*

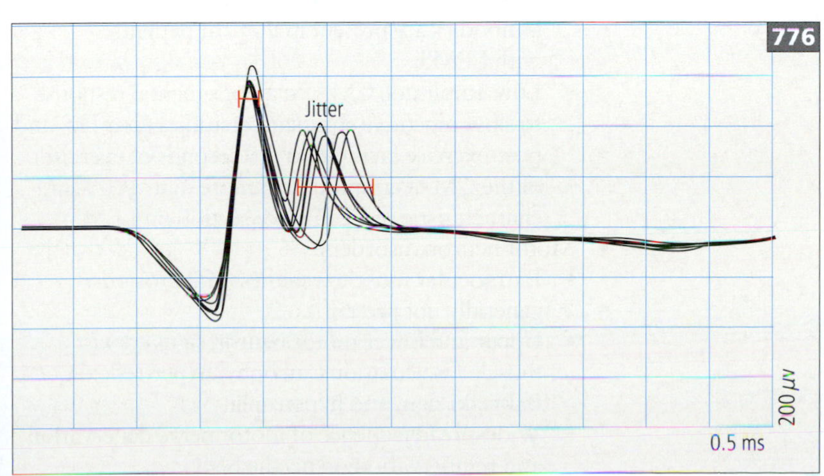

776 Single fiber EMG in a patient with myasthenia gravis showing increased jitter due to variable delay in neuromuscular transmission.

Antibody testing

Acetylcholine receptor binding antibody is the most specific serologic test and with current assays is positive in approximately 85% of patients with generalized disease and 50–65% of patients with ocular MG. Serum antibody titer does not correlate with clinical severity. High levels of acetylcholine receptor-modulating antibody may be associated with thymoma.

Striated muscle antibody has a high association with thymoma for patients between the ages of 20 and 50 years, but is nonspecific and can be seen in normal elderly. MuSK antibody is present in approximately 40% of patients who are negative for acetylcholine receptor binding antibody.

Low-affinity IgG antibodies to AChRs have been found in 66% of patients with MG who are antibody negative on conventional anti-AChR and anti-MuSK antibody assays[8].

Recently, antibodies to lipoprotein-related protein 4 (LRP-4) have been found in 2–50% of patients with MG who are anti-AChR and MuSK negative. LRP-4 is a receptor for agrin which activates MuSK and AChR clustering at the neuromuscular junction[9].

Chest imaging

Chest computed tomography (CT) or magnetic resonance imaging (MRI) should be done in every MG patient to evaluate for the presence of thymoma. Intravenous iodine contrast must be used with caution, as it may exacerbate MG symptoms.

Other tests

- Evaluation for associated disease: thyroid dysfunction.
- Pulmonary function test.
- Barium swallow.
- Prior to immunosuppressant therapy initiation:
  - Tuberculosis screening.
  - Hepatitis B screening.

Differential diagnosis

Ocular MG

- Thyroid ophthalmopathy:
  - Typical symptoms: proptosis, lid retraction, lid lag. Ptosis is usually not present.
  - MG and Graves disease can coexist.
- Chronic progressive external ophthalmoplegia:
  - Patients generally do not complain of diplopia in the presence of very restricted extraocular movements, which is typically more severe than seen in MG.
  - Retinal degeneration can coexist, and more generalized muscle weakness can occur later in the disease course.
- Cranial neuropathy:
  - MG never involves the pupil, distinguishing it from Horner's syndrome or a IIIrd nerve palsy.
  - MG may mimic VIth nerve palsy with isolated lateral rectus weakness, but may be distinguished by fatigability and lack of pain.
  - MG may produce a pseudo-internuclear ophthalmoplegia with isolated medial rectus weakness. Patients with true internuclear ophthalmoplegia usually have spared convergence.
- Brainstem pathology:
  - Tumors, strokes, aneurysms, carcinomatous meningitis, and so on.
  - Diagnosed with head imaging (CT, MRI) and cerebrospinal fluid (CSF) studies.

Generalized MG

- Lambert–Eaton myasthenic syndrome (LEMS):
  - LEMS has more prominent lower extremity weakness than MG. Ocular and bulbar symptoms are less prominent in LEMS than in MG and are seldom the presenting symptoms.
  - Autonomic symptoms are common: dry mouth, impotence, decreased sweating.
  - Voltage-gated calcium channel (VGCC) antibodies are present in 90% of patients with LEMS.
  - Low amplitude CMAPs, a decremental response to slow repetitive stimulation studies (2–5 Hz) and post-exercise facilitation (10 seconds of exercise) of the CMAP amplitude of more than 100% are characteristic of LEMS (see section on LEMS).
- Motor neuron disorders:
  - Extraocular muscle weakness and ptosis are generally not present.
  - Upper and lower motor neuron signs coexist: muscle fasciculations, atrophy, hyper-reflexia, Babinski sign, and hypertonia.
  - Widespread evidence of motor nerve denervation and reinnervation on needle EMG.

- Botulism:
  - Rapid onset of a descending pattern of weakness including ocular, bulbar, respiratory, and generalized weakness.
  - May have pupillary and autonomic involvement.
  - Low CMAP amplitudes and post-exercise facilitation of CMAP amplitude to a lesser degree than seen in LEMS are characteristic.
  - Needle EMG may demonstrate fibrillation potentials and short duration polyphasic motor unit action potentials (MUPs) as a result of chemodenervation.
- Drug-induced MG:
  - Penicillamine: induces production of acetylcholine antibodies; symptoms resolve within 3–12 months after withdrawal of the medicine.
- Congenital MG (see below):
  - Long history of symptoms (often from infancy or childhood) with gradual progression.
  - AChR or anti-MuSK antibodies are absent.
  - May have a positive family history.
  - May have characteristic findings on NCS (repetitive CMAP in slow channel syndrome or acetylcholineesterase deficiency).
  - Requires genetic testing or specialized electrophysiologic testing on intercostal or anconeus muscle.
  - Not responsive to immunotherapies.

Treatment

First-line

Cholinesterase inhibitors

- Increase the amount of acetylcholine available for binding at the NMJ.
- Provide symptomatic relief, but do not affect disease progression.
- Rarely provide complete or sustained benefit.
- Initial dose is 30 mg every 4–6 hours which is increased to maximize benefit and minimize side-effects. Dosages exceeding 120 mg every 3–4 hours are rarely beneficial and may place patient at risk for cholinergic overdose.
- Dose limiting side-effects include stomach cramps, diarrhea, excessive perspiration, salivation, bradycardia, nausea, vomiting, and increased bronchial secretions.
- Cholinergic overdose (dosages exceeding 450 mg daily) can induce worsening muscle weakness and is usually associated with muscarinic symptoms.

Tip

► *Vigilant monitoring of corticosteroid side-effects is indicated with serum glucose and vitamin D levels, bone density test, cataract screening, and so on. Most patients taking prednisone for >3 months should also take daily calcium, vitamin D, and a bisphosphonate.*

TABLE 117 **COMMON SIDE-EFFECTS OF CORTICOSTEROID TREATMENT**

Weight gain
Glucose intolerance
Hypertension
Osteoporosis
Bruising/thinning of the skin
Cataracts
Fluid retention

TABLE 118 **STEPS TO MINIMIZE SIDE-EFFECTS OF CORTICOSTEROIDS**

Calcium supplementation (1200–1500 mg daily)
Vitamin D supplementation (600–800 IU daily)
Bisphosphonates
Routine DEXA scans
Routine ophthalmologic examinations
Blood glucose monitoring
Blood pressure monitoring
Diet modification

DEXA:dual energy X-ray absorptiometry

Corticosteroids

- Prednisone is the most commonly used immune directed therapy:
  - Induces marked improvement or remission in >70% of patients[10,11].
  - Typically started at a high daily dose (0.75–1.0 mg/kg daily) and gradually tapered off over months or continued at a low daily or alternate day dose.
- One- third to one-half of patients experience a transient worsening of symptoms approximately 1–2 weeks after initiation. Some advocate gradual initiation of prednisone to reduce this risk.
- Beneficial effects start in 2–4 weeks and peak after 6–12 months.
- Side-effects are common (*Tables 117, 118*).

Thymectomy

- The only absolute indication for thymectomy is thymoma.
- Optimization of MG treatment should be obtained prior to thymectomy in all cases.
- Thymectomy is considered an option for patients with generalized disease who are less than 60 years of age.
- Although thymectomy may increase the likelihood for improvement or remission, rigorous clinical studies are lacking.
- There is no evidence to support thymectomy in MuSK myasthenia.

Second-line

Chronic immunotherapy (Table 119)

- Azathioprine (AZA):
  - Interferes with B- and T-cell proliferation by inhibiting purine synthesis.
  - Used for corticosteroid sparing.
  - Full benefit of treatment may not be reached until >1 year.
  - Initiated at 50 mg daily or twice daily and increased by 50 mg per week until maintenance dose of 2–3 mg/kg/day.
  - Major side-effects are hepatotoxicity and leukopenia. Therefore, liver function tests and white blood cell count should be monitored. A flu-like reaction may appear a few weeks after initiation (or in some cases much later) which may be severe and associated with neutropenia. AZA must be promptly discontinued.
  - Risk for certain malignancies, particularly hematopoietic malignancies, may increase in long-term treatment with AZA.
- Mycophenolate mofetil (MMF):
  - Interferes with B- and T-cell proliferation by inhibiting purine synthesis.
  - A double-blind, placebo-controlled pilot study showed a promising trend, favoring benefit of MMF compared to placebo[12]. However, two recent double-blind, placebo-controlled studies showed that there was no significant benefit of mycophenolate plus corticosteroids over corticosteroid treatment alone[13,14]. However, patients were only followed for 12 and 36 weeks in these two studies, and the mechanism of action of mycophenolate as well as experience with AZA and other immunosuppressive drugs suggest that longer treatment may be necessary for peak clinical effect.
  - Typical starting dose is 1000 mg twice daily.
  - A potentially serious side-effect is myelosuppression, and so complete blood cell count should be monitored.

Third-line

Cyclosporine

- Cyclosporine causes disruption of the calcineurin signaling pathway and blocking of interleukin-2 synthesis leading to disruption of T cell proliferation.
- Generally utilized as a corticosteroid-sparing agent if AZA or MMF fails. It has been demonstrated to be effective in both immunosuppressant-naïve patients and in combination with corticosteroid.
- The initial dose is 3–5 mg/kg divided to twice daily regimen. Onset of benefit may take 1–2 months
- Side-effects include tremor, excessive hair growth, anemia, nephrotoxicity, and hypertension; renal function should be monitored and trough cyclosporine levels should be followed regularly with a goal of 75–150 ng/ml.
- Cyclosporine may increase the risk of certain malignancies.

Tacrolimus

- Tacrolimus blocks T cell proliferation by inhibiting the calcineurin signaling pathway. In a pilot study, patients on tacrolimus required less plasma exchange and corticosteroid.
- Typical low-dose therapy is 3–5 mg/day divided into bid dosing.
- Side-effects: tremor, hyperglycemia, hypercholesterolemia, hypertension, nephrotoxicity, and hair loss.

Rituximab

- Monoclonal antibody that targets $CD20^+$ B lymphocytes.
- Both anti-AChR antibody-positive and anti-MuSK-positive refractory MG patients appear to respond to rituximab without significant adverse effects.
- Experience with this drug comes from small case series; a large randomized trial is needed to assess its effectiveness in MG.

TABLE 119 **IMMUNOTHERAPY IN MYASTHENIA GRAVIS**

Medication	Dosage	Onset	Indication	Mechanism	Major side-effects
LONG-TERM IMMUNOTHERAPY **First-line**					
Azathioprine	2–3 mg/kg/day	6–12 months	• Steroid-sparing	• Purine inhibition • B- and T-cell suppression	• Hepatotoxicity • Leukopenia • Flu-like reaction • Hematopoietic malignancy
Mycophenolate mofetil	500–1500 mg bid	4–8 months	• Steroid-sparing	• Purine inhibition • B- and T-cell suppression	• Myelosuppression • Flu-like reaction
Second-line					
Cyclosporine	3–5 mg/kg divided bid Serum trough goal 75–150 ng/ml	1–2 months	• Initial therapy • Steroid-sparing	• Disruption of calcineurin pathway • Decreased T-cell proliferation	• Drug interactions • Nephrotoxicity • Hypertension
Tacrolimus	3–5 mg daily divided bid	1–2 months	• Steroid-sparing • MG with thmoma?	• Disruption of calcineurin pathway	• Hyperglycemia • Hypertension • Hypercholesterolemia • Nephrotoxicity
Rituximab	1 g weekly × 3, repeat in 6 months as needed	12 weeks	• Refractory myasthenia • MuSK myasthenia?	• Monoclonal antibody to CD20+ cells	• Flu-like reaction
SHORT-TERM/ACUTE THERAPY					
Plasma exchange	3–4 l exchange QOD × 6	After 3–6 exchanges	• Respiratory crisis • Severe symptoms • High-dose steroid initiation • Pre-operatively	• Removes circulating antibodies	• Hypotension • Risks of vascular access
Intravenous immunoglobulin	1–2 g/kg divided over 1–5 days	3–4 days	• Same as plasmapheresis • Serially in refractory MG	• Competition with autoantibodies • Fc-receptor binding?	• Aseptic meningitis • Flu-like reactions • ATN, vascular events (rare)

ATN: acute tubular necrosis.

Short-term immunotherapy

Plasma exchange

Plasma exchange (PE) temporarily removes circulating antibodies. Improvement from PE is generally observed after three to six exchanges; typically a 3–4 liter exchange of plasma is given every other day for six exchanges. It is mainly used in patients who are in crisis, prior to thymectomy or in combination with high-dose corticosteroids to prevent a steroid-induced exacerbation. The effect of PE begins to taper after 2 weeks.

Adverse effects include hypotension, hypocalcemia, reduction in coagulation factors, thrombosis, and infection associated with central venous access.

Tip

▶ *Most serious adverse effects of PE are associated with the indwelling central venous catheter.*

IV immunoglobulin

IV immunoglobulin (IVIG) is used in a similar fashion to PE. It is also used serially in patients who have not obtained an adequate response with typical immunosuppressants. Initial dose is 1–2 g/kg divided over 1–5 days followed by 0.5–1 g/kg every 3–4 weeks as required.

The efficacy of IVIG was evaluated in a randomized, placebo-controlled trial in 2007; the IVIG-treated group had clinically significant improvement on the Quantitative Myasthenia Gravis (QMG) Score at 14 and 28 days[15]. IVIG and PE were shown to be equally efficacious in MG exacerbation, although IVIG was better tolerated. Arguably, suboptimal regimens of PE were utilized in the studies comparing PE and IVIG and the onset of effect was also not assessed. Experience would dictate that PE may be more efficacious in situations of crisis.

Side-effects include flu-like reaction, headache, aseptic meningitis, renal failure, and stroke.

Tip

▶ *Side-effects from IVIG infusion can be minimized by ample hydration, pre-treatment with antihistamines and acetaminophen (paracetamol), and utilizing a slow rate of infusion.*

Treatment of respiratory crisis

- MG crisis should be managed in the intensive care unit with close monitoring of pulmonary function. Elective intubation should be done if FVC <15 ml/kg or NIF <−30 mmH_2O.
- A precipitating factor can be identified in the majority of patients in crisis and include: bronchopulmonary infection, aspiration, surgical procedure including thymectomy, rapid tapering of immunotherapy, treatment with drug that can exacerbate myasthenic weakness including corticosteroid-induced worsening.
- Acute treatment with PE or IVIG; PE is preferable.
- Discontinue CIs as they can contribute to bronchopulmonary secretions. CIs will not protect a patient from respiratory crisis.
- Initiation of high-dose daily corticosteroid and immunosuppressant concomitantly with acute therapy.

Treatment of ocular MG

- The majority of patients have ocular symptoms at disease onset.
- If symptoms do not generalize within 2 years of the disease onset, then there is 90% likelihood that disease will remain restricted to the ocular muscles.
- CIs may be adequate in controlling ocular symptoms in some patients; however, corticosteroids are typically more effective, and in general, ocular MG can be controlled at a relatively low dose of prednisone (5–15 mg/day or the equivalent alternate day dose).

MG in pregnancy

- Course is unpredictable during pregnancy, but worsening of symptoms, if it occurs, tends to be in the first trimester or post-partum.
- Goal is to optimize MG treatment prior to delivery.
- CIs, corticosteroids, IVIG, and PE can be used during pregnancy.
- Immunosuppressant agents should generally be avoided due to potential teratogenic effects.
- Magnesium sulfate should not be used for premature labor due to its negative effect on neuromuscular transmission.
- Pregnancy-related changes in intestinal absorption and renal clearance may alter the amount of medication needed.
- Risk of pregnancy-related complications may be higher, but overall prognosis for MG is unchanged.

Transient neonatal MG

- Transient neonatal MG is caused by transplacental passage of maternal antibodies.
- Severity and duration of MG in the mother does not correlate with risk of development of neonatal MG.
- Two-thirds of cases develop within a few hours of birth (after maternal CIs are cleared by the infant).
- Signs: poor suck and swallow, generalized hypotonia, respiratory distress, and in rare cases arthrogryposis multiplex congenita.
- Occurs in approximately 5–20% of infants born to mothers with MG.
- Mothers with a previously affected child have a higher risk with subsequent births.
- These mothers may be treated with PE or IVIG prophylactically.
- Symptoms generally last less than 1 month, but may last much longer in some cases.
- Treatment: supportive care, such as assisted ventilation or tube feeding, CIs, and in severe cases, PE.

Medications that may exacerbate MG are listed in *Table 120*.

Prognosis

- Patients who present with ocular complaints have an 80–85% chance of generalizing.
- There is some evidence that treatment with corticosteroids may decrease this risk.
- The mortality rate from MG was more than 30% before the 1960s, but with the onset of modern critical care and immunosuppressive therapy life expectancy in MG now approaches normal.
- At least 80% of patients are able to experience significant improvement in their symptoms; however, fixed weakness may develop later in the disease course if muscle weakness is not treated optimally.
- Few patients are able to wean off immunotherapy completely.

TABLE 120 **MEDICATIONS THAT MAY EXACERBATE MYASTHENIA GRAVIS**

CONTRAINDICATED
Alpha-interferon, curare, D-penicillamine, botulinum toxin

USE WITH CAUTION
- Neuromuscular blocking agents:
  - Succinylcholine, D-tubocurarine
- Antibiotics:
  - Aminoglycosides (gentamicin, kanamycin, neomycin, streptomycin, tobramycin)
  - Macrolides (erythromycin, azithromycin)
  - Fluoroquinolones (ciprofloxacin, levofloxacin, norfloxacin)
- Quinine, quinidine, procainamide
- Magnesium salts
- Calcium channel blockers
- Beta-blockers
- Lithium
- Iodinated contrast agents

CONGENITAL MYASTHENIC SYNDROMES

Definition

Congenital myasthenic syndrome (CMS) is a heterogeneous group of disorders caused by various genetic mutations resulting in failed neuromuscular transmission. CMS should be considered in the differential diagnosis in seronegative myasthenia especially when there is a positive family history or the onset of symptoms is in infancy or at a young age.

Typical symptoms are similar to those seen in autoimmune MG, with fluctuating and fatigable muscle weakness resulting in ptosis, ophthalmoparesis, neck and limb, as well as respiratory muscle, weakness. There may be a history of decreased fetal movement *in utero*, and arthrogryposis is seen in some newborn infants. CMS may be classified according to the site of defect (*Table 121*).

TABLE 121 **CONGENITAL MYASTHENIC SYNDROMES**

Site of defect	Diagnostic clues	Electrophysiologic findings	Treatment
POSTSYNAPTIC DEFECTS			
AChR subunit mutations*	Multiple joint contractures	Decrement at low and high rates of RNS	Responds to CI, 3,4-DAP, and ephedrine
Rapsyn mutations	Multiple joint contractures; increased weakness/respiratory compromise by intercurrent infections	Decrement at slow and high rates of RNS (can be mild or absent)	Responds to CI, 3,4-DAP and ephedrine
Dok-7 mutations	Limb girdle and axial weakness; mild facial weakness and ptosis, but normal ocular movements	Decrement on RNS	Variable response to CI (may deteriorate), modest response to 3,4-DAP, and ephedrine
Slow-channel syndrome	Autosomal dominant inheritance Selective involvement of cervical, intrinsic hand muscles, wrist, and hand extensor muscles	Repetitive CMAPs with single supramaximal stimulation	CI worsens symptoms Responds positively to quinidine and fluoxetine
Fast-channel syndrome	Severe cases have multiple joint contractures	Decrement at slow rates of RNS, but repair of decrement after exercise or high rates of RNS	Responds to CI, 3,4-DAP
Sodium-channel syndrome	Recurrent episodes of bulbar and respiratory paralysis	No decrement with slow RNS, but decrement appears with sustained high frequency RNS[16]	Unknown
SYNAPTIC DEFECTS			
Endplate acetyl-cholinesterase deficiency	Sluggish pupillary reaction to light	Repetitive CMAPs with single supramaximal stimulation	No response to CI, which may make symptoms worse
Endplate choline acetyltransferase deficiency	Recurrent apneic episodes, spontaneous or with illness, excitement	Decrement with slow rates of RNS, post-exercise repair, and post-exercise exhaustion	Modest response to CI
PRESYNAPTIC DEFECTS			
Paucity of synaptic vesicles	Weakness onset in infancy	Decrement at slow RNS, with partial post-exercise repair	Modest response to CI
Congenital Lambert–Eaton-like CMS	Severe generalized and respiratory weakness in infancy	Low CMAP amplitude, with decrement at slow RNS and post-tetanic facilitation	Variable response to CI, 3,4-DAP and guinidine

*Most common congenital myasthenic syndrome (CMS).

CI: cholinesterase inhibitors; CMAP: compound muscle action potential; DAP: 3,4-diaminopyridine; RNS: repetitive nerve stimulation.

LAMBERT–EATON MYASTHENIC SYNDROME

Definition and epidemiology

Lambert–Eaton myasthenic syndrome (LEMS) is an autoimmune disorder caused by antibodies directed against the VGCC in the presynaptic motor nerve terminal. It is characterized by muscle weakness, fatigability, hyporeflexia, and autonomic dysfunction. LEMS is strongly associated with small-cell lung cancer (SCLC).

- LEMS is a rare disease with a reported incidence of 0.48 per million population.
- Patients are usually older than 40 years of age and there is a male predominance.
- LEMS occurs in 3% of patients with SCLC, and 60% of patients with LEMS have SCLC[17].
- SCLC can occur years after the onset of LEMS.
- Lymphoproliferative disease is less commonly associated with LEMS.

Pathophysiology

Antibodies develop against the VGCC on the presynaptic motor nerve terminal and autonomic nerve terminal. The majority of antibodies are against the P/Q-type VGCC while a small number of antibodies are against the N-type VGCC. The antibodies disrupt influx of calcium and release of acetylcholine.

Miniature end-plate potential amplitude in LEMS is similar to normal muscle. There is an adequate number of vesicles containing acetylcholine. AChR are also normal in number and function.

There is a significant reduction in acetylcholine release which can be facilitated by increased calcium concentration. SCLC cells express VGCC on the membrane surface.

Clinical features

- Progressive muscle weakness that preferentially affects the proximal lower extremities.
- Patients may report difficulty rising from a chair or climbing stairs; patients may also complain of muscle stiffness or aching.
- Facial, ocular, oropharyngeal, and respiratory muscle weakness occur in some patients.
- Most patients experience dry mouth. Other autonomic symptoms include: erectile dysfunction, less frequently blurred vision, and constipation.
- Absent or depressed deep tendon reflexes that may augment after brief, intense exercise.
- Some patients have paraneoplastic cerebellar degeneration occurring with LEMS concomitantly.

Tip

▶ *In LEMS patients, the degree of muscle weakness found on examination is often less than expected based on the patient's complaints.*

Investigations and diagnosis

Electrophysiology

- Low CMAP amplitude on routine NCS.
- Increment of CMAP amplitude immediately after brief, intense exercise or with high frequency (10–50 Hz) repetitive stimulation. The incremental response is usually >100%. This is called post-exercise or post-activation facilitation (777).
- An incremental response may not be present if baseline CMAP amplitude is normal and the disease is mild. An abnormal decrement is present in almost all patients and may be the only abnormal finding early in the disease course.
- LEMS patients typically have significant jitter with blocking on SFEMG that may improve with higher firing rates.

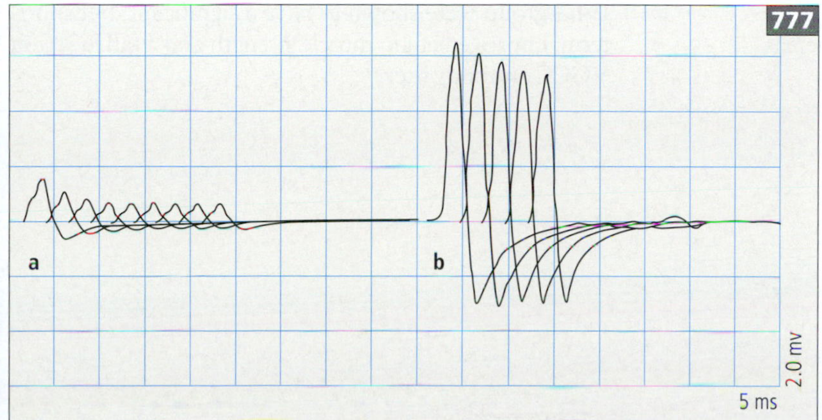

777 Post-exercise facilitation in LEMS. (a) Before exercise; (b) after brief, intense exercise.

Antibody testing

- Antibodies to P/Q-type VGCC are present in 90% of patients with LEMS and are confirmative of the diagnosis.
- 60% of LEMS patients have cancer; a low antibody titer may be present in those with other paraneoplastic disorders, autoimmune disorders, or amyotrophic lateral sclerosis (ALS).
- A recent study showed that anti-SOX1 antibody is found in 64% of patients with LEMS and SCLC, but none in SCLC patients without LEMS. It is a specific test that could be useful in the search for cancer in LEMS patients[18].

Other tests

CT of the chest should be done to evaluate for lung cancer. Positron emission tomography (PET) is able to detect a small tumor and should be considered in those with risk factors for cancer, most importantly a history of tobacco smoking and older age.

Differential diagnosis

Myopathy

- The most common misdiagnosis in LEMS patients is myopathy because patients frequently present with proximal lower extremity weakness. Therefore, a high index of suspicion is necessary.
- Muscle weakness does not fluctuate in myopathy and deep tendon reflexes are generally preserved.

MG

- Ocular and bulbar symptoms are more common and pronounced in typical MG.
- Autonomic symptoms and signs do not occur in MG.
- Reflexes are preserved in MG.

ALS

- ALS typically presents with asymmetric distal limb weakness, whereas in LEMS, weakness is symmetric and proximal.
- Muscle atrophy and fasciculations are not typical in LEMS.
- Brisk reflexes are expected in ALS whereas hyporeflexia is seen in LEMS.

Treatment

Treatment of cancer often improves symptoms. In patients who continue to have significant muscle weakness after cancer treatment, medications to improve neuromuscular transmission or immune therapy can be considered.

Medications that improve acetylcholine release

3,4-Diaminopyridine (3,4-DAP) is a potassium channel inhibitor and enhances acetylcholine release by enhancing calcium entry into the presynaptic nerve terminal. 3,4-DAP produces clinical benefit in the majority of patients with LEMS:

- Trials of 3,4-DAP in LEMS patients have demonstrated that it is effective in improving muscle strength and CMAP amplitude[19–21].
- Typical initial dose is 5 mg 3–4 times a day. Dose can be increased by 5 mg a day to a maximum of 80 mg daily.
- It is generally well-tolerated. Common side-effects are perioral tingling. Caution should be taken in patients who have history of seizure as it may lower seizure threshold.
- It is not available in the USA, but may be obtained from certain compounding pharmacies or through a pharmaceutical research protocol.
- Co-administration with a CI may potentiate the effect of 3,4-DAP.

Guanidine and 4-aminopyridine (4-AP) were shown to improve muscle strength and CMAP amplitude, but their use is limited by adverse side-effects (myelosuppression and renal failure in guanidine and seizure in 4-AP).

Immunotherapy

Use of immunomodulating therapies has been studied. IVIG, PE, prednisone, AZA, and myocophenolate have been reported to show benefit in small case series. PE and IVIG are generally used when there is severe weakness.

Only IVIG was studied in a randomized, double-blind, placebo-controlled study. The patients in the IVIG-group were shown to have a significant, but short-term, improvement in muscle strength and a fall in serum VGCC antibody titer.

BOTULISM

Definition and epidemiology

Botulism is caused by neurotoxins released by *Clostridium botulinum*, a Gram-positive, spore-forming anaerobic bacterium. The toxins can be transmitted via ingestion of contaminated food as in food-borne and infantile botulism, or via entry through a wound site. The toxins interfere with fusion of neurotransmitter-containing vesicles in the presynaptic nerve terminal. Disease manifestation and electrophysiologic findings can be variable.

- Over 100 cases of botulism are reported in the USA every year.
- Infantile botulism is the most common form, followed by food-borne and wound botulism.

Major forms

Food-borne botulism

- Caused by ingestion of food contaminated with *C. botulinum*, its spores, or neurotoxin.
- The toxins have accessory proteins that protect them from the proteolytic activity of the stomach acid.
- It is usually transmitted through inadequately prepared canned foods.
- Gastrointestinal symptoms (nausea, vomiting, diarrhea) may occur prior to onset of neurologic symptoms.
- Within 2–36 hours of ingestion, most patients develop cranial nerve dysfunction and autonomic symptoms. Typical presentations are ptosis, diplopia, blurred vision, dysarthria, nasal speech, and dysphagia. This is followed by upper limb and then lower limb and respiratory weakness in severe cases.
- Autonomic symptoms include: constipation, dry mouth, postural hypotension, urinary retention, and pupillary abnormalities. Fewer than 50% of patients have abnormal pupils.

Infantile botulism

- Most frequently reported form of botulism.
- Infants ingest toxin-containing spores of *C. botulinum*, which germinate and colonize the intestinal track. It occurs in infants less than 1 year of age and has been associated with ingestion of honey.
- Constipation is typically the initial sign followed by symmetric cranial nerve dysfunction (ptosis, impaired eye movement, poor suck and gag reflex). Limb weakness occurs next with generalized hypotonia.
- Autonomic symptoms also occur and manifest as decreased production of tears and saliva and pupillary abnormalities. Respiratory failure that requires mechanical ventilation can occur.
- Implicated as an explanation for some cases of sudden infant death syndrome. However, confirmatory bacteriologic evidence is lacking.

Wound botulism

- *Clostridium* bacteria, spores, or toxins inoculate wounds and gain access to the peripheral nerve terminal via blood.
- Symptoms are similar to those seen in food-borne botulism, except for lack of gastrointestinal symptoms.
- Higher incidence in intravenous drug users.

Inadvertent botulism

Clinical botulism, manifesting as generalized weakness, has been reported in patients who have received intramuscular injections of botulinum toxin for treatment of dystonia or spasticity. This is to be distinguished from inadvertent focal weakness, such as dysphagia after sternocleidomastoid injection, which occurs secondary to spread of toxin from the injected muscles into adjacent muscles.

Patients develop generalized weakness, likely from circulating botulinum toxin.

Pathophysiology

There are eight types of known botulinum toxin, among which types A, B, E, F, and G cause disease in humans. The toxins spread hematogenously to reach the presynaptic nerve terminal and the autonomic ganglia. The neurotoxins gain access into the nerve terminal via receptor-mediated endocytosis. When inside the nerve terminal, the toxins degrade SNARE (soluble N-ethylmaleimide-sensitive-factor attachment protein receptor) proteins, a superfamily of proteins that mediate the fusion of vesicles with the cell membrane. Acetylcholine release is reduced resulting in decreased EPP.

Differential diagnosis

Guillain–Barré syndrome (GBS) is the most important diagnosis to exclude. GBS patients have prominent sensory symptoms at presentation whereas the sensory nerves are spared in botulism. Late responses are normal in botulism, but they are frequently first to become abnormal in GBS.

Other diagnoses to consider include Miller–Fisher syndrome, tick paralysis, MG, LEMS, diphtheritic neuropathy, and periodic paralysis.

Investigations

Electrophysiology

- CMAP amplitudes are low in 85% of patients with botulism. After brief exercise the CMAP amplitude may increase.
- Nerve stimulation at high rates (50 Hz) or 10 seconds of isometric exercise, which is less painful for the patient, results in an incremental CMAP response (post-tetanic facilitation) in about 62% of patients.
- Typically the incremental response is 30–100% in botulism and can persist for several minutes, in contrast to LEMS, where the incremental response is typically over 100% and persists for 30–60 seconds.
- Infrequently there is a decrement to slow rates (3–5 Hz) of stimulation.
- Needle EMG may reveal spontaneous activity in the form of fibrillation potentials and positive sharp waves. Motor units may be myopathic in morphology. Significant jitter with blocking is seen on SFEMG.

Diagnosis

- Diagnosis is confirmed by testing for toxin in serum, stool, wound culture, or contaminated food.
- *C. botulinum* is found in the stool of 60% of patients with food-born botulism, if collected within 2 days of ingesting the toxin. *C. botulinum* is also found in the wound in approximately 60% of patients with wound botulism.

Treatment

The mainstay of treatment for severe botulism is intensive care unit monitoring with close observation of respiratory and cardiac functions. The use of antitoxin is controversial due to its lack of benefit in many cases and high risk of side-effects. It must be given within 24 hours of symptom onset when toxins are still in the circulation. Equine serum antitoxin is used in babies older than 1 year of age and adults. There is a 2% risk of anaphylaxis with equine serum antitoxin. A human-derived antitoxin is used in babies less than 1 year of age. The Center for Disease Control is the only source of antitoxin in the USA.

3,4-DAP and pyridostigmine can also be used for symptomatic control. Wound debridement should be performed in wound botulism.

Prognosis

Mortality rate was 8% in a retrospective review of 706 patients with food-borne botulism. Although recovery is expected, it could take months to years in patients with severe disease, because recovery is dependent on sprouting of new nerve terminals leading to the regeneration of new endplates.

REFERENCES

1 Meriggioli MN, Sanders DB (2009). Autoimmune myasthenia gravis: emerging clinical and biological heterogeneity. *Lancet Neurol* **8**:475–490.

2 Hoch W, McConville J, Helms S, Newsom-Davis J, Melms A, Vincent A (2001). Auto-antibodies to the receptor tyrosine kinase MuSK in patients with myasthenia gravis without acetylcholine receptor antibodies. *Nature Med* 7(3):365–368.

3 Castleman B (1966). The pathology of the thymus gland in myasthenia gravis. *Ann NY Acad Sci* **135**:496–505.

4 Drachman DB (1994). Myasthenia gravis. *N Engl J Med* **330**:1797–1810.

5 Evoli A, Tonali PA, Padua L, *et al.* (2003). Clinical correlates with anti-MuSK antibodies in generalized seronegative myasthenia gravis. *Brain* **126**(Pt 10): 2304–2311.

6 Vernino S (2009). Paraneoplastic disorders affecting the neuromuscular junction or anterior horn cell. *Contin Life Learn Neurol* **15**(1):132–146.

7 Golnik KC, Pena R, Lee AG, Eggenberger ER (1999). An ice test for the diagnosis of myasthenia gravis. *Ophthalmology* **106**(7):1282–1286.

8 Leite MI, Jacob S, Viegas S, *et al.* (2008). IgG1 antibodies to acetylcholine receptors in 'seronegative' myasthenia gravis. *Brain* **131**(7):1940–1952.

9 Zhang B, Tzartos JS, Belimezi M, *et al.* (2012). Autoantibodies to lipoprotein-related protein 4 in patients with double-seronegative myasthenia gravis. *Arch Neurol* **69**(4):445–451.

10 Pascuzzi RM, Coslett HB, Johns TR (1984). Long-term corticosteroid treatment of myasthenia gravis: report of 116 patients. *Ann Neurol* **15**(3):291–298.

11 Schneider-Gold C, Gajdos P, Toyka KV, Hohlfeld RR (2005). Corticosteroids for myasthenia gravis. *Cochrane Dat Syst Rev* **2**:CD002828.

12 Meriggioli, MN, Rowin J, Richman, JG, Leurgans S (2003). Myocophenolate mofetil for myasthenia gravis: a double-blind, placebo-controlled pilot study. *Ann NY Acad Sci* **998**:494–499.

13 The Muscle Study Group (2008). A trial of mycophenolate mofetil with prednisone as initial immunotherapy in myasthenia gravis. *Neurology* **71**(6):394–399.

14 Sanders DB, Hart IK, Mantegazza R, *et al.* (2008). An international, phase III, randomized trial of mycophenolate mofetil in myasthenia gravis. *Neurology* **71**(6):400–406.

15 Zinman L, Ng E, Bril V (2007). IV immunoglobulin in patients with myasthenia gravis. *Neurology* **68**:837–841.

16 Tsujino A, Maertens C, Ohno K, *et al.* (2003). Myasthenic syndrome caused by mutation of the SCN4A sodium channel. *Proc Nat Acad Sci USA* **100**(12): 7377–7382.

17 O'Neill JH, Murray NMF, Newsom-Davis J (1988). The Lambert–Eaton myasthenic syndrome: a review of 50 cases. *Brain* **111**(Pt3):577–596.

18 Sabater L, Titulaer M, Saiz A, Verschuuren J, Güre AO, Graus F (2008). SOX1 antibodies are markers of paraneoplastic Lambert–Eaton myasthenic syndrome. *Neurology* **70**(12):924–928.

19 McEvoy K M, Windebank A J, Daube J R, Low P A (1989). 3,4-Diaminopyridine in the treatment of Lambert–Eaton myasthenic syndrome. *N Engl J Med* **321**(23):1567–1571.

20 Sanders DB, Massey JM, Sanders LL, Edwards LJ (2000). A randomized trial of 3,4-diaminopyridine in Lambert–Eaton myasthenic syndrome. *Neurology* **54**(3):603–607.

21 Oh SJ, Claussen GG, Hatanaka Y, Morgan MB (2009). 3,4-Diaminopyridine is more effective than placebo in a randomized, double-blind, cross-over drug study in LEMS. *Muscle Nerve* **40**:795–800.

Further reading

Myasthenia gravis

Albers JW, Hodach RJ, Kimmel DW, Treacy WL (1980). Penicillamine-associated myasthenia gravis. *Neurology* **30**(11):1246–1249.

Amato AA, Russell JA (2008). Disorders of neuromuscular transmission. In: *Neuromuscular Disorders*. McGraw-Hill, New York. Ch 23, pp. 457–528.

Barohn RJ (2008) Treatment and clinical research in myasthenia gravis: how far have we come? *Ann NY Acad Sci* **1132**:225–232.

Ciafaloni E, Nikhar NK, Massey JM, Sanders DB (2000). Retrospective analysis of the use of cyclosporine in myasthenia gravis. *Neurology* **55**:448–450.

Farrugia ME, Weir AI, Cleary M, Cooper S, Metcalfe R, Mallik A (2009). Concentric and single fiber needle electrodes yield comparable jitter results in myasthenia gravis. *Muscle Nerve* **39**(5):579–585.

Gajdos P, Chevret S, Clair B, Tranchant C, Chastang C; Myasthenia Gravis Clinical Study Group (1997). Clinical trial of plasma exchange and high-dose intravenous immunoglobulin in myasthenia gravis. *Ann Neurol* **41**(6):789–796.

Hoff JM, Daltveit AK, Gilhus NE (2007). Myasthenia gravis in pregnancy and birth: identifying risk factors, optimizing care. *Eur J Neurol* **14**(1):38–43.

Jaretzki, A III (1997). Thymectomy for myasthenia gravis: analysis of the controversies regarding technique and results. *Neurology* **48**:52S–63S.

Keesey JC (2004). Clinical evaluation and management of myasthenia gravis. *Muscle Nerve* **29**(4):484–505.

Kouyoumdjian JA, Stalberg EV (2008). Concentric needle single fiber electromyography: comparative jitter on voluntary activated and stimulated extensor digitorum communis. *Clin Neurophysiol* **119**:1614–1618.

Kupersmith MJ (2009). Ocular myasthenia gravis; treatment successes and failures in patients with long-term follow-up. *J Neurol* **256**(8):1314–1320.

Matell G (1987). Immunosuppressive drugs: azathioprine in the treatment of myasthenia gravis. *Ann NY Acad Sci* **505**:589–594.

Mayer S (1997). Intensive care of the myasthenic patient. *Neurology* **48**(Suppl5):S70–S75.

Meriggioli MN (2009). Myasthenia gravis: immunopathogenesis, diagnosis, and management. *Contin Life Learn Neurol* **15**(1):35–62.

Meriggioli MN, Sanders DB (2005). Advances in the diagnosis of neuromuscular junction disorders. *Am J Phys Med Rehab* **84**(8):627–638.

Nagane Y, Utsugisawa K, Obara D, Kondoh R, Terayama Y (2005). Efficacy of low-dose FK506 in the treatment of myasthenia gravis – a randomized pilot study. *Eur Neurol* **53**(3):146–150.

Pascuzzi RM (2003). The edrophonium test. *Sem Neurol* **23**(1):83–88.

Phillips LH II (2003). The epidemiology of myasthenia gravis. *Ann NY Acad Sci* **998**:407–412.

Phillips LH II, Torner JC (1996). Epidemiologic evidence for a changing natural history of myasthenia gravis. *Neurology* **47**:1233–1238.

Phillips LH II, Torner JC, Anderson MS, Cox GM (1992). The epidemiology of myasthenia gravis in central and western Virginia. *Neurology* **42**(10):1888–1893.

Ponseti JM, Gamez J, Azem J, López-cano M, Vilallonga R, Armengol M (2008). Tacrolimus for myasthenia gravis. A clinical study of 212 patients. *Ann NY Acad Sci* **1132**:254–263.

Rowin J (2009). Approach to the patient with suspected myasthenia gravis or ALS: a clinician's guide. *Contin Life Learn Neurol* **15**(1):13–34.

Rózsa C, Mikor A, Kasa K, Illes Z, Komoly S (2009). Long-term effects of combined immunosuppressive treatment on myasthenic crisis. *Eur J Neurol* **16**(7):796–800.

Thomas CE, Mayer SA, Gungor Y, *et al.* (1997). Myasthenic crisis: clinical features, mortality, complications, and risk factors for prolonged intubation. *Neurology* **48**(5):1253–1260.

Tindall RS, Phillips JT, Rollins JA, Wells L, Hall K (1993). Clinical therapeutic trial of cyclosporine in myasthenia gravis. *Ann NY Acad Sci* **681**:539–551.

Tindall RS, Rollins JA, Phillips JT, Greenlee RG, Wells L, Belendiuk G (1987). Preliminary results of a double-blind, randomized, placebo-controlled trial of cyclosporine in myasthenia gravis. *N Engl J Med* **316**(12):719–724.

Wen JC, Liu TC, Chen YH, Chen SF, Lin HC, Tsai WC (2009). No increased risk of adverse pregnancy outcomes for women with myasthenia gravis: a nationwide population-based study. *Eur J Neurol* **16**(8):889–894.

Wolfe GI, Barohn RJ, Foster BM, *et al.*, Myasthenia Gravis-IVIG Study Group (2002). Randomized, controlled trial of intravenous immunoglobulin in myasthenia gravis. *Muscle Nerve* **26**(4):549–552.

Wolfe GI, Kaminski HJ, Jaretzki A III, Swan A, Newsom-Davis J (2003). Development of a thymectomy trial in nonthymomatous myasthenia gravis patients receiving immunosuppressive therapy. *Ann NY Acad Sci* **998**:473–480.

Congenital myasthenic syndromes

Engel AG, Sine SM (2005). Current understanding of congenital myasthenic syndromes. *Curr Opin Pharmacol* **5**(3):308–321.

Harper MC (2009). Congenital myasthenic syndromes. *Contin Life Learn Neurol* **15**(1):63–82.

Lambert–Eaton myasthenic syndrome

Argov Z, Shapira Y, Averbuch-Heller L, Wirguin I (1995). Lambert–Eaton myasthenic syndrome (LEMS) in association with lymphoproliferative disorders. *Muscle Nerve* **18**(7):715–719.

Bain PG, Motomura M, Newsom-Davis J, *et al.* (1996). Effects of intravenous immunoglobulin on muscle weakness and calcium-channel autoantibodies in the Lambert–Eaton myasthenic syndrome. *Neurology* **47**:678–683.

Elrington GM, Murray NM, Spiro SG, Newsom-Davis J (1991). Neurological paraneoplastic syndromes in patients with small cell lung cancer. A prospective survey of 150 patients. *J Neurol Neurosurg Psychiatry* **54**(9):764–767.

Wirtz PW, Nijnuis MG, Sotodeh M, *et al.*; Dutch Myasthenia Study Group (2003). The epidemiology of myasthenia gravis, Lambert–Eaton myasthenic syndrome, and their associated tumours in the northern part of the province of South Holland. *J Neurol* **250**(6):698–701.

Botulism

Cherington M (2008). Botulism. In: *Neuromuscular Disorders*. McGraw-Hill, New York. Ch 52, pp. 942–952.

Sharma SK, Singh BR (1998). Hemagglutinin binding mediated protection of botulinum neurotoxin from proteolysis. *J Nat Toxins* **7**(3):239–253.

Varma JK, Katsitadze G, Moiscrafishvili M, *et al.* (2004). Signs and symptoms predictive of death in patients with foodborne botulism – Republic of Georgia, 1980–2002. *Clin Infect Dis* **39**(3):357–362.

MUSCLE DISORDERS

Kourosh Rezania, Peter Pytel,
Betty Soliven

INTRODUCTION

Skeletal muscle tissue is unique in several regards. It is comprised of individual, large, multinucleated, tube-shaped syncytial structures called myofibers. These develop through fusion of mononucleated precursors. Myofibers are grouped into fascicles that, in turn, are arranged into individual muscles (**778**, **779**). The basic contractile units of myofibers are sarcomeres, composed of actin and myosin filaments, which give muscles their

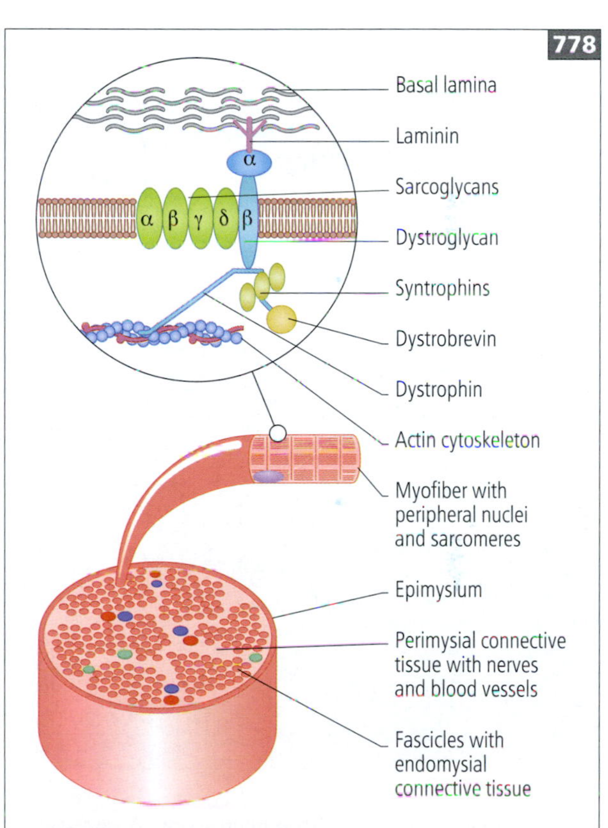

778 Diagram of myofiber architecture. In normal skeletal muscle, individual myofibers are tightly packed into fascicles. Within individual fascicles, only minimal delicate endomysial connective tissue separates myofibers. The perimysial connective tissue between fascicles contains larger blood vessels and nerve branches. Myofiber nuclei normally show a peripheral localization. Most of the cytoplasm is filled with the sarcomeres that make up the contractile apparatus (see 780). The dystrophin–glycoprotein complex includes dystrophin, sarcoglycans, and dystroglycans. It creates a link between the internal actin cytoskeleton and the basement membrane.

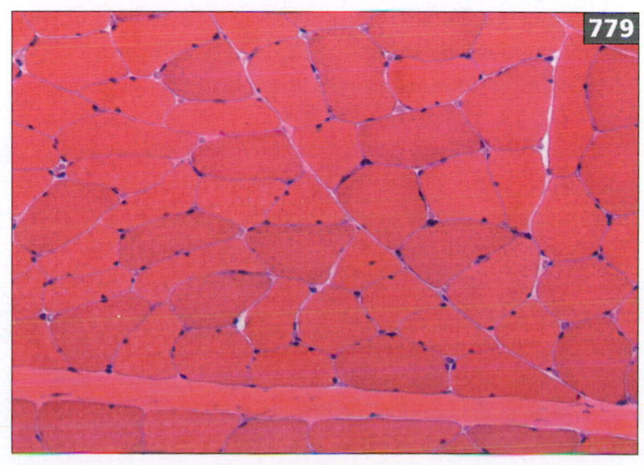

779 Normal muscle hematoxylin and eosin (H&E) histology. On cross-section, myofibers show polygonal profiles of relatively uniform size. Nuclei are peripherally placed. There is very little connective tissue between tightly packed myofibers within a fascicle. The lower half of the image shows a connective tissue septum separating fascicles.

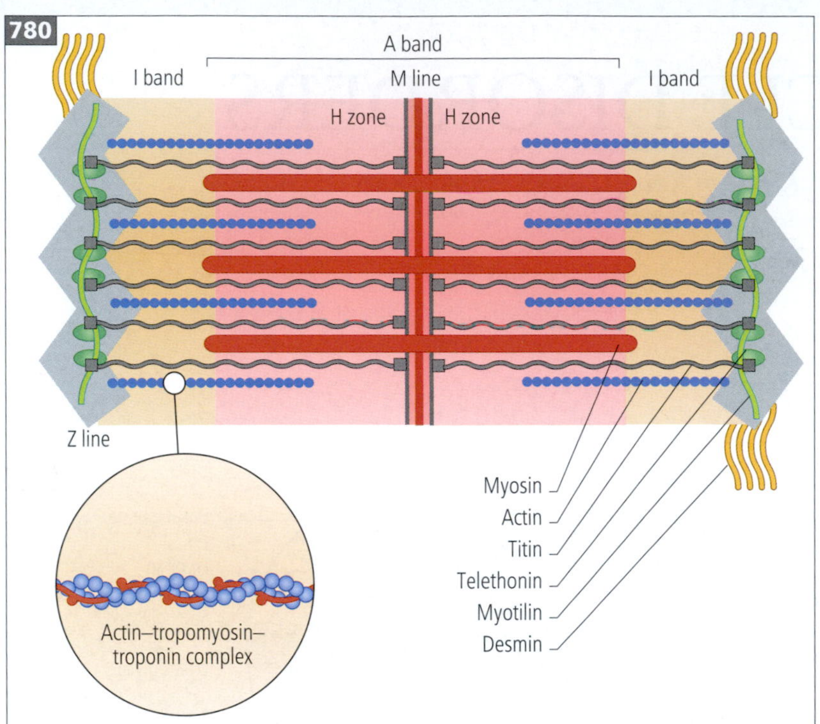

780 Major regions and proteins of a sarcomere. Muscle contraction is the result of interaction of actin and myosin heads. The Z line contains actin, α actinin, and a number of other proteins. Mutations of α actinin are associated with nemaline rod disease. Titin is the largest protein known; it stretches from the Z line to the M line. Mutations in titin are associated with limb-girdle muscular dystrophy (LGMD) 2J. Desmin is present in the peripheral part of the Z line and connects different sarcomeres. Desmin and myotilin mutations are associated with myofibrillar myopathy. Telethonin is another Z-line protein and has been linked to LGMD 2G.

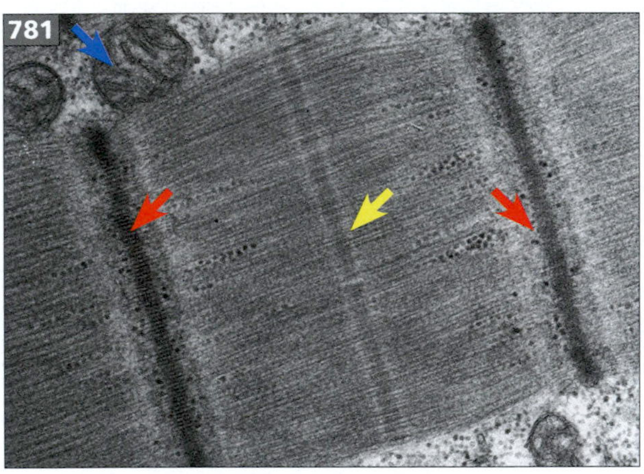

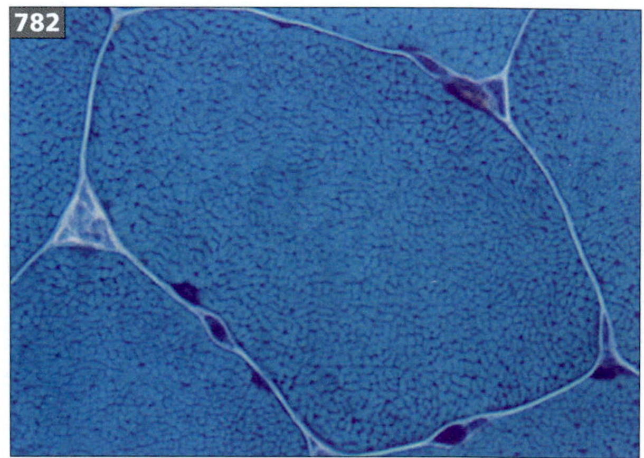

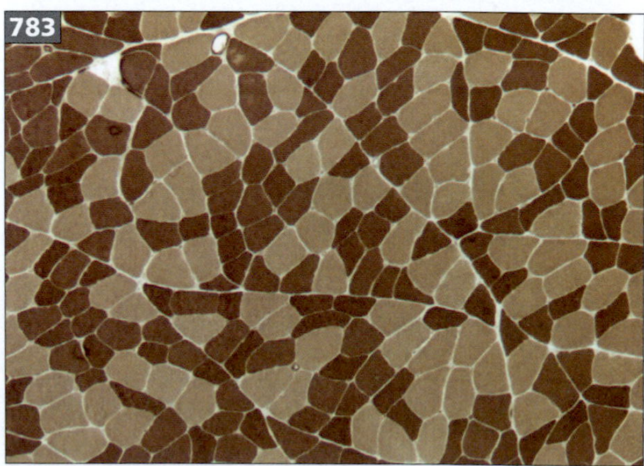

781 Normal histology, electron microscopy. A sarcomere is outlined by two Z bands (red arrows) that anchor the thin actin filaments. These overlap with the thick myosin filaments that extend outwards from the M band (yellow arrow). Mitochondria (blue arrow) are found between sarcomeres.

782 Normal histology, modified Gomori trichrome stain. Mitochondria and organelles stain in a delicate, dark, reticular pattern that outlines individual sarcomeres. Aggregates of mitochondria, lipids, or disease-related inclusions can be visualized with this stain.

783 Normal histology, ATPase. The ATPase reaction distinguishes fiber types. At pH 9.4, type I fibers are light and type II fibers are dark. Normally myofibers show the illustrated checkerboard type admixture.

striated appearance (**780, 781**). Organelles are arranged around the sarcomeres (**781, 782**). Different functional types of myofiber can be distinguished based on the expression of myosin isoforms and metabolic activity. The main distinction is between anaerobic fast-twitch type II fibers and aerobic slow-twitch type I fibers (**783**). There are other proteins besides sarcomeric ones that are essential for muscle function, including ion channels, metabolic enzymes, and the dystrophin–glycoprotein complex.

Tip

▶ *Histologically, type I fibers react strongly to stains for oxidative enzymes such as nicotinamide dinucleotide dehydrogenase (NADH), and weakly to ATPase and phosphorylase. Type II fibers exhibit the reverse reactivity, and can be further classified into type IIA, IIB, and IIC based on their ATPase reactions at different pH values. Type IIC fibers are fetal precursors and rarely seen in adult muscles. Type I fibers are innervated by small motor units, and type II fibers by large motor units.*

MYOPATHY

Definition

Weakness, fatigue and/or myalgia secondary to pathologic processes that primarily affect sarcolemma, contractile element, organelles, connective tissue, vasculature, and/or basement membrane.

Clinical features

- Negative symptoms: weakness, fatigue, contractures.
- Positive symptoms: pain (myalgia), cramps, myotonia (inability to relax), urine discoloration (due to myoglobinuria).
- Muscle atrophy, hypertrophy, or pseudohypertrophy.
- Normal or reduced deep tendon reflexes.
- Grip myotonia or percussion myotonia.

Diagnosis

- Pattern of weakness: usually proximal > distal with or without facial or bulbar involvement, but other patterns of weakness are also observed (*Table 122*).

TABLE 122 **PATTERNS OF WEAKNESS IN MYOPATHIES**

Pattern	Type of myopathy
Limb girdle (proximal > distal)	Inflammatory myopathies *Polymyositis* *Dermatomyositis* Endocrine *Hypothyroidism and hyperthyroidism* *Steroid myopathy* *Hyperparathyroidism* *Acromegaly* Toxic Metabolic *Glycogenoses* *Lipid storage* Muscular dystrophy: *Dystrophinopathies* *Limb-girdle muscular dystrophies* *Myotonic dystrophy type 2*
Distal > proximal	Myotonic dystrophy type 1 Some congenital myopathies Distal muscular dystrophies Hereditary inclusion body myopathy (hIBM)
Proximal arm/ distal leg (scapuloperoneal)	Scapuloperoneal dystrophy Fascioscapulohumeral dystrophy hIBM Emery–Dreifuss muscular dystrophy Lamin A/C deficient myopathy
Distal arm/ proximal leg	Sporadic inclusion body myopathy (sIBM)
Ptosis and/or ophthalmoparesis	Mitochondrial myopathy Myotonic dystrophy type 1 (only ptosis) Oculopharyngeal muscular dystrophy Nemaline rod myopathy (only ptosis)
Head drop (neck extension weakness)	Isolated neck extension myopathy sIBM, hIBM Polymyositis Myotonic dystrophy type 2 Carnitine deficiency Nemaline rod myopathy Hyperparathyroidism
Prominent respiratory muscle weakness	Acid maltase deficiency (adult onset) Critical illness myopathy Myotonic dystrophy Nemaline myopathy Centronuclear myopathy Myopathy with cytoplasmic bodies hIBM

- Muscle enzyme levels – creatine kinase (CK), aldolase:
  - Normal CK and aldolase do not exclude a myopathy.
  - Mild to moderately high CK is not specific for myopathy and can be seen in neurogenic disorders such as motor neuron disease.
  - Certain myopathies are associated with very high CK (*Table 123*).
- Electromyography (EMG) findings:
  - Spontaneous activity (fibrillation potentials and positive waves) is seen in myopathies with vacuolization, segmental myofiber necrosis, and fiber splitting. Examples are polymyositis, dermatomyositis, inclusion body myositis, necrotizing myopathy (toxic, medications), Intensive Care Unit (ICU) myopathy (some cases), muscular dystrophy, and acid maltase deficiency.
  - Absence of spontaneous activity does not exclude a myopathy. Examples are steroid myopathy, other endocrine myopathies, and some cases of ICU myopathy.
  - Activation of the muscle recruits short duration, sometimes polyphasic motor units. Early recruitment of motor units is usually seen.
- Muscle biopsy:
  - Selection of the muscles should be based on the distribution of muscle weakness, EMG findings, and sometimes MRI.
  - It is important to select a mild to moderately affected muscle (not severely affected or completely unaffected muscle).
  - Muscle biopsy should be processed in a specialized laboratory set up to snap freeze tissue.
  - Routine stains include hematoxylin/eosin (H&E), modified Gomori trichrome stain, and ATPase reaction (see **779, 782, 783**).
  - Enzyme histochemical studies, immunocytochemical tests and electron microscopy can be helpful.
  - Frozen muscle tissue can be utilized for biochemical testing and immunoblot (Western).
  - Biopsy allows distinction between neurogenic and myopathic processes, and often provides a specific diagnosis of the type of myopathy (**784**).
- Genetic testing.
- Others (e.g. biochemical studies)

TABLE 123 **DIFFERENTIAL DIAGNOSIS OF MYOPATHY BASED ON CREATINE KINASE (CK) LEVELS**

CK level	Type of myopathy
Very high (>10×)	Necrotizing myopathy Metabolic myopathy (during rhabdomyolysis) Severe trauma Muscular dystrophy *Duchenne's* *Dysferlinopathy* *Calpain deficiency* Polymyositis Hypothyroidism (some patients) ICU myopathy (acute stage)
Mild to moderate	Inclusion body myositis Metabolic myopathy (between episodes of rhabdomyolysis) Hypothyroidism Other (except hyperthyroidism) Idiopathic hyper-CKemia
Normal or low	Steroid myopathy *Iatrogenic* *Cushing's syndrome* Myopathy of disuse Alcoholism Hyperthyroidism End-stage muscle Multi-organ failure ICU myopathy (chronic stage)

ICU: Intensive care unit.

784 **Myopathic changes (H&E). A key feature of many myopathic processes is the presence of morphologic changes in myofibers, with individual fiber degeneration and regeneration. Necrotic amorphous cytoplasm (a) becomes progressively infiltrated and organized by inflammatory cells (b, c). The cytoplasm of regenerative myofibers (d) looks blue because of high ribonucleic acid content. Their nuclei are large, reflective of activation.**

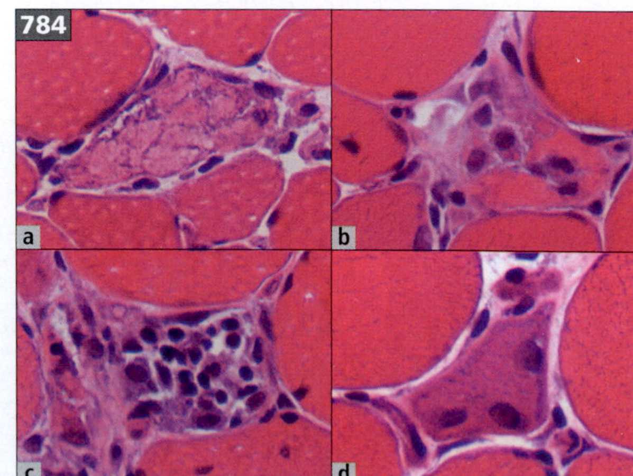

INFLAMMATORY MYOPATHY

Definition

Polymyositis, dermatomyositis, and inclusion body myositis (IBM) are the three major categories of idiopathic inflammatory myopathy[1]. This classification has its caveats. In contrast to polymyositis and dermatomyositis, IBM usually does not respond or is minimally responsive to immunosuppressive treatments. Although inflammation plays a role in the pathogenesis of IBM, it could be secondary to a primarily degenerative process.

IDIOPATHIC POLYMYOSITIS

Definition and epidemiology

An acquired inflammatory myopathy characterized by progressive muscle weakness and the presence of inflammatory infiltrates and degenerating or regenerating fibers in the muscle.

- Prevalence: about 1 in 100,000. However, this could be an overestimation, as many cases of polymyositis with older criteria turned out to have another type of myopathy (e.g. IBM and muscular dystrophy) when newer techniques such as immunohistochemistry were used.
- Age at onset: >18 years of age.
- Gender: F≥M.

Clinical features

- Slow onset (weeks to months).
- Usually symmetric weakness of proximal limb muscles, including the neck flexors; pelvic girdle muscles are involved more severely than the shoulder girdle.
- Occasionally pain and muscle tenderness.
- Weight loss, dysphagia, and hoarseness are common.
- No skin rash.
- Underlying cancer is less frequently associated with polymyositis (in contrast to dermatomyositis).

Differential diagnosis

- Dermatomyositis.
- IBM.
- Myositis associated with systemic autoimmune or connective tissue diseases.
- Muscular dystrophies:
  - Endomysial inflammatory infiltrate is often seen in fascioscapulohumoral dystrophy, dysferlinopathy, and some congenital myopathies.
  - Myotonic dystrophy type 2 typically presents with proximal > distal weakness.
- Viral myositis: human immunodeficiency virus (HIV), human T-cell lymphotropic virus type 1, influenza A, parainfluenza, adenovirus 2.
- Acute rhabdomyolysis: influenza A and B, Echo 9, adenovirus 21, herpes simplex, Epstein–Barr virus, Coxsackie B5 (also B1, 3, and 4).
- Bacterial myositis: acute suppurative myositis (*Staphylococcus aureus*, *Streptococcus* spp., *Yersinia* spp., anaerobic organisms).
- Fungal myositis.
- Parasitic myositis (e.g. toxoplasmosis, cysticercosis, trichinosis).
- Toxic myopathy:
  - Mitochondrial (zidovudine, germanium).
  - Lysosomal (colchicine, chloroquine, hydroxychloroquine).
  - Myofibrillar (emetine).
  - Myosin deficiency (steroids, vecuronium, atracuronium).
  - Rhabdomyolysis (statins, fibrates, cyclosporine, alcohol, cocaine, snake venoms).
  - Eosinophilia-myalgia syndrome (L-tryptophan).
  - Vacuolar (drugs that cause hypokalemia).
  - Inflammatory (D-penicillamine, α-interferon, statins).
  - Others (ε-amino caproic acid, amiodarone, valproic acid).
- Polymyalgia rheumatica:
  - Pain with limitation of movement.
  - CK is normal and muscle biopsy shows only minimal abnormalities, but erythrocyte sedimentation rate (ESR) is elevated.
- Endocrine myopathy.
- Other neuromuscular diseases (e.g. myasthenia gravis [MG]).

Investigations

- Blood tests:
  - Serum CK level: usually elevated (5–50 times normal). CK level often does not correlate with the severity of weakness; however, along with the clinical assessment of weakness, CK level is used in monitoring the response to therapy.
  - ESR: usually, though not invariably, elevated.
  - Anti Jo-1 antibody: found in about 30% of cases, is associated with interstitial lung disease and greater risk of cardiomyopathy. Other more myositis specific serological markers include antibodies to Mi-2, signal recognition particle, p155, and MJ[2].

- ECG: occasionally shows heart block.
- EMG (myopathic pattern) (See Introduction).
- Muscle MRI is often useful to differentiate active myositis from steroid myopathy, and to help choose an appropriate muscle for biopsy[1].
- Muscle biopsy: a muscle biopsy can help to confirm the diagnosis and exclude some other disease processes.

Diagnosis

Based on clinical features, supported by laboratory investigations (CK, EMG, and biopsy).

Pathology

Acute

- Predominantly endomysial inflammatory cell infiltrates, mainly of cytotoxic T cell ($CD8^+$) type, surrounding or partially invading individual muscle fibers (**785**).
- B cells are infrequent. Dendritic cells are frequently present, sometimes in contact with T cells.
- Myopathic changes in muscle morphology with degenerating/necrotic myofibers, regenerating myofibers, as well as variation in myofiber size, and internalized nuclei (**785**).

Chronic

- Endomysial and perifascicular fibrosis.
- Inflammatory cell exudates.
- Focally distributed architectural changes in individual fibers.

Treatment

See page 881 for treatment of polymyositis and dermatomyositis.

Prognosis

The response is less favorable than in dermatomyositis, particularly in those with a long duration of illness at presentation. Immunosuppressive therapy usually prevents further progression, but significant improvement may not occur. Antibody to signal recognition peptide, found in 5% of cases, is associated with a fulminant course and resistance to treatment.

DERMATOMYOSITIS

Definition and epidemiology

An inflammatory myopathy with characteristic cutaneous manifestations.

- Prevalence: 1 in 100,000.
- Age at onset: any age, affects children and adults. Comprises 95% of childhood myositis.
- Gender: F>M (2:1).

Etiology

- Unknown in most cases.
- Caused or exacerbated by drugs in a few patients:
  - Hydroxyurea (predominantly skin manifestations).
  - Quinidine.
  - Nonsteroidal anti-inflammatory drugs.
  - Penicillamine.
  - 3-Hydroxy-3-methylglutaryl coenzyme A-reductase inhibitors ('statins').

Pathophysiology

- A humorally mediated microangiopathy (e.g. antibodies against capillary endothelial cells with complement activation).
- Overexpression of type 1 interferons and their related proteins may play an important role in the pathogenesis of dermatomyositis[3,4].

Clinical features

Muscle disease

- Initial symptoms include subacute onset of myalgias, fatigue, and symmetric proximal weakness, manifested as difficulty climbing stairs and raising the arms for actions such as shaving or brushing hair.
- Pain and tenderness on palpation of the muscles is variable.
- The course is slowly progressive during a period of weeks to months.
- Difficulty swallowing (dysphagia) or symptoms of aspiration may reflect involvement of striated muscle in the pharynx or upper esophagus.
- Dysphonia.

Cutaneous manifestations

- Heliotrope rash (**786**): a violaceous to dusky erythematous rash, with or without edema, in a symmetric distribution involving the periorbital skin.
- Gottron's papules: slightly raised violaceous papules and plaques, with or without a slight scale and rarely a thick psoriasiform scale, over bony prominences, particularly the metacarpophalangeal joints, proximal interphalangeal joints, and distal interphalangeal joints. Papules may also be found overlying the elbows, knees, and feet.

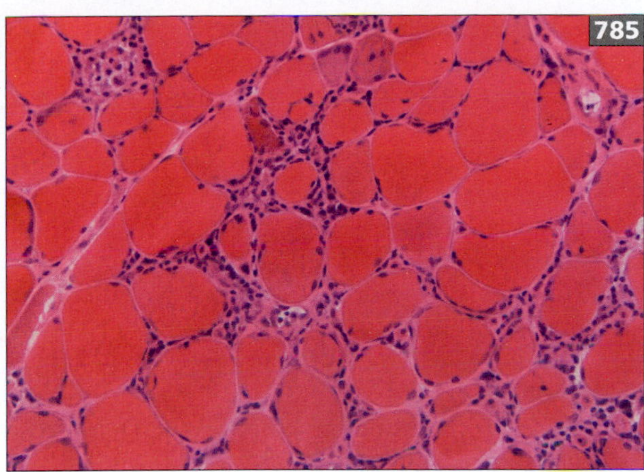

785 Polymyositis (H&E). Myopathic changes with myofiber necrosis/regeneration and variation in myofiber size are associated with focal mononuclear cell infiltrates. These tend to be most prominent in the endomysium.

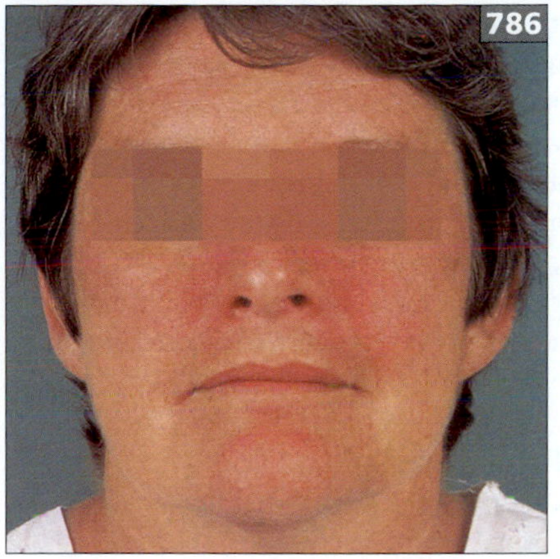

786 Heliotrope rash. Violaceous discoloration of the eyelids, cheeks, and nose in a patient with dermatomyositis.

- An erythematous to violaceous psoriasiform dermatitis involving the scalp.
- Malar erythema.
- Poikiloderma (which is the combination of atrophy, dyspigmentation, and telangiectasia) on sun exposed skin such as the extensor surfaces of the arms, the 'V' of the neck, and the upper back (shawl sign).
- Nailfold changes: periungual telangiectases and/or hypertrophy of the cuticle, and small hemorrhagic infarcts in the hypertrophic area.

Systemic features

- Raynaud's phenomenon.
- Generalized arthralgias, sometimes arthritis.
- Esophageal disease, manifested by dysphagia, occurs in about 15–50% of patients. There are two main forms:
  - Proximal dysphagia is caused by involvement of striated muscle of the pharynx or proximal esophagus, correlates with severity of the muscle disease, and responds to steroid treatment.
  - Distal dysphagia is due to involvement of non-striated muscle and is more common in patients who have an overlap with scleroderma or another collagen–vascular disorder.
- Pulmonary disease: occurs in about 15–30% of patients, particularly those with esophageal disease, and is usually due to an interstitial pneumonitis. Less common causes include the muscle disease itself (causing hypoventilation or aspiration), and treatments for the muscle disease (causing opportunistic infections or drug-induced hypersensitivity pneumonitis). Associated with a poor prognosis.
- Cardiac disease: present in up to 50% of patients but uncommonly symptomatic. Disorders include conduction defects and primary end-rhythm disturbances, and even less commonly congestive heart failure, pericarditis, and valvular disease. Associated with a poor prognosis.
- Calcinosis of the skin (firm, yellow or flesh-colored nodules, usually over bony prominences, and occasionally extruding through the surface of the skin) or muscle (generally asymptomatic) is unusual in adults, but may occur in up to 40% of children and adolescents with dermatomyositis.

Malignancy

- About 20–25% have associated malignancy, before the onset of myositis, concurrently with myositis, or after the onset of dermatomyositis.
- Malignancy is more common in older patients (>50 years) but may even occur in children.
- The site of malignancy can be predicted by the patient's age (e.g. testicular cancer in young men, colon and prostate cancer in elderly men).
- Gynecological malignancy, particularly ovarian carcinoma, is common.
- Nasopharyngeal carcinoma is common among Asians with dermatomyositis.

Childhood dermatomyositis

Childhood dermatomyositis is more common than childhood and adolescent polymyositis. Onset is usually subacute (over weeks), although it can be insidious (over months) or acute (over days and mistaken for a viral-type illness or dermatitis). Proximal weakness, neck flexion weakness occur, dysphagia in 30%, and sometimes chewing problems, or dysarthria. It is commonly characterized as a vasculitis and has greater potential for calcinosis than adult disease.

Differential diagnosis

- Muscle weakness (see the differential diagnosis of polymyositis, p. 877).
- Heliotrope rash and photosensitive poikilodermatous eruption:
  - Systemic lupus erythematosus (SLE): a heliotrope rash is rarely seen.
  - Scleroderma: a heliotrope rash is rarely seen.
- Gottron's papules:
  - SLE.
  - Psoriasis: distinct histopathology.
  - Lichen planus: distinct histopathology.
- Scalp erythematous to violaceous psoriasiform dermatitis:
  - Psoriasis.
  - Seborrheic dermatitis.
- Facial erythema:
  - SLE.
  - Rosacea.
  - Seborrheic dermatitis.
  - Atopic dermatitis.

Investigations

- Blood tests:
  - ESR is usually elevated.
  - Elevated serum muscle enzymes: CK, aldolase, lactate dehydrogenase, alanine aminotransferase (ALT).
  - CK levels may be raised up to 20 times normal, particularly in acute cases.
  - High antinuclear antibody titers.
  - Antibodies to Jo-1 are predictive of pulmonary involvement but are rare.
  - Antibodies to Ro (SS-A) are found in rare cases.
- EMG (myopathic pattern) (see Introduction, p. 873).
- Muscle MRI often shows signal abnormalities secondary to inflammation and edema. It may be useful in differentiating active myositis from steroid myopathy, and in helping to choose an appropriate muscle for biopsy[1].
- Muscle biopsy: may not be needed if skin biopsy confirms the diagnosis.
- Skin biopsy.
- Work-up for malignancy:
  - Depending on the patient's age and gender, appropriate work-up is necessary to assess for malignant disease.
  - Repeat each year for the first 3 years after diagnosis or whenever new symptoms arise.

Diagnosis

Based on clinical features, supported by laboratory investigations.

Pathology

- Infiltration of muscle by macrophages and T helper ($CD4^+$) and B lymphocytes.
- The inflammatory infiltrates are predominantly perivascular, around the interfascicular septa, rather than endomysial (in contrast to polymyositis).
- No invasion of inflammatory cells into non-necrotic myofibers.
- Microangiopathy: intramuscular blood vessels show endothelial hyperplasia with tubuloreticular inclusions, fibrin thrombi (particularly in children), and obliteration of capillaries.
- Capillary numbers are reduced; there are immunoglobulin deposits on vessel walls, and blood vessel endothelial cells. The capillary loss and consequent ischemia causes microinfarcts and may be responsible for the sometimes striking perifascicular atrophy seen.
- Perifascicular atrophy (787) is found in about 90% of children and at least 50% of adults with dermatomyositis and is diagnostic of dermatomyositis, even in the absence of inflammation.

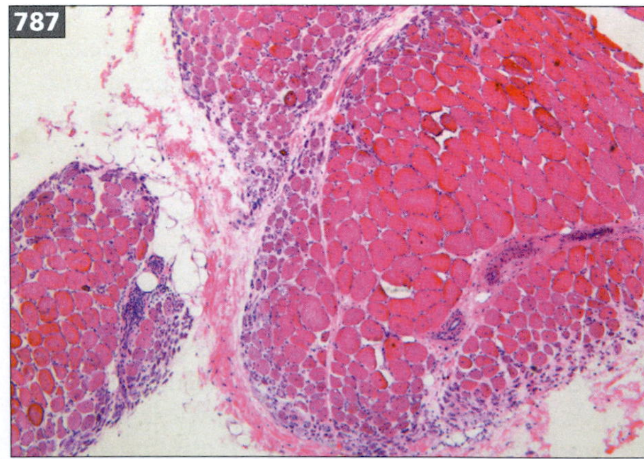

787 Dermatomyositis (H&E). Atrophic and myopathic changes show preferential involvement of periseptal/perifascicular myofibers.

Treatment[1,5]

General

- Encouragement of mobility (particularly in the elderly).
- Physiotherapy to prevent contractures is essential.
- Range-of-motion exercise program if patients have advanced weakness.
- Raise the head of the bed and avoid meals before bedtime in patients with dysphagia.
- A high protein diet is advisable.
- Attention to swallowing, adequacy of ventilation, and precautions against deep venous thrombosis must be considered.

Immunomodulatory treatment of myositis

Corticosteroids

- First-line of treatment in polymyositis and dermatomyositis. Patients with dermatomyositis generally respond better than those with polymyositis to steroids.
- In more severe cases, an initial course of IV methylprednisolone (1 g/day for 3 days) can be considered.
- In severe cases, oral prednisone 1.5 mg/kg/day up to 100 mg/day has been used.
- Tapering to alternate day regimen (up to 100 mg every other day) should be attempted over 1–3 months depending on the severity of the disease.
- In milder cases, oral prednisolone 0.5–1 mg/kg/day for at least 1 month after myositis has become clinically and enzymatically inactive. The dose is then gradually reduced over a period lasting 1.5–2 times the period of active intense treatment, depending on clinical progress and, to some extent, serum CK levels.
- Noticeable improvement is usually seen in 3–6 months. Diagnosis should be reassessed if there is no response to high-dose steroids (looking for IBM or muscular dystrophy for example).
- Complete response to steroids is seen in 30–60% of dermatomyositis and only 10–30% of polymyositis. A higher percentage of patients respond partially.

Second-line agents

- Consider starting a second-line agent with the steroids in cases with severe disease, underlying diabetes, osteoporosis, or post-menopausal state.
- Intravenous immunoglobulin (IVIG)[6]: starting dose is 2 g/kg divided over 4–5 days, every month for the first 2–3 months. This can be tapered to 0.5–1 g/kg every month depending on the individual response. IVIG is generally reserved for more severe and refractory cases and patients with significant adverse effects to steroids and immunosuppressants.
- Methotrexate: can be given as a single weekly oral dose, but not recommended in patients with underlying interstitial lung disease or those positive for anti-Jo antibodies.
- Azathioprine 2.5 mg/kg/day. Bone marrow suppression and hepatotoxicity are the most important side-effects.
- Mycophenolate: starting dose is 0.5 g twice a day, which is gradually increased (up to 3 g/day). The most common side-effect is diarrhea; patients should be monitored for leukopenia.

Third-line agents

- Cyclosporine: at a dose of 3–5 mg/kg/day in two divided doses, trough levels of 100–150 μg/ml are usually achieved. Common side-effects include nephrotoxicity, hypertension, headache, hirsutism, neurotoxicity, tremors, and hepatotoxicity.
- Tacrolimus: 3–5 mg/day in two divided doses to achieve a plasma trough level of 6–8 ng/ml. Side-effects are similar to cyclosporine but less frequent.
- Cyclophosphamide should be considered in patients refractory to immunosuppressants and IVIG. It can be given in monthly intravenous pulses (0.5–1 g/m^2 for 6–12 months) or oral (starting dose: 1 mg/kg/day). Side-effects include bone marrow suppression, infection, infertility, alopecia, and hemorrhagic cystitis.
- Tumor necrosis factor inhibitors such as etanercept and infliximab have been used with mixed results[2,5].
- Rituximab has shown efficacy in some refractory cases[1,2].
- Plasma exchange and leukopheresis: although uncontrolled studies have suggested improvement with plasma exchange and leukopheresis, a double blind study showed no efficacy[7].

Other 'last resort' forms of treatment

- Plasmapheresis.
- X-ray irradiation.
- Thoracic outlet drainage.
- Thymectomy.
- Stem cell transplant.

Treatment of skin disease

- Patients should avoid sunlight or use a broad-spectrum sunscreen with a high sun protective factor, if they are photosensitive.
- Hydroxychloroquine hydrochloric acid 200–400 mg/day is effective in about 80% of patients when used as a steroid-sparing agent.
- Chloroquine phosphate 250–500 mg/day can be used if patients are not responsive to hydroxychloroquine.
- Periodic ophthalmologic examinations and blood counts are required for patients on continuous anti-malarial therapy.
- Methotrexate 15–35 mg/week can also be used.

Prognosis

If treated early, most patients will respond well, with many showing full recovery of muscle function. Prognosis is adversely affected by:

- Increasing age.
- Severity of myositis.
- Dysphagia or dysphonia.
- Cardiopulmonary involvement.
- Malignant disease.
- Poor response to corticosteroid therapy

SPORADIC INCLUSION BODY MYOSITIS

Definition and epidemiology

Sporadic inclusion body myositis (SIBM) is a slowly progressive, often asymmetric myopathy. Degenerative and inflammatory factors may play a role in its pathogenesis.

- Prevalence: 5–10 per million.
- The most common cause of acquired myositis in patients over 50 years of age.
- Age at onset: after 50 years of age.
- Gender: M>F (3:1).
- Race: more common in whites than blacks.

Etiology and pathophysiology

- Although inflammatory and degenerative processes both contribute to the disease progression, it is uncertain which process comes first.
- Cytotoxic ($CD8^+$) T cells infiltrate myofibers which express MHC class I antigens.
- Deposition of amyloid precursor protein and amyloid β could play a role in vacuolar degeneration and myofiber atrophy.
- Many other proteins are also overexpressed, including prion protein, phosphorylated tau, ubiquitin, apolipoprotein E, and α synuclein.
- Multiple mitochondrial deoxyribonucleic acid (DNA) deletions are present in 75% of patients.

Clinical features

- Gradual onset with slow progression.
- Painless weakness starting in the proximal thigh and distal hand muscles, including long finger flexors, wrist flexors and quadriceps femoris, which may be asymmetric.
- Muscle wasting can be marked.
- Dysphagia in up to 30% of cases.
- Mild facial weakness, but extraocular muscles are spared.
- Early loss of deep tendon reflexes.

Tip

► *Most myopathies manifest as symmetric proximal weakness with some exceptions, such as SIBM where there is a often combination of proximal and distal weakness. SIBM should be suspected when there is prominent involvement of quadriceps, wrist flexors, and finger flexors.*

Differential diagnosis

- Polymyositis.
- Diabetic amyotrophy.
- Motor neuron disease.
- Myofibrillar myopathy.
- Nemaline rod myopathy.
- Hereditary IBM: the hereditary forms have rimmed vacuoles and filamentous inclusions, but usually lack inflammatory response and myofiber MHC class I expression:
  - IBM–Paget disease- frontotemporal dementia (mutations in valosin containing protein)[8]. Onset of weakness at 25–40 years.
    - Paget's disease is present in more than half the affected patients.
    - Dementia is present in more than one-third of patients usually manifesting as frontal lobe dysfunction in mid-50s.
  - IBM2: autosomal recessive, due to mutations in *GNE* (encoding UDP-acetylglucosamine 2-epimerase).
    - Predominantly in Middle Eastern Jewish population.
    - Onset in late teens or early adult life with distal weakness and foot-drop.
    - Weakness extends to the hands and thighs, but usually spares the quadriceps, even in advanced stages.
- Other forms of vacuolar myopathy, such as Welander distal myopathy.

Investigations

- Blood tests:
  - Serum CK level: often normal or mildly raised.
  - ESR: normal in 80% of cases.
- EMG:
  - Fibrillations and positive waves are usually seen.
  - Although myopathic units and recruitment are seen, the presence of large, neurogenic units can be misleading and suggests a primarily neurogenic disease such as neuropathy or motor neuron disease.
  - 30% of patients have EMG signs of axonal neuropathy.
- Muscle MRI: may reveal changes in the T2-weighted image in a characteristic pattern early in the disease: involvement of quadriceps, medial gastrocnemius, and flexor forearm muscles.
- Muscle biopsy: rimmed vacuoles and congophilic inclusions are probably late changes and may be not seen in early stages of the disease. If the clinical phenotype is present, diagnosis of IBM is not excluded in the absence of these findings.

Diagnosis

Highly likely if a clinical phenotype of asymmetric muscle weakness with prominent wrist flexor, finger flexor, and knee extensor muscle involvement is present. The diagnosis should be confirmed with a muscle biopsy.

Pathology

- Inflammatory infiltrates may vary in extent (788). They are most often endomysial and predominantly CD8+ T cells. They often surround or invade individual MHC class I-positive non-necrotic muscle fibers.
- Myopathic changes with some individual fiber degeneration/regeneration.
- Rimmed vacuoles are the hallmark of this disease (789). Ultrastructurally these correspond to myelinoid membranous debris and are often associated with aggregates of 15–21 nm filaments. The inclusions are congophilic, and contain proteins associated with neurodegenerative diseases including tau and ubiquitin.
- Often chronic changes in the form of endomysial fibrosis and fatty replacement (788).
- Sometimes clusters of atrophic angulated fibers may mimic neuropathic disease.
- Cytochrome oxidase (COX) negative and ragged red fibers are sometimes seen.

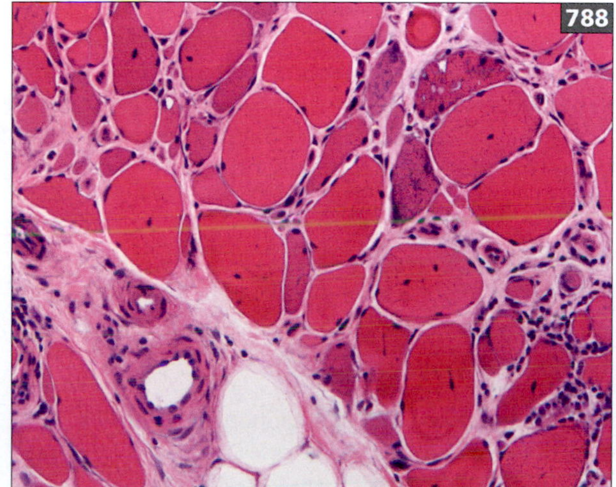

788 Inclusion body myositis (H&E). Myopathic changes in the form of myofiber degeneration/regeneration and increased variation in myofiber size are often associated with some chronic changes in the form of endomysial fibrosis and fatty replacement. Mononuclear inflammatory infiltrates tend to be endomysial.

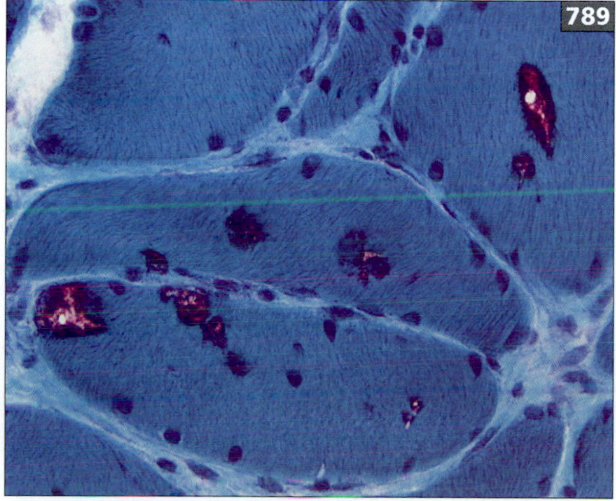

789 Inclusion body myositis (modified Gomori trichrome stain). Vacuoles with dense, somewhat red rimming are characteristic of inclusion body myositis, but can also be found in some familial 'inclusion body myopathies' that typically lack inflammatory changes.

Treatment

- Most patients are resistant to immunomodulatory treatment.
- In some younger patients, the condition may stabilize with a 3–6 month trial of prednisolone combined with methotrexate (or azathioprine).
- IVIG is used sometimes in patients with dysphagia.
- Immunosuppression directed against T cells (anti-thymocyte globulin and alemtuzumab) has shown promise in some preliminary studies, but larger studies have to be conducted.
- β-Agonist clenbuterol, which has anabolic effects, is used in some centers.
- A physiotherapy/strength training program and aerobic conditioning are advised.
- Besides IVIG treatment, patients with dysphagia may benefit from esophageal dilation or cricopharyngeal myotomy.

Prognosis

Gradual deterioration is usual, with increasing weakness of the neck, trunk, and distal arm muscles, and extensive weakness and wasting in the legs. The prognosis partly depends on the age of onset. The average time to need a walker is about 10 years in patients with age of onset of less than 60 years, and 5.7 years in those with onset of the disease later than 60. After 15–20 years into the disease, most of the patients are wheelchair bound.

CRITICAL ILLNESS MYOPATHY

Definition and epidemiology[9]

- Critical illness myopathy (CIM) is a major cause of severe and diffuse muscle weakness in the critically ill patients in the ICU.
- A concomitant critical illness polyneuropathy (CIP) is usually also present.
- 50% of ICU patients with a stay of more than 3 days have electrophysiologic evidence of CIM +/− CIP.
- 50–70% of patients with an ICU stay of more than 1 week develop clinical CIM +/− CIP; this figure may reach 100% in patients with long ICU stays with sepsis and end-organ damage.

Etiology and pathophysiology

Use of high doses of corticosteroids and neuromuscular blocking drugs (both typically used in severe asthma and chronic obstructive pulmonary disease) predispose to CIM, but CIM can occur in the absence of these factors. Other predisposing factors include:

- Long ICU stay.
- Sepsis.
- Multi-organ dysfunction.
- Vasopressor support.
- Central nervous system (CNS) disease (encephalopathy).

The pathophysiology is not completely elucidated. Increased levels of pro-inflammatory cytokines such as tumor necrosis factor α, interleukins-1 and -6, and interferon γ cause increased activity of proteolytic enzymes including calpain and lysosomal enzymes.

There is increased catabolism and breakdown of muscle proteins, with myosin heavy chains predominantly targeted for unknown reasons. Membrane depolarization and changes in the voltage-dependence of fast inactivation of Na^+ channels are observed in a rat model of CIM.

Clinical features

- Inability to wean from the ventilator in the absence of a pulmonary or cardiac explanation.
- Generalized muscle weakness and flaccidity.
- Reflexes are lost early.
- Facial weakness and ophthalmoparesis are rare.
- Muscle atrophy in chronic cases.

Differential diagnosis

- CIP (often coexists with CIM).
- Acquired inflammatory polyneuropathy.
- Prolonged neuromuscular block.

Investigations

- CK: elevated in at least 50%. It may peak in 2–5 days and then gradually normalize.
- Nerve conduction studies (NCS): sensory responses are normal (unless CIP is also present); motor response amplitudes can be normal or decreased; motor conduction velocity is normal (could be slow if a concomitant CIP is present).
- EMG: abnormal spontaneous activity (positive waves and fibrillations) is seen in some cases. Short duration and sometimes polyphasic motor units with early recruitment are sometimes noted.
- Direct muscle stimulation has been used to differentiate CIM from CIP.
- Muscle biopsy: the gold standard for the diagnosis, but is often not needed.

Pathology[9]

Three subtypes exist:

- Myosin deficient myopathy (**790, 791**).
- Cachectic myopathy (atrophic fibers, internalized nuclei, increased endomysial collagen tissue and fat cells).
- Necrotizing myopathy (myofiber vacuolization and phagocytosis).

Prevention and treatment

- Minimize the use of high doses of steroids and neuromuscular blocking agents.
- Some investigators suggest that sedation should be intermittent, and not continuous or prolonged to decrease the duration of immobility.
- Aggressive rehabilitation treatment may hasten recovery.
- Aggressive insulin treatment, keeping the blood sugar at 80–110 mg/dl (800–1100 mg/l), has been suggested to reduce the incidence of CIM and CIP.

Prognosis

- CIM +/− CIP increase the length of ICU and hospital stay, and the overall mortality rate.
- Spontaneous recovery can occur within weeks in mild cases and within months in moderate cases. Severe cases may result in chronic disability and lack of ambulation.
- Undetectable CMAP amplitude heralds a less favorable prognosis. CIM probably has a better prognosis than CIP.

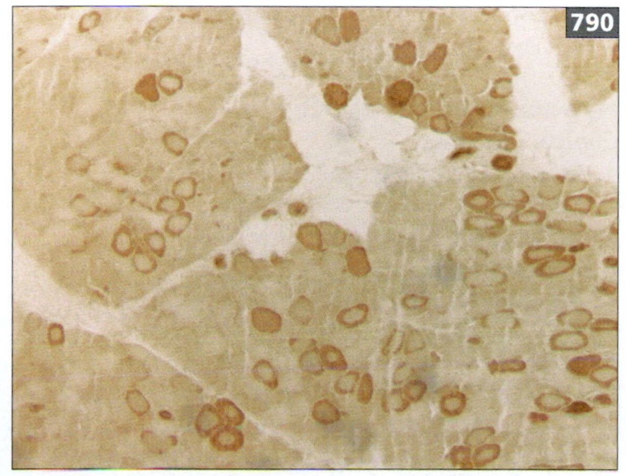

790 Critical illness myopathy/myosin deficient myopathy (ATPase reaction, pH 9.4). There is relatively selective loss of the myosin heavy chain. The ATPase activity of myosin is responsible for the color reaction in this stain. Critical illness/ICU myopathy is often associated with central loss of reactivity, resulting in a central, cleared, washed-out appearance, affecting type II fibers in particular.

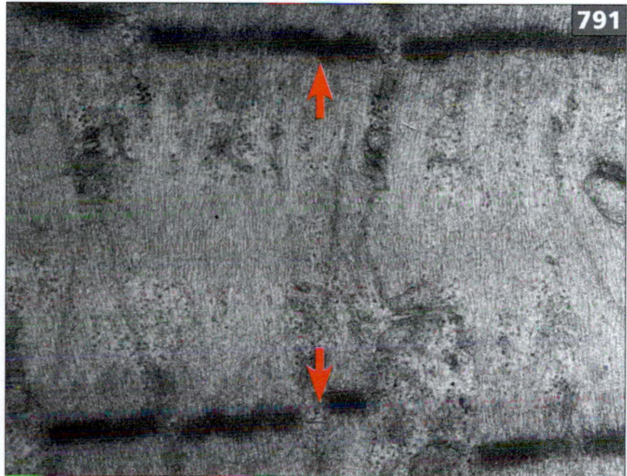

791 Critical illness myopathy/myosin deficient myopathy (electron microscopy). Ultrastructurally, the basic framework of sarcomeres may appear relatively preserved, but thick myosin filaments are lacking (see 781). No M line is seen between the Z bands (arrows).

ENDOCRINE AND METABOLIC MYOPATHIES

Definition

Metabolic and endocrine myopathies are a large, heterogeneous group of inherited and acquired disorders of muscle due to a disturbance of metabolism. Hormones such as thyroid tri-iodothyronine (T3) and thyroxine (T4) and steroids regulate many aspects of muscle biology. For example, thyroid hormone has a regulatory role on the transcription of numerous muscle genes encoding both myofibrillar and calcium-regulatory proteins.

Carbohydrates, lipids, and amino acids are the main fuels used by the muscle during rest and exercise. The relative contribution of each depends on the length and the intensity of exercise, sex, diet, and training status. Lipids (free fatty acids, intracellular lipid stores, and lipoprotein-derived triglycerol) contribute maximally during low and moderate intensity exercise, i.e. up to 60% maximal O_2 consumption. In higher levels of endurance exercise, carbohydrates (blood glucose and intracellular glycogen deposits) become the more important source. Endurance exercise training results in a switch from carbohydrate to fat consumption during a certain level of exercise.

ENDOCRINE MYOPATHIES

Myopathy can be part of the clinical manifestations, and sometimes the presenting symptom of a variety of endocrine diseases, including different diseases affecting the thyroid, adrenal, pituitary, and parathyroid glands.

In most cases, the weakness reverses when the metabolic defect is corrected, but improvement may take weeks to months. Typically, EMG shows a myopathic pattern, but only nonspecific findings of type II fiber atrophy are found on muscle biopsy.

Thyrotoxic myopathy

Clinical features

- Proximal muscle weakness and some wasting occurs.
- Occasionally only the bulbar and respiratory muscles are affected.
- Fatigue.
- Heat intolerance.
- Normal or augmented reflexes.
- Fasciculations, cramps.
- Rarely associated with hypokalemic periodic paralysis and MG.

Diagnosis

- Serum CK: normal or slightly elevated.
- EMG: myopathic units and recruitment, usually without positive waves, fibrillations, or fasciculations.
- Abnormal thyroid function tests.

Treatment

- Correct the hyperthyroidism.
- Symptomatic therapy with beta-blockers.
- Glucocorticoids can be used in thyroid storm to block the peripheral conversion of T4 to T3.

Dysthyroid eye disease (exophthalmic ophthalmoplegia)

Clinical features

- Can be quite asymmetric.
- Difficulty of upgaze initially (inferior rectus infiltrated early).
- Diplopia, ptosis often.
- Lid retraction.
- Exophthalmos.
- Conjunctival and lid edema.
- Exposure keratopathy.
- Often mild pain (grittiness or fullness).
- Eventually raised intraocular pressure and blindness may occur.

Diagnosis

- The patient is usually, but not necessarily, thyrotoxic.
- Thyroid antibodies: often positive.
- Computed tomography (CT) scan of the orbits: enlarged extraocular muscles.

Treatment

- Restore the euthyroid state.
- Tarsorrhaphy to protect the cornea.
- Surgical correction of diplopia if necessary.
- Severe cases: high doses of corticosteroids, cyclosporine, and even orbital decompression have been used to save sight.

Hypothyroid myopathy

Clinical features

- More common in women.
- Myalgia and muscle cramps.
- Muscle hypertrophy.
- Muscle weakness (rare).
- Myoedema (ridging of muscle on percussion).
- Slow-recovery reflexes.

Diagnosis

- Serum CK: may be grossly elevated.
- Thyroid function tests: low thyroxine. Thyroid stimulating hormone (TSH) may be elevated if primary hypothyroidism is present.
- Urine myoglobin: rhabdomyolysis may be present.

Treatment

Restore the euthyroid state.

Chronic steroid myopathy

Definition

Proximal weakness due to prolonged treatment with corticosteroids or less frequently, endogenous corticosteroid secretion (Cushing's syndrome). About 70% of patients with Cushing's syndrome have myopathy.

Fluorinated corticosteroids, such as dexamethasone and triamcinolone, have more myopathic potential. The dose required to cause myopathy varies among individuals.

Clinical features

- Proximal muscle weakness, earlier and worse in the lower limbs than upper limbs, and sometimes painful. Wasting is late.
- Cushingoid features may be present.
- Myalgia may or may not be present.

Investigations and diagnosis

- Serum CK: normal.
- EMG: normal insertional activity and no spontaneous activity. Myopathic units could be present.
- Muscle biopsy: type II myofiber atrophy (**792**).

Treatment

- Change to a nonfluorinated steroid.
- Reduce steroid dose to the lowest possible therapeutic level.
- Try to administer the steroid on an alternate daily basis.
- Adequate diet and exercise may assist recovery.

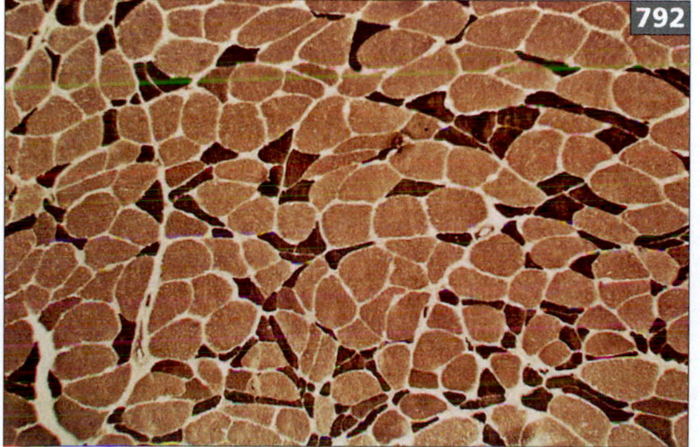

792 Type II fiber atrophy. The ATPase reaction at pH 9.4 shows a preferential atrophy of type II fibers (dark). This pattern of type II fiber atrophy is found with chronic steroid use, as well as disuse or cachexia.

Weakness due to Addison's disease and other forms of hypoadrenalism

Definition

Weakness due to diseases of adrenal gland or panhypopituitarism.

Clinical features

- Myalgia and muscle cramps.
- Although the patients may be generally weak, real myopathy generally does not occur.
- Fatigue and lassitude.
- Orthostatic hypotension.
- More severe cases may have confusional state, stupor, and coma.
- Skin hyperpigmentation may be present.

Diagnosis

- Serum electrolytes: hyponatremia and hyperkalemia.
- Panhypopituitarism may be present.
- CK may be mildly elevated.
- Low serum cortisol.

Treatment

- Cortisone (20–37.5 mg/day).
- Fludrocortisone.
- Increased salt intake.

Acromegaly

Clinical features

- Increased muscle bulk.
- Improved strength initially, but later muscle wasting and weakness occur.
- Nonspecific headache.
- Associated entrapment neuropathy (e.g. carpal tunnel syndrome).
- Sensorimotor peripheral neuropathy (sometimes with enlarged nerves).
- Visual field defects.
- Obstructive sleep apnea.
- Complications of diabetes and hypertension.

Diagnosis

- Hypopituitarism.
- Serum CK: sometimes elevated.

Treatment

- Resection of pituitary adenoma.
- Octreotide.

Hyperparathyroidism

Definition

Weakness associated with primary hyperparathyroidism (e.g. adenoma) or secondary hyperparathyroidism (e.g. renal disease).

Clinical features

Proximal and often painful muscle weakness, mainly affecting the legs and associated with mild wasting.

Investigations and diagnosis

- Serum CK: usually normal.
- Serum calcium, parathyroid hormone.

Treatment

- Primary hyperparathyroidism: remove the adenoma.
- Secondary hyperparathyroidism (typically to renal disease):
  - Partial parathyroidectomy.
  - 1, 25-dihydroxycholecalciferol.
  - 1-alpha tocopherol.
- Osteomalacia: vitamin D therapy.

DISORDERS OF GLYCOGEN METABOLISM

Glycogen is the main source of carbohydrates in the muscle; it is formed by a core protein called glyogenin and multiple branches of glucose chains. The concerted action of multiple enzymes is required for the synthesis, maturation, and degradation of the glycogen molecule. Several inherited disorders of glycogen metabolism (also called glycogenoses or glycogen-storage diseases) have been described (793). Acid maltase deficiency and McArdle's disease are typical examples that present predominantly with weakness and exercise intolerance, respectively. In the next sections the most common forms of glycogenoses associated with muscle involvement will be discussed.

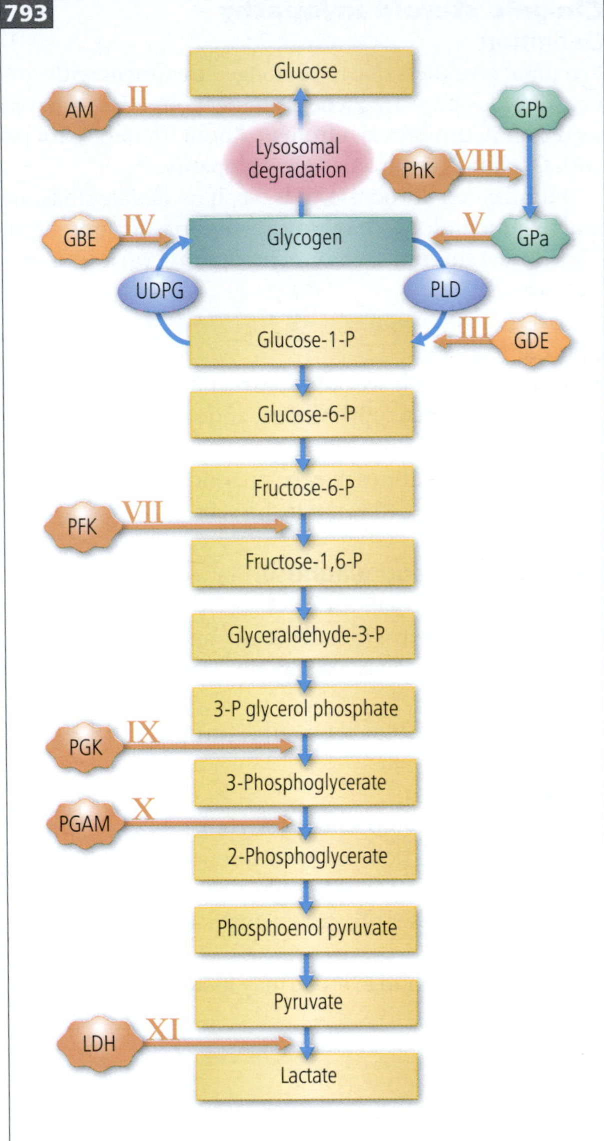

793 Schematic view of the glycogen metabolism pathway. Different types of glycogenosis (glycogen storage diseases) are caused by deficiency of different enzymes of the pathway. To date, 11 types of glycogenosis have been identified. Types II, III, IV, V, and VII are discussed in the text. Types I and VI do not cause a myopathy. PLD: phosphorylase limit dextrin; UDPG: uridine diphosphoglucose; AM: acid maltase; PhK: phosphorylase kinase; GPb, GPa: glycogen phosphorylase a, b; GBE: glycogen branching enzyme; GDE: glycogen debranching enzyme; PFK: phospho-fructokinase; PGK: phosphoglycerate kinase; PGAM: phosphoglycerate mutase; LDH: lactate dehydrogenase.

Acid maltase deficiency (Pompe disease, glycogen storage disease type II)

Definition and epidemiology

An autosomal-recessive glycogen storage disorder, with the genetic abnormality mapping to chromosome 17. Caused by a deficiency of lysosomal α-glucosidase (acid maltase) which results in impaired lysosomal conversion of glycogen to glucose so that glycogen accumulates in various organs depending on the disease form.

- Incidence (of all forms combined) is estimated to be 1/40,000.
- M=F.

Clinical features

- Infantile form: a generalized glycogenosis with severe cardiomyopathy, hypotonia, macroglossia, cardiomegaly, and hepatomegaly. Death occurs in infancy.
- Juvenile form: onset in teenage years, proximal > distal weakness:
  - Gower's sign, waddling gait.
  - Sometimes calf hypertrophy.
  - Hepatic and cardiac involvement uncommon, death occurs usually because of respiratory muscle weakness, in the third decade.
- Adult form: a slowly progressive myopathy that often predominantly affects the diaphragm and other respiratory muscles (hence respiratory failure):
  - Other muscles commonly involved are biceps, shoulder girdle, and thigh adductor muscles.
  - Scapuloperoneal pattern is rarely seen.
  - Symptoms typically begin in the third or fourth decades.
  - There is generally no hepatomegaly or cardiac involvement.
  - Sometime associated with intracerebral aneurysm.

Differential diagnosis

- Polymyositis.
- Other glycogen storage disease.
- Limb-girdle muscular dystrophies (LGMDs).
- Congenital myopathies for the infant form.
- Neuromuscular junction disease.

Investigations

- Serum CK: slightly to moderately elevated (1.5–15 times normal).
- EMG: myopathic motor units and recruitment. Myotonic discharges may be seen, but the patients do not have clinical myotonia.
- Blood leukocyte or urine α-glucosidase activity is reduced. Blood enzyme activity is simple, noninvasive, with high sensitivity and specificity.
- Muscle biopsy: a targeted truncal/paraspinal biopsy may be required for diagnosis; more distal muscles may lack diagnostic changes.
- Chorionic villi biopsy can be used for pre-natal diagnosis.
- Genetic testing

Diagnosis

Based on clinical features, biopsy and blood α-glucosidase activity.

Pathology (adult form)

- Affected muscles show features of a vacuolar myopathy (**794**). Vacuoles correspond to diastase-sensitive periodic-acid Schiff (PAS)-positive deposits of glycogen.
- There is increased activity of the lysosomal enzyme acid phosphatase.
- Electron microscopy typically shows glycogen accumulation that is partly located in membrane-bound lysosomal structures and associated with myelinoid lysosomal debris (**795**).

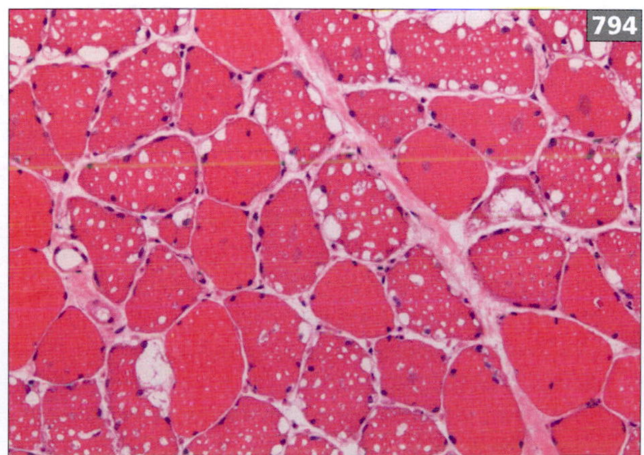

794 Adult acid maltase deficiency. H&E stained section of paraspinal muscle biopsy, showing a vacuolar myopathy pattern. The vacuoles have no prominent rimming. A deltoid biopsy showed no significant morphologic changes, illustrating the selective pattern of muscle involvement often seen in adult acid maltase deficiency.

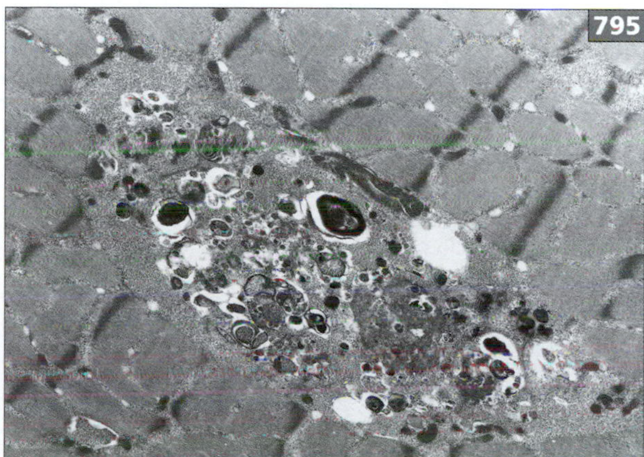

795 Acid maltase deficiency. Electron microscopy confirms that the vacuoles correspond to accumulations of glycogen in the cytoplasm of the myofibers and within membrane-bound structures that correspond to lysosomes. Additionally, there are deposits of membranous, partly lamellated myelinoid lysosomal debris.

Treatment[10,11]

- Enzyme replacement therapy (intravenous recombinant human α-glucosidase) has shown promising results in the infantile and adult forms of Pompe disease.
- Inspiratory exercises are useful.
- Two brands of recombinant human α-glucosidase (Myozyme and Lumizyme) are approved by the USA Food and Drug Administration, for infantile and adult onset acid maltase deficiency respectively.

McArdle's disease (Type V glycogenosis)

Definition and epidemiology

Autosomal recessive disorder characterized by post-exertional cramps or weakness. The gene for myophosphorylase (*PYGM*) maps to chromosome 11q13. It is caused by a myophosphorylase (α-1, 4-glucan orthophosphate glycosyltransferase) deficiency, which results in impaired conversion of glycogen to glucose-1-phosphate in muscle.

- Males are affected more than females (4:1).
- The prevalence of McArdle's disease is about 1 in 100,000.

Pathophysiology

Glycogen breakdown is impaired during a sudden burst of muscle activity, causing elevation in intracellular calcium and adenosine diphosphate, and lower inorganic phosphate; muscle cell pH is shown not to become acidotic, which increases the sensitivity of the contractile apparatus to calcium.

Clinical features

- Usually onset is in childhood or adolescence.
- Attacks of exercise intolerance with muscle pain (myalgia) and stiffness, often precipitated by brief, strong exercises.
- Muscle contractures and dark urine (myoglobinuria) usually do not develop until the second or third decades.
- Exercise which causes myalgia can be resumed at the same level after a brief period of exercise (second wind phenomenon).
- Often nonprogressive, but some patients develop fixed weakness after recurrent rhabdomyolysis.

Differential diagnosis of cramps +/– weakness

- Glycogen storage disease.
- Mitochondrial disease.
- Hypothyroid myopathy.
- Tetany secondary to hypocalcemia.
- Myotonia and neuromyotonia.
- Motor neuron disease.
- Medication-induced cramps.
- Electrolyte imbalance.

Investigations

- Serum CK: usually elevated even between periods of rhabdomyolysis.
- Urine: myoglobinuria occasionally.
- Routine NCS is normal, but repetitive nerve stimulation or stimulation following a short period of exercise may demonstrate decremental amplitude of the motor responses.
- EMG: can be normal, or show fibrillations, positive waves, myotonic discharges, or myopathic motor units. If needle study is done during a muscle contracture, it shows electrical silence.
- Forearm ischemic exercise: physiologic response to strenuous hand exercise is a 3–5-fold increase in serum lactate and ammonia, drawn from a vein in the forearm. In McArdle's disease, there is flat response (no increase) in venous lactate while the physiologic rise in serum ammonia is present.
- Muscle biopsy: histochemical and biochemical studies.
- Genetic testing: sequence analysis or assessment for targeted mutations of *PYGM*.

Diagnosis

Is usually based on clinical features and findings on the muscle biopsy.

Pathology

- A muscle may be morphologically normal (796) or show subsarcolemmal and intermyofibrillar deposits of glycogen.
- Sometimes there is evidence of individual fiber degeneration/regeneration.
- Enzyme histochemical staining shows significantly reduced or absent myophosphorylase (797). Staining for phosphorylase could be falsely positive soon after an episode of rhabdomyolysis, probably because of upregulation of a fetal isoenzyme.

Treatment

- Endurance exercise training: it has been shown that after a period of endurance training exercise, there is less reliance on glucose (and more on lipids) for a moderate intensity exercise.
- Oral sucrose supplementation before exercise increases exercise tolerance.
- Oral creatine supplementation may improve skeletal muscle function.

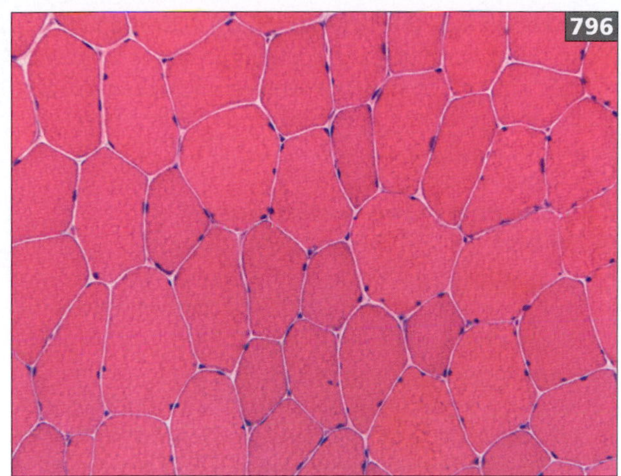

796 Myophosporylase deficiency. The H&E stained section from a patient with McArdle's disease shows no significant morphologic changes. In particular, there is no significant abnormal accumulation of glycogen. The enzyme histochemical studies (797) establish the diagnosis.

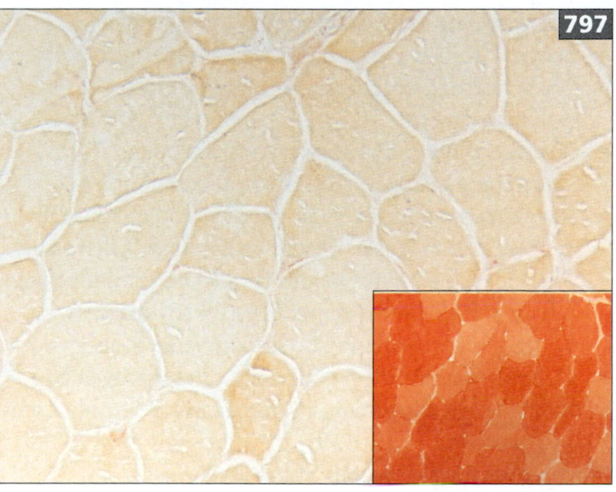

797 Myophosphorylase deficiency. This enzyme histochemical reaction on the biopsy illustrated in 796 shows lack of normal enzyme reactivity. The insert illustrates normal staining. Type II fibers are darker than type I fibers, but both show brown reaction product.

Phosphofructokinase (PFK) deficiency (Tarui's disease, glycogenosis type VII)

Definition and epidemiology

Autosomal recessive disorder due to PFK deficiency. PFK gene is mapped to chromosome 12. PFK catalyzes the conversion of fructose-6-phosphate to fructose-1, 6-diphosphate in muscle, which is the rate limiting step in the glycolytic pathway.

- Prevalent in Ashkenazi Jews and some Italian families.

Clinical features

- Onset: second to fourth decades.
- Exercise intolerance, muscle aches, contractures, myoglobinuria, and renal failure less frequent than McArdle's disease.
- Second wind phenomenon less prominent than that of McArdle's disease.
- A subgroup of PFK deficiency present with late onset progressive proximal (or less commonly scapuloperoneal) weakness without myoglobinuria or cramps.
- A mild hemolytic tendency is sometimes present, causing gout or jaundice.

Investigations and diagnosis

- Serum CK is usually elevated.
- Forearm ischemic exercise produces no increase in venous lactate levels (similar to McArdle's disease).
- In most patients, PFK activity is absent in the muscle and 50% reduced in the red blood cells.
- Muscle biopsy may be morphologically normal or show accumulation of normal glycogen and, less likely, accumulation of a diastase-resistant, PAS-positive material. Enzyme histochemical staining can confirm the lack of enzyme activity. Frozen tissue can be used for biochemical testing.

Debranching enzyme deficiency (type III glycogenosis, Cori–Forbes disease)

Definition

Autosomal recessive; the gene is localized to chromosome 1. Debranching enzyme catalyzes the hydrolysis of glycogen to glucose-1-phosphate.

Clinical features

- Infantile type:
  - Growth retardation, hepatomegaly, mild myopathy, and seizures which tend to improve after puberty.
  - Fasting hypoglycemia and ketonuria.
- Adult type: mild weakness of hands and legs. Cardiomyopathy is a late complication.

Investigations and diagnosis

- Serum CK: elevated 2–20 times.
- NCS: normal, or may show a sensorimotor polyneuropathy.
- Needle EMG: may show myopathic units, spontaneous activity and myotonic discharges.
- Forearm ischemic exercise produces no increase in venous lactate levels (similar to McArdle's disease).
- Muscle biopsy: cytoplasmic (not lysosomal) glycogen, which is PAS-positive and digestible by diastase. Glycogen deposits may be seen in nerve biopsy.
- Debranching enzyme deficiency can be proven by biochemical assessment of fibroblasts or lymphocytes.

Polyglucosan body disease (glycogenosis type IV, Andersen's disease, or amylopectinosis)

Definition

Autosomal recessive disorder caused by the deficiency of glycogen branching enzyme. This enzyme catalyzes the transfer of a glucose string from one glycogen chain to another while creating a new branch. The gene is localized to chromosome 3.

Clinical features

- The most common presentation is in childhood with liver involvement and cirrhosis.
- It can also present with neuronal involvement and hypotonia in infancy.
- Myopathy and cardiac involvement may occur in the childhood type.
- Myopathy is a rare manifestation of adult onset polyglucosan body disease.
- More common manifestations of polyglucosan body disease include upper and lower motor neuron disease, sensory neuropathy, extrapyramidal findings, dementia, and bladder involvement.

Investigations and diagnosis

- CK may be normal or mildly elevated.
- NCS: may be normal or show a neuropathy.
- Needle EMG may show spontaneous activity, neurogenic changes and myopathic units and early (myopathic) recruitment when myopathy is also present.
- Muscle biopsy shows polyglucosan bodies which are PAS-positive diastase-resistant inclusions.
- Polyglucosan bodies are also found in skin apocrine glands, peripheral nerves, and cardiac muscle, although mild accumulation of these structures can be seen with aging.
- Decreased or absent branching enzyme in skin fibroblasts.

DISORDERS OF LIPID METABOLISM

Long chain fatty acids are a major source of muscle energy and are consumed during muscular activity. Carnitine is involved in the transport of free fatty acids into mitochondria.

Muscle carnitine deficiency

Definition

- Myopathy secondary to lipid accumulation due to deficiency of carnitine, which may be primary or secondary.
- Secondary carnitine deficiency is seen in systemic diseases such as sepsis, malnutrition, hemodialysis, HIV infection (especially associated with zidovudine treatment), mitochondrial diseases, and treatment with valproic acid.

Clinical features

- Myopathy develops in infants, children or early adulthood.
- Limb-girdle pattern of weakness.
- Facial muscles or tongue may be affected.
- No pain or rhabdomyolysis.

Diagnosis

- CK moderately elevated. Normal blood level of carnitine.
- Muscle biopsy: accumulation of lipid which is deficient in carnitine.
- Biochemical testing on muscle tissue.

Treatment

Carnitine 2–4 g/day.

Carnitine palmitoyltransferase II (CPT2) deficiency

Definition

Autosomal recessive disorder caused by impaired transport of free fatty acids into mitochondria. The abnormal gene maps to chromosome 1. CPT2 deficiency is the most common inherited cause of recurrent myoglobinuria.

Clinical features

- Most patients are male.
- Onset in adolescence or early adulthood.
- Intermittent attacks occur without warning; precipitated by prolonged exertion, fasting, or a high fat diet.
- Muscle cramps, muscle pain, and dark urine (myoglobinuria) are present, with normal muscle strength between attacks.
- Exposure to cold, viral infections, general anesthesia, and valproic acid can also precipitate rhabdomyolysis.
- Renal failure (due to myoglobinuria) and respiratory failure may occur.
- Patients have a normal capacity to perform short, demanding exercise.
- Muscle weakness may occur later in life.

Investigations and diagnosis

- Urine: myoglobinuria.
- CK normal or mildly elevated between attacks and markedly elevated during attacks.
- High ratio of serum palmitoylcarnitine (C16:0) and oleoylcarnitine (C18:1) to acetylcarnitine (C2).
- Normal serum carnitine.
- During an acute episode the muscle shows myofiber degeneration and regeneration.
- Between attacks it shows normal morphology. Biochemical testing on frozen muscle tissue can confirm the diagnosis.

Treatment

- High-carbohydrate (70%) and low-fat (<20%) diet.
- Frequent meals; avoiding extended fasting and prolonged exercise.
- Oral carnitine.
- Infusion of glucose during periods of infection to prevent catabolism.
- Aggressive hydration during attacks of rhabdomyo–lysis to prevent renal failure.
- Caution should be exercised in the use of valproic acid, general anesthesia, ibuprofen, and diazepam in high doses.

MITOCHONDRIAL MYOPATHY

Definition

Mitochondrial diseases are systemic conditions resulting from mutations in nuclear or mitochondrial genes and present with very variable clinical features that may include myopathy[12] (see Chapter 8). This section focuses primarily on muscle involvement.

Etiology and pathophysiology

The mitochondrial DNA (mtDNA) encodes 13 structural proteins that are part of the respiratory chain, 2 rRNAs and 22 tRNAs. The genetics of mitochondrial disease vary in several aspects from those of other disease:

- mtDNA mutations are always inherited maternally, nuclear mutations follow Mendelian inheritance patterns.
- Common mtDNA mutations include large deletions as well point mutations disrupting individual tRNAs or rRNAs.
- A single cell may contain thousands of copies of mtDNA. In most cases a certain threshold of mutated mtDNA copies has to be exceeded to cause disease.
- The load of mutated mtDNA copies may vary between different tissues; this can explain differences in disease phenotypes. Some mutations are not detected unless diseased tissue is tested.
- Some mutations in nuclear DNA may lead to defects in individual components of the respiratory chain. Other mutations may disrupt mitochondrial function by disrupting the import of proteins into mitochondria, by changing the lipid composition of the inner mitochondrial membrane, or by changing intergenomic signaling to cause mtDNA depletion or multiple mtDNA mutations.
- Some mitochondrial mutations cause defects in individual proteins while others affect general function, for example by interfering with translation of mitochondrial genes.

Toxin exposure, treatment with zidovudine (azidothymidine [AZT]) and normal aging can result in acquired defects in mitochondrial function.

Clinical features

- The onset can vary from birth to adulthood.
- Clinically, skeletal muscle involvement can result in fixed weakness, exercise intolerance, premature fatigue, or myoglobulinuria.
- The disease course and presentation are extremely variable. The course can be rapidly progressive or static. The presentation can include generalized weakness, proximal weakness, extraocular eye muscle weakness, or rhabdomyolysis.
- Other features include cardiomyopathy, cataract, neurosensory hearing loss, and CNS involvement.

Investigations

- Serum CK: CK levels are often normal or mildly elevated.
- Electrocardiography (ECG) and echocardiogram: cardiologic evaluation is important and helpful in deciding on the timing for interventions including pacemaker placement.
- EMG: can vary from normal to nonspecific, to typically myopathic features.
- MRI: CNS imaging can be helpful in establishing the diagnosis of mitochondrial diseases associated with typical CNS involvement including MELAS (mitochondrial encephalomyopathy, lactic acidosis, and stroke-like episodes) and Leigh's disease.
- Muscle biopsy: a muscle biopsy can be helpful in establishing the diagnosis if the typical features discussed above are present. Some mitochondrial diseases are not associated with morphologic changes in the muscle.
- Genetic testing: can detect mtDNA mutations. Deciding on the most applicable mutations to screen and the appropriate tissue to use is important. A negative genetic study does not rule out a mitochondrial disease.

Pathology

Some mitochondrial diseases are associated with normal skeletal muscle morphology. There may be nonspecific changes including variation in myofiber size as well as evidence of individual myofiber degeneration and regeneration:

- The COX reaction may identify degeneration and regeneration. More specific features include myofibers lacking normal enzyme activity.
- The modified Gomori trichrome stain (798) and enzyme histochemical reactions for NADH and succinate dehydrogenase may identify myofibers with abnormal aggregates of mitochondria visible under light microscopy ('ragged red fibers').
- Electron microscopy can confirm the presence of abnormal mitochondrial aggregates as well as the presence of abnormal mitochondrial forms and mitochondria with paracrystalline inclusions (799).

Treatment

There are no specific therapies. Supportive therapy should address the presentation of the disease including seizure control, surgery for cataracts, management of endocrine disorders, and monitoring and treating cardiac involvement.

In specific cases supplementation with metabolites can be helpful including folic acid in Kearns–Sayre syndrome (KSS). CoQ10 has been used in KSS, myoclonic epilepsy with ragged red fibers, MELAS, or CoQ10 deficiency.

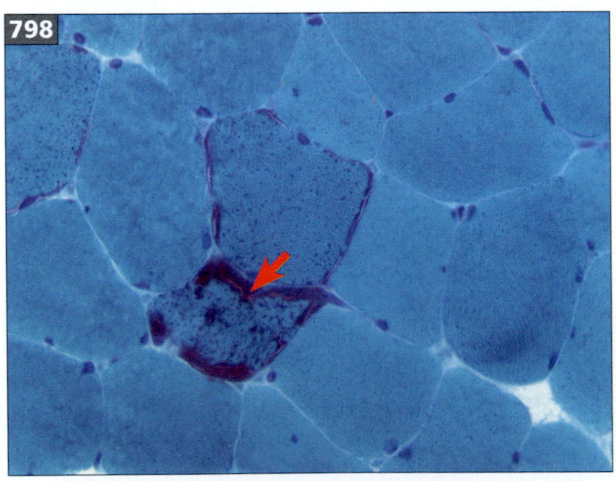

798 Mitochondrial myopathy (modified Gomori trichrome stain). Mitochondria cluster together in a preferentially subsarcolemmal distribution (arrow) instead of the normal fine stippled uniform distribution found on this stain (see 782). Myofibers with this morphology are referred to as ragged red fibers.

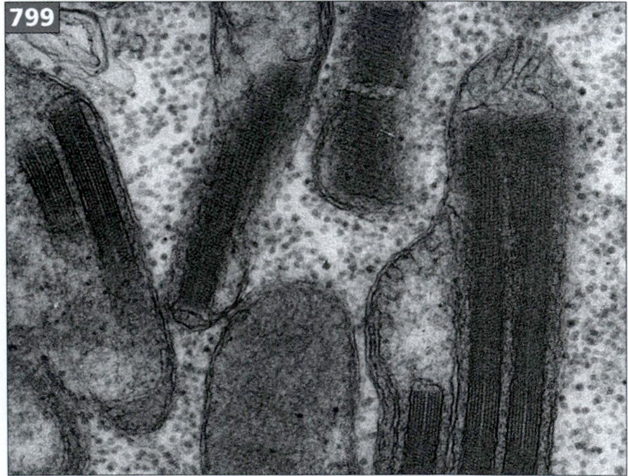

799 Mitochondrial myopathy (electron microscopy). Some of the abnormally aggregated mitochondria contain paracrystalline inclusions that show as electron-dense geometric structures within mitochondria.

MUSCULAR DYSTROPHIES

Definition

Defects in many of the proteins important for normal muscle function have been linked to disease. Some of these result in skeletal muscle specific phenotypes, while others additionally lead to cardiomyopathy or involvement of other organ systems. Clinical features like age of onset, muscle groups affected, pace of disease progression, and involvement of other organs can vary widely depending on the type of mutation, environmental factors, and genetic modifiers. In some instances family members that carry the same mutation present with distinctly different clinical phenotypes.

Important groups discussed below are dystrophinopathies, fascioscapulohumeral dystrophy, Emery–Dreifuss muscular dystrophy (EMD), LGMDs, and myotonic dystrophies. Other primarily pediatric diseases such as congenital myopathies (CMs) and congenital muscular dystrophies (CMDs) (summarized in *Tables 124* and *125*) are not discussed in detail, but may sometimes be considered in the differential diagnosis. In practice the distinction of these two entities is not always clear, but in principle the following features apply: CMs are typically characterized by: (1) childhood onset; (2) static or slowly progressive course; (3) association with specific structural abnormalities; (4) relative lack of ongoing degeneration/regeneration[13]. CMDs are characterized by: (1) childhood onset; (2) ongoing myofiber degeneration/regeneration and higher CK levels; (3) frequent CNS involvement[14]. In general, patients with muscular dystrophies are best cared for in a multidisciplinary setting that addresses the complex nature of their care.

DYSTROPHINOPATHIES

Definition

Dystrophinopathies include diseases of skeletal and cardiac muscle that are characterized by an X-linked inheritance pattern and mutations in the dystrophin (*DMD*) gene on Xp21[15]. The spectrum of clinical presentations include Duchenne's muscular dystrophy (DMD, incidence 1:3500) and Becker's muscular dystrophy (BMD, incidence 1:35,000).

Etiology and pathophysiology

Dystrophin is a large filamentous protein that is integral part of the dystrophin–glycoprotein complex (DGC) (see 778). The DGC is thought to provide structural integrity to individual myofibers during contraction by spanning the cell membrane and linking the actin cytoskeleton on the inside to the basement membrane on the outside. The DGC is also thought to play an important role in cell signaling. Both functions can be disrupted by mutations in dystrophin or other DGC components, including sarcoglycans and dystroglycans which are discussed below. Important components of dystrophin include the actin binding N-terminus, a long helical rod domain, and a highly conserved C-terminal domain that interacts with other proteins.

Tears in the cell membrane can lead to calcium influx, complement activation, and degeneration/necrosis of myofiber segments. Repeated episodes of degeneration and regeneration lead to chronic remodeling of muscle tissue with endomysial fibrosis and fatty replacement.

The dystrophin gene spans 2.5 million base pairs and is composed of 79 exons. The clinical disease severity depends on the underlying genetic defect and the amount of residual mutant protein made:

- BMD is a milder phenotype that typically shows expression of some residual dystrophin and is often linked to in-frame mutations in the rod domain that preserve the N- and C-terminal domains.
- DMD is more severe and typically linked to mutations that result in the virtually complete absence of any dystrophin protein. Often the underlying mutation disrupts the normal reading frame. Many result in an early stop codon.

Clinical features

General

- Cognitive impairment and mental retardation occur in a subset of DMD and BMD patients[16]. Typically these are nonprogressive and not related to the severity of the underlying muscle disease. Disruption of brain-specific splice variants may explain this part of the phenotype.
- Cardiac involvement with conduction defects as well as cardiomyopathy is common in BMD and DMD. The incidence in DMD patients is up to 90% at 18 years and nearly 100% in their 30s.
- Some patients have symptoms attributed to smooth muscle involvement including intestinal pseudo-obstruction, delayed gastric emptying as well as acute gastric dilatation, causing sudden episodes of vomiting and abdominal pain.

TABLE 124 **CONGENITAL MYOPATHIES (CM), PROTEIN AGGREGATE MYOPATHIES, AND AUTOPHAGIC VACUOLAR MYOPATHIES**

Disease group/ disease	Subgroup	Protein (gene)	Locus	Clinical features/allelic diseases/characteristic pathologic features
CONGENITAL MYOPATHIES				
Nemaline myopathies	NEM1*	Tropomyosin-3 (*TPM3*)	1q22–q23	Facial, bulbar, respiratory and proximal muscle weakness; wide range in clinical severity and presentation; cardiac involvement is rare but desenbed; ACTA1 mutations are also linked to CFTD and PAM; TPM3 mutations are also linked to CFTD/biopsy: nemaline rod type inclusions and variable degrees of chronic remodeling
	NEM2*	Nebulin (*NEB*)	2q22	
	NEM3*	Alplia-actin-1 (*ACTA1*)	lq42.1	
	NEM4*	Tiopomyosm-2 (*TPM2*)	9p13.2–13.1	
	NEM5*	Tioponin T1 (*TNNT1*)	19q13.4	
	NEM6*		15q15–q25	
	NEM7*	Cofilin-2 (*CFL2*)	14q12	
Central core disease		Ryanodine receptor 1 (*RYR1*)	19q13.1	Weakness, joint contractures, delayed motor development; allelic with malignant hyperthermia; biopsy: central areas of disorganized sarcomeres and disrupted myofiber architecture ('cores')
Multiminicore disease		Selenoprotein 1 (*SEPN1*)	lp36–p35	Axial myopathy, respiratory failure, scoliosis; biopsy: multiple short cores in most myofibers; mutations in SEPN1 are associated with a spectrum that includes desmin-related myopathy with Mallory bodies, CFTD and RSMD1; mutations in RYR1 are also associated with central core disease and malignant hyperthermia
		Ryanodine receptor 1 (RYR1)	19q13.1	
Centronuclear myopathy	X-linked, myotubular myopathy	Myotubularin (*MTM1*)	Xq28	Severe hypotonia requiring ventilation, normal cognition; biopsy: atropliic myofibers with central nuclei (geometric center) mimicking myotubes in development
Centronuclear myopathy	Autosomal dominant	Dynamin-2 (*DNM2*)	19p13.2	Weakness and wasting most prominent in neck and proximal muscles; DNM2 and RYR1 are linked to dominant inheritance, BIN1 to recessive; biopsy: central nuclei; DNM2 mutations also linked to CMT; mutations in RYR1 are also associated with multiminicore disease and central core disease
	Autosomal dominant	Ryanodine receptor 1 (*RYR1*)	19q13.1	
	Autosomal recessive	Amphyphysin 2 (*BIN1*)	2q14	

TABLE 124 continued

Disease group/ disease	Subgroup	Protein (gene)	Locus	Clinical features/allelic diseases/characteristic pathologic features
Congenital fiber type disproportion (CFTD)		Selenoprotein1 *(SEPN1)*	lp36–p35	Hypotonia, weakness, failure to thrive, facial and respiratory weakness, contractures; wide phenotypic spectrum; biopsy: predominance and atrophy of type I fibers (not specific); mutations in SEPN1 are associated with a spectrum that includes desmin-related myopathy with Mallory bodies, CFTD and RSMDl; mutations in ACTA1 are also associated with nemaline myopathy and PAM; mutations in TPM3 are also associated with nemaline myopathy
		Alpha-actin-1 (*ACTA1*)	lq42.1	
		Tropomyosin 3 (*TPM3*)	1q22–q23	
PROTEIN AGGREGATE MYOPATHIES (PAM)	Actin aggregate myopathy	Alpha-actin-1 (*ACTA1*)	lq42.1	ACTA1 mutations are also associated with nemaline myopathy and CFTD
	Mallory body myopathy	Selenoprotein 1 (*SEPN1*)	lp36–p35	Mutations in SEPN1 are associated with a spectrum that includes desmin-related myopathy with Mallory bodies, CFTD and RSMD1
	Myosin storage/hyaline body myopathy	Slow-skeletal beta cardiac myosin (*MYH7*)	14q12	Allelic with familial hypertrophic cardiomyopathy
	Desmin-related myopathy	Desmin (*DES*)	2q35	Also associated with cardiomyopathy and cardiac conduction defects
	Spheroid body myopathy	Myolilin (*TTID*)	5q31	Also associated with cardiomyopathy
AUTOPHAGIC VACUOLAR MYOPATHIES (AMV)	Danon's disease	Lysosome-associated protein 2 (*LAMP2*)	Xq24	Triad of hypertrophic cardiomyopathy, myopathy and mental retardation; biopsy: vacuolar myopathy associated with lack of LAMP2 expression
	X-linked autophagic vacuolar myopathy (XMEA or MEAX)	*VMA21*	Xq28	Slowly progressive atrophy and weakness of proximal muscles; sparing of cardiac and respiratory muscles; biopsy: morphology similar to Danon's disease; LAMP2 expression normal; deposition of complement C5b–9

* Nomenclature in Online Mendelian Inheritance in Man (OMIM). Abbreviations: CFTD: congenital fiber type disproportion; CMT: Charcot–Marie–Tooth disease; LGMD: limb-girdle muscular dystrophy; PAM: protein aggregate myopathy; RSMD1: rigid spine muscular dystrophy1

TABLE 125 **SUMMARY OF LIMB-GIRDLE DYSTROPHIES**

	Locus	Gene	Allelic diseases	Onset	Loss of ambulation	Muscles beyond limb girdle	Hypertrophy	Contractures	Other features or organs
1A	5q31	Myotilin		Adult	Late	+/− Distal; + resp.		+/− Ankle	Nasal dysarthric speech
1B	lq21.2	Lamin A/C	AD EMD; CMD 1A	Adult	–			+ Ankle; + elbow; +spinal rigidity	DCM; conduction defects; sudden cardiac death
1C	3p25	Caveclin 3	Rippling muscle disease	5 years	–		Calf hypertrophy		Muscle cramps, myalgia; +/− Cardiac
ID	7q			Adult	–	+/− Dysphagia			+/− Cardiac
1E	6q23				–				+/− Cardiac
1F	7q32.1–32.2			Juvenile or adult		+/− Distal LE; resp.			
2A	15q15.1–21.1	Calpain 3		2–40y (mean 14y)	5–39y (mean 17y)		Calf hypertrophy		In some eosinophilic fasciitis before presentation
2B	2p13.3–13.1	Dysferlin	Miyoshi myopathy; distal myopathy with tibial onset	15–26 (mean 18y)	30–55y	+/− Distal LE; +/− resp.	Transient early calf hypertrophy	Distal contractures	
2C	13q12	γ-Sarcoglycan		2–10y	<15y	Resp.	Calf hypertrophy; macroglossia		Cardiac

TABLE 125 continued

	Locus	Gene	Allelic diseases	Onset	Loss of ambulation	Muscles beyond limb girdle	Hypertrophy	Contractures	Other features or organs
2D	17q12–21.33	α-Sarcoglycan		2–15y	Late	Resp.	Calf hypertrophy; macroglossia		Cardiac
2F	5q33	β-Sarcoglycan		2–15y	15–25y	Resp.	Calf hypertrophy; macroglossia		Cardiac
2F	5q33	δ-Sarcoglycan		1–10y	15y	Resp.	Calf hypertrophy, macroglossia		Myalgia
2G	17q12	Telethonin		10–15y	30–35y	Distal LE			+/– Cardiac
2H	9q31–q34.1	*TRIM-32*	Sarcotubular myopathy	6–40y	60y	Distal LE; resp.; facial			Cardiac; +/– myalgia
2I	19q13.3	*FKRP*	Congenital muscular dystrophy 1C	1–40y	30–40y	+/– Resp.	Calf hypertrophy; +/– macroglossia	Ankle	Cardiac; myalgia
2J	2q31	Titin	CMD 1G	2–25y	20–50y	+/– Distal LE			+/– Cardiac
2K	9q34.1	*POMT1*		1–6y			Calf hypertrophy; macroglossia	Contractures	Microcephaly; mental retardation
2?	11p13–pl2			11–50y	20–60y	Often asymmetric quadriceps atrophy/ weakness			Myalgia
2?	9q31	Fukutin		<1y					

Abbrevations: CMD: dilated cardiomyopathy; AD: autosomal dominant; EMD: Emery–Dreifuss muscular dystrophy; Resp.: respiratory muscles; LE: lower extremity

Duchenne's muscular dystrophy

CK elevations of 10–100 times normal are present at birth even though infants usually show no clinical disease manifestation. Typically, delay in motor development is not noted until the age of 2–5 years. The skeletal muscle disease is relentlessly progressive.

Early (ages 2–6)

- Onset of walking delayed beyond 18 months.
- Abnormal gait with toe walking or waddling.
- Difficulty running.
- Frequent falls, difficulty rising from the floor (Gower's sign, **800, 801**).
- Prominent calf muscle bulge ('pseudo-hypertrophy').
- Hyperlordosis resulting in a protruding abdomen.
- Weakness in the lower extremities, pelvis, and lower trunk is clinically most apparent.
- In some patients there is global developmental delay, severe learning disabilities, failure to thrive.
- In some instances patients come to attention because of elevated ALT/aspartate aminotransferase (AST) during routine work-up, myoglobulinuria, or malignant hyperthermia-like episode with anesthesia.

Ages 7–10

- Progressive leg weakness leading to loss of walking and wheelchair dependence by mean age of 9.5 years.
- Joint contractures, especially of the iliotibial bands, hip flexors, and heel cords.
- Progressive scoliosis and thoracic deformities after loss of mobility.

Teenage years

- Development of more apparent upper extremity weakness.
- Worsening respiratory reserve and sleep hypoventilation, rapid eye movement-sleep related hypoxemic dips, and obstructive apnea.
- Scoliosis progresses rapidly with the pubertal growth spurt, with adverse effects on respiration, feeding, sitting, and comfort.
- In the past, most patients died in the late teens and early twenties. Improved therapy and supportive care has increased the mean survival over historical controls and will change the clinical problems facing these patients. Mean survival in the UK is now 27 years.

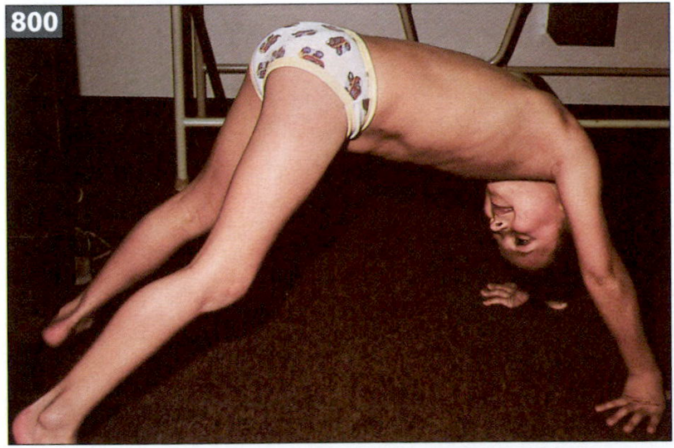

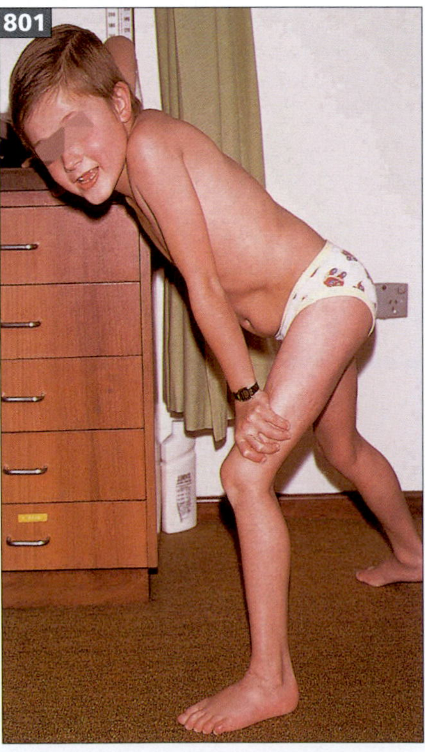

800, 801 A boy with Duchenne's muscular dystrophy rising from the floor, climbing up his legs, and pushing up against the legs to assist with straightening the trunk (Gower's sign). *Courtesy of Professor BA Kakulas, Neuropathology Department, Royal Perth Hospital, Australia.*

Becker's muscular dystrophy

- BMD is characterized by a later onset of symptoms and a slower rate of progression then that of DMD. The onset of disease is variable, but often not until teenage years, with the mean at 12 years and 90% before age 20. The patients often show similar but milder features than those found in DMD. The mean age at loss of ambulation is in the fourth decade, but patients may live for many decades. For some, cardiomyopathy dominates the clinical presentation.

Other dystrophinopathies

- Exercise intolerance with myalgias, muscle cramps, or myoglobulinuria.
- Asymptomatic elevation of CK levels.
- (Fatal) X-linked dilated cardiomyopathy without muscle weakness.
- Carriers may develop with mild to moderate muscle weakness (about 8%), cardiomyopathy, or asymptomatic CK elevation.

Differential diagnosis

- Spinal muscular atrophy.
- Congenital myopathies such as nemaline myopathy or central core disease (see *Table 124*).
- Congenital dystrophies such as fukutin or FKRP (fukutin related protein) deficiency (see *Table 124*) may have to be considered.
- X-linked or autosomal EMD can mimic DMD or BMD by also causing a presentation characterized by features of muscular dystrophy and cardiomyopathy. These patients typically show selective early involvement of distal leg muscles, triceps, and biceps, as well as contractures of elbows and neck.
- LGMD.
- Childhood onset acid maltase deficiency may result in proximal muscle weakness and calf enlargement by age 5 years.

Investigations and diagnosis

- CK: elevated CK levels in the thousands or tens of thousands IU/l precede clinical manifestation in DMD:
  - CK elevation is less prominent in older patients with loss of muscle mass.
  - BMD patients and female carriers also show variable CK level elevation.
- ECG and echocardiogram: to assess cardiac involvement.
- EMG: myopathic changes early in the disease course. Muscle tissue may become unexcitable as the number of activated muscle fibers decreases with disease progression.
- MRI: provides data on the degree of involvement of different muscle groups and establishes the presence of a typical pattern of involvement.
- Muscle biopsy with immunohistochemical studies and sometimes immunoblot analysis can be helpful in confirming the diagnosis.
- Genetic testing is the most efficient way to confirm the diagnosis in typical cases of DMD with a positive family history.
  - Multiplex polymerase chain reaction (PCR) has now largely replaced Southern blotting. It can detect the underlying mutation in some 65% of DMD cases as well as those in BMD patients. Other techniques include partially automated single-stranded conformational polymorphism (SSCP) analysis and high-throughput direct sequencing of all dystrophin exons can aid the discovery of point mutations.
  - In some cases, mRNA analysis performed on cDNA obtained through reverse transcriptase (RT)-PCR can help to confirm unusual mutations or duplications.
  - 30–40% of dystrophin mutations are new spontaneous mutations.
  - Pedigree analysis and CK analysis may help to identify possible carriers; however, CK levels are only elevated in 45–70% of definite carriers. In many cases a carrier state can be confirmed by available genetic tests.
  - Up to 20% of new DMD cases may result from gonadal mosaicism that would be missed by genetic testing on somatic cells of the mother, but could be confirmed by carrier detection analysis on the mother's daughters and sisters.
  - Prenatal diagnosis can be achieved through chorionic villous sampling at 8 weeks of gestation or through preimplantation DNA testing on embryos.

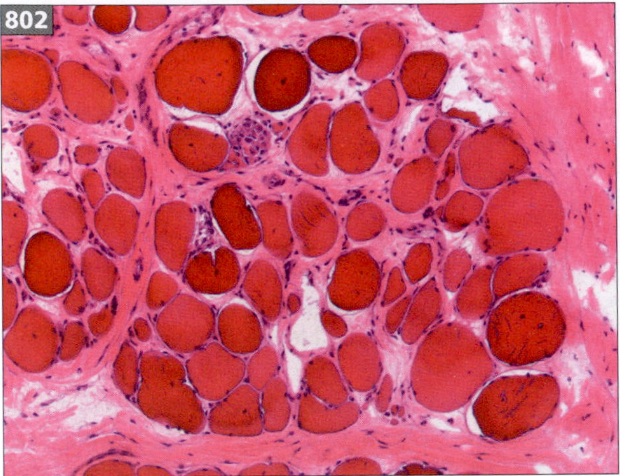

802 Duchenne's muscular dystrophy (H&E). There are myopathic changes with necrotic myofibers and variation in fiber size. Some fibers are hypercontracted and appear bright dark red. Individual myofibers are no longer tightly packed together, but separated by endomysial fibrosis, a sign of disease chronicity.

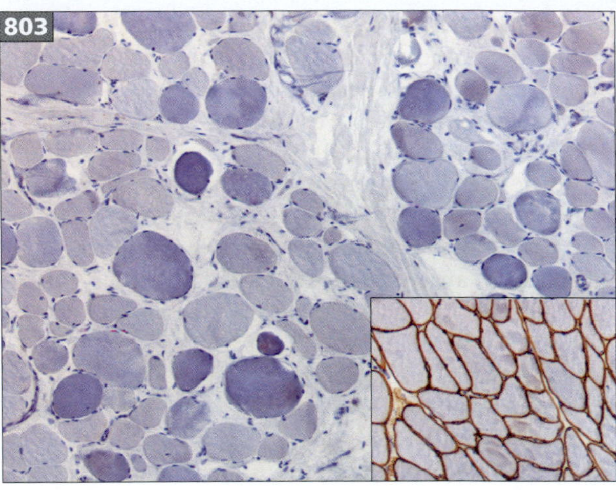

803 Duchenne's muscular dystrophy (immunohistochemistry for dystrophin). In normal muscle (insert) this stain uniformly outlines individual myofibers. This patient's sample lacks dystrophin expression that would show up as brown rimming of myofibers.

Pathology

- Muscle biopsies show myopathic changes with evidence of individual fiber degeneration and regeneration (802).
- With progression there is increasing variation in myofiber size with atrophy, hypertrophy, and fiber splitting. Endomysial fibrosis and fatty replacement cause disruption of normal fascicular architecture.
- Beyond macrophages in degenerating myofibers, inflammatory infiltrates are usually absent.
- BMD patients may show changes that are similar in principle but much milder than those in DMD patients of comparable age.
- In DMD immunocytochemical studies typically show absence of staining with antibodies specific for all main domains of dystrophin (803). BMD patients often show less severe disruption of dystrophin expression with patchy staining or complete absence of only one of the domains.

Treatment

Current management

Corticosteroids or the prednisone derivative deflazocort are effective in delaying loss of mobility by 6 months to 2 years. This therapy may have an especially high long-term impact if it can decrease the development of scoliosis by allowing some of the pubertal growth spurt to occur before loss of mobility. Patients are typically started on 0.75 mg/kg/day to 1.5 mg/kg/day in the early ambulatory phase (4–6 years). Some regimens include intermittent courses. Weight gain and vertebral body fractures are common complications. Calcium and vitamin D supplementation are therefore also given.

Rehabilitation with knee–ankle–foot orthoses can prolong walking for some 18–24 months. Passive exercise, stretching of joints, and night-time splints can help to prevent or reduce joint contractures. Surgery may be considered for management of scoliosis and release of contractures of the ankle and hip.

Respiratory therapy includes inspiratory resistive exercises that may increase the endurance of respiratory muscles. Cough assist devices may aid respiratory function. Noninvasive ventilation at night may help to improve respiration during sleep. Long-term assisted ventilation in advanced muscular dystrophy raises ethical questions and is controversial.

Angiotensin-converting enzyme (ACE) inhibitors and/or beta-adrenergic blockers may be beneficial in treating and potentially preventing/delaying cardiomyopathy.

Future strategies for therapy

- Correction of genetic alterations: these are specific for certain types of mutations.
  - Antisense oligonucleotides can be used to induce exon skipping. Inducing the skipping of individual exons or pairs of exons can restore a disrupted reading frame and lead to the expression of a shortened but functional dystrophin protein. This in turn can ameliorate the clinical phenotype[17].
  - Aminoglycosides and newer drugs like PTC124 cause preferential stop-codon read-through in premature stop codons[17].
- Gene replacement:
  - Use of viral vectors to replace a mutated dystrophin gene.
  - Muscle tissue is unique because fusion of stem cells or stem cell-like cells to existing myofibers is a process of normal muscle repair. Bone marrow-derived stem cells as well as engineered muscle tissue-derived stem cells may therefore offer possible ways to replace a mutated dystrophin gene.
- Others:
  - Utrophin is a protein that is expressed at neuromuscular and musculotendinous junctions. It shows homology to dystrophin. Upregulation of utrophin may be able to compensate for some of the effects of dystrophin loss.
  - Inducing muscle hypertrophy by upregulating genes involved in muscle growth, such as insulin-like growth factor 1 (IGF-1) or L-arginine, may help to fight muscle wasting.
  - Blocking the effect of myostatin as a negative regulator of muscle mass could have a similar beneficial effect.

FACIOSCAPULOHUMERAL MUSCULAR DYSTROPHY

Definition

Facioscapulohumeral muscular dystrophy (FSHD) is the third most common muscular dystrophy after DMD and myotonic dystrophy, with an incidence of about 1/20,000. It is an autosomal dominant disease characterized by weakness and atrophy of facial, scapulohumeral, as well as anterior tibial muscles.

Etiology and pathophysiology

FSHD has been linked to genetic alterations in the subtelomeric portion of chromosome 4q35. This region normally contains 11 to over 100 so-called D4Z4 repeat elements[18]. FSHD patients show a contraction in the number of these D4Z4 repeats to fewer than 11. This results in inefficient repression of a retrogene *DUX4* and inappropriate DUX4 protein expression in muscle cells. The mechanisms underlying DUX4-induced muscle toxicity remain unclear.

Patients with one to three repeats remaining may show most severe disease, but in contrast to nucleotide repeat diseases, there is no clear anticipation and no strong correlation between the number of repeats and the clinical phenotype. The change in D4Z4 repeats is thought to result in complex changes in gene expression rather than simply alteration of a single gene.

Clinical features

- Asymmetry in weakness and muscle atrophy.
- Stepwise progression that may include long periods of stable disease. Often the disease shows a downwards progression with early involvement of facial muscles and late effects on pelvic girdle and leg muscles (**804, 805**).

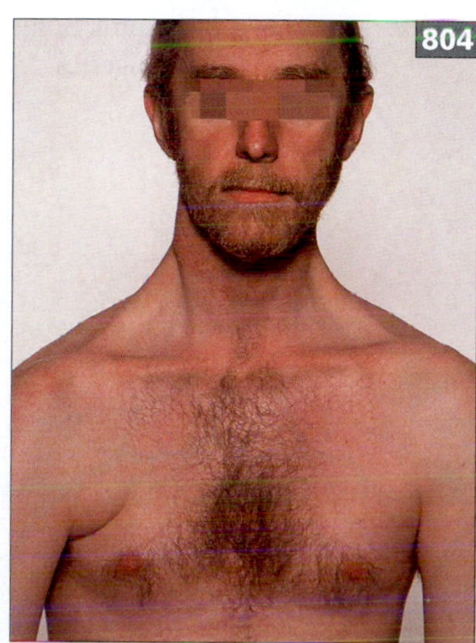

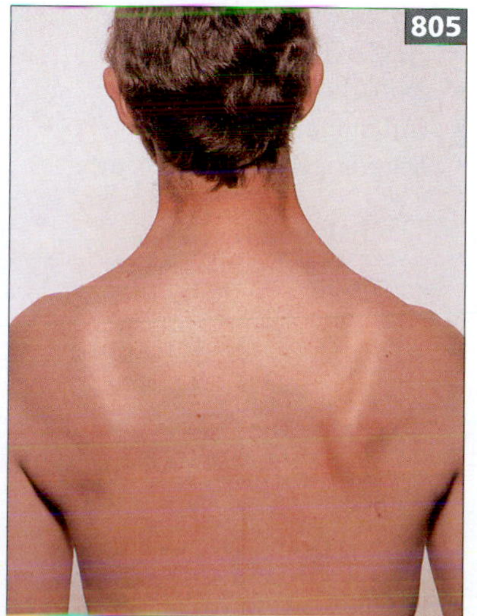

804, 805 Fascioscapulohumeral muscular dystrophy. Wasting and weakness of the muscles of the face, upper arms, and shoulders, with prominent atrophy of the pectoral muscles and winging of the scapulae.

- Facial weakness affecting the orbicularis oculi and orbicularis oris but sparing the masseter, temporalis, extraocular eye muscles, and oropharyngeal muscles.
- The muscles that fix the scapula to the chest, including the latissimus dorsi, lower trapezius, rhomboid, and serratus anterior, are prominently affected, leading to scapular elevation when raising the arms.
- Sternocleidomastoid, biceps, brachioradialis, and pectoralis muscles are typically weak and atrophic, while the deltoids and other distal arm muscles are relatively spared.
- Abdominal muscle weakness may lead to marked lumbar lordosis. If asymmetric it can lead to lateral positioning of the umbilicus when sitting up from a supine position (Beevor's sign).
- The tibialis anterior is often affected early, even when other pelvic and leg muscles are spared. This leads to foot drop in some patients. Only about 25% of all patients develop lower extremity weakness severe enough to require a wheelchair.
- Respiratory muscle involvement is uncommon.
- Clinically significant cardiac involvement is unusual. Some patients show evidence of cardiac arrhythmia.
- Pain is a frequent finding in FSHD patients.
- Subclinical retinal vasculopathy is relatively common but only rarely associated with clinically significant visual impairment.
- High-tone hearing loss is found in 25–65% of patients.

Differential diagnosis

The diagnosis of facial weakness in the patient or in family members is very helpful. A number of conditions may present with scapuloperoneal weakness:

- EMD (typically associated with contractures).
- Dsyferlin deficiency.
- Reducing body myopathy.
- Hyaline body myopathy.
- Acid maltase deficiency.
- Mitochondrial disease.
- Inflammatory myopathy.
- Scapuloperoneal syndrome.

Investigations and diagnosis

- Serum CK: normal or mild elevation (2–7 times normal).
- EMG: myopathic pattern.
- Muscle biopsy: as discussed below, the muscle biopsy may show myopathic changes with or without inflammation, but lacks specific features.
- Genetic testing: typically done by EcoRI/BlnI double digest. With a cutoff of 35 kb of DNA for the lower limit of normal, this test is 100% specific and 95% sensitive.

Pathology

- Morphologic findings vary widely, depending on the severity of the patient's phenotype and the site of the muscle biopsy.
- Muscle biopsies may show nonspecific myopathic changes with degeneration and regeneration of individual myofibers.
- There may be evidence of chronic remodeling in the form of endomysial fibrosis and fatty replacement
- Biopsies on FSHD patients may show significant perimysial or endomysial inflammatory infiltrates. This feature is shared with dysferlin deficiency and merosin deficiency, but is unusual in other muscular dystrophies.

Treatment

- Mild aerobic exercise may help to improve muscle tone.
- Ankle–foot orthoses are helpful in the management of foot-drop.
- The use of steroids during time of disease progression and the utility of scapular fixation surgery is debatable.
- For many FSHD patients, neck and back pain is the most limiting factor to their quality of life. Nonsteroidal anti-inflammatory agents are often helpful. Some patients require long-acting narcotic analgesics.

EMERY–DREIFUSS MUSCULAR DYSTROPHY

Definition

Emery–Dreifuss muscular dystrophy (EMD) is a condition that historically was characterized by the triad of: (1) slowly progressive muscle weakness and atrophy in a humeroperoneal distribution; (2) cardiomyopathy with conduction defects; (3) early contractures in Achilles tendon, spine muscles, and elbows.

Etiology and pathophysiology

- X-linked EMD (EMD1) is linked to mutations in the *STA* gene encoding emerin.
- Autosomal dominant (EMD2) and autosomal recessive (AR-EMD) presentations are linked to mutations in the *LMNA* gene encoding lamin A/C. Mutations in lamin A/C can also result in other clinical phenotypes that include LGMD1B, dilated cardiomyopathy with conduction defects, familial partial lipodystrophy, autosomal recessive axonal neuropathy (CMT2B1), and Hutchinson–Gilford progeria syndrome.
- Lamin A/C and emerin are part of the inner nuclear envelope. They are thought to have a role in maintaining nuclear shape and to be important for scaffolding DNA in the nucleus. Through DNA binding these proteins may influence gene expression.

Clinical features

- Muscle weakness and contractures precede the development of cardiac manifestations in most but not all cases.
- The degree of muscle involvement can vary from asymptomatic to debilitating between and even within families.
- Muscle weakness typically has humeroperoneal (EMD1) or scapulohumeroperoneal (EMD2) pattern. With progression, patients may develop some weakness of facial, thigh, and hand muscles. Loss of ambulation is more common with EMD2.
- Affected patients invariably develop cardiac disease manifestations during their adult life. Cardiac conduction defects typically progress from prolonged PR interval and sinus bradycardia to complete heart block and atrial paralysis. There is a risk of sudden cardiac death.
- Female carriers of EMD1 typically do not show evidence of skeletal muscle disease, but are at risk of cardiac involvement including sudden cardiac death.

Investigations and diagnosis

- Serum CK levels vary from normal to 10 times normal.
- ECG and echocardiogram: ECG can identify early cardiac involvement in younger patients. Arrhythmias are more severe during sleep; 24-hour monitoring may therefore be helpful. Annual Holter monitoring is advised for all patients with ECG abnormalities or those older than 17 years.
- EMG: myopathy pattern or normal.
- Genetic testing: can confirm the presence of an *STA* gene or *LMNA* gene mutation.

Pathology

The skeletal muscle may show nonspecific myopathic changes including an increase in myofiber size, an increased number of myofibers with internalized nuclei, and mild features of myofiber degeneration/regeneration.

EMD1 cases usually indicate a loss of emerin expression on immunocytochemical analysis. *LMNA* gene mutations, however, typically show preserved expression of lamin A/C.

Some studies have described irregularities of the nuclear membrane and the peripheral arrangement of heterochromatin by electron microscopy.

Treatment

- Pacemaker insertion is recommended for patients with a ventricular heart rate below 50 beats per minute. Implantation of an implantable cardioverter defibrillator helps to reduce the risk of sudden cardiac death.
- Prophylactic anticoagulation can reduce the risk of embolization.
- ACE inhibitors and diuretics are helpful in patients with symptomatic ventricular involvement.
- Cardiac transplantation may be considered in patients with dilated cardiomyopathy.
- Orthopedic surgery may help to alleviate symptoms from foot deformities and marked neck hyperextension.

LIMB-GIRDLE MUSCULAR DYSTROPHY

Definition

The LGMDs are a group of clinically as well as genetically heterogeneous diseases that share an autosomal inheritance pattern and predominant weakness of the proximal limb-girdle muscles. Some of the associated genes have been linked to other allelic diseases. The overall incidence is around 1:25,000–1:50,000. Cases with mutations in calpain3, dysferlin, FKRP, or one of the sarcoglycans are the most common forms.

Etiology and pathophysiology

LGMDs are inherited as autosomal dominant (LGMD1) or autosomal recessive (LGMD2) traits and are linked to a growing number of some 19 individual loci or genes as summarized in *Table 125*. The proteins encoded by these genes fall into several functional categories: (1) proteins of the cell membrane important for function of the dystrophin–glycoprotein complex; (2) other cell membrane proteins; (3) proteins associated with the contractile apparatus; (4) proteins with enzymatic functions; (5) proteins of the inner nuclear membrane[19].

TABLE 126 **CONGENITAL MUSCULAR DYSTROPHIES (CMDS)**

Disease group/ disease	Subgroup	Protein (gene)	Locus	Clinical features/allelic diseases/ characteristic pathologic features
Congenital muscular dystrophy with defects in extracellular matrix	Ullrich's congenital muscular dystrophy (UCMD)	Collagen VI A1, A2 or A3 (*COL6A1, COL6A2, COL6A3*)	2q37/ 21q22.3/ 21q22.3	Hypotonia, proximal contractures, distal hyperextensibility, scoliosis, proximal weakness; Bethlem is a milder allelic disease; biopsy: mismatched expression of perlecan and collagen VI by immunofluorescent microscopy
	Congenital muscular dystrophy 1A (MDCIA)	Merosin (*LAMA2*)	6q22–q23	Congenital muscular dystrophy; some LGMD-like; some with mostly subclinical cardiac disease; some have seizures or mental retardation
Congenital muscular dystrophies with the abnormalities in the receptors for extracellular matrix	Fukuyama congenital muscular dystrophy	Fukutin (*FKTN*)	9q31	Hypotonia; defects in CNS development, seizures, mental retardation
	Congenital muscular dystrophy 1C	Fukutin related protein, FKRP (*FKRP*)	19q13.3	Some with congenital muscular dystrophy; some with LGMD, some with cardiac disease, some with changes on brain MRI
	Congenital muscular dystrophy ID	Acetylglucosaminyl-transferase-like protein (*LARGE*)	22q12.3–q13.1	Congenital muscular dystrophy; mental retardation; structural brain changes
	Muscle–eye–brain disease (MEB)	Protein O-mannose beta-1,2-N-acylglucosaminyl-transferase (*POMGNT1*)	lp34–33	Congenital muscular dystrophy; congenital myopia, glaucoma, retinal hypoplasia; mental retardation
	Walker–Warburg syndrome (WWS)	Protein O-mannosyl-transferase-1 and 2 (*POMT1* and *POMT2*)	9q34.1 and 14q24.3	Congenital muscular dystrophy; structural brain changes and hydrocephalus; POMT also linked to LGMD2K
	Integrin alpha-7 deficiency	Integrin alpha-7 (*ITGA7*)	12q13	Delayed psychomotor milestones associated with dystrophic changes on biopsy
Congenital muscular dystrophy with abnormal endoplasmic reticulum protein	Rigid spine with muscular dystrophy 1 (RSMD1)	Selenoprotein1 (*SEPN1*)	1p36–p35	Hypotonia, neck weakness, early scoliosis, respiratory insufficiency; mutations in SEPN1: spectrum that includes desmin-related myopathy with Mallory bodies, congenital fiber type disproportion and RSMD1

Abbreviations: CMT: Charcot–Marie–Tooth disease; LGMD: limb-girdle muscular dystrophy.

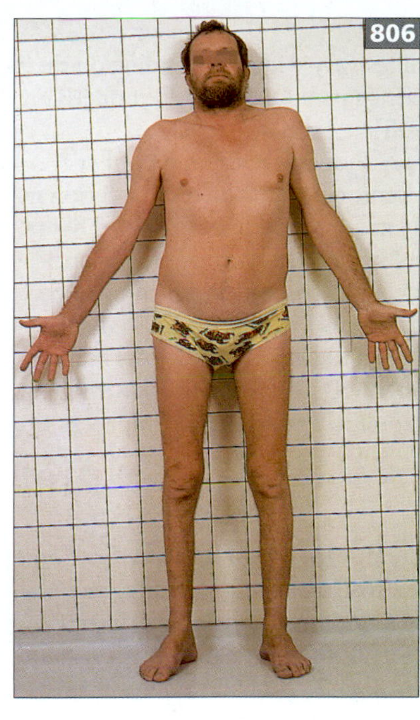

806 The limb-girdle muscular dystrophy phenotype: Note wasting of the proximal two-thirds of the deltoid (with pseudohypertrophy of the distal third), forearm flexors, thigh adductors, and medial heads of the gastrocnemius muscles.

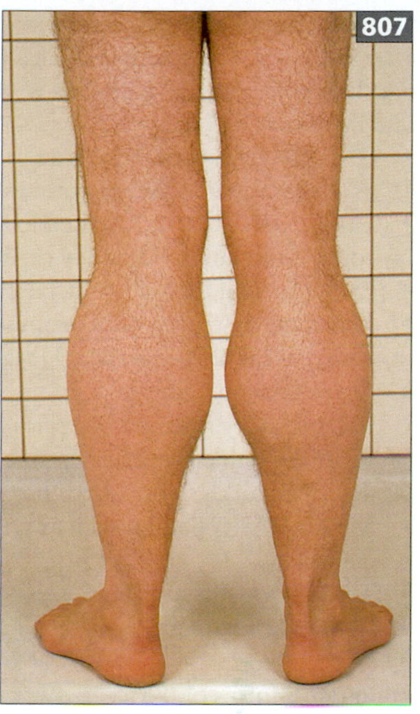

807 Calf hypertrophy in a 30-year-old man with sarcoglycanopathy.

Protein types

1. The dystrophin–glycoprotein complex (see 778) includes the sarcoglycans and dystroglycans. It is discussed above under dystrophinopathies (*Table 126*). Defects in sarcoglycans present as LGMD2C, 2D, 2E, 2F. Mutations in FKRP, POMT1, and Fukutin disrupt the function of glycosyl transferases that are important for the post-translational modification of alpha-dystroglycan in the DGC (778).
2. Caveolin 3 (LGMD1C) is the principal component of caveolae in striated muscle. Caveolin 3 oligomers are important in establishing membrane domains involved in cell signaling. Mutations affect oligomerization and therefore have a dominant negative effect. Dysferlin (LGMD2B) is a transmembrane protein that is thought to mediate the fusion of vesicles to the cell membrane to repair sites of injury and the fusion of vesicles during cell trafficking.
3. Mutations in sarcomeric (see 779) thin filaments are linked to nemaline myopathy (*Table 124*), and mutations in thick filaments to hypertrophic cardiomyopathy. LGMD has been linked to mutations of Z-disk proteins telethionin and myotilin as well as to mutations in titin. Beyond a pure mechanical role these proteins may also play important signaling functions.
4. Calpain 3 (LGMD2A) is a muscle-specific protease that has an important role in regulating other proteases as well as signaling pathways. It also interacts with dysferlin and may have a role in membrane resealing. TRIM32 (LGMD2H) is thought to play a role in the ubiquitin–proteasome pathway that is important for protein degradation.
5. Mutations in lamin A/C are linked to an LGMD phenotype (type 1B) in addition to other presentations discussed above under EDMD.

Clinical features

Table 125 summarizes some of the important specifics about individual LGMDs. The phenotype of different LGMDs is highly variable (**806, 807**). Features such as geographic location and ethnicity, cardiac involvement, calf or tongue hypertrophy, contractures, age of onset, and disease severity vary and can be suggestive of certain types. Patients typically have sparing of facial muscles and extraocular muscles. They typically lack cognitive changes found in some DMD patients. The autosomal recessive variants tend to have a more severe phenotype. Mutations in the sarcoglycans, particularly, are linked to early onset aggressive disease that may mimic DMD.

Differential diagnosis

Due to the wide spectrum in clinical phenotype, the general list of differential diagnoses to consider is also wide and includes:

- DMD/BMD especially in cases of early onset disease as seen with sarcoglycanopathies.
- Early cases of classic X-linked EDMD still lacking contractures and evidence of cardiac involvement.
- FSHD lacking prominent facial involvement.
- Myotonic dystrophy with prominent proximal muscle weakness, especially DM2. EMG is helpful.
- Congenital myopathies.
- Inflammatory myopathies especially in cases with relatively sudden onset in teenage years or later as described for dysferlin deficiency.
- Metabolic myopathies such as juvenile acid maltase deficiency.
- Toxic myopathy.
- Endocrine myopathy.
- Mitochondrial myopathy.
- Familial forms of IBM.

Investigations and diagnosis

- Serum CK is typically elevated:
  - In autosomal dominant cases the CK levels typically vary between normal and mild elevation.
  - Autosomal recessive patients more often show high CK levels, especially in cases of dysferlin deficiency and sarcoglycanopathies. These latter variants may be associated with 50- or 100-times normal levels. CK levels may drop with disease progression.
- ECG and echocardiogram: many types of LGMD are associated with cardiac involvement in the form of cardiac arrhythmia and/or cardiomyopathy.
- EMG: myopathic pattern, nonspecific changes or normal.
- MRI: can confirm the selective involvement of specific muscle groups.
- Muscle biopsy: the results of immunocytochemical studies can be helpful in guiding molecular tests.
- Genetic testing: establishes the definite classification and provides the basis for genetic counseling. It allows the assessment of risk of cardiac involvement that may require therapy.

Pathology

- Morphologic findings vary widely depending on the severity of the patient's phenotype and the underlying type of LGMD (808).
- Muscle biopsies may show evidence of myofiber degeneration/regeneration. Often there is variation in myofiber size with atrophic and hypertrophied fibers. Split fibers and lobulated fibers may be prominent.
- There may be evidence of chronic remodeling in the form of endomysial fibrosis and fatty replacement.
- Immunocytochemical studies may be helpful in the diagnosis of some LGMDs including those with defects in the dystrophin–glycoprotein complex and dysferlin.

Treatment

There is no curative therapy for any of the LGMDs. Some of the modalities used to treat DMD patients may also benefit sarcoglycanopathy patients, including surgery for scoliosis and ventilatory support for nocturnal respiratory failure. Because of smaller patient numbers there are only limited data on the use of corticosteroids in sarcoglycanopathy patients.

Depending on the underlying mutations patients should be followed and treated by a cardiologist. Placement of a cardiac pacing device will help to prevent sudden cardiac death in patients with *LMNA* mutation.

In general, future therapeutic strategies being considered for DMD patients may also apply for some LGMD patients. Smaller patient numbers complicate the study of these therapies.

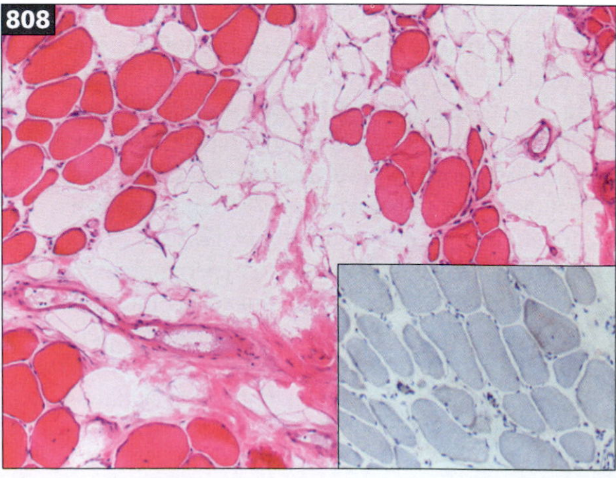

808 LGMD2B, dysferlin deficiency. This biopsy shows chronic remodeling with fatty replacement and increased variation in myofiber size. Normal immunohistochemical staining for dysferlin outlines myofibers in a pattern similar to staining seen with dystrophin (803). In this sample, expression of dysferlin is lacking (insert).

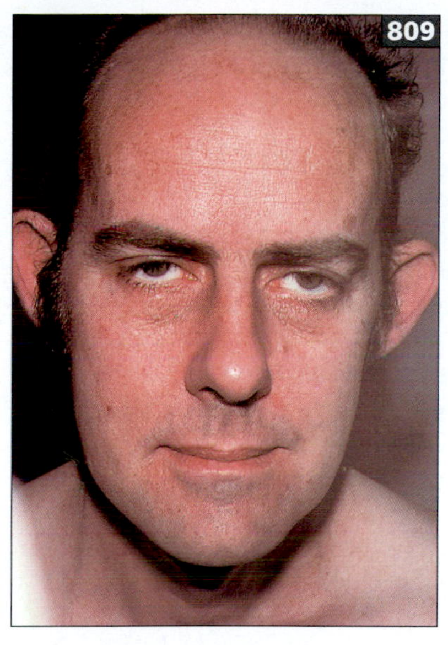

809 Myotonic dystrophy. Frontal alopecia and myopathic facies, with ptosis and wasting of temporalis, masseters, and sternocleidomastoids.

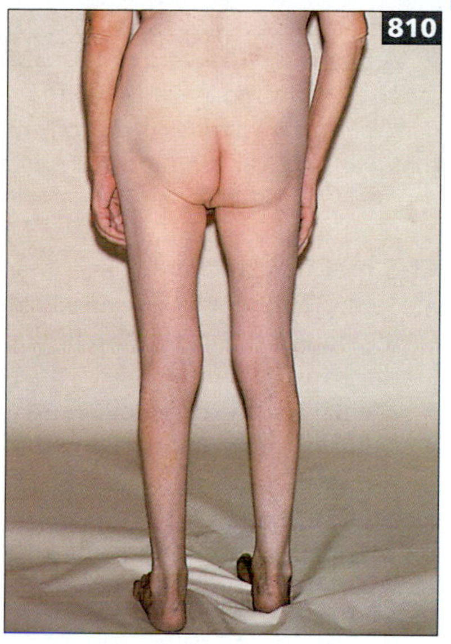

810 Myotonic dystrophy. Wasting of the distal limb muscles such as forearm, anterior tibial muscles, and calf muscles.

MYOTONIC DYSTROPHY

Definition and epidemiology

An autosomal dominant multi-system disorder characterized by myotonia, weakness, muscle wasting, typical facies, cataracts, cardiac arrhythmias, and endocrinopathies. Myotonic dystrophy type 1 is due to a mutation causing an expanded CTG repeat in the *DMPK* gene on chromosome 19 which encodes for a putative serine threonine protein kinase; myotonic dystrophy type 2 is due to an expanded CCTG repeat of the zinc finger protein 9 (*ZNF9*) gene on chromosome 3.

- The most common form of muscular dystrophy in adults.
- Incidence: 12–14/100,000 live births.
- Prevalence: 1 in 20,000.
- Age: any age.
- Gender: M=F.

Etiology and pathophysiology

Myotonic dystrophy is a RNA-mediated disease where long expansion of CUG or CCUG RNA repeats leads to abnormal regulation of alternative splicing, thereby affecting multiple pathways. Other postulated mechanisms in DM1 include *DMPK* reduction, and effect on neighboring genes such as *SIX5* (implicated in cataracts).

Expanded CUG repeats fold into ds(CUG) hairpins that sequester nuclear proteins including human Muscleblind-like (MBNL) and hnRNP H alternative splicing factors. Myotonia results from reduced expression of chloride channel (CLC-1) either due to dysregulated splicing of the CLC-1 premRNA or decreased transcription of the CLC-1 gene.

The disease range of CTG repeat numbers is 50 to 4000. The length of the repeat correlates directly with the severity of the disease and inversely with the age of onset. Anticipation occurs due to tendency of repeats to expand with successive generations.

Clinical features

Systemic symptoms

- Cardiac arrhythmias (e.g. first degree block, bundle branch block, tachyarrhythmia particularly during perioperative period).
- Subcapsular cataracts (Christmas tree cataracts).
- Gastrointestinal dysfunction (e.g. dysphagia, vomiting, diarrhea).
- Endocrinopathies (e.g. diabetes, thyroid disease, testicular atrophy).
- Early frontal balding.
- Skull abnormalities (hyperostosis, small pituitary fossa).
- Respiratory defects (hypoventilation, reduced response to hypoxia).

Neuromuscular symptoms and signs

- Ptosis and occasional diplopia.
- Hatched and thin face (weakness of facial muscles with temporalis and masseter atrophy), dysarthria, and weakness of sternocleidomastoid muscles (**809**).
- Limb weakness which is predominantly distal in myotonic dystrophy type 1 (**810**), and proximal in myotonic dystrophy type 2. The latter usually has milder neuromuscular and nonneuromuscular symptoms compared to myotonic dystrophy type 1.
- Diaphragmatic weakness.
- Grip or percussion myotonia, muscle stiffness, or cramps.

Tip

▶ *Myotonia is characterized by inability to relax a muscle after voluntary movement or with percussion. EMG correlates of myotonia consist of rhythmic discharges that wax and wane in amplitude and frequency.*

CNS manifestations

- Somnolence due to a disturbance of central mechanisms, but may also be due to obstructive sleep apnea.
- Mental apathy or mental retardation.
- White matter changes on brain MRI.

Special forms

Congenital myotonic dystrophy

- Present since birth.
- The abnormal gene is transmitted exclusively through maternal inheritance. CTG repeats range from 730 to 4300. There may be aberrant methylation of dinucleotide CpGs in the region of the CTG repeat at DM1 locus.
- The fetus shows hydramnios and reduced fetal movements.
- Neonates show respiratory distress, bilateral facial weakness, and hypotonia.
- In children mental retardation is a major feature; 75% of patients need special education, and 75% of the remainder at mainstream schools require further assistance to achieve minimum standards in reading and counting.
- There is a high prevalence of cardiac and gastrointestinal involvement.
- 25% die before 18 months of age, and 50% survive into the mid-30s.

Differential diagnosis of myotonia

- Myotonic dystrophies type 1 and 2.
- Myotonia congenita (dominant and recessive forms).
- Paramyotonia congenita.
- Hyperkalemic periodic paralysis.
- Hypothyroid myopathy.
- Drugs: lipid lowering agents, beta-blockers, and depolarizing muscle relaxants (e.g. succinylcholine) may cause or exacerbate myotonia.

Investigations and diagnosis

- Blood: fasting glucose, thyroid function tests, serum IgG reduced, CK (normal or mildly elevated).
- Slit lamp examination: cataracts.
- ECG:
  - An annual ECG is recommended because ECG changes are often a predictor of development of cardiac symptoms.
  - Ventricular late-potentials may be predictive of ventricular arrhythmias. However, potentially fatal heart block or rhythm disturbances can occur despite a normal ECG.
  - As the perioperative period is a particularly dangerous time with respect to development of tachyarrhythmias and heart block, the anesthesiologist must always be made aware of the diagnosis of myotonic dystrophy.
  - A 24-hour Holter is indicated if cardiac symptoms are present or a significant change occurs on the ECG.
  - EMG: myotonic discharges with or without myopathic changes.
  - Molecular DNA analysis: CTG triplet or CCTG quadruplet repeat expansion.

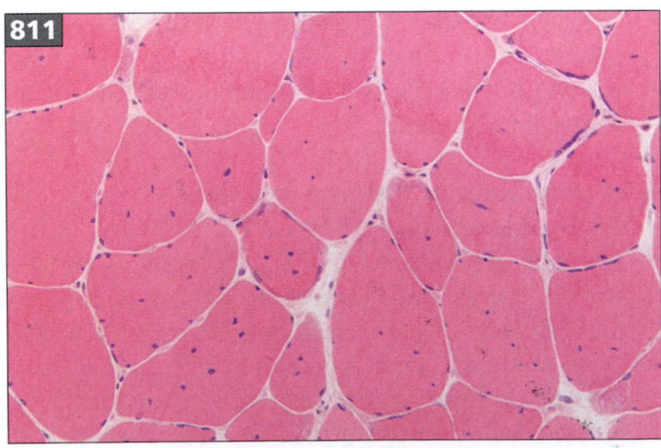

811 Myotonic dystrophy. H&E section showing increased variation in myofiber size, with atrophic and hypertrophied fibers. There is prominent internalization and random location of nuclei throughout the fiber cytoplasm.

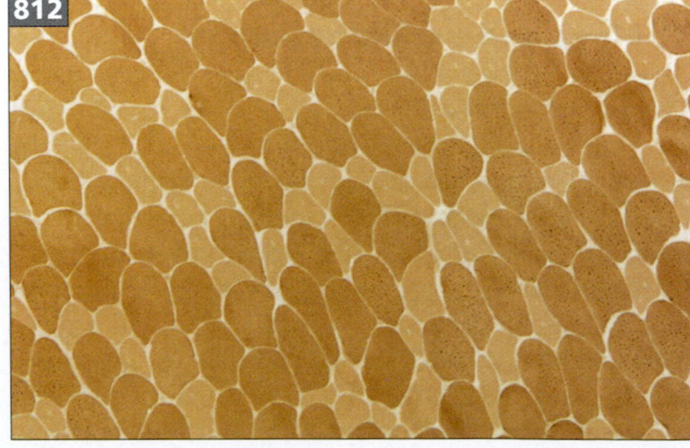

812 Myotonic dystrophy. The ATPase reaction at pH 9.4 shows preferential atrophy of light-stained type I fibers, with relative sparing of type II fibers.

Diagnosis is clinical and from EMG, but is confirmed by genetic testing.

Pathology

- Large numbers of internal nuclei (**811**), often occurring in long chains, together with sarcoplasmic masses and ring-fibers.
- Increased variability in fiber size.
- Increased endomysial and interfascicular fibrous tissue.
- Moth-eaten fibers.
- Individual necrotic and regenerating fibers are rare.
- Type I fibers appear smaller than Type II fibers (**812**).

Treatment

The main goals are prevention and treatment of systemic disease. In general, patients do not complain much about myotonia. Any improvement in myotonia may not necessarily translate to functional benefit for patients whose symptoms are more as a result of weakness than myotonia.

Medications for myotonia

- Phenytoin 100–200 mg bid orally can alleviate disabling and bothersome myotonia with reasonable efficacy and safety.
- Topiramate 50–100 mg bid.
- Antimyotonic drugs such as quinine sulfate, disopyramide (100–200 mg three times daily) and procainamide (250–500 mg four times daily) prolong the PR interval and can impair cardiac conduction. Other medications to avoid include amitriptyline, digoxin, propranolol, and sedatives.

Treatment of excessive daytime sleepiness

- Life-style advice: take short naps at convenient times, such as after meals, to minimize disruption of daily activities.
- Methylphenidate or modafinil may be helpful.
- Continuous positive airway pressure if there is sleep apnea or hypercapnia.

Prognosis

Sudden death is well recognized, and may be due to heart block, other arrhythmia, or respiratory failure.

MUSCLE CHANNELOPATHIES (DISORDERS OF MEMBRANE EXCITABILITY)

MYOTONIA CONGENITA

Definition and epidemiology

- Myotonia congenita, the most common muscle channelopathy, is caused by mutations in the skeletal muscle chloride channel gene *CLCN1*, and is distinguished from myotonic dystrophy by the absence of progressive weakness and systemic features. The autosomal dominant form is called Thomsen's disease, while the recessive form is called Becker's disease.

The world wide prevalence is estimated to be approximately 1 in 100,000, but varies depending on the region (7–10 per 100,000 in Scandinavia). Myotonic symptoms are generally more severe in males than in females.

Etiology and pathophysiology

Normal muscle requires a high resting chloride conductance for stabilization of membrane excitability and for fast repolarization of transverse tubules. Mutations in *CLCN1* result in decreased chloride current at the physiologic range, predisposing it to the hyperexcitability induced by K^+ accumulation in the T-tubules[20–22]. An approximately 80% decrease in chloride conductance is required to cause myotonia.

Recessive mutations lead to loss of function, while dominant mutations exert a dominant negative effect on co-expressed wild type, and shift the voltage-dependence of *CLCN1* to more positive voltages. The same mutation (e.g. R894X) can cause recessive or dominant myotonia congenita in different families.

Different allelic expression and dosage effect contribute to the intrafamilial and interfamilial variability.

Clinical features

- Age of onset is variable (childhood to after 40), but is generally later in Becker's disease than in Thomsen's disease.
- Myotonia may involve grip, eyelid, tongue (mild to moderate in Thomsen's, moderate to severe in Becker's). Symptoms are not or mildly aggravated by cold and reduced by repetitive contractions (warm-up phenomenon).
- Muscle hypertrophy is common.
- Weakness has been reported in the recessive form.

Differential diagnosis

Similar to the ones listed under myotonic dystrophies above.

Investigations and diagnosis

- CK: slightly elevated or normal.
- EMG: myotonic discharges: motor units are normal in Thomsen's, but may be mildly myopathic in Becker's.
- Repetitive nerve stimulation: decrement at high frequency.
- Genetic testing for *CLCN1* mutations.

Diagnosis is based on clinical features and EMG, but is confirmed by genetic testing. The histopathologic findings are minimal or nonspecific.

Treatment

- Dilantin (300–400 mg/day).
- Quinine (200–1,200 mg/day).
- Topiramate (50–100 mg bid).
- Mexiletine (150 mg bid to 300 mg tid)[23].
- Procainamide (125–1000 mg/day).
- Tocainide (bone marrow suppression is a side-effect).
- Acetazolamide (125–750 mg/day).

PARAMYOTONIA CONGENITA (EULENBURG'S DISEASE) AND POTASSIUM AGGRAVATED MYOTONIAS

Definition

Paramyotonia congenita is an autosomal dominant disorder characterized by episodic cold-induced or exercise-induced myotonia in exposed areas lasting minutes to hours. Potassium aggravated myotonias (PAMs) are characterized by worsening of myotonia with potassium ingestion and include myotonia fluctuans, myotonia permanens, and acetazolamide-sensitive myotonia.

Etiology and pathophysiology

Mutations of the skeletal muscle Na^+ channel gene *SCN4A* produce a spectrum of disorders characterized by myotonia and periodic paralysis, depending on the magnitude of membrane depolarization[24,25]. Mild membrane depolarization (5–10 mV) causes repetitive firing of action potentials (myotonia), while strong depolarization (20–30 mV) causes inactivation of Na^+ channels and electrical silence (paralysis).

Functional defects in mutant Na channels cause impaired inactivation and abnormal voltage-dependence.

Clinical features

- Paradoxical myotonia (stiffness worsens rather than improves with repetitive contractions).
- Myotonia worsens with cold exposure in paramyotonia congenita, but may or may not do so in PAMs.
- Usually no persistent weakness occurs, although paramyotonia congenita may progress later in life to weakness.
- Muscle hypertrophy is less frequent than in myotonia congenita.

Differential diagnosis

Similar to those listed for myotonia under myotonic dystrophy.

Investigations and diagnosis

- EMG: myotonic discharges are less prominent than in other myotonic disorders and may be absent at normal temperature.
- Cooling: initially induces myotonic discharges which disappear with prolonged or increased cooling in paramyotonia congenita. The effect of cooling is absent or mild in PAMs.
- Genetic testing for *SCN4A* mutations.

Diagnosis is based on clinical features and EMG, but is confirmed by genetic testing. Muscle biopsy may show variation in fiber diameter or increase in central nuclei (nonspecific changes).

Treatment

Same as listed for myotonia congenita.

HYPERKALEMIC PERIODIC PARALYSIS

Definition

Hyperkalemic periodic paralysis (HyperPP) is an autosomal dominant disorder characterized by episodes of flaccid muscle weakness associated with hyperkalemia and is caused by mutations in *SCN4A*[25,26].

Etiology and pathophysiology

Extracellular K^+ increases → mild depolarization → opening of normal and mutant Na^+ channels → persistent inward current from noninactivating mutant Na^+ channels → sustained depolarization → inactivation of normal Na^+ channels → further membrane depolarization → paralysis.

A small fraction of noninactivating Na^+ channels (2%) causes myotonia, while a larger fraction causes paralysis. T704M and M1592V mutations in *SCN4A* account for most of th e cases.

Clinical features

- Attacks of limb paralysis usually begin in childhood (first decade) and increase in frequency during puberty.
- Triggers include ingestion of K^+ rich foods, rest after strenuous exercise, cold exposure, stress, fasting; relieved by carbohydrate intake and mild exercise.
- Episodes of paralysis last 15 min to 1 hr.
- Permanent weakness may ensue.
- Myotonia may be present in between attacks of weakness.

Differential diagnosis

- Hypokalemic periodic paralysis.
- Thyrotoxic periodic paralysis.
- MGand other NMJ disorders.
- Guillain–Barré syndrome.
- Sleep disorders (cataplexy or sleep paralysis).
- Multiple sclerosis.
- Transient ischemic attack.

Investigations

- Serum K^+.
- CK may be normal to slightly increased.
- EMG: exercise test shows increased CMAP amplitude during and immediately after sustained (5 min) maximal contraction, which progressively reduces (by 40%) during rest 20–40 min after initial increment[27,28].
- Provocative test: oral K^+ load only if serum K^+, cardiac and renal functions are normal.
- Genetic testing.

Diagnosis

Diagnosis is based on clinical features and EMG, plus results of genetic testing or provocative test.

Muscle biopsy may show vacuolar changes, tubular aggregates, or nonspecific changes.

Treatment

- Carbohydrate ingestion may be given during attacks, though most attacks are brief and do not require treatment.
- Acetazolamide or thiazide is given for prophylaxis.

HYPOKALEMIC PERIODIC PARALYSIS

Definition and epidemiology

Hypokalemic periodic paralysis (HypoPP) is an autosomal dominant disorder characterized by episodes of flaccid muscle weakness associated with hypokalemia. Types of hypoPP include:

- HypoPP1 (mutations in calcium channel gene [*CACNA1S*] dihydropyridine receptor) (most common).
- HypoPP2 (*SCN4A* mutations).
- HypoPP3 (*KCNE3*).
- Thyrotoxic periodic paralysis (*KCNJ18*).
- Andersen syndrome (*KCNJ2*).
- Distal renal tubular acidosis (*SLC4A1*).

HypoPP is the most common type of periodic paralysis, with prevalence of 1 in 100,000.

- Age: young adults.
- Gender: M>F.
- Thyrotoxic periodic paralysis is most common in Asians, Latin Americans, and native Americans.

Etiology and pathophysiology

- Mutations in the voltage sensor (S4) of the CACNA1S channel impair the transduction of the depolarization signal to the ryanodine receptors and, as a result, there is a defect in excitation–contraction coupling.
- Mutations in the voltage sensor of SCN4A result in enhanced channel inactivation and lead to slow and small action potentials.
- In thyrotoxic periodic paralysis, KCNJ18 is transcriptionally regulated by thyroid hormones.

Clinical features

- Onset: early childhood to 30s.
- Attacks begin in early morning hours, and triggered by physical activity, carbohydrate-rich meal, and alcohol in the preceding day.
- Truncal musculature is weak; cranial nerves are spared except in thyrotoxic periodic paralysis where bulbar muscles and respiratory muscles may be involved.
- Duration of attack: hours to days (longer than hyperPP).
- Myotonia: focal in eyelids, usually not in limbs.
- Older patients may have proximal myopathy.
- In hypoPP2, myalgias are prominent.
- Rhabdomyolysis may occur in some patients.
- Attacks are aggravated by acetazolamide in hypoPP2 and thyrotoxic PP.

Differential diagnosis

Same as listed for hyperPP.

Investigations and diagnosis

- Serum K^+, TSH.
- CMAP is small during attacks, but similar results with exercise test as in hyperPP.
- Provocative tests: glucose plus insulin.
- Genetic testing for mutations in *CACNA1S*, *SCN4A*, *KCNJ18*.

Diagnosis is based on clinical presentation and laboratory investigations, including genetic testing.

Pathology

Muscle biopsy may show predominance of vacuolar changes in hypoPP1, and tubular aggregates in hypoPP2. Other changes include internal nuclei and vacuolar dilatation of sarcoplasmic reticulum.

Treatment

- Oral potassium supplement.
- Correct thyrotoxicosis if present.
- Acetazolamide except in hypoPP2 and thyrotoxic PP.

MALIGNANT HYPERTHERMIA

Definition

An autosomal dominant disorder characterized by susceptibility to a number of drugs, particularly anesthetics such as halothane and succinylcholine. Other drugs, including tricyclic antidepressants, monoamine oxidase inhibitors, methoxyflurane, ketamine, enflurane, diethyl ether, and cyclopropane, can cause malignant hyperthermia.

Etiology and pathophysiology

- Due to a malfunction of the calcium channel of the sarcoplasmic reticulum (the ryanodine receptor). The abnormal ryanodine receptor may accentuate calcium release.
- The gene for the ryanodine receptor (*RYR1*) maps to chromosome 19 (13–1). Some mutations in *RYR1* cause malignant hyperthermia, some central core disease, and some both.
- Fast, uncontrolled increase in skeletal muscle metabolism associated with rhabdomyolysis may also occur in association with dystrophinopathies.

Clinical features

- Rapid elevation of temperature which may rise to 43°C (109°F).
- Tachycardia.
- Muscle rigidity (e.g. begins with trismus).
- Areflexia.
- Coma.

Differential diagnosis

- Neuroleptic malignant syndrome: also presents with high fever, rigidity, tachycardia, and rhabdomyolysis, but it is of slower onset over days to weeks, is not familial, and is usually triggered by drugs that block central dopaminergic pathways, such as phenothiazines, lithium, and haloperidol, or can occur after discontinuation of L-dopa for Parkinson's disease.
- Sepsis.
- Hyperthyroid crisis.
- Heat stroke.
- Pheochromocytoma crisis.

Investigations

- Arterial blood gases: metabolic acidosis.
- Serum CK: precipitous rise, sometimes to 10,000 times the normal values.
- Blood coagulation profile: may show evidence for disseminated intravascular coagulation.
- Urine: myoglobinuria.

Diagnosis

RYR1 gene mutations are identified in up to 80% of individuals with confirmed malignant hyperthermia[29,30].

- Halothane and caffeine contracture tests.
- Contracture of muscle (obtained from a fresh muscle biopsy) when exposed to 3% halothane or increasing concentrations of caffeine.
- This test may be considered to diagnose MH when genetic testing is not available or comes back negative in clinically suspected cases.

Pathology

- There are no specific morphologic changes.
- *In vitro* contracture testing with halothane, caffeine, and ryanodine on fresh muscle has been used to confirm the diagnosis.
- Central core disease and malignant hyperthermia are both linked to mutations in the ryanodine receptor. Some patients with central core disease (see *Table 124*) have malignant hyperthermia and some patients with malignant hyperthermia show central cores on muscle biopsy.

Treatment

- Mild cases: discontinue the anesthetic (succinylcholine and inhalational anesthetic).
- More severe cases:
  - Dantrolene 2 mg/kg IV q 5 min, up to 10 mg/kg: inhibits calcium release from the sarcoplasmic reticulum.
  - Treat associated hyperkalemia.
  - Increase ventilation.
  - Correct the acid–base disturbance: give IV sodium bicarbonate 2–4 mg/kg.
  - Cool the patient: cooling blankets and cold IV fluids until temperature reaches 38°C (100°F).
  - Intravenous hydration with or without diuretics if myoglobinuria is present.
  - Give steroids for the acute stress reaction.

Prevention and prognosis

- If the disease-related mutation is known, the relatives of affected patients should be tested for that mutation.
- Barbiturate, nitrous oxide, and opiate nondepolarizing relaxant anesthesia should not induce malignant hyperthermia.
- There is a high mortality rate unless the patient is immediately diagnosed and treated.
- The patients may also have complications such as myoglobinuria, renal failure, and disseminated intravascular coagulation.
- With immediate diagnosis and treatment, mortality and morbidity is less than 5%.

REFERENCES

1 Amato AA, Barohn RJ (2009). Evaluation and treatment of inflammatory myopathies. *J Neurol Neurosurg Psychiatry* **80**(10):1060–1068.

2 Miller FW (2012). New approaches to the assessment and treatment of the idiopathic inflammatory myopathies. *Ann Rheum Dis* **71**(Suppl 2):i82–i85.

3 Greenberg SA (2008). Proposed immunologic models of the inflammatory myopathies and potential therapeutic implications. *Neurology* **69**(21):2008–2019.

4 Greenberg SA (2010). Dermatomyositis and type 1 interferons. *Curr Rheumatol Rep* **12**(3):198–203.

5 Gordon PA, Winer JB, Hoogendijk JE, Choy EH (2012). Immunosuppressant and immunomodulatory treatment for dermatomyositis and polymyositis. *Cochrane Dat Syst Rev* **8**:CD003643.

6 Dalakas MC, Illa I, Dambrosia JM, *et al.* (1993). A controlled trial of high-dose intravenous immune globulin infusions as treatment for dermatomyositis. *N Engl J Med* **329**(27):1993–2000.

7 Miller FW, Leitman SF, Cronin ME, *et al.* (1992). Controlled trial of plasma exchange and leukapheresis in polymyositis and dermatomyositis. *N Engl J Med* **326**(21):1380–1384.

8 Barohn RJ, Watts GD, Amato AA (2009). A case of late-onset proximal and distal muscle weakness. *Neurology* **73**(19): 1592–1597.

9 Zink W, Kollmar R, Schwab S (2009). Critical illness polyneuropathy and myopathy in the intensive care unit. *Nat Rev Neurol* **5**(7):372–379.

10 Van Den Hout JM, Kamphoven JH, Winkel LP, *et al.* (2004). Long-term intravenous treatment of Pompe disease with recombinant human alpha-glucosidase from milk. *Pediatrics* **113**(5): e448–e457.

11 Cupler EJ, Berger KI, Leshner RT, *et al.*; AANEM Consensus Committee on Late-onset Pompe Disease (2012). Consensus treatment recommendations for late-onset Pompe disease. *Muscle Nerve* **45**(3): 319–333.

12 Taylor R, Schaefer A, Barron M, Mcfarland R, Turnbull D (2004). The diagnosis of mitochondrial muscle disease. *Neuromuscul Disord* **14**(4):237–245.

13 Laing N (2007). Congenital myopathies. *Curr Opin Neurol* **20**(5):583–589.

14 Mendell J, Boue D, Martin P (2006). The congenital muscular dystrophies: recent advances and molecular insights. *Pediatr Dev Pathol* **9**(6):427–443.

15 Hoffman E, Kunkel L (1989). Dystrophin abnormalities in Duchenne/Becker muscular dystrophy. *Neuron* **2**(1):1019–1029.

16 D'angelo M, Bresolin N (2006). Cognitive impairment in neuromuscular disorders. *Muscle Nerve* **34**(1):16–33.

17 Hoffman EP, Bronson A, Levin A, *et al.* (2011). Restoring dystrophin expression in Duchenne muscular dystrophy muscle – progress in exon skipping and stop codon read through. *Am J Pathol* **179**(1):12–22.

18 Richards M, Coppee F, Thomas N, *et al.* (2012). Facioscapulohumeral muscular dystrophy (FSHD): an enigma unravelled? *Hum Genet* **131**:325–340.

19 Broglio L, Tentorio M, Cotelli MS, *et al.* (2010). Limb-girdle muscular dystrophy-associated protein diseases. *Neurologist* **16**:340–352.

20 Koch MC, Steinmeyer K, Lorenz C, *et al.* (1992). The skeletal muscle chloride channel in dominant and recessive human myotonia. *Science* **257**(5071):797–800.

21 Pusch M, Steinmeyer K, Koch MC, Jentsch TJ (1995). Mutations in dominant human myotonia congenita drastically alter the voltage dependence of the CIC-1 chloride channel. *Neuron* **15**(6):1455–1463.

22 Platt D, Griggs R (2009). Skeletal muscle channelopathies: new insights into the periodic paralyses and nondystrophic myotonias. *Curr Opin Neurol* **22**(5):524–531.

23 Statland JM, Bundy BN, Wang Y, *et al.*; Consortium for Clinical Investigation of Neurologic Channelopathies (2012). Mexiletine for symptoms and signs of myotonia in nondystrophic myotonia: a randomized controlled trial. *JAMA* **308**(13):1357–1365.

24 Cannon SC, Strittmatter SM (1993). Functional expression of sodium channel mutations identified in families with periodic paralysis. *Neuron* **10**(2):317–326.

25 Jurkat-Rott K, Lehmann-Horn F (2005). Muscle channelopathies and critical points in functional and genetic studies. *J Clin Invest* **115**(8):2000–2009.

26 Cannon SC, Brown RH Jr, Corey DP (1991). A sodium channel defect in hyperkalemic periodic paralysis: potassium-induced failure of inactivation. *Neuron* **6**(4):619–626.

27 Kuntzer T, Flocard F, Vial C, *et al.* (2000). Exercise test in muscle channelopathies and other muscle disorders. *Muscle Nerve* **23**(7):1089–1094.

28 Fournier E, Arzel M, Sternberg D, *et al.* (2004). Electromyography guides toward subgroups of mutations in muscle channelopathies. *Ann Neurol* **56**(5):650–661.

29 MacLennan DH, Duff C, Zorzato F, *et al.* (1990). Ryanodine receptor gene is a candidate for predisposition to malignant hyperthermia. *Nature* **343**(6258):559–561.

30 Seo MD, Velamakanni S, Ishiyama N, *et al.* (2012). Structural and functional conservation of key domains in InsP3 and ryanodine receptors. *Nature* **483**(7387):108–112.

Further reading

General

Dubowitz V, Sewry CA (2007). *Muscle biopsy: a Practical Approach*, 3rd edn. Saunders/Elsevier, Philadelphia.

Engel A, Franzini-Armstrong C (2004). *Myology*, 3rd edn. McGraw-Hill Medical Pub Div, New York.

van Adel BA, Tarnopolsky MA (2009). Metabolic myopathies: update 2009. *J Clin Neuromuscul Dis* **10**(3):97–121.

Inflammatory myopathies

Amato AA, Griggs RC (2003). Treatment of idiopathic inflammatory myopathies. *Curr Opin Neurol* **16**(5):569–575.

Callen JP (2000). Dermatomyositis. *Lancet* **355**(9197):53–57.

Dalakas MC (1998). Controlled studies with high-dose intravenous immunoglobulin in the treatment of dermatomyositis, inclusion body myositis, and polymyositis. *Neurology* **51**(6 Suppl 5):S37–S45.

Dalakas MC, Hohlfeld R (2003). Polymyositis and dermatomyositis. *Lancet* **362**(9388):971–982.

Gordon PA, Winer JB, Hoogendijk JE, Choy EH (2012). Immunosuppressant and immunomodulatory treatment for dermatomyositis and polymyositis. *Cochrane Dat Syst Rev* **8**:CD003643.

Needham M, Mastaglia FL (2007). Inclusion body myositis: current pathogenetic concepts and diagnostic and therapeutic approaches. *Lancet Neurol* **6**(7):620–631.

Peng A, Koffman BM, Malley JD, Dalakas MC (2000). Disease progression in sporadic inclusion body myositis: observations in 78 patients. *Neurology* **55**(2):296–298.

Van Der Meulen MF, Bronner IM, Hoogendijk JE, *et al.* (2003). Polymyositis: an overdiagnosed entity. *Neurology* **61**(3):316–321.

Metabolic, endocrine, and mitochondrial myopathies

Amato A (2000). Acid maltase deficiency and related myopathies. *Neurol Clin* **18**(1):151–165.

Andersen ST, Haller RG, Vissing J (2008). Effect of oral sucrose shortly before exercise on work capacity in McArdle disease. *Arch Neurol* **65**(6):786–789.

Devries MC, Tarnopolsky MA (2008). Muscle physiology in healthy men and women and those with metabolic myopathies. *Neurol Clin* **26**(1):115–148.

Klein I, Ojamaa K (2000). Thyroid (neuro) myopathy. *Lancet* **356**(9230):614.

Rosenow EC IIIrd, Engel AG (1978). Acid maltase deficiency in adults presenting as respiratory failure. *Am J Med* **64**(3): 485–491.

Vorgerd M, Grehl T, Jager M, *et al.* (2000). Creatine therapy in myophosphorylase deficiency (McArdle disease): a placebo-controlled crossover trial. *Arch Neurol* **57**(7):956–963.

Critical illness myopathy

Khan J, Harrison TB, Rich MM (2008). Mechanisms of neuromuscular dysfunction in critical illness. *Crit Care Clin* **24**(1):165–177.

Lacomis D, Zochodne DW, Bird SJ (2000). Critical illness myopathy. *Muscle Nerve* **23**(12):1785–1788.

Muscular dystrophies and congenital myopathies

Brook JD, Mccurrach ME, Harley HG, *et al.* (1992). Molecular basis of myotonic dystrophy: expansion of a trinucleotide (CTG) repeat at the 3' end of a transcript encoding a protein kinase family member. *Cell* **68**(4):799–808.

Chakkalakal J, Thompson J, Parks R, Jasmin B (2005). Molecular, cellular, and pharmacological therapies for Duchenne/Becker muscular dystrophies. *FASEB J* **19**(8): 880–891.

Cossu G, Sampaolesi M (2007). New therapies for Duchenne muscular dystrophy: challenges, prospects and clinical trials. *Trends Mol Med* **13**(12):520–526.

Den Dunnen J, Beggs A (2006). Multiplex PCR for identifying DMD gene deletions. *Curr Protoc Hum Genet* Chapter 9 (Unit 9.3).

Den Dunnen J, Grootscholten P, Bakker E, *et al.* (1989). Topography of the Duchenne muscular dystrophy (DMD) gene: FIGE and cDNA analysis of 194 cases reveals 115 deletions and 13 duplications. *Am J Hum Genet* **45**(6):835–847.

Dubowitz V (1975). Neuromuscular disorders in childhood. Old dogmas, new concepts. *Arch Dis Child* **50**(5):335–346.

Goebel H (2003). Congenital myopathies at their molecular dawning. *Muscle Nerve* **27**(5):527–548.

Groh WJ, Groh MR, Saha C, *et al.* (2008). Electrocardiographic abnormalities and sudden death in myotonic dystrophy type 1. *N Engl J Med* **358**(25):2688–2697.

Guglieri M, Straub V, Bushby K, Lochmuller H (2008). Limb-girdle muscular dystrophies. *Curr Opin Neurol* **21**(5):576–584.

Jiang H, Mankodi A, Swanson MS, Moxley RT, Thornton CA (2004). Myotonic dystrophy type 1 is associated with nuclear foci of mutant RNA, sequestration of muscleblind proteins and deregulated alternative splicing in neurons. *Hum Mol Genet* **13**(24): 3079–3088.

Koenig M, Hoffman E, Bertelson C, *et al.* (1987). Complete cloning of the Duchenne muscular dystrophy (DMD) cDNA and preliminary genomic organization of the DMD gene in normal and affected individuals. *Cell* **50**(3):509–517.

Meola G, Moxley RT IIIrd (2004). Myotonic dystrophy type 2 and related myotonic disorders. *J Neurol* **251**(10):1173–1182.

Mercuri E, Jungbluth H, Muntoni F (2005). Muscle imaging in clinical practice: diagnostic value of muscle manetic resonance imaging in inherited neuromuscular disorders. *Curr Opin Neurol* **18**(5):526–537.

Nishino I (2006). Autophagic vacuolar myopathy. *Semin Pediatr Neurol* **13**(2):90–95.

Norwood F, De Visser M, Eymard B, Lochmuller H, Bushby K (2007). EFNS guideline on diagnosis and management of limb girdle muscular dystrophies. *Eur J Neurol* **14**(12):1305–1312.

Ranum LP, Day JW (2004). Myotonic dystrophy: RNA pathogenesis comes into focus. *Am J Hum Genet* **74**(5):793–804.

Ranum LP, Rasmussen PF, Benzow KA, Koob MD, Day JW (1998). Genetic mapping of a second myotonic dystrophy locus. *Nat Genet* **19**(2):196–198.

Roux K, Burke B (2007). Nuclear envelope defects in muscular dystrophy. *Biochim Biophys Acta* **1772**(2):118–127.

Schoser BG, Ricker K, Schneider-Gold C, *et al.* (2004). Sudden cardiac death in myotonic dystrophy type 2. *Neurology* **63**(12): 2402–2404.

Tawil R (2008). Facioscapulohumeral muscular dystrophy. *Neurotherapeutics* **5**(4): 601–606.

Tubridy N, Fontaine B, Eymard B (2001). Congenital myopathies and congenital muscular dystrophies. *Curr Opin Neurol* **14**(5):575–582.

Wheeler TM, Thornton CA (2007). Myotonic dystrophy: RNA-mediated muscle disease. *Curr Opin Neurol* **20**(5):572–576.

Toxic myopathies

Kuncl RW (2009). Agents and mechanisms of toxic myopathy. *Curr Opin Neurol* **22**(5):506–515.

Sieb JP, Gillessen T (2003). Iatrogenic and toxic myopathies. *Muscle Nerve* **27**(2):142–156.

Skeletal muscle channelopathies

Colding-Jorgensen E (2005). Phenotypic variability in myotonia congenita. *Muscle Nerve* **32**(1):19–34.

Matthews E, Labrum R, Sweeney MG, *et al.* (2009). Voltage sensor charge loss accounts for most cases of hypokalemic periodic paralysis. *Neurology* **72**(18): 1544–1547.

Miller TM (2008). Differential diagnosis of myotonic disorders. *Muscle Nerve* **37**(3):293–299.

Ptacek LJ, Tawil R, Griggs RC, *et al.* (1994). Dihydropyridine receptor mutations cause hypokalemic periodic paralysis. *Cell* **77**(6):863–868.

Ptacek LJ, Tawil R, Griggs RC, *et al.* (1994). Sodium channel mutations in acetazolamide-responsive myotonia congenita, paramyotonia congenita, and hyperkalemic periodic paralysis. *Neurology* **44**(8): 1500–1503.

SLEEP DISORDERS

John H. Jacobsen, Michael Kohrman

INTRODUCTION

Surveys have reported sleep-related complaints occurring at least several times per month in approximately 30% of the population. It is estimated that sleep disorders' cost to the USA economy in 2004 was 109 billion USA dollars, including direct medical costs and indirect costs due to accidents, illness, and decreased productivity[1]. The rising level of obesity in the developed world is predicted to result in an increased prevalence of sleep-disordered breathing and insomnia, which are already commonplace. Sleep disorders often result in impaired daytime functioning, affecting work performance and increasing the likelihood of motor vehicle accidents. These disorders may cause or worsen medical and psychiatric conditions, such as cardiovascular disease, metabolic disorders, depression, and anxiety. Recent studies also demonstrate long-term health implications of insufficient sleep, which add to the need to identify and treat these common problems.

Six major categories of sleep disorders in the International Classification of Sleep Disorders[2] are discussed in this chapter:
- Insomnias.
- Hypersomnias of central origin.
- Sleep-related movement disorders.
- Sleep-related breathing disorders.
- Circadian rhythm disorders.
- Parasomnias.

An exhaustive treatment of all sleep disorders is beyond the scope of this chapter. The focus will be on frequently encountered disorders, and those of greater interest to the neurologist.

NORMAL SLEEP

Definition

Early concepts of sleep considered it to be a state intermediate between wakefulness and death. The current definition is more specific, and characterizes sleep as:
- A *physiologic* state of reduced consciousness.
- Recurrent.
- Reversible.
- Accompanied by *physiologic* cycles of neuronal activity involving brainstem, cortex, and spinal cord.

Sleep is thereby distinguishable from encephalopathy, coma, or anesthesia, as none of these are physiologic. Furthermore, encephalopathy or coma may or may not be reversible.

Sleep stages

Rules for staging of sleep and wakefulness were established by Rechtschaffen and Kales and were widely used for many years[3]. A stage is assigned to each 30-second epoch of a polysomnogram. The rules were modified in a manual published by the American Academy of Sleep Medicine in 2007[4], as a result of reviews of the literature and the need for standards of digital recording and for new rules for scoring arousals, respiratory events, cardiac events, and movements. The main difference in terminology for sleep staging in the modified system of 2007 concerns non rapid eye movement (REM) stages. Stages S1, S2, S3, and S4 have been replaced by N1, N2, and N3, as explained below, in the descriptions of the stages. Stages S3 and S4 have been collapsed into a single stage, N3, because there appears to be no need to divide slow-wave sleep into two separate stages.

Wakefulness (813)

- Electroencephalogram (EEG): alpha (8–13 Hz) in quiet wakefulness with eyes closed.
- High muscle tone.
- Rapid eye movements (REMs).
- Irregular respirations and heart rate.

N1 (formerly S1 or Stage 1)

Non-REM light sleep; defines sleep onset (**814**).

- EEG: low-voltage, mixed frequency pattern (mostly 4–7 Hz) for more than 50% of the 30-second epoch; vertex waves (sharply contoured waves over the central region lasting <0.5 seconds).
- Muscle tone intermediate.
- Slow rolling eye movements.
- Respirations and heart rate becoming regular.

N2 (formerly S2 or Stage 2)

The major stage of non-REM sleep in adults (**815**).

- EEG: K-complexes (negative sharp wave followed immediately by a positive component) and/or sleep spindles (11–16 Hz activity lasting ≥0.5 seconds).
- Muscle tone intermediate.
- No or a few slow eye movements.
- Regular respirations and heart rate.

N3 (replaces S3 and S4)

Deep non-REM sleep: slow-wave sleep (**816**).

- EEG: 20% or more of a 30-second epoch consists of 0.5–2 Hz waves, of amplitude >75µV, predominant over the frontal regions.
- Muscle tone intermediate.
- Mostly no eye movements.
- Regular respirations and heart rate.

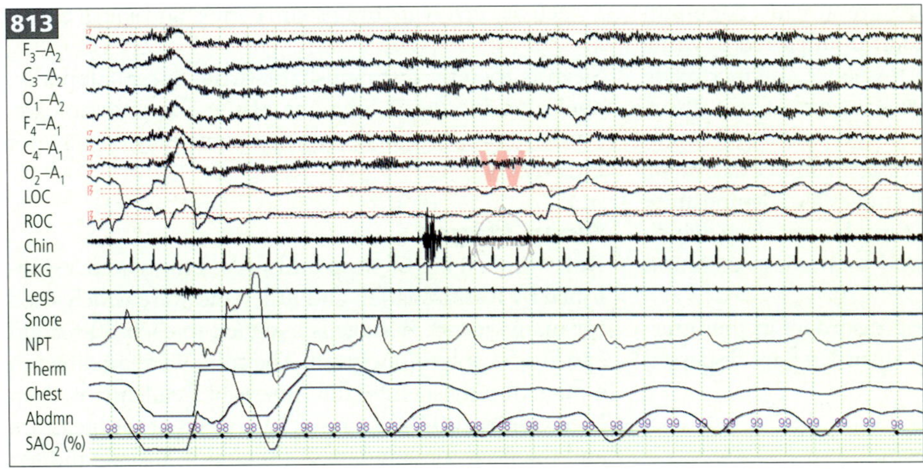

813 30-second epoch of wakefulness. Note prominent alpha activity, rapid eye movements, high chin EMG tone, and irregular respirations. LOC: L outer canthus; ROC: R outer canthus; Chin: chin EMG; Legs: leg EMG; NPT: nasal pressure transducer; Therm: thermistor; SAO_2: oxygen saturation.

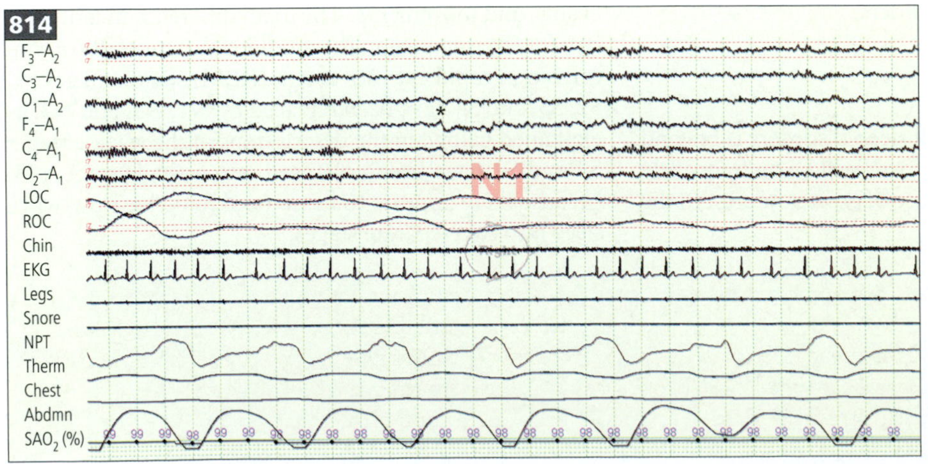

814 30-second epoch of stage N1 sleep. Note vertex sharp wave near center of epoch (asterisk), dropout of alpha activity, and slow rolling eye movements. LOC: L outer canthus; ROC: R outer canthus; Chin: chin EMG; Legs: leg EMG; NPT: nasal pressure transducer; Therm: thermistor; SAO_2: oxygen saturation.

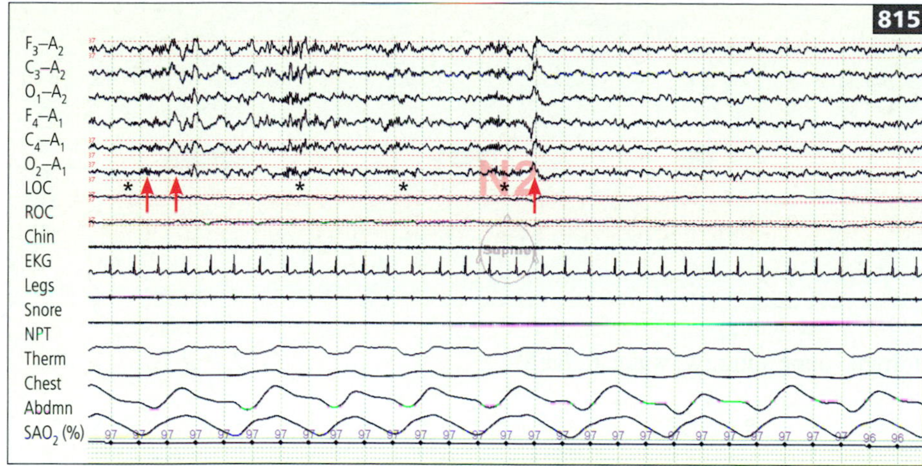

815 30-second epoch of stage N2 sleep. Note K complexes (arrows), sleep spindles (asterisks), and regular respirations. LOC: L outer canthus; ROC: R outer canthus; Chin: chin EMG; Legs: leg EMG; NPT: nasal pressure transducer; Therm: thermistor; SAO_2: oxygen saturation.

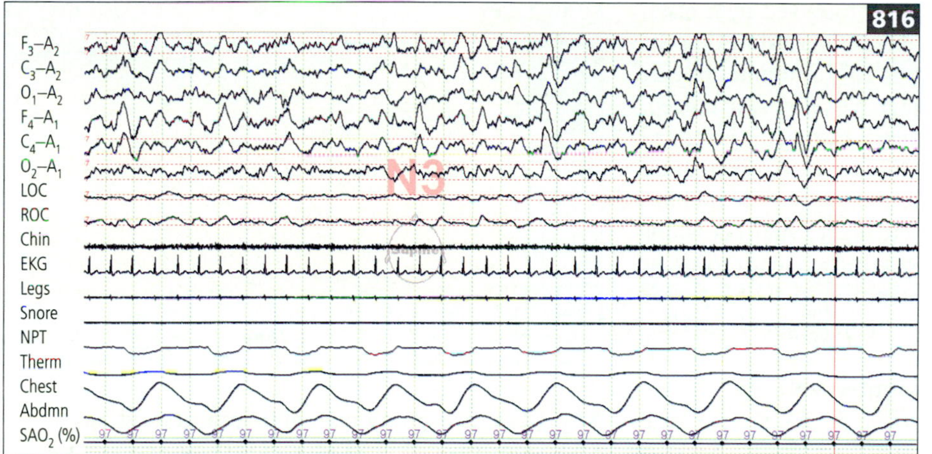

816 30-second epoch of stage N3 sleep. Note high-amplitude delta waves and very regular respirations. LOC: L outer canthus; ROC: R outer canthus; Chin: chin EMG; Legs: leg EMG; NPT: nasal pressure transducer; Therm: thermistor; SAO_2: oxygen saturation.

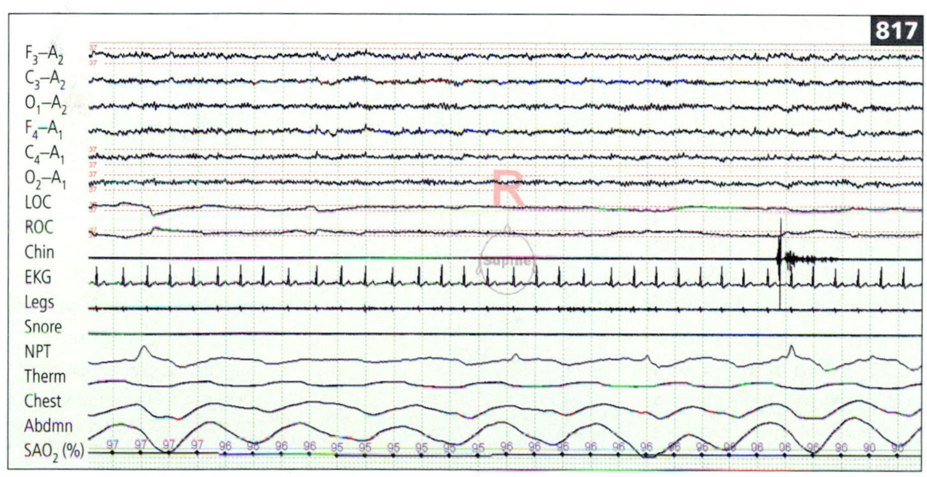

817 30-second epoch of stage REM. Note low-amplitude EEG, rapid eye movements at beginning of epoch, phasic EMG twitch in chin at end of epoch, and irregular respirations. LOC: L outer canthus; ROC: R outer canthus; Chin: chin EMG; Legs: leg EMG; NPT: nasal pressure transducer; Therm: thermistor; SAO_2: oxygen saturation.

R (REM sleep, also known as paradoxical sleep) (817)

- EEG: low-amplitude, mixed frequency EEG.
- Muscle tone low (tonic electromyography [EMG]), except for short bursts of EMG activity lasting <0.25 seconds (phasic EMG).
- REMs, resembling those observed in wakefulness (phasic REM) or no eye movements (tonic REM).
- Irregular respirations and heart rate.
- Penile or clitoral tumescence.
- Poikilothermia.

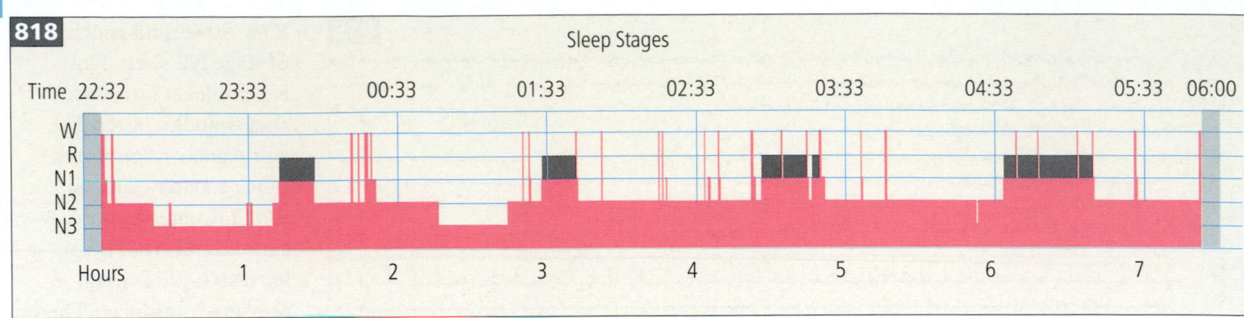

818 Typical hypnogram of a normal young adult. W: wake; R: REM.

Sleep cycles

A typical night in an adult or adolescent begins with 70–80 minutes of non-REM sleep followed by a brief, several-minute REM period. There is a rapid descent from stage N1 to stage N2. After 10–25 minutes of N2, there may be deepening into stage N3, slow-wave sleep, for a number of minutes, particularly during the first third of the night in younger subjects. Sleep cycles of alternating non-REM and REM periods occur every 60–120 minutes throughout the night. A complete night usually contains four or five sleep cycles. Slow-wave sleep tends to occur during the first third of the night, and REM period duration tends to lengthen as the night progresses (**818**).

Total sleep requirement changes with age

Infants require 16–18 hours of sleep per 24 hours, young children 9–10 hours, and adults 7–8 hours. Surveys of sleep habits by the National Sleep Foundation have shown that our society is becoming increasingly sleep-deprived[5,6]. Insufficient sleep now is present in growing numbers of pre-adolescents and is the most common sleep problem today.

Effect of aging

A full-term infant spends about one-half of the total sleep time in REM sleep. By age 5, the amount of REM sleep has decreased to 20–25%, and remains remarkably constant through life, with only very limited decline with aging (**819**). Slow-wave sleep, in contrast, declines markedly with age[7]. This decline is most marked in males, who may exhibit only a few percent or less slow-wave sleep at ages over 50 years.

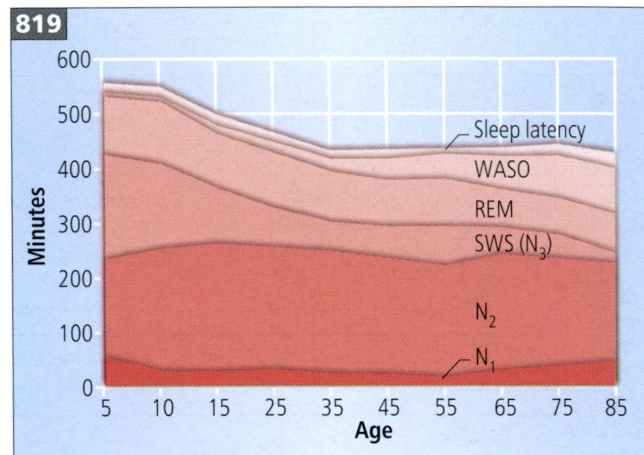

819 Changes in proportions of sleep stages with aging. SWS: slow-wave sleep; REM: rapid eye movement sleep; WASO: wake after sleep onset.

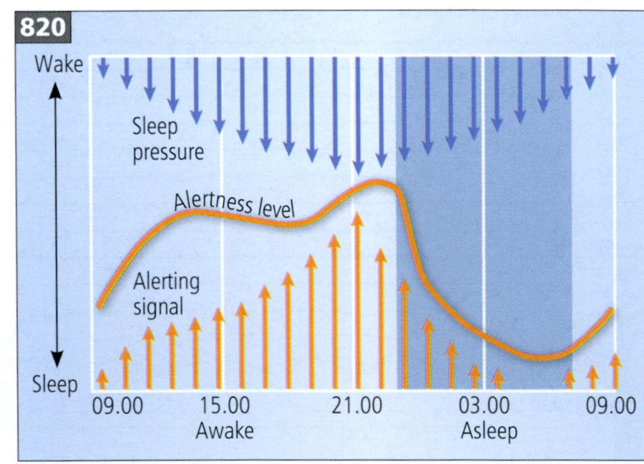

820 Homeostatic sleep pressure (top) and circadian drive to wakefulness (bottom) during the 24-hour cycle.

Control of sleep–wake behavior

According to a proposed two-process model of sleep regulation[8], sleep is controlled by a homeostatic mechanism (process S, sometimes also referred to as process H) and a circadian mechanism (process C). These two mechanisms exist independently but interact with each other (**820**).

Homeostatic mechanism

- Sleepiness increases in proportion to prior awake time; alertness increases in proportion to prior sleep time.
- There is a 'pressure' to keep awake and sleep time balanced.
- There is a need for recovery sleep after sleep deprivation, despite the lack of a circadian influence.
- The substrate that mediates the pressure to sleep is unknown, but adenosine has been proposed as a prime candidate. Caffeine, an agent well known to enhance wakefulness, is an adenosine receptor antagonist.

Circadian mechanism

- Circadian rhythmicity arises from within the organism.
- Genes functioning in relation to the circadian rhythm are found in virtually all cells of the body.
- The mammalian 'master clock' is located within the suprachiasmatic nucleus (SCN) in the anterior hypothalamus.
- This rhythm is influenced through environmental cues called 'zeitgebers', that set the 'master clock'.
- Feeding and activity may act as environmental cues but the principal zeitgeber is light.
- Light information is relayed to the SCN mainly through the retinohypothalamic tract (**821**). The SCN relays information to the pineal gland through the superior cervical ganglion. Light stimulation inhibits the secretion of melatonin, a hormone that promotes sleep.

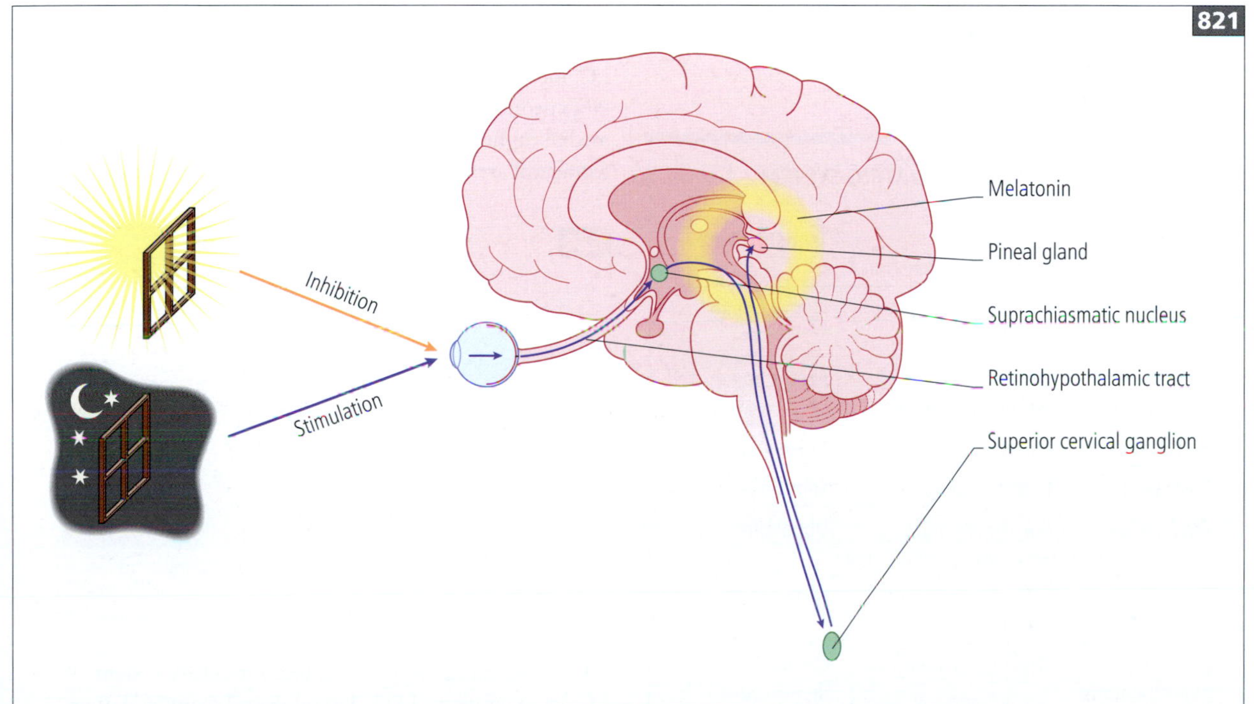

821 Regulation of the production of melatonin by the retinohypothalamic tract. The secretion of melatonin by the pineal gland in response to darkness is mediated by photosensitive postganglionic nerve fibers that pass through the retinohypothalamic tract, and is controlled by the suprachiasmatic nucleus.

Neural networks

- Ascending reticular activating system: wakefulness (822) (*Table 127*):
  - Location: brainstem, lateral/posterior hypothalamus, basal forebrain.
  - The orexin- (also known as hypocretin) secreting neurons are key to maintenance of wakefulness (823). These neurons have wide-ranging projections to the brain and brainstem and are thought to be stimulatory to most of the other cell groups in the reticular activating system, and inhibitory to the preoptic nuclei (see below).
- Descending inhibitory system: sleep-promoting (824):
  - Inhibitory projections arise from the ventrolateral preoptic area and associated neuronal groups, such as the median preoptic nucleus, to initiate and maintain sleep.
  - Inhibitory projections synapse on multiple nuclei of the reticular activating system.
  - Neurotransmitters are gamma-aminobutyric acid (GABA) and galanin.

Relative activation of the ascending, wake-promoting system *vs*. the descending, sleep-promoting system is thought to be under the control of the circadian and homeostatic processes. The ascending and descending systems are mutually inhibitory, creating a 'flip–flop' switch that enables sudden transitions from wakefulness to sleep and *vice versa* (825).

TABLE 127 **RETICULAR ACTIVATING SYSTEM**

Location	Nucleus/ cell structure	Transmitter
Brainstem	Pedunculopontine nucleus	Acetylcholine
Brainstem	Lateral dorsal tegmental nucleus	Acetylcholine
Brainstem	Locus ceruleus	Norepinephrine
Brainstem	Raphe nuclei	Serotonin
Brainstem	Substantia nigra Ventral tegmental area	Dopamine
Posterior hypothalamus	Tuberomamillary nucleus	Histamine
Lateral hypothalamus	Orexogenic neurons	Orexin (hypocretin)
Basal forebrain	Basal forebrain nuclei	Acetylcholine, γ-aminobutyric acid

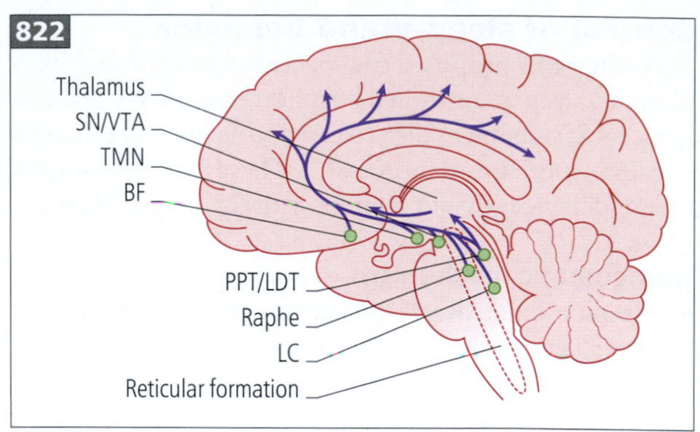

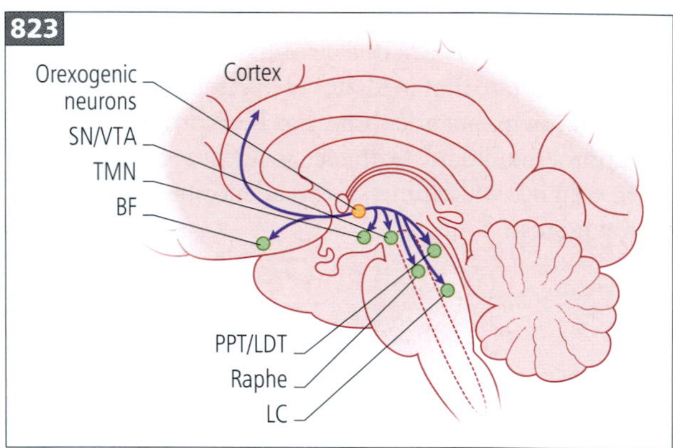

822, 823 Ascending reticular activating system (822) and connections of the wake-promoting orexin/hypocretin-secreting neurons (823). BF: basal forebrain; LC: locus ceruleus; LDT: lateral dorsal tegmental area; PPT: pedunculopontine tegmental area; Raphe: dorsal and medial raphe nuclei; SN/VTA: substantia nigra and ventral tegmental area; TMN: tuberomammillary nucleus.

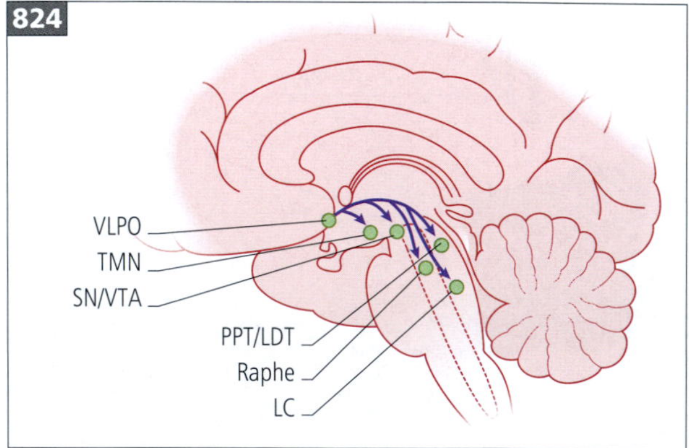

824 Descending sleep-promoting inhibitory system. LC: locus ceruleus; LDT: lateral dorsal tegmental area; PPT: pedunculopontine tegmental area; Raphe: dorsal and medial raphe nuclei; SN/VTA: substantia nigra and ventral tegmental area; TMN: tuberomammillary nucleus; VLPO: ventrolateral preoptic area.

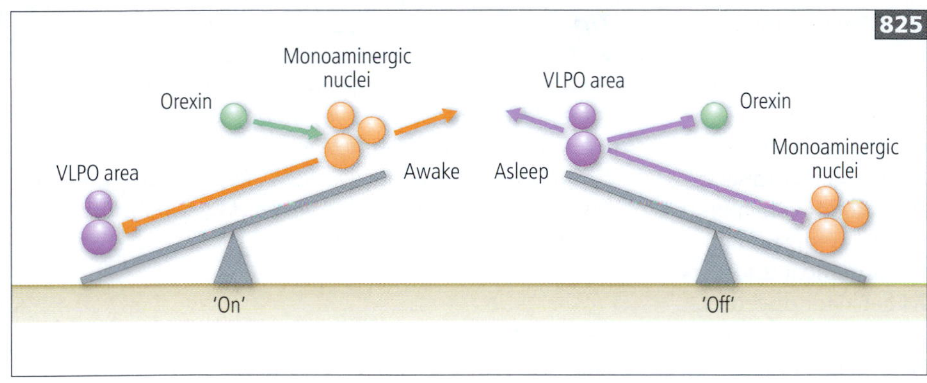

825 The putative 'flip–flop' switch, that allows sudden transitions between wakefulness and sleep and *vice versa*. During the waking state, monoaminergic neurons inhibit the sleep-promoting ventrolateral preoptic (VLPO) neurons. Maintenance of wakefulness is reinforced by stimulation of the monoaminergic neurons by orexin neurons (ORX). During sleep, the VLPO neurons inhibit both orexin and monoaminergic neurons.

COMMONLY PERFORMED SLEEP TESTS

Polysomnography[4]

Recommended channels include:

- EEG: minimum three-channel derivations include either frontal, central, and occipital scalp regions referred to the contralateral mastoid (F4–M1, C4–M1, and O2–M1 according to the International 10–20 System), or C4–M1 and two midline bipolar derivations (Fz–Cz and Cz–Oz). Expanded EEG montages are frequently used when nocturnal seizures are suspected (**826**).
- Electro-oculogram (EOG).
- Chin EMG.
- Leg EMG.
- Airflow monitoring: thermal sensor and nasal pressure transducer. End-tidal carbon dioxide monitoring is often added in pediatric studies or when neuromuscular conditions or obesity–hypoventilation syndromes are a consideration.
- Respiratory effort: inductance plethysmography is currently recommended. Less commonly, esophageal manometry is used.
- Pulse oximetry.

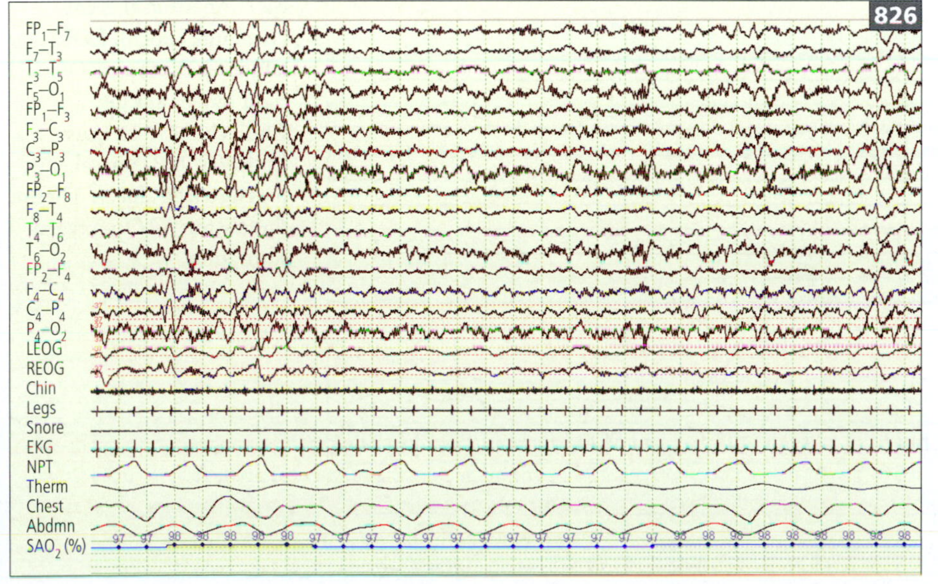

826 Example of an expanded EEG montage, 30-second epoch. Note multifocal sharp waves at the beginning of the epoch.

- Microphone for recording of snoring sounds.
- Electrocardiogram (ECG).
- Body position: recorded by the sleep technologist or by position sensors.
- Video recording: most state-of-the-art laboratories now use time-locked audiovisual recording to correlate behaviors and body position with polygraphic findings. This information is most useful for evaluation of sleep-related movement disorders, parasomnias (including REM behavior disorder), and suspected seizures.
- Other monitors are occasionally employed:
  - Intraesophageal pH probe: in suspected gastroesophageal reflux disease.
  - Intraesophageal balloon: for pressure measurement, as an aid to distinguish obstructive from central respiratory events.
  - EMG of the upper extremities: in cases where upper body movements are reported.
  - Nocturnal penile tumescence: monitoring with strain gauges, in cases of suspected erectile dysfunction – now rarely used.

Definitions of terms used in standard polysomnogram reports

Arousal events

An arousal event is defined as an abrupt shift of EEG from any sleep stage to theta (4 Hz) or higher frequencies, not including sleep spindles, lasting at least 3 seconds, with at least 10 seconds of stable sleep preceding (**827**). An arousal during REM requires a concurrent increase in submental EMG lasting at least 1 second.

Tip

► *The reason for the extra requirement of increased EMG activity in order to score an arousal in REM sleep is that faster frequencies, including alpha frequencies, are frequently observed in the EEG in normal REM sleep. Do NOT score an arousal in REM sleep if only a shift to faster EEG frequencies is observed. In non-REM sleep, a shift to faster frequencies alone is sufficient.*

Respiratory events (adult)

Apnea is defined as a drop in peak thermal sensor airflow ≥90% of baseline, lasting at least 10 seconds, with 90% of the event's duration meeting the amplitude reduction criteria. Obstructive apneas are apneas associated with continued or increased inspiratory effort (**828**). Central apneas are apneas without inspiratory effort (**829**). Mixed apneas have absent inspiratory effort in the initial portion of the event, followed by resumption of respiratory effort but continued absence of detectable airflow (**830**). Hypopneas are defined as a drop in peak nasal pressure transducer airflow ≥30% of baseline, lasting at least 10 seconds, with ≥4% oxygen desaturation from the pre-event baseline, and at least 90% of the event's duration meeting the airflow amplitude reduction criteria.

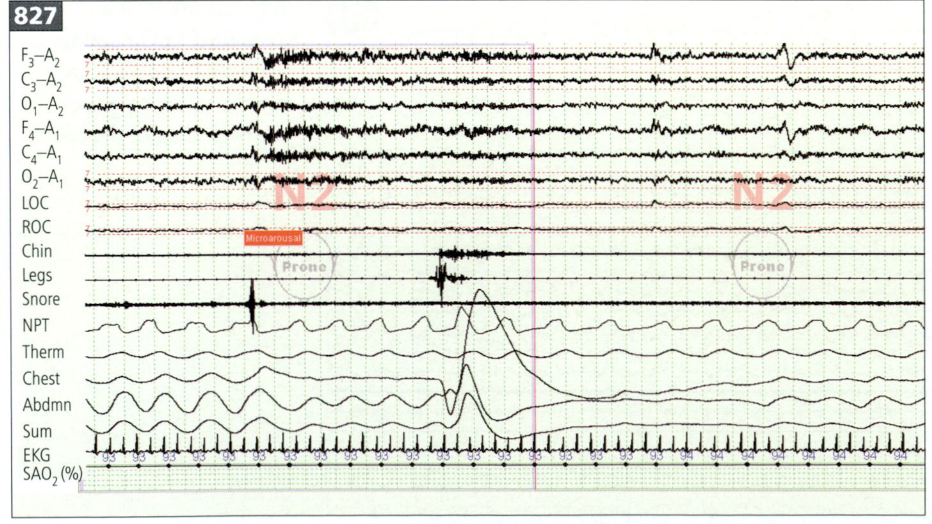

827 An arousal event (1-minute epoch). LOC: left outer canthus; ROC: right outer canthus; Chin: chin EMG; Legs: leg EMG; NPT: nasal pressure transducer; Therm: thermistor; SAO_2: oxygen saturation.

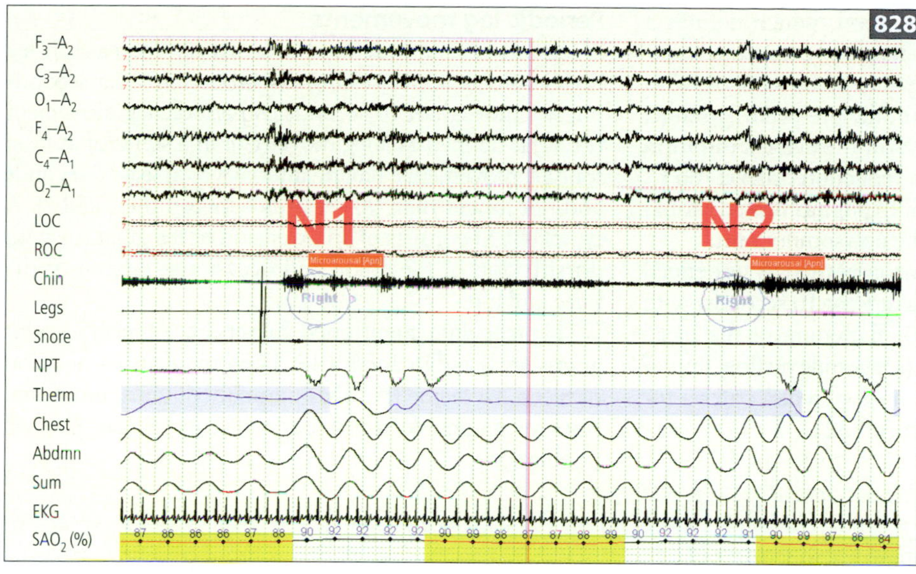

828 Obstructive apneas (1-minute epoch). Note cessation of airflow as measured by both NPT and thermistor, with continuing respiratory effort. Arousals and oxygen desaturations occur at the end of the events. LOC: left outer canthus; ROC: right outer canthus; Chin: chin EMG; Legs: leg EMG; NPT: nasal pressure transducer; Therm: thermistor; SAO_2: oxygen saturation.

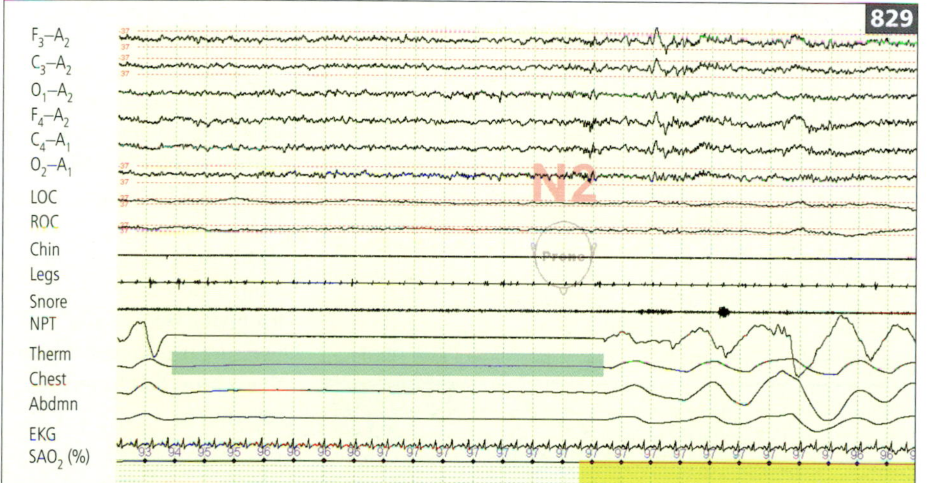

829 Central apnea (30-second epoch). LOC: left outer canthus; ROC: right outer canthus; Chin: chin EMG; Legs: leg EMG; NPT: nasal pressure transducer; Therm: thermistor; SAO_2: oxygen saturation.

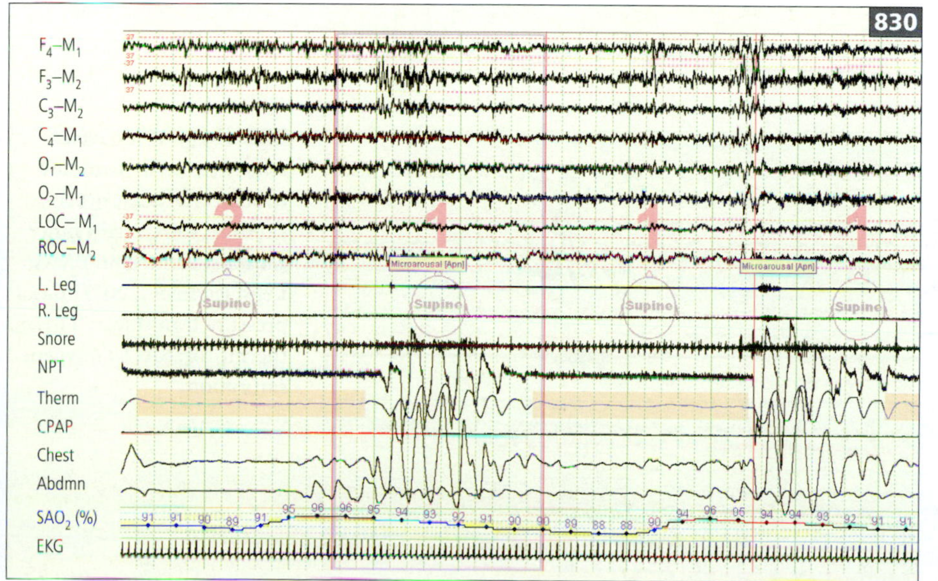

830 Mixed apneas (2-minute epoch). LOC: left outer canthus; ROC: right outer canthus; Chin: chin EMG; Legs: leg EMG; NPT: nasal pressure transducer; Therm: thermistor; SAO_2: oxygen saturation.

There is an alternative definition, which defines a hypopnea as a drop in peak nasal pressure transducer airflow ≥50% of baseline, lasting at least 10 seconds, with ≥3% oxygen desaturation from the pre-event baseline, or an arousal, and at least 90% of the event's duration meeting the airflow amplitude reduction criteria (**831**). Which of the two definitions for hypopnea is used should be mentioned in the report of the polysomnogram.

A respiratory event-related arousal (RERA) is defined as a sequence of breaths lasting at least 10 seconds, with increasing respiratory effort or flattening of the nasal pressure transducer waveform (suggesting airflow limitation) leading to an arousal from sleep, when criteria for an apnea or hypopnea are not met (**832**).

Tip

▶ *Differing criteria for scoring of hypopneas are a source of much confusion in the literature. Close scrutiny of these criteria is necessary in any attempt to compare different studies.*

Periodic leg movements

A leg movement is defined as a ≥8 μV increase in leg EMG voltage above resting EMG, lasting >0.5 seconds but not more than 10 seconds. A periodic leg movement (PLM) is defined as a leg movement in a series of at least four leg movements, having intervals of at least 5 seconds and not longer than 90 seconds between them (**833**). A typical PLM consists of an extension of the great toe with dorsiflexion of the ankle and occasional flexion of the knee and hip.

Typical data mentioned in reports of polysomnograms are listed in *Table 128*. The American Association of Sleep Medicine (AASM) manual contains additional rules for staging sleep and scoring events for the pediatric population.

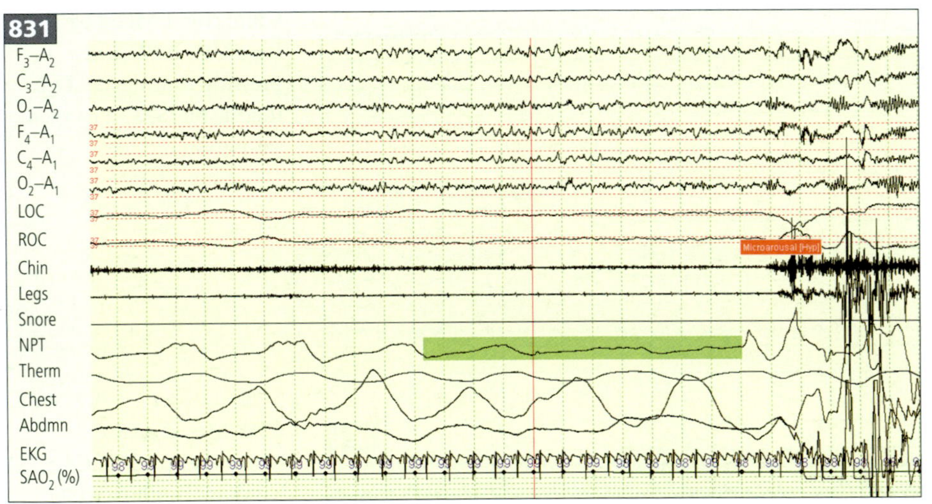

831 Obstructive hypopnea with an arousal (1-minute epoch of REM sleep). LOC: left outer canthus; ROC: right outer canthus; Chin: chin EMG; Legs: leg EMG; NPT: nasal pressure transducer; Therm: thermistor; SAO_2: oxygen saturation.

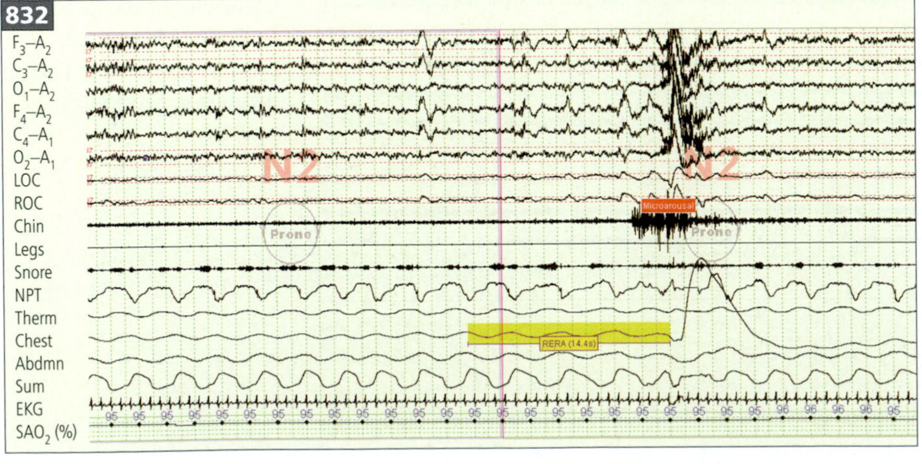

832 Respiratory event-related arousal (1-minute epoch). LOC: left outer canthus; ROC: right outer canthus; Chin: chin EMG; Legs: leg EMG; NPT: nasal pressure transducer; Therm: thermistor; SAO_2: oxygen saturation.

TABLE 128 **TYPICAL DATA INCLUDED IN POLYSOMNOGRAPHY REPORTS**

Category	Parameter	Definition/comments
Staging	Lights out (hr:min)	
	Lights on (hr:min)	
	Total sleep time (TST) (min)	
	Time in bed (min)	Time in bed = lights on minus lights out (min)
	Sleep latency (SL) (min)	Lights out to lights on
	REM (rapid eye movement) latency (min)	Lights out to first epoch of any stage
	Wake after sleep onset (WASO) (min)	Sleep onset to first epoch of REM
	Sleep efficiency (%)	Wake during time in bed, minus SL
	Time in each stage (min)	TST/time in bed
	% of TST in each stage	
Arousal events	Number of arousals	Number of arousals/hour of sleep
	Arousal index	
Respiratory events	Number of obstructive, mixed and central apneas	
	Number of hypopneas	
	Number of apneas + hypopneas	
	Apnea index (AI)	Number of all types of apneas/hour of sleep
	Apnea + hypopnea index (AHI)	Total number of all apneas and hypopneas/ hour of sleep
	Mean oxygen saturation (%)	
	Minimum oxygen saturation during sleep (%)	
	Occurrence of Cheyne–Stokes breathing, if present	
	Number of RERAs	Optional
	Respiratory disturbance index	Total number of apneas, hypopneas and RERAs/hour of sleep (optional)
	Number of oxygen desaturations (could be defined as 3% or 4%)	Optional
	Oxygen desaturation index (ODI)	Total number of desaturations/hour of sleep (optional)
	Hypoventilation, if present	Optional
Cardiac events	Average heart rate during sleep (beats/min)	
	Tachcardia, bradycardia, or other arrhythmias, if present	
Periodic leg movements (PLMs)	Number of PLMs	
	PLM index	Number of PLMs/hour of sleep
	Number of PLMs accompanied by arousals	
	PLM arousal index	Number of PLMs with arousal/hour of sleep

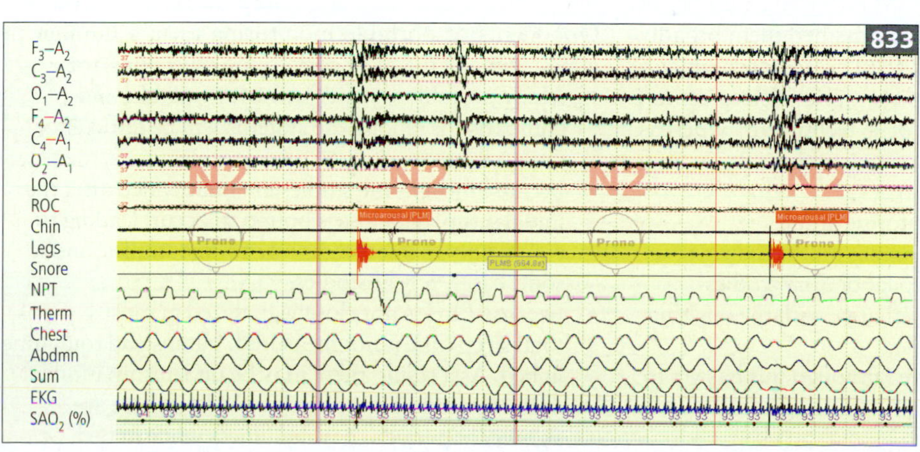

833 Periodic leg movements. Note arousals in association with these leg movements. LOC: left outer canthus; ROC: right outer canthus; Chin: chin EMG; Legs: leg EMG; NPT: nasal pressure transducer; Therm: thermistor; SAO_2: oxygen saturation.

TABLE 129 **LEVELS OF PORTABLE POLYSOMNOGRAPHY**

Level	I	II	III	IV
Number of channels	≥7	≥7	≥4	≤2*
Specific channels	EEG, EOG, chin EMG, ECG, airflow, respiratory effort, oxygen saturation	EEG, EOG, chin EMG, ECG or heart rate, airflow, respiratory effort, oxygen saturation	2 channels of respiratory movement (or 1 channel of respiratory movement + 1 channel of airflow), ECG or heart rate, oxygen saturation	Minimum of oxygen saturation, ± airflow or chest movement
Body position	Documented or objective	Possibly	Possibly	No
Leg movements	EMG or motion sensor desirable but optional	EMG or motion sensor desirable but optional	Possibly	No
Technician in constant attendance	Yes	No	No	No
Interventions	Possible	No	No	No

*For covered services, the USA Centers for Medicare and Medicaid Services in 2007 broadened the definition of Level IV to a monitor that uses three channels, but did not further specify the channels.

ECG: electrocardiogram; EEG: electroencephalogram; EMG: electromyogram; EOG: electro-oculogram.

Portable polysomnography

'Portable monitoring' refers to polysomnography that can be performed outside of the sleep laboratory, usually in the patient's home. In recent years, due to realization that there are many patients with undiagnosed sleep apnea, and a perceived shortage of sleep laboratory resources, there has been a proliferation of devices developed to perform such studies. Portable monitoring is widely used outside of the USA for diagnosis of obstructive sleep apnea (OSA).

There has been considerable debate, however, concerning exactly what sort of monitoring, if any, is appropriate, and what types of patients are appropriate for these studies[9]. In 1994, the AASM reviewed a number of portable monitoring devices and classified them broadly into four categories (*Table 129*)[10]. Level I approximates what occurs during a polysomnogram in a sleep center, with continuous attendance of a technician, whereas Level IV incorporates only oximetry plus one or two other channels.

Advocates of portable monitoring argue:

- Portable monitoring is sometimes more readily available than in-house sleep laboratory studies (although the situation may change with the ongoing proliferation of sleep centers).
- It may be more cost-effective (although this has yet to be proven).
- It can be effectively used to diagnose and rule out severe forms of OSA.
- Several limited studies and a multi-site randomized trial[11] have shown outcomes comparable with in-laboratory studies in terms of continuous positive airway pressure (CPAP) treatment with an auto-titrating device after diagnosis of sleep apnea by portable monitoring.
- Furthermore, a USA government agency (Center for Medicare Services)[12] issued a memorandum concluding that either in-house sleep laboratory studies or home portable monitoring are 'reasonable and necessary' for diagnosis of OSA.

Opponents of portable monitoring raise a number of issues. Some of the most concerning objections are:

- Many portable systems are now available, and comparisons among the systems will be difficult or impossible.
- Because most home studies are unattended after the initial setup, data loss is bound to occur, leading to complexity in interpretation of some studies, and in some cases, repeat studies.
- Because EEG is not closely analyzed in most systems, total sleep time is not measured, but instead total time in bed. As a result, there may be underestimation of the apnea/hypopnea index (AHI) if there are significant periods of wakefulness while in bed.

- Portable monitoring cannot diagnose other sleep-related disorders, such as upper airway resistance syndrome, central sleep apnea, complex sleep apnea, PLMs, or nocturnal epilepsy.
- Portable monitoring has not yet been validated for:
  - Mild to moderate OSA.
  - Patients with comorbidities, such as cardiac or pulmonary disease, and neuromuscular conditions.

The AASM has issued guidelines for performance of portable monitoring[13]. Some of the more salient recommendations included:

- Patients should have a high pre-test probability of moderate to severe obstructive sleep apnea.
- Portable monitoring is most appropriate for those for whom sleep laboratory testing is difficult due to immobility, safety, or critical illness.
- Portable monitoring is appropriate for measuring response to non-CPAP treatments for OSA, including oral appliances, upper-airway surgery, and weight loss.
- Monitoring parameters should include: air flow (ideally both nasal–oral thermistor and nasal pressure transducer), respiratory effort (inductance plethysmography), and pulse oximetry.
- Home studies are not recommended for patients with comorbidities.
- Home studies are not validated for, or intended to be used for, screening asymptomatic subjects.

Although it seems highly likely that portable monitoring will be increasingly used, partly due to increasing demand for sleep studies and partly due to budgetary constraints, further validation of its utility and cost-effectiveness is needed. The field will undoubtedly evolve in coming years.

Tip

▶ *Indications for and reimbursement criteria for portable polysomnography are evolving at an increasingly rapid pace. It is likely that in the near future, portable polysomnography will take the place of at least some routine in-house polysomnography. The ultimate outcome is currently unclear.*

Multiple sleep latency test

The multiple sleep latency test (MSLT)[14,15] is useful in assessment of disorders of excessive somnolence, and in measurement of somnolence in research experiments, such as studying the effect of various drugs on wakefulness, or quantifying the effects of sleep restriction. It is also useful in identifying the premature appearance of REM sleep after sleep onset, as may occur in narcolepsy. The procedure consists of a series of opportunities to nap at 2-hour intervals across the day. The montage used is a modification from standard polysomnography, with employment of only EEG, EOG, mental/submental EMG, ECG, respiratory flow, and snore channels. The patient is encouraged to sleep while resting in a comfortable position. A minimum of four naps is recommended, but the test is often continued for a fifth nap, particularly when narcolepsy is suspected and REM sleep has occurred in one or fewer previous naps. During each nap opportunity, if definite sleep has not occurred after 20 minutes, the test is terminated and the patient is instructed to remain awake until the next nap. If, on the other hand, sleep onset does occur in the first 20 minutes, the test is continued for another 15 minutes of clock time (not necessarily sleep time) before termination of the nap. Sleep onset latencies and occurrence of REM sleep (sleep onset REM periods, or SOREMPs) or lack thereof during each nap are recorded (**834**).

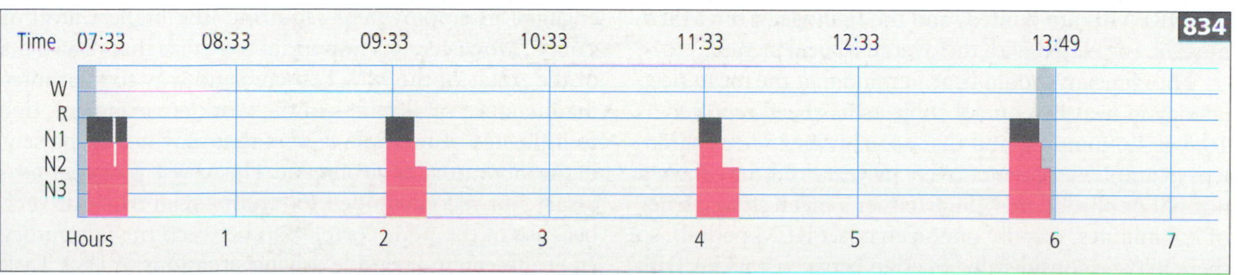

834 Hypnogram of a multiple sleep latency test, demonstrating sleep-onset REM periods.

The results of the MSLT may be confounded by a number of factors, and every effort must be made to prevent these influences. Prior sleep habits, sleep duration the night before the MSLT, and sleep quality the night before may significantly alter the results. A sleep diary for 1–2 weeks prior to the test is recommended, as well as full-night polysomnography on the night immediately preceding the MSLT.

Documentation of at least 6 hours of sleep on the prior polysomnogram is recommended before proceeding with the MSLT. Sleep disruption, as may occur in the setting of sleep-disordered breathing, movement disorders, and in other conditions, may shorten the mean sleep latency in the MSLT and may even result in SOREMPs. In the event that confounding factors such as these are discovered on the prior polysomnogram, the MSLT may be deferred until the disrupting conditions are adequately treated.

Multiple drugs such as hypnotics, sedatives, stimulants, and antidepressants, or withdrawal from these agents, may affect sleep latency and/or REM latency. Ideally, these drugs should be discontinued at least 2 weeks prior to the MSLT, although the situation can be complicated due to factors such as risk of exacerbation of depression during withdrawal from antidepressant medication. Urine drug screening may be useful if the medication history is unclear.

In general, a mean sleep latency <5 minutes is considered pathologic, indicating excessive daytime sleepiness, and can be found in patients with disorders of excessive sleepiness, such as narcolepsy, as well as sleep-deprived normal control subjects. SOREMPs occurring during two out of five naps is considered highly unusual, suggestive of narcolepsy. This pattern has also been observed in sudden withdrawal from REM-suppressant medication, or in association with sleep deprivation, or with sleep disruption as may occur in OSA. If the MSLT is performed during usual hours on a subject with sleep phase delay syndrome (described in the section on circadian rhythm disorders), appearance of REM sleep during the first or second nap may merely reflect physiologic REM cycles during a sleep period that has been prematurely terminated at the end of the prior night's polysomnogram. As with any guideline, the sensitivity and specificity of these cutoff points relating to mean sleep latency and number of SOREMPs are limited, and the findings of the MSLT must be correlated with the overall clinical picture.

The clinician should bear in mind that the mean sleep latency in healthy control subjects has been reported as 10.5 ± 4.6 minutes, and that as many as 25% of narcolepsy/cataplexy patients over 36 years old may have a normal or borderline MSLT (either a mean sleep latency of ≥8 minutes, or only one sleep onset REM period), so there may be considerable overlap between patients with pathologic disorders and normal subjects.

Maintenance of wakefulness test

The maintenance of wakefulness test (MWT)[15,16] is the opposite of the MSLT, in that the subject is asked to remain awake and resist sleep, in the circumstance of a sleep-promoting environment. Whereas the MSLT is intended to measure a subject's ability to fall asleep, the MWT is intended to measure a subject's ability to stay awake. Most of the concerns regarding sleep habits, conditions causing sleep disruption, and medication use that may affect the results of the MSLT also apply to the MWT. The test is often used to assess the effectiveness of interventions to improve daytime alertness (for example, CPAP therapy for OSA, or stimulant therapy for narcolepsy). Patients are usually highly motivated to demonstrate daytime alertness, because such demonstration may support continued employment. Sleep logs are generally not required prior to the MWT, and routine polysomnography on the prior night is not essential, though it may be employed depending on clinical circumstances.

A variety of protocols for performance of the MWT have been used. Currently the AASM practice parameters recommend four trials consisting of 40 minutes for each trial, with 2 hours between each trial. The patient is asked to lie in a comfortable bed in a darkened room, with the head supported by a pillow. A light breakfast is recommended 1 hour before the first trial, and smoking cessation 30 minutes prior. A light lunch is recommended after the second trial. The recording setup is the same as for the MSLT. Sleep latencies, sleep stages, and total sleep time are recorded. Each trial ends after 40 minutes if no sleep has occurred, or after unequivocal sleep, defined as three consecutive epochs of N1 or one epoch of any other stage of sleep.

There is a relative lack of normative data for the MWT. One study on healthy subjects revealed a mean sleep latency of 30.4 ± 11.2 minutes, and 97.5% of healthy subjects had a mean sleep latency ≥8 minutes. Furthermore, 42% of the healthy subjects remained awake for the entire duration of each of the four trials. Currently a mean sleep latency of ≤8 minutes is considered 'abnormal', whereas values between 8 and 40 minutes are regarded to have uncertain significance. Staying awake for the entire duration of all four trials is considered to be an appropriate expectation for individuals engaged in employment requiring 'the highest level of safety'. However, it is important to realize that regardless of the result of the MWT, there is no way to guarantee maintenance of alertness in the work environment, due to influence of multiple factors that may not be present in the laboratory environment. The MWT is neither necessary nor recommended for commercial truck drivers, because of the poor correlation between the laboratory environment and real-life driving situations. A USA Task Force comprised of members of several organizations, including the National Sleep Foundation, did recommend clearance for work for truck drivers with OSA, based on demonstrated compliance with positive airway pressure and/or a documented AHI of ≤10[17].

In view of concerns about sensitivity and specificity of the MSLT and MWT in measuring sleepiness or alertness in various patient groups, the clinical utility of these tests has been questioned[18]. Nonetheless, both tests remain in use for research and patient care, with the MSLT more frequently employed as a measure of sleepiness.

INSOMNIAS

Definition

Insomnia is a syndrome rather than a single clinical disease. Its definition is comprised of two parts[2]:

- Complaint of prolonged sleep latency, difficulty maintaining sleep, or the experience of unrefreshing or poor sleep.
- Impairment in daytime functioning, experienced as lack of concentration, dysphoria, or other symptoms.

The patient must have adequate opportunity and circumstances to allow sleep. Therefore the definition does not include either voluntary sleep deprivation or circadian rhythm disorders.

Epidemiology

The complaint of insomnia is very common in the general population. Reported prevalences range between 5 and 30%, depending on the criteria used[19]. 10% or more of the adult population meet diagnostic criteria for an insomnia disorder[20,21]. A population-based longitudinal study of 388 adults found a remission rate of 54% over 3 years, but 27% of those with remission eventually experienced a relapse, suggesting that insomnia is often a persistent, relapsing condition[22]. A study of incidence of insomnia over 1 year found that out of 464 good sleepers, 7% would develop the insomnia syndrome[23].

Individuals suffering from insomnia have an increased rate of absenteeism from their employment, and decreased efficiency when at work. Untreated insomnia is estimated to result in a high economic burden[24]. Comorbidities of hypertension, diabetes, and depression have been found in association with chronic insomnia[25,26]. The direction of causality, however, has yet to be established.

Etiology and pathophysiology

Traditionally, insomnias have been divided into categories of 'primary' and 'secondary' (due to an acute stressor, poor sleep hygiene, psychiatric disease, substance abuse, or a medical condition), though this distinction may be misleading. The USA National Institutes of Health[27] proposed that the term comorbid insomnia should replace secondary insomnia because: 1) the term secondary places a focus on the comorbid condition and may result in undertreatment of the insomnia; 2) a true etiologic relationship between the various associated comorbidities and the insomnia has not been well established; and 3) all insomnias are probably a result of multiple interacting factors. Patients with insomnias associated with comorbid disease often will give a history of sleep problems antedating onset of the comorbid disorder.

Numerous models of insomnia have been proposed, including a physiologic state of hyperarousal, cognitive models, behavioral models, and an integrated neurocognitive model[28]. Several lines of evidence support the concept of a hyperarousal state in insomnia. For example, EEG spectral analysis reveals increased high-frequency activity in patients with primary insomnia[29]. In a positron emission tomography (PET) study, seven patients with chronic insomnia exhibited increased global glucose metabolism during wakefulness and non-REM sleep when compared to 20 good-sleeper controls[30].

A *cognitive model*[31] posits that insomnia is a result of interaction of:

- Dysfunctional cognition (ruminative thinking or worry).
- Concern about the consequences of sleep loss (cognitive, emotional, physical).
- Arousal (emotional, cognitive, physiologic).

A *behavioral model*[32] (the 3-P model) introduces a behavioral component to explain how acute insomnia becomes chronic:

- A person may be disposed toward insomnia due to innate traits (predisposing factors).
- Subsequent life stressors (precipitating factors) bring on acute insomnia.
- Then maladaptive coping strategies (perpetuating factors) convert acute insomnia to the chronic form. Perpetuating factors include:
  - Staying in bed while awake.
  - Extending the time for sleep opportunity, either by going to bed earlier or by staying in bed later, in an attempt to 'recover' what has been lost. This maladaptive behavior actually results in more time spent lying awake in bed.

Evidence for the validity of these theories comes mainly from the success of cognitive and behavioral treatments for insomnia, which are discussed in following sections. Genetic studies to identify genes or receptor polymorphisms related to insomnia have not yet been undertaken. Higher concordance rates of insomnia in monozygotic twin pairs than for dizygotic twins have been reported[33]. Intriguing candidates for investigation of genetic susceptibility to insomnia include the adenosine receptor and systems related to the neurotransmitter GABA.

Clinical features

Primary insomnias

- Idiopathic insomnia: onset in infancy or childhood, no known cause, unremitting course through adult life. Patients with this type of insomnia have distressing symptoms, in contrast to physiologic short sleepers.
- Psychophysiologic insomnia ('learned insomnia'): due to a maladaptive response to the bed environment. Patients come to associate the bedroom with a wakeful state, and attempts to sleep create frustration, tension, and more arousal. This insomnia often begins with a sleepless response to an acute stressor, but due to perpetuating factors, the insomnia persists despite remission of the stressor. Patients sometimes report improvement in sleep outside of their normal bedroom environment, as during travel or even in the sleep laboratory.
- Paradoxical insomnia (sleep state misperception): complaints of being awake most of the night, despite demonstration of fairly normal sleep by polysomnography or actigraphy. The etiology of this insomnia is poorly understood and is under investigation.

Comorbid insomnias

- Adjustment insomnia: associated with an acute stressor. This insomnia is usually short-lived, and resolves after removal of the stressor.
- Inadequate sleep hygiene: due to varying sleep and wake times, frequent napping, or inappropriate stimulus control, such as watching television in bed, or inappropriate timing of caffeine use.
- Insomnia due to a psychiatric disorder: commonly associated with depression and/or bipolar disorder, but also may occur with anxiety disorders and psychotic disorders such as schizophrenia or schizoaffective disorders.
- Insomnia due to a drug or substance: includes use of some medications (e.g. selective serotonin reuptake inhibitors [SSRI] antidepressants, venlafaxine, duloxetine, monoamine oxidase inhibitors, dopamine/dopamine agonists, beta blockers, diuretics, and theophylline), and abuse of other drugs (e.g. alcohol, amphetamine-like stimulants, caffeine, opiates, and aminergic decongestants).
- Insomnia due to a medical condition: encompasses a large variety of disorders, including but not limited to those with neurologic (e.g. Parkinson's disease, epilepsy, stroke, peripheral neuropathy, chronic pain disorders, neuromuscular disorders, dementias, and fatal insomnia), cardiopulmonary (e.g. chronic obstructive pulmonary disease, congestive heart failure), genitourinary (e.g. benign prostatic hypertrophy, incontinence), endocrine (e.g. thyroid disorders, diabetes), rheumatologic (e.g. arthritis, fibromyalgia), and reproductive (e.g. pregnancy, menstrual cycle variations, menopause) etiologies. Many sleep disorders, such as OSA, restless legs syndrome (RLS)/periodic leg movement disorder (PLMD), circadian rhythm sleep disorders, and parasomnias, may present with the primary complaint of insomnia.

Diagnosis and differential diagnosis

Distinction between the various types of insomnia described above is based on careful history-taking and the physical examination. Circadian rhythm sleep disorders (described in a separate section below) and behaviorally induced insufficient sleep syndrome (described in the hypersomnias of central origin section) should be ruled out.

Corroborating history from a family or household member can be extremely useful. In cases of progressive extreme insomnia accompanied by alteration of vigilance and hallucinations during wakefulness, the differential diagnosis includes fatal insomnia, the very rare Morvan's fibrillary chorea (a limbic encephalitis due to antibodies binding to potassium channels or neuronal acetylcholine presynaptic receptors), and delirium tremens[34]. The syndrome of delirium tremens usually can be easily identified by clinical presentation.

Investigations

A detailed history should include at a minimum: specific insomnia complaints, sleep–wake patterns, pre-sleep conditions, daytime symptoms, evolution of the insomnia, perpetuating factors, and comorbid medical, substance-related, or psychiatric conditions.

There should also be assessment for dysfunctional beliefs and attitudes, such as the patient's opinions about the consequences of the insomnia. Physical and mental status examinations should be directed toward detection of comorbid conditions.

Some subjective measurement of sleepiness, such as the Epworth Sleepiness Scale (an eight-item questionnaire to assess subjective sleepiness, score range 0–24, normal <10)[35] should be obtained. Some other potentially useful questionnaires include the Pittsburgh Sleep Quality Index, Beck Depression Inventory, Short Form Health Survey (SF-36) and Dysfunctional Beliefs and Attitudes about Sleep Questionnaire[36]. One or more of these tools can be applied during treatment to assess outcomes.

Sleep diary data in the form of a sleep log is recommended prior to and during the course of active treatment. Polysomnography and MSLT testing are not routinely indicated in the evaluation of chronic insomnia. Polysomnography may be useful when there is a question of interrupted sleep due to sleep-disordered breathing, a movement disorder, parasomnia, nocturnal epilepsy, or in cases of treatment failure.

Additional studies such as brain imaging and blood testing are not indicated unless they are needed for diagnosis of a suspected comorbid disorder.

Pathology

The common insomnias do not have any major central nervous system (CNS) pathology that has been identified to date. An important exception is fatal insomnia, a prion disease which can occur in both sporadic and familial forms. It was first recognized in the familial form[37], which is caused by a mis-sense GAC to AAC mutation at codon 178 of the prion protein gene, in association with a methionine polymorphism at codon 129 on the mutant allele. Interestingly, if codon 129 on the mutant allele codes for valine instead of methionine, the phenotype of familial Creutzfeldt–Jakob disease (CJD) results, rather than fatal familial insomnia[38]. Sporadic fatal insomnia does not have a known mutation, but does have a homozygous methionine polymorphism at codon 129. Clinical presentation of both forms of fatal insomnia is similar, with initially insidious onset of difficulties with vigilance and initiating and maintaining sleep, followed by hypertension, evening hyperpyrexia, autonomic dysfunction, ataxia, myoclonus, and worsening dream-like stupor and hallucinations. Patients die usually in 8–72 months, either suddenly or from concomitant respiratory failure or infection. No effective therapy has been found.

The hallmark of prion diseases is the deposition of abnormally folded, protease-resistant prion protein. Compared with CJD, the deposition in fatal insomnia is 5 to 10 times less. The most common neuropathologic feature of fatal insomnia is in the thalamus, where >50% loss of neurons is observed in the anterior, ventral, and mediodorsal nuclei (835, 836).

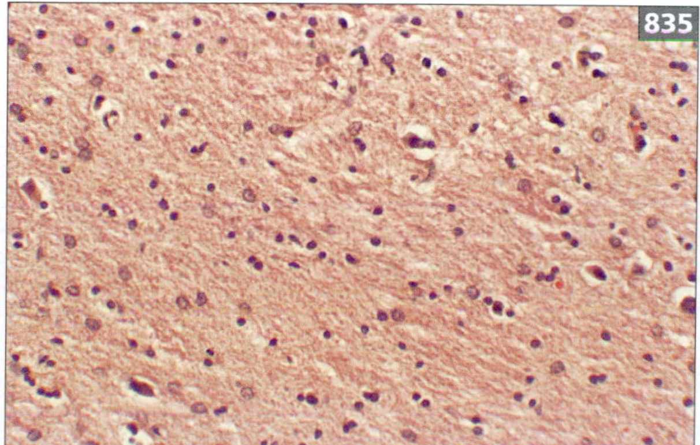

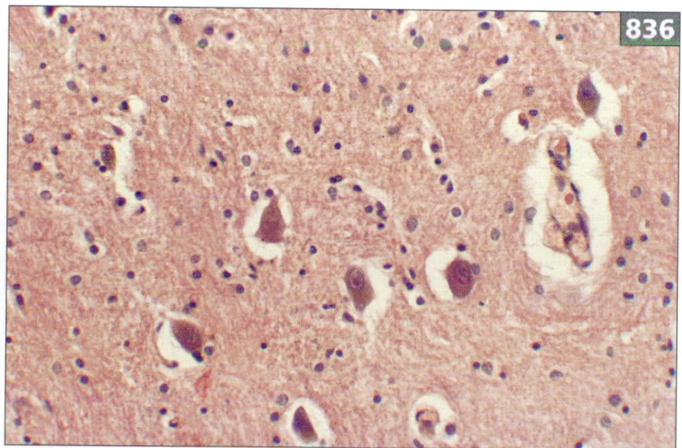

835, 836 Thalamic neuronal loss in fatal insomnia. (835) H&E stained paraffin section of medial thalamus, region of mediodorsal nucleus, demonstrating loss of neurons and proliferation of astrocytes; (836) H&E stained paraffin section of lateral thalamus at same coronal level as image 835, region of reticular nuclei, demonstrating preservation of neurons and background.

Treatment

Cognitive behavioral therapy (CBT) and pharmacotherapy (with benzodiazepine receptor agonists or benzodiazepines) are the only two modalities that have adequate supporting evidence for efficacy in the treatment of insomnia. They are often used in combination. There have been relatively few trials of the two therapies in head-to-head comparison, but those that have been performed seem to indicate relative superiority of CBT.

Pharmacotherapy produces benefits during the acute phase, but CBT seems to result in the most enduring remissions, especially when pharmacotherapy is discontinued during CBT[39]. However, CBT is time-consuming[40] and the patient is sometimes unable to come in for frequent visits for a several-week period, and not all medical facilities have the resources to offer this therapy.

In comorbid insomnias, it is appropriate to direct therapy towards the comorbidity as well. For pharmacotherapy, over-the-counter antihistamines remain popular with the public, but evidence for their efficacy is lacking and they are not recommended due to substantial side-effects. Sedating antidepressants, especially trazodone, have been widely prescribed for treatment of insomnia in patients without depression, but because of lack of evidence for efficacy and because of their side-effect profile, they are recommended only for patients with comorbid depression.

The basic elements of CBT are as follows:

- Stimulus control therapy:
  - Go to bed only when sleepy.
  - Do not engage in other activities such as watching television, eating, or reading while in bed.
  - If you are unable to sleep after 20 minutes, leave the bed and engage in a relaxing activity until drowsy, then return to bed – repeat as necessary.
  - Leave the bed when you have a subjective impression that 20 minutes of wakefulness have elapsed. Do not watch the clock.
- Sleep restriction therapy:
  - Limit time in bed to the estimated total sleep time (but not less than 5 hours).
  - Establish a consistent wake-up time.
  - Increase bed time by 15 minutes when estimated sleep efficiency has reached 90% by sleep log.

TABLE 130 **SELECTED USA FDA-APPROVED DRUGS FOR INSOMNIA**

Drug	**Class**	**Time to maximum plasma concentration** (min)	**Elimination half-life** (hours)	**Dose**	**Predominant type of insomnia for which drug is recommended**
Ramelteon	MRA	0.5–1.5	1–3	16–64 mg	Sleep-onset
Zaleplon	NBBRA	60	1	5–20 mg	Sleep-onset, or maintenance (taken on awakening during night)
Zolpidem	NBBRA	90	1.5–2.4	5–10 mg	Sleep-onset
Triazolam	BZD	60–120	2–5	0.125–0.25 mg	Sleep-onset
Zolpidem, controlled release	NBBRA	Variable	4–5	6.25–12.5 mg	Sleep-maintenance
Eszopiclone	NBBRA	60	5–7	1–3 mg	Sleep-maintenance
Temazepam	BZD	Variable	10–20	7.5–30 mg	Sleep-maintenance
Estazolam	NBBRA	30–360	10–24	0.5–2 mg	Sleep-maintenance

BZD: benzodiazepine; FDA: Food and Drug Administration; NBBRA: nonbenzodiazepine receptor agonist; MRA: melatonin receptor agonist.

- Sleep hygiene therapy:
  - Keep a regular schedule.
  - Remove environmental noise, television, and other disturbances from the bedroom.
  - Avoid napping.
  - Avoid caffeine, alcohol, nicotine, excessive fluids, exercise, or other stimulating activities before bedtime.
- Relaxation training: utilize progressive muscle relaxation training, guided imagery, or abdominal breathing to reduce elevated levels of arousal.
- Paradoxical intention: aimed to reduce performance anxiety:
  - Lie quietly awake.
  - Avoid conscious efforts to fall asleep.
- Cognitive therapy:
  - Correct faulty beliefs about insomnia.
  - Reduce catastrophic thinking about consequences of sleep loss.

Drugs recommended for pharmacotherapy of insomnia are presented in *Table 130*. Ramelteon, a melatonin MT1 and MT2 receptor agonist, has shown only a modest decrease in sleep latency, occasionally relieves sleep-initiation insomnias, but may have limited benefits for treatment of most insomnias. Melatonin is available over-the-counter as a hypnotic, but its manufacture is not regulated, and conclusive studies of its efficacy are lacking. Zaleplon is a very short-acting benzodiazepine agonist that may be used on nocturnal awakening if at least 4 more hours of subsequent sleep are anticipated. The controlled-release form of zolpidem has not been directly tested for efficacy against the immediate-release form, so its exact role is unclear. Two other benzodiazepines, flurazepam and quazepam, are older benzodiazepines approved by the USA Food and Drug Administration as hypnotics, but these are rarely used today, due to their elimination half-lives of over 48 hours. The benzodiazepine and nonbenzodiazepine agonists have all been approved for short-term use of 7–10 days. No clear limitations on length of treatment have been applied to eszopiclone or zolpidem. All these agents except ramelteon have distinct sedative properties and should not be combined with other sedatives such as alcohol, or used with drugs that may inhibit their metabolism. Relatively low doses are appropriate for the elderly.

HYPERSOMNIAS OF CENTRAL ORIGIN

These disorders all have a primary complaint of daytime somnolence, which cannot be attributed to disruption of nocturnal sleep or misaligned circadian rhythms.

Narcolepsy with cataplexy

Definition

The term *narcolepsy* was coined by Gelineau in 1880 from the Greek *narcosis* (drowsiness) and *lambanein* (to seize or take)[41]. Westphal had described a syndrome consistent with narcolepsy with cataplexy earlier in 1877, but did not use those specific terms, and in fact the term *cataplexy* was not used to describe attacks of loss of muscle tone without loss of consciousness until the 20th century by Henneberg[42].

Epidemiology

The prevalence of narcolepsy with cataplexy varies depending on country and ethnic group[43]. European and North American studies estimate the prevalence to be 0.02–0.067%. Narcolepsy in Israel is very uncommon, perhaps as low as 0.002%, whereas the prevalence in Japan is much higher (0.16–0.18%). Although familial cases occur in 4.3–9.9%, twin studies indicate a poor concordance, suggesting an environmental factor in the development of the disease. Age of onset can be from early childhood (rarely before age 5) to the 50s, with a peak at age 15 years and a smaller peak around age 36, with a slight male predominance.

Pathophysiology

Associations between several human leukocyte antigen (HLA) types and narcolepsy have been reported since 1984, prompting speculation that the pathophysiology of narcolepsy may be immune-mediated. The most specific marker of narcolepsy with cataplexy is HLA-DQB1*0602[44], occurring in about 90% of patients. However, this antigen occurs in up to 34% of the general population, depending on ethnicity, so the usefulness of HLA testing in diagnosis of narcolepsy is limited. The discovery of the hypocretin/orexin neurons in the lateral hypothalamus contributed greatly to the understanding of the pathogenesis of narcolepsy[45,46]. The peptides hypocretin-1 and hypocretin-2 (also known as orexin

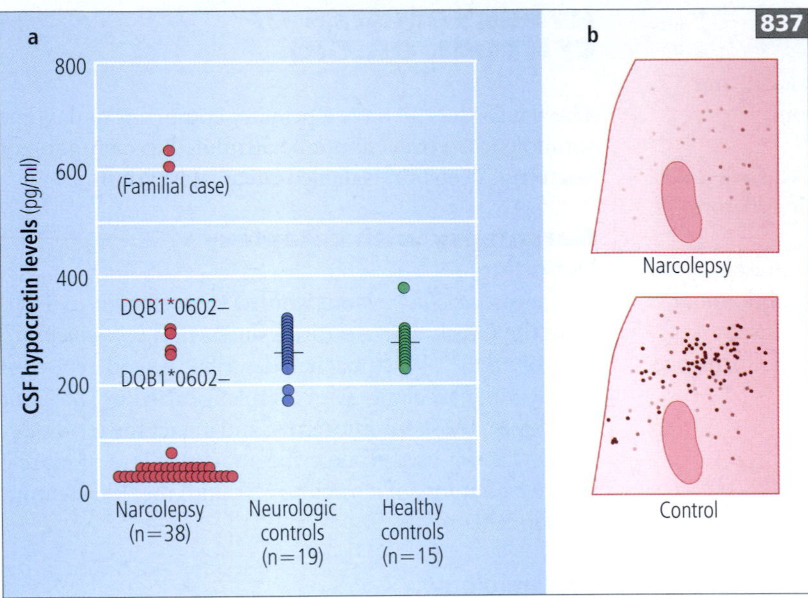

837 (a) A study of cerebrospinal fluid (CSF) hypocretin-1 levels in narcoleptic and control subjects. CSF hypocretin-1 levels are undetectably low in most narcoleptic subjects (84.2% in this study). Note that two HLA DQB1*0602-negative and one familial case have normal or high CSF hypocretin levels. (b) Preprohypocretin messenger ribonucleic acid *in situ* hybridization in the hypothalamus of control and narcoleptic subjects. Preprohypocretin transcripts are detected in the hypothalamus of control but not narcoleptic subjects. *Adapted from Nishino S (2007). 'Clinical and neurobiological aspects of narcolepsy'. Sleep Med 8(4): 373–399 with permission.*

A and orexin B) secreted by these neurons are stimulatory and promote wakefulness by binding to receptors on a wide diversity of neuronal groups in the CNS. Most patients with narcolepsy with cataplexy have low or undetectable levels of hypocretin-1 in the CSF (837). Although autopsy studies on large numbers of narcolepsy patients have not been performed, studies to date have revealed significant loss of hypocretin/orexin neurons in the lateral hypothalamus[47]. This neuronal loss does not appear to be congenital, because narcolepsy usually develops in adolescents or young adults. Immunologically mediated destruction of these neurons has long been suspected. Abnormalities in total serum immunoglobulins and immunoglobulin subsets in patients with narcolepsy and other patients with idiopathic hypersomnolence *vs.* normal controls have been reported[48]. Elevated serum antistreptococcal antibodies have been found in patients with recent narcolepsy onset[49]. Furthermore, a spike in patients presenting with new onset narcolepsy with cataplexy occurred about 6 months after the 2009 H1N1 influenza pandemic in China[50]. However, direct evidence of an immune attack, such as demonstration of inflammation in the lateral hypothalamus of narcoleptic patients, is currently lacking. A narcolepsy phenotype ('secondary narcolepsy') may occasionally emerge in association with other disorders, such as certain inherited disorders, tumors, encephalitis, and head trauma resulting in hypothalamic dysfunction.

Tip

▶ *In 2010, three independent investigative teams found that some narcolepsy patients, especially those tested shortly after onset of disease, have elevated serum antibodies to the protein Tribbles homolog 2, which is highly expressed in orexin neurons, but of unknown function[51]. The significance of this finding is an area of active investigation.*

Clinical features

Excessive daytime sleepiness

Irresistible urges to sleep are experienced, usually several times during the day. Sleep attacks may occur during unusual circumstances such as while talking, eating, or driving. Naps tend to be of short duration (10–30 minutes or less) and are usually refreshing. The symptom of excessive sleepiness is often the first to occur. In cases of severe sleepiness, episodes of 'automatic behavior' may occur, during which the patient performs an activity (such as taking notes or driving), in a semi-automatic fashion, without full consciousness or memory of the event.

Cataplexy

This phenomenon is thought to be caused by intrusion of the atonia of REM-sleep into the wakeful state. Extraocular muscles and muscles of respiration are not affected. Attacks are often triggered by positive emotions, such as amusement, surprise, and elation, but may also occur with negative emotions such as anger or fear. The distribution of weakness from the atonia is variable, ranging from total postural collapse to minor forms involving focal muscle groups: buckling of the knees, dropping of the head, sagging of the face or jaw, or merely slurred speech. Consciousness is preserved and the duration is short, ranging from a few seconds to a few minutes. Recovery is rapid and complete.

Sometimes attacks are followed by sleep, and patients sometimes report dreams immediately after cataplectic episodes. The most severe form of cataplexy involves attacks in rapid succession (termed status cataplecticus) that are usually triggered by very strong emotion, or by withdrawal from medication used to treat cataplexy (see section on treatment below).

Tip

▶ *The manifestations of cataplexy may be subtle. Questions such as, 'Do you ever fall down when someone tells a joke?' are, in isolation, inadequate for a proper history. In-depth questioning regarding jaw sagging, head nodding, slurred speech, a feeling of weakness in the knees, and similar subtle symptoms occurring during periods of strong emotion is necessary.*

Sleep paralysis

This event occurs at sleep onset or on awakening, and is also thought to be due to an intrusion of REM sleep atonia into wakefulness. It is characterized by a terrifying feeling of being unable to move or speak despite being awake, and there is often a feeling of suffocation. Sleep paralysis rarely lasts more than a few seconds or minutes. 40–80% of narcoleptic patients experience sleep paralysis, but in order for it to be considered a significant symptom, it must occur repeatedly, as it is also commonly reported as a rare event in the general population. Hypnagogic or hypnopompic hallucinations may occur along with the episode of sleep paralysis, thereby enhancing the frightening aspect of these spells.

Tip

▶ *Patients with isolated sleep paralysis, without any other underlying sleep disorder, occasionally present to a sleep clinic, as the experience can be terrifying.*

Hallucinations

During transitions from wakefulness to sleep (hypnagogic events) or from sleep to wakefulness (hypnopompic events), vivid dream-like hallucinations thought to be related to sleep-onset REM sleep occur repeatedly in 40–80% of patients with narcolepsy with cataplexy. These are distinguished from hallucinations in other psychotic states by their exclusive association with wake/sleep transitions. Similar to sleep paralysis, hypnagogic hallucinations also occur sporadically in the normal population.

Disturbed nocturnal sleep

Although this feature is not a part of the classical tetrad (sleep attacks, cataplexy, sleep paralysis, and hallucinations) of narcolepsy, patients often complain of fragmented nocturnal sleep. Total sleep time in a 24-hour period, however, is similar for narcoleptic patients and normal subjects.

Tip

▶ *Occasionally a patient with narcolepsy with cataplexy will present with the most prominent complaint of insomnia and fragmented sleep, rather than sleep attacks or cataplexy, although these other features should also be present to support the diagnosis.*

Other associated conditions

- PLMs of sleep.
- REM behavior disorder.
- Increased body mass index, occasional obesity.
- OSA. Because OSA is relatively common, and because narcoleptic patients are often overweight, obstructive apnea may coexist with narcolepsy.

Narcolepsy without cataplexy

Major features are similar to narcolepsy with cataplexy, except for the absence of cataplexy. These patients constitute a minority (probably less than half, possibly as low as 10%) of the narcoleptic population.

- Onset is usually in adolescence.
- True prevalence is unknown, because 1–3% of adults may have multiple SOREMPs during random MSLTs, and up to 30% of the general population may have a mean sleep latency of ≤8 minutes. Furthermore, conditions such as OSA, PLMs during sleep, and insufficient sleep may cause decreased mean sleep latency on the MSLT, and multiple SOREMPs, resulting in diagnostic confusion.
- Pathogenesis and pathophysiology are largely unknown. Loss of orexogenic neurons in the hypothalamus has been demonstrated in only a minority of cases. The etiology of this condition is likely heterogeneous.

Idiopathic hypersomnolence with long/short sleep time

- Prevalence is uncertain. Estimates range from 10% as common as narcolepsy, to almost as prevalent as narcolepsy.
- Usually diagnosed in adults. There is no clear gender predominance.
- Mainly distinguished from narcolepsy by:
  - Tendency for naps to be long and unrefreshing.
  - Absence of REM-associated phenomena, such as cataplexy, hypnagogic hallucinations, or sleep paralysis.
  - Absence of SOREMPs on the MSLT.
- Pathogenesis/pathology is not known. There is no known HLA association or any abnormality in the hypocretin/orexin system.

Long sleepers are currently defined as those with average sleep time >10 hours (usually >11–12 hours) in a 24-hour period. These patients tend not to be overweight, and may complain of difficulty awakening to an alarm in the morning. Confusional behavior on arousal and intermittently during the day is common. Although current criteria specify a mean sleep latency <8 minutes on the MSLT, some authorities suggest that a subset of patients with idiopathic hypersomnolence with long sleep time may have a normal mean sleep latency on the MSLT, and should be allowed to sleep *ad libitum* for another 24 hours after the MSLT in order to assess better the typical total sleep time in a 24-hour period[52].

The diagnosis is basically one of exclusion, after narcolepsy and other causes of fatigue and excessive daytime sleepiness (especially depression) have been ruled out.

Differential diagnosis of narcolepsy and idiopathic hypersomnias

Diagnosis is based on a careful history and physical, and the results of nocturnal polysomnography and a MSLT performed the following day. HLA typing and CSF analysis for low hypocretin-1 (<110 pg/ml) are not routinely performed, but may be useful to aid in diagnosis of atypical cases. Distinguishing characteristics are presented in *Table 131*.

Treatment of narcolepsy and idiopathic hypersomnias

- Behavioral adaptations:
  - Encouragement of good sleep hygiene (avoid sleep deprivation).
  - Daytime structured naps, if permissible in the work environment.
- Pharmacologic stimulants for excessive daytime sleepiness. Dopamine enhancement is the mechanism of action of most of these agents, though the exact mechanism for modafinil and armodafinil remains unclear.
- Agents for suppression of cataplexy. These drugs act as REM suppressants and enhance mostly the norepinephrine and serotonin systems. One exception is sodium oxybate, whose exact mechanism of action is unknown. Sodium oxybate appears to consolidate the fragmented sleep of narcoleptics and can treat both cataplexy and excessive daytime sleepiness in these patients.

Examples of commonly used agents are given in *Table 132*.

TABLE 131 **DIFFERENTIAL DIAGNOSIS OF NARCOLEPSY AND IDIOPATHIC HYPERSOMNIA**

Diagnosis	Nap duration	Refreshed after nap	Other symptoms	MSLT latency	MSLT SOREMPs	HLA DQB1*0602	Low hypocretin
Narcolepsy with cataplexy	Short (10–30 min)	Yes	Sleep paralysis, hallucinations	<8 min	≥2	>90%	85–90%
Narcolepsy without cataplexy	Short (10–30 min)	Yes	Sleep paralysis, hallucinations	<8 min	≥2	40–50%	10–20%
Idiopathic hypersomnia with long sleep time	Long (>30 min)	No	Prolonged nocturnal sleep (>10 h)	<8 min	≤1	No increased frequency	No
Idiopathic hypersomnia without long sleep time	Variable	No	No prolonged nocturnal sleep	<8 min	≤1	No increased frequency	No

MSLT: Multiple Sleep Latency Test; SOREMP: sleep onset REM period.

TABLE 132 **PHARMACOLOGIC AGENTS FOR NARCOLEPSY AND IDIOPATHIC HYPERSOMNOLENCE**

Target	Drug	Enhanced neurotransmitter(s)	Common adverse events	Comments	Starting dose–maximum dose/24 hr
Excessive daytime sleepiness	Modafanil (R and S racemic mixture)	Dopamine?; mechanism poorly understood	Headache, nausea	Relatively benign adverse events; interferes with oral contraceptives	100–400 mg; may be given in divided doses, on awakening and at midday
	Armodafanil (R enantiomer of modafinil)	Dopamine?	Same as for modafinil	Longer-acting than racemic modafanil; interferes with oral contraceptives	150–300 mg, once on awakening
	Methyl-phenidate	Norepinephrine, dopamine, and serotonin	Irritability, mood changes, hyper-tension, anorexia, insomnia	Long-acting forms are available; abuse potential	10–60 mg; short-acting forms may be given in divided doses
	Dextroampheta-mine	Norepinephrine, dopamine, and serotonin	Same as for methyl-phenidate, but potentially more intense	Addictive potential	5–50 mg
	Pemoline	Norepinephrine, dopamine, and serotonin	Same as for methyl-phenidate, but less intense; potentially hepatotoxic	Requires periodic hepatic function monitoring; not available in the USA	20–115 mg; may be given in divided doses
	Selegiline	Monoamine oxidase inhibitor	Hypertension, palpitations at higher doses	Not often used; adverse reaction with tricyclic anti-depressants and SSRIs	5–40 mg
Cataplexy	Imipramine	Norepinephrine and serotonin	Anticholinergic	Tricyclic antidepres-sants are second-line, due to side-effects	10–150 mg at bedtime
	Clomipramine	Norepinephrine and serotonin	Anticholinergic	As for imipramine	25–150 mg at bedtime
	Protriptyline	Norepinephrine and serotonin	Anticholinergic	As for imipramine	5–20 mg at bedtime
	Fluoxetine	Serotonin	Nausea, insomnia, headache, sexual dysfunction		10–40 mg in the morning
	Venlafaxine	Serotonin, norepinephrine, and dopamine	Nausea, dizziness, dry mouth, constipation, and sedation	Long-acting forms are available	75–375 mg; may be given in divided doses
Cataplexy and excessive daytime sleepiness	Sodium oxybate	Gamma-hydroxybutyrate	Nausea, headaches, sedation, respiratory depression, salt load	Abuse potential at higher doses	4.5–9 g nightly in two divided doses

SSRI: selective serotonin reuptake inhibitor.

Tip

▶ *Addition of sodium oxybate to a regimen of pharmacologic stimulants given to a narcolepsy patient will often allow reduction of dosage (occasionally even elimination) of the stimulant medications.*

Kleine–Levin syndrome

This is a rare syndrome of recurrent hypersomnia, with the first episode lasting 7–21 days and recurrences lasting usually 5–10 days.

- Prevalence is estimated at 1:1,000,000.
- Male predominance is 2–4:1. Age of onset is usually in the second decade, though cases have been described at ages 4–80 years.
- No consistent pathology has been demonstrated in the few autopsy cases. Brain MRI is normal.
- Etiology and pathophysiology are unknown. Single-photon emission computed tomography (SPECT) analysis has demonstrated thalamic hypoperfusion in several cases during the symptomatic period. Prevalence in Ashkenazi Jews, and reports of a few familial cases suggests a genetic predisposition. Frequent association with a prodromal febrile illness, particularly upper respiratory infection, suggests a possible immune-mediated etiology.
- Clinical features:
  - Hypersomnia, usually over 12 hours (often 16–18 hours) in each 24-hour period, with waking only for eating or voiding.
  - Megaphagia with compulsive eating.
  - Hypersexuality with inappropriate behaviors (most often in males).
  - Other behavioral abnormalities, including confusion, hallucinations, irritability, and aggressiveness when aroused.
  - Normal alertness, cognitive ability, and mental status between episodes.
  - Gradual decrease in duration and severity of recurrences, with resolution after 1 to several years.
- Diagnosis is based on the above clinical features. In the differential diagnosis, it is particularly important to rule out primary psychiatric disease. An infectious or post-infectious etiology may be considered if the first episode occurs shortly after a febrile illness. Polysomnography is not required, and is often impractical due to agitated behavior.
- Treatment trials have in general been disappointing. The best-tolerated stimulant has been modafanil, 200 mg/day, but it does not appear to decrease the frequency of relapses. Some benefit of valproic acid and/or amantadine therapy has been reported[53].

Behaviorally induced insufficient sleep syndrome

- Exact prevalence is unknown, but this condition is relatively common in adolescence, when sleep requirement is high but social and cultural pressures to curtail sleep and a normal age-dependent shifting of sleep phase, delaying sleep onset, combine to produce insufficient sleep.
- Excessive daytime sleepiness is present for 3 months or more, and may be accompanied by other symptoms, including irritability, fatigue, difficulty concentrating, and malaise.
- Symptoms develop as psychologic and physiologic responses of a normal individual to sleep deprivation.
- When the habitual short sleep schedule is not maintained, as may occur on weekends or vacation, the patient will sleep longer than usual.
- The patient is unaware of the obvious cause of the sleepiness and fatigue.
- Diagnosis is established by a sleep log or by actigraphy, which confirm a sleep time shorter than normal, or in individuals with long habitual sleep time, an insufficient sleep period.
- Extension of the habitual sleep period results in amelioration of symptoms and confirms the diagnosis.
- The differential diagnosis is wide and includes all other causes of excessive daytime sleepiness or short duration of the sleep period. These causes should not explain the patient's hypersomnia.
- Polysomnography is not necessary, but if done should demonstrate a short sleep latency and a high (>90%) sleep efficiency.

SLEEP-RELATED MOVEMENT DISORDERS

Introduction

These disorders are characterized by stereotyped, repetitive, relatively simple movements that occur predominantly during sleep, or by less stereotyped movements that interfere with sleep onset (i.e. RLS). The movements should cause either nocturnal sleep disturbance or daytime symptoms. Otherwise, the movements are not considered as the hallmark of a disorder. For example, nocturnal periodic leg movements are common in the asymptomatic elderly. Some movements, such as hypnic jerks occurring during the transition from wakefulness to sleep, are typical of normal physio logic sleep.

Restless legs syndrome (RLS)/ periodic leg movement disorder (PLMD)

Definition

Because of their close association, these will be discussed together. RLS diagnostic criteria were established by the International RLS Study Group in 1995[54], then modified in 2003[55].

- Essential criteria for RLS (necessary for diagnosis):
  - An urge to move the legs, usually accompanied by or caused by uncomfortable sensations.
  - Onset or worsening during periods of rest or inactivity.
  - Total or partial relief by moving the legs or walking.
  - Onset or worsening in the evening or at night.
- Supportive criteria for RLS (not required, but if present, assist in diagnosis):
  - Positive family history.
  - Occurrence of periodic limb movements (PLMs) in sleep, and possibly wakefulness.
  - Clinical response to dopaminergic agents.

PLMs are defined as 'periodic episodes of repetitive and highly stereotyped limb movements that occur during sleep'. PLMs are very common in the general population, increasing in prevalence with age to over 50% in the elderly[56]. Rules for polysomnographic scoring of periodic leg movements are described on p. 926. PLMs with an index ≥5 are found in 80–90% of RLS patients during one or two nights of polysomnography. Conversely, only a minority (<20%) of subjects with polysomnographically documented PLMs complain of RLS symptoms. Therefore, most patients with RLS exhibit PLMs on polysomnography, but most individuals with PLMs do not have RLS. Nonetheless, the two conditions appear to be highly correlated.

- Criteria for PLMD diagnosis:
  - Demonstration of PLMs on polysomnography.
  - Elevated PLM index (>15 for adults and >5 for children is recommended), though emphasis is placed on clinical context rather than absolute numbers.
  - Clinical sleep disturbance or daytime fatigue must be present.
  - Disruption of a bed-partner's sleep by PLMs is not a criterion for diagnosis.

Tip

► *The finding of PLMs on polysomnography, in the absence of symptoms of nocturnal sleep disruption or daytime dysfunction, is often regarded as incidental, not warranting treatment.*

Epidemiology

- Several surveys show a RLS prevalence of approximately 10% in Caucasian populations.
- Prevalence estimates are less for Mediterranean populations, and may be around 1% or less in Asian populations.
- Although RLS may occur in children, prevalence is much higher in those over 40 years old. There are modified diagnostic criteria for children.
- Prevalence in women is 1.5–2 times higher than men.
- In 40–60% of patients, there is a positive family history.
- Most pedigrees suggest an autosomal dominant pattern.
- The genetics of RLS/PLMs appears to be complex. Over 12 chromosomal regions have been identified as possible loci contributing to risk for RLS and/ or PLMs. Interestingly, no mutation has yet been identified as a frequent cause of familial RLS.
- The prevalence of PLMD (PLMs with sleep disruption and absence of RLS symptoms) is unknown, but it is thought to be rare.

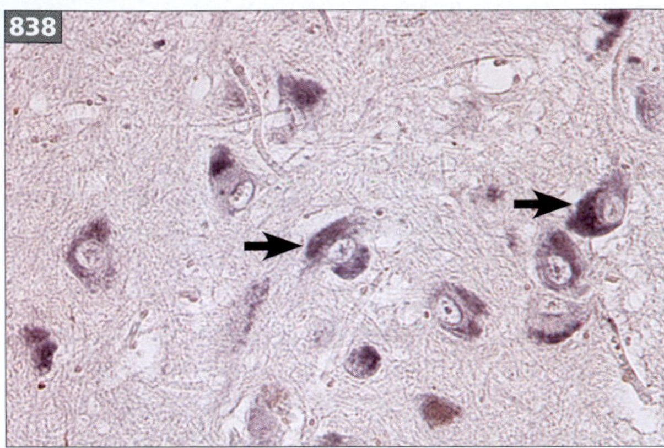

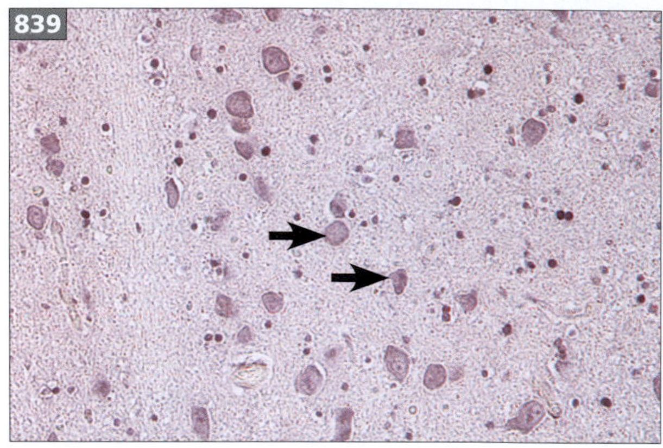

838, 839 **H-ferritin immunostaining in the substantia nigra in control (838) and restless legs syndrome (839) autopsy tissue after bleaching of neuromelanin. Arrows denote neurons, and the small round cells that immunostain strongly in the RLS tissue are glia. The H-ferritin immunoreaction product is more robust in control neurons as compared to RLS, which is consistent with the notion of decreased iron levels in neurons in RLS and the diminished need for iron storage.** *Courtesy of Dr. Amanda Snyder and Dr. James R. Connor, Penn State College of Medicine.*

Pathophysiology

The pathophysiology of RLS is poorly understood. Besides genetic factors mentioned above, abnormal iron metabolism and dopaminergic dysfunction have been implicated. CSF studies, brain imaging[57], and studies of postmortem brain pathology[58] have demonstrated brain iron deficiency (**838, 839**). Evidence that dopaminergic systems are involved comes mostly from pharmacologic observations that dopaminergic agents often dramatically relieve RLS symptoms, and that dopamine blocking agents may exacerbate or trigger RLS. Opioid pathways are also implicated by clinical improvement with narcotics. A clear anatomic substrate has yet to be identified.

Possible secondary causes of RLS and disease associations include:

- Iron deficiency.
- Renal failure.
- Pregnancy.
- Peripheral neuropathy: a recent case–control study of 245 patients and 245 controls revealed a higher prevalence of RLS in hereditary neuropathies, but not in acquired neuropathies[59]. The degree to which peripheral neuropathy is a risk factor for RLS remains somewhat controversial.
- Parkinson's disease.
- Essential tremor.
- Multiple sclerosis.
- Hereditary ataxias.
- Some rheumatologic diseases.
- Spinal cord injury.
- Repeated blood donations (causing iron deficiency).
- Some medications:
  - Most antidepressants except for bupropion, which has dopamine-promoting activity
  - Sedating antihistamines.
  - All central dopamine receptor antagonists, including various antiemetic and antipsychotic medications.

Although pathology in other organ systems is not classically described with RLS/PLMD, there is accumulating evidence that autonomic activation associated with these conditions may contribute to risk of cardiovascular disease or stroke.

Differential diagnosis

RLS

- Nocturnal leg cramps: associated with painful muscle contractions, unlike the dysesthesias in RLS.
- PLMD: occurs only during sleep; absence of symptoms during wakefulness.
- Painful peripheral neuropathy: symptoms present also during the day, and not relieved by walking.
- Arthritis of lower limbs: pain localized to joint areas; circadian pattern absent.
- Positional discomfort after prolonged sitting or lying in one position: resolves by changing position; does not require continual movement.
- Drug-induced akathesia: entire body is often involved; circadian pattern absent; no relief with movement; positive history of neuroleptic drug exposure.
- Painful feet and moving toes: feet prominently involved; continuous slow writhing of toes.

PLMD

- Hypnic jerks: brief (20–100 ms, briefer than PLMs) at transitions from wakefulness to sleep; not periodic.
- REM phasic activity: variable duration, usually associated with rapid eye movements; lack periodicity.
- Leg movements associated with arousal from sleep-disordered breathing: occur towards the end of apneas or hypopneas. Differentiation of arousals due to sleep-disordered breathing from arousals due to PLMs at times can be difficult.
- Spinal cord dysfunction (myelopathy) causing flexor spasms in the lower extremities: usually distinguished by careful neurologic examination.
- Nocturnal epilepsy or myoclonic epilepsy: associated EEG abnormalities; events often occur as well in wakefulness.

Investigations

- For diagnosis of RLS, polysomnography is not required, unless there is suspicion of a superimposed disorder, such as sleep-disordered breathing or epilepsy, or if the diagnosis is questionable.
- Serum ferritin, iron, and total iron-binding capacity as a screen for iron deficiency.
- Further evaluation for the etiology of iron deficiency, including causes of blood loss, are warranted if the ferritin is low.
- EMG, nerve conduction studies, and screening for common causes of neuropathy, if peripheral neuropathy or radiculopathy is suspected. Skin biopsy may be considered if small-fiber neuropathy is suspected. Further investigations may be needed if neuropathy is confirmed.
- For diagnosis of PLMD, polysomnography is necessary.

Treatment

Nonpharmacologic measures have variable success, depending on the individual patient:

- Avoidance of alcohol, which usually exacerbates RLS.
- Massage.
- Application of heat (e.g. hot baths) or cold.
- Moderate exercise, such as walking, prior to bedtime.

TABLE 133 **COMMON PHARMACOLOGIC AGENTS USED FOR TREATMENT OF RESTLESS LEGS SYNDROME**

Medication class	Drug	Dose	Common side-effects	Comments
Iron (indicated if serum ferritin is $< 50\ \mu g/l$)	Ferrous sulfate (oral)	325 mg + 100–200 mg vitamin C, twice a day	Nausea	Follow ferritin levels
	Iron dextran	1000 mg	Anaphylaxis; long-term safety unknown; usually not repeated before 3 months	Infrequently used; some reports of response in patients with 'normal' ferritin
Dopaminergic drugs	Pramipexole	0.125–1.0 mg	Nausea, orthostatic hypotension, insomnia, sleep attacks, compulsive behavior; augmentation	Longer duration than levodopa
	Ropinirole	0.25–4.0 mg	Same as for pramipexole	Slow-release preparations available
	Rotigotine	0.5–6.0 mg	Same as for pramipexole	Transdermal delivery by patch
	Carbidopa/ levodopa	25/100–50/200 mg	Same as for promipexole	Augmentation more likely than with agonists
Anticonvulsants	Gabapentin	300–1200 mg	Weight gain, somnolence, pedal edema	Helpful if painful paresthesias are present
	Gabapentin enacarbil	600–12,000 mg	Same as for gabapentin	Gabapentin prodrug
Opiates	Hydrocodone	5–10 mg	Constipation	
	Methadone	2–15 mg		Latency to benefit
Benzodiazepines	Clonazepam	0.5–2.0 mg	Sedation	Tolerance
	Temazepam	15–30 mg	Sedation	Tolerance

Pharmacologic treatments are presented in *Table 133*. Some, but not all, iron-deficient patients respond to iron supplementation. Trials of various intravenous iron preparations are ongoing. A recent randomized double-blind placebo-controlled trial of intravenous iron sucrose for RLS failed to demonstrate improvement[60]. Subjects in this trial, however, had a wide range of serum ferritin levels, including some in the normal range. Iron dextran, which has a longer half-life, may be more effective, though there is the risk of anaphylaxis during administration[61].

Dopaminergic agents, clonazepam, and gabapentin are sometimes repeated once during the night if needed. Monotherapy is preferred, but some patients with severe symptoms require multiple agents. With use of dopaminergic agents, especially levodopa, care must be taken to avoid the phenomenon of augmentation, in which escalating doses of drug are accompanied by increasing intensity of symptoms, earlier onset of symptoms, and sometimes involvement of additional limbs. The mechanism causing the appearance of augmentation in some patients is poorly understood. If augmentation occurs with levodopa, a switch to a dopamine agonist may be considered. If augmentation occurs during treatment with an agonist, a switch to a different medication class should be considered.

Sleep-related bruxism

Definition

The International Classification of Sleep Disorders defines sleep-related bruxism as 'an oral activity characterized by grinding or clenching of the teeth during sleep, usually associated with sleep arousals'. Tonic activity may occur in the form of sustained jaw clenching. Phasic activity in the form of repetitive muscle contractions may also occur and is sometimes termed 'rhythmic masticatory muscle activity'.

Epidemiology

According to surveys of verbal reports by patients, parents, or bed-partners, sleep-related bruxism is most prevalent in childhood, estimated at 14–17%, with decreasing prevalence associated with aging.

- Approximately one-third of affected children will have sleep-related bruxism persist into adulthood.
- There are no reported sex differences.
- A high concordance rate in dizygotic twins and an even higher concordance rate in monozygotic twins (based on questionnaires or estimation of tooth wear), as well as reports of dominance of the condition in a familial distribution, suggest a possible genetic component.

Etiology and pathophysiology

The exact etiology of sleep-related bruxism remains controversial. Studies providing compelling evidence are sparse. Factors that have been proposed include[62]:

- Problems with dental occlusion ('occlusional interferences').
- Stress and anxiety.
- Presence of excess systemic catecholamines/sympathetic activation.
- Conditions associated with increased arousals, such as smoking, caffeine use, and sleep-disordered breathing.

Clinical features

The hallmark feature is the report by the patient or family members of tooth-grinding sounds or tooth clenching during sleep. On routine polysomnography, sleep-related bruxism is suggested by a polygraphic microarousal (90% of episodes), followed by EMG artifact in EEG derivations (**840**). This artifact consists of either: 1) a phasic pattern at about 1 Hz; 2) tonic activity lasting longer than 2 seconds; or 3) a mixed pattern. Episodes may occur in all stages of sleep, but are most common in stages N1 and N2.

Polysomnographic diagnosis requires monitoring of EMG over at least one masseter muscle, and auditory (and preferably also video) monitoring. Conclusive diagnosis by polysomnography requires at least four episodes of bruxism per hour of sleep, or 25 individual muscle bursts per hour of sleep and at least two audible tooth-grinding episodes during the night, in the absence of epileptiform EEG activity. Polysomnography may be relatively insensitive in mild sleep-related bruxism.

Differential diagnosis

This diagnosis is usually not difficult. Other conditions that may be considered include:

- Facio-mandibular myoclonus: myoclonic jerks of the jaw resulting in brief dental occlusion without tooth-grinding (usually a benign condition).
- Daytime dyskinesias persisting in sleep.
- Sleep-related epilepsy (rarely results in bruxism).
- REM behavior disorder or confusional arousals.

Investigations

- Dental examination in those with severe or frequent bruxism to monitor tooth wear.
- EEG if seizures are suspected.

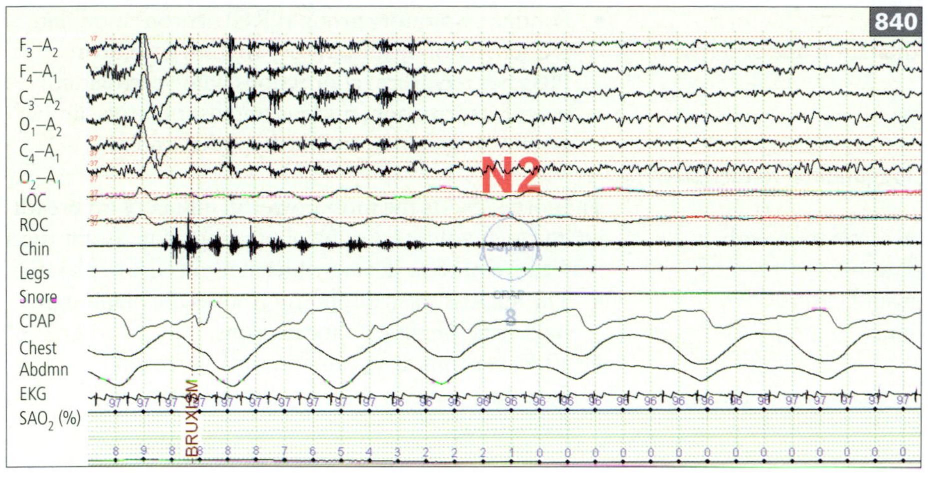

840 Bruxism (30-second epoch). LOC: Left outer canthus, ROC: Right outer canthus; Chin: chin EMG; Legs: leg EMG; NPT: nasal pressure transducer; Therm: thermistor; SAO_2: oxygen saturation.

Diagnosis

The diagnosis of sleep bruxism is usually clinical, based on the following criteria:

- Reports of tooth-grinding sounds or jaw-clenching during sleep.
- One or more of the following:
  - Abnormal wear on the teeth.
  - Jaw muscle discomfort, fatigue, or pain and difficulty opening jaw on awakening.
  - Masseter muscle hypertrophy as demonstrated on voluntary jaw clenching.
- No better explanation by another sleep disorder, neurologic disorder, medication, or substance abuse.

Pathology

- No clear central nervous system pathology has been demonstrated in sleep-related bruxism.
- Tooth wear, fractured teeth, and occasional buccal lacerations may occur.

Treatment

The best treatment for sleep bruxism is controversial[63,64]. Varying success rates have been described for:

- Clonidine.
- Occlusal splints.
- Clonazepam.

Occlusal splints appear to be best tolerated, with fewest side-effects, and protect teeth from future wear. At present, occlusal splints appear to be the treatment of choice. Further research is needed.

SLEEP-RELATED BREATHING DISORDERS

Introduction

Sleep-related breathing disorders (SBDs) are the most common group of sleep disorders treated today. As the general population ages and the current obesity epidemic continues, these disorders, especially obstructive sleep apnea, will continue to increase in frequency and severity (**841**)[65]. Commonly encountered sleep-related breathing disorders include:

- Obstructive sleep apnea (OSA) (see **828**).
- Central sleep apnea (CSA) (see **829**).
- Cheyne–Stokes respiration (see **846**).
- Sleep-related hypoventilation.

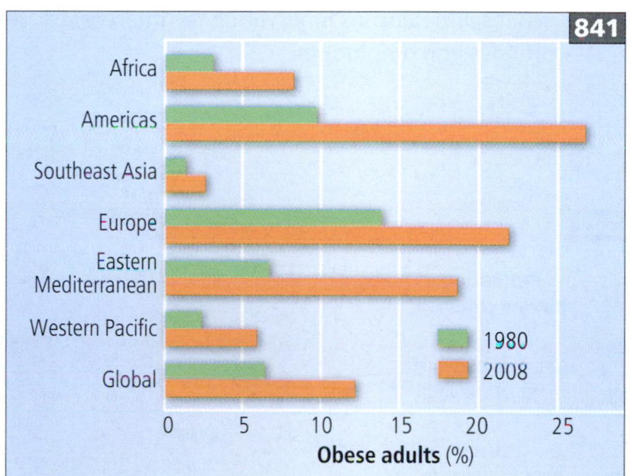

841 The percentage of obese (BMI ≥30) adults aged 20 years and over in World Health Organization (WHO) regions. By 2008, more than 1.4 billion adults were overweight and 500 million were obese. Worldwide obesity has nearly doubled since 1980.

Pathophysiology[66]

Airway anatomy effects both dilatation and collapse of the airway (**842**).

- Airway patency is affected by:
  - Pharyngeal dilator muscle constriction
  - Lung volume producing longitudinal retraction of the neck.
- Airway constriction occurs in association with:
  - Negative pressure of inspiration.
  - Extraluminal positive pressure.
  - Extraluminal fat deposition.
  - Small mandible.
  - Muscle and bone factors affecting generation of negative pressure:
    - Diaphragm and intercostal muscles.
    - Stability of rib cage.

Control of respiration[67].

The ventilatory control mechanism autonomously generates a rhythm for contraction of the respiratory muscles. Sensory input is not required (**843**).

Brainstem neurons involved include:

- Nucleus tractus solitarius, contains: (1) afferent chemo- and pulmonary stretch receptors; and (2) dorsal respiratory neurons that fire during inspiration to stimulate the phrenic motor neurons innervating the diaphragm.
- Ventrolateral medulla (VLM), contains pacemaker cells of respiration that generate bursts of spikes that are the source of the respiratory rhythm:
  - Vagal motor neurons innervate laryngeal and pharyngeal muscles through the dorsal nucleus ambiguus.
  - Ventral lateral reticular formation neurons synapse on neurons innervating the intercostal muscles and diaphragm.
- Pontine respiratory group (PRG) neurons modulate the activity of the respiratory rhythm generator. PRG has reciprocal connections with ventrolateral reticular formation, nucleus tractus solitarius, limbic system (amygdala), and the hypothalamus.

The cortex exerts the most powerful influence on breathing through voluntary control of respiration. Inspiration is an active process during which neurons fire *in* phase:

- The nucleus tractus solitarius moves the diaphragm by driving phrenic motor neurons.
- VLM neurons drive phrenic and intercostal motorneurons via the ventrolateral reticular formation.

Both groups are further modulated:

- Chemoreceptors in the carotid body, under conditions of low O_2 saturation, stimulate the petrosal ganglion and the nucleus tractus solitarius to increase inspiratory activity.
- Pulmonary stretch receptors act through the nodose ganglion to inhibit inspiration (Hering–Breuer reflex).

Expiration is a passive process during which neurons fire *out* of phase, but may become active during increased ventilatory drive (e.g. exercise):

- Ventrolateral medullary expiratory neurons inhibit inspiratory neurons and increase firing in response to decreased pCO_2.
- pCO_2 is sensed within the central nervous system in the ventral medulla via connections to the nucleus tractus solitarius.

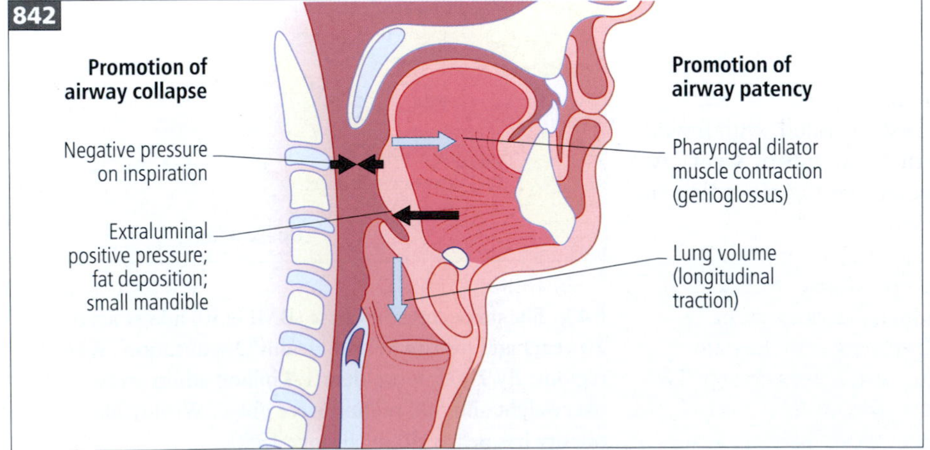

842 Airway anatomy effects both dilatation and collapse of the airway. The sum of these factors affects the critical pressure.

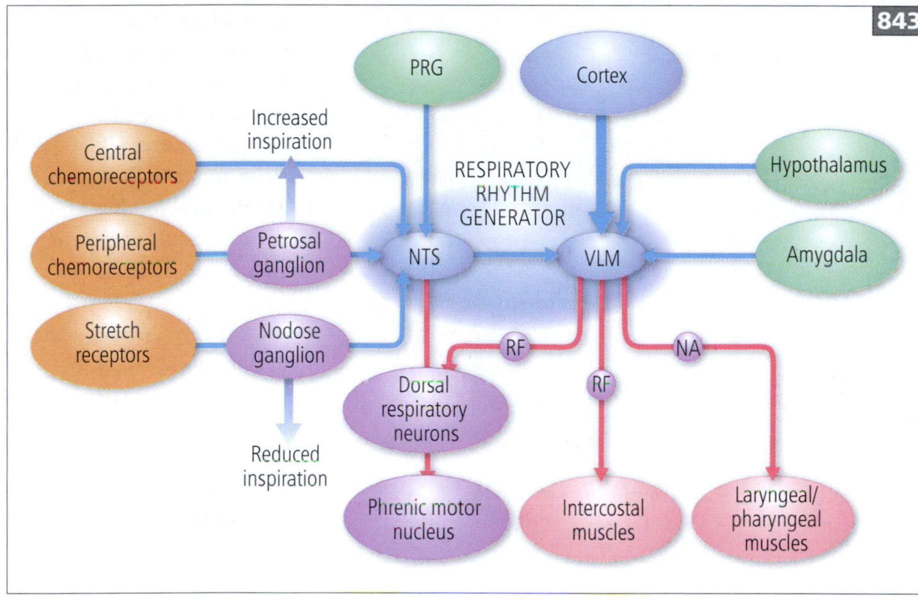

843 Mechanisms of respiratory control. PRG: pontine respiratory group; NTS: nucleus tractus solitarius; VLM: ventrolateral medulla; RF: reticular formation; NA: nucleus ambiguus.

Obstructive sleep apnea syndrome

Definition and clinical features

The hallmark of OSA syndrome is airway obstruction causing apneas and/or hypopneas. In addition, multiple medical consequences result in the symptom complex identified as obstructive sleep apnea *syndrome*[68]. The primary effects of obstructive apnea are on the cardiovascular, pulmonary, endocrine, and central nervous systems. Patients with OSA syndrome may complain of a variety of symptoms including but not limited to:

- Snoring.
- Apnea witnessed by caregivers.
- Nocturnal choking episodes.
- Daytime hypersomnolence.
- Difficulty maintaining sleep.
- Morning headache.

Epidemiology and risk factors

The prevalence of OSA in males is approximately three times that in females. In middle age the prevalence of OSA (as defined by AHI >5, with hypopnea defined as >50% reduction in effort accompanied by oxygen desaturation of 4% or more) is 24% for males and 9% for females, whereas the prevalence of symptomatic OSA *syndrome* (as defined by AHI >5 with complaint of excessive daytime sleepiness) in middle-aged adults is estimated to be 4% in men and 2% in women.

- Obesity: over 70% of patients with OSA are overweight or obese[65]. The prevalence of OSA in overweight or obese individuals is twice that in normal individuals. Mild OSA patients who gain 10% of their bodyweight are at six times greater risk for progression of symptoms. The loss of 10% of body weight decreases OSA severity by 20%.
- Age: there is a two to three-fold increased incidence of OSA above age 60.
- Endocrine:
  - Metabolic syndrome as manifested by decreased insulin sensitivity is seen in 26.7–43% of patients with OSA.
  - 2.4% of patients with OSA have hypothyroidism.
- Race: risk for severe apnea in African Americans is 2.33 times risk in Caucasians. Higher prevalence at lower body mass indices is observed for East Asian populations.
- Genetic: increased risk with multiple affected relatives.
- Craniofacial morphology.

Pathophysiology[67]

The airway can be modeled as a Starling resistor, a tube having infinite compliance (totally collapsed) at one transmural pressure and low compliance (not collapsed) at other pressures. The pressure at which the tube closes due to external pressure equaling the intralumenal pressure is called the critical pressure or *P*crit:

- Pharyngeal dilator muscle activity (tensor palatine, genioglossus) is diminished during sleep, increasing airway compliance.
- As airway collapse increases, increased negative inspiratory pressure is necessary to maintain airflow and results in additional collapse. Eventually *P*crit is reached and the airway occludes.

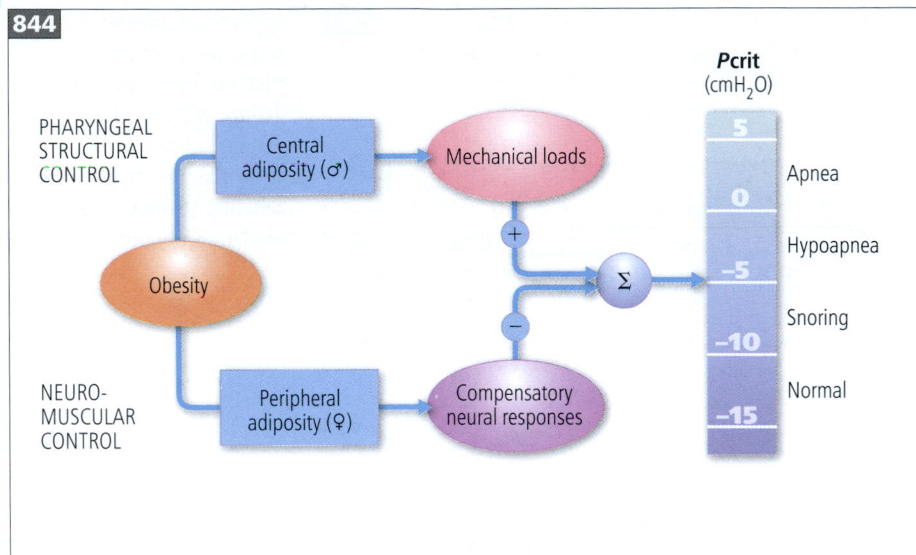

844 **Illustration relating obesity, body fat distribution, upper airway collapsibility critical pressure (*P*crit), and sleep apnea pathogenesis. Mechanical loads and neuromuscular responses sum (∑) to increase (+) and decrease (–) *P*crit, respectively. Mechanical and humoral effects of regional adipose depots can affect these components, which can mediate differences in sleep apnea susceptibility between men and women.**

- Interaction between pharyngeal structural properties and neuromuscular regulation determines pharyngeal airway collapsibility. Obesity impacts on this balance by reducing lung volume and narrowing the pharyngeal airway, with neural compensation for these abnormalities being lost during sleep (**844**).

Intrinsic airway obstruction increases airway resistance and increased negative inspiratory pressure is required to maintain airflow:

- Anatomic abnormalities: micrognathia or macroglossia.
- Adenotonsillar hypertrophy is the most common cause of OSA in young children.

Airway obstruction may also result from extrinsic factors:

- Para-airway adipose tissue: neck size correlates with increased risk of apnea.
- Decreased airway dilator muscle activity, as may occur in the setting of neuromuscular disease.

Other pathology associated with OSA syndrome[69]

- Hypertension: 30–40% of hypertensive patients have OSA. Approximately 50% of patients with OSA are hypertensive. Patients with an AHI >15 have a risk of hypertension 2.89 times that of normal controls.
- Stroke: Post-stroke, 60–80 % of patients have OSA with a respiratory disturbance index (RDI) greater than 10. Risk of stroke in patients with OSA increases with increasing AHI, rising from 1.75 relative risk if AHI is <12, to 3.30 if the AHI is >36. 54% of strokes occur at night in OSA patients, whereas stroke incidence is greatest in the first few hours after awakening in the general population[70].
- Congestive heart failure: sleep apnea is seen in over 50% of patients with heart failure. OSA increases the risk of heart failure by an odds ratio of 2.38. Treatment with CPAP increases left ventricular ejection fraction by 25–33%[71].
- Coronary artery disease: 30–58% of patients with coronary artery disease have OSA.
- Neurocognitive effects: neurocognitive dysfunction correlates with sleep disruption/deprivation, and especially if intermittent hypoxia occurs in association with respiratory events[72]. Patients with hypersomnolence have poorer cognitive functioning than those who do not have daytime sleepiness. OSA has been shown to have negative effects on:
  - Cognitive processing.
  - Working memory.
  - Executive function.
  - Vigilance.

Diagnosis

Polysomnography demonstrates an AHI >5. Current USA Medicare criteria for diagnosis and reimbursement of therapy for OSA require that events scored as apneas and hypopneas are accompanied by ≥3% oxygen desaturation. Differential diagnosis in a patient observed to snore and have possible observed apneas includes primary snoring (without clinically significant OSA), Cheyne–Stokes respiration, obstructive hypoventilation, obesity hypoventilation syndrome, sleep-related hypoventilation due to a medical or neuromuscular condition, and CSA syndromes.

Treatment

Weight reduction is the primary long-term therapy for all patients with elevated body mass index. However for acute treatment, positive airway pressure (PAP) is the standard of care[73]. Positive pressure is delivered by a mask or similar device (**845**):

- Pressure provides a physiologic stent to the airway to relieve obstruction.
- CPAP provides a constant inspiratory and expiratory pressure to stent the airway.
- Bi-level positive airway pressure (BiPAP) delivers increased inspiratory pressure and a decreased expiratory pressure. The goal of decreased expiratory pressure is to preserve the stenting effect while making expiration easier, and allowing therapy to be better tolerated, especially at high inspiratory pressures. This mode may also provide better ventilation for patients with neuromuscular conditions that cause difficulty with expiration against a continuous pressure.
- Another option is an auto titrating machine, which automatically adjusts pressure within a range of pressures set by the physician, as needed throughout the night.

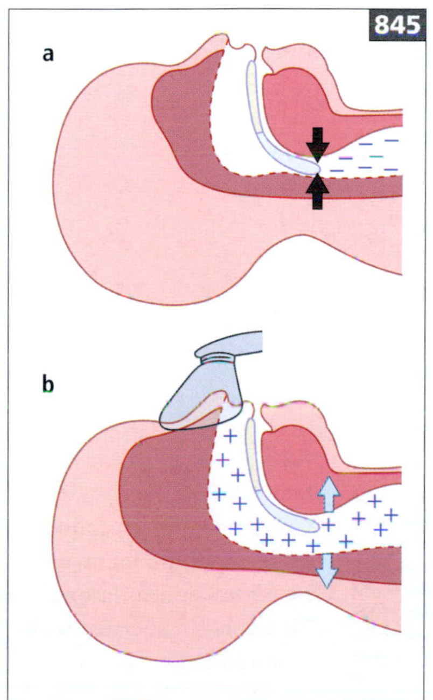

845 Positive airway pressure. (a) Demonstrates the anatomy of airway collapse. Note negative pressure in airway and extrinsic forces on airway causing collapse. (b) Effect of positive airway pressure opening the airway and restoring patency.

Oxygen alone or in addition to CPAP therapy is indicated for hypoxemia not resolved by CPAP and may occasionally be used as primary therapy for patients unable to tolerate CPAP. For severe OSA refractory to treatment with PAP, tracheostomy may be required.

Systemic processes including hypertension, coronary artery disease, and metabolic syndrome must also be addressed.

Primary central sleep apnea

CSA, while common in preterm infants, is rare in children and adults.

- Pathophysiology: in primary sleep apnea, there is a high ventilatory response to rising pCO_2, resulting in an increased respiratory rate and excessive lowering of pCO_2, that in turn causes apnea. These apneas produce little oxygen desaturation.
- Diagnosis: excessive daytime sleepiness and arousals, awakenings or insomnia complaints are the presenting symptoms. Diagnosis is confirmed by polysomnography demonstrating five or more central apneas per hour greater than 10 seconds in duration.
- Treatment for central apnea and hypoventilation syndromes[74]:
  - Assisted ventilation is the most effective and safest treatment for primary CSA.
  - Noninvasive BiPAP with a backup rate or newer machines employing 'adaptive servo-ventilation', with proprietary software designed to maintain a tidal volume and rate, may be options for some patients.
  - Respiratory stimulants such as acetazolamide, caffeine, progesterone, or doxapram may be effective in some patients.
  - Oxygen therapy may be sufficient in mild cases.

Sleep-related hypoventilation/ hypoxemia due to neuromuscular and chest wall disorders

Obesity hypoventilation syndrome is the most common manifestation of this multi-causal problem.

- Pathophysiology: reduced contractility of ventilatory muscles is the major cause of hypoventilation. The cause can be at any level of the neuromuscular system, or may result from mechanical factors such as morbid obesity. Anatomic abnormalities of the thorax can also cause chest wall restriction, or lung collapse resulting in hypoventilation. Baseline elevation in the pCO_2 set point limits pCO_2 response and leaves only the hypoxemic response to drive respiration[67].

- Etiologies:
  - Obesity.
  - Chest wall abnormalities.
  - Kyphoscoliosis.
  - Neuromuscular abnormalities:
    - Anterior horn cell disease.
    - Myopathy.
    - Neuropathy.
    - Stroke.
    - Genetic.
- Diagnosis: polysomnography demonstrates oxygen saturation <90% for more than 5 min at night and a nadir of at least 85%, or oxygen saturation <90% for more than 30% of the night.
- Treatment: assisted ventilation and tracheostomy may be necessary in severe cases, as for primary CSA. Milder cases may be managed with noninvasive strategies as detailed above for milder forms of primary CSA.

Central sleep apnea due to drug or substance use

- Pathophysiology: chronic substance abuse, especially abuse involving opioids, decreases the response of central chemoreceptors in the ventral medulla, so that there is decreased ventilatory drive to rising pCO_2.
- Clinical features: variable breathing patterns:
  - Central apnea.
  - Obstructive apnea.
  - Periodic breathing.
  - Biot's breathing.
- Treatment of primary substance abuse is key[2]. Supportive intervention may be indicated, based on the severity and type of breathing pattern. Apnea usually resolves spontaneously over a few months.

Cheyne–Stokes breathing

- Definition: Cheyne–Stokes respirations are recurrent periods of central apneas and hypopneas, alternating with respiratory periods having a pattern of crescendo–decrescendo tidal volumes (**846**).
- Etiologies:
  - Congestive heart failure.
  - Stroke.
  - Renal failure.
- Pathophysiology of Cheyne–Stokes: increased vagal tone and increased sensitivity of peripheral and central chemoreceptors are thought to play a role. In addition, circulatory delay causes a delayed response of respiratory drive to changes in pO_2 or pCO_2, resulting in the characteristic crescendo–decrescendo respiratory pattern[75].
- Predisposing factors:
  - Male, >60 years.
  - Atrial fibrillation.
  - Awake pCO_2 ≥38 torr.
- Diagnosis: polysomnography demonstrates ≥10 central apneas per hour. Central apneas associated with crescendo–decrescendo respirations are demonstrated.
- Treatment:
  - Noninvasive assisted ventilation at night.
  - Treatment of heart failure.
  - Supplemental oxygen alone is effective for some patients.

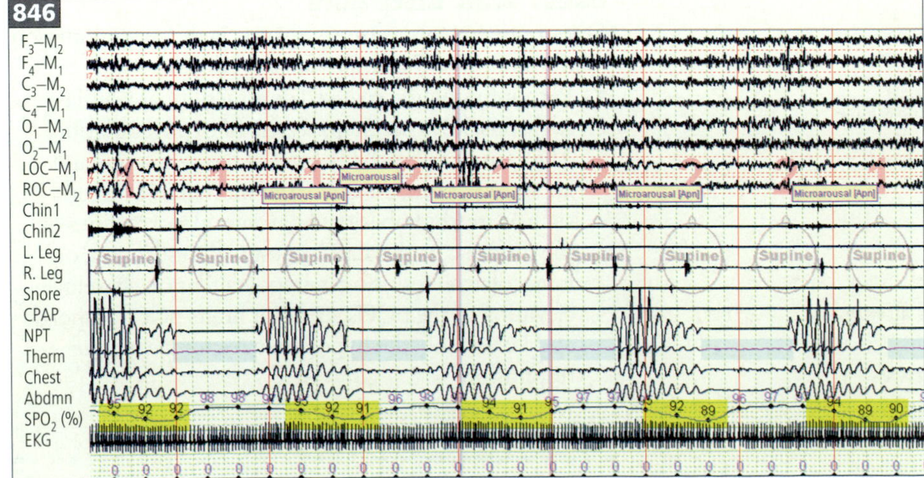

846 Example of Cheyne–Stokes respiration. Crescendo–decrescendo respirations are followed by central apneas lasting 20 seconds associated with desaturation.

Congenital central hypoventilation syndrome

- Definition: a respiratory pattern characterized by the persistence of fetal breathing into the extrauterine environment. Patients hypoventilate or in severe cases completely stop breathing when the transition from waking to non-REM sleep occurs[74].
- Epidemiology: over 200 cases have been reported world-wide.
- Clinical features and pathophysiology: congenital central hypoventilation syndrome is present from birth. The syndrome is caused by mutations in the *Phox2B* gene. In addition to hypoventilation, the syndrome is often associated with autonomic nervous system dysfunction.
- Differential diagnosis includes:
  - Apnea of prematurity.
  - Apnea of infancy.
  - Apparent life threatening events.
  - Diaphragmatic paralysis.
  - Muscular dystrophy.
  - Congenital myopathies.
  - Sepsis, periodic breathing.
  - Metabolic disorders.

All of these disorders can produce central apneas, but they are usually more severe during REM sleep. Arnold–Chiari malformations can also produce central apneic spells; however, these are of short duration and occur in wakefulness and all sleep stages.

- Diagnosis:
  - Polysomnography: central hypoventilation or sleep-onset apnea is the classic finding. Ventilation improves during REM sleep. During the initial non-REM sleep period and any transition from wake to non-REM sleep, central hypoventilation can again be demonstrated. In infants the transition from wake to REM sleep is normal. The absence of respiratory drive in non-REM transitions and the presence of respiratory drive in REM transitions is pathognomonic for this syndrome.
  - Gene testing for *Phox2B* mutation is confirmatory.
- Treatment:
  - Nocturnal ventilation supplementation to maintain gas exchange is the primary therapy; home ventilation is now common practice. Invasive options include tracheostomy with nocturnal ventilation or a diaphragmatic pacemaker.
  - In milder cases, noninvasive ventilation can be provided with BiPAP at a constant rate, negative pressure ventilation, or a rocking bed.
  - Respiratory stimulants, including theophylline, progesterone, and doxapram, have been tried with limited success.

CIRCADIAN RHYTHM SLEEP DISORDERS

Introduction

Circadian rhythm disorders can be produced by extrinsic or intrinsic disruption of the natural synchrony between our external environment and our innate biological clock. Extrinsic factors include shift work and travel across time zones. Intrinsic circadian disturbances include advanced sleep phase, delayed sleep phase, a free-running cycle, and an irregular sleep–wake cycle[76].

Neuroanatomy and physiology of the circadian system[77]

The suprachiasmatic nucleus (SCN) is the central biological clock. Synchronization with the external environment occurs through light stimuli that travel from the retina via the retinohypothalamic tract to the SCN, ultimately to the pineal gland. Light stimulus inhibits the pineal secretion of the sleep-promoting hormone melatonin, thereby providing synchronization of wakefulness to daytime in humans (see **821**). The result of the actions of the SCN also produces day and night differences in many biological functions, including body core temperature and cortisol levels, which can be measured and correlated with the phase of the sleep–wake cycle (**847**). These circadian phases can be altered with light, melatonin, or behavioral therapies.

847 Melatonin phase response curve (orange line) demonstrating delayed and advanced sleep phase shifts, depending on the timing of melatonin administration. For bright light exposure (red line), the most significant phase delay shift occurs with exposure in the late evening, and the most significant phase advance shift occurs with exposure in the early morning, after the nadir of core body temperature.

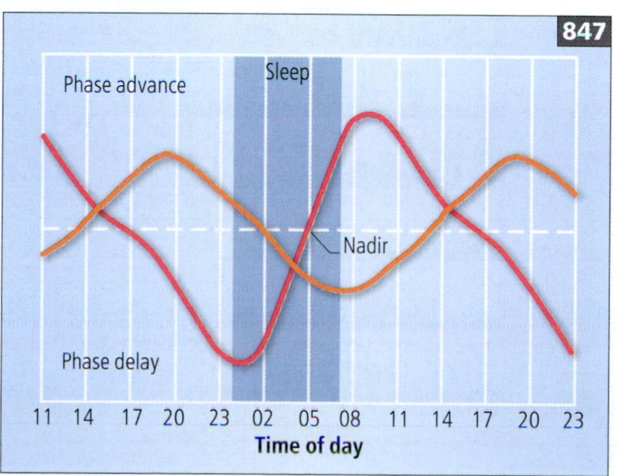

Consequences of disruption of circadian rhythms include:

- Cognitive impairment.
- Impaired motor skills.
- Loss of vigilance.
- Risks of errors and accident.
- Mood disturbance, irritability, low energy.

Diagnosis

Diagnosis of these disorders is accomplished with the use of sleep diaries or actigraphy. An actigraph, a noninvasive device resembling a wristwatch, detects body movements and has been well correlated with polysomnographic measures of sleep. As can be seen in the normal sleep actigram (**848**) there is a marked decrease in movements recorded in the sleep state.

Treatment[78]

Melatonin

Melatonin has phase shift effects and hypnotic effects. Early evening dosing causes sleep phase advance. Late night or early morning dosing causes sleep phase delay. If it is used for its hyypnotic effect:

- It has a half-life of 45 min.
- It can be given 15–30 min prior to desired bedtime.
- 0.1–0.5 mg is a physiologic dose.
- 1–6 mg is a pharmacologic dose.

Light therapy[79]

- Exposure to bright light during the evening causes sleep phase delay.
- Exposure to bright light during the morning causes sleep phase advance.

Chronotherapy

Chronotherapy is used to resynchronize the body clock. The patient gradually shifts the sleep time over a period of weeks. Once the shift is completed, the patient must adhere to the new schedule to maintain the effect.

Regularization of sleep–wake schedule is mandatory. Adherence to a fixed wake-up time is most important. Napping should not be permitted for intrinsic circadian disorders. Napping may improve function acutely. Planned naps for extrinsic circadian disorders can lessen the impact of sleep loss and circadian imbalance.

The advent of the 80-hour work week for USA medical housestaff (less in UK and Europe) has forever changed medical education. Sleep loss is additive. Total sleep deprivation for 2 days is equal to 12 days of 6 hours of sleep. The cognitive effects of sleep loss are often not perceptible to the individual suffering deprivation. One night of sleep deprivation is equivalent to a blood-alcohol level of between 0.05% and 0.10% in driving simulators. The consequences of sleep loss include drowsy driving and increased auto accidents. Increased rates of medical errors are well documented in sleep-deprived housestaff[80].

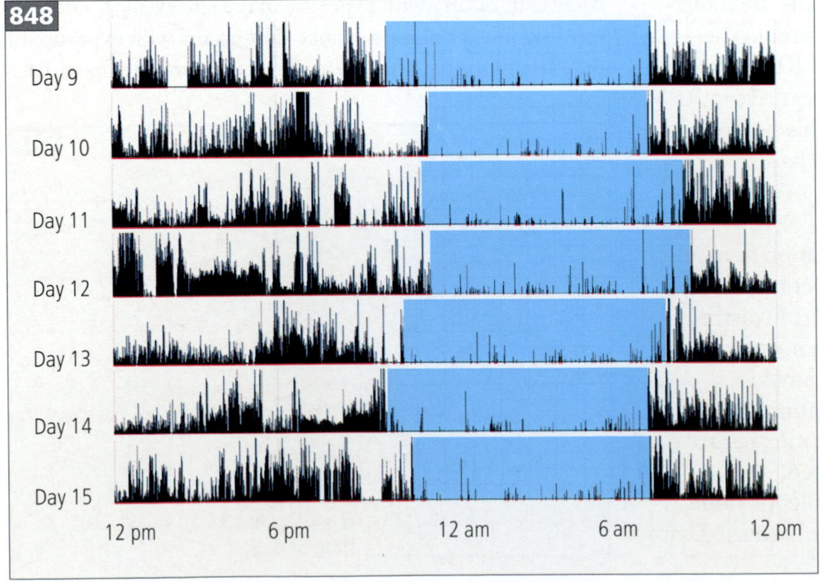

848 Normal sleep pattern demonstrated with actigraphy. Note the lack of high amplitude movements during the sleep periods (shaded blue) recorded by the actigraph.

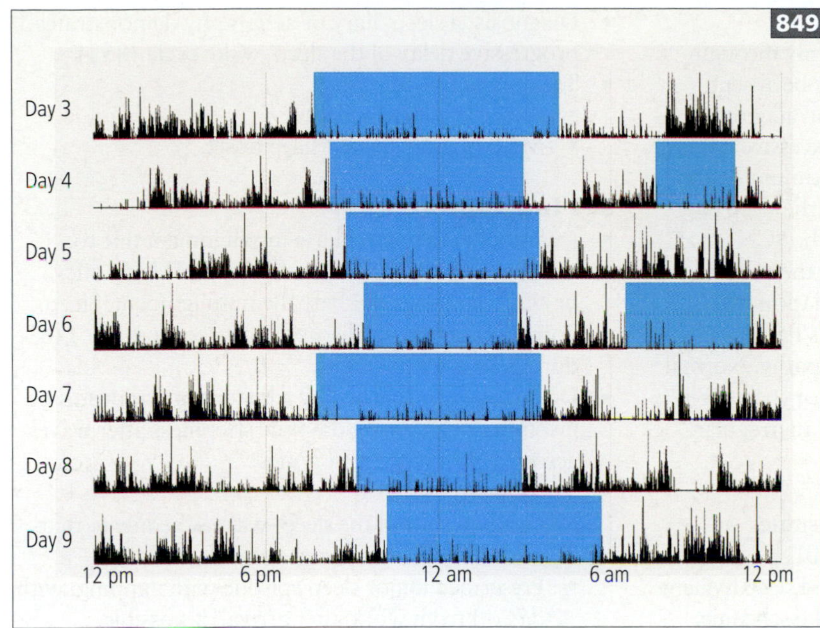

849 **Actigraphy demonstrates nightly early onset (advance) of the major sleep phase with normal duration.**

Delayed sleep-phase syndrome type

- Definition: onset of sleep is delayed in relationship to the environment. Symptoms include difficulty falling asleep and difficulty awakening in the early morning. This syndrome is extremely common in adolescents.
- Diagnosis is established by a detailed history, supplemented by a sleep diary and/or actigraphy. Other behavioral and sleep-hygiene issues should be excluded. The differential diagnosis includes non-24 hour and irregular sleep–wake cycle syndromes.
- Treatment options:
  - Melatonin at desired sleep onset.
  - Early morning light.
  - Sleep scheduling consisting of a progressive shift of sleep–wake schedule and adherence to the desired schedule once it is achieved.

Tip

▶ *Delayed sleep-phase syndrome is extremely common among teenagers and young adults. Reassurance that appearance of the syndrome in this age group usually does not signify a serious medical problem is often helpful. Emphasis on principles of good sleep hygiene is also very useful, in addition to the approaches mentioned above.*

Advanced sleep-phase type[81]

- Definition: onset of sleep is early in relationship to the environment. Symptoms include difficulty staying awake in the evening, and early morning insomnia.
- Diagnosis is established by a detailed history and a sleep diary and/or actigraphy (849). The differential diagnosis is the same as for sleep-phase delay syndrome. Depression should be excluded.
- Treatment options:
  - Evening light.
  - Sleep scheduling consisting of a progressive shift of sleep–wake schedule and adherence to the desired schedule once it is achieved.

Irregular sleep–wake type[81]

- Definition: sleep periods occur randomly throughout the day. A major sleep period may be absent and multiple daily naps may be seen on actigraphy. Symptoms include insomnia and/or excessive daytime sleepiness and variable periods of maximum sleepiness. Sleep in these patients resembles the sleep of experimental animals with lesions in the SCN.
- Etiologies may involve dysfunction of the SCN or its connections, as may occur in association with dementia, movement disorders such as Parkinson's disease, trauma, or hepatic encephalopathy. Normal individuals without compelling work or social obligations, such as retirees, may develop an irregular sleep–wake schedule.
- Diagnosis and treatment:
  - A sleep diary or actigraphy demonstrates disturbed rhythmicity of sleep (**850**).
  - Treatment involves practice of good sleep hygiene and adherence to a fixed sleep–wake schedule.

Free-running type[81]

- Definition: in the absence of light/dark input, the SCN runs free at its intrinsic period, which is slightly greater than 24 hours in humans. Most commonly this syndrome occurs in congenital or acquired blindness, pituitary tumors, or when there is inadequate light–dark exposure or continuous low-light exposure. Symptoms may include either excessive daytime sleepiness or insomnia.
- Diagnosis: a sleep diary or actigraphy demonstrates progressive delay of the sleep–wake cycle (**851**).
- Treatment:
  - Prescribed sleep schedule.
  - Melatonin at desired sleep onset.

Jet lag type[77]

- Definition: circadian phase misalignment due to travel across time zones. In-flight use of hypnotics or alcohol may exacerbate the misalignment. Sleep homeostasis may be disrupted by sleep loss prior to, during, or after the flight.
- Diagnosis is established by a history of symptoms of insomnia or excessive daytime sleepiness after travel across two or more time zones.
- Treatment:
  - Gradual shift of the sleep–wake schedule to that of the destination prior to travel.
  - Prescribed major sleep episode with napping, with day off from work after arrival, if possible.
  - Melatonin or a short-acting hypnotic at desired sleep onset for eastward destinations.
  - Timed light exposure to advance or delay the circadian clock:
    - Westward travel: morning light at the destination and avoidance of evening light.
    - Eastward travel: afternoon and early evening light at the destination and avoidance of morning light.

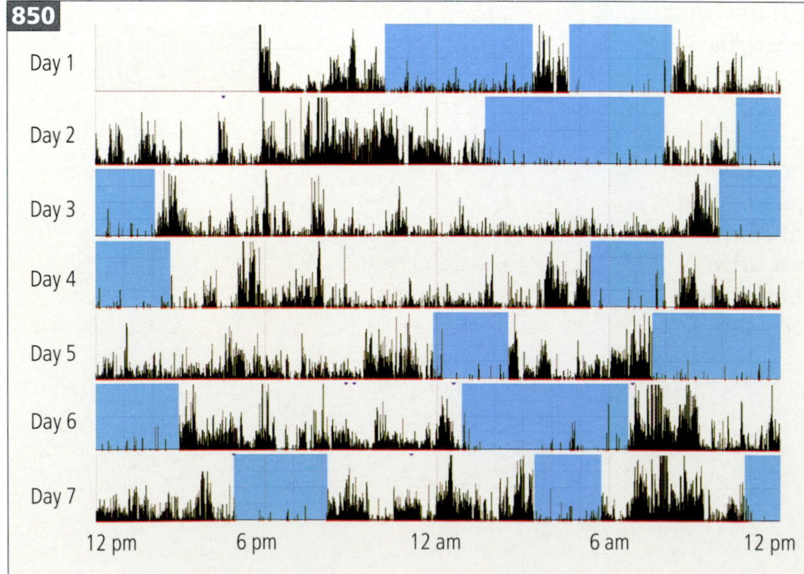

850 Actigraph recording demonstrates fragmented sleep unrelated to external cues, without circadian organization. Note the difficulty initiating and maintaining sleep and frequent daytime naps.

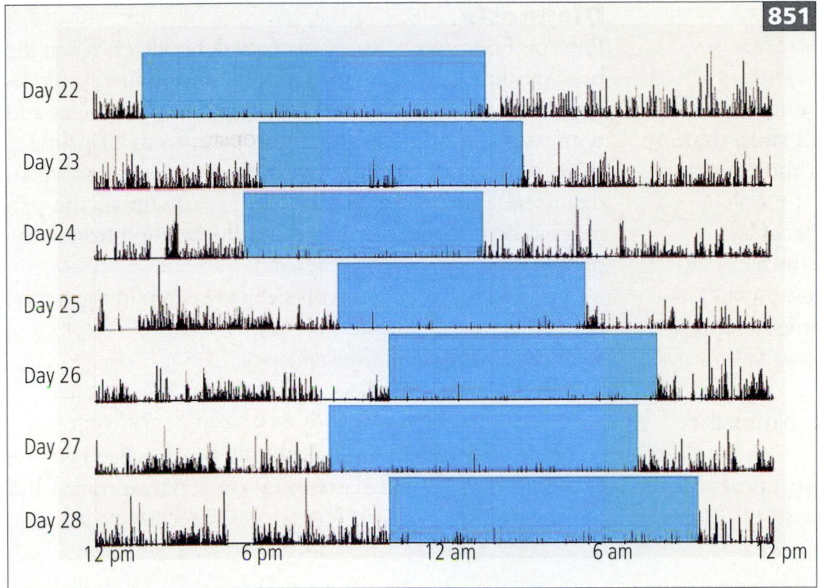

851 Actigraphy of an example of a free-running pattern, demonstrating a constant duration of the major sleep phase with short delay each night. This delay is caused by the intrinsic circadian rhythm which is longer than the external 24-hour clock. This pattern demonstrates the impact of the loss of synchronization of the clock with external cues.

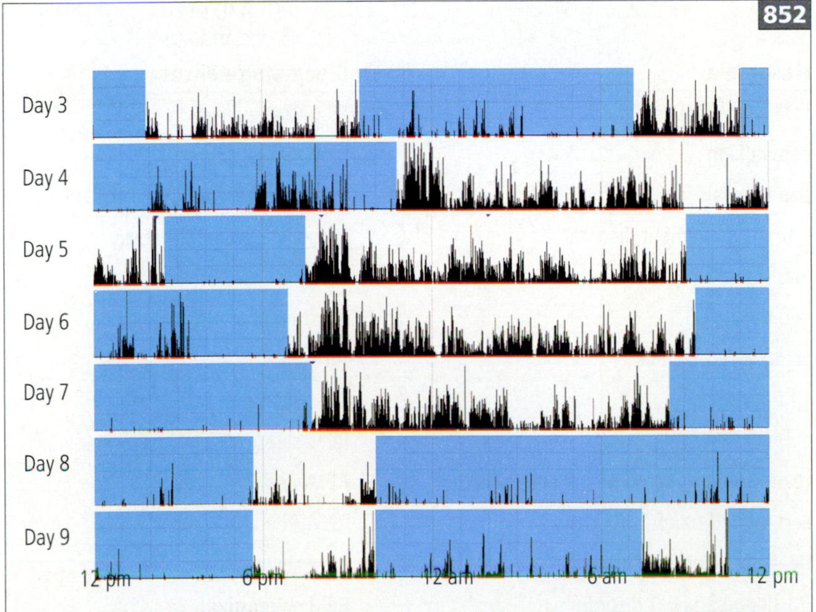

852 Actigraphy demonstrates effects of shift work on the sleep pattern. The night shift occurs between days 4 and 7, with recovery sleep on days 8 and 9.

Shift work type[77]

- Definition: shift work produces a forced desynchronization of circadian rhythms from the external environment (852). While prolonged shift changes may lessen the effects and allow for resynchronization of circadian rhythms, short work stints and the need for socialization during off days often interfere with this process and cause added sleep loss. Some individuals are never able to adjust fully to shift work.
- Diagnosis is established by a history of insomnia or excessive daytime sleepiness associated with a recurring work schedule that overlaps the habitual sleep time.
- Treatment:
  - A prescribed major sleep episode with napping prior to work may be useful.
  - Hypnotics or melatonin may aid in inducing sleep at the desired time.
  - Bright light exposure during the shift may improve performance.
  - Stimulants such as modafinil during the shift also enhance performance.

PARASOMNIAS

Introduction

In the broadest sense, parasomnias encompass all behaviors or experiences associated with sleep that are undesirable or unpleasant to the sleeper or those nearby[82]. Parasomnias:

- Are associated with the normal sleep process.
- Arise predominately out of sleep.
- Are associated with specific sleep stages.
- Involve behaviors that have at least some stereotypy.

Types of parasomnias include[2]:

- Arousal disorders.
- Parasomnias associated with REM sleep disorders.
- Other parasomnias.
- A list of the parasomnias in each group appears in *Table 134*.

Diagnosis

Polysomnography is rarely necessary; however, when the presentation is atypical, then a polysomnogram is recommended. For all the arousal parasomnias, the patient and witnesses should be asked about symptoms of primary sleep disorders associated with arousals, such as sleep-disordered breathing or PLMD. Treatment of the primary sleep disorder sometimes results in resolution of the parasomnia.

Epilepsies associated with sleep are often in the differential diagnosis:

- Nocturnal frontal lobe epilepsy.
- Other partial epilepsies.

A minimum of 10 EEG leads should be recorded because of the overlap of clinical presentation of parasomnias and the epilepsies[83].

TABLE 134 **TYPES OF PARASOMNIAS**

Group	Parasomnia	Sleep-stage onset
Arousal disorders	Confusional arousals	Slow-wave sleep
	Sleepwalking	Slow-wave sleep
	Sleep terrors	Slow-wave sleep
Sleep–wake transition disorders	Rhythmic movement disorder	Stage 1, 2 non-REM sleep
	Sleep starts	Stage 1 non-REM sleep
	Sleep talking	All stages
	Nocturnal leg cramps	All stages
Parasomnias associated with REM sleep	Nightmares	REM sleep
	Sleep paralysis	REM sleep
	Impaired sleep-related penile erections	REM sleep
	Sleep-related painful erections	REM sleep
	REM sleep-related sinus arrest	REM sleep
	REM sleep behavior disorder	REM sleep
Other parasomnias	Sleep bruxism	Stage 2 non-REM sleep
	Sleep enuresis	All stages
	Sleep-related abnormal swallowing syndrome	Stages 1, 2 non-REM sleep
	Nocturnal paroxysmal dystonia	Stages 2, 3, 4 non-REM sleep
	Sudden unexplained nocturnal death syndrome	
	Sudden infant death syndrome	
	Benign neonatal sleep myoclonus	Quiet sleep
	Sleep-related eating disorder	
	Catathrenia	
	Other parasomnia NOS	

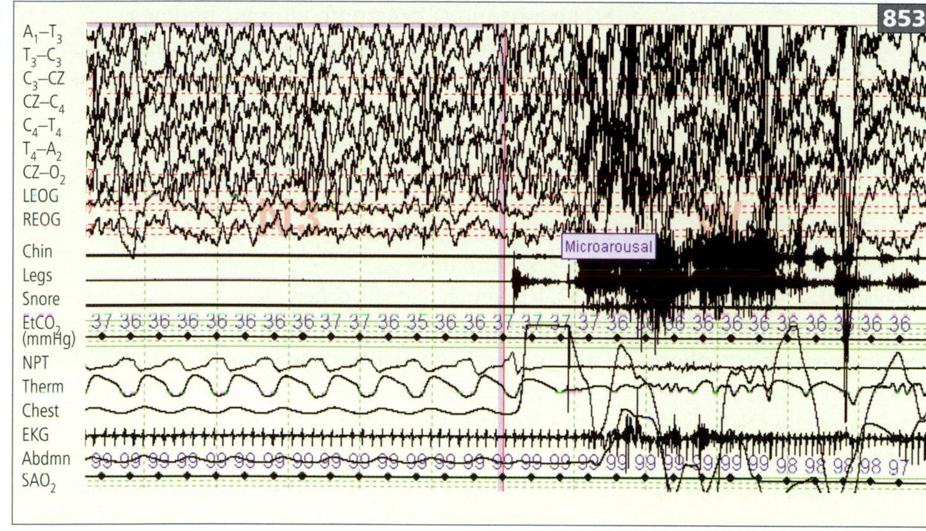

853 Arousal from slow-wave sleep. This is the typical finding associated with confusional arousal, night terrors, and sleepwalking.

Treatment

Treatment of the parasomnias is symptomatic:

- Prevention of injury to the patient or bed-partner.
- Discussion and reassurance to the patient and family that these events are common and are not a sign of other sleep problems or pathology.
- The secondary goal of treatment is to improve sleep quality and decrease sleep disruption for the patient, bed-partner, and family.

Non-REM arousal parasomnias (853)[84]

Confusional arousals

- Clinical features: short arousals associated with crying and or being frightened and disoriented are the typical presentation of confusional arousals. The arousals usually last less than 5 minutes. The child is typically easily consoled and returns to sleep quickly. When asked, the child does not usually describe events or a memory causing the arousal. Confusional arousals are nearly universal in young children.
- Diagnosis and treatment:
  - The diagnosis is made on clinical history.
  - There should be no other symptoms associated with a primary sleep disorder.
  - A sleep study should be obtained if daytime episodes are reported.
  - Patients beyond age 7–8 years should have a sleep study to exclude other sleep disorders producing arousals, including seizure disorders, sleep-related breathing disorders, or RLS/PLMD.
  - Reassurance for parents is typically the only treatment that is required with confusional arousals.

Sleepwalking (somnambulism)

- Definition: a partial arousal from sleep that is associated with ambulation.
- Epidemiology:
  - Sleepwalking occurs occasionally in approximately 40% of children and rarely in adults.
  - Sleepwalking peaks in incidence between 10 and 12 years of age.
  - About 2–3% of children are frequent sleep walkers, having episodes more than once per month.
- Clinical features: the patient arises from bed, may walk throughout the residence, unlock doors, and may even be found wandering outside the house. Sleepwalkers may mistake windows for doors and fall from windows. Sleepwalkers are very difficult to awaken. They may return to their normal sleeping location or may be found in other rooms or on a floor sleeping.
- Investigations: polysomnographic findings:
  - Because most patients have infrequent episodes, the polysomnogram is often unremarkable.
  - Sleepwalking occurs out of slow-wave sleep, with faster rhythms superimposed on slow waves during the arousal. Video monitoring shows the patient arising from bed and beginning to walk around. He or she may pull off leads, open doors, and pull equipment along.
  - If a polysomnogram is clinically indicated, an extended EEG montage should be utilized which includes bilateral frontal, temporal, and anterior temporal electrodes, as seizure disorders of frontal and temporal origin are included in the differential diagnosis.
  - Capability to review 10-second epochs is necessary to identify seizure activity.

- Differential diagnosis:
  - Complex partial seizures.
  - Nocturnal frontal lobe epilepsy.
  - Nocturnal paroxysmal dystonia.
  - REM behavior disorder.
- Diagnosis and treatment:
  - A typical clinical history as described above obtained from family members establishes the diagnosis.
  - Polysomnography is rarely needed.
  - Episodes that have atypical presentation, occurring at sleep onset, associated with complex movements and vocalizations that appear purposeless or occur more than once per week, raise the question of seizure disorder.
  - Early morning episodes raise the question of REM behavior disorder.
  - If the presentation is atypical, then polysomnography with extended EEG leads or overnight video EEG should be performed.
  - For treatment, patient safety is most important. Windows and doors should be securely locked in severe cases to prevent injury. Clonazepam is used to suppress events if they occur frequently.

Sleep terrors

- Definition and clinical features:
  - Sleep terrors are also called night terrors or pavor nocturnus.
  - Events are partial arousals out of slow-wave sleep and are therefore observed mostly during the first third of the night.
  - Events are characterized by the child screaming out, with accompanying autonomic symptoms of fright, such as tachycardia, elevated blood pressure, and diaphoresis.
  - The child appears terrified, is inconsolable and does not seem to be fully awake. After 20 –30 minutes the child becomes consolable and may awaken.
  - There is little recall for the event, and little detail of what was producing the frightening emotion. Typically there is no recall of the event in the morning.
- Epidemiology:
  - Most children presenting with night terrors are under the age of 10 years.
  - Less than 10% of children will have a night terror.
  - Patients will often have later somnambulism.
  - Sleep terrors may occur less commonly in adults.
- Investigations: polysomnographic findings:
  - An arousal from slow-wave sleep is associated with screaming, increased heart rate, mydriasis, and diaphoresis.
  - Features of a waking background EEG are superimposed on slow waves.
  - This state may persist for 20–30 minutes.
- Differential diagnosis:
  - Nightmares.
  - REM behavior disorder.
  - Both nightmares and REM behavior disorder occur in the early morning hours when REM-sleep predominates.
  - Nightmares and REM behavior disorder are associated with vivid dream recall, unlike sleep terrors.
  - Complex partial seizures: these tend to be associated more with automatisms than with episodes of terror, although certain types, especially frontal lobe seizures, can be confused with night terrors. Frontal lobe seizures often occur several times per night, whereas night terrors usually occur only once per night.
- Diagnosis and treatment:
  - The clinical description is usually sufficient to diagnose this parasomnia.
  - Events typically occur sporadically.
  - Intervention typically is reassurance.
  - If frequent events interfere with the sleep of caregivers or bed-partner, a small dose of diazepam or clonazepam is given at bedtime. Benzodiazepines are thought to prevent the events by decreasing slow-wave sleep and/or increasing arousal threshold.

Sleep-related eating disorder[85]

- Definition: recurrent episodes of involuntary eating and drinking during the main sleep period. Patients usually have fragmentary or no recall of the event, but reduced awareness and amnesia are not required for diagnosis.
- Epidemiology:
  - Occurs in 8–16% of patients with eating disorders, and in one series, 4.6% of university students.
  - Commonly associated with other sleep disorders that cause arousal or disrupt sleep, including sleepwalking.
  - Also associated with use of sedating and hypnotic medications, particularly in the setting of patient escalation of hypnotic medication dosing.

- Clinical features may include:
  - Consumption of peculiar, inedible, or toxic substances.
  - Symptoms referable to disrupted sleep, such as fatigue or somnolence.
  - Sleep-related injury or potentially dangerous behaviors, as may occur during food preparation.
  - Morning anorexia.
  - Adverse health consequences referable to binge eating and weight gain.
- Diagnosis is usually based on the history. Screening for possible primary sleep disorders associated with arousals should be performed.
- Treatment:
  - Treatment of any underlying primary sleep disorder, if present.
  - Discontinuation of sedating or hypnotic medication.
  - Pharmacologic options: all are given at bedtime. The mechanisms of efficacy are poorly understood:
    - Dopaminergic agents.
    - Topiramate.
    - Selective serotonin reuptake inhibitors.

REM-related arousal disorders

Nightmares[86]

- Definition and clinical features:
  - Nightmares are dreams that awaken the individual, associated with frightening or disturbing content.
  - Typical of dream recall, there is vivid memory of events, colors, movement, and passage of time.
  - Like pleasant dreams they may recur and continue along a similar theme over a single night or recur across multiple nights without apparent pattern.
  - Like all dreams, nightmares are a REM-sleep related phenomena.
- Epidemiology:
  - Like dreams, nightmares are essentially universal events.
  - Nightmares can begin in infancy, but confirmation may not be possible without the child being able to describe the dream.
  - 50% of children will have nightmares between ages 3 and 6.
  - The incidence decreases with age.
  - Frequent nightmares occur in 1% of adults.
- Differential diagnosis:
  - Night terrors.
  - Confusional arousals.
  - REM behavior disorder.
- Investigations; polysomnographic findings:
  - REM-sleep is associated with dreaming.
  - Typical nightmares are preceded by a REM period and followed by an arousal.
- Diagnosis and treatment:
  - Diagnosis is usually obtained by the history of a frightening dream awakening the individual from sleep in the early morning hours.
  - There is usually vivid recall of the frightening dream.
  - Nightmares associated with movements that increase with intensity over time raise the question of REM behavior disorder and in these cases a polysomnogram is required for diagnosis.
  - Typically nightmares require only reassurance to the patient.
  - If insomnia develops then occasional hypnotic use may be helpful.
  - Use of relaxation techniques prior to sleep onset and 'worry time' reviewing stressors in the early evening, a number of hours prior to sleep onset, may also help limit nightmares.

REM sleep behavior disorder[87]

- History and clinical features:
  - As part of the work to characterize the physiology of REM sleep, Jouvet in the late 1950s lesioned the REM motor off center in cats. The result was that these cats acted out their dreams (during REM sleep they would pounce, fight and play with nonexistent objects).
  - It was not until 1986 that Schenck and Mahowald first described similar behavior in humans.
  - Typically patients report increasingly violent dream content in the months prior to the onset of motor behaviors during sleep.
  - During an event, the patient may be noted to swing his arms wildly, talk, appear to fight, and may even get out of bed and run down the hall screaming.
  - The bed-partner may be attacked. In one study of 93 patients, 32% injured self and 64% injured the bed-partner[88].

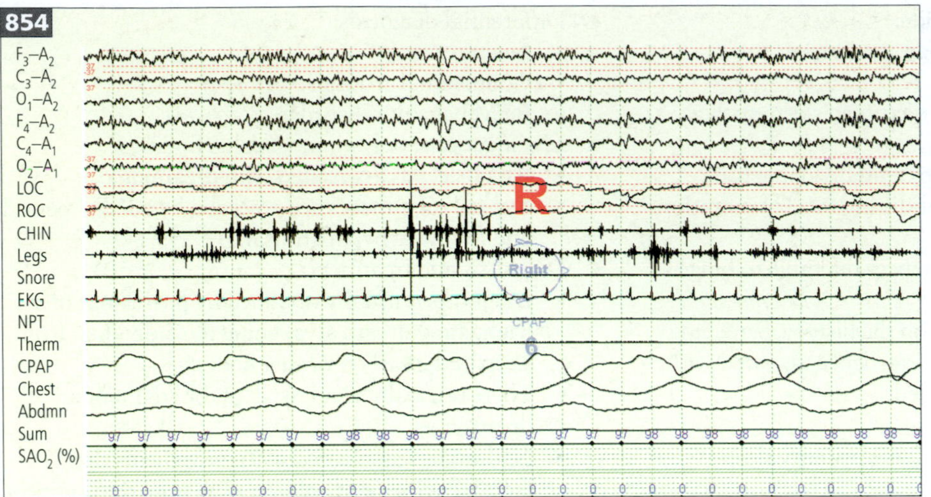

854 Period of REM sleep during which muscle activity persists. This lack of REM atonia is a hallmark of REM sleep behavior disorder.

- Epidemiology:
  - Mean age of onset is 61 years. Children with REM behavior disorder as young as 4 years have been reported.
  - In two large studies almost 87% of patients are males[88,89]. Almost one-half of patients with REM behavior disorder have other neurologic conditions[88]. An association with Parkinson's disease was found in 27%, dementia in 7.5%, multiple system atrophy in 15%, and narcolepsy in 4.3% of the cases[88].
- Pathology and pathophysiology: poorly understood. Recently the association of parkinsonism and multiple system atrophy with REM sleep behavior disorder has been linked to decreased dopamine transporter activity in the striatum. REM sleep behavior disorder may precede other symptoms of the synucleinopathies by years. However, there may be a subset of patients with isolated REM behavior disorder unassociated with neurodegenerative disease.
- Investigations: polysomnographic findings (854):
  - In a series of 93 patients 97% had excessive phasic or tonic EMG during REM sleep[88].
  - Abnormal gross motor behavior was noted in 45%.
  - Obstructive apnea was observed in 34%.
  - Periodic leg movements in 47%.
  - Mean REM percentage was 17% and slow-wave sleep mean percentage was 12.5%, both normal for age.
- Differential diagnosis:
  - Nocturnal frontal lobe epilepsy may produce unusual motor manifestations but seizures rarely occur in REM sleep.
  - Sleepwalking, confusional arousals, and sleep terrors are also non-REM phenomena.

Tip

► *If REM behavior disorder is suspected, a careful neurologic examination for signs of parkinsonism is indicated. For the patient with established idiopathic REM behavior disorder, serial follow-up neurologic examinations over time are appropriate.*

- Diagnosis: polysomnography that demonstrates epochs of REM-sleep with excessive amounts of phasic or tonic EMG tone is required. One of the following must also be present:
  - A history of sleep-related injurious, potentially injurious, or disruptive behavior.
  - Abnormal REM-sleep behaviors documented during the polysomnogram:
    - Absence of associated EEG epileptiform behavior.
    - No better explanation for the sleep disturbance.
- Treatment:
  - Clonazepam 0.25–1.5 mg at bedtime is the standard treatment for this disorder.
  - If the patient does not tolerate clonazepam, melatonin or pramipexole have also been shown to be effective in some patients.
  - Safety measures such as placing the mattress on the floor or sleeping in separate beds should be employed if the patient has injured themself or their bed-partner.

Nocturnal paroxysmal dystonia[90]

- Definition: episodes of dyskinetic or dystonic posturing that occur during non-REM sleep. At present time most groups believe that this disorder is a manifestation of nocturnal frontal lobe epilepsy (NFLE):
  - An autosomal dominant form of NFLE has recently been mapped to the neuronal nicotinic acetylcholine receptor.
  - Association with loci on chromosome 20 has been identified in three cohorts and on chromosome 15 in another family.
  - Patients are often unaware of motor activity but come to attention because of excessive daytime sleepiness or bed-partner complaints.
- Epidemiology of the syndrome is unknown, but patients often present from childhood.
- Differential diagnosis:
  - Other forms of hereditary dystonias; however, these are typically seen during the waking state.
  - Other movement disorders such as Wilson's disease and Huntingon's disease should be excluded. However, the most common presenting symptom in juvenile Huntington's disease is seizures.
- Investigations: polysomnographic findings:
  - Video monitoring with full electrode placement for long-term EEG monitoring is required for definitive diagnosis.
  - Frontal lobe discharges, especially medial and inferior discharges, are often difficult to record.
  - Video recordings demonstrate bizarre stereotyped motor behaviors that may include dystonic posturing, ballistic activity, or wandering around the laboratory.
  - Several events may occur in a single night.
- Diagnosis and treatment:
  - Diagnosis is based on semiology of the event and EEG findings.
  - Carbamazepine is the drug of choice for these patients. There are no studies utilizing newer anticonvulsants.

Tip

▶ *The exception to the general rule that polysomnography is unnecessary for diagnosis of parasomnias occurs when frontal lobe epilepsy is part of the differential diagnosis. This is particularly true when episodes involve hypermotor behavior and/or dramatic vocalizations. Diagnosis may be impossible from observation of a single episode (even by video-EEG monitoring), as epileptiform activity may not be evident on the scalp EEG because the focus may be deep, and the recording is often obscured by muscle artifact. Video-EEG monitoring over multiple nights may be necessary, and the monitoring should be interpreted in light of the overall clinical features of the episodes.*

CONCLUSION

The growing awareness of the general public about sleep disorders coupled with the obesity epidemic requires every physician to review sleep issues with patients on a regular basis. A basic sleep history, including questions about snoring, sleep habits, sleep initiation and continuity, daytime fatigue or sleepiness, leg symptoms, and bed-partner complaints, should become a part of every neurologic evaluation. Identification of sleep disorders and issues related to sleep hygiene will improve patient quality of life and medical outcomes in many neurologic and systemic diseases. Neurologists are uniquely positioned to assess sleep disorders from a more global patient perspective than that of other medical specialists.

REFERENCES

1 Hillman DR, Murphy AS, Pezzullo L (2006). The economic cost of sleep disorders. *Sleep* **29**(3):299–305.
2 American Academy of Sleep Medicine (2005). *International Classification of Sleep Disorders: Diagnostic and Coding Manual*, 2nd edn. American Academy of Sleep Medicine, Westchester.
3 Rechtshaffen A, Kales A (eds) (1968). *A Manual of Standardized Terminology, Techniques and Scoring System for Sleep Stages of Human Subjects*. UCLA Brain Information Service/Brain Research Institute, Los Angeles.
4 Iber C, Ancoli-Israel S, Chesson A, Quan SF (eds) (2007). *The AASM Manual for the Scoring of Sleep and Associated Events: Rules, Terminology, and Technical Specification*, 1st edn. American Academy of Sleep Medicine, Westchester.
5 National Sleep Foundation (2005). Sleep in America Poll 2005. Adult sleep habits and styles. http://www.sleepfoundation.org/article/sleep-america-polls/2005-adult-sleep-habits-and-styles.
6 National Sleep Foundation (2009). Sleep in America Poll 2009. Health and safety. http://www.sleepfoundation.org/article/sleep-america-polls/2009-health-and-safety.
7 Ohayon MM, Carskadon MA, Guilleminault C, Vitiello MV (2004). Meta-analysis of quantitative sleep parameters from childhood to old age in healthy individuals: developing normative sleep values across the human lifespan. *Sleep* **27**(7):1255–1273.
8 Borbely AA (1982). A two process model of sleep regulation. *Human Neurobiol* **1**(3):195–204.
9 Gay PC, Selecky PA (2010). Are sleep studies appropriately done in the home? *Respiratory Care* **55**(1):66–75.
10 Ferber R, Millman R, Coppola M, *et al.* (1994). Portable recording in the assessment of obstructive sleep apnea. ASDA standards of practice. *Sleep* **17**(4):378–392.
11 Rosen CL, Auckley D, Benca R, *et al.* (2012). A multisite randomized trial of portable sleep studies and positive airway pressure autotitration versus laboratory-based polysomnography for the diagnosis and treatment of obstructive sleep apnea: the HomePAP Study. *Sleep* **35**(6):757–767.
12 Services CfMaM (2009). Decision memo for sleep testing for obstructive sleep apnea (CAG-00405N) http://www.cms.hhs.gov/mcd/viewdecisionmemo.asp?id=227.
13 Collop NA, Anderson WM, Boehlecke B, *et al.* (2007). Clinical guidelines for the use of unattended portable monitors in the diagnosis of obstructive sleep apnea in adult patients. Portable Monitoring Task Force of the American Academy of Sleep Medicine. *J Clin Sleep Med* **3**(7):737–747.
14 Carskadon MA, Dement WC, Mitler MM, Roth T, Westbrook PR, Keenan S (1986). Guidelines for the multiple sleep latency test (MSLT): a standard measure of sleepiness. *Sleep* **9**(4):519–524.
15 Littner MR, Kushida C, Wise M, *et al.* (2005). Practice parameters for clinical use of the multiple sleep latency test and the maintenance of wakefulness test. *Sleep* **28**(1):113–121.
16 Mitler MM, Gujavarty KS, Browman CP (1982). Maintenance of wakefulness test: a polysomnographic technique for evaluation of treatment efficacy in patients with excessive somnolence. *Electroenceph Clin Neurophysiol* **53**(6):658–661.
17 Hartenbaum N, Collop N, Rosen IM, *et al.* (2006). Sleep apnea and commercial motor vehicle operators: Statement from the joint task force of the American College of Chest Physicians, the American College of Occupational and Environmental Medicine, and the National Sleep Foundation. *Chest* **130**(3):902–905.
18 Bonnet MH (2006). ACNS clinical controversy: MSLT and MWT have limited clinical utility. *J Clin Neurophysiol* **23**(1):50–58.
19 Ohayon MM (2002). Epidemiology of insomnia: what we know and what we still need to learn. *Sleep Med Rev* **6**(2):97–111.
20 Morin CM, LeBlanc M, Daley M, Gregoire JP, Merette C (2006). Epidemiology of insomnia: prevalence, self-help treatments, consultations, and determinants of help-seeking behaviors. *Sleep Med* **7**(2):123–130.
21 Buysse DJ, Angst J, Gamma A, Ajdacic V, Eich D, Rossler W (2008). Prevalence, course, and comorbidity of insomnia and depression in young adults. *Sleep* **31**(4):473–480.
22 Morin CM, Belanger L, LeBlanc M, *et al.* (2009). The natural history of insomnia: a population-based 3-year longitudinal study. *Arch Internal Med* **169**(5):447–453.
23 LeBlanc M, Merette C, Savard J, Ivers H, Baillargeon L, Morin CM (2009). Incidence and risk factors of insomnia in a population-based sample. *Sleep* **32**(8):1027–1037.
24 Daley M, Morin CM, LeBlanc M, Gregoire JP, Savard J (2009). The economic burden of insomnia: direct and indirect costs for individuals with insomnia syndrome, insomnia symptoms, and good sleepers. *Sleep* **32**(1):55–64.
25 Vgontzas AN, Liao D, Bixler EO, Chrousos GP, Vela-Bueno A (2009). Insomnia with objective short sleep duration is associated with a high risk for hypertension. *Sleep* **32**(4):491–497.
26 Vgontzas AN, Liao D, Pejovic S, Calhoun S, Karataraki M, Bixler EO (2009). Insomnia with objective short sleep duration is associated with type 2 diabetes: A population-based study. *Diabetes Care* **32**(11):1980–1985.
27 National Institutes of Health (2005). National Institutes of Health State of the Science Conference Statement on Manifestations and Management of Chronic Insomnia in Adults, June 13–15, 2005. *Sleep* **28**(9):1049–1057.
28 Perlis ML, Pigeon WR, Drummond SP (2006). The neurobiology of insomnia. In: Gilman S (ed). *Neurobiology of Disease*. Elsevier, Burlington, pp. 735–744.
29 Perlis ML, Merica H, Smith MT, Giles DE (2001). Beta EEG activity and insomnia. *Sleep Med Rev* **5**(5):363–374.
30 Nofzinger EA, Buysse DJ, Germain A, Price JC, Miewald JM, Kupfer DJ (2004). Functional neuroimaging evidence for hyperarousal in insomnia. *Am J Psychiatry* **161**(11):2126–2128.
31 Morin CM (1993). *Insomnia: Psychological Assessment and Management*. Guilford, New York
32 Spielman AJ, Caruso LS, Glovinsky PB (1987). A behavioral perspective on insomnia treatment. *Psychiatr Clin North Am* **10**(4):541–553.
33 Watson NF, Goldberg J, Arguelles L, Buchwald D (2006). Genetic and environmental influences on insomnia, daytime sleepiness, and obesity in twins. *Sleep* **29**(5):645–649.
34 Montagna P, Lugaresi E (2002). Agrypnia excitata: a generalized overactivity syndrome and a useful concept in the neurophysiopathology of sleep. *Clin Neurophysiol* **113**(4):552–560.
35 Johns MW (1991). A new method for measuring daytime sleepiness: the Epworth sleepiness scale. *Sleep* **14**(6):540–545.
36 Schutte-Rodin S, Broch L, Buysse D, Dorsey C, Sateia M (2008). Clinical guideline for the evaluation and management of chronic insomnia in adults. *J Clin Sleep Med* **4**(5):487–504.
37 Lugaresi E, Medori R, Montagna P, *et al.* (1986). Fatal familial insomnia and dysautonomia with selective degeneration of thalamic nuclei. *N Engl J Med* **315**(16):997–1003.
38 Goldfarb LG, Petersen RB, Tabaton M, *et al.* (1992). Fatal familial insomnia and familial Creutzfeldt–Jakob disease: disease phenotype determined by a DNA polymorphism. *Science* **258**(5083):806–808.
39 Morin CM, Vallieres A, Guay B, *et al.* (2009). Cognitive behavioral therapy, singly and combined with medication, for persistent insomnia: a randomized controlled trial. *JAMA* **301**(19):2005–2015.
40 Morgenthaler T, Kramer M, Alessi C, *et al.* (2006). Practice parameters for the psychological and behavioral treatment of insomnia: an update. An American Academy of Sleep Medicine report. *Sleep* **29**(11):1415–1419.
41 Schenck CH, Bassetti CL, Arnulf I, Mignot E (2007). English translations of the first clinical reports on narcolepsy and cataplexy by Westphal and Gelineau in the late 19th century, with commentary. *J Clin Sleep Med* **3**(3):301–311.
42 Henneberg R (1916). Ueber genuine narkolepsie. *Neurologisches Centralblatt* 30:282–290.

43 Nishino S (2007). Clinical and neurobiological aspects of narcolepsy. *Sleep Med* **8**(4):373–399.

44 Mignot E (1998). Genetic and familial aspects of narcolepsy. *Neurology* **50**(2 Suppl 1):S16–S22.

45 de Lecea L, Kilduff TS, Peyron C, *et al.* (1998). The hypocretins: hypothalmus-specific peptides with neuroexcitatory activity. *Proc Nat Acad Sci USA* **95**(1):322–327.

46 Sakurai T, Amemiya A, Ishii M, *et al.* (1998). Orexins and orexin receptors: a family of hypothalamic neuropeptides and G protein-coupled receptors that regulate feeding behavior. *Cell* **92**(4):573–585.

47 Blouin AM, Thannickal TC, Worley PF, Baraban JM, Reti IM, Siegel JM (2005). Narp immunostaining of human hypocretin (orexin) neurons: loss in narcolepsy. *Neurology* **65**(8):1189–1192.

48 Tanaka S, Honda M (2010). IgG abnormality in narcolepsy and idiopathic hypersomnia. *PLoS One* **5**(3):e9555.

49 Aran A, Lin L, Nevsimalova S, *et al.* (2009). Elevated anti-streptococcal antibodies in patients with recent narcolepsy onset. *Sleep* **32**(8):979–983.

50 Han F, Lin L, Warby SC, *et al.* (2011). Narcolepsy onset is seasonal and increased following the 2009 H1N1 pandemic in China. *Ann Neurol* **70**(3):410–417.

51 Lim ASP, Scammell TE (2010). The trouble with tribbles: do antibodies against TRIB2 cause narcolepsy? *Sleep* **33**(7):857–858.

52 Vernet C, Arnulf I (2009). Idiopathic hypersomnia with and without long sleep time: a controlled series of 75 patients. *Sleep* **32**(6):753–759.

53 Arnulf I, Lin L, Gadoth N, *et al.* (2008). Kleine–Levin syndrome: a systematic study of 108 patients. *Ann Neurol* **63**(4): 482–493.

54 Walters AS (1995). Toward a better definition of the restless legs syndrome. The International Restless Legs Syndrome Study Group. *Mov Disord* **10**(5):634–642.

55 Allen RP, Picchietti D, Hening WA, Trenkwalder C, Walters AS, Montplaisi J (2003). Restless legs syndrome: diagnostic criteria, special considerations, and epidemiology. A report from the restless legs syndrome diagnosis and epidemiology workshop at the National Institutes of Health. *Sleep Med* **4**(2):101–119.

56 Coleman RM, Miles LE, Guilleminault CC, Zarcone VP, Jr, van den Hoed J, Dement WC (1981). Sleep–wake disorders in the elderly: polysomnographic analysis. *J Am Geriatr Soc* **29**(7):289–296.

57 Allen RP, Barker PB, Wehrl F, Song HK, Earley CJ (2001). MRI measurement of brain iron in patients with restless legs syndrome. *Neurology* **56**(2):263–265.

58 Connor JR, Boyer PJ, Menzies SL, *et al.* (2003). Neuropathological examination suggests impaired brain iron acquisition in restless legs syndrome. *Neurology* **61**(3):304–309.

59 Hattan E, Chalk C, Postuma RB (2009). Is there a higher risk of restless legs syndrome in peripheral neuropathy? *Neurology* **72**(11):955–960.

60 Earley CJ, Horska A, Mohamed MA, Barker PB, Beard JL, Allen RP (2009). A randomized, double-blind, placebo-controlled trial of intravenous iron sucrose in restless legs syndrome. *Sleep Med* **10**(2):206–211.

61 Ondo WG (2010). Intravenous iron dextran for severe refractory restless legs syndrome. *Sleep Med* **11**(5):494–496.

62 Lavigne GJ, Khoury S, Abe S, Yamaguchi T, Raphael K (2008). Bruxism physiology and pathology: an overview for clinicians. *J Oral Rehabil* **35**(7):476–494.

63 Huynh N, Manzini C, Rompre PH, Lavigne GJ (2007). Weighing the potential effectiveness of various treatments for sleep bruxism. *J Can Dent Assoc* **73**(8): 727–730.

64 Klasser GD, Greene CS (2009). Oral appliances in the management of temporomandibular disorders. *Oral Surg, Oral Med, Oral Pathol, Oral Radiol Endod* **107**(2):212–223.

65 Romero-Corral A, Caples SM, Lopez-Jimenez F, Somers VK (2010). Interactions between obesity and obstructive sleep apnea: implications for treatment. *Chest* **137**(3):711–719.

66 Schwartz AR, Patil SP, Squier S, Schneider H, Kirkness JP, Smith PL (2010). Obesity and upper airway control during sleep. *J Appl Physiol* **108**(2):430–435.

67 White DP (2005). Pathogenesis of obstructive and central sleep apnea. *Am J Respir Crit Care Med* **172**(11):1363–1370.

68 Shahar E, Whitney CW, Redline S, *et al.* (2001). Sleep-disordered breathing and cardiovascular disease: cross-sectional results of the Sleep Heart Health Study. *Am J Respir Crit Care Med* **163**(1):19–25.

69 Calhoun DA, Harding SM (2010). Sleep and hypertension. *Chest* **138**(2):434–443.

70 Dyken ME, Im KB (2009). Obstructive sleep apnea and stroke. *Chest* **136**(6):1668–1677.

71 Kasai T, Narui K, Dohi T, *et al.* (2008). Prognosis of patients with heart failure and obstructive sleep apnea treated with continuous positive airway pressure. *Chest* **133**(3):690–696.

72 Findley LJ, Barth JT, Powers DC, Wilhoit SC, Boyd DG, Suratt PM (1986). Cognitive impairment in patients with obstructive sleep apnea and associated hypoxemia. *Chest* **90**(5):686–690.

73 Kushida CA, Chediak A, Berry RB, *et al.* (2008). Clinical guidelines for the manual titration of positive airway pressure in patients with obstructive sleep apnea. *J Clin Sleep Med* **4**(2):157–171.

74 Vanderlaan M, Holbrook CR, Wang M, Tuell A, Gozal D (2004). Epidemiologic survey of 196 patients with congenital central hypoventilation syndrome. *Pediatr Pulmonol* **37**(3):217–229.

75 Bordier P (2009). Sleep apnoea in patients with heart failure: part II: therapy. *Arch Cardiovasc Dis* **102**(10):711–720.

76 Bjorvatn B, Pallesen S (2009). A practical approach to circadian rhythm sleep disorders. *Sleep Med Rev* **13**(1):47–60.

77 Sack RL, Auckley D, Auger RR, *et al.* (2007). Circadian rhythm sleep disorders: part I, basic principles, shift work and jet lag disorders. An American Academy of Sleep Medicine review. *Sleep* **30**(11): 1460–1483.

78 Morgenthaler TI, Lee-Chiong T, Alessi C, *et al.* (2007). Practice parameters for the clinical evaluation and treatment of circadian rhythm sleep disorders. An American Academy of Sleep Medicine report. *Sleep* **30**(11):1445–1459.

79 Fahey CD, Zee PC (2006). Circadian rhythm sleep disorders and phototherapy. *Psychiatr Clin North Am* **29**(4):989–1007; abstract ix.

80 Olson EJ, Drage LA, Auger RR (2009). Sleep deprivation, physician performance, and patient safety. *Chest* **136**(5): 1389–1396.

81 Sack RL, Auckley D, Auger RR, *et al.* (2007). Circadian rhythm sleep disorders: part II, advanced sleep phase disorder, delayed sleep phase disorder, free-running disorder, and irregular sleep-wake rhythm. An American Academy of Sleep Medicine review. *Sleep* **30**(11):1484–1501.

82 Avidan AY 2009 Parasomnias and movement disorders of sleep. *Semin Neurol* **29**(4):372–392.

83 Tinuper P, Provini F, Bisulli F, *et al.* (2007). Movement disorders in sleep: guidelines for differentiating epileptic from non-epileptic motor phenomena arising from sleep. *Sleep Med Rev* **11**(4):255–267.

84 Kohrman MH (1999). Pediatric sleep disorders. In: Swaiman K, Ashwal S (eds). *Pediatric Neurology*. Mosby, St. Louis.

85 Howell MJ, Schenck CH (2009). Treatment of nocturnal eating disorders. *Curr Treat Options Neurol* **11**(5):333–339.

86 Kotagal S (2009). Parasomnias in childhood. *Sleep Med Rev* **13**(2):157–168.

87 Iranzo A, Santamaria J, Tolosa E (2009). The clinical and pathophysiological relevance of REM sleep behavior disorder in neurodegenerative diseases. *Sleep Med Rev* **13**(6):385–401.

88 Olson EJ, Boeve BF, Silber MH (2000). Rapid eye movement sleep behaviour disorder: demographic, clinical and laboratory findings in 93 cases. *Brain* **123**(Pt 2):331–339.

89 Schenck C, Hurwitz T, Mahowald M (1993). Symposium: Normal and abnormal REM sleep regulation: REM sleep behaviour disorder: an update on a series of 96 patients and a review of the world literature. *J Sleep Research* **2**:224–231.

90 Provini F, Plazzi G, Montagna P, Lugaresi E (2000). The wide clinical spectrum of nocturnal frontal lobe epilepsy. *Sleep Med Rev* **4**(4):375–386.

Further reading

Overviews

Panossian LA, Avidan AY (2009). Review of sleep disorders. *Med Clin North Am* **93**(2):407–425, ix.

Thorpy MJ (2004). Approach to the patient with a sleep complaint. *Sem Neurol* **24**(3):225–235.

Normal sleep

Brzezinski A (1997). Melatonin in humans. *N Engl J Med* **336**(3):186–195.

Espana RA, Scammell TE (2004). Sleep neurobiology for the clinician. *Sleep* **27**(4):811–820.

Richardson GS (2005). The human circadian system in normal and disordered sleep. *J Clin Psychiatry* **66**(Suppl 9):3–9; quiz 42–43.

Saper CB, Scammell TE, Lu J (2005). Hypothalamic regulation of sleep and circadian rhythms. *Nature* **437**(7063): 1257–1263.

Commonly performed sleep tests

Collop NA (2008). Portable monitoring for the diagnosis of obstructive sleep apnea. *Curr Opin Pulm Med* **14**(6):525–529.

Doghramji K, Mitler MM, Sangal RB, *et al.* (1997). A normative study of the maintenance of wakefulness test (MWT). *Electroenceph Clin Neurophysiol* **103**(5):554–562.

Mulgrew AT, Fox N, Ayas NT, Ryan CF (2007). Diagnosis and initial management of obstructive sleep apnea without polysomnography: a randomized validation study. *Ann Internal Med* **146**(3):157–166.

Quality AfHRa (2007). Technology assessment: home diagnosis of obstructive sleep apnea-hypopnea syndrome.

Insomnias

Benca RM, Peterson MJ (2008). Insomnia and depression. *Sleep Med* **9**(Suppl 1):S3–S9.

Reder AT, Mednick AS, Brown P, *et al.* (1995). Clinical and genetic studies of fatal familial insomnia. *Neurology* **45**(6):1068–1075.

Hypersomnias of central origin

Ali M, Auger RR, Slocumb NL, Morgenthaler TI (2009). Idiopathic hypersomnia: clinical features and response to treatment. *J Clin Sleep Med* **5**(6):562–568.

Anderson KN, Pilsworth S, Sharples LD, Smith IE, Shneerson JM (2007). Idiopathic hypersomnia: a study of 77 cases. *Sleep* **30**(10):1274–1281.

Dahlitz M, Parkes JD (1993). Sleep paralysis. *Lancet* **341**(8842):406–407.

Frenette E, Kushida CA (2009). Primary hypersomnias of central origin. *Sem Neurol* **29**(4):354–367.

Garnock-Jones KP, Dhillon S, Scott LJ (2009). Armodafinil. *CNS Drugs* **23**(9):793–803.

Huang YS, Lakkis C, Guilleminault C (2010) Kleine–Levin syndrome: current status. *Med Clin North Am* **94**(3):557–562.

Morgenthaler TI, Kapur VK, Brown T, *et al.* (2007). Practice parameters for the treatment of narcolepsy and other hypersomnias of central origin. *Sleep* **30**(12): 1705–1711.

Nishino S, Kanbayashi T (2005). Symptomatic narcolepsy, cataplexy and hypersomnia, and their implications in the hypothalamic hypocretin/orexin system. *Sleep Med Rev* **9**(4):269–310.

Ribstein M (1976). Hypnagogic hallucinations. In: Guilleminault C, Dement WC, Passouant P (eds). *Narcolepsy*. Spectrum, New York, pp. 145–160.

Tsujino N, Sakurai T (2009). Orexin/hypocretin: a neuropeptide at the interface of sleep, energy homeostasis, and reward system. *Pharmacol Rev* **61**(2):162–176.

Wise MS, Arand DL, Auger RR, Brooks SN, Watson NF (2007). Treatment of narcolepsy and other hypersomnias of central origin. *Sleep* **30**(12):1712–1727.

Sleep-related movement disorders

Abele M, Burk K, Laccone F, Dichgans J, Klockgether T (2001). Restless legs syndrome in spinocerebellar ataxia types 1, 2, and 3. *J Neurol* **248**(4):311–314.

Earley CJ, Allen RP, Connor JR, Ferrucci L, Troncoso J (2009). The dopaminergic neurons of the A11 system in RLS autopsy brains appear normal. *Sleep Med* **10**(10):1155–1157.

Ekbom KA (1945). Restless legs: a clinical study. *Acta Medica Scand Suppl* **158**:1–123.

Manconi M, Govoni V, De Vito A, *et al.* (2004). Pregnancy as a risk factor for restless legs syndrome. *Sleep Med* **5**(3):305–308.

Manconi M, Rocca MA, Ferini-Strambi L, *et al.* (2008). Restless legs syndrome is a common finding in multiple sclerosis and correlates with cervical cord damage. *Multiple Sclerosis* **14**(1):86–93.

Montplaisir J, Boucher S, Poirier G, Lavigne G, Lapierre O, Lesperance P (1997). Clinical, polysomnographic, and genetic characteristics of restless legs syndrome: a study of 133 patients diagnosed with new standard criteria. *Mov Disord* **12**(1):61–65.

Ondo WG (2009). Restless legs syndrome. *Neurologic Clin* **27**(3):779–799, vii.

Ondo WG, Lai D (2006). Association between restless legs syndrome and essential tremor. *Mov Disord* **21**(4):515–518.

Taylor-Gjevre RM, Gjevre JA, Skomro R, Nair B (2009). Restless legs syndrome in a rheumatoid arthritis patient cohort. *J Clin Rheumatol* **15**(1):12–15.

Walters AS, Rye DB (2009). Review of the relationship of restless legs syndrome and periodic limb movements in sleep to hypertension, heart disease, and stroke. *Sleep* **32**(5):589–597.

Sleep-related breathing disorders

Epstein LJ, Kristo D, Strollo PJ, Jr, *et al.* (2009). Clinical guideline for the evaluation, management and long-term care of obstructive sleep apnea in adults. *J Clin Sleep Med* **5**(3):263–276.

Yaggi HK, Concato J, Kernan WN, Lichtman JH, Brass LM, Mohsenin V (2005). Obstructive sleep apnea as a risk factor for stroke and death. *N Engl J Med* **353**(19):2034–2041.

Parasomnias

Combi R, Dalpra L, Tenchini ML, Ferini-Strambi L (2004). Autosomal dominant nocturnal frontal lobe epilepsy – a critical overview. *J Neurol* **251**(8):923–934.

Giglio P, Undevia N, Spire JP (2005). The primary parasomnias. A review for neurologists. *Neurologist* **11**(2):90–97.

Mason TB, 2nd, Pack AI (2007). Pediatric parasomnias. *Sleep* **30**(2):141–151.

INDEX

Note: Page references in **bold** indicate major discussion of topics; those in *italic* refer to tables, or figures where these are not included in the page range.

A

B

C

D

N

O

P

Q

R

S

T

U

V

W

X

Z